Pharmacology for Rehabilitation Professionals

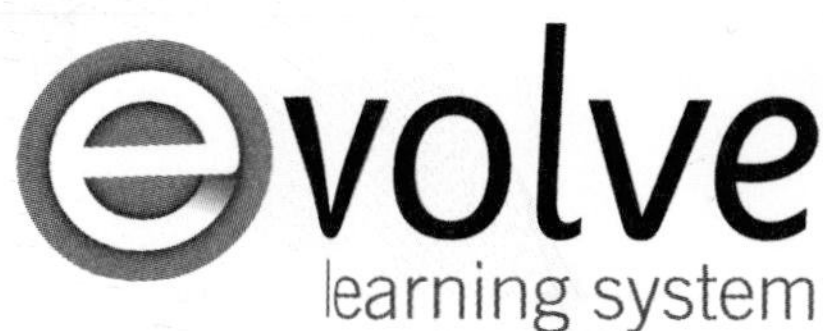

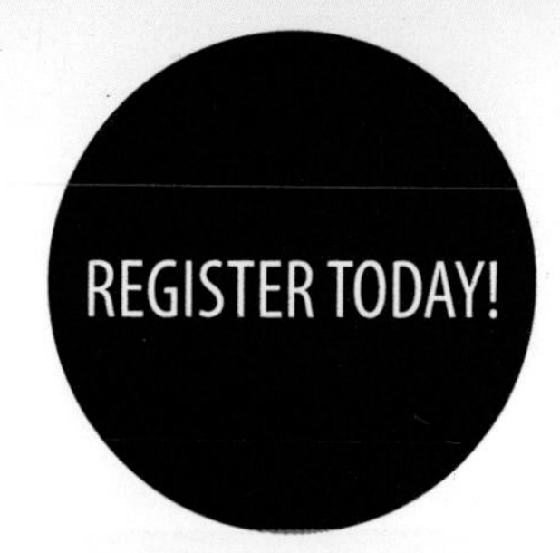

To access your Online Resources, visit:

http://evolve.elsevier.com/Gladson/

Evolve Student Learning Resources for Gladson: Pharmacology for Rehabilitation Professionals, second edition, offers the following features:

- **Activities**
  Printable Version of End of Chapter Activities including answers and answer guidelines
- **Additional Resources**
  Printable information including a list of online sources of drug information and a printable version of generic and trade names of commonly used drugs
- **Content Updates**
  Provides the most current information on the latest drugs
- **References**
  End of chapter References linked to Medline
- **Weblinks**
  An exciting resource that lets you link to hundreds of websites carefully chose to supplement the content of the textbook.
- **Image collection**
  All of the illustrations from *Pharmacology for Rehabilitation Professionals* appear here for use in the classroom.
- **Test bank**
  Over 500 multiple choice questions, including answers and answer rationales, have been included on Evolve to help instructors prepare for exams.

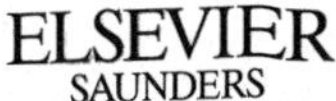

Pharmacology for Rehabilitation Professionals

SECOND EDITION

Barbara Gladson PT, OTR, PhD
Director
Biopharma Education and Curriculum Development
Associate Professor of Pharmacology and Physiology
Professor of Physical Therapy
University of Medicine and Dentistry of New Jersey
Newark, New Jersey

ELSEVIER
SAUNDERS

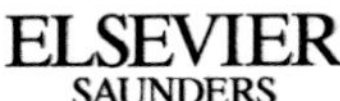

3251 Riverport Lane
St. Louis, Missouri 63043

PHARMACOLOGY FOR REHABILITATION PROFESSIONALS ISBN: 978-1-4377-0757-1

Library of Congress Cataloging-in-Publication Data

Gladson, Barbara.
Pharmacology for rehabilitation professionals / Barbara Gladson. -- 2nd ed.
p. ; cm.
Rev. ed. of: Pharmacology for physical therapists / Barbara Gladson. c2006.
Includes bibliographical references and index.
ISBN 978-1-4377-0757-1 (pbk. : alk. paper)
1. Pharmacology. 2. Medical rehabilitation. 3. Physical therapists. I. Gladson, Barbara. Pharmacology for physical therapists. II. Title.
[DNLM: 1. Pharmacology, Clinical. 2. Physical Therapy Modalities. QV 38 G5425pa 2011]
RM301.G63 2011
615'.1--dc22
2010024796

Vice President and Publisher: Linda Duncan
Executive Editor: Kathryn Falk
Senior Developmental Editor: Christie M. Hart
Publishing Services Manager: Catherine Albright Jackson
Associate Project Manager: Sara Alsup
Senior Book Designer: Paula Catalano

Printed in the United States of America

Last digit is the print number: 9 8 7 6 5 4 3 2 1

To my husband, Jim, and my children, Sam and Carly,
you give me tremendous support and unconditional love
no matter how many ball games or school events I miss.

To Pat whose thoughtful and kind lessons have meant so much to me.

To my fitness buddies who keep me healthy in mind and body with their empowering challenges and no-fail attitudes.

To Jen whose high standards make me constantly strive to be the best.

Giovanni Caracci, M.D., F.A.P.A.
Interim Chairman, Department of Psychiatry
Associate Professor of Psychiatry
University of Medicine & Dentistry of New Jersey
New Jersey Medical School
Newark, New Jersey

Lisa R. Dehner, PT, PhD
Associate Professor of Physical Therapy
College of Mount St. Joseph
Cincinnati, Ohio

Lee Dibble, PT, PhD, ATC
Assistant Professor of Physical Therapy
University of Utah
Salt Lake City, Utah

Najeeb U. Hussain, MBB
Assistant Professor
Department of Psychiatry
University of Medicine & Dentistry of New Jersey
Newark, New Jersey

Carlos Jordan, MD
Child and Adolescent Psychologist
Los Angeles, California

Leslie-Faith Morritt Taub, ANP-C, GNP-BC, CDE, C.BSM, DNSc
Assistant Professor
Division of Graduate Studies
School of Nursing
University of Medicine & Dentistry of New Jersey
Newark, New Jersey

Mary Jane Myslinski, PT, MA, EdM, EdD
Associate Professor
Doctoral Program in Physical Therapy
University of Medicine & Dentistry of New Jersey
Newark, New Jersey

Sue Paparella-Pitzel, PT, MS, DPT
Assistant Professor of Physical Therapy
University of Medicine & Dentistry of New Jersey
Newark, New Jersey

Lillian F. Pliner, M.D., F.A.C.P.
Assistant Professor of Medicine
Interim Director, Division of Hematology/Oncology
University of Medicine & Dentistry of New Jersey
Newark, New Jersey

Tracie K. Saunders RN, MS, CCRC, OCN
Director, Clinical Research Unit
Center for Translational and Clinical Sciences
New Jersey Medical School
Newark, New Jersey
Director, Oncology Nursing Services
NJMS-UH Cancer Center
Newark, New Jersey

Sue Ann Sisto, PT, MA, Ph.D.
Professor, Physical Therapy
Research Director, Division of Rehabilitation Sciences
School of Health Technology & Management
Research and Development Park
Rehabilitation Research and Movement Performance (RRAMP) Laboratory
Development Drive
Stony Brook University
Stony Brook, NY

Wolfgang Vogel, MS, PhD
Professor Emeritus
Department of Pharmacology
Jefferson Medical College
Thomas Jefferson University
Philadelphia, Pennsylvania
Adjunct Professor
Florida Gulf Coast University
Fort Meyers, Florida

Arnold Williams, MD
PGY-4 Resident
Department of Psychiatry
University of Medicine and Dentistry of New Jersey
New Jersey Medical School
Newark, New Jersey

Jane E. Ziegler, DCN, RD, LDN, CNSD
Assistant Professor
Department of Nutritional Sciences-School of Health Related Professions
University of Medicine and Dentistry of New Jersey
Newark, New Jersey

PREFACE

The second edition of Pharmacology for Rehabilitation Professionals presents basic pharmacological principles along with the mechanism of action and side effects of major drug categories seen in rehabilitative practice. Similar to the first edition, the chapters are organized using the systems approach. Each section begins with the pathophysiology and continues with a discussion of the drug groups used for treatment. Most sections end with a discussion about how drugs affect rehabilitation and how therapeutic interventions may affect drug effectiveness. Drug-exercise interactions, when known, are discussed. The chapters conclude with discussion activities that help the student learn the material and apply it to practice. The title has been changed to reflect the inclusion of coverage of other rehabilitation professionals.

New to this edition are chapters on vitamins and minerals (including their interactions with drugs), complementary and alternative agents, drugs used to facilitate wound healing, and drugs of abuse and doping agents. In particular the chapter on alternative medicine (chapter 26), provides an in-depth review of the supporting evidence, or lack thereof, of the supplements commonly used by patients with cardiovascular disease and women undergoing menopause. The chapter on wound healing (chapter 25), specifically discusses venous stasis ulcers, and arterial and diabetic ulcers. Cleansing agents, antimicrobials for wounds, and enzymatic agents are discussed as are pressure dressings. The chapter on abuse (chapter 27) reviews the physiological effects of alcohol, heroin, marijuana, and hallucinogenic agents and the pharmacological management of these addictions. An extensive review of methadone treatment has been added to the chapter on pain.

In addition to the new chapters, all original chapters have been updated with the newest drug information with emphasis on marketed drugs as opposed to those in the pipeline. The discussion activities have also been expanded with new cases and questions that will spur some debate and promote integration into practice. Boxes have been inserted providing generic and brand names of drugs along with special comments for easy reference, and many figures have been redrawn. Specifically the cardiovascular pharmacology chapters and the diabetes section have been expanded and further debate has been provided on the affects of non-steroidal anti-inflammatory agents on the cardiac system and even the role that diuretics and β blockers may have in increasing the risk of diabetes. The chapter, "Exploring Drug-Exercise Interaction" (chapter 28) follows the model presented in the first edition by specifically reviewing exercise-drug implications for cardiovascular disease, pulmonary disease, and diabetes, discussing red flags particularly related to drug treatment and exercise, and presenting sample exercise prescriptions. Additionally the chapters on chemotherapeutic drugs and antimicrobials/antiviral agents have been expanded. There is further discussion on monoclonal antibodies in the prescription of exercise while cycling on chemotherapy. Treatment sections for HIV disease and hepatitis have also been expanded to reflect the newest drug regimens.

The book continues to be written on a level commensurate with rehabilitation education, while offering a mix of basic and clinical science following the knowledge requirements of a Doctorate in Physical Therapy. The website companion to the book offers answers to many of the discussion activities, sample test questions, image library, updates, and links to supplemental resources.

ACKNOWLEDGMENTS

I wish to acknowledge the continuing efforts of the staff at Elsevier who managed to keep calm when the author did not always display proper decorum. A special thanks also goes to my contributing authors who brought expert knowledge and practical experience to their chapters. Additionally I would like to thank my colleagues at the University of Medicine & Dentistry whose scholarship continues to amaze me and provides me with everlasting goals.

Barbara Gladson

SECTION ONE
Principles of pharmacology

SECTION TWO
Autonomic and Cardiovascular Pharmacology

SECTION THREE
Pain Control

SECTION FOUR
Endocrine Pharmacology

SECTION FIVE
Neurologic Pharmacology

SECTION SIX
Anti-Infective and Anti-Cancer Agents

SECTION SEVEN
Special Topics in Pharmacology

SECTION I

Principles of Pharmacology

1

Introduction

Barbara Gladson

WHAT IS PHARMACOLOGY?

Pharmacology is defined as the study of how chemical substances affect living tissue, and it includes the monitoring of how these agents bind to receptors to enhance or inhibit normal function.[1,2] The study of pharmacology may be divided into two main areas: pharmacotherapeutics (also known as medical pharmacology) and toxicology. Pharmacotherapeutics is the use of chemical agents to prevent, diagnose, and cure disease, whereas toxicology is the study of the negative effects of chemicals on living things, including cells, plants, animals, and humans. Pharmacology is separate from pharmacy, which refers to the mixing and dispensing of drugs, as well as to clinical functions, including monitoring drug prescriptions for appropriateness and monitoring patients for adverse drug interactions.[3]

Pharmacotherapeutics may be further divided into two domains: pharmacokinetics and pharmacodynamics. When we think of the word *kinetics*, we think of mathematical formulas and rates. When the word *kinetics* is applied to pharmacology, it refers to the study of how fast and how much of a drug is absorbed into the body, how it is distributed to the various organs, and how it is ultimately metabolized and excreted by the body. Computing the concentration of drug absorbed or excreted is part of a pharmacokinetic study.

Pharmacodynamics describes what the drug does to the body and its beneficial or adverse effects at the cellular or organ level. Pharmacodynamic studies identify the mechanism of action and compare effects of different drugs for potency and efficacy. Pharmacodynamic principles are often presented in a graphic form called a *dose-response curve*.[2] This curve demonstrates the effect of increasing drug doses on a particular response (see Figures 2-10 and 2-11). The dose-response curve helps explain the nature of the drug-receptor interaction and is useful for comparing drugs in similar categories for strength and effectiveness (see Chapter 2).

Although this schema for describing the basis of pharmacology is simple and easily understood, it should, in fact, be expanded to include not only the traditional areas of pharmacology driven by a systems approach but also some new specialty areas such as pharmacogenomics, pharmacoepidemiology, and pharmacoeconomics.[4]

Pharmacogenomics examines how our genetic makeup produces unexpected and peculiar reactions to drugs and helps direct therapeutics according to a person's genotype.[5,6] The science of pharmacogenomics has its roots as far back as 1948 when it was descovered that some patients suffered fatal reactions to the local anesthetic drug procaine. It was later discovered that these individuals had a genetic alteration that produced a low affinity between the drug and its metabolizing enzyme. We now know that there are many variations in both gene sequence and expression that alter responses to drugs and that these variabilities appear more common in certain races and ethnicities. It has been accepted that genetic variations exist in drug receptors, ion channels, and other drug targets. And, in fact, genetic tests are available that help identify if a patient will respond to certain medications or not.[7] Tests can help determine whether a woman with breast cancer would respond to either of the breast cancer drugs tamoxifen and trastuzumab (Herceptin) and if a patient with a coagulation disorder would receive adequate anticoagulation from the drug warfarin. From a clinical perspective, genetics is why Asians and Hispanics diagnosed with schizophrenia have significantly higher serum drug levels than white individuals, which results in a greater incidence of extrapyramidal symptoms, and why angiotensin-converting enzymes are less effective in blacks than in whites.[8] The recognition of these genetic polymorphisms has led to the development and marketing of pharmacodiagnostic tests to help determine which drug to choose for an individual patient.[9]

Pharmacoepidemiology is concerned with the effectiveness of a drug in large populations compared with that in individuals.[10] This discipline utilizes all the tools for studying epidemics and chronic diseases to evaluate the use and effectiveness of medicines. Particular emphasis is placed on determining the frequency of adverse drug reactions by adopting a systematic approach after spontaneous postmarketing reporting. The true value of pharmacoepidemiology is that it provides information about drug effectiveness and safety.

Pharmacoeconomics is the area of pharmacology that quantifies in dollar amounts the cost versus benefit of therapeutics.[11] Pharmacoeconomic studies have been used to contain health care costs and are favored by governments and insurance companies to encourage changes in prescribing patterns. These entities have placed limits on the amount of reimbursable dollars for medications and encourage generic substitutions.

WHY SHOULD PHYSICAL THERAPISTS STUDY PHARMACOLOGY?

The field of pharmacology is constantly changing. Almost daily, new drugs appear on the market, and new information about older drugs is presented in medical journals. Drug therapy is pervasive among our physical therapy patients, and therefore we must have some understanding of mechanisms of action and adverse reactions of drugs. Perhaps even more important is an understanding of how drugs affect physical therapy practice. Some beneficial effects of drugs may be enhanced by our interventions, and in some cases, our interventions may be able to lessen some of the negative effects of medication. However, we must also be aware that physical therapy intervention may exacerbate some of the adverse effects of drugs and necessitate a change in treatment. Excellent examples of interventions that may produce adverse effects include massage procedures and strengthening exercises performed in an area recently injected with insulin.[12,13]

There are four specific reasons that physical therapists should study pharmacology. First, physical therapists must understand patients' responses to different drugs. Drugs often cause fatigue and can interfere with cognitive and motor functions. Examples of drugs that cause fatigue are sedatives, opioids, and muscle relaxants; however, many other drugs also produce sedation and affect muscle strength.[14,15] A second reason to study pharmacology is to determine the ideal treatment schedule. A therapist may want to see a patient when the patient's pain medication has reached its peak effect; however, the therapist would not want to *treat* a patient at peak sedation. The same is true for a patient taking antiparkinsonian medication; the patient may be experiencing the peak antitremor effect during the scheduled therapy session. The third reason for studying pharmacology is to learn to recognize drug–therapy interactions. Whirlpool treatments and other heat-related modalities produce peripheral vasodilation, which can exacerbate the orthostatic hypotension produced by certain antihypertensive agents and lead to syncope.[16,17] Lastly, from 1998 to 2005, the number of serious adverse drug reactions (ADRs) reported to the U.S. Food and Drug Administration (FDA) increased approximately 2.6 times to 89,842 cases and the number of fatal adverse drug events was reported to be 15,107.[18] Many of these ADRs are preventable, and therapists must recognize these reactions and report them immediately to the patient's physician.

DRUG DEVELOPMENT AND REGULATION PROCESS

The FDA is the administrative arm of the U.S. government that directs the drug development process and gives approval for marketing a new drug or approves a new use for an older drug. The FDA's power comes from a series of legislation enacted since the passage of the Pure Food and Drug Act of 1906.[19] This Act represented the U.S. government's earliest attempts to protect public health, following the discovery of unsanitary practices in the meat-packing industry. Next came the Sherley Amendment of 1912 which prohibited companies from making fraudulent claims for drug products. Later on, the Food, Drug, and Cosmetic Act of 1938 was passed. This was prompted by the deaths of 107 individuals (mostly children) who ingested a medication, diethylene glycol solution that was mixed with the powdered antibiotic sulfanilamide, which was marketed for the treatment of streptococcal infections. The sweet raspberry taste of the liquid was thought to be appealing to children. This new formulation was tested for flavor, appearance, and fragrance but not toxicity. The victims were sick for about 7 to 21 days showing signs of kidney failure, abdominal pain, nausea, vomiting, and convulsions. Numerous letters from parents who lost their children arrived at President's Franklin Roosevelts's office and also at the FDA. The result was the new Food, Drug, and Cosmetic Act, which mandated that drugs be safe and of good quality but did not require evidence of efficacy. It was not until the Kefauver-Harris Amendments to the Food, Drug, and Cosmetic Act were signed in 1962 that drug approval was contingent upon both safety and efficacy. This legislation was a reaction to the evidence that thalidomide, a supposedly nontoxic hypnotic, when taken during pregnancy was responsible for phocomelia, a rare birth defect involving the shortening or absence of limbs.

Additional legislative Acts that have since been passed include the Comprehensive Drug Abuse Prevention and Control Act of 1970, which limits access to drugs of abuse, and the Expedited Drug Approval Act of 1992, fueled by the acquired immune deficiency syndrome (AIDS) crisis, which helped shorten the drug development process for certain life-saving medications. However, it was not until 1997 that legislation requiring pharmaceutical companies to provide information on the adverse effects of drugs to consumers was passed (Agriculture, Rural Development, Food and Drug Administration and Related Agencies Appropriations Act, 1997).[20] Senator Edward Kennedy, in his amendment speech to this bill, said, "Millions of Americans are affected and billions of dollars are spent on medical problems caused by prescription drugs. The nation spends as much to cure the illnesses caused by prescription drugs as we spend on the drugs themselves."[21]

Drug regulation is essential to ensure a safe and effective product. The purposes of regulation include balancing the need of the pharmaceutical companies to show a profit with the need of patients to have easy access to safe medications, especially nonprofitable drugs or "orphan drugs" (drugs for rare diseases). The regulatory process is designed to ensure drug safety and efficacy by a detailed review of all research studies, both preclinical and clinical, to scrutinize product labeling to prevent fraud and to make sure directions are accurate and easily understood by patients, and to ensure quality in the manufacturing process.[22] In the United States, the FDA is charged with this responsibility, but in Europe and the rest of the world, there are both centralized and decentralized procedural methods for drug approval. In the European Union, the European Medicines Evaluation Agency (EMEA), has replaced the previously individual country approval process.[23] Individual countries still have the authority to grant national licenses, but there is a significant "harmonization of practice" at the global level. Harmonization of regulations was more formally accepted in 1990 with the establishment of the International Conference on Harmonisation of Technical Requirements for Registration of Pharmaceuticals for Human Use (ICH).[24] The ICH is a group of pharmaceutical regulators and companies from Europe, the United States, and Japan that produce guidance documents addressing how clinical trial data obtained in one country might be used to support the regulatory application in another country so that trials need not be duplicated. There are, however, exceptions to harmonization. The Japanese Pharmaceutical Affairs Bureau requires most prescription drugs to be first studied in Japan prior to regulatory approval. The reason for this tighter control is due to differences in the metabolism and body size of Japanese individuals compared with those of individuals who originate from the United States or Europe.

Although some centralized control over drug regulation is exercised, individual countries have their own rules regarding possession and prescription of drugs, and these rules vary greatly. In some countries, patients can obtain drugs without a prescription, whereas in others purchase of drugs by individuals is tightly controlled. In addition, vitamins, dietary supplements, and herbal remedies are not regulated as drugs in the United States and many other countries, so manufacturers of these items do not have to abide by the strict regulations for safety, purity, and efficacy governing prescription drugs.[25]

Drug Development

The first step in the drug development process is the determination of a target market by the drug company. For example, let us say that Drug Company X decides that there is a need for an oral form of insulin. Insulin is commonly delivered by means of a subcutaneous injection, a form of drug delivery that is less desirable to patients. First, the drug company enlists some chemists to perform research on and provide support to the new proposal. The chemists recruited have knowledge of the structure of the insulin receptor and develop chemical compounds that bind to the receptor. These compounds are then passed along to the pharmacologist for drug screening. A variety of biological assays are used to test the compounds at the molecular and cellular levels as well as at the organ and animal levels. The tissues selected for testing are those influenced by insulin, and the animals chosen for testing are those that have insulin receptors similar to those of humans. An evaluation of cardiovascular and renal functions are performed on healthy animals for safety. Specifically, acute and chronic toxicity tests are performed; as well, the drug's effect on reproduction and its mutagenic and carcinogenic potentials are evaluated. Efficacy testing is conducted on animals bred to become diabetic. Additional testing on the respiratory, gastrointestinal, reproductive, and central nervous systems is performed. These experiments constitute the preclinical testing phase, usually lasting 2 to 6 years.[26] At the end of this phase, representatives from Drug Company X take the data on their lead compound to the FDA and seek approval to begin testing the oral insulin in humans. If the compound is believed to be safe for humans, a Notice of Claimed Investigational Exemption for a New Drug (IND) is filed with the FDA. Human testing begins once the FDA approves the investigational new drug (IND) and consists of four phases as described below.

Phase 1 is the safety assessment study. In this study, the oral insulin is given to a small number of healthy volunteers (about 25 to 50), and a safety profile is established.[27] These studies are conducted to identify any toxic effects and to begin to establish a safe dosage range. Pharmacokinetic studies are also performed. If the drug is thought to have significant toxic effects, testing will be conducted on volunteer patients with the disease being targeted instead of on healthy control subjects. This is often the case for AIDS drugs or drugs designed for resistant types of cancers. This phase lasts up to 2 years.

Phase 2 is the drug effectiveness study.[27] In this phase, a small number of patients (approximately 200) who have the targeted disease receive the new drug. The study design is usually single-blinded, and the new drug is compared with a placebo (a nonactive compound) or with an older active agent with known safety and efficacy. Therefore a phase 2 study using the above example would compare glucose levels in patients administered the gold standard, that is, injectable insulin, with those in patients taking the experimental version. The questions that would be addressed by this study include: Is the experimental drug safe for patients with diabetes, and is it more effective than the injectable form of the drug in lowering blood glucose levels? This phase may last for another 1 to 2 years but the duration can vary, depending on the specific endpoint being studied. In our example, lowered blood glucose level is the endpoint, but the study might track the time to development of cardiovascular complications or other secondary sequela of the disease, such as retinal damage, which would extend the length of the study.

Phase 3 is a much larger study, including many more subjects with diabetes than in the previous phase (5000 to 10,000 subjects or more).[28] In addition, the duration of the study is usually extended, perhaps up to as long as 3 to 6 years. Investigators and study sites for these trials are chosen from all over the world. Safety and effectiveness are again studied but on a much larger scale. Phase 3 trials tend to be double-blinded randomized controlled trials (RCTs) that are either parallel or crossover in design. Parallel designs test at least two therapies at the same time, but each patient group is assigned only one drug. In studies with crossover designs, patients act as their own control subjects by receiving therapies in sequence. Some patients may receive Drug A first and then Drug B, and other patients may receive Drug B first and then Drug A. Phase 3 studies tend to be performed in larger tertiary care centers by experts in the targeted disease. Again, in our example of oral insulin, test sites would be set up around the country and in Europe and Japan, preferably at centers for the study of diabetes. These centers receive funding from the pharmaceutical company to recruit and pay subjects, set up data collection systems, and obtain any other supplies or equipment needed to support the research. Clinical researchers from the drug company will closely monitor all the data to make sure that the oral insulin is effective and safe throughout phase 3.

If phase 3 studies are successful, the drug company files a New Drug Application (NDA) with the FDA.[28] As part of this application, the company submits all preclinical and clinical data on the oral insulin. The FDA then reviews the materials, and if the drug seems to be effective and without significant adverse effects, the FDA gives permission to the company to market the oral insulin to the public.

Phase 4 begins when the drug is approved for public use. It is called the postmarketing surveillance phase and is a much larger study than any previously performed.[29] This phase constitutes monitoring the drug for safety in large numbers of patients under real-life conditions. During this phase, members of the public who have diabetes become study subjects without their knowledge. If many adverse drug reactions are discovered during this phase, and if they present significant health risks, the drug may be recalled. Technically, phase 4 has infinite duration because the drug company will continue monitoring for any problems throughout the marketing process. However, even though the drug has been released for public consumption after phase 3, it is prudent to wait until it has been on the market for at least 2 years before using it. It is responsible health care to prescribe an older drug with a proven track record first and then to switch to a newer drug after all the adverse drug reactions (ADRs) have been identified. This process underscores the attitude among many health care professionals that every drug prescription should be viewed as a therapeutic experiment and that we are all subjects in drug studies.

The time it takes to bring a drug to market is long, as just the clinical phases (phases 1 to 3) take, on average, 8.6 years and the entire process may take between 10 and 15 years in the United States.[30,31] In 2001, the total cost from molecule to marketing was estimated to be $802 million, and there is no evidence that this cost has been reduced.[30] It is a labor-intensive process that does not always lead to success. One of the major bottlenecks in the process is subject recruitment. Trials are often delayed or abandoned due to poor enrollment of subjects. Eighty-six percent of studies conducted in the United States do not recruit the required number of subjects in a timely manner.[32] In addition, the United States ranks behind Asia, Western Europe, Eastern Europe, and South America in the number of subjects recruited into trials per month.[33] Between 2003 and 2006, the average trial time increased by 74%, compared with data collected between 1999 and 2003.[34] This delay has led to a growing number of trials being conducted abroad.[35]

Due to the tremendous costs and time involved in drug discovery, pharmaceutical companies maintain some exclusivity on their products through patents. Patents are filed usually around the end of the preclinical studies and are in place for 20 years.[28] However, since the clinical phases take time, the patent owner has only a limited amount of time to market the drug before the generic forms begin to appear in pharmacies. The drug companies therefore fight hard to extend their patents by coming up with new uses for their drugs to balance out the lengthy review process and the cost of failed compounds.

When the patent expires, any company may produce and sell the drug as a generic without having to pay any fees to the original company, but the licensed trade name given to the drug remains the property of the original drug maker. In the case of a lengthy FDA review process, the patent may be extended for up to 5 years.

Although the FDA approves drugs for specific indications, which then become listed on the package insert, it does not limit the use of drugs to these described conditions. Physicians have the final say on how a drug may be used. Prescribing a drug for off-label or unapproved uses is common and legally permitted.

Orphan Drugs and Treatment Investigational New Drugs

Because drug development is an extremely expensive and lengthy process, drugs for rare diseases, the so-called "orphan drugs," tend not to be researched or marketed by drug companies. Therefore, in 1983, the Orphan Drug Act was passed to provide research grants for the study of diseases affecting fewer than 200,000 patients in the United States.[19] This Act provides special financial incentives to companies to help offset their development costs.

However, lack of profit is not the only reason that orphan drugs are rarely studied. These drugs present some scientific dilemmas because it is difficult to establish safety and effectiveness in small numbers of patients. In addition, many rare diseases occur in children, and investigators prefer not to include children in early clinical trials.

The FDA has also provided guidelines to streamline the development of certain drugs for life-threatening conditions such as AIDS and certain cancers.[36] These drugs receive Treatment Investigational New Drugs (IND) status, allowing them special priority throughout the review procedure. This status also allows patients outside the ongoing studies to be treated with investigational drugs. Treatment IND status is issued for a drug designed to treat serious life-threatening illnesses when no other acceptable alternative is available in the market. The drug must already be involved in a clinical trial, and the pharmaceutical company must show that it is proceeding with the normal steps involved in the drug approval process. If a physician wants to prescribe a drug that is in clinical study but lacks the treatment IND status, the drug may still be obtained for a patient under a "compassionate use" clause.

Barriers to Drug Development

Many barriers to development of new drugs exist, particularly for diseases that progress over time, such as multiple sclerosis and Parkinson's disease. Foremost among the barriers, of course, is the issue of funding. This barrier affects studies of rare diseases much more than studies of the more common diseases; but the discovery of new drugs even for common illnesses is risky and quite expensive. Drug researchers suggest that charity organizations and government support programs continue to be emphasized as funding sources.[37]

Another barrier to development is the fact that many diseases lack specific markers of identification or there is lack of consensus regarding clinical trial endpoints, which makes it difficult to document treatment progress. Examples include Alzheimer's disease and some mental illnesses such as bipolar disorder and schizophrenia. Mental illness tends to be a multifactorial condition demonstrating impairments in language, memory, motor planning, and cognitive domains.[38] Functional testing in all these areas is necessary to prove that a medication is effective. Even when markers have been identified, researchers in the field do not always agree on the level of significance that these markers provide in terms of documenting improvement. For example, manufacturers of arthritis drugs may claim that their drugs are effective by showing a reduction in the signs and symptoms of rheumatoid arthritis (e.g., redness, swollen joints), but others may insist that effectiveness claims be based on a slowing of disease progression as determined by radiography.[39] Because the lack of a specific drug target or marker is a result of our incomplete understanding of pathophysiology, we can hope that in the future further study in this area will lead to more effective drugs.

Another problem with the drug discovery process, in the case of many diseases, is the lack of animal models for drug screening.[37] Even though there are animals that can grow specific tumors, animals that are bred to have diabetes, and even animal models for epilepsy, animal models are lacking for many other illnesses. Again, mental illness is a good example because no animal model exists for the testing of different compounds.

Reluctance to include women and children in clinical trials, largely because of differences in pharmacokinetics and pharmacodynamics in these populations, represents another impediment to clinical trials. One solution to this has been the establishment of the Office of Women's Health within the FDA in 1994.[40] This office has promoted the development and approval of drugs for diseases affecting women. In addition, this office is dedicated to identifying how drugs affect women because traditionally most clinical trials have been conducted only on men. Governmental groups have attempted to provide incentives to the pharmaceutical industry to include more minorities and women into clinical trials. The National Institutes of Health (NIH) Revitalization Act of 1993 (Public Law 103-43) requires that all studies funded by the NIH include representations of women and minority groups.[41] However, despite this legislation, several populations remain under-represented in clinical trials.[42-45] Minorities and women are still less likely to enroll in studies compared with white males, particularly in cancer and HIV clinical trials. In the future, the U.S. House of Representatives is expected to consider legislation that would extend patent rights to companies that run clinical trials that are ethically and racially focused.[46] Additional barriers include the lack of experienced principal investigators, and lack of coordinated data collection systems, greater protocol complexity.[47,48]

Drug development is a labor-intensive, expensive, risky, and time-consuming process. Although this process is widely accepted and adhered to, there is growing discussion regarding alternative methods to prove drug safety and efficacy.[49] Improved postmarketing surveillance, which involves a coordinated data collection system from around the world, has been suggested to detect unanticipated events, both positive and negative, that could lead to greater accuracy in identifying treatment options.[50,51] The use of meta-analyses for analyzing many trials simultaneously has also been suggested as a way of improving therapy. In some cases, a meta-analysis of multiple small trials can be used to identify a drug effect not previously recognized by individual trials. Pharmacoeconomics, which consists of studies that determine the cost/benefit ratio of drugs, is likely to become a growing field as research dollars continue to shrink. Pharmacoeconomic studies examine overall outcome in clinical practice and are used to inform changes in practice. These suggestions are not likely to become standard operating procedures in the drug delivery process yet, but the FDA has instituted a number of changes that will ultimately benefit patients. Approvals of drugs via the "fast-track" and greater inclusion of women in clinical trials represent two recent changes in the drug discovery process. In addition, the FDA has begun using outside help, groups of clinical specialists in a variety of fields, in evaluating studies to hasten the review process. Further changes focused on streamlining the process and improving data collection are expected as time goes on.

ELEMENTS OF A PRESCRIPTION

The prescription is an order written by a licensed practitioner (e.g., physician, dentist, veterinarian, or podiatrist, and, in some states, the physician assistant and nurse practitioner) to instruct the pharmacist to provide a specific medication needed by a patient. The elements contained in the prescription include the following[52] (Figure 1–1):

1. The prescribing physician's name, credentials, address, and telephone number.
2. The date the prescription was written and the patient's full name and address.
3. Rx, called the superscription, which tells how the drug is to be administered to the patient (e.g., orally or by injection). Rx is an abbreviation of the Latin word for "recipe" and "receive thou."
4. Inscription, which includes the drug name (either brand or generic), dose, and quantity to dispense.
5. Subscription, which gives directions to the pharmacist regarding the mixing instructions (compounding), IF NEEDED.

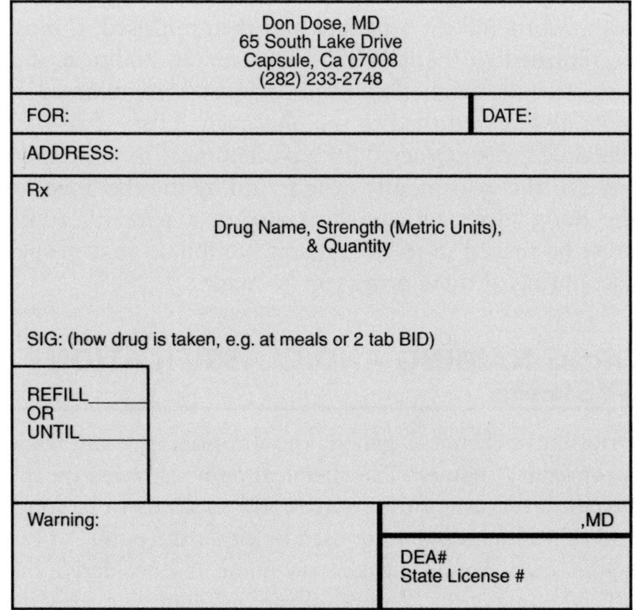
Don Dose, MD
65 South Lake Drive
Capsule, Ca 07008
(282) 233-2748
FOR:
DATE:
ADDRESS:
Rx
Drug Name, Strength (Metric Units), & Quantity
SIG: (how drug is taken, e.g. at meals or 2 tab BID)
REFILL____
OR
UNTIL____
Warning:
,MD
DEA#
State License #

FIGURE 1-1 Sample drug prescription.

6. The Signa or Sig, which gives directions to the patient, including how often to take the drug, how much drug to take, and additional instructions such as "shake well" or "take with food." Signa is Latin for "label." The patient instructions are usually written with Latin abbreviations.
7. Refill information.
8. Prescriber's signature.
9. Drug Enforcement Administration (DEA) number, which is required for controlled substances, as well as for insurance claims processing.

In the past, many adverse drug events have occurred due to prescribing errors. Quickly scribbled prescriptions that omit important information are illegible or contain the wrong dose or dose units and can be disastrous. A misplaced decimal point is not uncommon and can lead to a 10-fold difference in dose, which is why, for example, ".1 mg" should always be preceded by a zero, "0.1 mg". Another recommendation is to avoid using the abbreviated form of micrograms, "μg" since this can be read as "mg" which would produce a 1000-fold error. U for Units should also not be used since it may be mistaken as a zero, and QD, QOD, and qd can all be mistaken for one another, so these instructions should be written out as "daily" and "every other day." Box 1–1 lists acceptable abbreviations.

CONTROLLED SUBSTANCES

Controlled substances are drugs classified according to their potential for abuse. They are regulated under the Controlled Substances Act (CSA), which classifies these compounds into schedules (levels) from I to V.[52] This law, which was enacted in 1971, also makes provisions for research into drug abuse and treatment programs for dependency. This Act, along with assistance from the DEA, controls the manufacture, distribution, and dispensing of drugs that have the potential to be abused.

Schedule I

Schedule I drugs are available only for research. They have the highest abuse potential, leading to dependence without any acceptable medical indication. Some examples include heroin, LSD (lysergic acid diethylamide), and mescaline. Special approval is necessary before any of these agents can be used.

Schedule II

Schedule II drugs also have a high abuse potential with the likelihood of physical and psychological dependence, but unlike schedule I drugs, they have accepted medical uses. Drugs classified at this level include stimulants such as amphetamines; opioids, including morphine, fentanyl, and oxycodone; and some barbiturates. Automatic refills

BOX 1-1 Common Abbreviations used in Prescription Writing

ā	before
ac	before meals
bid	twice a day
cap	capsule
dil	dissolve, dilute
disp, dis	dispense
elix	elixir
g	gram
gtt	dros
h	hour
hs	at bedtime
IA	intra-arterial
IM	intramuscular
IV	intravenous
IVPB	IV piggyback
kg	kilogram
mEq, meq	milliequivalent
mg	milligram
mcg, μg	microgram (always write)
OD	right eye
OS, OL	left eye
OTC	over-the-counter
OU	both eyes
p	after
pc	after meals
PO	by mouth
PR	per rectum
prn	when needed
q	every
qam, om	every morning
ad	every day (write "daily")
qh, q1h	every hour
q2h, q3h, etc	every 2 hours, every 3 hours, etc
qhs	every night at bedtime
qid	
qod (do not use) every other day	
qs	sufficient quantity
rept, repet	may be repeated
Rx	take
SC, SQ	subcutaneous
Sig, S	label
Sos	if needed
stat	at once
sup, supp	suppository
susp	suspension
tab	tablet
tbsp, T	tablespoon (write out 15 ml)
tid	three times a day
tsp	teaspoon (write out 5 ml)
U	units (write out units)

are not allowed, and the prescriber must write a new prescription each time a refill is needed. In the hospital setting, if an order is written on an as-needed basis, it is only valid for 72 hours. Prescription scripts older than 6 months cannot be filled.

Schedule III

Schedule III drugs have a lower abuse potential than those in schedules I or II; however, they may also be abused, resulting in some physical and psychological dependence. Refills are allowed, but no more than five refills are permitted within a 6-month period. Mild to moderately strong opioids, barbiturates, and steroids are categorized at this level. Opioids that are formulated with aspirin and acetaminophen as well as anabolic steroids are also included under schedule III.

Schedule IV

Schedule IV drugs have less abuse potential than those in schedule III; however, this does not mean that they are not popular among drug abusers. They include opioids such as propoxyphene (Darvon), benzodiazepines such as diazepam (Valium), and some stimulants. No more than five refills within 6 months are allowed under one prescription.

Schedule V

Schedule V drugs have the lowest abuse potential and may even be available without a prescription. Actual availability without a prescription is state regulated, so laws governing their use vary. Various cold and cough medicines containing codeine are listed in this category.

Rules Governing Narcotics

It is against the law for any person to possess a scheduled drug unless it has been obtained with a prescription. It is also illegal to transfer possession of any scheduled drug to another person.[53] In the hospital setting if a narcotic is ordered for a patient and then not used, it must be returned to the hospital pharmacy. In addition, if a narcotic falls on the floor and becomes contaminated, it must also be returned to the pharmacy. Every dose of a schedule II drug ordered for a patient must be accounted for. For this reason, any drug found by the therapist on the floor, table, or anywhere else in a patient's room must be turned in to the nursing station so that proper accounting of these drugs can be made.

DRUG NAMING AND CLASSIFICATION SYSTEMS

Drugs have chemical, generic (nonproprietary), and trade (proprietary) names. The chemical name is based on the specific structure of the compound.[54] It tends to be long, and this name is often not used by either the public or the health care team. The generic name is considered the official name of the compound and may have some resemblance to the names of other drugs that fall within the same category or have the same purpose. It is the name listed in the official drug compendia, *The United States Pharmacopeia*, and stays with the compound, no matter how many trade names it accumulates. The generic names are also the only names recognized for use in scientific journals, although these names, too, can vary from one country to another; for example, acetaminophen in the United States is known as paracetamol in the United Kingdom. The trade name or brand name is the name given to the drug by the pharmaceutical company and is copyrighted to that company. In recent years, there has been a push for trendy names that the public will recognize. An example is the drug Singulair. Singulair, taken from the word "single," is supposed to remind the public that it has once-a-day dosing and is thus a more desirable drug than one that must be administered several times a day. These names, although they are helpful in steering the public toward a particular drug, actually add more confusion to the system of naming and increase the possibility that someone might make a mistake when writing a prescription. Once a patent expires, other pharmaceutical companies have a right to market the drug and assign their own trade names. Because there may be several trade names given to one generic drug, use of trade names should be avoided while writing prescriptions.

Drug Classification

Drugs are often classified into specific categories. These categories do not represent a universally accepted system, and one drug may be placed into a variety of different classes.[55] The classes do, however, provide a useful framework for studying pharmacology. Drugs may be classified according to the body system being treated, for example, cardiovascular drugs, pulmonary drugs, and gastrointestinal drugs. Drugs may also be classified according to their pharmacotherapeutic actions, or the overall pharmacologic actions of the drugs on specific disease processes. Examples of drugs classified in this manner are antidepressants and antihypertensives. A mistake that is often made when medicines are delineated in this manner is the assumption that all the drugs classified under the same heading act in the same manner. However, this is not always true. Diuretics and calcium channel blockers are both antihypertensives, but they have very different mechanisms of action.

Drugs may also be categorized according to their pharmacological actions, for example, arterial vasodilators. Some of these drugs act directly on smooth muscle and others act by blocking specific receptors. The result is the same (dilation of the arterioles), but their mechanisms of action are different. A fourth way in which drugs may be classified is according to their molecular actions. Molecular action is described by identifying the molecular target of the drug. These targets consist of receptors for hormones, enzymes, ion channels, and cell membrane transporters. Examples include calcium channel blockers, beta blockers, and angiotensin-converting enzyme inhibitors. The last method for categorizing drugs is a classification based on either the chemical makeup or the source for the drug. Plant material provides a good natural source for many compounds. Atropine is named after the plant species Atropa. Penicillin is part of a group of compounds described as β-lactam antibiotics because they contain a β-lactam ring, a four-member nitrogen-containing carbon structure.

The system that is currently in place for classifying and naming drugs is imprecise, confusing, and implies that all drugs within the same classification group act in a similar manner.[56] In light of the potential for mistakes when trade or proprietary names are used and the inaccuracies implied in using functional categories for naming, there is a push toward using the official or generic names of drugs when speaking to patients and health care professionals or when writing prescriptions. However, pharmaceutical companies continue to market their drugs with trendy trade names.

ACTIVITIES 1

1. This chapter has reviewed the phases of clinical drug development. Outline some elements that must be taken into consideration to ensure that this is an ethical process.
2. Discuss the key questions that should be answered concerning a drug during the development process.
3. Look-alike/sound-alike drugs are responsible for many medication errors.
   A. Name a few sound-alike drugs, and give their indications.
   B. Discuss some strategies that can be used to reduce look-alike and sound-alike medication errors.
4. Describe the following drugs using the pharmacotherapeutic, pharmacologic, and molecular categories of drug naming:
   Propranolol
   Prazosin
   Captopril
   Losartan
   Nifedipine
   Hydrochlorothiazide

REFERENCES

1. Katzung BG: Introduction. In Katzung BG, editor: Basic & clinical pharmacology, New York, 2007, McGraw-Hill.
2. Sutter MC, Walker MJ: Introduction. In Page CP et al, editors: Integrated Pharmacology, Philadelphia, 2006, Mosby.
3. Carmichael JM, O'Connell MB, Devine B, et al: Collaborative drug therapy management by pharmacists. Pharmacotherapy, 17(5):1050–1061, 1997.
4. Rang HP Dale MM, Ritter, JM: What is pharmacology? In Rang HP Dale MM, Ritter, JM, editors: Pharmacology, New York, 2007, Churchill Livingstone.
5. Kalow W: Historical Aspects of Pharmacogenetics. In Kalow W, Meyer UA, Tyndale RF, editors: Pharmacogenomics, Boca Raton, Fl, 2005, Taylor & Francis.

6. Fargher EA, Eddy C, Newman W, Qasim F, et al: Patients' and healthcare professionals' views on pharmacogenetic testing and its future delivery in the NHS. Pharmacogenomics, 8(11): 1511–1519, 2007.
7. Pollack A: Patient's DNA may be signal to tailor medication, New York, 2008, The New York Times.
8. Tate SK, Goldsstein DB:Will tomorrow's medicines work for everyone? Nat Genet, 36(11): S34–S41, 2004.
9. Jorgensen JT: From blockbuster medicine to personalized medicine. Personalized Med, 5(1): 55–63, 2008.
10. Strom BL: What is pharmacoepidemiology? In Strom BL, Kimmel SE, editors: Textbook of pharmacoepidemiology, Hoboken, NJ, 2006, John Wiley & Sons, Ltd.
11. Hennessy S: Basic principles of clinical pharmacology relevant to pharmacoepidemiology studies. In Strom BL, Kimmel SE, editors: Textbook of pharmacoepidemiology, Hoboken, NJ, 2006, John Wiley & Sons, Ltd.
12. Koivisto VA, Felig P: Effects of leg exercise on insulin absorption in diabetic patients. N Engl J Med, 298(2):79–83, 1978.
13. Linde B: Dissociation of insulin absorption and blood flow during massage of a subcutaneous injection site. Diabetes Care, 9(6): 570–574, 1986.
14. Allen GJ, Hartl TL, Duffany S, Smith SF, et al: Cognitive and motor function after administration of hydrocodone bitartrate plus ibuprofen, ibuprofen alone, or placebo in healthy subjects with exercise-induced muscle damage: A randomized, repeated-dose, placebo-controlled study. Psychopharmacology, 166(3): 228–233, 2003.
15. Bower EA, Moore JL, Moss M, et al: The effects of single-dose frexofenadine, diphenhydramine, and placebo on cognitive performance in flight personnel. Aviat Space Environ Med, 74(2): 145–152, 2003.
16. Nagasawa Y, Komori S, Sato M, et al: Effects of hot bath immersion on autonomic activity and hemodynamics—Comparison of the elderly patient and the healthy young. Jpn Circ J, 65: 587–592, 2001.
17. Allison TG, Maresh CM, Armstrong LE: Cardiovascular responses in a whirlpool bath at 40 degrees C versus user-controlled water temperatures. Mayo Clin Proc, 73(3): 210–215, 1998.
18. Moore T, Cohen MR, Furberg C: Serious adverse drug events reported to the Food and Drug Administration, 1998–2005. Arch Int Med, 167(16): 1752–1759, 2007.
19. Food and Drug Administration: History of the FDA (website). www.fda.gov/oc/history/default.htm. Accessed May 5, 2009.
20. Making appropriations for Agriculture, Rural Development, Food and Drug Administration, and Related Agencies programs for the fiscal year ending September 30, 1997, and for other purposes, In H.R.3603, 1996.
21. Gray J: Senate backs bill to require data on drugs for consumers, New York, 1996, The New York Times, p. 19.
22. Lal R, Kremzner M: Introduction to the new prescription drug labeling by the Food and Drug Administration. Am J Health-Syst Pharm, 64(23): 2488–2494, 2007.
23. European Medicines Agency (website). www.emea.europa.eu/htms/aboutus/emeaoverview.htm. Accessed May 5, 2009.
24. International Conference on Harmonisation (website). www.ich.org/cache/compo/276-254-1.html. Accessed May 6, 2009.
25. Barrett S: How the Dietary Supplement Health and Education Act of 1994 weakened the FDA, June 8, 2000 (website). www.quackwatch.org. Accessed May 6, 2009.
26. Berkowitz BA, Katzung BG: Development & regulation of drugs. In Katzung BG, editor: Basic & clinical pharmacology, New York, 2007, McGraw-Hill.
27. Machin D: General issues. In Machin D, Day S, Green S, editors: Textbook of clinical trials, Hoboken, NJ, 2004, John Wiley & Sons, Ltd.
28. Rang HP, Dale MM, Ritter JM: Drug discovery and development. In Rang HP, Dale MM, Ritter JM: Rand & Dale's pharmacology, New York, 2007, Churchill Livingstone.
29. Fontanarosa PB, Rennie D, DeAngelis C: Postmarketing surveillance—Lack of vigilance, lack of trust. JAMA, 2004, 292(1): 2647–2650.
30. Kaitin KI et al: Tufts CSDD Outlook 2009. 2009, Tufts Center for the Study of Drug Development.
31. Christel MD: Patient recruitment. In R & D Directions, 2008, PharmaLive, pp 1–13.
32. Getz KA, Wenger J, Campo RA, et al: Assessing the impact of protocol design changes on clinical trial performance. Am J Ther, 15(5): 450–457, 2008.
33. Getz K: Overview of the global clinical trial landscape. In Global R & D Congress. Philadelphia, 2007, Cambridge Healthtech Institute.
34. Getz K: First things first. In Focus On, 2008, Informa UK Ltd. III-IV.
35. Glickman SW, McHutchison JG, Peterson ED, et al: Ethical and scientific implications of the globalization of clinical research. N Engl J Med, 360(8): 816–823, 2009.
36. Expanded access and expedited approval of new therapies related to HIV/AIDS (website). www.fda.gov/oashi/aids/expanded.html. Accessed May 6, 2009.
37. Fillit HM, O'Connell AW, Brown WM, et al: Barriers to drug discovery and development for Alzheimer disease. Alzheimer Dis Assoc Disord, 16(Supplement 1): S1–S8, 2002.
38. Carpenter WT, Koenig JI: The evolution of drug dvelopment in schizophrenia: Past issues and future opportunities. Neuropsychopharmacology, 33: 2061–2079, 2008.
39. Witter J: Drug development in rheumatoid arthritis. Curr Opin Rheumatol,14: 276–280, 2002.
40. Sheppard A: US Food and Drug Office of Women's Health: Update. J Am Med Womens Assoc, 54(2): 97–98, 1999.
41. Freedman LS, et al: Inclusion of women and minorities in clinical trials and the NIH Revitalization Act of 1993—The perspective of NIH clinical trialists. Control Clin Trials, 16(5): 277–285, 1995.
42. Murthy VH, Krumholz HM, Gross CP: Participation in cancer clinical trials. JAMA, 291(22): 2720–2727, 2004.
43. Stewart JH, Bertoni AG, Staten JL, Levine EA, Gross CP: Participation in surgical oncology clinical trials: Gender, race/ethnicity, and age-based disparities. Ann Surg Oncol, 14(12): 3328–3334, 2007.
44. Mouton CP, Harris S, Rovi S, Solorzano P, Johnson MS: Barriers to black women's participation in cancer clinical trials. J Natl Med Assoc, 89(11): 721–727, 1997.
45. Gifford AL, Cunningham WE, Heslin KC, et al: Participation in research and access to experimental treatments by HIV-infected patients. N Engl J Med, 346(18): 1373–1382, 2002.
46. Getz K, Faden L: Racial disparities among clinical research investigators. Am J Ther,15: 3–11, 2008.
47. Sung NS, Crowley WF Jr, Genel M, et al: Central challenges facing the nation clinical research enterprise. JAMA, 289(10): 1278–1287, 2003.
48. Getz K: First things first, 2008, Informa UK Ltd. 3–4.
49. Carpenter WT: From clinical trial to prescription. Arch Gen Psychiatry, 59: 282–285, 2002.
50. Czarnecki A, Voss S: Safety signals using proportional reporting ratios from company and regulatory authority databases. Drug Inform J, 42(3): 205–209, 2008.
51. Oliva A et al: Bioinformatics modernization and the critical path to improved benefit-risk assessment of drugs. Drug Inform J, 42(3): 273–279, 2008.
52. Lofholm PW, Katzung BG: Rational prescribing and prescription writing. In Katzung BG, editor: Basic and clinical pharmacology, New York, 2007, McGraw Hill.

53. Roach SS, Ford SM: General principles of pharmacology. In Introductory clinical pharmacology, Philadelphia, 2008, Lippincott Williams & Wilkins.
54. Kwo EC, Kamat P, Steinman MA: Physician use of brand versus generic drug names in 1993–1994 and 2003–2004. Ann Pharmacother, 43(3): 459–468, 2009.
55. Berman A: Reducing medication errors through naming, labeling, and packaging. J Med Syst, 28(1): 9–29, 2004.
56. Santell JP, Cousins DD: Medication errors related to product names. Jt Comm J Qual Patient Saf, 31(11): 649–654, 2005.

2

Pharmacodynamics: Mechanism of Action

Barbara Gladson

TARGETS FOR DRUG ACTION

As discussed in the previous chapter, drugs are classified according to their actions. The main emphasis of this chapter will be to describe these actions on both molecular and cellular levels. Later chapters will deal with the effects of these actions at tissue and system levels. When a drug acts at a molecular level, its target is usually a protein molecule containing a binding site for the drug. Previously, a receptor was considered to be a distinct protein channel imbedded in the cell's phospholipid membrane whose function was to open and close in response to drug binding (Figure 2–1). However, not all drugs have this type of distinct receptor. Other molecular targets or receptors include transport molecules, enzymes that catalyze chemical reactions, nucleic acids, some miscellaneous targets such as metal ions, or gastrointestinal contents.[1] There are also drugs for which a distinct single molecular or chemical binding entity has yet to be descovered.[2] But, in general, the sites for drug action include specific binding sites on proteins that undergo a conformational change in the presence of a ligand (drug) to initiate a cascade of events leading to the drug's action called *transduction*. Identifying the drug–receptor interaction has been critical to the understanding of how a drug works.

Receptor Types

Four receptor superfamilies have been identified: ion channel–linked receptors (ligand-gated and voltage-gated), G-protein–coupled receptors, deoxyribonucleic acid (DNA)-coupled receptors, and kinase-linked receptors.[1] All except the intracellular DNA-coupled receptor are transmembrane receptors in that they contain receptors responding to ligands outside the cell but contain structural proteins that link this region to the intracellular domain.

Ligand- and voltage-gated receptors are transmembrane proteins arranged around a central aqueous channel (pore). The channel opens in response to a ligand or a voltage change in the membrane, allowing the selective transfer of ions from a greater concentration to a lesser concentration.[3,4] Ion specificity is determined by the structural configuration of the amino acids (pore size) and the charge on the molecule. Both the charge and size of the pore vary for each type of ion channel. Common voltage-gated channels include sodium (Na^+) and calcium (Ca^{2+}) channels in which these cations diffuse into the cell, causing a depolarization (Figure 2–2). When potassium (K^+) channels open, the ion tends to flow out of the cell causing the cytosol to become more negative. A well-known ligand-gated receptor is the nicotinic acetylcholine (ACh) receptor consisting of five protein subunits arranged around a central pore. When two ACh molecules bind to the α subunit, the channel opens (Figure 2–3). Other ligand-gated channels include γ-aminobutyric acid (GABA), glycine, and serotonin receptors. Several different subtypes exist for each of these main types of channels; however, they all share a property for quick activation, that is, the channel opens in a millisecond timescale. The patch-clamp technique developed by Neher and Sakmann is a way to measure the ion flow that occurs through the channel during opening. Neher, E., *Ion channels for communication between and within cells*. Science, 1992. **256**: p. 498-502.

A tight seal is formed between a micropipette containing an electrode and a cell membrane (Figure 2–4). When the cell is exposed to a neurotransmitter or to a voltage change, the pipette is able to measure the current passing through a single channel. Many drugs are tested in this manner to determine their effects on specific ion channels. This has become a very important tool in the drug discovery process because there is evidence to support ion-channel mutations in a number of diseases (e.g., cystic fibrosis, long QT syndrome, and several types of myopathies).[5,6] In addition, targeting ion channels for treatment in cardiovascular and neurodegenerative diseases has become common. Examples of drugs that bind to ion channels include vasodilator drugs that inhibit the opening of L-type calcium channels in cardiac and smooth muscles and the benzodiazepine tranquilizers that bind to the $GABA_A$ receptor.

G-protein–linked receptors consist of a transmembrane receptor coupled to an intracellular system by a special

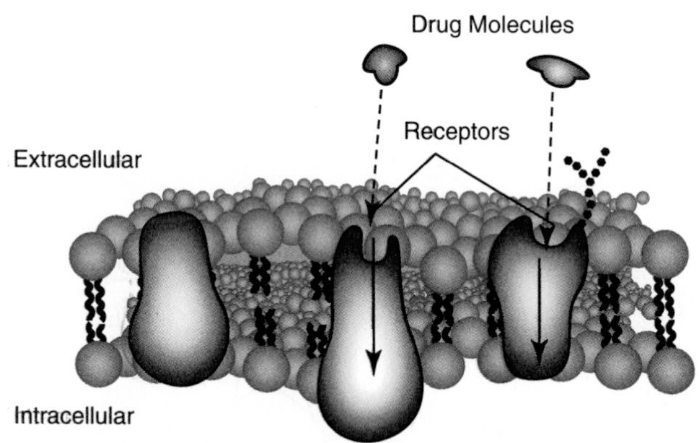

FIGURE 2-1 A protein embedded in a cell membrane containing an extracellular binding site for a drug.

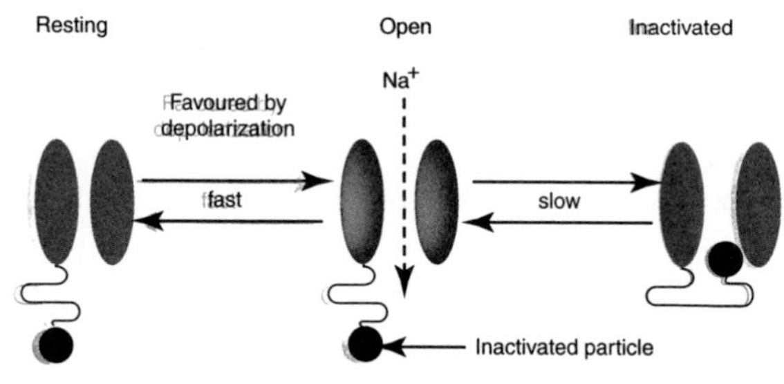

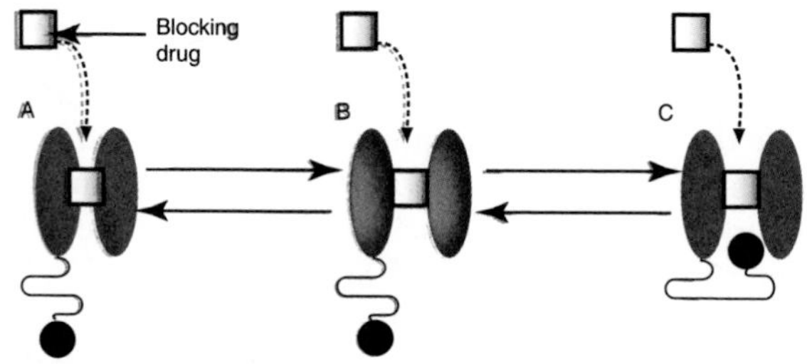

FIGURE 2-2 Resting, activated, and inactivated states of voltage-gated channels, exemplified by the sodium channel.

protein called guanosine-binding protein (G-protein).[1,7] The actual receptor crosses the membrane seven times, with the outer loops containing the active site for ligand binding (Figure 2–5). The inner loops are involved in activating of the G-protein. Once the appropriate ligand or drug binds to the extracellular side, a change occurs in the three-dimensional structure of the receptor that activates the G-protein, which then activates other effectors such as ion channels and enzymes. G-proteins consist of three protein subunits: α-, β-, and γ-subunits. Once activated, the α-subunit binds guanosine triphosphate (GTP) and loses its affinity for the βγ-subunit (joined subunit). The α-subunit bound to GTP dissociates from the βγ-subunit, and each exerts its influence on a second messenger system. There are several types of G-proteins, the functions of which are determined by the type of α-subunit. The ultimate effects may be seen on enzyme activity, contractile proteins, ion channels, and cytokine production. Examples of receptors that are linked to G-proteins include subtypes of the muscarinic acetylcholine receptor, dopamine receptor, and norepinephrine receptor, as well as a variety of hormone receptors.[8-10] In addition, G-protein–linked receptors function as targets for drugs for approximately 30 currently available medications, including montelukast (Singulair), losartan (Cozaar), and loratadine (Claritin). It is expected that therapeutic intervention with these receptors will have a major impact on a variety of diseases in the future.

DNA-coupled receptors are intracellular receptors that stimulate gene transcription, leading to the synthesis of proteins and enzymes.[11-13] Because most are located intracellularly in the nucleus, the ligands must be lipophilic to facilitate crossing the cell membrane. Many of the ligands that activate this type of receptor are steroid hormones, including estrogen, progesterone, cortisol, and thyroid hormone. Each receptor contains two regions, one for binding to DNA and the other for binding to the hormone. When the hormone binds to the receptor on the nuclear membrane, it interacts with a hormone response element on the genome to either activate or depress gene expression. If gene expression is activated, an increase in ribonucleic acid (RNA) polymerase activity is detected within a few minutes. The result is altered protein synthesis. Mineralocorticoids act at these receptors to stimulate the production of new carrier proteins involved in transport of ions through the kidney tubules.[14]

The last type of receptor to be discussed is the kinase-linked receptor. Kinase-linked receptors have a single transmembrane helical region with a larger extracellular domain for ligand binding.[1,15] The size of the extracellular region is related to the size of the endogenous ligand, an example of which is the insulin molecule.[16] Insulin binding produces a dimerization, that is, a linkage of two kinase receptors that then phosphorylate each other. The autophosphorylation of the tyrosine amino acids further provides strong binding sites for other intracellular proteins. These intracellular proteins vary, depending on the receptor involved, but are usually related to cell division and growth, with the final product being transcription of genes. Tyrosine kinase receptors have become recent targets for new and innovative treatments for cancer, including lung, breast, and gastrointestinal stromal tumors.[17-20]

Other Sites of Drug Action

In addition to the receptors discussed previously, drugs may bind to several other specific sites. In the kidney tubules, in particular, specific cell membrane ion pumps and carrier proteins act as sites of drug action. Many diuretics bind to Na^+ transporters in the renal tubules to block reabsorption of NA^+.[21] If Na^+ is not reabsorbed, water is lost (excreted), and plasma volume is decreased, resulting in a lowering of blood pressure. Digoxin binds to the Na^+/K^+-adenosine triphosphatase pump in

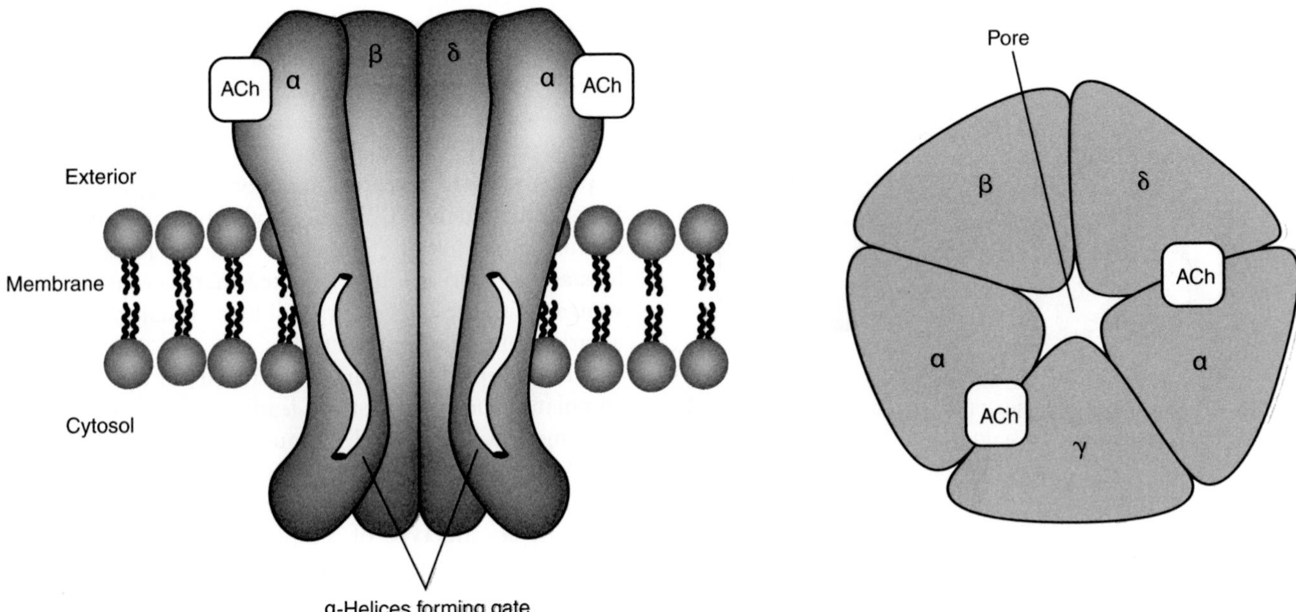

FIGURE 2-3 The structure of the nicotinic acetylcholine (Ach) receptor. The five receptor subunits (α, β, γ, σ) surround a central transmembrane pore, with the luminal amino acids being negatively charged. This negative charge attracts positively charged ions. When two acetylcholine molecules bind to the extracellular portion of the receptor, then the channel opens and ions flow into the cell.

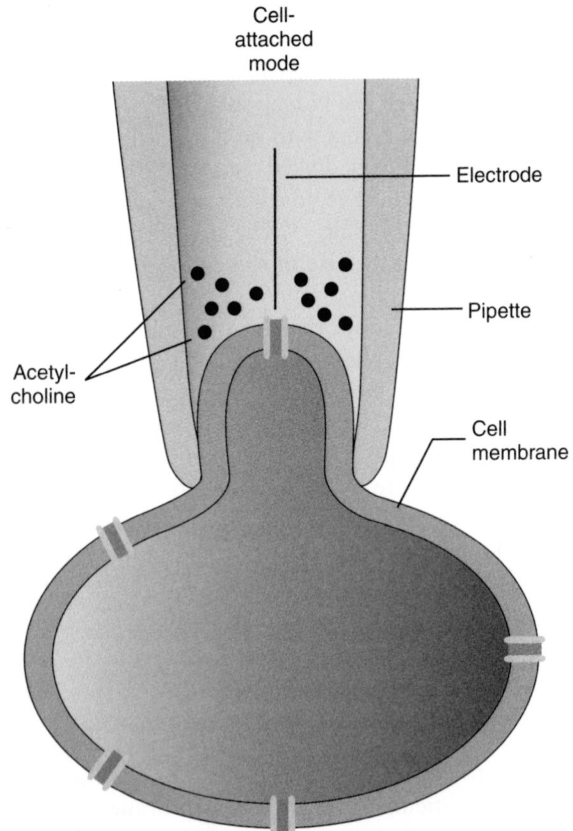

FIGURE 2-4 Patch-clamp technique to measure the flow of ions through an acetylcholine-sensitive potassium channel (I_{KACh}) used as an example. A pipette is pressed tightly against the cell membrane, suction is applied, and a tight seal is formed between the pipette and the membrane. Acetylcholine in the pipette activates the channel, and electrodes in the pipette measure the flow of ions.

cardiac tissue to inhibit it, ultimately resulting in greater contractility of the ventricles.[22]

Enzymes represent another target for drugs. Drugs that bind to acetylcholinesterase to inactivate it have been developed. This function of the drugs allows active acetylcholine to remain longer at the synaptic cleft to activate the neuromuscular junction.[23] Drugs used in the treatment of myasthenia gravis work in this manner.

Other targets for drugs include molecular targets that are not part of human cells.[24] Some antibiotics bind to the bacterial ribosome and not to the similar organelle in humans. The same is true for antiviral agents in that they bind to viral DNA and RNA but not necessarily to the human nucleotides.

DRUG–RECEPTOR INTERACTIONS

The binding of drugs to receptors has a certain specificity and selectivity. Drugs that act on only one type of receptor are considered specific for that receptor. For example, norepinephrine (a neurotransmitter released by sympathetic nerve terminals) is specific for binding only to a sympathetic adrenergic receptor and not to the muscarinic cholinergic receptor. However, norepinephrine is not selective for only one subtype of adrenergic receptor. It has affinity for many sympathomimetic receptors, α_1, α_2, β_1, β_2, and β_3.[25] The β-adrenoceptor blocker propranolol is also specific for β-receptors but is not selective because it can bind both β_1- and β_2-adrenoceptors.[25] Metoprolol, another β-adrenoceptor blocker, is selective in that it will bind preferentially to β_1- and not to β_2-receptors.[25] However, as the concentration of a nonselective drug is increased, it will begin to bind to all subtypes

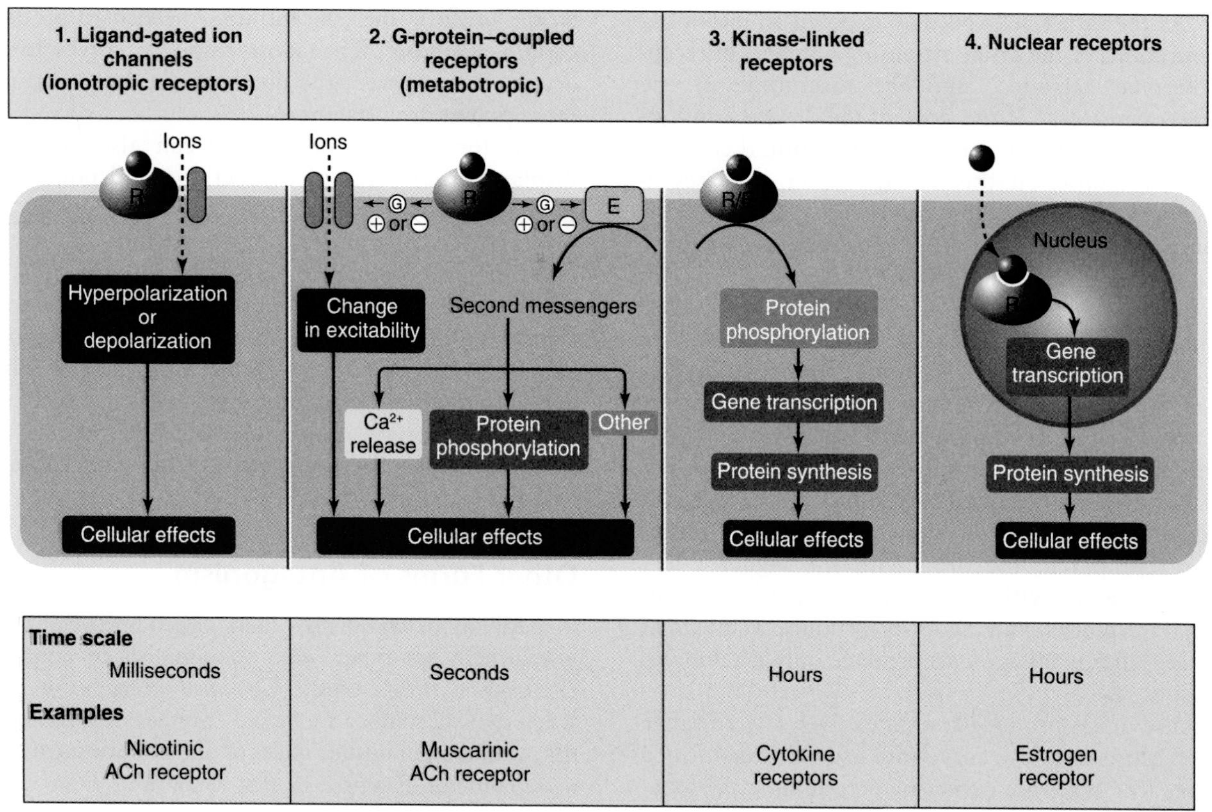

FIGURE 2-5 Major receptor types demonstrating activation times.

of receptors. These concepts of specificity and selectivity are important because the more specific and selective a drug is, the more targeted the therapeutic approach can be. In addition, selective drugs tend to have fewer adverse effects than do nonselective drugs.

Agonists and Antagonists

The strength of binding of a drug to a receptor can be illustrated both quantitatively and qualitatively. In drug binding experiments, a radioactive ligand is used to measure binding affinity. In these experiments, varying concentrations of the radioactive drug are incubated with the tissue containing the receptor of interest. The tissue is then removed and analyzed for its radioactivity. A binding curve that shows the relationship between concentration and the amount of drug bound is then created.[26] If two drugs are incubated with the receptor of interest, they may compete for occupation in the same receptor. In this case, each drug will reduce the binding affinity of the other drug. The first drug may be called the agonist in that it binds to the receptor and produces a change that triggers a response. When all the receptors are occupied by the agonist, a maximum response is seen. When a second drug is added, it may compete for receptor occupation with the first drug by blocking its access to the receptor which also blocks the response. In this case, the second drug is labeled as the antagonist. However, an antagonist is strictly defined as a ligand that binds to the receptor but does not cause the usual conformational change in the receptor. It simply blocks the channel, thus preventing the flow of ions into or out of the cell.

Antagonists may be divided into two categories: *competitive antagonist* and *noncompetitive antagonist*.[27] The competitive antagonist binds at the same site as the agonist, but it can be displaced by the agonist as its concentration increases. Thus it is also known as a *reversible antagonist*. A noncompetitive antagonist cannot be reversed by additional agonist, since it blocks receptors permanently. A noncompetitive angtagonist also can bind to other locations on the receptor, but its end result is to diminish or block completely the effect of the agonist.

Another drug–receptor interaction can be described by the action of a partial agonist. The partial agonist is a drug that might demonstrate both agonist and antagonist properties toward a receptor. At low concentrations it will trigger a response, but at high concentrations it will compete with the natural ligand by physically preventing access of that ligand to its receptor; therefore only a partial or submaximal response will be attained.

Dose-Response Curves

The relationship among agonists, partial agonists, and antagonists can be illustrated graphically. When a drug is administered to a patient, a certain response will occur. As the target cells become exposed to increasing concentrations of the drug, increasing numbers of receptors become activated, and the magnitude of the response increases.[28] If the dose of the drug is continuously increased, the response grows until there is a maximal response. At this point, further increases in drug concentration produces no further response. Pharmacologists demonstrate this "drug receptor theory" with a dose-response curve (Figure 2–6).

In the dose-response curve, by convention, the dose is plotted on the x-axis and the response is plotted on the y-axis. These curves resemble rectangular hyperbolas. The plateau portion of this curve represents the Emax, or the maximum response, that can occur despite infinite concentrations. The Emax is also a measure of drug efficacy or strength of the response. If two drugs that occupy the same proportion of receptors are compared, the drug with the higher Emax represents the one with greater efficacy, that is, greater maximal response. Full agonists produce a maximal response, but partial agonists produce only a submaximal response.

Because drugs produce responses over a wide range of doses, dose-response curves are usually transformed into log–dose-response curves by determining the logarithm of the dose (see Figure 2–6). The new curve then approximates a sigmoid curve. The Emax is still obvious on the sigmoid curve, and the linear portion of this curve makes it easy to determine other parameters such as the Kd or the median effective dose (ED_{50}). The Kd is the dose that produces one half of the expected maximum, Emax, or the dose that produces 50% of the expected response. For the purposes of this book, Kd_{50} and ED_{50} can be viewed as representing the same concept.

The Kd_{50} and ED_{50} are measures of potency. Potency is a measure of binding affinity. The more potent a drug is, the lower is the concentration needed to produce a certain response. When dose–response curves for two drugs are compared, the one with the lower Kd is the more potent drug (Figure 2–7).

The log–dose-response curve can also be used to display the concepts of competitive and noncompetitive antagonists and partial agonists (Figure 2–8). Competitive antagonists compete with the agonists for available receptors and make the agonists look less potent (shift of the log–dose-response curve to the right) (see Figure 2–8). Noncompetitive antagonists cannot be displaced from the receptor and will block agonist effects permanently, thus reducing the Emax. Log–dose-response curves for the partial agonist look similar to those for the noncompetitive antagonist in that the Emax is lowered.

Other Forms of Antagonism

In addition to competitive and noncompetitive antagonism, there are other ways to diminish or completely eliminate a drug's effect. *Chemical antagonism* occurs when two substances are mixed together in solution, and the result is a diminished effect of one or both agents.[1] The most common example of this is the use of antacids to neutralize acid and increase gastric pH. Another example is the use of chelators that form complexes with metal ions and maintain them in an inactive form. Chelation therapy is used to treat heavy metal poisoning.

Physiologic antagonism refers to the administration of two different drugs that have opposite effects. Diuretics are drugs that reduce blood pressure by forcing the excretion of sodium causing a diuresis. Nonsteroidal anti-inflammatory drugs (NSAIDs) reduce pain in inflamed joints but also increase sodium reabsorption through the kidney tubules. Therefore administration of an NSAID will make a diuretic less effective.[29]

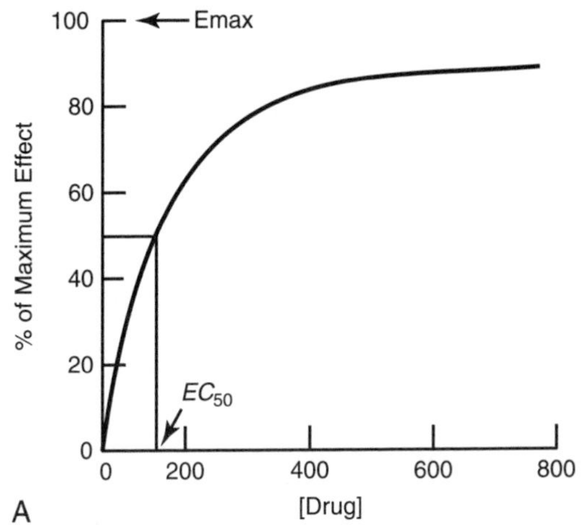

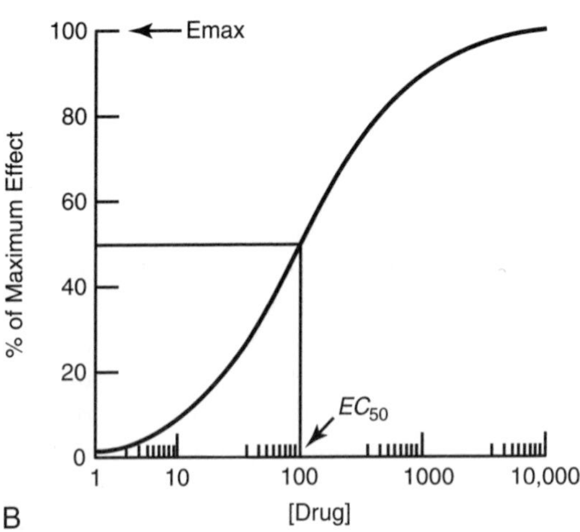

FIGURE 2-6 Dose-effect curves plotted using a linear (**A**) or logarithmic (**B**) scale for drug dose concentration on the x-axis.

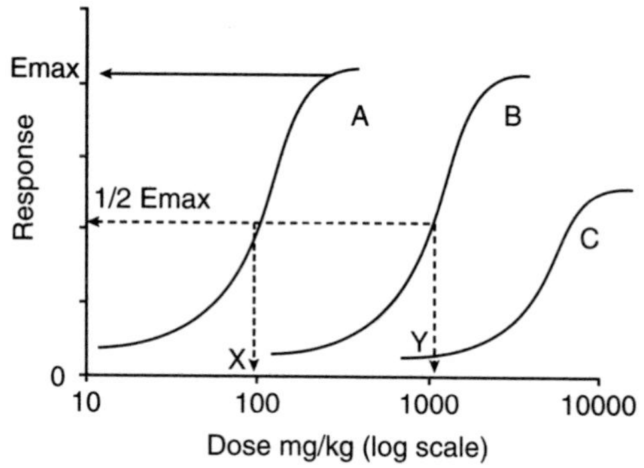

FIGURE 2-7 Graded dose-response curves for three drugs differing in affinity and maximal efficacies. The doses indicated by X and Y represent the dose of drug required to cause 50% of that drug's maximal effect. Drug A is about 10 times more potent than Drug B. Drug A and Drug B have greater efficacies than Drug C. *(Redrawn from Flynn EJ: Pharmacodynamic and pharmacokinetic principles of pharmacology,* J Neurol Phys Ther, *27:94, 2003.)*

Another type of antagonism is referred to as *pharmacokinetic antagonism*. This occurs when an agent increases or induces the activity of an enzyme used to metabolize another drug. Phenobarbital induces the activity of an enzyme involved in the metabolism of many drugs including itself.[30] Long-term administration induces its own metabolism, thus leading to drug tolerance (see Chapter 3).

Changes in receptors may also be viewed as another type of drug antagonism.[31] Receptors that are directly coupled to an ion channel can undergo desensitization. This desensitized state is characterized by a change in the shape of the receptor without either opening or closing of the channel. This may occur rapidly for ion channels, or more slowly for a G-protein–linked receptor through uncoupling with its second messengers. And lastly, an internalization or loss of receptors may occur following prolonged exposure to an agonist, possibly due to "internalization" of the receptor.

DRUG SAFETY

Data obtained from studies examining dose-response relationships may be manipulated to reflect how drugs affect populations in terms of efficacy and safety. Pooling drug responses across many subjects and evaluating the final outcomes in terms of effectiveness help determine how safe a drug is expected to be. Quantal dose-response curves for effectiveness and for toxic effects are used to determine a therapeutic and safety index.

Quantal Dose-Response Curves

Dose-response curves represent graded responses to a drug taken by a single subject or by many subjects from a single population. A *quantal dose-response curve* is a variation on the dose-response curve that is used to examine discrete outcomes (patient is either cured or not cured) instead of a gradation of responses.[26] These curves are used to assess outcomes in heterogeneous populations and also help assess the safety of drugs. Typically, two curves are established. The first is used to examine the beneficial effects of the drug and the second to examine the toxic or lethal effects of the drug. An example is a drug that is used to treat migraines. Increasing doses of the drug are given until all subjects have been cured of their headache (in our example n = 100 patients). For each dose, the number of subjects cured by the drug is recorded. Dosing begins at 1 mg/kg which cures only one subject. Increasing the dose to 2 mg/kg may cure an additional 12 subjects. By the time the dose is increased to 3 mg/kg, roughly half the patients are cured. And when the dose is increased to as high as 5 mg/kg, all 100 subjects are free of headaches (Figure 2–9). Plotting these data as a frequency curve yields a bell-shaped curve. This bell-shaped curve can then be replotted as a cumulative percentage responding (y-axis) versus dose (x-axis). The second curve is determined by repeating the experiment,

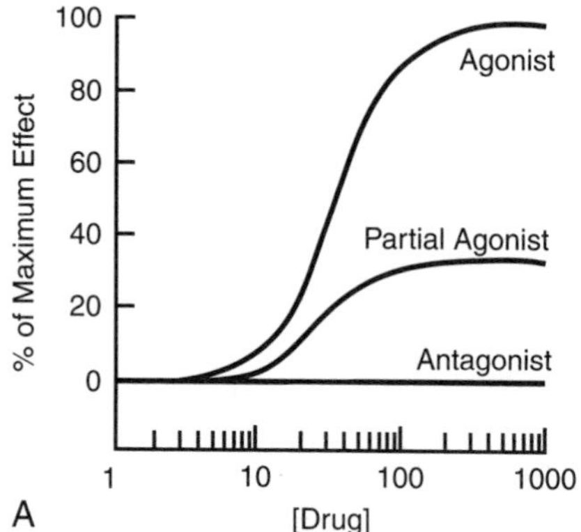

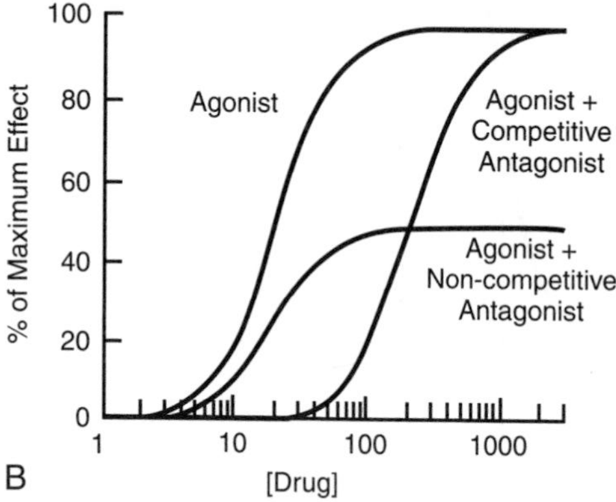

FIGURE 2-8 **A**, Dose-effect curves describing the types of pharmacologic effects produced when a drug interacts with its receptor. An agonist produces the maximum stimulatory effect, a partial agonist produces less than the maximum stimulator effect, and an antagonist elicits no effect, but inhibits the effect of an agonist. **B**, Dose-effect curves for the combination of an agonist and antagonist. A competitive antagonist reduces the potency of the agonist but not the maximum effect. A noncompetitive agonist reduces the efficacy (maximum effect) but does not alter the potency of the agonist. *(From Atkinson AJ, Abernethy DR, et al:* Principles of clinical pharmacology, *2e, Burlington, MA, Academic Press, 2007.)*

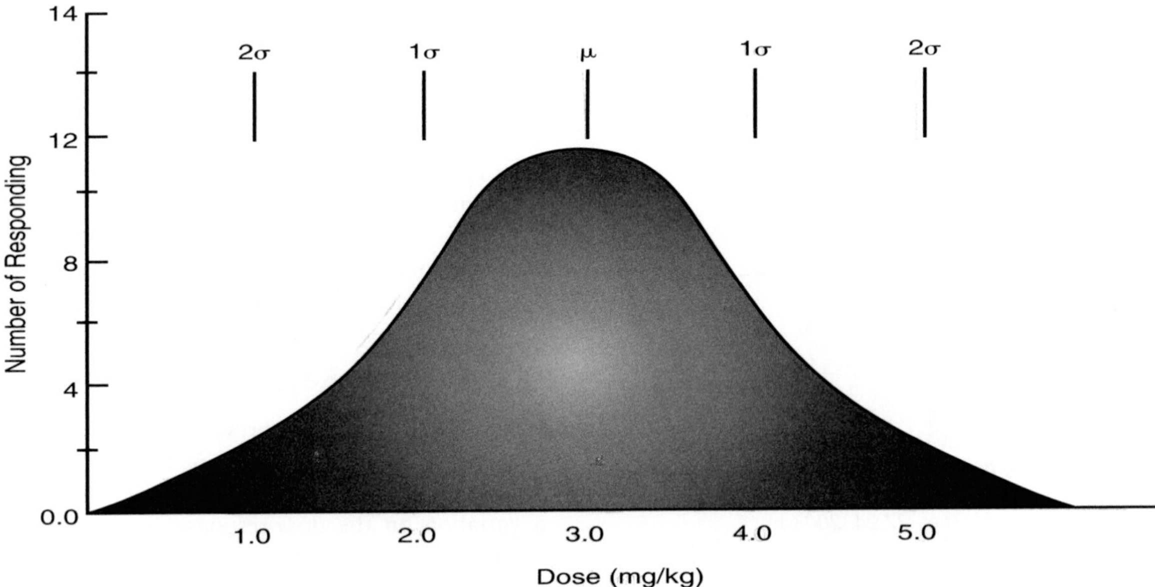

FIGURE 2-9 A quantal dose-response curve after administering increasing amounts of a drug to 100 subjects.

but this time with greater drug concentrations. The outcome in this case is an unwanted effect, possibly death (theoretically only). The ED_{50} is determined for the first curve, but for the curve representing unwanted effects, the lethal dose that kills 50% of the subjects taking the drug (LD_{50}) is determined. The bell-shaped curves are transformed into sigmoid curves and then graphed together on the same x- and y-axes, and the ED_{50} and LD_{50} are compared (Figure 2–10). If the two curves are far apart from each other, then the drug is considered relatively safe. This means that a much greater amount of the drug would have to be taken to kill the patient than that to help the patient. Pharmacologists may also determine the toxic dose at 50% (TD_{50}), the dose that produces adverse effects as opposed to lethal effects in half the population, so that the doses producing adverse effects are known.

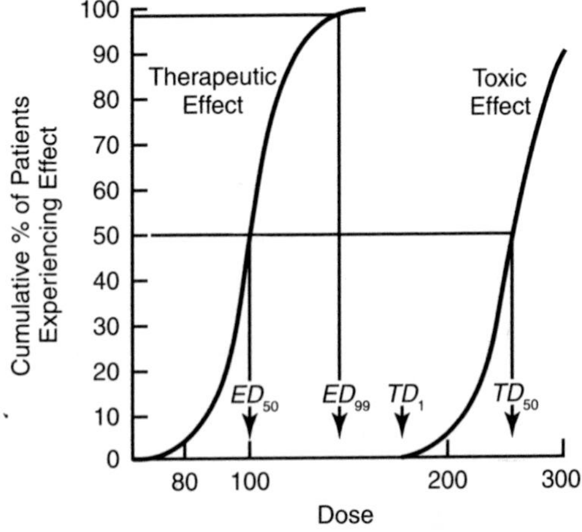

FIGURE 2-10 Cumulative quantal dose-effect curves for a drug's therapeutic and toxic effects. The ED_{50} and the ED_{99} are the doses required to produce the drug's therapeutic effect in 50% and 99% of the population, respectively. The TD_1 and TD_{50} are the doses that cause the toxic effect in 1% and 50% of the population respectively. *(From Atkinson AJ, Abernethy DR, Daniels CE, editors:* Principles of clinical pharmacology, *2e, Burlington, MA, Academic Press, 2007.)*

Therapeutic Index

The *therapeutic index* (TI) describes the distance between a quantal dose-response curve for a desired effect and a quantal dose-response curve for the undesired drug effect.[32] It is calculated as the ratio of the LD_{50} to the ED_{50}. The greater this value, the less lethal is the drug. Some drugs have very low TIs (e.g., lithium and digoxin). Patients taking drugs with low TIs, less than 2.5, must be monitored for adverse reactions. Because it is likely that adverse events will occur, instead of some observable or toxic event, a "defined target plasma concentration" is used to determine proper dosing. An additional parameter, called the *safety margin*, is calculated as the ratio of the LD_{01} (dose that kills 1% of the subjects) to the ED_{99} (dose that is effective in 99% of the subjects). The safety margin is a more conservative measure of safety than the TI.

These measures of safety have some specific limitations. First, patient response to medications is highly individual. The TI does not take into consideration other drugs that a patient may be taking that could lead to a drug-to-drug interaction. Second, it is not always easy to determine a measure of effectiveness. Patients and the medical community may not share the same definition of what is effective. Patients may want complete cessation of their migraine headaches, whereas physicians may interpret the drug as being successful if a patient is able to return to work even if some discomfort is still present. Third, data from toxicity studies come from experiments with animals, and thus the findings cannot be readily applied to the human population. Some social and economic factors also diminish the significance of the TI. Patient compliance issues such as failure to take prescribed medications as specified and borrowing or taking friends' drugs that are expired or issued at different doses are factors that may render a drug dangerous but which is otherwise presumed safe.

New methods are now being explored to help quantify the benefits and risks associated with drug use. One method is called the number-needed-to-treat (NNT). This method calculates the number of patients who must be exposed to a drug for one patient to experience the desired effect. It is hoped that this method will take into consideration individual variations among patients and provide a more realistic measure of drug safety, at least one that can be more easily explained to patients.

ACTIVITIES 2

Constructing a Quantal Dose-response Curve

1. Groups of mice will receive varying doses of a drug used to lower heart rate. Some of the mice will have some bradycardia, and some will have excessive bradycardia leading to death. Refer to the table and plot the percentage responding at each dose level for its therapeutic effect and its lethal effect and calculate the therapeutic index. Discuss whether the drug is safe. Describe a situation in which the therapeutic index may be misleading.

Dose (mg/kg)	Bradycardia	Death
1	0%	0%
2	3%	0%
3	13%	0%
4	45%	3%
5	80%	23%
6	100%	68%
7	100%	100%
8	100%	100%

2. Discuss the difference between a medication's mechanism of action and its therapeutic effect.
3. If a patient must take a drug with a low therapeutic index, what must happen to ensure that the patient does not experience a toxic event?
4. What cognitive, behavioral, and physical factors in a patient could reduce a drug's therapeutic index and reduce the safety of the agent?

REFERENCES

1. Page C, Curtis, MJ, Sutter, MC, Walker, MJ, Hoffman, BB et al: The general mechanisms of drug action. In Clive PP, Brian H, Michael C, Michael W, editors: Integrated pharmacology, Philadelphia, 2006, Mosby.
2. Carmody JJ: Some scientific reflections on possible mechanisms of general anaesthesia.(Clinical report), Anaesth Intensive Care, 37(2):175(15), 2009.
3. Gadsby DC: Ion channels versus ion pumps: The principal difference, in principle, Nat Rev Mol Cell Biol, 10(5): 344–352, 2009.
4. Swartz KJ: Sensing voltage across lipid membranes. Nature, 456(7224): 891–897, 2008.
5. Verkman AS, Galietta LJV: Chloride channels as drug targets, Nat Rev Drug Discov, 8(2):153–171, 2009.
6. Zareba W, Cygankiewicz I: Long QT syndrome and short QT syndrome, Prog Cardiovasc Dis, 51(3):264–278, 2008.
7. Milligan G, et al: Novel pharmacological applications of G-protein-coupled receptor—G protein fusions, Curr Opin Pharmacol, 7(5):521–526, 2007.
8. Yeagle PL, Albert AD: G-protein coupled receptor structure. Biochemica et Biophysica Acta (BBA) - Biomembranes, 1768(4):808–824, 2007.
9. David P, Yongsheng L, Krassimira A, Demarg G, Meehan TP, Fanelli F, Narayan P: Structure-function relationships of the luteinizing hormone receptor, Ann N Y Acad Sci, 1061 (Testicular Cell Dynamics and Endocrine Signaling):41–54, 2005.
10. Filardo EJ, Thomas P: GPR30: A seven-transmembrane-spanning estrogen receptor that triggers EGF release, Trends Endocrinol Metab, 16(8):362–367, 2005.
11. Ma WW, Adjei AA: Novel agents on the horizon for cancer therapy, CA Cancer J Clin, 59(2):111–137, 2009.
12. McEwan IJ: Nuclear receptors: One big family, Methods Mol Biol, 505:3–18, 2009.
13. Novac N, Heinzel T: Nuclear receptors: Overview and classification, Current Drug Targets—Inflammation & Allergy, 3(4):335–346, 2004.
14. Funder JW, Mihailidou AS: Aldosterone and mineralocorticoid receptors: Clinical studies and basic biology, Mol Cell Endocrinol, 301(1-2):2–6, 2009.
15. Jones JI, Clemmons DR: Insulin-like growth factors and their binding proteins: Biological actions, Endocr Rev, 16(1):3–34, 1995.
16. Pollak M: Insulin and insulin-like growth factor signalling in neoplasia, Nat Rev Cancer, 8(12):915–928, 2008.
17. Belinsky MG, Rink L, Cai KQ, et al: The insulin-like growth factor system as a potential therapeutic target in gastrointestinal stromal tumors, Cell Cycle, 19:2949–2955, 2008.
18. Gralow J, Ozols RF, Bajorin DF, et al. Clinical cancer advances 2007: Major research advances in cancer treatment, prevention, and screening—a report from the American Society of Clinical Oncology, J Clin Oncol, 26(2):313–325, 2008.
19. Stockmans G, et al. Triple-negative breast cancer. Current Opinion in Oncology, 20:614–620, 2008.
20. Herbst RS, Heymach JV, Lippman SM: Lung cancer. N Engl J Med, 359(13):1367–1380, 2008.
21. Ecelbarger CA, Tiwari S: Sodium transporters in the distal nephron and disease implications, Curr Hypertension Rep, 8:158–165, 2006.
22. Newman RA, Yang P, Pawlus AD, Block KI: Cardiac glycosides as novel cancer therapeutic agents. Mol Interv, 8(1):36–49, 2008.
23. Martyn JAJ, Eriksson L: M.J.F.L.I.E., Basic principles of neuromuscular transmission, Anaesthesia, 64(s1):1–9, 2009.
24. Rang HP, et al: Antibacterial drugs. In Rang HP, Dale MM, Ritter JM, Flower R, editors: Rang and Dale's pharmacology, Philadelphia, 2007, Churchill Livingstone.
25. Rang HP, et al: Noradrenergic transmission. In Rang HP, Dale MM, Ritter JM, Flower R, editors: Rang and Dale's pharmacology, Philadelphia, 2007, Churchill Livingstone.
26. Lowe ES, Balis FM: Dose-effect and concentration-effect analysis. In Atkinson AJ. Jr, Daniels CE, Dedrick RL, Grudzinskas

CV, Markey SP, editors:: Principles of clinical pharmacology, New York, 2007, Academic Press.
27. Vauquelin GI, Van Liefde I, Birzbier BB, Vanderheyden P: New insights in insurmountable antagonism, Fundam Clin Pharmacol, 16(4):263–272, 2002.
28. Tallarida RJ: Interactions between drugs and occupied receptors, Pharmacol Ther, 113(1):197–209, 2007.
29. Gurwitz JH, Everitt DE, Monane M, et al: The impact of ibuprofen on the efficacy of antihypertensive treatment with hydrochlorothiazide in elderly persons, J Gerontol: A: Biol Sci Med Sci, 51(2):M74–M79, 1996.
30. Sueyoshi T, Negishi M: Phenobarbital response elements of cytochrome P450 genes and nuclear receptors, Ann Rev Pharmacol Toxicol, 41:123-143, 2001.
31. Rang HP, et al: How drugs act: General principles. In Rang HP, Dale MM, Ritter JM, Flower R, editors: Rang and Dale's pharmacology, Philadelphia, 2007, Churchill Livingstone.
32. Bennett PN, Brown MJ: General pharmacology. In Bennett PN, Brown MJ, editors: Clinical pharmacology, New York, 2008, Churchill Livingstone.

3

Pharmacokinetics and Drug Dosing

Barbara Gladson

WHAT IS PHARMACOKINETICS?

Strictly defined, *pharmacokinetics* refers to the rate at which drug concentrations accumulate in and are eliminated from various organs of the body. It is what the body does to the drug and, in the liberal sense, encompasses how a drug is absorbed, distributed, metabolized, and ultimately eliminated from the body.[1] This chapter examines pharmacokinetics in the broad sense and includes discussion of the movement of drugs across cell membranes, routes of administration, and volume of distribution, as well as the more literal definition of pharmacokinetics—breakdown reactions and elimination. Each of these concepts may be explained both physiologically and mathematically. The mathematic description of pharmacokinetics determines the dosing schedules, but because of the complex nature of the equations, our discussion on this topic will be a simplified one.

MOVEMENT OF DRUGS ACROSS CELL MEMBRANES

As drugs move from their site of administration to their target tissue, they cross many biologic barriers. These barriers, or cell membranes, are commonly bilayers of lipid molecules with hydrophilic regions on both the outside and inside layers of the membrane and a hydrophobic region between the two layers.[2] Lipid-soluble molecules are able to diffuse readily into cells across this membrane. Water-filled channels are also found, through which water-soluble substances of small size may cross. In addition, special proteins called *carrier proteins* that allow passage of specific substances are interspersed throughout the membrane. Depending on the location, more or less of these water-soluble channels and carrier proteins exist; for example, the jejunum contains many channels and carriers, whereas the urinary bladder has only a few.

Drugs cross membranes in five main ways: (1) endocytosis, (2) pinocytosis, (3) diffusion through the water-filled channels or specialized ion channels, (4) carrier-mediated processes that include facilitated diffusion or active transport, and (5) passive diffusion through the lipid membrane (Figure 3-1).[3,4] The methods of endocytosis and pinocytosis have limited usefulness for drug transport because they are primarily concerned with the uptake of macromolecules. However, certain drugs have been incorporated into a lipid vesicle or liposome, necessitating the use of this method for drug transfer, particularly across the blood–brain barrier.[5,6] Passage of drugs through ion channels occurs for very small molecules such as therapeutic ions (e.g., lithium and radioactive iodide).[7] If such small molecules pass through the water-filled pores, they must be water soluble. The impetus for drug transfer for this process is a concentration gradient. Carrier-mediated processes are involved in movement of drugs across the blood–brain barrier, the gastrointestinal (GI) epithelium, and the renal tubules. Drug entry via passive diffusion was previously believed to be the primary mode of entry into cells, but now uptake by transporter proteins is thought to be more significant as well as possibly being a site for drug interactions.[8] This method involves a transmembrane protein that binds to a drug, changes conformation (shape), and then releases the molecule on the other side of the membrane. When this process is passive, it is called *facilitated diffusion*. The drug in this case must resemble a natural ligand and travel from an area of high concentration to one of low concentration. Levodopa, a drug used for the treatment of Parkinson's disease, is transferred through the duodenum and jejunum and across the blood–brain barrier by facilitated diffusion by means of a large neutral amino acid–specific carrier system.[9] In the renal tubules, many drugs act by binding to carrier proteins.[10] When binding is strong, the molecule is released slowly; therefore the actual drug action is to block carrier function. Many diuretics act in this manner and prevent the reabsorption of sodium. When a drug requires transport against a concentration gradient, energy is required and it is called active transport.

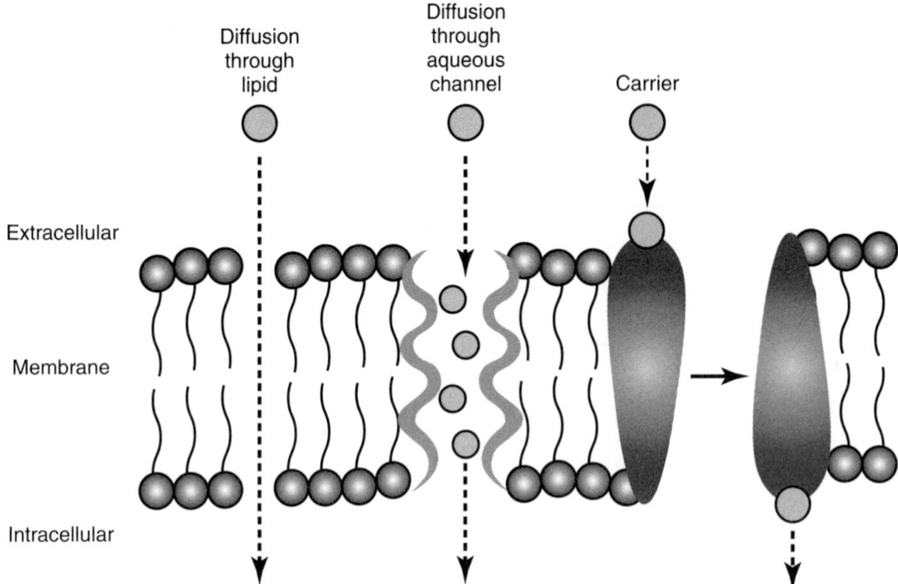

FIGURE 3-1 Routes by which drugs can pass through cell membranes.

Passive Diffusion of Drugs Across Lipid Membranes

Passive diffusion down a concentration gradient is one of the primary methods by which drugs cross membranes.[4,11] Nonpolar neutral molecules dissolve easily in lipids and therefore traverse cell membranes without difficulty. Fick's law describes this passive diffusion as a function of the concentration difference across the membrane, the thickness of the membrane, and the permeability coefficient, P. The greater the concentration difference between the two sides of the membrane, the greater will be the rate of diffusion. In addition, the thicker the membrane, the more slowly will the drug cross.

The permeability coefficient is unique to each drug and depends on certain physicochemical factors such as its lipid solubility and degree of ionization. Lipid solubility is determined by the molecule's partition coefficient.[11] There is a close correlation between the partition coefficient and the compound's solubility, and this correlation is an important factor in determining the drug's rate of absorption and elimination. Thiopental is a sedative-hypnotic agent that is used as an anesthetic. It has an effective partition coefficient value of 2000.[11] This drug is extremely soluble in lipids, allowing for rapid diffusion across the lipid-rich blood–brain barrier to produce a quick loss of consciousness (within seconds). Pentobarbital is also a sedative–hypnotic agent that has a coefficient of 42. It is less lipid soluble and therefore diffuses into the brain at a slower rate than does thiopental. It has been used for its preanesthetic effect of reducing anxiety and facilitating anesthesia induction when given along with other barbiturates. Barbital, another sedative–hypnotic agent, has a coefficient value of 1.1. This drug is much less membrane soluble than either thiopental or pentobarbital, and thus diffusion is slower. It used to be prescribed for people who could fall asleep but had trouble staying asleep. Barbital and pentobarbital are rarely used now for sleep disturbances or anxiety because of their addictive quality, but the issue of lipid solubility is well illustrated by these drugs.

Even if a drug is lipid soluble, its molecular weight may preclude absorption from the gastrointestinal (GI) tract. Molecules of drugs such as insulin are simply too large to pass through the GI mucosa; therefore these drugs must be administered by injection.[12]

Many drugs are weak acids or bases and therefore can exist in both un-ionized (electrically neutral) and ionized (either a positive or negative charge) forms. The problem is that ionized molecules have very low lipid solubility. However, the degree of ionization depends on the pH of the local environment and the negative logarithm of the acid ionization constant (pKa) of the compound.[3] In an acidic environment such as the stomach, weak acids will exist in an uncharged or neutral state (Figure 3-2).

Thus drugs that are acidic, such as aspirin, will be absorbed from this area. However, in the intestine where the pH is greater, the compound would tend to give off hydrogen and thus exist in an ionized state. In the stomach, basic drugs will more likely exist in a charged form but will be neutral in the intestine. The loss of protons in the small intestine will increase the percentage of neutral molecules and thus aid in drug absorption into the circulation. However, in the intestine, neutrality is not the only parameter influencing absorption because the very large surface area for

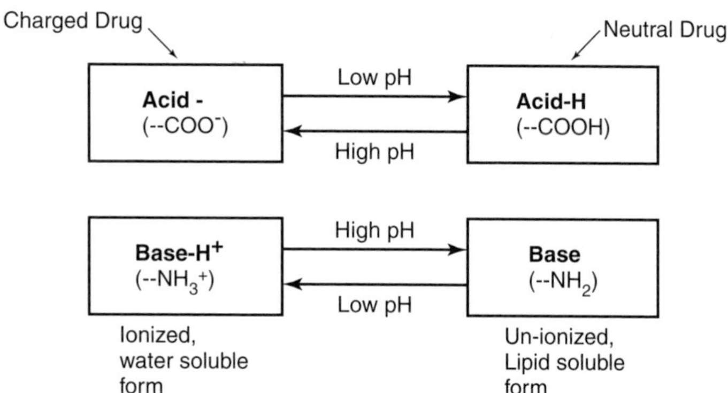

FIGURE 3-2 The direction of ionization varies with pH. In a low pH environment, an acid will be predominately neutral while a base will be charged. The reverse is true in a high pH environment.

absorption is also a determining factor in how a drug gets through the mucosal surface. The degree of ionization can be determined by using the Henderson-Hasselbalch equation, which relates the ratio of protonated (containing hydrogen H^+) to the unprotonated form of a weak acid or base to the pH of the environment and the pKa of the molecule. This equation is used to calculate the degree of ionization of both acidic and basic drugs and demonstrates that the lower the pH relative to the pKa, the more of the drug is protonated than unprotonated. An acidic drug passing through the stomach will therefore primarily exist in the protonated (neutral) form. Artificially controlling the pH of a particle body compartment has some clinical significance. Drugs that alkalinize the urine can be used to treat aspirin overdose. Consuming bicarbonate will cause the pH of the urine to increase, thus maintaining salicylate ionization. The charged compound will undergo elimination rather than being reabsorbed through the kidney tubules and into the systemic circulation.

$$\log \frac{(\text{Protonated})}{(\text{unprotonated})} = pK_a - pH$$

DRUG ABSORPTION AND ROUTES OF ADMINISTRATION

Drug *absorption*, the first phase of pharmacokinetics, is the process by which the drug is transferred from its site of administration to the systemic circulation. The efficiency and ease of this process depends on the physicochemical properties of drugs as discussed previously but also depends on the route of administration, including oral, intravenous (IV), intramuscular, inhalation, sublingual, subcutaneous, and topical applications.[13]

Absorption from the Gastrointestinal Tract

Oral administration of drugs with absorption occurring from the GI tract is the most convenient route of administration and most favored by patients. Medicines that are absorbed in this manner are dispensed in tablet, capsule, or syrup form. However, a number of factors make this method one of the most complex ways of giving medications. Drugs can be absorbed via simple lipid diffusion or as in the case of levodopa be taken across via carrier-mediated transporters.

Drug formulation influences rate of absorption because the tablet or capsule must disintegrate, releasing the drug into the GI contents before absorption can take place.[14] Most tablets will dissolve quickly; however, considerable research is being conducted on fast orally disintegrating systems. These formulations use different excipients as well as new manufacturing processes that promote disintegration almost immediately upon entering the oral mucosa.[14-17] These are especially useful for patients with dysphagia or emesis or for any individual who does not have water available immediately. These quick-dissolving drugs are available in a variety of forms, including tablets, wafers, gums, and films.

Some drug formulations are specially designed to delay disintegration so that absorption can occur slowly over time. This is the principle behind slow-release agents. Tablets coated with a semipermeable membrane will demonstrate delayed absorption. Additionally, tablets may be formulated to dissolve only in the intestines to prevent gastric irritation. Aspirin coated in an acid-insoluble layer (enteric-coated) has delayed absorption until the drug reaches the intestine. A new technology is under study that uses mucoadhesive microspheres to delay drug absorption and to increase efficiency of locally applied agents.[18] The microspheres coupled with the drug can adhere to mucosal surfaces and maintain the drug's contact with the absorbing surface for an extended period. This technique promises improved drug absorption not only in oral administration of drugs but also in buccal, nasal, ocular, vaginal, and rectal modes of administration.

Gastric emptying also influences the rate at which drugs are absorbed.[14] When gastric emptying is hastened, the drug is delivered to the small intestine more quickly, which enhances absorption. Coadministration of cholinomimetic agents (drugs that stimulate the parasympathetic system) will speed gastric emptying. However, excessive motility will decrease absorption. The presence of food in the GI tract tends to delay absorption, although there are exceptions, for example, drugs such as propranolol that undergo greater absorption with food, probably as a result of increased splanchnic blood flow after a meal. Research has shown that transit time for a drug taken on an empty stomach is less than 2 hours compared with 10 hours if consumed after a large meal.[19] Transit time through the small intestine is approximately 3 hours in spite of being taken with or without food.

Breakdown of drugs may occur in the GI tract before or during absorption.[14] The intestinal lumen and wall contain many enzymes such as monoamine oxidase and L-aromatic amino acid decarboxylase, which are responsible for the breakdown of many drugs.[20] The GI bacteria and the very acidic environment of the stomach also contribute to reduced absorption.[21] Penicillin G is unstable in the low pH of the stomach, and therefore very large oral doses would need to be given to patients if this were the preferred route of administration. Instead, this drug is administered intravenously. Efflux pumps pose another hazard to drug absorption. These drug transporters (adenosine triphosphate (ATP)-binding cassette drug transporters and solute carrier transporters) actually pump the drug back out into the intestinal tract for subsequent elimination in the feces.[22]

Because there is considerable loss of the drug in the GI tract before absorption, only a fraction of the given oral dose actually enters the systemic circulation. The term that describes this fraction is *bioavailability*.[23] Bioavailability refers to the percentage of the drug that makes it into the systemic circulation from the site of administration, taking into consideration early degradation. It is more of a conceptual image than an exact percentage because bioavailability is variable and can be altered by the local pH, intestinal motility, and presence of food. However, drugs that typically exhibit low bioavailability are either given by injection or administered to the patient with special instructions. Alendronate is a drug that reduces bone absorption, commonly given to postmenopausal women to treat osteoporosis. This drug is only 1 to 10% bioavailable, and for this reason, patients are asked to take the drug on an empty stomach, 30 minutes before eating a meal.[24] When a drug is administered intravenously, 100% of it is bioavailable because all of it enters the systemic circulation.

Even if a compound makes it through the intestinal wall into the portal circulation, a significant amount of drug may undergo metabolism in the liver before it ever arrives at the target organ. This is referred to as *first-pass metabolism* or *first-pass elimination*.[24] When a drug is administered orally, its next stop after the GI tract, via the portal circulation, is the liver. Because the liver is considered the primary organ of drug metabolism, some of the drug is degraded before it makes its systemic entrance. In fact, every time the drug cycles through the liver, approximately 20% is potentially metabolized because that is the percentage of cardiac output that enters the organ.[2] Therefore oral doses must be much greater than intravenous doses. First-pass metabolism can be avoided if a drug is administered by any route other than the oral route (e.g., through a topical patch, intranasal administration, or IV infusion).

Enteral Drug Administration

Enteral administration refers to drugs being administered anywhere along the GI tract. This includes oral, sublingual, and rectal administration. However, some pharmacologists do not consider sublingual and rectal administration as enteral administration because both those methods avoid intestinal absorption.[2] *Sublingual absorption* refers to the passage of a drug through the buccal or sublingual mucosa. The classic example is sublingual nitroglycerin, which is placed under the tongue and absorbed rapidly into the venous drainage from the mouth to enter the superior vena cava within 1 to 3 minutes.[25,26] However, the patient must be able to tolerate the taste and also the irritation to the mucous membranes.

Rectal drugs are usually in the form of solutions, suspensions, or suppositories. The rectal mucosa are rich in blood and lymph vessels and offer absorption free from first-pass metabolism.[14] An advantage of this route of administration is that it can be used in a patient who is vomiting or experiencing a migraine. It is also a good choice for a patient who has diffculty swallowing or for a child who is uncooperative. The disadvantage is that rectal absorption is inconsistent.

Administering Oral Drugs

It will never be the responsibility of the therapist to administer medications to a patient, but since most of us are consumers of prescription and over-the-counter drugs, a discussion of some important precautions is relevant in this text. In the presence of difficulty swallowing, there is the tendency to crush the tablet and then to mix the contents in soft food such as apple sauce. Patients should, however, refrain from this practice unless the physician's or the manufacturer's instructions indicate that this method of administration is acceptable.[13] Enteric-coated tablets or sustained-release agents should never be crushed, and capsules should never be opened. These special formulations are designed to protect the stomach from irritation. Opening the capsule or crushing the tablet will release all the medication at once, which may cause gastric irritation, inactivation of the medication by gastric acids, and toxic effects caused by total release of a dose designed for slow release.

Properly positioning the patient for medication administration is another important consideration. Patients should be either sitting or side-lying to avoid aspiration. Sitting, standing, and lying on the left side (recumbent left) have been shown to also increase absorption of orally administered drugs resulting in a shorter time to peak plasma drug level.[27] Four to six ounces of water is also recommended for proper disintegration of the drug and to ensure that it reaches the stomach. Occasionally drugs will need to be administered through a nasogastric or gastrostomy tube. Before patients receive the medications, they must be positioned in either the semi-Fowler's or Fowler's position and remain in this position for 30 minutes after administration to prevent aspiration. Many drugs interact with tube feedings, and therefore tube feedings must be discontinued and the tubes fully flushed before drug administration.

Sublingual and buccal medications have their own set of rules. Sublingual forms of medication should be placed under the tongue, and buccal drugs are placed between the upper or lower molars and the cheek. Patients should refrain from drinking until the tablet has fully dissolved, and they should, of course, resist the temptation to swallow the pill.

Parenteral Drug Administration

Parenteral administration refers to administration of drugs in any manner other than through the GI tract; however, some pharmacologists exclude topical as well as inhalation administration from this category.[28] The parenteral route is, then, the route that requires some type of injection, including IV, subcutaneous, intramuscular, epidural, and intrathecal injections. Absorption from all but the IV method occurs by passive diffusion along the drug's concentration gradient but is limited by the density of the absorbing capillaries and the solubility of the drug in the interstitial fluid. IV administration of drugs avoids the absorption phase because the correct concentration of medication is injected immediately into the blood. However, the major disadvantage of this method is that if the wrong amount of drug is injected, there is no recourse. Pumping the stomach or administering an emetic drug will not change the outcome of an overdose given intravenously. However, to avoid a catastrophe, it is recommended that IV push (or bolus) injections be performed slowly, preferably over a period of 1 to 5 minutes.[13] The circulation time between the antecubital vein and the brain is about 10 to 15 seconds, so if a sudden loss of consciousness occurs, the infusion can probably be stopped before the complete dose enters the circulation.[11] Other problems that may occur include local venous thrombosis with prolonged infusion and infection at the site of an IV catheter.

A subcutaneous injection is given under the skin into the fat. This method is effective only for drugs that are nonirritating to the tissues. It is a useful method for self-administration, but if repeated injections are given at the same site, lipoatrophy may occur, as in the case of insulin injections.[29] Subcutaneous injections produce a faster effect than do orally administered drugs, but the rate is variable and depends on the site of injection, how quickly the drug can diffuse through the tissues, and on the local blood flow. In addition, absorption may be slowed by immobilization of the limb or vasoconstriction from cooling of the area. In contrast, heating, exercise, and massage of an area will facilitate absorption of an injected drug.[30,31] This necessitates caution when heat-modalities are used near an area that has recently been injected.

An intramuscular injection administers a drug directly into skeletal muscle. Because muscles have greater blood flow, absorption is more rapid than with subcutaneous injections.[32] The disadvantage of this method is that the drug cannot be injected into an exercising muscle because the increase in blood flow with activity will unduly hasten absorption. In addition, this method is painful and often difficult to self-administer. Too rapid absorption, particularly of insulin, could lead to fatal hypoglycemia.[33]

Intrathecal injections use cerebrospinal fluid for drug transport.[34] An intrathecal injection is given directly into the spinal subarachnoid space, facilitating drug entry into the central nervous system. This type of drug administration may be used to treat brain infections, since many of the available antibiotics are not lipid soluble enough to diffuse across the blood–brain barrier. Baclofen, a drug used to reduce spasticity, may also be administered in this manner.[35] Epidural injections deliver medication into the spinal column but outside the dura. Other parenteral routes include intra-articular (delivery into a synovial cavity), intraosseous (delivery into the bone marrow), intra-arterial (delivery into an artery), and intraperitoneal (delivery into the peritoneal cavity).

Implanted delivery systems consist of a pump and drug reservoir implanted in the belly. Insulin, morphine, and baclofen may be delivered in this manner.

Other Routes of Drug Administration

The lungs have a large surface area and an extensive capillary network, which is excellent for drug absorption.[36] Inhaled anesthetics can be rapidly taken up into the circulation and distributed to the brain for quick induction of sleep. In addition, drugs such as bronchodilators that are used to stop an asthma attack can be inhaled directly into the bronchiole tubules, the target tissue, for effective treatment.

Topical applications of drugs are useful for the treatment of skin, ear, nose, and eye disorders.[36] The advantage of this method is treatment that does not have a systemic effect, although if the agent is applied in a great enough concentration, these effects will occur.[37]

Special transdermal delivery systems have been engineered with a "rate-controlling membrane" specifically to introduce the drug through the skin into the circulation, bypassing the liver.[38] Scopolamine skin patches for the prevention of motion sickness and fentanyl skin patches for the treatment of pain are examples. Transdermal systems are also used to administer estrogen and nitroglycerin.

Exercise and Drug Absorption

For many drugs, neither the effects of exercise on pharmacologic action nor the impact of the drug on the body's response to exercise and exercise performance have been well studied. The impact of exercise on drugs is not typically assessed during clinical trials; hence data on dosing with exercise does not become apparent until after the drug has been approved. For example, antibiotic-induced Achilles tendinopathy specifically associated with ciprofloxacin did not receive attention until years after the drug was out of clinical trials.[39,40]

Data on exercise studies are presented throughout this text as individual drugs are considered. However, we can discuss here a few points regarding absorption. Exercise does appear to affect drug absorption, but this is variable. Theoretically, exercise should reduce absorption of orally administered drugs due to a reduction in splanchnic blood flow. However, the effect on absorption may depend on whether the drug is a weak acid or a weak base. It has been shown that maximum aerobic exercise for more than 30 minutes lowers the pH of blood and of the gastric mucosa.[41] In the case of acidic drugs, this means a greater proportion of the dose will be non-ionized and that drug absorption might be increased. The opposite would occur for drugs that are basic in nature. However, research has not supported this notion. In a study of 10 patients with Parkinson's disease receiving levodopa, absorption was decreased in 5 patients, increased in 3 patients, and unchanged in 2 patients during cycling exercise.[42] In another study, blood levodopa levels were related to unified Parkinson's disease rating scales with and without exercise in 10 patients with the disease.[43] This study revealed that exercise begun at 1 hour after levodopa ingestion did not influence motor scores or the plasma level of the drug, indicating that absorption was not affected. Yet another study on levodopa indicated improved absorption after 2 hours of cycling exercise in 12 patients with Parkinson's disease.[44] Therefore, at least for levodopa, we cannot state with any certainty that exercise has an effect on the absorption of this drug. Exercise, however, was shown to reduce absorption of midazolam (an anxiolytic agent) in six healthy volunteers after 50 minutes of treadmill running.[45] Therefore the effect of exercise on absorption of orally administered drugs is variable and probably depends on the intensity and mode of exercise, the fitness of the patient, drug properties, and the presence or absence of any other medical condition.

Other reports in the literature indicate that exercise has no significant effect on the absorption of oral drugs but does increase absorption from intramuscular, subcutaneous, transdermal, and inhalation sites of administration.[46] Intramuscular, subcutaneous, and transdermal preparations will show increased absorption when applied near an exercising muscle, and absorption may be delayed if preparations are applied farther from an exercising muscle because of the shift in blood flow toward the exercising limb. One hour of intermittent moderate cycling has been shown to increase regular insulin absorption from the thigh but not when the insulin is injected into the arm.[47]

Research has confirmed that exercise increases the absorption of several drugs applied transdermally, including glyceryl trinitrate, fentanyl, nicotine, and hormones used for birth control. Glyceryl trinitrate (nitroglycerin) is a powerful arterial and venous vasodilator used to treat angina. Cycling at a workload adjusted to maintain a heart rate of 110 beats/min, alternating with a workload that increases heart rate to 150 beats/min (sustained for 1 minute every 10 minutes) for a total of 1 hour of exercise, produced a 93% increase in plasma level of the drug.[48] In another study conducted on 12 healthy individuals, a 20-minute sauna treatment resulting in peak skin temperature of 39 °C significantly increased plasma concentration of nitroglycerin from 2.3 to 7.3 nmol/L compared with a control group at room temperature. Nine of the 12 subjects experienced a significant drop in diastolic blood pressure as well as significant reflex tachycardia.[49] This demonstrates that the increased absorption of transdermal drug applications is, in part, due to an increase in skin temperature. Similar results have been obtained by others.[49,50] Increased skin temperature and skin hydration occurring with exercise may be helpful to the patient with a transdermal nitroglycerin patch, especially if the patient experiences angina with activity. However, there is also the risk that exercise-induced vasodilation will lead to hypotension and syncope because of more rapid absorption of the drug.[51] Another point to consider is that nitroglycerin undergoes high hepatic extraction, and when this is combined with the redistribution of blood flow away from the liver during exercise, an elevated plasma drug level would be expected.

DISTRIBUTION OF DRUGS

Once a drug enters the systemic circulation, it is distributed throughout the body. This begins the second phase of pharmacokinetics called *distribution*.[23] The drug may be distributed to different parts of the body, interstitial and intracellular fluids, and extravascular tissues. The rate at which this occurs depends on a variety of factors including organ blood flow, degree of drug ionization in the different compartments, binding to plasma proteins, molecular weight, lipid solubility, and any local metabolism that takes place at any tissue other than the target organ.

If a drug is given intravenously, the initial distribution is related to blood flow. The brain, heart, liver, and kidneys are among the most highly perfused organs and therefore receive most of the drug soon after it is administered.[36] Distribution to the muscle, skin, and fat takes longer, and the drug may not reach equilibration for several hours in these tissues (Figure 3-3). Agents that are very lipid soluble are initially distributed to the brain and then slowly diffuse out into the body to reach other lipid tissues. Later, the drug may diffuse out of the fat and back into the brain. This produces the hungover feeling that patients experience after awakening from anesthesia. Patients who have the same body mass but more fat tissue may need to have their dose adjusted for very-lipid-soluble medications because at one time there may be more drug in the fat tissue than free drug available to act at the target tissue. At some later time, however, the drug will diffuse back into the circulation, prolonging some of its effects.

The distribution of a drug may be described mathematically by dividing the total amount of drug in the body by the plasma drug concentration. This is not a true volume but rather is a way to relate the concentration of a drug in the plasma to the total amount of drug in the body.

$$Vd = \frac{\text{Total Drug Concentration in Body}}{\text{Plasma Concentration}}$$

If the volume of drug in the plasma is greater than that in the tissues, the drug is presumed to be highly bound to the plasma proteins (see below) in the circulation, and the volume of distribution (Vd) will be small and close to blood volume (approximately 3 L).[23] These drugs which are essentially confined to the plasma compartment include heparin and warfarin, two anticoagulants. When Vd is large, the amount of drug bound to

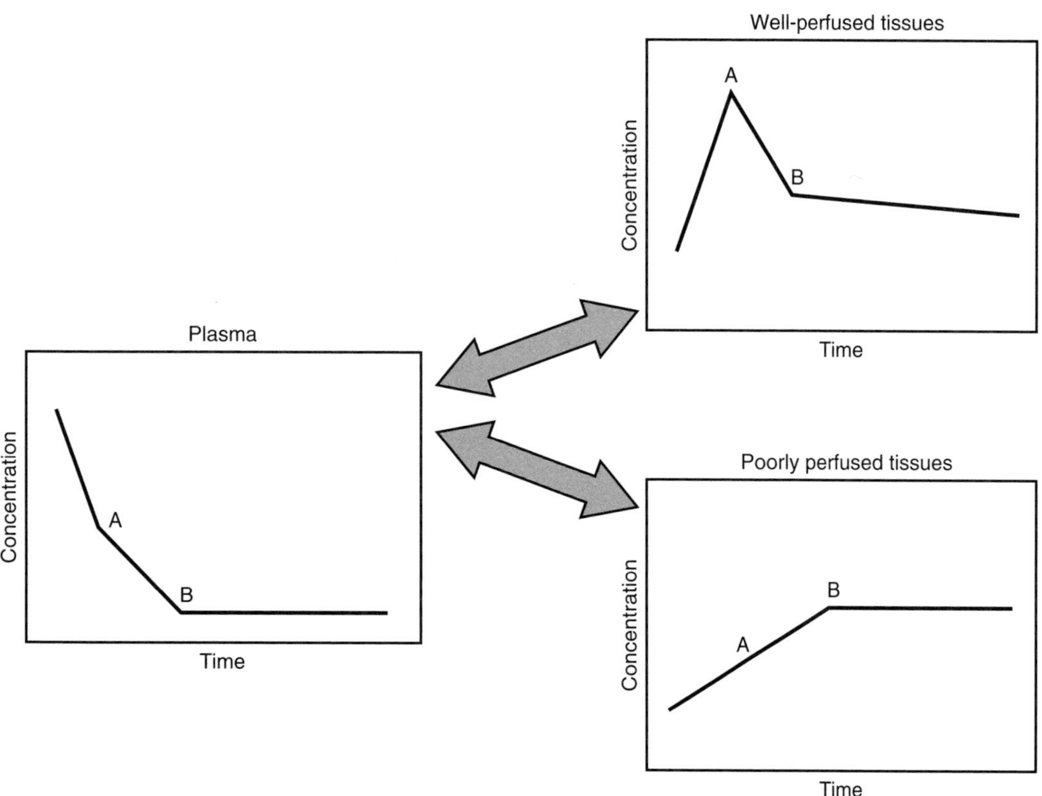

FIGURE 3-3 The redistribution of drugs between tissues. There is an initial decrease in drug concentration in the plasma as drug perfuses into the well-perfused tissues, which reaches equilibrium at point A. Between points A and B, the drug enters poorly perfused tissues, which results in a decrease in the concentrations in both plasma and well-perfused tissues. At point B, all tissues are in equilibrium.

the tissues is much higher than that in the blood. This indicates that the drug can easily pass through the lipid membranes of the cells and distribute widely around the body. Drugs with larger Vd tend to take longer to clear from the body.

Proper drug dosing takes into consideration the fact that while the drug is undergoing absorption, it is also undergoing elimination. So while the drug is accumulating in the body, a fraction is always being cleared. After repeated dosing, steady state at some predetermined therapeutic plasma level is achieved such that the amount going into the body is equal to the amount being cleared. In most cases, this occurs over several dosing periods. However, at certain times, steady state drug level must be achieved immediately, for example, when amiodarone or digoxin is needed to stop life-threatening arrhythmias. Under these circumstances, a loading dose of the drug is administered. The Vd of a drug is used to determine this loading dose.[52] The Vd then is the volume that must be filled with the drug to achieve equilibrium between the vascular compartment and the tissues, all the time accounting for drug elimination.

BOX 3-1 Examples of Drugs That are Highly Bound to Plasma Proteins

	Bound to Albumin
Bound to α_1-Acid	**Glycoprotein**
Clofibrate	Chlorpromazine
Digitoxin	Propranolol
Furosemide	Quinidine
Ibuprofen	Tricyclics
Indomethacin	Lidocaine
Phenytoin	
Salicylates	
Sulfonamides	
Thiazides	
Tolbutamide	
Warfarin	

(Adapted from Waller DG, Renwick AG, Hillier K: *Medical pharmacology and therapeutics*. New York, 2002, WB Saunders.)

Binding to Plasma Proteins

Distribution also depends on the presence of plasma proteins. Albumin is a plasma protein that binds particularly to acidic drugs.[36] Once a drug binds to albumin, it is temporarily unable to interact with the target tissue because only free drug can produce a response. Drugs that bind to plasma proteins tend to have more drug–drug interactions because of competition for binding sites. In addition, proteins act as drug depots. Warfarin, an anticoagulant, binds readily to albumin.[53] If a second drug that also exhibits strong binding to albumin is taken with it, the warfarin will be displaced, and a greater than normal amount of drug warfarin will be suddenly free to act on its target tissue, causing the patient to hemorrhage.

Many basic drugs bind to α_1-acid glycoprotein.[53] Unfortunately, the concentration of this globulin is variable and increases with age, inflammation, and other illnesses. Box 3-1 presents examples of drugs that show extensive binding to plasma proteins.

The presence of disease may alter the protein binding of many drugs. In cirrhosis of the liver, hypoalbuminemia will exist, leaving more drugs in their free, unbound state to exert harmful influences. Therefore it is important that drug dose be adjusted in the presence of chronic illness.

Blood–Brain and Placental Barriers

Lipid-soluble drugs, such as the anesthetic agent thiopental, easily pass into the brain. However, water-soluble drugs have a very difficult time entering this organ. This fact has led to the concept of a blood–brain barrier.[54] Many areas of the brain have tight junctions between capillary endothelial cells and fewer and smaller aqueous pores available for drug diffusion. The only way for a water-soluble drug to enter the brain is via a specific carrier or by injection into the cerebrospinal fluid. However, some new drug delivery systems under study specifically target getting a drug into the brain. Some of these systems utilize nanotechnology. Nanoparticles are very small molecules (diameter less than 100 nm) that can be adhesed to drugs. These particles can be made to form shells with hollow spheres that can carry nonlipid soluble drugs across the capillary endothelial cell.[55] These shells are expected to be especially useful in oncology, since they can be engineered to attach to specific receptors on tumor cells and release a drug with minimal toxicity to surrounding areas. Greater understanding of carrier systems that traverse brain capillary endothelial cells have also led to the development of immunoliposomes. These liposomes bind to a receptor on the luminal membrane of the brain capillary and undergo endocytosis.[6]

The placenta is much less of a barrier than the brain. It is assumed that essentially all drugs cross over from the maternal circulation to that of the fetus, but not all drugs exert harmful influences.[56] Drug diffusion, however, is delayed as a result of limited placental blood flow. This means that if a woman receives a drug during pregnancy, the drug would not be detected in the fetal circulation for several minutes. The mother then can receive drugs just before delivery without the risk of the drug crossing over to the baby.

METABOLISM

Metabolism, also called *biotransformation*, is the third phase of pharmacokinetics and refers to how a drug is inactivated and prepared for elimination.[57] This phase primarily takes place in the liver with the goal of decreasing the drug's pharmacologic activity and lipid solubility. Reducing lipid solubility is crucial to this process because the compound must be polar to be excreted via the kidney tubules. If this were not the case, the compound would be reabsorbed into the circulation and be redistributed to target tissues. Drug metabolism involves two processes that usually occur sequentially and are labeled phase I and phase II reactions (Figure 3-4).

Phase I Metabolism

Phase I reactions are catabolic and involve oxidation, reduction, or hydrolysis reactions, with oxidation occurring most frequently. Most of these reactions are catalyzed by a group of enzymes known as the cytochrome P450 monooxygenases.[58] Several hundred isoforms of these enzymes are found primarily in the liver, although they are active in the lungs, kidneys, and the GI tract as well. A specific nomenclature has been developed to help identify these P450 enzymes, beginning with the capital letters CYP. The next few numbers indicate the isoform family, subfamily, and gene product (Box 3-2). The CYP3A family appears to be the most prevalent enzyme in both the liver and the small intestine. The CYP2C family is next in line.

Although the goal of metabolism is to inactivate a drug, sometimes a more active metabolite is created in the process. A good example of this is the sedative diazepam, which converts to desmethyldiazepam during phase I reactions and increases the overall duration of drug activity.[59] Some drugs are administered in a prodrug form, which is then converted into the active substance only after it interacts with the enzymes.

A variety of individual variations in P450 enzymes influence drug development and therapeutics. Differences between species limit the types of animals that can be used for testing.[57] Differences in these enzymes exist among the human population, resulting in variations in responses to drugs. In addition, enzyme inhibitors and inducers in the environment and diet may have huge effects on therapeutic outcomes. For example, cigarette smoke and cruciferous vegetables (e.g., broccoli and cabbage) are inducers of these enzymes.[60] This essentially means that the activity of the microsomal enzymes is increased, which, in turn, hastens drug metabolism. Grapefruit juice acts to inhibit the P450 enzymes, specifically CYP3A4, which, in turn, inhibits drug metabolism.[61,62] The risk in this case is that plasma levels of the drug will increase and might reach a toxic level. In addition, sometimes two drugs will compete for the same P450 enzyme and slow the rate of metabolism for one or both drugs, which is also considered enzyme inhibition. This will result in higher than normal drug plasma levels, producing an adverse event. Some drugs, such as phenobarbital, when given on a long-term basis, can induce their own metabolism, thus producing drug tolerance.[63] *Tolerance* is defined as needing increasing amounts of a drug to produce an effect. Patients presenting with variations in their P450 enzymes are referred to as either "fast metabolizers" or "slow metabolizers."

Phase II Metabolism

In phase II, the drug undergoes conjugation reactions.[57] Hydrophilic groups such as glucuronic acid, glutathione, acetate, and sulfate groups become attached to the drug

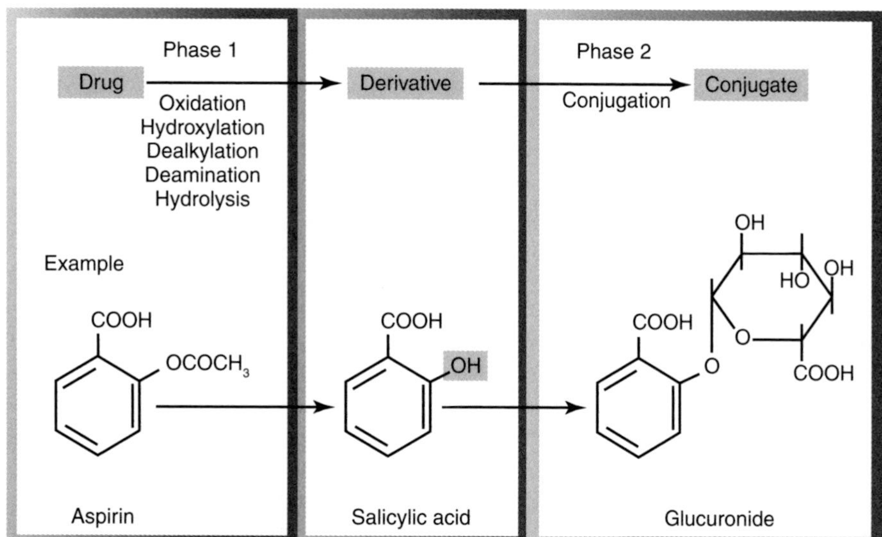

FIGURE 3-4 Metabolism of aspirin. *(From Rang HP, Dale MM, Ritter JM, Moore PK:* Pharmacology, *ed 6. New York, 2007, Churchill Livingstone.)*

BOX 3-2 Examples of Common Drugs That are Substrates for P450 Isoenzymes

Isoenzyme P450	Drug
CYP1A1	Theophylline
CYP1A2	Caffeine, paracetamol, tacrine, theophylline
CYP2A6	Methoxyflurane
CYP2C8	Taxol
CYP2C9	Ibuprofen, phenytoin, tolbutamide, warfarin
CYP2C19	Omeprazole, diazepam, naproxen, propranolol
CYP2D6	Clozapine, codeine, fluoxetine, haloperidol, metoprolol
CYP2E1	Alcohol, enflurane, halothane
CYP3A4/5	Cyclosporine, losartan, nifedipine, diltiazem, indinavir

molecule. In general, these reactions inactivate the compound and make it less lipid soluble; however, there are some exceptions.

DRUG ELIMINATION

Drugs are eliminated from the body by various routes. Elimination in fluids occurs through urine, breast milk, saliva, tears, and sweat. Drugs can also be eliminated through the GI tract in the feces and expelled in exhaled air through the lungs. Renal and fecal excretions are the most common ways in which drugs are excreted from the body.

Renal Excretion

Many drug molecules undergo glomerular filtration to enter the tubular fluid. In addition, a small amount of drug may be secreted into the tubular fluid by nonselective carriers, especially if glomerular filtration is compromised, as it is in renal diseases. Penicillin, which is highly protein bound, is cleared from the kidneys through the glomerulus in a small amount but is almost completely cleared by secretion into the proximal convoluted tubule.[64] If a compound is sufficiently polar, it remains in the tubular fluid and is excreted with urine. However, lipid soluble compounds in the tubular fluid are often reabsorbed into the circulation for another go-around and travel back to the liver for additional metabolism.

The degree of drug ionization also influences renal excretion. Basic drugs will become ionized in the acidic urine and will be readily excreted. Acidic drugs will become neutral in this environment and will be subject to reabsorption. However, urine can be artificially alkalinized with oral or parenteral doses of bicarbonate to facilitate excretion in an overdose situation.

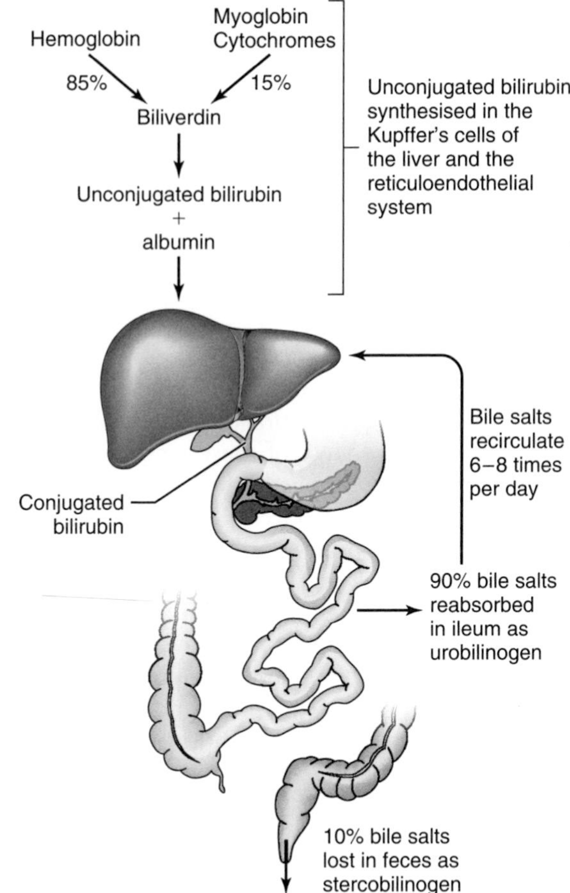

FIGURE 3-5 Enterohepatic circulation and excretion from the liver.

Fecal Excretion

Uptake of drug into the hepatocytes with elimination through bile is the favored route of elimination for large-molecular-weight compounds. Once a drug has entered the intestine with the bile fluids, it will be eliminated in feces. Enterohepatic recycling may occur if the drug escapes once again to the portal vein (Figure 3-5).

MATHEMATIC BASIS OF PHARMACOKINETICS

Half-Life (t½)

It is important clinically to determine the time required for drug effects to be manifested, as well as the concentrations of the drug in a variety of body compartments and at variable times and the elimination rate, in order to determine the proper dosing schedule. Most drugs follow "first order elimination" in which elimination is an exponential or logarithmic process.[52] This means that a *constant proportion* of the drug is eliminated consistently within a specified period. For simplicity, the constant proportion referred to is "50%" of the original concentration in the plasma. The period for elimination can then be determined by measuring the concentration of drug in the plasma over time and determining the time necessary for the concentration to drop by half. For example, if a patient is taking a drug with a t½ of 4 hours and 10 mg/L of the drug is given initially, then in 4 hours, the plasma concentration will be equal to 5 mg/L. In another 4 hours, the concentration will be down to 2.5 mg/L, and in 4 more hours (total of 12 hours since drug administration), the plasma concentration will be down to 1.25 mg/L. This is illustrated in Figure 3-6, which graphs both linear and semilogarithmic scales. When the data are plotted as a log of the plasma concentration versus time, a straight line results, with the proportionality constant (slope) representing the proportion of drug in the body eliminated per unit time and has units "per hour."[57] Most drugs are considered to have been removed from the body in about five half-lives. The remainder of the drug at that point is considered too small to produce either a therapeutic or a toxic effect.

The factors that most determine a drug's half-life are clearance and volume of distribution (Vd). Clearance from the body represents elimination through the kidney, sweat, lungs, and so on and also elimination by metabolism. If it takes longer to clear the drug from the body, then it is easy to understand why half-life would be increased. The larger the Vd, the more drug is concentrated in tissues than in blood. This will increase t½ since clearance by the kidney and liver depends on the amount of drug arriving to these organs via the circulation. When the Vd is small, more drug is present in blood and therefore subject to metabolism in the liver or filtering through the kidney renal glomerulus.

FIRST-ORDER ELIMINATION AND DOSING

Appropriate dosing must take into consideration the level of drug necessary to produce an effective response versus the level of drug that produces toxic effects. Usually, the dose given to patients is the one necessary to produce a response. However, because elimination is always going on, it takes time for the drug level to reach steady state, that is, when the amount excreted in a specified period is equal to the amount of drug administered. Steady state is usually achieved within four or five half-lives. Therefore a drug with a t½ of 6 hours will reach its steady state in approximately 24 to 30 hours. If this waiting period is unacceptable, then the effective response may be achieved sooner with a loading dose, as discussed previously. The maintenance dose then reflects plasma clearance and the desired interval between doses.

In general, a drug with a t½ of 6 to 12 hours can be given in repeated doses every 6 to 12 hours. A drug with a longer t½ can be given only once a day, which is the desired dosage. However, the longer the dosing interval, the greater are the fluctuations in plasma concentration (Figure 3-7). If the t½ is short, 3 hours or less, the drug would have to be given more frequently than is compatible with patient compliance and should preferably be given by continuous IV infusion. Another option is the development of a modified-release formulation so that the frequency of dosing can be reduced. The sustained-release formulas are designed to mimic continuous infusion and therefore reduce the peaks and troughs in drug levels during the dosing interval.

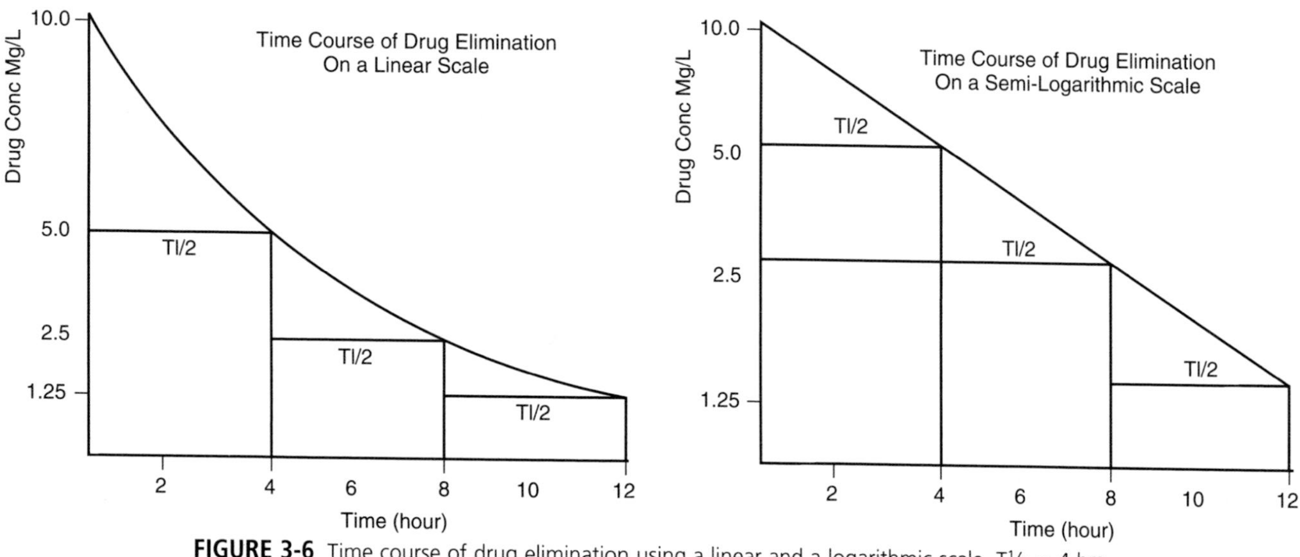

FIGURE 3-6 Time course of drug elimination using a linear and a logarithmic scale. T½ = 4 hrs.

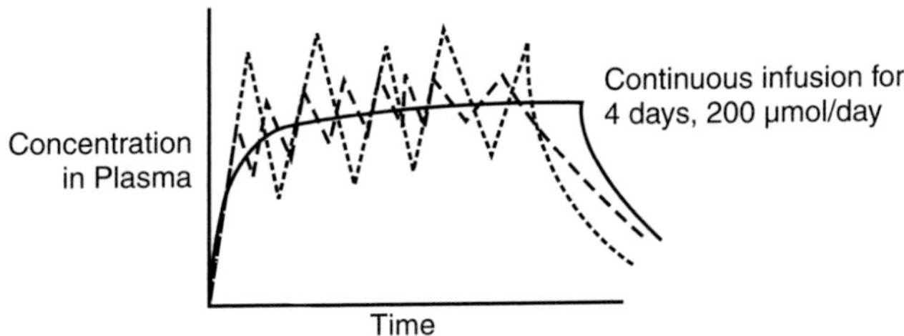

FIGURE 3-7 Fluctuation in plasma concentration during intermittent and continuous dosing. *(Adapted from Rang HP, Dale MM, Ritter JM, Moore PK:* Pharmacology, *ed 6. New York, 2007, Churchill Livingstone.)*

Zero-Order Elimination

For a few drugs, such as ethanol, phenytoin, and aspirin, elimination does not follow the patterns discussed earlier.[14] These drugs demonstrate a linear loss, in which a constant amount of the drug is lost per unit of time as opposed to being based on a percentage of plasma concentration. In other words, elimination is independent of concentration.

FACTORS AFFECTING PHARMACOKINETICS

Clinicians have long noted that patients demonstrate great variability in their responses to identical drug treatments.[65] To understand where these individual responses come from, we need to discuss factors that affect pharmacokinetics and dynamics, such as genetics, age, environmental factors, and the presence of other disease processes.

Changes in Pharmacokinetics with Age

The incidence of adverse drug reactions increases with age.[66] Some reasons are discussed below. Older adults take many more drugs than do their younger counterparts. The more drugs one takes, the greater is the likelihood of either a drug–drug interaction or an interaction with one or more other disease states. Competition for P450 enzymes may slow metabolism, leaving a higher level of active drug in the system. In addition, the serum albumin concentration decreases with age, resulting in increases in free drug concentration. Lean body mass also decreases with age, and this will affect how certain drugs are distributed, particularly fat-soluble drugs. Additionally, renal and liver functions may be reduced, slowing down drug elimination and prolonging the t½. All of these factors would lead to greater-than-expected levels of active drug in the system. This is particularly problematic for drugs with narrow therapeutic margins. On the other hand, reduced blood flow to the GI tract may limit overall absorption, but this is not viewed as being very significant.

Although most of the changes in the older adult affect the kinetics of drug action, some pharmacodynamic changes also occur with aging.[67] Older adults appear to be more sensitive to drugs, in part because of changes in drug–receptor interactions. Changes in receptor number or sensitivity, or even changes in signal transduction, may be to blame. Specifically, older adults react more profoundly to sedative-hypnotics and analgesic medications. These drugs are likely to produce sedation, respiratory depression, and confusion. Changes in the blood–brain barrier may allow these drugs to enter the central nervous system more easily. In addition, baroreceptor sensitivity is reduced, leading to orthostatic hypotension caused by these drugs as well as by drugs for hypertension. As a result of all these changes, an older adult can be expected to have many more adverse drug events compared with a younger patient. Every drug has a risk/benefit ratio, and this ratio becomes greater with age.

Changes in Pharmacokinetics Caused by Genetics

Inherited factors may cause different responses to drugs.[68] Single genes tend to control the production of enzymes. Gene mutations are inheritable, leading to abnormal enzymes producing increased, decreased, or completely unexpected responses to drugs.[69] *Pharmacogenetics* is the study of drug responses that are produced by genes. Genetic polymorphisms of cytochrome CYP2D6 results in poor, intermediate, efficient, or ultrarapid metabolizers of drugs inactivated by this enzyme. This gives rise to some concern, since CYP2D6 is responsible for the metabolism of approximately 20 to 25% of clinically useful medications, including haloperidol, hydrocodone, metoprolol, and codeine, to name a few. Some of the clinically relevant consequences noted have been higher serum levels of haloperidol and a greater incidence of extrapyramidal symptoms in Asians compared with whites, and a higher incidence of nonresponders to antidepressants among Europeans.[69] Individuals who also are deficient in CYP2D6 activity are unable to convert codeine to its active metabolite morphine, thus greatly reducing pain control in affected patients.

Polymorphisms also exist in genes coding for drug transporters as well as for drug receptors.[70,71] A well-recognized alteration exists in the α_2 adrenoreceptor. Some individuals with asthma who have this mutation will show increased bronchodilator desensitization. Another significant genetic defect affecting drug response is a cholinesterase deficiency. Succinylcholine is a neuromuscular blocking agent that is used to induce paralysis during certain major surgical procedures. The action of this drug is terminated by the enzyme cholinesterase. Affected individuals may produce so little cholinesterase that the metabolism of succinylcholine is slowed, necessitating assisted ventilation for the patient for a certain period after the surgery is over.[72]

Changes in Pharmacokinetics with Disease

As discussed previously, diseases of the liver and kidneys have profound effects on the t½.[73] Metabolism and elimination are reduced, leaving the active drug around longer. In addition, other illnesses, such as viral infections, reduce the activity of the P450 enzymes, also producing a longer t½. Perhaps the greatest problem associated with the presence of multiple disease processes and drug action is a patient's need for multiple drugs. Administration of multiple drugs increases the risk for drug–drug interactions, either because of competition for P450 enzymes or due to competing responses to different drugs. An example of a competing drug response is when a patient taking a diuretic for hypertension is also prescribed a nonsteroidal anti-inflammatory drug (NSAID) for arthritis.[74] This occurrence is unfortunately common among older adults. The NSAID blocks the production of prostaglandins (pain-mediating substances) in the periphery and also in the kidneys. However, prostaglandins are needed in the kidneys for maintaining adequate renal perfusion. The result of this interaction is diminished excretion from the kidneys, producing increased blood volume, which, in turn, raises blood pressure.

Changes in Pharmacokinetics with Exercise

Exercise affects a number of factors involved in drug pharmacokinetics, including vascular flow, pH, temperature, GI function, metabolism, and excretion. The drug propranolol can be used to illustrate the changes that occur with exercise.

Exercise has been shown to affect the pharmacokinetics of propranolol.[75,76] This drug is a β-adrenergic blocker that reduces blood pressure by blocking the access of catecholamines to β-receptors in the heart. The net effect is lowered heart rate and contractility, which, in turn, reduces blood pressure. Propranolol is quite lipophilic and also shows high first-pass metabolism. In a study performed on healthy volunteers, propranolol was administered before prolonged exercise (25 minutes) at 70% workload maximum (Wmax) on a cycle ergometer and during a 10-minute exercise period at 50% Wmax. Plasma concentrations of propranolol were determined at rest, during exercise, and during recovery. Oral propranolol was given for 1 week before testing with the more strenuous exercise protocol but was given intravenously by continuous infusion during testing with the light exercise protocol. Plasma concentrations of propranolol were significantly increased in both tests. However, after corrections were made for changes in the plasma volume (lost fluid) during exercise, drug elevation in plasma was significant only during exhaustive exercise, the protocol that required oral administration of propranolol. The increase in plasma level above the pre-exercise level suggests better absorption, changes in the volume of distribution (reduced drug in peripheral compartments), or reduced drug clearance. Because propranolol normally undergoes significant first-pass metabolism, it can be speculated that during exhaustive exercise, with oral dosing, hepatic blood flow is reduced, resulting in a smaller first-pass effect. This is a more plausible explanation when the results are compared with the IV study in which there was no first-pass effect and plasma concentration was not elevated. However, the irreconcilable findings between the two studies could also have been due to the differences in exercise. Increases in lactic acid production and a lowering of pH during the high-intensity exercise could be responsible for an increase in lipid solubility and, hence, better absorption through the GI tract. This better absorption, combined with diminished blood flow to the liver in vigorous exercise, is a reasonable explanation for the greater plasma level. Changes in metabolism and excretion were ruled out because comparisons with another β-blocker, atenolol, did not show any change in plasma concentration during exercise performed with the IV-administered drug. In addition, atenolol concentration was not affected by vigorous exercise with oral dosing, suggesting that it was the degree of ionization associated with pH changes with exercise that produced the elevated propranolol level. Drug-receptor changes were also ruled out because there was no change in concentration with atenolol, which interacts with the same receptors as propranolol. One other explanation proposed was that because propranolol binds to skeletal muscles, it is conceivable that greater muscle perfusion is responsible for a "washout of the drug" from this area. This rather lengthy discussion regarding the pharmacokinetics of propranolol with exercise was designed to illustrate the complexities that researchers face when performing drug–exercise studies. In fact, these studies are not done with most drugs, which leaves the therapist without guidance. Many variables appear to be involved in pharmacokinetics—including type and intensity of exercise, route of administration, dosing schedule, issues related to the methods of separating the processes of metabolism from those of elimination, and examination of what is happening at the target organ and receptor levels.

It is important to mention that many drug–exercise studies are performed on healthy volunteers, and the results of these studies therefore do not always translate to our patient populations. Designing a series of studies to explore the interactions of drugs with exercise and applying this method consistently to test a variety of different drugs, particularly those that are likely to be given to patients desiring exercise, continue to be a challenge.

ACTIVITIES 3

1. Discuss factors that affect gastrointestinal absorption.
2. You are treating a 70-year-old man for wrist drop caused by radial nerve dysfunction. The patient also has a host of other medical problems related to alcoholic liver disease: anemia, thrombocytopenia, jaundice, and hypoalbuminemia. How is each phase of pharmacokinetics influenced by the patient's medical condition? What should be done to ensure that the patient does not experience any adverse drug reactions?
3. Interview a relative, neighbor, or patient who is over 65 years old about his or her medication use. List all prescribed and over-the-counter medicines (use generic names), including herbal medications, that have been taken within the past 6 months. Ask your subject about any adverse effects, the number of pills he or she takes per day, and his or her compliance with the regimen. Discuss your findings with other students to determine the 10 drugs most commonly used in this age group.
4. How does oral administration of a drug compare with IV administration of the same drug? Draw a hypothetical plasma concentration curve versus time after a single oral drug dose and a single IV injection.
5. Describe the mechanisms involved in the renal elimination of drugs.

REFERENCES

1. Atkinson AJ: Background. In Atkinson AJ. Jr, Daniels CE, Dedrick RL, Grudzinskas CV, Markey SP, editors: Principles of clinical pharmacology, New York, 2007, Elsevier.
2. Bennett PN, Brown MJ: General pharmacology. In Bennett PN, Brown MJ, editors: Clinical pharmacology. Philadelphia, 2008, Churchill Livingstone.
3. Ganong WF: The general and cellular basis of medical physiology, Rev Med Physiol: http://www.accessmedicine.com/content.aspx?aID=701440. Accessed September 22, 2005.
4. Katzung BG: Introduction. In Katzung BG, editor: Basic and clinical pharmacology, New York, 2007, McGraw-Hill.
5. Lu J, Jeon E, Lee BS, Onyuksel H, Wang ZJ: Targeted drug delivery crossing cytoplasmic membranes of intended cells via ligand-grafted sterically stabilized liposomes, J Control Release, 110(3):505–513, 2006.
6. Cornford EM, Cornford ME: New systems for delivery of drugs to the brain in neurological disease, Lancet Neurol, 1(5):306–315., 2002.
7. Sachs GS, Renshaw PF, Lafer B, et al: Variability of brain lithium levels during maintenance treatment: A magnetic resonance spectroscopy study, Biol Psychiatry, 38:422–428, 1995.
8. Dobson PD, Lanthaler K, Oliver SG, Kell DB: Implications of the dominant role of transporters in drug uptake by cells, Curr Top Med Chem, 9(2):163–181, 2009.
9. Stocchi F: The hypothesis of the genesis of motor complications and continuous dopaminergic stimulation in the treatment of Parkinson's disease, Parkinsonism & Related Disorders, 2009, 15(Supplement 1):S9–S15.
10. Somogyi A: Renal transport of drugs: Specificity and molecular mechanisms, Clin Exp Pharmacol Physiol, 23(10/11):986–989, 1996.
11. Pratt WB: The entry, distribution, and elimination of drugs. In Pratt WB, Taylor P, editors: Principles of drug actions: The basis of pharmacology, New York, 1990, Churchill Livingstone.
12. Delie F, Blanco-Prieto MJ: Polymeric particulates to improve oral bioavailability of peptide drugs, Molecules, 31(1):65–80, 2005.
13. Lilley LL, Harrington S, Snyder JS: Photo atlas of drug administration, In Lilley LL, Harrington S, Snyder JS, editors: Pharmacology and the nursing process, Philadelphia, 2007, Mosby.
14. Lilley LL, Harrington S, Snyder JS: Pharmacologic principles. In Lilley LL, Harrington S, Snyder JS, editors: Pharmacology and the nursing process, Philadelphia, 2007, Mosby 4–34.
15. Goel H, Rai P, Rana V, Tiwary AK: Orally disintegrating systems: Innovations in formulation and technology, Recent Pat Drug Deliv Formul, 2(3):258–274, 2008.
16. Yamanaka YJ, Leong KW: Engineering strategies to enhance nanoparticle-mediated oral delivery, J Biomater Sci Polym Ed, 19(12):1549–1570, 2008.
17. Fu Y, Yang S, Jeong SH, Kimura S, Park K: Orally fast disintegrating tables: Developments, technologies, taste-masking and clinical studies, Crit Rev Ther Drug Carrier Syst, 21(6):433–476, 2004.
18. Patil SB, Sawant KK: Mucoadhesive microspheres: A promising tool in drug delivery, Curr Drug Deliv, 5(6):312–318, 2008.
19. Davis SS, Hardy JG, Fara JW: Transit of pharmaceutical dosage forms through the small intestine, Gut, 27(8):886–892, 1986.
20. Nakamura T, Yamamori M, Sakaeda T: Pharmacogenetics of intestinal absorption, Curr Drug Deliv, 5(3):153–169, 2008.
21. Sousa T, Paterson R, Moore V, et al: The gastrointestinal microbiota as a site for the biotransformation of drugs, Int J Pharmaceutics 363(1-2):1–25, 2008.
22. Oostendorp RL, Beijnen JH, Schellens JHM: The biological and clinical role of drug transporters at the intestinal barrier, Cancer Treat Rev, 35(2):137–147, 2009.
23. Winter ME: Basic clinical pharmacokinetics. New York, 2004, Lippincott Williams & Wilkins.
24. Black DM, Thompson DE, Bauer DC, et al: Fracture risk with alendronate in women with osteoporosis: The Fracture Intervention Trial, J Clin Endocrinol Metab, 85(11):4118–4124, 2000.
25. Hashimoto S, Kobayashi A: Clinical pharmacokinetics and pharmacodynamics of glyceryl trinitrate and its metabolites, Clin Pharmacokinet, 42(3):205–221, 2003.
26. Pather SI, Rathbone MJ, Senel S: Current status and the future of buccal drug delivery systems, Expert opin Drug Deliv, 5(5):531–542, 2008.
27. Queckenberg C, Fuhr U: Influence of posture on pharmaokinetics, Eur J Clin Pharmacol, 65(2):109–119, 2009.
28. Somogyi A: Clinical pharmacokinetics and dosing schedules. In Brody TM, Larner J, Minneman KP, editors: Human pharmacology: Molecular to clinical, Philadelphia, 1998, Mosby.
29. Beltrand J, Guilmin-Crepon S, Castanet M, et al: Insulin allergy and extensive lipoatrophy in child with type 1 diabetes, Horm Res, 65(5):253–260, 2006.

30. Koivisto VA, Felig P: Effects of leg exercise on insulin absorption in diabetic patients. N Engl J Med, 298(2):79–83, 1978.
31. Linde B: Dissociation of insulin absorption and blood flow during massage of a subcutaneous injection site, Diabetes Care, 9(6):570–574, 1986.
32. Prettyman J: Subcutaneous or intramuscular? Confronting a parenteral administration dilemma, MEDSURG Nursing, 14(2):93–99, 2005.
33. Ludvigsson J, Samuelsson U: Continuous insulin infusion (CSII) or modern type of multiple daily injections (MDI) in diabetic children and adolescents: A critical review on a controversial issue, Pediat Endocrinol Rev, 5(2):666–678, 2007.
34. Patel MM, Goyal BR, Bhadada SV, Bhatt JS, Amin AF: Getting into the brain: Approaches to enhance brain drug delivery, CNS Drugs, 23(1):25–58, 2009.
35. Brochard S, Remy-Neris O, Filipetti P, Bussel B: Intrathecal baclofen infusion for ambulant children with cerebral palsy, Pediat Neurol, 40(4):265–270, 2009.
36. Rang HP, et al: Absorption and distribution of drugs. In Rang HP, Dale MM, Ritter JM, Flower R, editors: Rang and Dale's pharmacology, Philadelphia, 2007, Churchill Livingstone.
37. Bewley A: Expert consensus: Time for a change in the way we advise our patients to use topical corticosteroids, Br J Dermatol, 158(5):917–920, 2008.
38. El Maghraby GM, Barry BW, Williams AC: Liposomes and skin: From drug delivery to model membranes, Eur J Pharm Sci, 34(4-5):203–222, 2008.
39. Greene BL: Physical therapist management of fluoroquinolone-induced Achilles tendinopathy, Phys Ther, 82(12):1224–1231, 2002.
40. Williams RJ III, Attia E, Wickiewicz TL, Hannafin JA: The effect of ciprofloxacin on tendon, paratendon, and capsular fibroblast metabolism, Am J Sports Med, 28(3):364–369, 2000.
41. Nielsen HB, Svendsen LB, Jensen TH, Secher NH: Exercise-induced gastric mucosal acidosis, Med Sci SportsExerc, 27(7):1003–1006, 1995.
42. Carter JH, Nutt JG, Woodward WR: The effect of exercise on levodopa absorption, Neurology, 42(10):2042–2045, 1992.
43. Goetz CG, Thelen JA, MacLeod CM, et al: Blood levodopa levels and unified Parkinson's disease rating scale function: With and without exercise. Neurology, 43(5):1040–1042, 1993.
44. Reuter I, Harder S, Engelhardt M, Baas H: The effect of exercise on pharmacokinetics and pharmacodynamics of levodopa, Mov Disord, 15(5):862–868, 2000.
45. Strömberg C, Vanakoski J, Olkkola KT, et al: Exercise alters the pharmacokinetics of midazolam, Clin Pharmacol Ther, 51(5):527–532, 1992.
46. Khazaeinia T, Ramsey AA, Tam YK: The effects of exercise on the pharmacokinetics of drugs, J Pharm Pharmaceut Sci, 3(3):292–302, 2000.
47. Koivisto VA, Felig P: Effects of leg exercise on insulin absorption in diabetic patients, N Engl J Med, 298(2):79–83, 1978.
48. Weber S, de Lauture D, Rey E, et al: The effects of moderate sustained exercise on the pharmacokinetics of nitroglycerine, Br J Clin Pharmacol, 23(1):103–105, 1987.
49. Barkve TF, Langseth-Manrique K, Bredesen JE, Gjesdal K: Increased uptake of transdermal glyceryl trinitrate during physical exercise and during high ambient temperature, Am Heart J, 112(3):537–541, 1986.
50. Lefebvre RA, et al: Influence of exercise on nitroglycerin plasma concentrations after transdermal application, Br J Clin Pharmacol, 30(2):292–296, 1990.
51. Vanakoski J, Seppälä T: Heat exposure and drugs. A review of the effects of hyperthermia on pharmacokinetics, Clin Pharmacokinet, 34(4):311–322, 1998.
52. Atkinson AJ: Clinical Pharmacokinetics. In Atkinson AJ. Jr, Daniels CE, Dedrick RL, Grudzinskas CV, Markey SP, editors: Principles of clinical pharmacology, New York, 2007, Academic Press.
53. Reine PA, U. E. Kongsgaard A. Andersen A. K. ThØGersen H. Olsen: Infusion of albumin attenuates changes in serum protein binding of drugs in surgical patients compared with volume replacement with HAES, Acta Anaesthesiol Scand 52(3):406–412, 2008.
54. Bernacki J, Dobrowolska A, Nierwińska K, Małecki A: Physiology and pharmacological role of the blood–brain barrier, Pharmacol Rep 60:600–622, 2008.
55. Staggers N, McCasky T, Brazelton N, Kennedy R: Nanotechnology: The coming revolution and its implications for consumers, clinicians, and informatics, Nurs Outlook 56(5):268–274, 2008.
56. Myllynen P, Pasanen M, Vahakangas K: The fate and effects of xenobiotics in human placenta, Expert Opin Drug Metab Toxicol 3(3):331–346, 2007.
57. Rang HP, et al: Drug elimination and pharmacokinetics. In Rang HP, Dale MM, Ritter JM, Flower R, editors: Rang & Dale's pharmacology, New York, 2007, Churchill Livingstone. Text does not specify.
58. Dressntan JB, Thelen K, Jantratid E: Towards quantitative prediction of oral drug absorption. Clin Pharmacokinetics 47(10):655–667, 2008.
59. Liu LL, Gropper MA: Postoperative analgesia and sedation in the adult intensive care unit: A guide to drug selection, In Drugs ADIS International Limited 755–767, 2003.
60. Steinkellner H, et al: Effects of cruciferous vegetables and their constituents on drug metabolizing enzymes involved in the bioactivation of DNA-reactive dietary carcinogens. Mutat Res 480–481, 2001; 285–297 (abstract).
61. Veronese ML, Gillen LP, Burke JP,, et al: Exposure-dependent inhibition of intestinal and hepatic CYP3A4 in vivo by grapefruit juice, J Clin Pharmacol 43(8):831–839, 2003.
62. Kane GC, Lipsky JJ: Drug-grapefruit juice interactions, Mayo Clin Proc 75(9):933–942, 2000.
63. Sueyoshi T, Negishi M: Phenobarbital response elements of cytochrome P450 genes and nuclear receptors, Ann Rev Pharmacol Toxicol 41:123–443, 2001.
64. VanWert AL, Bailey RM, Sweet DH: Organic anion transporter 3 (Oat3/Slc22a8) knockout mice exhibit altered clearance and distribution of penicillin G, Am J Physiol Renal Physiol 293(4):F1332-F1341, 2007.
65. McDowell SE, Coleman JJ, Ferner RE: Systematic review and meta-analysis of ethnic differences in risks of adverse reactions to drugs used in cardiovascular medicine, Br Med J 332:1177–1181, 2006.
66. Hughes SG: Prescribing of the elderly patient: why do we need to exercise caution? Br J Clin Pharmocol 46(6):531–533, 1998.
67. MacLaughlin EJ, Raehl CL, Treadway AK, et al: Assessing medication adherence in the elderly. Which tools to use in clinical practice? Drugs Aging 22(3):231–255, 2005.
68. Chen ML: Ethnic or racial differences revisited. Clin Pharmacokinet 45(10):957–964, 2006.
69. Ingelman-Sundberg M: Genetic polymorphisms of cytochrome P450 2D6 (CYP2D6): Clinical consequences, evolutionary aspects and functional diversity, Pharmacogenomics J 5:6–13, 2005.
70. Preusch P: Equilibrative and concentrative transport mechanisms. In Atkinson AJ, et al, editors: Principles of clinical pharmacology, New York, 2007, Elsevier.
71. Flockhart D, Bertilsson L: Clinical pharmacogenetics. In Atkinson AJ. Jr, Daniels CE, Dedrick RL, Grudzinskas CV, Markey SP, editors: Principles of clinical pharmacology, New York, 2007, Elsevier.

72. Ries CR, Quastel DMJ: Drug use in anesthesia and critical care. In Page CP, Hoffman B, Curtis M, Walker M, editors: Integrated pharmacology. Philadelphia, 2002, Mosby.
73. Li YF, Fu S, Hu W, et al: Systemic anticancer therapy in gynecological cancer patients with renal dysfunction, Int J Gynecol Cancer 17:739–763, 2007.
74. Hughes S: AHA updates NSAID advice for heart disease patients. Medscape Medical News 2007: http://www.medscape.com/viewarticle/552845. Accessed 2007.
75. van Baak MA: Hypertension, beta-adrenoceptor blocking agents and exercise. Int J Sports Med 15(3):112–115, 1994.
76. van Baak MA, Mooij JMV, Schiffers PMH: Exercise and the pharmacokinetics of propranolol, verapamil and atenolol, Eur J Clin Pharmacol 43:547–550, 1992.

4

Adverse Drug Reactions

Barbara Gladson

RISK/BENEFIT RATIO

As mentioned in the previous chapters, every drug has a risk/benefit ratio, and this ratio increases as a patient ages.[1] However, the risks are not only experienced by older adults but also pose a threat to people of all ages. These risks may result from drug–drug interactions, food–drug interactions, patient-related factors, allergic reactions, and side effects from medications caused by their pharmacodynamic properties.

CLASSIFICATION OF ADVERSE DRUG REACTIONS

The term *adverse drug reactions (ADRs)* is defined by the World Health Organization (WHO) as any unintended or unwanted effects of a drug that may occur even at acceptable dose levels.[2] This is a rather exclusionary definition because it does not include human errors in drug administration and patient compliance issues. Nevertheless, as defined here, the numbers of ADRs are astounding. A meta-analysis of 39 prospective studies, beginning in 1964 and ending in 1996, revealed that serious ADRs occurred in 6.7% of hospitalized patients.[2] This figure represents patients who were admitted solely because of an ADR as well as patients who were already hospitalized for a different reason and experienced their ADRs in the hospital. This figure includes serious ADRs only, ones for which hospitalization was necessary and death may have been a final outcome. Specifically, in 1994, ADRs were among the six leading causes of death. According to this information, it is estimated that 1 in 10 hospital admissions is drug related. If ADRs caused by human error and compliance issues are included, ADRs grow to an even more alarming number. Criticism of this study included the fact that some of the numbers were taken from large tertiary care hospitals that attract the more seriously ill patients, the ones more likely to have ADRs.

The term *adverse drug events (ADEs)* refers to anything that can go wrong when a person is administered a drug. It is a much more expansive term and includes prescribing, dosing, and formulation errors, plus ADRs as defined above. The National Electronic Injury Surveillance System–Cooperative Adverse Drug Event Surveillance Project (NEISS–CADES) pools data on ADEs from 63 hospitals, which provide a nationally representative sample of all hospitals, and is used to record ADEs.[3] Data obtained from this surveillance system between January 1, 2004, and December 31, 2005, estimated that over 700,000 patients were seen in the emergency room annually, and out of these, 1 in 6 patients required hospitalization. Those individuals who were 65 or older were found to be responsible for one quarter of these events with warfarin, insulin, and digoxin producing nearly one third of these incidences. Another study performed by the Institute for Safe Medication Practices examined all voluntary reports submitted directly to the Adverse Event Reporting System (AERS) of the U.S. Food and Drug Administration (FDA) and found that in the 8-year period between 1998 and 2005, serious ADEs increased 2.6-fold from 34,966 to 89,842. Fatal ADEs increased 2.7-fold from 5519 to 15,107.[4] Box 4-1 lists the most frequent drugs suspected in death or serious injury during this period.

The United Kingdom (UK) also has unacceptably high numbers of ADEs. ADEs were responsible for 6.5% of all hospital admissions that resulted in approximately an 8-day stay.[5] Another study in the UK found that 25% of ambulatory patients experienced ADEs, and 13% of these were considered serious.[6]

Definitions

The term *side effects* has traditionally been reserved for minor effects of drugs, and the term *adverse reactions* has been used to label the serious effects of drugs at therapeutic doses.[7] The term *adverse event*, however, refers to a negative outcome that occurs while a patient is taking a drug but does not imply causality as does the term *adverse reaction*. For the purposes of this book, the phrases "adverse drug events" and "adverse drug reactions" will be used interchangeably and will include both major and minor drug effects. The term *toxicity* refers to an adverse drug event that occurs at a high dose, and *carcinogenicity* (causing cancer) and *teratogenicity* (causing fetal damage) refer to special cases of toxicity.[8]

BOX 4-1 Most Frequent Drugs Suspected in Producing Death or Injury Reported to the FDA, 1998–2005

Drug Name	Drug Class
Drugs Producing Death	
Oxycodone	Opioid analgesic
Fentanyl	Opioid analgesic
Clozapine	Antipsychotic
Morphine	Opioid analgesic
Acetaminophen	Analgesic
Methadone	Opioid analgesic
Infliximab	Antirheumatic
Risperidone	Antipsychotic
Etanercept	Antirheumatic
Paclitaxel	Chemotherapy
Acetaminophen-hydrocodone	Combination analgesic
Olanzapine	Antipsychotic
Rofecoxib	NSAID
Paroxetine	Antidepressant
Drugs Producing Injury	
Estrogens	Hormone
Insulin	Antidiabetic
Infliximab	Antirheumatic
Interferon-beta	Immunomodulator
Paroxetine	Antidepressant
Rofecoxib	NSAID
Warfarin	Anticoagulant
Atorvastatin	Cholesterol-lowering
Etanercept	Antirheumatic
Celecoxib	NSAID
Phentermine	Weight loss
Clozapine	Antipsychotic
Interferon-alpha	Immunomodulator
Simvastatin	Cholesterol-lowering
Venlafaxine	Antidepressant

NSAID, nonsteroidal anti-inflammatory drug.
(Adapted from Moore TJ, Cohen MR, Furberg CD: Serious adverse drug events reported to the Food and Drug Administration, 1998–2005, *Arch Intern Med* 167(16):1752–1759, 2007.)

Reasons for ADRs

Most ADRs may be classified as an extension of the expected or desired pharmacologic action. Variations exist in the pharmacokinetics and pharmacodynamics of drugs as reviewed earlier. Drugs with a narrow therapeutic index, such as warfarin or digoxin, are responsible for most ADRs, and older adults and pediatric patients are most at risk.[9] It is estimated that older adults suffer 60 ADRs per every 10,000 patients.[10] Polypharmacy along with comorbidities such as diminished liver and kidney functions are particular culprits. Genetic polymorphisms in metabolizing enzymes and drug–drug interactions are other reasons for ADRs.

ADRs may also come from a variety of clinician-related factors. Besides the obvious reason, that of writing a prescription for the wrong drug or dosage, a physician may err by not prescribing the appropriate dose for fear that this would produce toxicity, particularly in the case of drugs that have a narrow therapeutic index.[11] Two examples that have been cited include intravenous (IV) aminoglycosides and heparin. Underdosing of these two medications can lead to the development of resistant bacteria and thromboembolism, respectively.

Noncompliance with treatment is another major reason for the development of ADRs and also for lack of treatment efficacy. As with drug toxicity, noncompliance with treatment is considered an ADR, since it, too, may result in hospitalization. It is estimated that patients taking drugs for chronic diseases have a noncompliance rate of about 50%.[12,13] This is particularly problematic among patients with human immunodeficiency virus (HIV) infection, since maintaining a low viral load depends on 95% compliance.[14] Most noncompliance is due to a dose lapse as opposed to taking extra doses. It has also been observed that patients' compliance improves 5 days prior to a scheduled appointment but then lapses again a month after the visit.[15] Similar patterns of compliance are noted among patients taking antihypertensive agents, antiseizure medications, and cholesterol-reducing agents.[16,17] Dose omissions create problems with some drugs, since sudden withdrawal can produce a rebound of symptoms as well as some life-threatening consequences. This is particularly true for beta-blockers, antiseizure medications, and benzodiazepines.

Simplification of treatment regimens has been suggested as one strategy to reduce noncompliance. Studies using electronic monitoring have shown that compliance is reduced as the number of dosages increases.[18] A study conducted in Canada showed better compliance in patients with hypertension who received once a day amlodipine versus twice a day diltiazem.[19] However, some individuals on a once daily dose may be more likely to skip days without treatment, especially over a weekend.

Other sources of medication errors include problems with the transcribing, documenting, and dispensing of drugs. Medications have several names as described earlier in the text. Generic names are assigned by the United States Adopted Name Council (USAN) using some very specialized set of guidelines that incorporate the chemical characteristic or indication for a drug.[20] The proprietary name is chosen by the manufacturer. The result is that drugs with completely different chemical characteristics and indications with similar names exist, as do multiple names for the same active ingredient or drug. Verapamil, a drug used for arrhthymia, has the brand names Calan, Calan SR, Isoptin, and others. In addition, the same medication may have different names when used for different indications, for example, bupropion is marketed as Wellbutrin for depression and as Zyban for smoking cessation. Another example is finasteride (Proscar) for benign prostatic hyperplasia, which is called Propecia when used to treat baldness. The FDA uses a risk analysis system developed by the University of Illinois to review and evaluate proposed names and rejects those that might be easily confused. In addition, other computerized systems in physicians' offices and at pharmacies are also becoming more sensitive to picking up medication errors attributed to look-alike drugs as well as look-alike packaging.

Identifying ADRs

Identifying an ADR can be very difficult, and often new symptoms that arise are attributed to disease progression rather than to prescribed drugs. A symptom may also be perceived as an unrelated, new condition, not as an ADR. In this case, the physician will most likely prescribe a new drug to treat the unrecognized ADR, which leads to polypharmacy.

Several algorithms have been used to identify ADRs. They all have some common themes and include using the following questions:

- Have the patient's symptoms been previously reported for the same drug?
- Is the timing of the reaction consistent with the dosing schedule of the drug and its time course of action?
- Did the symptoms disappear when the dose was reduced or the drug was withdrawn?
- Did the symptoms return upon rechallenge with the drug?
- Was the correct dose given, taking into consideration the patient's age, weight, and health status?

These questions aim to establish causality for the reaction.

If using the algorithm above does not establish a cause-and-effect relationship between the drug and the symptom, then a probability assessment tool such as the Naranjo Probability Scale (Box 4-2) can be used.[21] The Naranjo Algorithm consists of 10 questions, which are scored 0, $^{+}1$, or -1. A $^{+}1$ is assigned if the question can be answered with a yes and a -1 is given for a no answer. Zero is assigned for a "do not know" answer. Scores of 9 or 10 indicate that the patient is definitely experiencing an ADR. Scores of 5 to 8 indicate that an ADR is "probable." Scores of 1 to 4 indicate a "possible" relationship between the drug and the symptom, whereas a score of less than 1 indicates that this relationship is "doubtful."

Another approach to detecting ADRs assesses the patient's risk of developing an ADR. The Medication Risk Assessment Questionnaire is a self-administered survey that asks patients about the quantity of medications they receive as well as their pill burden.[22] In addition, it asks patients to check off the drugs they are receiving from a list of high-alert medications. The questionnaire is based on the fact that the more medications the patient is taking, the more likely is the patient to have a reaction. In addition, the greater number of doses a patient is receiving per day, the higher is the risk of an event.

When a health care practitioner suspects that an ADR may have occurred, it is imperative that the reaction be documented. ADRs need to be reported to the governing regulatory agencies, the FDA in the United States, the Ministry of Health, Labour, and Welfare (MHLW) in Japan, and the European Medicines Evaluation Agency (EMEA) in Europe to ensure that other similar ADRs are prevented. Specifically in the United States, ADRs can be reported by any health care practitioner or lay person using the FDA MedWatch Web site http://www.fda.gov/Safety/MedWatch/default.htm.

BOX 4-2 Probability Method for the Estimation of ADRs

Question	Yes	No	Do Not Know	Score
1. Are there previous conclusive reports on this reaction?				
2. Did the adverse event appear after the suspected drug was given?				
3. Did the adverse reaction improve when the drug was discontinued or a specific antagonist was given?				
4. Did the adverse reaction reappear when the drug was re-administered?				
5. Are there alternative causes (other than the drug) that could on their own have caused the reaction?				
6. Did the reaction reappear when a placebo was given?				
7. Was the drug detected in the blood in high concentrations known to be toxic?				
8. Was the reaction more severe when the dose was increased, and lessened when the dose was reduced?				
9. Did the patient have a similar reaction to the same or similar drugs in the past?				
10. Was the adverse event confirmed by any other objective testing?				

(Adapted from Naranjo CA, Busto U, Seller EM, et al: A method for estimating the probability of adverse drug reactions, *Clin Pharmacol Ther* 30: 239–245, 1982.)

Collecting Information on ADRs

In 1993, the FDA introduced MedWatch, which is the FDA's national pharmacovigilance program.[23] The main goal of this Web site is to provide a way for individuals to submit suspicions of drug side effects and to distribute this information to both the public and the professionals. MedWatch provides information on safety issues involving prescription and over-the-counter (OTC) drugs, cosmetics, infant formulas, biologics, vaccines, medical devices, radiation-emitting agents, and nutritional and dietary supplements. This Web site consists of a "What's New" section that reports safety alerts, recalls, withdrawals, and labeling changes. In addition, it provides an index to drug-specific information, drug shortages, product safety educational resources, and, of course, instructions on how to file a report. The site also links to DailyMed, which contains the FDA-approved package insert and label for each drug, and "Join the E-list," where individuals can sign up for MedWatch e-mail updates.

Once the FDA receives a negative report on a drug, it assigns a group of safety evaluators to explore more fully the potential risk involved. These evaluators search patient databases and review the drug's history in clinical trials to determine whether other adverse reports exist and to identify any common trends. In addition, it is necessary to establish a causal relationship between the drug and the adverse event and to assign a possible physiologic reason for the event. These evaluators look at other drugs in the same class as well as at dose-response relationships to prove association.

The ultimate action by the FDA depends on the seriousness of the adverse event and the number of events recognized. The agency might require the drug maker to inform prescribers about the hazard and add a boxed warning label to the drug's packaging. In addition, the FDA may require patient information material to accompany every prescription. Some recent warnings sent out from MedWatch include a warning against using a topical anesthetic agent over a large area of the body to numb the skin for certain procedures such as light/laser procedures and mammograms.[24] Another safety alert included a recommendation to the public to discontinue using Zicam cold remedy nasal products and swabs because they could produce long-lasting or permanent loss of the sense of smell.[25]

MedWatch's Adverse Event Reporting System (AERS) is a very large database of adverse event reports with many new reports being submitted each year. In 2004, approximately 400,000 reports were submitted compared with 150,000 in 1996.[26-28] Even though this appears to be a robust database that can suggest causality, it is considered a "passive system." The primary reason for this is that reporting is voluntary by consumers and prescribers.[29] It is estimated that only 20% of reports come from prescribers.[30] Reporting by manufacturers, distributors, and drug packagers is, however, mandatory. The major weaknesses of a passive surveillance system include under-reporting, reports containing misinformation, and the difficulty encountered in obtaining follow-up information on patients who experienced the reported reaction.

Pharmaceutical companies, along with regulatory agencies, have been working diligently to develop active surveillance systems to complement the passive spontaneous reporting of ADRs. Data mining techniques using statistical methods to identify "safety signals" are being evaluated. These systems utilize databases containing spontaneous reports of adverse events and calculate the number of expected ADRs for a particular drug. In very simple terms, the spontaneous reports data are compared with actual events observed to quantify any disproportionality present. The use of registries is another means of active surveillance. Registries offer an organized system to collect specific data related to drug use or disease. The drug registries monitor patients over a period and collect specific data related to drug use, dose, date of prescribing and dispensing, ADRs, and expenditures. Patients are regularly sent survey questionnaires to capture new events, or data may be collected through the national health care registry electronically, as it is done in Sweden.[31]

Another form of active surveillance is the use of "sentinel sites." Patient information is collected at preselected sites by electronic monitoring with specialized software that uses "action-oriented triggers," and the information is then analyzed for adverse events.[32] This type of monitoring is most suitable for institutional settings such as hospitals or nursing homes. However, there is some selection bias present, and the data collected only reflect the number of patients enrolled in selected facilities. Postmarketing surveillance for ADRs is a very difficult endeavor. In addition, it is quite clear that there is no one solution for obtaining these data, and a collection of strategies are probably necessary to ensure that drugs are as safe as they can be.

Risk Management in Pharmacology

In 2007, Congress passed the Food and Drug Administration Amendments Act (FDAAA). This law requires, on a selective basis, that pharmaceutical companies submit a Risk Evaluation and Mitigation Strategy (REMS) around the time of drug approval. This document must contain specific strategies or tools to minimize adverse reactions produced by the approved drug. The REMS identifies the risks to be minimized and the methods that will be used to minimize these specific risks.[33] Some of the tools used include a Medication Guide and a Patient Package Insert, that is, something that shows that the sponsor is communicating the risks to the potential patient.[34] Other tools include provisions on the dispensing of the drug that mandate that only subspecialists administer the product and even specific lab tests based on which the product can be given safely. The REMS must also include a timeline for assessment, which is usually at 18 months, 3 years, and 7 years after drug approval.

Alphabetic Classification of Adverse Drug Events

Adverse reactions may be classified into a number of different categories by using an alphabetic classification system (Table 4-1).[8,35] An *augmented response* (A) is a dose-related response. This response is related to the pharmacologic action of the drug, which is usually predictable. Examples include a hypoglycemic reaction associated with insulin and hemorrhage caused by the anticoagulant warfarin. This type of reaction is managed by reducing or withholding the dose. *Bizarre effects* (B) are non–dose-related and unpredictable reactions. An anaphylactic reaction to penicillin and liver toxicity associated with inhaled anesthetic agents fall into this category. These effects are managed by eliminating the use of the drug and avoiding it in the future. *Chronic effects* (C) are related to dose and time. These events occur during prolonged administration or as the result of a cumulative dose. Examples include movement disorders that occur with antipsychotics and suppression of the hypothalamic–pituitary–adrenal axis by steroids. Management consists of reduction of the dose or withdrawal of the drug. *Delayed effects* (D) are carcinogenic, such as secondary cancers that occur years after use of chemotherapy agents. The last category is *end-of-treatment effects* (E). Abrupt withdrawal from many drugs can lead to adverse events. A good example of this is opiate withdrawal. Management includes reintroduction and subsequently slow withdrawal of the drug.

A simpler classification system, one more commonly used, consists of the following categories: Adverse Drug Events type A, which include dose-related reactions; Adverse Drug Events type B, which include idiosyncratic or unpredictable reactions: and Adverse Drug Withdrawal Events.[36]

DRUG–DRUG INTERACTIONS

A drug–drug interaction occurs when a second drug is added to a first drug, resulting in a diminished response to either drug, or when the combined effect of the two drugs is additive or synergistic.[37] Drug interactions

TABLE 4-1 Alphabetical Classification of Adverse Drug Effects

Type	Type of Effect	Definition	Examples
A	Augmented pharmacologic effects	Adverse effects that are known to occur from the pharmacology of drug and are dose related	Hypoglycemia caused by insulin injection Bradycardia caused by β-adrenoceptor antagonists Hypotension caused by calcium channel blockers Hemorrhage caused by anticoagulants
B	Bizarre effects	Adverse effects that occur unpredictably and often have a high rate of morbidity and mortality; uncommon	Anaphylaxis caused by penicillin Acute hepatic necrosis caused by halothane Tendon rupture with statin drugs Tendon rupture with ciprofloxacin Bone marrow suppression by chloramphenicol
C	Chronic effects	Adverse effects that occur only during prolonged treatment and not with single doses	Iatrogenic Cushing's syndrome with prednisolone Orofacial dyskinesia caused by phenothiazine tranquilizers Colonic dysfunction caused by laxatives
D	Delayed effects	Adverse effects that occur remote from treatment, either in the children of treated patients or in patients themselves years after treatment	Secondary cancers in those treated with alkylating agents for Hodgkin's disease Craniofacial malformations in infants whose mothers took isotretinoin Clear-cell carcinoma of the vagina in the daughters of women who took diethylstilbestrol during pregnancy
E	End-of-treatment effects	Adverse effects that occur when a drug is stopped, especially when it is stopped suddenly (so called withdrawal effects)	Unstable angina after β-adrenoceptor antagonists are suddenly stopped Adrenocortical insufficiency after glucocorticosteroids such as prednisolone are stopped Withdrawal seizures when anticonvulsants such as phenobarbital or phenytoin are stopped

(Adapted from Page C, Curtis MJ, Sutter MC, Walker MJ, Hoffman BB, editors: *Integrated pharmacology*, ed 2. Philadelphia, 2002, Mosby.)

may be beneficial or harmful. An example of a desired drug–drug interaction is the combination of two pain medications so that pain is controlled better than when either drug is used alone, producing an additive response. Synergistic interactions result from combining two drugs to produce a response greater than the sum of the responses to both drugs. Examples include combining a diuretic and a β-adrenergic blocking agent to lower blood pressure.[38] Another example is the "HIV cocktail," a combination of two or more antiviral drugs that attack the virus at various stages in its replication process.[39] A harmful synergistic reaction occurs when a sedative is combined with either alcohol or an analgesic. Both these combinations produce excessive central nervous system (CNS) depression.[40]

Antagonistic drug relationships result in a combined effect that is less than the response produced by each drug alone. Some of these relationships are beneficial, such as when naloxone is given to reverse an opiate overdose or when flumazenil is used to treat a benzodiazepine overdose.[41] These drugs are competitive antagonists. However, many antagonistic relationships are not desirable. When an aspirin-type drug is added to a diuretic for hypertension, the diuretic becomes less effective.[41] The aspirin inhibits prostaglandin production in the kidneys, and prostaglandin synthesis is important for maintaining renal perfusion and appropriate reabsorption and secretion of ions.

Pharmacokinetic and Pharmacodynamic Basis for Drug–Drug Interactions

Pharmacokinetic reasons for drug interactions include many of the issues discussed in the previous chapter. Slowing of gastrointestinal (GI) motility by drugs such as opioids and tricyclic antidepressants (the antimuscarinic effects) may increase the absorption of other drugs.[42] Laxatives, which increase GI motility, have the opposite effect by allowing less time for absorption.[43]

Interactions during distribution occur with drugs that readily bind to plasma proteins.[44] The antiseizure drugs sodium valproate and phenytoin interact when valproate causes phenytoin to be displaced from albumin and also inhibits the metabolism of phenytoin.[45]

Enzyme inhibition and enzyme induction produce interactions that occur during metabolism. For example, birth control pills are metabolized more quickly when phenytoin is administered, leading to a diminished contraceptive effect and a possible pregnancy.[46] Boxes 4-3 and 4-4 present additional examples of enzyme-inducing and enzyme-inhibiting drugs.

The process of renal excretion is not free from drug interactions. A helpful interaction is the use of probenecid to compete with the renal transport of penicillin and other antibiotics into the tubular fluid.[47] This is a useful method of prolonging the action of antibiotics for the treatment of certain infections.

BOX 4-3 Examples of Drugs That Inhibit Drug-Metabolizing Enzymes

Drugs Inhibiting Enzyme Action	Drugs with Metabolism Affected
Allopurinol	Mercaptopurine, azathioprine
Chloramphenicol	Phenytoin
Cimetidine	Amiodarone, phenytoin, pethidine
Ciprofloxacin	Theophylline
Corticosteroids	Tricyclic antidepressants, cyclophosphamide
Ciprofloxacin	Theophylline
Disulfiram	Warfarin
Erythromycin	Cyclosporine, theophylline
Monoamine oxidase inhibitors	Pethidine
Ritonavir	Saquinavir

(From Rang HP, Dale MM, Ritter JM, Moore, PK: *Pharmacology*, ed 5. New York, 2003, Churchill Livingstone.)

BOX 4-4 Examples of Drugs That Induce Drug Metabolizing Enzymes

Drugs Inducing Enzyme Action	Drugs with Metabolism affects
Phenobarbital	Warfarin
Rifampicin	Oral contraceptives
Griseofulvin	Corticosteroids
Phenytoin	Cyclosporine
Carbamazepine	Drugs listed in left-hand column will also be affected

(From Rang HP, Dale MM, Ritter JM, Moore PK: *Pharmacology*, ed 5. New York, 2003, Churchill Livingstone.)

FOOD–DRUG INTERACTIONS

The coadministration of certain drugs with acidic beverages such as Coca-Cola Classic and Pepsi, which have a pH under 3, can alter the absorption of some drugs. A weak base administered with these drinks will cause ionization of the drug and diminish absorption. Food and liquid in the stomach also affect the dissolution rate of drugs which can slow the absorption rate. Transit time through the GI tract is also slowed by food and liquid. However, it is important to realize that slowed absorption does not necessarily mean a decrease in the amount of drug absorbed. When aspirin and food are taken together, there is a delay in the onset of pain relief but the overall bioavailability of the drug remains the same.

Since cytochrome P450 enzymes are also involved in the metabolism of food and food can induce or inhibit these enzymes, it is easy to understand why certain combinations of food and drugs should be avoided. Grapefruit juice, unlike other citrus juices, is a well-known inhibitor of P450 enzymes and therefore increases the bioavailability of many drugs (e.g., cyclosporine, calcium channel blockers, and statins).[48] Repeated exposures to grapefruit juice inhibits not only these enzymes but also the expression of the genes that control their production. Therefore grapefruit juice should be avoided entirely when these drugs are taken. In other cases of nutrient–drug interactions, ingestion of the food and administration of the drug need only be separated for a few hours. Another well-recognized food–drug interaction involving the P450 enzymes includes the interaction between cruciferous vegetables and warfarin.[49] Indoles in the cabbage, brussels sprouts, and broccoli significantly induce the metabolisms of certain medications, particularly warfarin, leading to a lowered serum level and less efficacy. Charbroiled food is an inducer of CYP1A2 and 3A4 and decreases the efficacy of acetaminophen and naproxen.[50,51]

Foods rich in vitamin K interfere with anticoagulation, although not through a P450 mechanism. Warfarin is a vitamin K antagonist that reduces the enzymatic reduction of the active form of vitamin K necessary for the production of clotting factors. However, a diet high in vitamin K will interfere with the anticoagulant's effectiveness and lowers the International Normalized Ratio (INR).[52]

Administration of a number of formulas via enteral feeding tubes has been implicated in drug–nutrient interactions. Absorption of warfarin, tetracycline, and phenytoin is decreased when these drugs are administered with enteral feedings.[53] Chelation reactions, in which divalent cations and drug molecules bind to each other, are particularly problematic. The macronutrients in enteral feedings, especially protein, may also reduce bioavailability.[48] Certain drugs, such as phenytoin, may bind to the plastic tubing, which also reduces bioavailability. The location of drug delivery can influence drug absorption as well. A drug that requires an acidic environment for activation will show diminished efficacy if it is administered with tube feedings into the distal portion of the small intestine where the environment is not acidic.

The management of drug–nutrient interactions becomes clear once the mechanism of the reaction is understood. If interactions occur as a result of mixing the feeding formulas with the drug, formulas can be withheld for at least 2 hours before or after drug administration.[48] If the issue is the binding of the drug to the plastic tubing, the tubes can be flushed with saline solution. However, most of the interactions involving metabolism cannot be stopped by a time separation, so the interacting nutrient will have to be avoided completely by the patient.

DRUG ALLERGY AND DRUG-INDUCED ILLNESSES

Drug allergies or hypersensitivities range from mild presentations (urticaria) to very severe life-threatening events (anaphylaxis). For a drug to produce a reaction, it must have antigenic effects, and it must stimulate antibody formation, or the formation of sensitized T lymphocytes, which is immune related. It is estimated that up to one third of all ADRs are attributed to drug allergy.[54,55] In most instances of allergy, the drug combines with some protein and forms a complex that has antigenic activity. The synthesis of antibodies may take 1 to 2 weeks. When the patient is re-exposed to the drug, manifestations of the allergy develop. Specifically, drug allergies are classified into four types, although classifying a drug into a specific category can present a challenge.

Type I (Anaphylactic Reactions)

Anaphylaxis is the most severe allergic reaction. It involves the skin and the pulmonary and cardiovascular systems, producing cardiovascular and respiratory collapse. The mechanism of this reaction is degranulation of mast cells, basophils, or both after exposure to a specific antigen in sensitized individuals. In general, immunoglobulin E (IgE) antibodies are formed and attach to basophils and circulating mast cells in connective tissue, skin, and mucous membranes during the initial exposure. On re-administration of the antigen, the basophils and mast cells release large amounts of histamine, which results in bronchoconstriction, peripheral vasodilation, increased vascular permeability, and increased mucus production. Specifically, this results in some of the following signs and symptoms:[56]

- Neurologic—dizziness, weakness, seizures
- Ocular—pruritus, lacrimation, edema around the eyes
- Upper airway—nasal congestion, hoarseness, stridor, laryngeal edema, cough, obstruction
- Lower airway—dyspnea, tachypnea, cyanosis, bronchospasm, accessory muscle use to assist respiration, respiratory arrest
- Cardiac—tachycardia, hypotension, arrhythmias, myocardial infarction, cardiac arrest
- Skin—flushing, erythema, pruritus, angioedema, urticaria, maculopapular rash
- GI—nausea, vomiting, diarrhea

These symptoms generally occur within minutes after antigen exposure but may occur even up to 1 hour later. This reaction may have two phases. In about 20% of cases, the initial symptom presentation is followed by a second phase of reactivity 10 hours later.[57] The condition is treated initially with parenteral epinephrine, the establishment of an airway, and supplemental oxygen. Histamine blockers (diphenhydramine and ranitidine) are also given once the patient's condition has stabilized, followed by administration of steroids to prevent the second phase of the reaction. Prevention strategies include use of self-injectable epinephrine and wearing a medical alert bracelet. Certain drug desensitization protocols (e.g., for penicillin) have also been used, but patient avoidance of the offending agent is recommended. In addition, the patient must be instructed to avoid drugs that exhibit cross-reactivity with the offending agent.

Type II (Cytotoxic Reaction)

In a type II reaction, the antigen adheres to the target cell. Antibodies (IgG and IgM) are formed and attach to the target tissue with subsequent antigen–antibody complex formation and activation of complement.[58] This complex then begins to destroy the target tissue. Essentially, the drug combines with a protein that the body no longer recognizes as self. Drugs known to produce this reaction include penicillin, cephalosporins, salicylates, and phenytoin. This reaction takes some time (several days to a week) as the levels of IgG and IgM increase and the antibodies begin to attach themselves to red blood cells, platelets, and basophils. Clinical manifestations include fever, arthralgia, rash, splenomegaly, and lymph node enlargement. This group of symptoms is known as a *serum sickness–like reaction*, but when there is specific internal organ involvement, it is referred to as *drug hypersensitivity syndrome* (multiorgan dysfunction). More severe manifestations may include hemolytic anemia, glomerulonephritis, thrombocytopenia, and leukopenia.[7] The reaction is self-limiting and resolves within several days to weeks after the drug is discontinued.

Type III (Autoimmune Reaction)

A type III reaction is a complex-mediated hypersensitivity reaction, in which the body has difficulty eliminating antigen–antibody complexes.[7] These complexes attach to normal tissue and activate a cascade, creating an inflammatory response. This same mechanism governs autoimmune disorders such as drug-induced lupus and rheumatoid arthritis. Manifestations include serum sickness, glomerulonephritis, vasculitis, and pulmonary disorders. Drug-induced SLE may be caused by isoniazid, methyldopa, or chlorpromazine.[59] Once the drug has been discontinued, the lupus resolves in 4 to 6 weeks.

Type IV (Cell-Mediated Hypersensitivity)

A type IV reaction is mediated through T lymphocytes as opposed to antibodies. The response is a local or tissue reaction such as contact dermatitis.[7]

Clinical Manifestations of Drug-Induced Reactions

Urticarial rashes constitute an eruption of itchy wheals. The reaction may be general but is usually worse around the area where a drug has been injected or applied topically. The reaction can also occur with oral administration. Along with angioedema, urticaria is seen in type I and III reactions.[7] Angioedema refers to edema of the lips and face. Nonurticarial rashes are seen in type I, II, and IV reactions. This category can include severe skin disorders such as exfoliative dermatitis and Stevens-Johnson syndrome (in which lesions involve both the oral and anogenital mucosa, and systemic symptoms of fever, headache, arthralgia, and conjunctivitis are present).[60] Exudative lesions are also present. Drugs that have produced these skin disorders include carbamazepine, phenytoin, penicillin, and sulfonamides. These conditions respond to epinephrine, antihistamines, and steroids.

Other drug-induced disorders include diseases of the lymphoid tissues, ocular toxicity, hepatotoxicity, ototoxicity, pulmonary toxicity, and nephrotoxicity.[7] Infectious mononucleosis, when present with a maculopapular rash, is probably an allergic reaction. Erythromycin and penicillins may cause this reaction. Pulmonary manifestations such as asthma are seen in type I reactions; pulmonary fibrosis may be seen in a type III reaction. Blood disorders such as thrombocytopenia, granulocytopenia, and aplastic anemia are seen in type II reactions. Medications may, at times, affect the ears, producing dizziness, hearing loss, and balance difficulties. Antibiotics that have reduced clearance from the kidneys accumulate in other tissues such as the cranial nerves.

Many drugs cause liver damage which may manifest in a mild form as elevated liver enzymes or as full blown hepatic failure.[61] Hepatotoxicity, producing increased transaminase levels, jaundice, and pruritus can be a type II reaction but can also be present as a general adverse reaction because the liver is susceptible to both parenchymal hepatic damage and bile channel injury by the chemicals processed there. Reactive metabolites such as hydrogen peroxide and other hydroxyl radicals are cytotoxic to the membrane lipids of cells. In addition, glutathione, a chemical involved in phase II metabolism, may be exhausted by the accumulation of normal metabolic products or toxic chemicals. With an overdose of acetaminophen, the enzymes involved in conjugation are saturated and cannot metabolize the phase I product, N-acetyl-p-benzoquinone imine (NAPBQI). As the NAPBQI accumulates, it has a toxic effect on the liver, which is made even worse with concomittant chronic alcohol use.

Nephrotoxicity is another common drug-induced problem.[62] Nonsteroidal anti-inflammatory drugs (NSAIDs) and angiotensin-converting enzyme inhibitors (ACE inhibitors) both can cause acute renal failure, especially in those individuals who already have compromised renal function. NSAIDs inhibit vasodilator prostaglandins important for maintaining glomerular filtration and renal blood flow. Allergic interstitial nephritis can also be caused by NSAIDs. ACE inhibitors block an enzyme needed for aldosterone release, and decreased aldosterone can lead to hyperkalemia. Another mechanism for neprotoxicity is exposure to high concentrations of drug metabolites as fluid undergoes reabsorption through the kidney tubules.

Diagnostic Tests for Drug Allergy

A number of diagnostic tests may be helpful in determining whether a reaction is drug related. General lab tests such as liver function tests, determination of blood urea nitrogen and creatinine levels, and complete blood counts are useful; and chest radiography can help determine which organs are involved in the reaction. In addition, some more specific tests such as determination of antinuclear antibodies (for drug-induced lupus) and a urine histamine test (for anaphylaxis) may be performed. When mast cells are involved, tryptase, a protease that is contained in mast cell granules, is a useful biochemical marker.[56]

Skin tests for large polypeptides such as insulin and streptokinase are available and measure IgE-mediated reactions to determine whether the agent can be given again safely. However, the tools available are limited because drug allergy and the different mechanisms involved are not yet completely understood.[56] Skin patch testing may show no evidence of IgE antibodies, which can mean either that they are not present or that they are present in amounts too small to be detected. However, even a very low, undetectable concentration can cause a reaction. The antigenic component of the skin test may not be the agent that necessarily triggers a reaction in all patients allergic to it.

ACTIVITIES 4

1. You are treating a patient for lateral epicondylitis. During today's session, you notice a red rash over the lateral aspect of the involved elbow. The patient tells you that she is using a herbal cream designed to reduce pain, which she had purchased from a general nutrition store. Outline some questions you should ask to determine whether this rash is a drug-induced disorder.
2. You suspect an adverse drug reaction in a patient you are treating. List some sources for drug safety that you can consult to verify your suspicion.
3. You are asked to evaluate a 70-year-old woman who had been admitted to the hospital with muscle weakness, dehydration, and anorexia. Her medical history is significant for type 2 diabetes and osteoporosis. Her medications prior to hospital admission included insulin and glyburide, both of which lower the blood glucose level. These two medications have been continued while she is in hospital. You arrive at her room at 10 A.M. for the evaluation and find her unresponsive and diaphoretic. Her blood glucose level is 40 mg/dL. Her medications are discontinued, and she is treated with dextrose. Additionally, continuous monitoring of carbohydrate intake is initiated. The patient's mental status improves, and she is ready for therapy. Is this an adverse drug event, and should this be reported to the FDA?
4. You are seeing a new outpatient for evaluation and treatment of weakness secondary to a stroke. During your interview, you realize that the patient is taking several sound-alike or look-alike drugs. How might you counsel your patient so that adverse drug events could be prevented?

REFERENCES

1. Chutka DS, Evans JM, Fleming KC, Mikkelson KG: Symposium on Geriatrics Part I: Drug prescribing for elderly patients, Mayo Clin Proc 70(7):685-693, 1995.
2. Lazarou J, Pomeranz BH, Corey PN: Incidence of adverse drug reactions in hospitalized patients, JAMA 279(15):1200-1205, 1998.
3. Budnitz DS, Pollock DA, Weidenbach KN, et al: National surveillance of emergency department visits for outpatient adverse drug events, JAMA 296(15):1858-1866, 2006.
4. Moore T, Cohen MR, Furberg C: Serious adverse drug events reported to the Food and Drug Administration, 1998–2005, Arch Intern Med 167(16):1752-1759, 2007.
5. Pirmohamed M, James S, Meakin S: Adverse drug reactions as a cause of admissions to hospital: Prospective analysis of 18,820 patients, Br Med J 329:15-19, 2004.
6. Gandhi TK, Weingart SN, Borus J: Adverse events in ambulatory care, N Engl J Med 348:1556-1564, 2003.
7. Bennett PN: Unwanted effects and adverse drug reactions, In Bennett PN, editor: Clinical pharmacology, Philadelphia, 2008, Curchill Livingstone.
8. Edwards IR, Aronson JK: Adverse drug reactions: Definitions, diagnosis, and management. Lancet 356:1255-1259, 2000.
9. Raebel MA, Carroll NM, Andrade SE: Monitoring of drugs with a narrow therapeutic range in ambulatory care, Am J Manag Care 12:268-274, 2006.
10. Ghose K: The need for a review journal of drug use and the elderly, Drugs Aging 1(1):2-5, 1991.
11. Lenert LS, Markowitz DR, Blaschke TF: Primum non nocere? Valuing of the risk of drug toxicity in therapeutic decision making, Clin Phamacol Ther 53:285-291, 1993. (abstract).
12. Haynes RB, McDonald JP, Garg AX: Helping patients follow prescribed treatment: Clinical applications, JAMA 288:2880-2883, 2002.
13. Benner JS, Glynn RJ, Mogun H, et al: Long-term persistence in use of statin therapy in elderly patients, JAMA 288:455-461, 2002.
14. Holmes WC, Bilker WB, Wang H, Chapman J, Gross R: HIV/AIDS-specific quality of life and adherence to antiretroviral therapy over time, J Acquir Immune Defic Syndr 46(3):323-327, 2007.
15. Cramer JA, Scheyer RD, Mattson RH: Compliance declines between clinic visits, Arch Intern Med 150:1509-1510, 1990.
16. Eisen SA, Miller DK, Woodward RS, Spitznagel E, Przybeck TR: The effect of prescribed daily dose frequency on patient medication compliance, Arch Intern Med 150:1881-1884, 1990.
17. Jackevicius CA, Mamdani M, Tu JV: Adherence with statin therapy in elderly patients with and without acute coronary syndromes, JAMA 288:462-467, 2002.
18. Kruse W, Rampmaier J, Ullrich G, Weber E: Patterns of drug compliance with medications to be taken once and twice daily assessed by continuous electronic monitoring in primary care, Int J Clin Pharmacol Ther 32:452-457, 1994.

19. Leenen FH, Wilson TW, Bolli P: Patterns of compliance with once versus twice daily antihypertensive drug therapy in primary care: A randomized clinical trial using electronic monitoring, Can J Cardiol 13:914-920, 1997.
20. Berman A: Reducing medication errors through naming, labeling, and packaging, J Med Sys 28(1):9-29, 2004.
21. Naranjo CA, Busto U, Sellers EM, et al: A method for estimating the probability of adverse drug reactions, Clin Pharmacol Ther 30:239-245, 1981.
22. Langford BJ, Jorgenson D, Kwan D, Papoushek C: Implementation of a self-administered questionnaire to identify patients at risk for medication-related problems in a family health center, Pharmacotherapy 26(2):260-268, 2006.
23. MedWatch: The FDA Safety information and Adverse Event Reporting Program (website). http://www.fda.gov/medwatch/. Accessed June 29, 2009.
24. MedWatch: Safety Alerts for Human Medical Products: Topical Anesthetics (website). http://www.fda.gov/Safety/MedWatch/SafetyInformation/SafetyAlertsforHumanMedicalProducts/ucm092082.htm. Accessed February 8, 2010.
25. MedWatch: Safety Alerts for Human Medical Products: Zicam Cold Remedy Nasal Products: (website). http://www.fda.gov/Safety/MedWatch/SafetyInformation/SafetyAlertsforHumanMedicalProducts/ucm166996.htm. Accessed February 8, 2010.
26. Ahmed SR: Spontaneious reporting in the United States, In Strom BL, editor: Pharmacoepidemiology, Chichester, UK, 2005, John Wiley and Sons.
27. Sharrar RG, Hostelley LS, Mussen F: Regulations and pharmacovigilance. In Waldman SA, Terzic A, editors: Pharmacology and therapeutics: Principles to practice, Philadelphia, 2009, W.B. Saunders.
28. Strom BL: How the US drug safety system should be changed, JAMA 295:2072-2075, 2006.
29. Bennett CL, Nebeker JR, Yarnold PR, et al: Evaluation of serious adverse drug reactions: A proactive pharmacovigilance program (RADAR) vs safety activities conducted by the Food and Drug Administration and pharmaceutical manufacturers, Arch Intern Med. 167(10):1041-1049, 2007.
30. Cobert B: Manual of drug safety and pharmacovigilance, Boston, 2007, Jones and Bartlett Publishers.
31. Wettermark B, Hammar N, Fored CM, et al: The new Swedish Prescribed Drug Register—Opportunities for pharmacoepidemiological research and experience from the first six months, Pharmacoepidemiol Drug Saf 16:726-735, 2007.
32. Rozich J, Haraden CR, Resar RK: Adverse drug event trigger tool: A practical methodology for measuring medication related harm, Qual Saf Health Care 12:194-200, 2003.
33. FDA: Title IX of FDAAA: REMS Authorities (website). www.fda.gov/downloads/Drugs/DrugSafety/InformationbyDrugClass/UCM163674.pdf. Accessed July 1, 2009.
34. FDA: Approved Risk Evaluation and mitigation Strategies (REMS) (website). http://www.fda.gov/Drugs/DrugSafety/PostmarketDrugSafetyInformationforPatientsandProviders/ucm111350.htm. Accessed July 1, 2009.
35. Ferner R, Mann RD: Drug safety and pharmacovigilance. In Page CP, Curtis M, Sutter M, Hoffman B, editors: Integrated pharmacology, Philadelphia, 2002, Mosby.
36. Bates DW, Leape L: Adverse drug reactions. In Carruthers S, Hoffman B, Melmon K, Nierenberg D, editors: Melmon and Morrelli's clinical pharmacology, New York, 2000, McGraw-Hill.
37. Huang SM, Lesko LJ, Temple R: Adverse drug reactions and interactions. In Waldman SA, Terzic A, editors: Pharmacology and therapeutics: Principles to practice, Philadelphia, 2009, Saunders.
38. Elghozi JL, Azizi M, Plouin PF: Hypertension. In Waldman SA, Terzic A, editors: Pharmacology and therapeutics: Principles to practice, Philadelphia, 2009, Saunders.
39. Pham PA, Flexner CW: HIV Infections and AIDS. In Waldman SA, Terzic A, editors: Pharmacology and therapeutics: Principles to practice, Philadelphia, 2009, Saunders.
40. Choi DS, Karpyak VS, Frye MA, Hall-Flavin DK, Mrazek DA.: Drug Addiction. In Waldman SA, Terzic A, editors: Pharmacology and therapeutics: Principles to practice, Philadelphia, 2009, Saunders.
41. Dedier J, Stampfer MJ, Hankinson SE, et al: Nonnarcotic analgesic use and the risk of hypertension in US women, Hypertension 40:604-608, 2002.
42. Davis SS, Hardy JG, Fara JW: Transit of pharmaceutical dosage forms through the small intestine, Gut 27(8):886-892, 1986.
43. Sullivan SN, Wong C: Runners' diarrhea. Different patterns and associated factors. J Clin Gastroenterol 14(2):101-104, 1992.
44. Larsen FG, Larsen CG, Andersen S, et al: Warfarin binding to plasma albumin, measured in patients and related to fatty acid concentrations, Eur J Clin Invest 16(1):22-27, 1986.
45. Johannessen CU, Johannessen SI: Valproate: Past, present, and future, CNS Drug Rev 9(2):199-216, 2003.
46. Harden CL, Leppik I: Optimizing therapy of seizures in women who use oral contraceptives, Neurology 26(67[suppl 4]): S56-S58, 2006.
47. Spina SP, Dillon EC: Effect of chronic probenecid therapy on cefazolin serum concentrations. Ann Pharmacother 37:621-624, 2003.
48. Lingtak-Neander C: Drug-nutrient interaction in clinical nutrition, Curr Opin Clin Nutr Metab Care 5:327-332, 2002.
49. Michalets EL: Update: Clinically significant cytochrome P-450 drug interactions, Pharmacotherapy 18(1):84-112, 1998.
50. Fujita K: Food-drug interactions via human cytochrome P450 3A (CYP3A), Drug Metabol Drug Interact 20(4):195-217, 2004.
51. McCabe BJ, Frankel EH, Wolfe JJ: Handbook of food-drug interactions, Boca Raton, 2003, CRC Press.
52. Rohde LE, Silva de Assis C, Rabelo ER: Dietary vitamin K intake and anticoagulation in elderly patients, Curr Opin Clin Metab Care 10:1-5, 2007.
53. Hornsby LB, Hester EK, Donaldson AR: Potential interaction between warfarin and high dietary protein intake, Pharmacotherapy 28(4):536-539, 2008.
54. Thong BY, Leong KP, Tang CY, Chng HH: Drug allergy in a general hospital: Results of a novel prospective inpatient reporting system, Ann Allergy Asthma Immunol 90:342-347, 2003.
55. Akdis CA, Akdis M: Mechanisms and treatment of allergic disease in the big picture of regulatory T cells, J Allergy Clin Immunol 123(4):735-746, 2009.
56. Gruchalla RS: Drug allergy. J Allergy Clin Immunol 11(2):S548-S559, 2003.
57. Ellis AK, Day JH: Diagnosis and management of anaphylaxis, CMAJ 169(4):307-312, 2003.
58. Schnyder B, Pichler WJ: Mechanisms of drug-induced allergy. In Mayo Clinic Proceedings, 84(3) , 2009, Mayo Foundation for Medical Education & Research.
59. Knowles SR, Uetrecht J, Shear NH: Idiosyncratic drug reactions: The reactive metabolite syndromes, Lancet 356:1587-1591, 2000.
60. Chia FL, Leong KP: Severe cutaneous adverse reactions to drugs, Curr Opin Allergy Clin Immunol 7(4):304-309, 2007.
61. Park BK, Kitteringham NR, Maggs JL, Pirmohamed M, Williams DP: The role of metabolic activation in drug-induced hepatotoxicity, Ann Rev Pharmacol toxicol 45: 177-202, 2005.
62. Taber SS, Pasko DA: The epidemiology of drug-induced disorders: The kidney, Expert Opin Drug Saf 6(6):679-690, 2008.

SECTION II

Autonomic and Cardiovascular Pharmacology

5

Drugs Acting on the Autonomic Nervous System

Barbara Gladson

AUTONOMIC NERVOUS SYSTEM

The autonomic nervous system (ANS) is divided into two main anatomical divisions: (1) the sympathetic nervous system (SNS) and (2) the parasympathetic system (PNS). Some authors, however, include the enteric nervous system as a third division, describing the intrinsic nerve plexuses of the gastrointestinal (GI) tract.[1] The enteric system is closely aligned with the other two divisions with interconnections between them. The ANS is responsible for many involuntary functions such as contraction and relaxation of smooth muscle, exocrine and some endocrine secretions, heart rate and contractility, blood pressure, and digestion.

Anatomy and Physiology of the Autonomic Nervous System

The most significant anatomic difference between the ANS and the somatic system is that the ANS requires two neurons in sequence, whereas the somatic system uses a single motor neuron to relay information from the central nervous system (CNS) to the skeletal muscles. The two neurons comprising the autonomic pathway are known as preganglionic and postganglionic neurons.

Preganglionic sympathetic fibers originate with their cell bodies in the lateral horn of the gray matter of the thoracic and lumbar segments (from T1 to L2) (Figure 5-1).[2] Hence, they are also called the thoracolumbar system. The fibers leave the spinal cord in the spinal nerves and then synapse in the paravertebral chain of the sympathetic ganglia lying bilaterally on either side of the spinal cord. The short preganglionic fiber then synapses on the cell body of the postganglionic fiber and rejoins some of the spinal nerves to reach their destination. Nerves for the abdominal and pelvic viscera have their cell bodies in unpaired prevertebral ganglia in the abdomen.

In the SNS, the postganglionic neuron is long, extending to the glands and viscera, but the opposite is true of the PNS (Figure 5-2).[3] The preganglionic fibers originate in the cranial area of the spinal cord and travel a long distance to synapse in ganglia on or near their effector organs. The cranial nerves containing PNS fibers include the oculomotor, facial, glossopharyngeal, and vagus nerves. Input destined for the pelvic and abdominal viscera emerge from the sacral area and also traverse a significant distance to reach their ganglia. Thus the postganglionic fibers for the PNS are rather short compared with the postganglionic fibers for the SNS.

The adrenal medulla is a part of the SNS but provides an exception to the two-neuron rule.[4,5] It receives preganglionic fibers but lacks postganglionic neurons. Instead, it influences the target organs by secreting epinephrine, also known as adrenaline, directly into the blood.

Neurotransmitters for the Autonomic Nervous System

The preganglionic neurotransmitter for both the sympathetic and parasympathetic systems is acetylcholine (ACh).[2] When released, ACh binds to nicotinic receptors on the postganglionic cell. However, the neurotransmitter for the postganglionic neuron for each system is different. The postganglionic neuron for the sympathetic system is norepinephrine, also known as *noradrenaline*. At the target organ, norepinephrine interacts with adrenergic receptors. Release occurs when depolarization of the nerve terminal opens calcium channels in the terminal membrane. Calcium flowing into the terminal triggers fusion and release of the synaptic vesicle containing norepinephrine. The action of norepinephrine is terminated by reuptake into the neuron and is either stored in vesicles again or is metabolized by monoamine oxidase in mitochondria. Norepinephrine can also diffuse away from the receptor into extraneuronal cells and then can be inactivated by another enzyme, catechol-O-methyl-transferase (see Figure 5-2).

The natural endogenous catecholamines are norepinephrine, epinephrine, and dopamine. The precursor for the synthesis of norepinephrine and all the catecholamines is the amino acid tyrosine, which is acted on by several enzymes in the nerve terminal to form dopamine and then norepinephrine (Figure 5-3).[6] In the adrenal medulla, the norepinephrine is further converted to epinephrine.

ACh is the neurotransmitter for the postganglionic neuron of the parasympathetic system.[6] Release of a

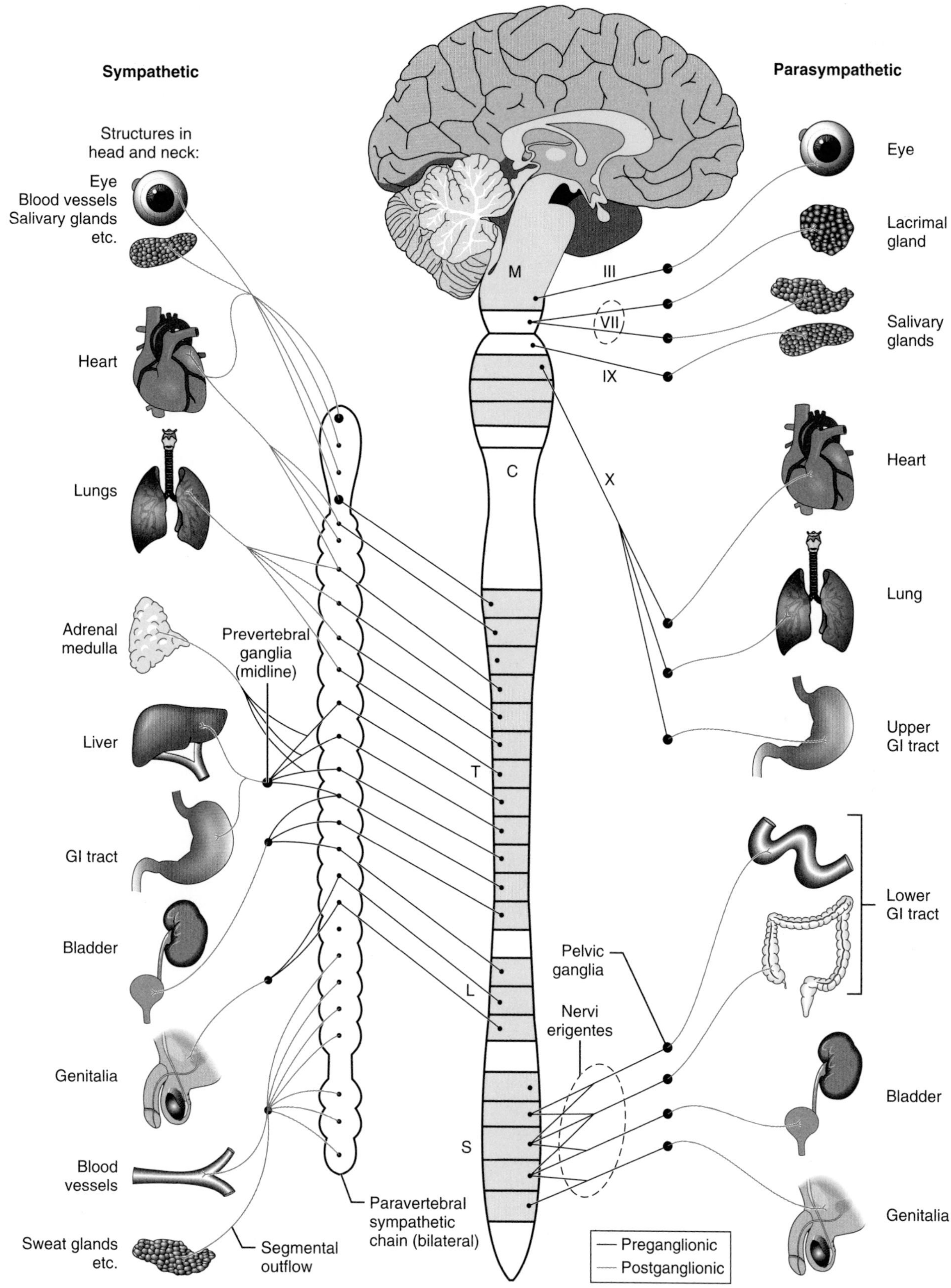

FIGURE 5-1 Anatomic organization of the autonomic nervous system.

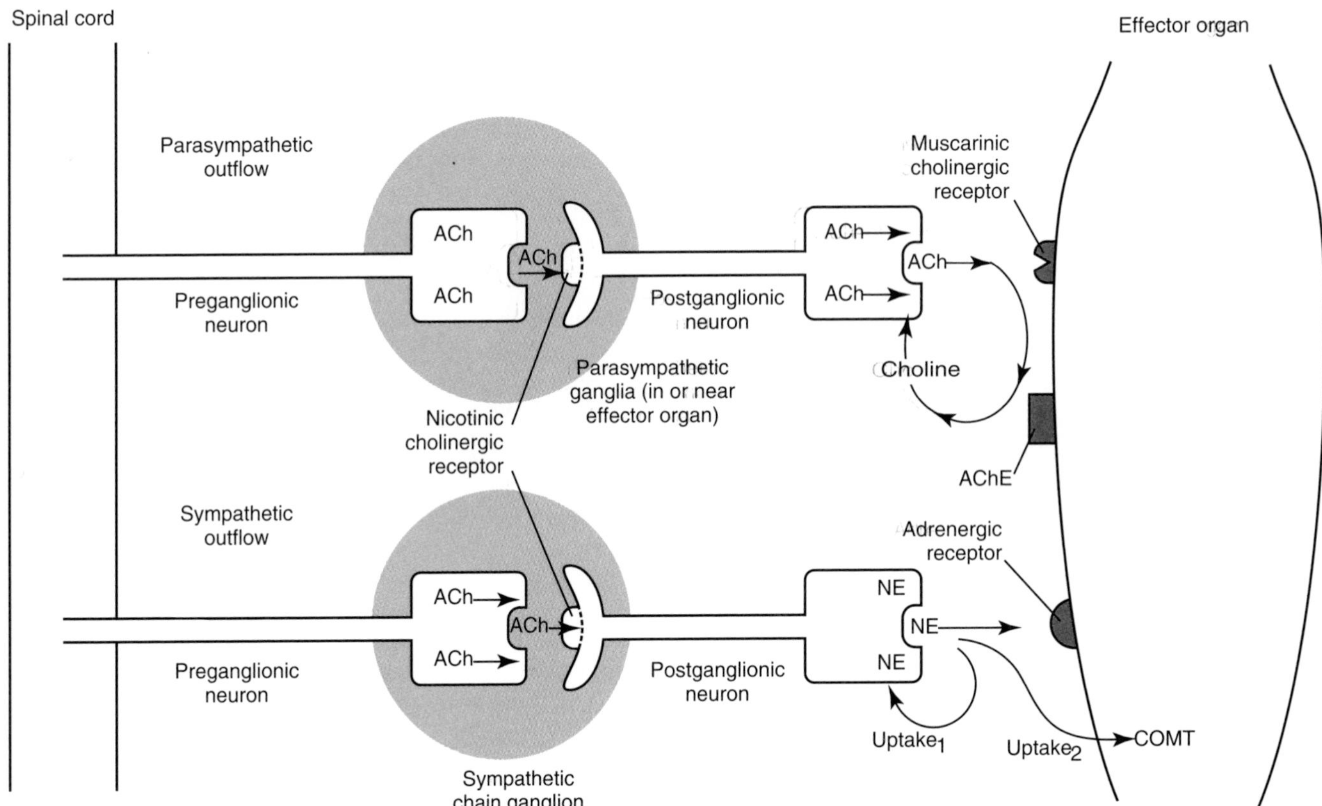

FIGURE 5-2 Neurochemical transmission in the parasympathetic divisions of the peripheral autonomic nervous system. The neurotransmitter liberated in both parasympathetic and sympathetic ganglia is acetylcholine (ACh), which is released upon the arrival of an action potential at the preganglionic nerve terminal. ACh liberated from preganglionic neurons in the parasympathetic and sympathetic ganglia diffuses across the synaptic cleft to interact with nicotinic cholinergic receptors on the cell bodies of postganglionic neurons. The interaction of ACh with ganglionic cholinergic receptors results in the generation and propagation of action potentials that elicit the release of a neurotransmitter at the postganglionic nerve terminal (neuroeffector junction). The neurotransmitter liberated from postganglionic parasympathetic nerves is ACh, which diffuses across the synaptic cleft and activates muscarinic cholinergic receptors on the effector organ. The liberated ACh is rapidly metabolized by acetylcholinesterase (AChE) into choline. Choline is taken up into the parasympathetic nerve terminal and used to resynthesize ACh, which is subsequently stored. A similar process occurs at the postganglionic sympathetic neuroeffector junction, except that the neurotransmitter released is norepinephrine (NE), which diffuses across the neuroeffector junction to stimulate the adrenergic receptors and elicit the end-organ response. Most of the liberated NE is taken back up into the sympathetic nerve terminal (uptake1) and is either stored in the adrenergic storage vehicles or is metabolized by monoamine oxidase (MAO) located in the mitochondria. A smaller amount of the liberated NE may diffuse away from the adrenergic receptors and be accumulated by extraneuronal cells (uptake2), after which it may be metabolized by catechol-O-methyltransferase (COMT).

neurotransmitter from the PNS is quite similar to release from the SNS. An action potential passes down an axon to the terminal, resulting in a change in membrane potential. This voltage change triggers the influx of calcium into the cell, triggering the fusion of a vesicle to the cell membrane and release of ACh into the synaptic cleft. The neurotransmitter diffuses across the cleft and either binds to the muscarinic receptor or is inactivated by the enzyme acetylcholinesterase (AChE), splitting ACh into acetate and choline (Figure 5-4). Choline is then taken back into the neuron by a special choline transport system.

Receptors for the Autonomic Nervous System

There are three main types of nicotinic ACh receptors: (1) those located on the neuromuscular junction of skeletal muscle, (2) ganglionic receptors responsible for communication between preganglionic and postganglionic fibers of the sympathetic and parasympathetic systems, and (3) CNS-type receptors widely dispersed throughout the neural system. All muscle nicotinic receptors consist of five protein subunits and contain two binding sites for ACh that need to be filled for the channel to open.[7]

The muscarinic receptors are divided into five types: M_1 to M_5.[8] M_1 is found mainly in the CNS and has excitatory effects. These receptors exert an excitatory effect by causing depolarization. Diminished ability to upregulate during adrenergic neuron loss in Alzheimer's disease has led to speculation that the progressive decline in cognition may be caused, in part, by problems with this receptor. M_1 receptors are also thought to inhibit dopaminergic neurotransmission in the striatum, and therefore M_1 agonists might be helpful in treating the overactive dopaminergic transmission that occurs in

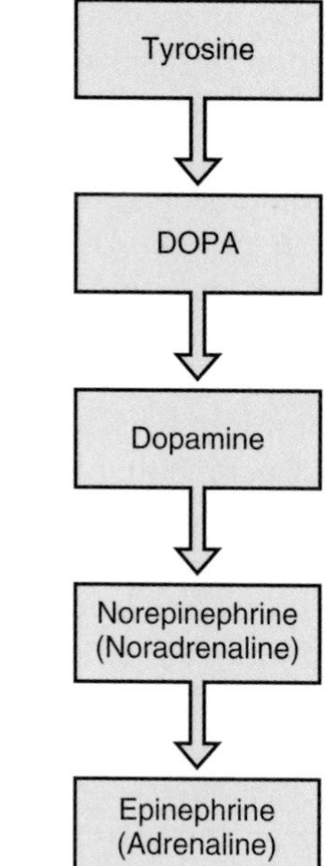

FIGURE 5-3 Biosynthesis of catecholamines.

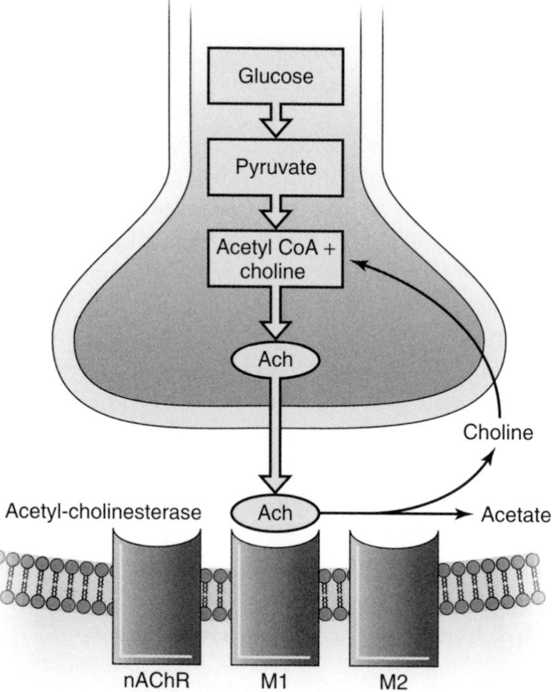

FIGURE 5-4 Action potential–induced release of the neurotransmitter acetylcholine (ACh) and its metabolism at the neuromuscular junction. *nAChR*, nicotinic receptor; M_1-type muscarinic receptor; M_2type muscarinic receptor.

schizophrenia. M_1 receptors are also located in the gastrointestinal (GI) tract and are involved in the secretion of gastric acid after vagal stimulation during a meal. M_2 receptors are located in the heart and produce an increase in potassium (K^+) conductance and block calcium channels, thus reducing heart rate and contractility. These receptors are also located in the CNS, where they produce neural inhibition. Other M_2 receptors expressed in the stomach, intestine, and bladder are responsible for smooth muscle contraction. M_3 receptors are primarily located in the glands and smooth muscle. Release of glandular secretions such as saliva, bronchial secretions, and sweat result from stimulation of M_3 receptors. GI smooth muscle contraction is also stimulated by M_3. M_3 receptors produce vasodilation of vascular smooth muscle by producing the release of nitric oxide from endothelial cells. M_2 and M_3 receptors are also located in the bladder.

Adrenergic receptors are divided primarily into alpha (α)- and beta (β)-receptors, and each of these receptor types is subdivided further.[9] There are two main α-adrenoceptors, α_1 and α_2, and three β-adrenoceptors, β_1, β_2, and β_3, as well as subtypes of each. All of these receptors are G-protein–linked receptors but have different second messengers. α_1-Receptors increase phospholipase C, which stimulates release of intracellular calcium. These receptors function to produce constriction of blood vessels and bronchi and to relax the GI tract and the genitourinary (GU) tract; α_2-receptors decrease cyclic adenosine monophosphate formation and inhibit calcium release, which reduces sympathetic activity by acting as an autoreceptor; and the three β-receptors stimulate cyclic adenosine monophosphate formation and produce increases in cardiac rate and contractility, bronchodilation, and lipolysis. Dopamine (D) receptors are another subclass of adrenoceptors. D_1-receptors are located on renal vascular smooth muscle and mediate vasodilation of the renal artery. D_2-receptors are found on presynaptic nerve terminals. Other types of dopamine receptors also exist in the CNS.

Functions of the Autonomic Nervous System and Specific Innervations

The SNS mediates the fight-or-flight response, and the PNS tends to place the body in a more calm state. However, some authors state that no generalization can be used to explain whether the SNS or PNS causes excitation or inhibition.[3]

The SNS response is triggered by direct sympathetic stimulation of the effector organs and by stimulation of the adrenal medulla to release epinephrine and norepinephrine into the circulation. This system functions as a "unit," producing a set of reactions that occur together. The SNS functions to dilate the pupils, increase the heart rate and contractility, raise the serum glucose level for energy, dilate the bronchioles, increase skeletal blood flow, and relax the GI and GU tracts.[10] Blood is shunted from the GI system and skin to the muscles by constriction of the arterioles and dilation of the muscular vasculature. We can remember these actions by thinking that in the fight-or-flight response, a human being needs to see better (pupil dilation), breathe better (bronchodilate), and get blood to the muscles (increase cardiac output) but does not need to look for a rest room (limited GI and GU activity). Some specific innervations and their receptors associated with the sympathetic system include the following:

1. Contraction of the radial muscle of the iris causing mydriasis: α_1
2. Pilomotor reflex: α_1
3. Prostate contraction: α_1
4. Vasoconstriction of vascular smooth muscle: α_1
5. Adrenergic inhibition: α_2
6. Increased heart rate and contractility: $\beta_1 > \beta_2$
7. Renin secretion: β_1
8. Skeletal muscle blood vessel dilation, bronchiole dilation, uterine relaxation, gluconeogenesis: β_2
9. Glycogenolysis: α_1 and β_2
10. Bladder wall relaxation and detrusor relaxation: β_2; trigone contraction: α_1 (net effect is decreased urination)
11. Decreased GI motility: α_2 and β_2

The PNS functions to conserve energy and is involved in rest and digestion. Some specific innervations associated with the PNS include the following:[11]

1. Contraction of the constrictor pupillae muscle of the eye, causing miosis
2. Decreased rate and contractility of the heart via the vagus nerve
3. Constriction of the trachea and bronchioles
4. Increased muscle motility and tone of the GI tract
5. Bladder wall contraction, detrusor contraction, and trigone relaxation, resulting in urination
6. Release of endothelial-derived relaxing factor in response to stimulation of muscarinic receptors, resulting in relaxation of vascular smooth muscle (vasodilation)
7. Smooth muscle (other than vascular smooth muscle) contraction in response to muscarinic stimulation

Refer to Table 5-1 for more specific innervations.

Many organs are innervated by both the sympathetic and parasympathetic systems, and most of the time they have opposing effects. However, exceptions do exist because both systems perform similar secretory functions and increase salivation. Also, some organs are innervated by only one system. The sweat glands and most blood vessels receive only sympathetic input, and the bronchial smooth muscle has only parasympathetic innervation. However, the bronchioles are extremely sensitive to circulating catecholamines because they contain β_2-receptors.

Enteric Nervous System

The enteric nervous system controls the exocrine and endocrine functions of the GI tract and motility, microcirculation, and immune and inflammatory processes.[12] It can function independently from the CNS, although it maintains connections to the brain via the SNS and PNS. It contains two major plexuses: (1) the myenteric plexus, which innervates the two muscle layers of the entire gut and the secretory portion of the mucosa with extensions to the gallbladder and pancreas, and (2) the submucous plexus in the small intestine, which innervates the muscularis mucosa, glandular epithelium, and submucosal blood vessels. A similar plexus is found in the gallbladder, pancreas, cystic duct, and common bile duct.

The neurotransmitters involved in the enteric system were originally thought to include only ACh and serotonin. However, recent research has shown that adenosine triphosphate, gamma (γ)-aminobutyric acid, substance P, vasoactive intestinal polypeptide, nitric oxide, and a variety of other peptides are active in this system.[1,12] The stimulatory motor neurons use ACh and substance P as their main neurotransmitters, whereas the inhibitory motor neurons contain vasoactive intestinal polypeptide and nitric oxide. Connections to these nerves include parasympathetic motor pathways through the vagus nerve that innervate the motor and secretomotor functions of the upper GI tract and the sacral nerves that control the distal colon and rectum. Postganglionic sympathetic fibers containing vasoactive intestinal polypeptide target the secretomotor neurons, submucosal blood vessels, and GI sphincters. Sensory information is carried through the vagus and splanchnic nerves.

Problems with the enteric nervous system have been implicated in a number of GI disorders.[13] Severe vomiting caused by chemotherapy has been linked to excessive serotonin release by damaged mucosal enterochromaffin cells. High levels of serotonin activate receptors on the vagal primary afferents that extend to the vomiting center in the brainstem. Defective enteric neurons can cause a slowing of intestinal propulsion, leading to bowel obstruction. Another example is achalasia—difficulty swallowing—which is related to a loss of inhibitory myenteric neurons innervating the lower esophageal sphincter. This sphincter tonically contracts and fails to let food cross into the stomach. Drugs that act on the nervous system to help normalize motility and secretions have been developed and are now available.

Nonadrenergic, Noncholinergic System of the Autonomic Nervous System

ACh and norepinephrine are not the only neurotransmitters associated with the ANS. It has been demonstrated that nonadrenergic, noncholinergic transmission can occur from the neurons that were thought to contain only the usual sympathetic and parasympathetic transmitters.[1] Apparently, other neurotransmitters, nitric oxide, vasoactive intestinal peptide, adenosine triphosphate, and neuropeptide Y can exist side by side with ACh and norepinephrine and be secreted by the same neuron. This complicates drug development because some drugs designed to facilitate or block the ANS would also have to exert action on these other transmitters.

TABLE 5-1 The Main Effects of the Autonomic Nervous System

Organ	Sympathetic Effect	Adrenergic Receptor Type	Parasympathetic Effect	Cholinergic Receptor Type
Heart				
Sinoatrial node	Rate ↑	β_1 β_2	Rate ↓	M_2
Atrial muscle	Force ↑	β_1 β_2	Force ↓	M_2
Atrioventricular node	Automaticity ↑	β_1 β_2	Conduction velocity ↓	M_2
			Atrioventricular block	M_2
Ventricular muscle	Automaticity ↑ Force ↑	β_1	No effect	
Blood Vessels				
Arterioles				
Coronary	Constriction	α		
Muscle	Dilatation	β_2	No effect	
Viscera	Constriction	α	No effect	
Skin	Constriction	α	No effect	
Brain	Constriction	α	No effect	
Erectile tissue	Constriction	α	Dilatation	? M_3
Salivary gland	Constriction	α	Dilatation	? M_3
Veins	Constriction	α	No effect	
	Dilatation	β_2	No effect	
Viscera				
Bronchi				
Smooth muscle	No sympathetic innervation, but dilated by circulating epinephrine	β_2	Constriction	M_3
Glands		No effect	Secretion	M_3
Gastrointestinal tract				
Smooth muscle	Motility ↓	α_1, α_2, β_2	Motility ↑	M_3
Sphincters	Constriction	α_1, α_2, β_2	Dilatation	M_3
Glands	No effect		Secretion	M_3
			Gastric acid secretion	M_1
Bladder Wall	Relaxation	β_2	Contraction	M_3
	Sphincter contraction	α_1		
Uterus				
Pregnant	Constriction	α	Variable	
Nonpregnant	Relaxation	β_2		
Male Sex Organs	Ejaculation	α	Erection	? M_3
Eye				
Pupil	Dilatation	α	Constriction	M_3
Ciliary muscle	Relaxation (slight)	β	Constriction	M_3
Skin				
Sweat glands	Secretion (mainly cholinergic)	α	No effect	
Pilomotor	Piloerection	α	No effect	
Salivary Glands	Secretion	α, β	Secretion	M_3
Lacrimal Glands	No effect		Secretion	
Kidney	Renin secretion	β_1	No effect	
Liver	Glycogenolysis Gluconeogenesis	α, β_2	No effect	

(Adapted from Rang HP, Dale MM, Ritter JM, Moore, PK: *Pharmacology*, ed 5, New York, 2003, Churchill Livingstone.)

DRUGS THAT MIMIC THE PARASYMPATHETIC NERVOUS SYSTEM

Drugs that affect the PNS are divided into two categories: (1) those that act directly on the cholinergic (muscarinic) receptors and (2) those that act indirectly by inhibiting the enzyme AChE. AChE rapidly hydrolyzes ACh in the synaptic cleft by cleaving ACh to acetate and choline. Inhibitors of AChE stimulate cholinergic action by prolonging the lifetime of ACh.

Clinical Applications for Muscarinic Agonists

Drugs that mimic the actions of the PNS are used to reduce intraocular pressure in glaucoma, to increase the motility of the GI tract in paralytic ileus, to increase tone of the detrusor muscle for the treatment of urinary retention, and to improve cognition in Alzheimer's disease. Discussions of the drugs for the GI system and for Alzheimer's disease are included in later chapters.

Effects on the Eye. Parasympathetic input to the eye contracts both the constrictor pupillae and the ciliary muscles.[14,15] Contraction of this muscle allows the lens to accommodate for near vision. The constrictor pupillae muscle runs circumferentially around the iris and by contracting produces miosis (Figure 5-5). The ciliary muscle relaxes the suspensory ligaments, allowing the lens to bulge and adjusting the curvature of the lens, which reduces the focal length of the lens.

Aqueous humor is normally secreted slowly and continuously from the ciliary body. The fluid drains through the canal of Schlemm. However, in acute glaucoma, the canal of Schlemm becomes blocked by a dilated pupil, and the fluid cannot drain. The intraocular pressure is raised, which damages the eye and can lead to blindness. Pupil constriction under these circumstances can improve drainage by moving the pupil away from the pathway for aqueous humor, allowing the fluid to drain into the canal.

Effects on Myasthenia Gravis. Myasthenia gravis is an autoimmune disorder caused by antibodies specific for the nicotinic ACh receptor at the neuromuscular junction.[16-19] Patients demonstrate muscle weakness and easy fatigability, being unable to sustain muscular contractions. Areas of involvement may include the eyelids, extraocular muscles, extremities, diaphragm, and neck extensor muscles. Occasionally, however, the only manifestation of the disease may be drooping eyelids (ptosis). Diagnosis is made by using sensitive electromyography and by administering a short-acting intravenous drug (edrophonium) to prolong the effects of ACh at the junction. A positive test result for the disease consists of a rapid (within 2 minutes) but short-lived improvement (less than 5 minutes) in muscle strength. Dynamometer testing and lung vital capacity testing are used to monitor strength. Other treatments for myasthenia gravis include immunosuppressant drugs such as azathioprine, cyclosporine, and prednisone. These drugs are covered in later chapters.

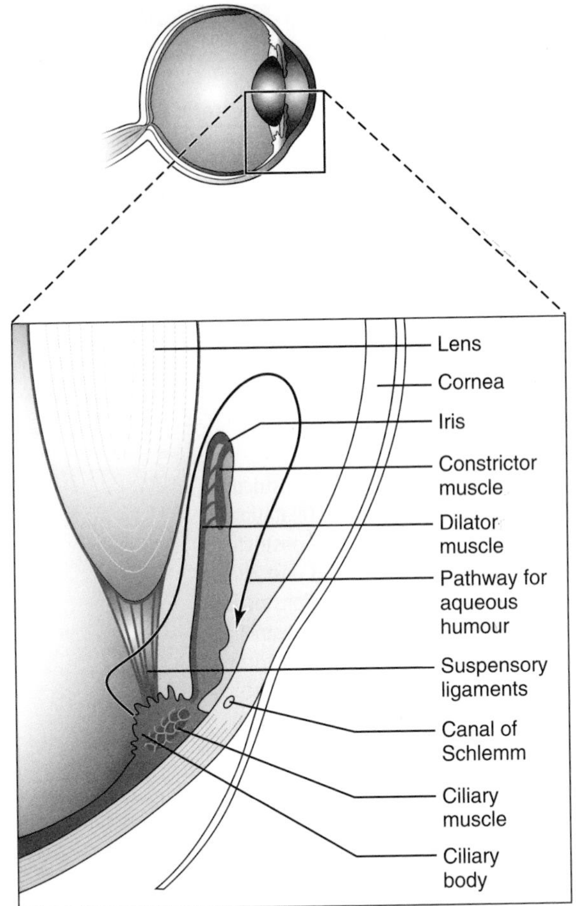

FIGURE 5-5 The anterior chamber of the eye, showing the pathway for secretion and drainage of the aqueous humor.

Direct-Acting Muscarinic Agonists

Direct-acting agonists bind directly to the muscarinic receptors, functioning just like ACh, to mimic the actions of the PNS (Table 5-2).[9] Pilocarpine and bethanechol are the two most commonly used direct-acting agents. Pilocarpine is obtained from the Pilocarpus shrubs of South America and is applied topically to the cornea to produce miosis in acute glaucoma. The duration of action is 24 hours. With topical application, there is a reduced chance of the drug producing a systemic adverse effect. Due to its ability to increase secretions, it is also used in the treatment of xerostomia (dry mouth) in Sjögren's syndrome and after radiation therapy for head and neck cancers.

Bethanechol stimulates the PNS with a particular selectivity for the detrusor muscle in the bladder (see discussion of the physiology and function of the bladder) and the smooth muscle of the GI tract. It is used to treat urinary retention or to reduce urethral resistance in detrusor-trigone dyssynergia. It is particularly useful to treat postpartum or postoperative urine retention. In the

GI tract, the drug stimulates gastric motility and restores peristaltic activity in the paralytic ileus. It may also be used in the treatment of reflux esophagitis, particularly in children experiencing projectile vomiting, but has more recently been replaced by proton pump inhibitors.[20] Unlike ACh, it is not inactivated by AChE and therefore has a longer duration of action than the endogenous transmitter. It is available in an oral form and as a subcutaneous injection. With the oral formulation, onset of action is within 30 to 90 minutes, and the duration of action may be up to 6 hours.

Indirect-Acting Muscarinic Stimulants

Indirect-acting muscarinic stimulants act by inhibiting AChE to prolong the action of ACh. There are actually two types of cholinesterases that are seen in the body, (1) AChE and (2) butyrylcholinesterase (plasma cholinesterase located at non-neuronal sites). Both these enzymes produce a very rapid breakdown of ACh—10^4 molecules of ACh in 1 second by a single enzyme.[21] The drugs appear to inhibit both forms of the enzyme with equal potency.

In general, the indirect-acting agents fall into three categories: (1) short-acting anticholinesterases, (2) medium-duration anticholinesterases, and (3) irreversible anticholinesterases. Edrophonium is a very short-acting compound used in the diagnosis of myasthenia gravis. Neostigmine and pyridostigmine are medium-duration anticholinesterases. In fact, pyridostigmine is the treatment of choice for patients with mild myasthenia gravis because it has greater bioavailability and a half-life of 4 hours.[21]

Irreversible anticholinesterases contain an organic group; hence, they are called organophosphate compounds.[22] These agents have been developed into war gases (sarin) and insecticides (malathion). These bind to AChE irreversibly, producing weakness and sensory loss. Depolarizing neuromuscular blockade occurs, in which the muscle initially contracts but is quickly followed by a phase of nondepolarizing blockade with marked muscle weakness because there is no longer free ACh to act on the muscle junction.[11] Other signs are related to muscarinic excess and include miosis, sweating, salivation, bronchial constriction, vomiting, and diarrhea. Death may occur as result of paralysis of the respiratory muscles and excessive bronchial secretions. These agents are highly lipid soluble and are rapidly absorbed through the mucous membranes and even through intact skin. Because these compounds are absorbed rapidly through the cuticles of insects, they are used in agriculture for pest control.

Therapeutic Concerns with Direct-Acting and Indirect-Acting Muscarinic Agents

Direct-acting and indirect-acting muscarinic agents can produce significant cardiovascular effects, including bradycardia and decreased cardiac output. The reduction in cardiac output results from a decrease in contractility, particularly in the atria, caused by the relative denseness of the muscarinic receptors in this area.[23] Therapists must monitor the patient's heart rate and notify the physician if the resting heart rate drops below 60 beats/min. Further dosing may be contraindicated, but the physician will make this determination.

Cholinesterase inhibitors are now recognized to cause some serious adverse effects in older adults with dementia.[24] In particular, they are associated with syncope leading to pacemaker insertion. Drug-induced syncope has been responsible for several events related to falls, such as hip fractures.

Another adverse effect that may occur with these drugs is generalized vasodilation, producing a marked decrease in blood pressure. Nitric oxide and endothelial-derived relaxing factor mediate this effect.[25]

Smooth muscles in the lungs and GI tract are also affected by excess muscarinic activity. This produces abdominal pain, diarrhea, vomiting, frequent urination, bronchoconstriction, and increased secretions (increased sweating and salivation).[11] These drugs are therefore contraindicated for anyone with a history of allergy and asthma. Urinary incontinence, which places the patient at risk for integumentary issues and causes the inconvenience of having to visit the bathroom frequently, presents additional problems that need to be addressed.

MUSCARINIC ANTAGONISTS

Drugs that block the muscarinic receptors are often labeled as parasympatholytic because they block the action of parasympathetic nerve activity. They all function as competitive antagonists of ACh.

Clinical Application for Antimuscarinic (Anticholinergic) Drugs

Antimuscarinic drugs are used to treat motion sickness, relieve symptoms of Parkinson's disease, dilate pupils for an ocular exam, reduce motility of the GI and GU tracts, and dilate the airways.[26] In addition, because they reduce secretions, they can be used preoperatively to prevent excessive salivation and reduce bronchiole tract secretions associated with anesthesia.

Anticholinergic Drugs

Atropine is the prototypical anticholinergic agent. It is the primary alkaloid found in the plant *Atropa belladonna* (or "deadly nightshade"). It is both a central and a peripheral cholinergic antagonist, although it appears to have little effect at the nicotinic receptor sites, so the autonomic ganglia are not usually affected unless high doses are given.[26] The same is true of the nicotinic receptors at the neuromuscular junction. Atropine is primarily used to produce mydriasis in the eye for an

TABLE 5-2 Summary of Drugs that Affect Noradrenergic Transmission

Type	Drug*	Main Action	Uses/Function	Unwanted Effects	Pharmacokinetic Aspects	Notes
Sympathomimetic (direct-acting)	Norepinephrine†	α/β-Agonist	Not used clinically Transmitter at post-ganglionic sympathetic neurons, and in CNS Hormone of adrenal medulla	Hypertension, vasoconstriction, tachycardia (or reflex bradycardia), ventricular arrhythmias	Poorly absorbed by mouth. Rapid removal by tissues. Metabolized by MAO and COMT. Plasma $t\frac{1}{2} \sim 2$ min	
	Epinephrine†	α/β-Agonist	Asthma (emergency treatment), anaphylactic shock, cardiac arrest. Added to local anesthetic solutions. Main hormone of adrenal medulla	As norepinephrine	Given IM or SC. As norepinephrine	
	Isoprenaline	β-Agonist (nonselective)	Astham (obsolete)	Tachycardia, arrhythmias	Some tissue uptake, followed by inactivation (COMT) Plasma $t\frac{1}{2} \sim 2$ h	Now replaced by salbutamol in treatment of asthma
	Dobutamine	β_1-Agonist (nonselective)	Not an endogenous substance	Arrhythmias	Plasma $t\frac{1}{2} \sim 2$ min Given IV	
	Salibutamol	β_2-Agonist	Asthma, premature labor	Tachycardia, arrhythmias, tremor, peripheral vasodilation	Given orally or by aerosol Mainly excreted unchanged Plasma $t\frac{1}{2} \sim 4$ h	
	Salmeterol	β_2-Agonist	Asthma	As salbutamol	Given by aerosol Long acting	Formoterol is similar
	Terbutaline	β_2-Agonist	Asthma	As salbutamol	Poorly absorbed orally Given by aerosol Mainly excreted unchanged Plasma $t\frac{1}{2} \sim 4$ h	
	Clenbuterol	β_2-Agonist	"Anabolic" action to increase muscle strength	As salbutamol	Active orally; long-acting	Illicit use in sports
	Phenylephrine	α_1-Agonist	Nasal decongestion	Hypertension, reflex bradycardia	Given intranasally Metabolized by MAO Short plasma $t\frac{1}{2}$	
	Methoxamine	α-Agonist (nonselective)	Nasal decongestion	As phenylephrine	Given intranasally Plasma $t\frac{1}{2} \sim 1$ h	
	Clonidine	α_2-Agonist	Hypertension, migraine	Drowsiness, orthostatic hypotension, edema and weight gain, rebound hypertension	Well absorbed orally Excreted unchanged and as conjugate Plasma $t\frac{1}{2} \sim 12$ h	
Sympathomimetic (indirect-acting)	Tyramine	NA release	No clinical uses; present in various foods	As norephinephrine	Normally destroyed by MAO in gut; does not enter brain	

	Amphetamine	NA release, MAO inhibitor, uptake 1 inhibitor, CNS stimulant	Used in CNS stimulant in narcolepsy, also (paradoxically) in hyperactive children Appetite suppressant Drug of abuse	Hypertension, tachycardia, insomnia Acute psychosis with overdose Dependence	Well absorbed orally Penetrates freely into brain Excreted unchanged in urine Plasma t½ ~ 12 h, depending on urine flow and pH	Methylphenidat is similar
	Ephedrine	NA release, β-agonist, weak CNS stimulant	Nasal decongestion	As amphetamine, but less pronounced	Similar to amphetamine	Contraindicated if MAO inhibitors are given
Adrenoceptor antagonists	Phenoxybenzamine	α-Antagonist (nonselective, irreversible) Uptake 1 inhibitor	Pheochromocytoma	Hypotension, flushing tachycardia, nasal congestion, erectile dysfunction	Absorbed orally Plasma t½ ~ 12 h	Action outlasts presence of drug in plasma because of covalent binding to receptor
	Phentolamine	α-Antagonist (nonselective, vasodilator)	Rarely used	As phenoxybenzamine	Usually given IV Metabolized by liver Plasma t½ ~ 2 h	Tolazoline is similar
	Prazosin	α_1-Antagonist	Hypertension	As phenoxybenzamine	Absorbed orally Metabolized by liver Plasma t½ ~ 4 h	Doxazosin and terazosin are similar but longer-acting
	Tamsulosin	α_1-Antagonist ("uroselective")	Prostatic hyperplasia	Failure of ejaculation	Absorbed orally Plasma t½ ~ 5 h	Selective for α_{1A}
	Yohimbine	α_2-Antagonist	Not used clinically; claimed to be aphrodisiac	Excitement, hypertension	Absorbed orally Metabolized by liver Plasma t½ ~ 4 h	Idazoxan is similar
	Propranolol	β-Antagonist (nonselective)	Angina, hypertension, cardiac arrhythmias, anxiety tremor, glaucoma	Bronchoconstriction, cardiac failure, cold extremities, fatigue and depression, hypoglycemia	Absorbed orally Extensive first-pass metabolism About 90% bound to plasma protein Plasma t½ ~ 4 h	Timolol is similar and used mainly to treat glaucoma
	Alprenolol	β-Antagonist (nonselective) (partial agonist)	As propranolol	As propranolol	Absorbed orally Metabolized by liver Plasma t½ ~ 4 h	Oxprenolol and pindolol are similar
	Practolol	β_1-Antagonist	Hypertension, angina, arrhythmias	As propranolol, also oculomucocutaneous syndrome	Absorbed orally Metabolized by liver Plasma t½ ~ 4 h	Withdrawn from clinical use
	Metoprolol	β_1-Antagonist	Angina, hypertension, arrhythmias	As propranolol, less risk of bronchoconstriction	Absorbed orally Mainly metabolized in liver Plasma t½ ~ 3 h	Atenolol is similar with a longer half-life
	Butoxamine	β_2-Antagonist	No clinical uses			

*For chemical structures, see Hardman et al (2001).
†Note that norepinephrine and epinephrine are the recommended drug names for noradrenaline and adrenaline, respectively.

Continued

TABLE 5-2 Summary of Drugs that Affect Noradrenergic Transmission—cont'd

Type	Drug	Main Action	Uses/Function	Unwanted Effects	Pharmacokinetic Aspects	Notes
	Labetalol	α/β-Antagonist	Hypertension in pregnancy	Postural hypotension, broncho-constriction	Absorbed orally; conjugated in liver Plasma t½ ~ 4 h	
	Carvedilol	α/β-Antagonist	Heart failure	As for other β-blockers Exacerbation of heart failure Renal failure	Absorbed orally t½ ~ 10 h	Additional actions may contribute to clinical benefit
Drug Affecting Noradrena-line Synthesis	α -Methyl-*p*-tyrosine	Inhibits tyrosine hydroxylase	Occasionally used in pheochromocytoma	Hypotension, sedation		
	Carbidopa	Inhibits DOPA decarboxylase	Used as adjunct to levodopa to prevent peripheral effects		Absorbed orally; does not enter brain	
	Methyldopa	Flase transmitter precursor	Hypertension in pregnancy	Hypotension, drowsiness, diarrhea, erectile dysfunc-tion, hypersensitivity reactions	Absorbed slowly by mouth Excreted unchanged or as conjugate	
	Reserpine	Depletes NA stores by inhibiting vesicular uptake of NA	Hypertension (obsolete)	As methyldopa. Also depression, parkinsonism, gynecomastia	Plasma t½ ~ 6 h Poorly absorbed orally Slowly metabolized Plasma t½ ~ 100 h Excreted in milk	Antihypertensive effect develops slowly and persists when drug is stopped
Drugs Affecting Noradrena-line Release	Guanethidine	Inhibits NA release; also causes NA depletion and can damage NA neurons irreversibly	Hypertension (obsolete)	As methyldopa Hypertension on first administration	Poorly absorbed orally Mainly excreted unchanged in urine Plasma t½ ~ 100 h	Action prevented by uptake 1 inhibitors. Bethanidine and debrisoquin are similar
Drugs Affecting Noradrena-line Uptake	Imipramine	Blocks uptake 1; also has atropine-like action	Depression	Atropine-like adverse effects Cardiac arrhythmias in overdose	Well absorbed orally 95% bound to plasma protein Converted active metabo-lite (desmethyl-imipramine) Plasma t½ ~ 4 h	Desipramine and amitriptyline are similar
	Cocaine	Local anesthetic; blocks uptake CNS stimulant	Rarely used local anesthetic Major drug of abuse	Hypertension, excitement, convulsions, dependence	Well absorbed orally	

(From Rang HP, Dale MM, Ritter JM, Moore, PK: *Pharmacology.* ed 5, New York, 2003, Churchill Livingstone.)
NA, Noradrenaline; *MAO,* monoamine oxidase; *CNS,* central nervous system; *COMT,* catechol-*O*-methyltransferase; *IM,* intramuscular; *SC,* subcutaneous; *IV,* intravenous; t½ half-life.

ocular exam by blocking contraction of the papullary constrictor muscle. During the Renaissance period, dilated pupils were considered desirable, and therefore, despite reduced vision, women used these eye drops as a cosmetic treatment, hence the name "belladonna," or beautiful woman in Italian. Atropine is also used as an adjunct to anesthesia to reduce respiratory secretions. The tissues most sensitive to atropine's action include the exocrine glands, particularly the salivary glands, and the tissue least sensitive is the parietal cell of the stomach. However, atropine can produce a variety of effects because of the large number of parasympathetic cholinergic nerves that exist within the body, limiting the drug's usefulness.

Scopolamine, another anticholinergic drug,[27] has an effect similar to that of atropine but produces greater CNS depression causing drowsiness, memory loss, and sleep. Its primary use is to prevent motion sickness and vertigo caused by depression of vestibular function. It is available in a parenteral preparation as an adjunct to anesthesia and in a transdermal form for prevention of motion sickness. The patch is applied behind the ear for 3 days, preferably 4 hours before a trip begins.

Ipratropium is an inhaled anticholinergic agent, available alone or in combination with albuterol (a β_2-agonist), for the treatment of bronchospasm related to asthma and other chronic obstructive lung diseases. Because this drug is inhaled directly into lung tissue rather than administered orally, there are fewer systemic effects compared with other anticholinergic agents. Dry mouth and pharyngeal irritation are the major complaints with ipratropium, but it can also increase intraocular pressure in patients with glaucoma. This drug and similar ones are reviewed in Chapter 9.

Therapeutic Concerns with Anticholinergic Drugs

At low doses, atropine affects the salivary glands, producing dry mouth; larger doses block accommodation of the eyes, causing blurred vision. Vagal effects become blocked as the drug level increases, producing tachycardia, diminished bronchial secretions, and sweating. Parasympathetic tone of the gut and the urinary tract is blocked, which produces constipation and urinary retention. In fact, after surgery, many patients given atropine complain that they have the sensation that they must urinate but are unable to relax the sphincter to initiate urinary flow. At still higher doses, atropine produces effects on the CNS, including restlessness, confusion, hallucinations, and coma.

Most patients seen in therapy will not be receiving anticholinergic drugs, with the exception of those designed to reduce urinary incontinence and frequency. However, it is important to recognize that many drugs, particularly mood-altering medications, have anticholinergic adverse effects. Most patients complain of sedation and fatigue, which reduce exercise capacity. Two other concerns include increased heart rate and the inability to cool oneself (especially in young children and older adults). Vital signs, including the patient's temperature, should be monitored frequently, particularly if there is a history of cardiac issues.

DRUGS AFFECTING THE SYMPATHETIC (ADRENERGIC) NERVOUS SYSTEM

Drugs that mimic the SNS are labeled sympathomimetic (see Table 5-2). They are designed to either facilitate norepinephrine and epinephrine release or to activate the adrenergic receptors. Figure 5-6 is a diagram of a noradrenergic nerve terminal and shows the sites of drug action. Specifically, sympathomimetic drugs constrict arterioles to reduce bleeding, slow diffusion of local anesthetics, decongest mucous membranes, and raise blood pressure in shock and hypotensive states.

Pharmacologic Effects of Catecholamines

Cardiac Effects. Catecholamines produce a significant increase in myocardial contractility (positive inotropic effect) and a significant increase in heart rate (positive chronotropic effect).[10,28] Both these factors improve cardiac output because

$$\text{Heart Rate} \times \text{Stroke Volume} = \text{Cardiac Output.}$$

The increase in contractility results from an increase in calcium influx into cardiac fibers. The increase in heart rate is produced by increasing the rate of membrane depolarization in the sinus node. Catecholamines also hasten cardiac conduction. Atrioventricular conduction improves, so some physicians use catecholamines to treat heart blocks.

Vascular Effects. The vascular effects of catecholamines vary because net effect depends on dose given.[10] At low doses, epinephrine will decrease peripheral vascular resistance via β_2-receptor–mediated dilation of skeletal muscle blood vessels.[29] At higher doses, the α_1-receptor influence balances the β_2-receptor influence, and at even higher doses, the α_1-receptor influence predominates, producing vasoconstriction (elevated peripheral vascular resistance) and hypertension. Norepinephrine produces predominantly an α-effect at all doses, thus elevating blood pressure.

Central Nervous System Effects. The natural catecholamines are relatively polar, and therefore they do not enter the CNS easily.[10] However, in larger doses, they are still capable of producing anxiety, tremors, and headaches. The noncatecholamine adrenergic agonists such as phenylephrine, ephedrine, and amphetamine have greater lipid solubility and produce more CNS effects.

Nonvascular Smooth Muscle Effects. Catecholamines are capable of relaxing the smooth muscle of the GI

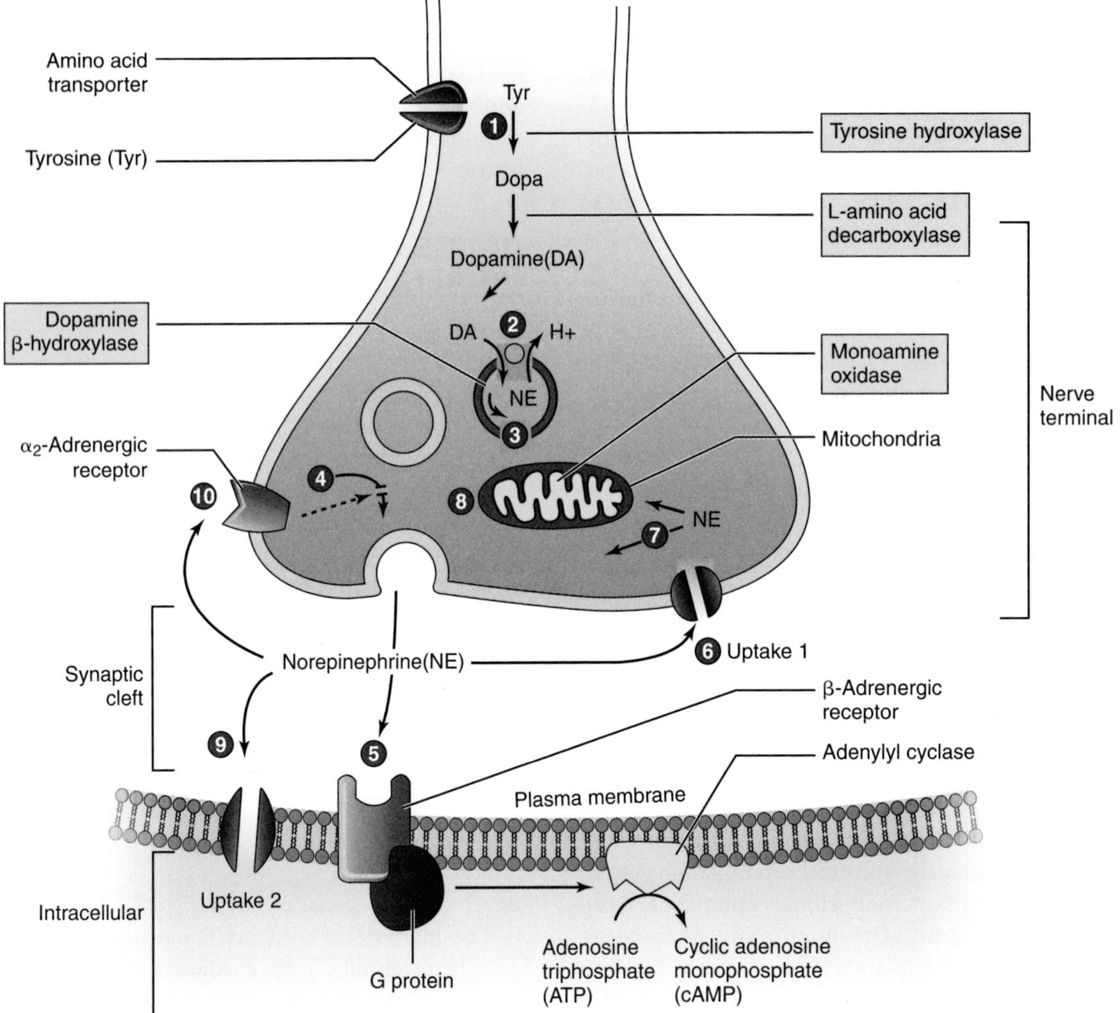

FIGURE 5-6 Generalized diagram of a noradrenergic nerve terminal showing sites of drug action. Action of indirect-acting sympathomimetic drugs is not shown. *NA*, Noradrenaline; *MAO*, monoamine oxides; *MeNA*, methylnoradrenaline.

tract, thus reducing the strength of intestinal peristalsis.[10] In the bladder, epinephrine will cause urinary retention by trigone sphincter constriction and detrusor relaxation. In the lungs, bronchial smooth muscle dilates in response to catecholamines acting on β_2-receptors.

Effects on Nerve Terminals. α_2-Receptors are present presynaptically on cholinergic and adrenergic nerve terminals. These are autoreceptors that act to inhibit neurotransmitter release.[30] These receptors act as the safety valve for turning off sympathetic outflow when there is excessive stimulation. Clinically, they have primarily been used to reduce sympathetic outflow as a treatment for hypertension but are also being used as analgesics and for reducing spasticity.

Metabolic Effects. Epinephrine acts to increase blood glucose and fatty acid levels to supply the needed energy for activity. Insulin secretion is inhibited, and glycogenolysis and gluconeogenesis are enhanced.

Direct-Acting Nonselective Adrenergic Agents

Three catecholamines occur naturally in the human body: (1) norepinephrine, (2) epinephrine, and (3) dopamine.[9] Norepinephrine and epinephrine interact directly with α- and β-receptors. Even though dopamine is the precursor of both norepinephrine and epinephrine, it is also a neurotransmitter, binding to and affecting dopamine receptors, as well as α- and β-receptors.

As mentioned previously, epinephrine has effects on all α- and β-receptors, but its net effect depends on the dose. Epinephrine activates β_1-receptors to increase the strength and rate of cardiac contractions; on β_2-receptors to relax bronchiole smooth muscle, activate glycogenolysis in the liver, and dilate skeletal muscle blood vessels; and on β_3-receptors to activate lipolysis in fat cells. Epinephrine activates α_1-receptors to constrict vascular smooth muscle and also on α_2-receptors presynaptically. The net effect is that epinephrine is a potent vasoconstrictor and a cardiac stimulant, although in some cases, a drop in peripheral vascular resistance is seen, producing a fall in diastolic pressure.[31]

Epinephrine is predominantly used in the emergency department to treat anaphylactic or cardiogenic shock. Therapists may find this drug in the form of Ana-Guard or EpiPen in the homes of patients at risk for anaphylaxis. Pressor-type drugs are critical during cardiopulmonary resuscitation (CPR) to stimulate heart contraction, raise arterial pressure, and redistribute blood flow to important organs, with peripheral α-receptor stimulation being the crucial component.[32] Epinephrine is also used to treat acute exacerbations of asthma and has a role in the treatment of allergy to relieve bronchospasm and decrease pulmonary congestion by constricting the nasal mucosal blood vessels. Small amounts of epinephrine are given along with local anesthetics to reduce circulation to the site of injection, thus preventing diffusion of the anesthetic.[33] This is a common practice in dentistry because it helps prolong the effect of the anesthetic agent.

Epinephrine is given by inhalation or by subcutaneous injection. It has a rapid onset, within 6 to 15 minutes, if given by injection and even sooner if given by inhalation. The duration of action is 1 to 3 hours. In cases of severe asthma or shock, the doses may be repeated.

Norepinephrine activates α_1-adrenergic receptors to a greater extent than α_2-and β_1-receptors. It has little effect on β_2-receptors.[10] Increases in peripheral resistance and both diastolic and systolic blood pressure occur. Cardiac output does not increase as much as it does with a comparable dose of epinephrine because the vascular resistance increases considerably. In addition, heart rate may not increase as much as one would expect, since there are compensatory vagal reflexes in response to the elevated blood pressure. These vagal reflexes overcome the chronotropic effects, but the positive inotropic effects on the heart remain.

Dopamine, the immediate precursor of norepinephrine, activates α_1-and β_1-receptors and D_1 and D_2 dopaminergic receptors. These dopamine receptors exist in the renal vascular beds, and activation produces vasodilation of renal and splanchnic arterioles. At low doses, dopamine stimulates β_1-receptors, producing inotropic and chronotropic effects; but at very high doses, α-receptors are stimulated, causing vasoconstriction. Dopamine has been the drug of choice for the treatment of shock in renal failure, as it raises blood pressure by increasing heart rate and contractility and at the same time facilitates perfusion of the kidneys.[32]

Indirect-Acting Adrenergic Agents: Sympatholytic and Sympathomimetic

Indirect-acting sympathomimetic drugs include ephedrine and amphetamine. They are structurally related to norepinephrine but have weaker actions on the adrenergic receptors. Amphetamine is taken up into the nerve terminal by the norepinephrine uptake mechanism and enters the vesicles in exchange for norepinephrine, which is then freed to act on the postsynaptic receptors. It also blocks the action of monoamine oxidase, which, in itself, raises catecholamine levels. So the net effect is enhanced release of norepinephrine, producing an increase in blood pressure and cardiac contractility. Amphetamine readily enters the CNS where it facilitates the release of dopamine, producing euphoria. It also causes increased alertness, decreased fatigue, decreased appetite, and a marked increase in sympathetic activity. Some forms of the drug have been used in the treatment of narcolepsy and attention deficit disorder and are currently being studied in patients with brain injury for the purpose of improving motor and cognitive performances.[34]

Ephedrine was introduced to the West in 1924 from China.[10] It is now made synthetically and can be found in many herbal medications under the name *ma-huang*. It is an orally active sympathomimetic with a longer duration of action than that of epinephrine, but it has a milder effect. Ephedrine facilitates the release of norepinephrine, activates adrenergic receptors, and easily enters the CNS. It increases systolic and diastolic blood pressure and cardiac contractility, and is capable of producing effects similar to those of amphetamine.

α-Agonists

Phenylephrine is a drug that is used topically to produce mydriasis and nasal decongestion by constricting the mucosal blood vessels. It is a direct-acting synthetic adrenergic drug that primarily stimulates α_1-receptors and produces hypertension. It also may be used for severe hypotension, especially in treating unwelcome tachycardia. Phenylephrine is found in many over-the-counter cold preparations.

Clonidine, unlike phenylephrine, lowers blood pressure. It reduces sympathetic tone by activating the α_2-receptor peripherally and in the CNS. This drug is reviewed more fully in the cardiac chapters.

β-Agonists

β-Agonists are either nonselective and stimulate both β_1-and β_2-receptors or are selective for either receptor. Isoproterenol is a potent nonselective β-agonist with positive chronotropic and inotropic actions. It is primarily used to increase the contractility of the heart during congestive heart failure. Dobutamine is a β_1-selective agonist that increases cardiac contractility with little β_2-agonist effects. It is also used to treat shock or acute congestive heart failure and is used to induce stress to the heart as an alternative to exercise in patients undergoing myocardial perfusion studies.[35,36] Both isoproterenol and dobutamine are administered parenterally.

Selective β-agonists such as terbutaline and salmeterol are used in the treatment of asthma and other obstructive lung diseases. In addition, because β_2-receptors relax uterine contractions in a pregnant uterus, they have been instrumental in stopping premature labor and prolonging gestation.[37] The β_2-agonist drugs are covered more extensively in the pulmonary chapter.

Drugs Used to Treat Shock

For more than 60 years, epinephrine has been the primary drug used as a vasopressor during treatment for cardiac arrest. However, the evidence supporting its efficacy has been largely anecdotal. In recent randomized controlled studies, epinephrine has been compared with placebo and with other vasopressors in both animals and humans; the findings suggest that other drugs might be more effective during resuscitation. Research in this area has been ethically difficult to perform because drugs are crucial to recovery from cardiac standstill, so comparison with placebo is not an option. In addition, standardizing doses of the drugs while someone is in the throes of a cardiac arrest is not easy because the drugs are injected rapidly and without regard for certain pharmacokinetic variables that influence bioavailability, such as the volume of intravenous tubing or site of injection. In addition, some decrement in concentration occurs with storage of this drug.[38] The challenge is to restore cardiac contractions and increase blood pressure while maintaining cerebral and renal perfusion. Many times, cardiac function returns, but postresuscitation problems occur. There is concern about epinephrine's ability to revive patients after a prolonged arrest, which often results in irreversible brain damage. Other concerns include the risks of severe hypertension and epinephrine overdose.

Laboratory evidence indicates that α-adrenergic agents might be extremely useful in treating cardiac arrest. Phenylephrine has the ability to increase aortic pressure without extreme myocardial excitation, which is particularly useful in the treatment of a cardiac arrest with ventricular fibrillation.[32,39] A comparison between phenylephrine and epinephrine showed no difference in the overall rates of successful resuscitation, but further studies are needed before phenylephrine becomes part of standard practice.

Vasopressin, also known as *antidiuretic hormone*, is a vasoactive peptide that acts on vasopressin receptors (V_1-receptors), leading to contraction of vascular smooth muscle cells. Several animal studies show greater vital organ blood flow during resuscitation with this drug compared with epinephrine.[40,41] In addition, one study has shown improved survival rate when vasopressin and a steroid was added to epinephrine.[42] However, further study is needed before this combination becomes standard practice. The current guidelines for resuscitation in adult patients recommend using either vasopressin or epinephrine. However, dobutamine can be used when cardiac contractility is the primary requirement, as well as in treating renal failure. Occasionally, norepinephrine is used when vasoconstriction is top priority, as might be the case in septic shock, but this depends on underlying basal microcirculation.[43]

α- and β-Adrenergic Blockers

Because α- and β-adrenergic blockers are largely used to lower blood pressure and reduce angina, they are covered in the cardiac chapters.

Therapeutic Concerns about Sympathomimetics

With the exception of the β_2-agonists used in the treatment of pulmonary disease, therapists will have little contact with patients administered sympathomimetic drugs. This is, in part, due to their use in the treatment of shock in the emergency department. However, because a significant number of over-the-counter cold remedies contain phenylephrine, therapists should be alert to the cardiac adverse effects of these medications. Given that one of the primary functions of the sympathetic system is to increase heart rate and contractility and peripheral resistance, these drugs increase the overall workload of the heart and have the potential to induce hypertension, cardiac arrhythmias, and angina, even at the lower doses contained in nasal decongestants and cold tablets. Other adverse effects have included cerebral hemorrhage, seizures, and deaths, particularly among ephedra users.[44] In 2004, the U.S. Food and Drug Administration (FDA) demanded elimination of ephedra from weight loss products and herbal remedies because of the high numbers of adverse events.[45] Use of any of these products should be contraindicated for patients with hypertension, hyperthyroidism, ischemic heart disease, arrhythmias, and cerebrovascular insufficiency.

PHYSIOLOGY AND FUNCTION OF THE BLADDER

Bladder anatomy and innervation will be briefly reviewed here because drugs that act on the SNS or PNS are used to treat bladder dysfunction. The lower urinary tract includes the detrusor muscle (smooth muscle of the bladder wall), trigone, and the urethra.[46] The detrusor muscle receives a dominating cholinergic innervation, and when it contracts, it opens the bladder and causes it to empty. This muscle also has β_2-receptors, which, when stimulated, allow the bladder to relax and fill. The trigone (sphincter) and urethra have α_1-receptor input. In summary, sympathetic stimulation keeps the bladder from emptying, whereas parasympathetic activity, via M_2 and M_3 muscarinic receptors, allows it to empty. The urethra also contains striated muscle that forms the external urethral sphincter and is under voluntary control.

Overactive bladder (OAB) is a condition characterized by the "sudden desire to urinate that cannot be postponed."[47] Patients with OAB complain of urgent and frequent urination as well as nocturia. The immediate consequences of this condition include quality-of-life issues as well as increased risk of falls, particularly in older adults with limitations of mobility. Anticholinergics, such as oxybutynin and tolterodine, have an antispasmodic effect on the lower urinary tract and are used to treat OAB. These are potent antimuscarinics that suppress detrusor reflex contractions and increase bladder capacity in patients who have incontinence issues.

However, in older adults, these drugs can exacerbate existing conditions such as dry mouth, constipation, tachycardia, glaucoma, gastroesophageal reflux, and dementia. None of the currently available drugs selectively block only the M_2 and M_3 receptors of the bladder.[48] In addition, particularly worrisome is the M_2-blocking effect of these drugs on the heart, which leads to hypertension, tachycardia, and other more serious arrhythmias. New drug delivery systems, such as an oxybutynin-impregnated ring implanted intravaginally and transdermal preparations, may enhance effectiveness and reduce systemic effects.[49] Darifenacin is one of the newer drugs in this category, which appears to be more selective for the M_3-receptor than the M_2-receptor, thus reducing the cardiac adverse effects; however, it increases the occurrence of constipation.[47]

One of the more disturbing outcomes from the development of drugs for OAB has been the use of these anticholinergic agents among those patients who are already on cholinesterase inhibitors. Cholinesterase inhibitors are prescribed to patients with dementia to improve cognition or to slow the decline in memory and thought processes associated with Alzheimer's disease. Three large studies, two in the United States and one in Sweden, have shown that a high number of individuals (30%) take an anticholinergic drug and a cholinesterase inhibitor drug at the same time.[50-52] While it is not surprising that older adults suffering from various degrees of dementia also suffer from urinary incontinence, it is very surprising that these drugs are being prescribed together. Clearly, these two categories of drugs produce opposite effects and, from a pharmacological point of view, should not be taken together. The fact that they are prescribed concurrently points to an earlier contention that some prescribers give little thought to the mechanisms of action and adverse effects of prescription medications. It is important that the concurrent use of these agents should be minimized as much as possible.

Other types of bladder dysfunction may also be improved with medications. Patients with bladder retention problems and those with suprasacral spinal cord injury may be treated with cholinergic agonists such as bethanechol.[53] The drug is administered subcutaneously every 4 to 6 hours, and patients are asked to try to void 20 to 30 minutes after each dose. Bethanechol also may be combined with a bladder-decompression regimen. As the residual urine diminishes, the patient may be switched to an oral dose administered four times a day. Those who have a tonically active trigone (inability to relax the sphincter) may be given an α-adrenergic blocker such as phenoxybenzamine to facilitate flow. Botulinum toxin, which inhibits ACh release at the neuromuscular junction of striated muscle, also has been used to treat dyssynergia and flow resistant conditions; some other antispasticity agents (baclofen, dantrolene, and benzodiazepines) have also been used for these purposes.[54] Calcium channel blockers can increase bladder capacity and decrease leakage in detrusor hyperactivity. This classification of drugs is discussed in Chapter 6.

ACTIVITIES 5

1. Drugs that mimic the PNS may produce bradycardia and urinary and fecal incontinence. What is the impact that these adverse effects have on the patient and also on physical therapy intervention? What suggestions do you have for the patients taking these drugs to help minimize possible adverse effects?
2. Interview a relative, neighbor, or patient who is over 65 years old about his or her medication use. List all prescription and over-the-counter medicines (use generic names) that have been taken within the past 6 months. Ask your subject about adverse effects, number of pills he or she takes per day, and compliance. Look up information on the adverse effects, and determine whether any are considered "anticholinergic." Discuss the impact that these effects have on the older adult population and how they may affect physical therapy intervention.
3. You are treating a 65-year-old man in the homecare setting following a total knee replacement 12 weeks ago. Your patient is a landscape contractor, who has been off work during this time but has still been able to supervise his employees. You arrive at his home for the therapy session but the patient is nowhere to be seen. The patient's wife thinks he is in the garage preparing some lawn application for his employees to put down at a customer's house. She reports he has been out there for the past week preparing solutions and has not been performing his exercises. You then find him unconscious in the garage. The patient is immediately transported to the hospital. At the hospital, the wife reports that her husband had abdominal discomfort and loose and frequent stools over the past week. He has no history of mental illness or alcohol abuse and was not taking any medications. His skin is warm and moist, and copious amounts of saliva is noted. Blood pressure and pulse are within normal limits WNL, but respirations are rapid and shallow. Pupils are constricted and auscultation of

the chest reveals wheezing. Muscle fasciculations are noted but then the tone diminishes. There is no evidence of trauma. What type of symptoms is this patient displaying? What do you think has happened to this patient? What drug might be used in this patient's treatment?

4. Compare and contrast norepinephrine, phenylephrine, and isoproterenol (a β_1-agonist) in terms of their effects on systolic and diastolic blood pressure and heart rate.
5. Discuss the general effects of anticholinergic drugs and their implications with regard to therapy.

REFERENCES

1. Rang HP, Dale MM, Ritter JM, Flower: Chemical mediators and the autonomic nervous system. In Rang HP, Dale MM, Ritter JM, Flower R, editors: Rang and Dale's pharmacology, Philadelphia, 2007, Churchill Livingstone.
2. Guyton AC, Hall JE: Textbook of medical physiology, ed 10, Philadelphia, 2000, WB Saunders.
3. Katzung BG: Introduction to autonomic pharmacology. In Katzung BG, editor: Basic and clinical pharmacology, New York, 2007, McGraw-Hill.
4. Kerwin R, Travis MJ, Page CP, Hoffman BB, Walker MJA, Simons OR, Moore PK., et al: Drugs and the nervous system. In Page CP, Curtis M, Sutter MC, Walker M, editors: Integrated pharmacology, Philadelphia, 2002, Mosby.
5. Wong DL: Why is the adrenal adrenergic? Endocr Pathol 14(1):25-36, 2003.
6. Benarroch EE: Neurotransmitters. In Waldman SA, Terzic A, editors: Pharmacology and therapeutics: Principles to practice, Philadelphia, 2009, WB Saunders.
7. Martyn JAJ, Fagerlund MJ, Eriksson LI: Basic principles of neuromuscular transmission, Anaesthesia 64(Suppl. 1):1-9, 2009.
8. Eglen RM: Muscarinic receptor subtypes in neuronal and non-neuronal cholinergic function, Autonomic Autacoid Pharmacol 26:219-233, 2006.
9. Lympeooulos A, Koch WJ: Autonomic pharmacology. In Waldman SA, Terzic A, editors: Pharmacology and therapeutics: Principles to practice, Philadelphia, 2009, WB Saunders.
10. Hoffman BB: Adrenoceptor-activating and other sympathomimetic drugs. In Katzung BG, editor: Basic and clinical pharmacology, Philadelphia, New York, 2007, McGraw Hill.
11. Pappano AJ: Cholinoceptor-activating and cholinesterase-inhibiting drugs. In Katzung BG, editor: Basic and clinical pharmacology, Philadelphia, New York, 2007, McGraw Hill.
12. Goyal RK, Hirano I: Mechanisms of disease: The enteric nervous system, N Engl J Med 334(17):1106-1115, 1996.
13. Gan TJ: Mechanisms underlying postoperative nausea and vomiting and neurotransmitter receptor antagonist-based pharmacotherapy, CNS Drugs 21(10):813-833, 2007.
14. Schuman JS: Short- and long-term safety of glaucoma drugs, Exp Opin Drug Saf 1(2):181-194, 2002.
15. Kanner E, Tsai JC: Glaucoma medications: Use and safety in the elderly population, Drugs Aging 23:321-332, 2006.
16. Vincent A, Palace J, Hilton-Jones D: Myasthenia gravis, Lancet 357:2122-2128, 2001.
17. Rang HP, Dale MM, Ritter JM, Flower R: Cholinergic Transmission. In Rang HP, Dale MM, Ritter JM, Flower R, editors: Rang and Dale's `pharmacology, Philadelphia, 2007, Churchill Livingstone.
18. Brenner T, Nizri E, Irony-Tur-Sinai M, et al. Acetylcholinesterase inhibitors and cholinergic modulation in Myasthenia Gravis and neuroinflammation, J Neuroimmunol 201-202: 121-127, 2008.
19. Gilhus NE: Autoimmune myasthenia gravis, Expert Rev Neurother 9(3):351-358, 2009.
20. Cucchiara S, Franco MT, Terrin G, et al. Role of drug therapy in the treatment of gastro-oesophageal reflux disorder in children, Paedriat Drugs 2(4):263-272, 2000.
21. Ehlert FJ: Drugs affecting the parasympathetic nervous system and autonomic ganglia. In Brody MJ, Larner J, Minneman KP, editors: Human pharmacology: Molecular to clinical, Philadelphia, 1998, Mosby.
22. Newmark J: Nerve agents, Neurologist 13(1):20-32, 2007.
23. Brodde OE, Michel MC: Adrenergic and muscarinic receptors in the human heart, Pharmacol Rev 51:681-690, 1999.
24. Gill SS, Anderson GM, Fischer HD, et al: Syncope and its consequences in patients with dementia receiving cholinesterase inhibitors, Arch Intern Med 169(9):867-873, 2009.
25. Moncada S, Palmer RM, Higgs EA: Nitric oxide: Physiology, pathophysiology, and pharmacology, Pharmacol Rev 43: 109-142, 1991.
26. Pappano AJ, Katzung BG: Cholinoceptor-blocking drugs. In Katzung BG, editor: Basic and clinical pharmacology, Philadelphia, New York, 2007, McGraw Hill.
27. Kranke P, Morin AM, Roewer N, Wulf H, Eberhart LH: The efficacy and safety of transdermal scopolamine for the prevention of postoperative nausea and vomiting: A quantitative systematic review, Anesth Analg 95:133-143, 2002.
28. Esler M, Lambert G, Brunner-La Rocca HP, Vaddadi G, Kaye D: Sympathetic nerve activity and neurotransmitter release in humans: Translation from pathophysiology into clinical practice, Acta Physiol Scand 177:275-284, 2003.
29. Joyner MJ, Dietz NM: Sympathetic vasodilation in human muscle, Acta Physiol Scand 177(3):329-336, 2003.
30. Ruffolo RR: Pharmacologic and therapeutic applications of alpha 2 adrenoceptor subtypes, Annu Rev Pharmacol toxicol 33:243-279, 1993.
31. de Diego AM, Gandia L, Garcia AG: A physiological view of the central and peripheral mechanisms that regulate the release of catecholamines at the adrenal medulla, Acta Physiol Scand192:287-301, 2008.
32. Coons JC, Seidl E: Cardiovascular pharmacotherapy update for the intensive care unit, Crit Care Nurs30(1):44-57, 2007.
33. Conrado VC, de Andrade J, de Angelis GA, et al: Cardiovascular effects of local anesthesia with vasoconstrictor during dental extraction in coronary patients, Arq Bras Cardiol 88(5):446-452, 2007.
34. Flanagan SR, Kane L, Rhoades D: Pharmacological modification of recovery following brain injury, J Neurol Phys Ther 27(3):129-137, 2003.
35. Sicari R, Nihoyannopoulos P, Evangelista A, et al: Stress echocardiography expert consensus statement: European Association of Echocardiography (EAE) (a registered branch of the ESC). Eur J Echocardiogr 9(4):415-437, 2008.
36. Elhendy A, Bax JJ, Poldermans D: Dobutamine stress myocardial perfusion imaging in coronary artery disease, J Nucl Med 43(12):1634-1646, 2001.
37. Berkman ND, Thorp JM Jr, Lohr KN, et al. Tocolytic treatment for the management of preterm labor: A review of the evidence,. Am J Obstet Gynecol 188(6):1648-1659, 2003.
38. Bonhomme L, Benhamou D, Comoy E, Preaux N: Stability of epinephrine in alkalinized solutions, Ann Emerg Med 19(11):1242-1244, 1990.
39. Silfvast T, Saarnivaara L, Kinnunen A, et al: Comparison of adrenaline and phenylephrine in out-of-hospital cardiopulmonary resuscitation. A double-blind study, Acta Anaesthesiol Scand 29(6):610-613, 1985.
40. Zed PJ, Abu-Laban RB, Shuster M, et al: Update on cardiopulmonary resuscitation and emergency cardiovascular care

guidelines, Am J Health Syst Pharm 65(24):2337-2346, 2008.
41. Ornato JP: Optimal vasopressor drug therapy during resuscitation, Crit Care 12(2):123-126, 2008.
42. Mentzelopoulos SD, Zakynthinos SG, Tzoufi M, et al: Vasopressin, epinephrine, and corticosteroids for in-hospital cardiac arrest, Arch Intern Med 169(1):15-24, 2009.
43. Dubin A, Pozo MO, Casabella CA, et al: Increasing arterial blood pressure with norepinephrine does not improve microcirculatory blood flow: A prospective study, Crit Care 13(3):R92, 2009.
44. Bent S, Tiedt TN, Odden MC, Shlipak MG: The relative safety of ephedra compared with other herbal products, Ann Intern Med 138(6):468-471, 2003.
45. Flanagan CM, Kaesberg JL, Mitchell ES, Ferguson MA, Haigney MC: Coronary artery aneurysm and thrombosis following chronic ephedra use, Int J Cardiol August 19 2008.
46. Michel MC, Barendrecht MM: Physiological and pathological regulation of the autonomic control of urinary bladder contractility, Pharmacol Ther 117:297-312, 2008.
47. Chughtai B, Levin R, De E: Choice of antimuscarinic agents for overactive bladder in the older patient: Focus on darifenacin, Clin Interven Aging 3(3):503-509, 2008.
48. Chapple CR, Yamanishi T, Chess-Williams R: Muscarinic receptor subtypes and management of the overactive bladder, Urology 60(Suppl 5A):82-89, 2002.
49. Gupta S, Sathyan G, Mori T: New perspectives on the overactive bladder: Pharmokinetics and bioavailability, Urology 60(Suppl 5A):78-81, 2002.
50. Carnahan RM, Lund BC, Perry PJ: The concurrent use of antichoinergics and cholinesterase inhibitors: Rare event or common practice? J AmGeriat Soc 52(12):2082-2087, 2004.
51. Roe CM, Anderson MJ, Spivack B: Use of anticholinergic medications by older adults with dementia, J Am Geriat Soc 50(5):836-842, 2002.
52. Johnell K, Fastbom J: Concurrent use of anticholinergic drugs and cholinesterase inhibitors: Register-based study of over 700,000 elderly patients, Drugs Aging 25(10):871, 2008.
53. Wein AJ, Saini R, Staskin DR: Voiding dysfunction. In Waldman SA, Terzic A, editors: Pharmacology and therapeutics: Principles to practice, Philadelphia, 2009, WB Saunders.
54. Flynn MK, Amundsen CL, Perevich M, Liu F, Webster GD: Outcome of a randomized, double-blind, placebo controlled trial of botulinum, a toxin for refractory overactive bladder, J Urol 181(6):2608-2615, 2009.

6

Antihypertensive Agents

Barbara Gladson

HYPERTENSION

Hypertension is a leading cause of cardiovascular morbidity and mortality and affects more than one in six adults worldwide.[1] Data from the National Health and Nutrition Examination Survey (NHANES) showed that in the United States, during 2005–2006, the percentage of adults living with hypertension was 29%, with the highest prevalences (41%) in non-Hispanic blacks followed by non-Hispanic whites (28%) and then Mexican Americans (22%).[2] Of the total number of patients with at least stage 1 hypertension, 6.6% had never found out that they had the disease. Sixty-eight percent of those patients who were aware of the disease, were currently being treated, but just 64% had their blood pressure (BP) controlled. In addition, the majority of American adults with other cardiac issues such as coronary artery disease, congestive heart failure, stroke, or diabetes also have hypertension; yet, despite more thoughtful treatment compared with uncomplicated hypertension, only a third of these individuals had their BP under control.[3] These studies highlight some of the problems involved in the treatment of elevated BP—lack of awareness, poor compliance, complexities of treatment, and lack of effectiveness.

There are certain specific causes for high blood pressure, but in most cases there is no one definitive etiology, that is, the etiology is multifactorial. This type of hypertension is referred to as primary or essential hypertension. Secondary hypertension is more easily understood because it is produced by a specific cause such as an adrenal tumor secreting epinephrine, head trauma, or renal artery stenosis. However, more than 90% of patients with high blood pressure have primary hypertension.[4] It is suspected that environmental factors, also known as acquired factors, such as stress, poor diet, smoking, and obesity predispose individuals to hypertension. Specifically, it is thought that these factors produce an increase in sympathetic activity. The increase in sympathetic output produces excitatory effects on the heart and peripheral vasculature to increase blood pressure. Cardiac output is increased, and adaptive changes begin to occur in the vasculature. The vessels become less compliant and more reactive to pressor substances such as norepinephrine and angiotensin II. Persistent hypertension leads to hypertrophy of the left ventricle and also of the medial layer of resistance vessels, leading to narrowing of the lumen.[4,5] In later stages of hypertension, cardiac output may return to normal, but increased vascular resistance remains.

PHYSIOLOGY AND PATHOPHYSIOLOGY OF BLOOD PRESSURE

The two main equations that describe how some hemodynamic variables influence blood pressure are as follows:

$$\text{Cardiac output} = \text{Heart rate} \times \text{Stroke volume}$$
$$\text{Mean arterial pressure} = \text{Cardiac output} \times \text{Peripheral resistance}$$

The first equation describes cardiac output as a function of heart rate and stroke volume. Increased cardiac output is a function of increased heart rate, increased contractility, or both.[6,7] As rate and contractility increase, so does the amount of blood that is pumped out of the heart each minute (cardiac output). Venous return (preload) also increases cardiac output unless the heart is so damaged that it cannot accommodate the additional flow (Frank-Starling law).[8] Heart rate, stroke volume, and venous return can all be increased by the sympathetic nervous system.

The second equation describes the relationship between cardiac output and blood pressure. This equation is analogous to Ohm's law, in which $V = IR$ (voltage = current × resistance), except hemodynamically, V is related to pressure in the vasculature, I is blood flow, and R is resistance in the artery that impedes flow.[9,10] See Figure 6-1 for a summary of the factors involved in blood pressure control.

We have several pharmacologic means of controlling blood pressure by using these equations. Certain drugs act to block the sympathetic system to reduce heart rate through β-receptors, which, in turn, will reduce cardiac output and arterial pressure. Drugs can also decrease stroke volume by decreasing contractility. This alteration will also decrease the blood pressure. The diameter of blood vessels can be increased, which results in a lowering of peripheral resistance and reduced blood pressure. Reducing overall plasma volume with diuretics is also a

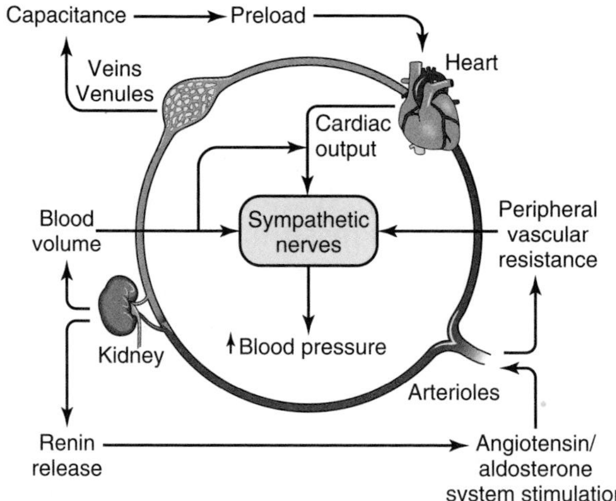

FIGURE 6-1 Factors involved in blood pressure control. One of the determinants of blood pressure is cardiac output, based on heart rate and stroke volume. Cardiac output depends on the amount of blood returning to the heart, which, in turn, depends on vein and venule capacitance (preload) and blood volume (under the control of kidneys). Peripheral vascular resistance is determined by the diameter of the arterioles.

way to decrease the pressure because there will be a concomitant reduction in stroke volume.

Acquired Factors Producing Hypertension

Genetic factors and several acquired factors can lead to hypertension. Hemodynamic changes such as increased cardiac output may be seen in younger individuals with hypertension. Over time, cardiac output normalizes but the set elevated BP is maintained by increasing peripheral resistance. This fact is being debated, but on the basis of this observation, some have reasoned that an exaggerated response to vasoconstrictor influences is maintained as a person ages. The kidney also plays an important role in the development of hypertension. Renal blood flow is reduced early in hypertension, and the relative increase in resistance of the renal vessels surpasses that of other vascular beds. Glomerular filtration decreases as the hypertension progresses. And a defect in sodium excretion, resulting from elevated aldosterone concentration and abnormalities in the renal tubules, is present. As blood volume increases as a result of elevated plasma sodium levels, a pressure-natriuresis occurs.[11] However, over time, the BP at which this natriuresis occurs becomes elevated, that is the blood pressure needed to balance sodium excretion with intake is raised. If a patient is salt sensitive, it means that the BP required for natriuresis is greater than for non–salt-sensitive individuals with hypertension and normotensive individuals.

Abnormalities in potassium, magnesium, and calcium are also implicated in causing hypertension.[1] Potassium has direct and indirect effects one vascular dilation and increases the sensitivity of baroreceptors (see below). Calcium has a similar effect on vascular dilation by enhancing the secretion of vasodilator peptides. Also, a reduction in magnesium produces smooth muscle contraction. Low levels of these ions speak to the need for a well-balanced diet to lower the risk of hypertension.

Essential hypertension is characterized by thickening of the arterial wall, which narrows the lumen and raises resistance.[12] Over time, the vessels become stiff and noncompliant, and they appear more reactive to vasoconstrictor influence, such as circulating epinephrine. Frequent spikes in blood pressure have been shown to activate pathways, leading to arterial remodeling and cardiac hypertrophy, at least in an animal model.[13] A combination of factors is responsible—sympathetic hyperactivity, abnormal balance between angiotensin II (a vasoconstrictor) and nitric oxide (a vasodilator), and genetics.[14,15]

Hyperinsulinism and insulin resistance have been shown to be related to hypertension as well. Often metabolic syndrome precedes hypertension, and correction of this, along with a reduction in weight or blocking of insulin release, will lower blood pressure. Under these circumstances, the sympathetic nervous system via α- and β-receptors will increase glycogenolysis in an attempt to provide necessary nutrients to working muscles. In addition, high levels of insulin stimulate renal sympathetic outflow.[16] Other acquired factors include abnormal neural and hormonal controls over blood pressure. Primarily, these relate to the sympathetic nervous system, baroreflexes, and the renin–angiotensin system as described below.

Control of Blood Pressure through Baroreceptors and Chemoreceptors

The body makes an effort to maintain blood pressure within a narrow range not only to allow for adequate organ perfusion but also to make sure that pressure does not rise to a level at which it becomes injurious to the arterials. Quick adjustments in pressure can be made through the baroreceptor reflex.[7] Afferent nerves located in the walls of the internal carotid arteries and the aortic arch are stimulated by high pressure via stretch. Impulses are then transmitted to the medullary cardiovascular control center to inhibit central sympathetic discharge. If a fall in pressure is detected, these same neurons send fewer impulses to this vasomotor center. This will initiate an increased sympathetic output, resulting in vasoconstriction and increased cardiac output to raise pressure. Chronic stimulation of baroreceptors has led to a reduced sensitivity in patients with hypertension.

Peripheral chemoreceptors also play a role in the regulation of blood pressure.[7] They are located in the carotid body (between the external and internal carotid arteries) and the aortic bodies (under the concavity of the aortic arch). These organelles are sensitive to the arterial blood gases PO_2 (partial pressure oxygen) and

Pco_2 (partial pressure carbon dioxide) and to pH. An increase in carbon dioxide or a drop in Po_2 or in pH triggers an increase in the afferent firing to the medulla. The hypoxia and high Pco_2 stimulate respiration to improve oxygenation. This increase in ventilation helps blow off the carbon dioxide, raising the pH, which is actually inhibitory to the cardioinhibitory center, and in tachycardia. A high Pco_2 acting on the central chemoreceptor area produces an increase in sympathetic output, which leads to generalized vasoconstriction.

Vascular Endothelium and Intermediate Control of Blood Pressure

The vascular endothelium contains plasma within a specific compartment and is also a source of many chemical mediators that affect blood pressure. These agents affect the release of intracellular calcium (Ca^{2+}), leading to the contraction or relaxation of the vascular smooth muscle. Prostaglandins are derivatives of arachidonic acid released from damaged endothelial cells after they have been acted on by the cyclooxygenase enzyme. Prostacyclin (PGI_2) and prostaglandin E_2 (PGE_2) tend to be strong vasodilators. PGI_2 also inhibits platelet aggregation, and PGE_2 inhibits the release of norepinephrine from sympathetic nerve terminals. Levels of PGI_2 and PGE_2 are noticeably reduced in hypertension. Other prostaglandins are endothelium-derived contracting factors, specifically thromboxane A_2. Cyclooxygenase inhibitors such as aspirin can prevent this vasoconstrictor response.

Endothelium-derived relaxing factor, also known as nitric oxide, is released continuously, producing vasodilator tone and relaxation of vascular smooth muscle. It also inhibits the adaptive changes and the vascular smooth muscle cell proliferation that stiffens the arteries, including those in the kidney.[17] Inhibition of platelet adhesion and aggregation is another function that is very important in preventing thrombosis. Additionally, many vasodilator substances such as bradykinin and even acetylcholine act by producing nitric oxide. Currently, several mediators of nitric oxide are being studied for their effectiveness in relaxing vascular tone.

Several peptides are secreted by the endothelium and these include C natriuretic peptide, endothelium-derived hyperpolarizing factor, and adrenomedulin, all of which are vasodilators.[18] Natriuretic peptides cause diuresis, decrease aldosterone release, decrease cell growth in the vascular wall, and inhibit the renin–angiotensin system (see the following section).[19] Vasoconstrictive peptides include angiotensin-converting enzyme (ACE) and endothelin. ACE exists on the surfaces of endothelial cells, especially those of the lungs, and is extremely important in producing angiotensin II, a powerful vasoconstrictor. Endothelins are responsible for extremely strong and long-lasting vasoconstriction.[19] Several endothelin inhibitors and endothelin-receptor blockers and their role in controlling hypertension are now under study.

Renin–Angiotensin System and Long-Term Control of Blood Pressure

The renin–angiotensin system works in concert with the sympathetic nervous system, producing very potent vasoconstriction. It also is responsible for the stimulation of aldosterone release, which enhances the reabsorption of sodium (Na^+) and the secretion of hydrogen (H^+) from renal tubules, resulting in a rise in plasma volume. Renin is an enzyme secreted by the kidney juxtaglomerular apparatus, which is located in the distal convoluted tubule. It is secreted in response to diminished renal perfusion or a decrease in Na^+ concentration. Flow may be reduced because of fluid loss (dehydration or bleeding), or the kidney may sense decreased flow caused by an atherosclerotic renal artery or a sympathetically vasoconstricted artery.

Renin converts angiotensinogen (secreted by the liver) to angiotensin I, which is subsequently converted to angiotensin II with the help of ACE in the lungs (Figure 6-2). As mentioned previously, angiotensin II is a very powerful vasoconstrictor (40 times more potent than norepinephrine in elevating blood pressure).[20] Other enzymes further cleave angiotensin II into angiotensin III and IV but appear to be somewhat less vasoactive than angiotensin II.

Prostaglandins and Renal Function

The prostaglandins that are produced in the kidneys affect the hemodynamics of the renal system. PGE_2 is produced in the kidney medulla, and PGI_2 comes from the glomeruli.[21] Prostaglandin synthesis is stimulated by ischemia, trauma, angiotensin II, catecholamines, and antidiuretic hormone. When these sympathomimetic chemicals are present, PGE_2 and PGI_2 are produced and counteract the vasoconstrictive effect on the kidneys.[22] Vasodilation, particularly of the renal artery, is maintained to ensure that the kidneys are well perfused. The significance of renal prostaglandins becomes apparent when patients with cirrhosis of the liver, heart failure, nephritic syndrome, or hypertension take nonsteroidal anti-inflammatory drugs (NSAIDs), which inhibit prostaglandin synthesis. Under these conditions, NSAIDs can produce renal failure and exacerbate hypertension or cardiac failure.[23]

Secondary Hypertension

Certain substances and conditions directly lead to hypertension. Nephropathy, polycystic kidney, hyperaldosteronism, excess glucocorticoids and pheochromocytomas

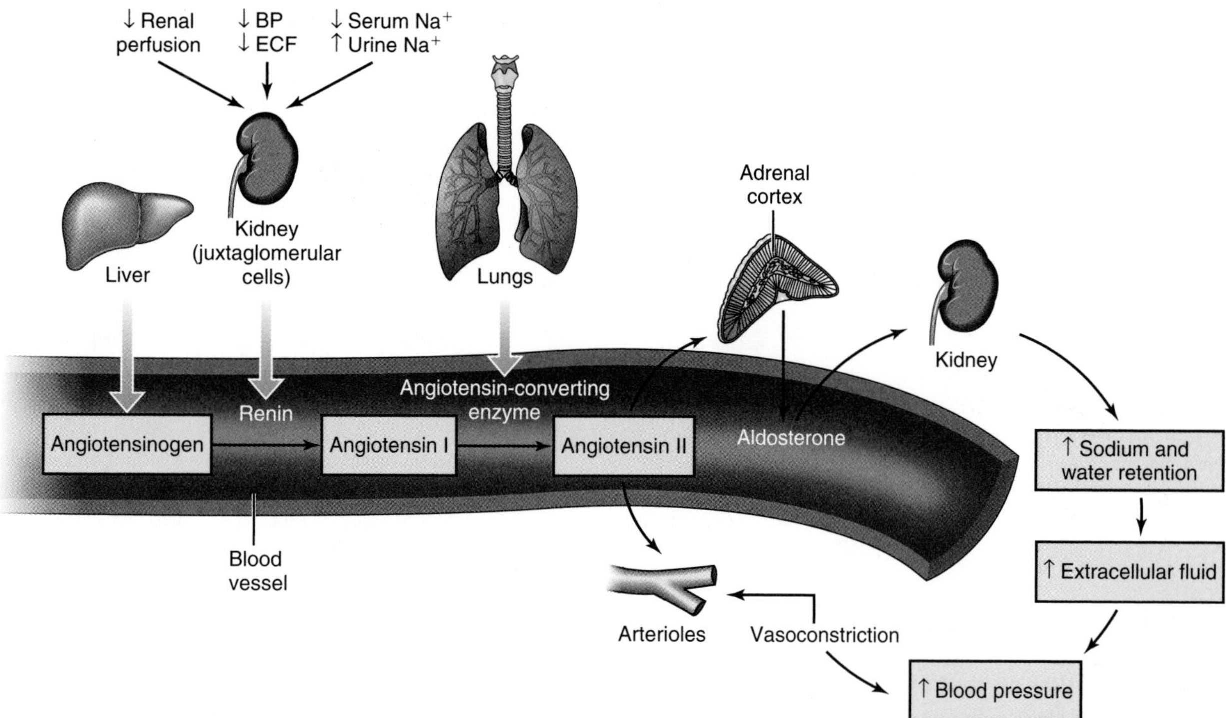

FIGURE 6-2 Renin–angiotensin–aldosterone system. Release of renin stimulates conversion of angiotensinogen (from the liver) to angiotensin I, which, in turn, is converted to angiotensin II under the influence of angiotensin-converting enzyme. Angiotensin II leads to vasoconstriction, release of aldosterone (adrenal cortex), and sodium (Na^+) retention. Sodium retention increases blood pressure but reduces renin release; thus the renin–angiotensin–aldosterone system is a homeostatic process.

(a catecholamine secreting tumor) are just a few of the conditions that lead to elevated blood pressure.[1] Many of these conditions can be treated and the hypertension reversed. In addition, pressor substances, when consumed, can elevated blood pressure, for example, alcohol, oral contraceptives, and licorice.

Classification of Blood Pressure

The seventh report of the Joint National Committee on Prevention, Detection, Evaluation, and Treatment of High Blood Pressure (JNC 7) provides guidelines for the classification and management of blood pressure (Table 6-1).[24] The JNC 7 report was published in 2003 as a joint effort between the National Heart, Lung, and Blood Institute of the U.S. National Institutes of Health (NIH) and the American Society of Hypertension. The original publication, JNC 1, came out in 1976 and has been regularly updated every 4 to 5 years since that year. The JNC 8 report is expected to be published in the summer of 2010.[25] Along with this release will be other guidelines such as those for the prevention, detection, evaluation and treatment of high blood cholesterol (an updated Adult Treatment Panel (ATP) IV) and guidelines on obesity.[26]

Normal blood pressure is classified as a systolic reading <120mm Hg and a diastolic reading <80mm Hg. The JNC 7 report also introduced a new classification labeled *prehypertension*, with a systolic reading between 120 and 139mm Hg or diastolic reading between 80 and 89mm Hg. At this stage, no antihypertensive drug is recommended, but patients are encouraged to follow a healthy lifestyle. The prehypertension stage is followed by stage 1 hypertension with a systolic reading between 140 and 159mm Hg or a diastolic reading between 90 and 99mm Hg. It is at this stage that drug treatment begins. Therapy may begin with one drug; however, more physicians nowadays are beginning treatment with combination drugs, particularly if the patient is at high risk for cardiac morbidities. Patients with a systolic reading of 160mm Hg or above or a diastolic reading of 100mm Hg or above will definitely require two or more antihypertensive drugs to control blood pressure. This report stresses tighter controls on blood pressure than recommended by previous reports, especially in patients with diabetes or chronic kidney disease, with the recommendation that their blood pressure be less than 130/80mm Hg.

Although lower BP is more efficacious than high BP, exactly how low one should go is a matter of debate. The Valsartan in Acute Myocardial Infarction Trial (VALIANT) demonstrated that either high or low BP following myocardial infarction was associated with a poor outcome.[27] High BP was defined as a systolic level above 140 mm Hg and low blood pressure as a systolic level below 100 mm Hg. The trial demonstrated that

TABLE 6-1 Classification and Management of Blood Pressure in Adults Aged 18 Years or Older

			Management Initial Drug Therapy*		
BP Classification	**Systolic BP, mm Hg***	**Diastolic BP, mm Hg***	**Lifestyle Modification**	**Without Compelling Indications**	**With Compelling Indications**
Normal	<120 and	<80	Encourage	—	—
Prehypertension	120–139 or	80–89	Yes	No antihypertensive drug indicated	Drug(s) for the compelling indications†
Stage 1 hypertension	140–159 or	90–99	Yes	Thiazide-type diuretics for most; may consider ACE inhibitor, ARB, β-blocker, CCB, or combination	Drug(s) for the compelling indications Other anti-hypertensive drugs (diuretics, ACE inhibitor, ARB, β-blocker, CCB) as needed
Stage 2 hypertension	≥160 or	≥100	Yes	Two-drug combination for most (usually thiazide-type diuretic and ACE inhibitor or ARB or β-blocker or CCB)‡	Drug(s) for the compelling indications Other anti-hypertensive drugs (diuretics, ACE inhibitor, ARB, β blocker, CCB) as needed

From Joint National Committee on Prevention, Detection, Evaluation, and Treatment of High Blood Pressure: Classification and management of blood pressure in adults aged 18 years or older: the 7th report of the Joint National Committee on Prevention, Detection, Evaluation, and Treatment of High Blood Pressure, *JAMA* 289:2560–2572, 2003.

ACE, Angiotensin-converting enzyme; *ARB*, angiotensin receptor blocker; *BP*, blood pressure; *CCB*, calcium channel blocker.

*Treatment determined by highest BP category.

†Treat patients with chronic kidney disease or diabetes to BP goal of less than 130/80 mm Hg.

‡Initial combined therapy should be used cautiously in those at risk for orthostatic hypotension.

patients with the higher BP were more likely to develop cardiovascular death, another myocardial infarction, or stroke, and those with low pressure were more likely to develop heart failure. So the target BP depends on multiple factors, one of which is the actual BP following a cardiac event.

Nondrug treatment for hypertension is always the first choice for therapy and includes exercise, reduction in weight, restriction of salt intake, cessation of smoking, and a reduction in alcohol intake.[4] When these steps are not successful, a variety of drugs can be used to reduce blood pressure. The major categories include diuretics, sympatholytics, direct-acting vasodilators, calcium antagonists, and renin–angiotensin inhibitors. Specific actions include regulating electrolyte and fluid level through the kidney tubules, altering the rate and contractility of the heart, dilating arterioles, inhibiting angiotensin II production, and reducing central sympathetic output.

DIURETICS

In general, diuretics result in an increased excretion of sodium (Na^+) and water by the kidneys.[28] However, the manner in which diuretics reduce blood pressure has not been clearly delineated. It is assumed that they reduce pressure by reducing plasma volume. However, in general, their action as antihypertensive agents is poorly related to their diuretic activity. Loop diuretics are moderate antihypertensive drugs but strong diuretics. Thiazide diuretics are powerful antihypertensive agents but moderate diuretics. The three major classifications of diuretic drugs are named on the basis of location of action.

Loop Diuretics

Loop diuretics are often used along with other diuretics in cases of salt and water overload. Specific conditions include pulmonary edema, congestive heart failure, ascites caused by liver failure, hypercalcemia, and renal failure. They are often combined with thiazide diuretics in the treatment of hypertension.

The mechanisms of action of loop diuretics include inhibiting the sodium/potassium/chloride ($Na^+/K^+/2Cl^-$) Okay co-transporter on the luminal membrane of the ascending loop of Henle, blocking the reabsorption of these electrolytes from the tubular fluid (Figure 6-3).[29] When this co-transporter is functioning, it creates a hypertonic interstitial segment in the kidney medulla, which provides the osmotic pressure needed for the reabsorption of water from the collecting tubules. When the transporter is blocked by the drug, the luminal fluid stays hypertonic, facilitating water loss into the tubules.

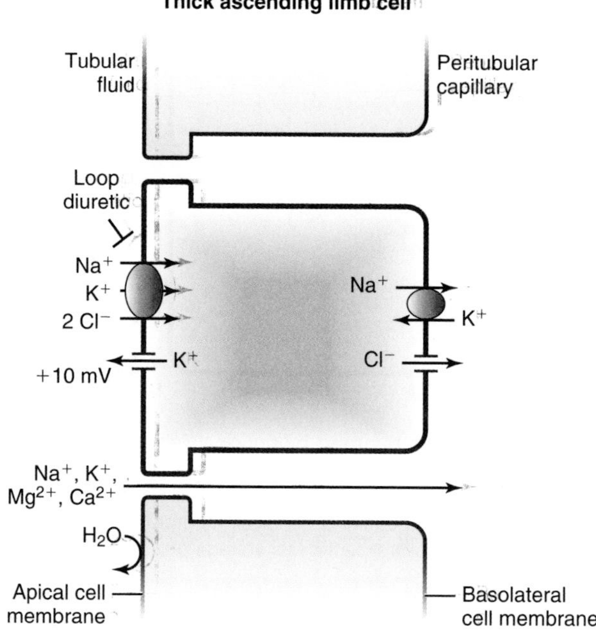

FIGURE 6-3 Cellular transport by thick ascending limb cells. Cell model for ion transport by a thick ascending limb. This segment, also referred to as the diluting segment, is impermeable to water, and thus the tubular lumen concentration of ions decreases.

A greater concentration of Na^+ in the lumen then facilitates the loss of hydrogen (H^+) and K^+ via exchange with Na^+ in the distal portion of the nephron.

Intravenous loop diuretics produce short-term vasodilation secondary to the facilitating release of prostaglandins.[29] This is the mechanism of action responsible for the almost immediate relief in acute pulmonary edema before any diuresis has begun. Venodilation produced by the prostaglandins decreases cardiac preload, resulting in a fall in pulmonary artery wedge pressure and a decrease in symptoms.

The prototypical loop diuretic is furosemide. Some other examples are bumetanide and ethacrynic acid, both of which are more easily absorbed from the gastrointestinal tract (>80%) than furosemide (50%).[29] Because they are strongly bound to plasma proteins, they are not freely filtered through the glomerulus. They reach their sites of action by being actively transported into the proximal convoluted tubule. Their onset of action is approximately 1 hour, with duration from 3 to 6 hours. In renal disease, less of the drug reaches the proximal convoluted tubule, so larger doses need to be administered.

Loop diuretics are useful in the treatment of hypercalcemia because less solute is reabsorbed.[29] However, they should not be given to patients who are prone to renal stones because greater calcium excretion in the tubules can lead to precipitation.

Adverse drug reactions (ADRs) associated with loop diuretics include dehydration, hypokalemia, hyponatremia, hypocalcemia, ototoxicity, hyperglycemia, and increased levels of low-density lipoproteins (LDLs).[30] Hypokalemia and metabolic alkalosis from H^+ loss can occur, so supplemental K^+ or K^+-sparing diuretics are often given along with these drugs. The ototoxicity is associated with loss of cochlear hair cells but is not fully understood yet.[29] This ADR is more common at high doses, when given by rapid intravenous injection, in patients with renal disease, and when used in combination with other ototoxic drugs.

Thiazide Diuretics

Thiazide diuretics are the prime diuretics used to reduce blood pressure. They are also given along with loop diuretics in cases of congestive heart failure and severe edema. They are the diuretics of choice for patients who are prone to renal calculi.

Thiazide diuretics inhibit the Na^+/Cl^- co-transporter on the luminal membrane of the distal convoluted tubule and proximal collecting duct (Figure 6-4).[29] Reduction in intracellular Na^+ enhances the sodium/calcium (Na^+/Ca^{2+}) pump located on the basolateral cell membrane, facilitating calcium reabsorption. Thus these drugs are favored over other diuretics for older adults in terms of reducing calcium loss and maintaining bone mass.[31,32] These drugs also enhance K^+ excretion in the collecting duct. In summary, thiazide diuretics promote Na^+ and K^+ excretion and reabsorption of Ca^{2+}.

Hydrochlorothiazide is the prototypical thiazide diuretic. In addition, it is the most widely prescribed diuretic in the United States, with 135 million prescriptions written in 2008. It is well absorbed through the gastrointestinal tract after oral administration and is actively secreted into the tubules. Its maximum effect occurs in about 4 hours, with duration of action between 8 and 12 hours. However, at the recent European Meeting on Hypertension in June 2009, it was reported that hydrochlorothiazide was found to be significantly inferior to angiotensin receptor blockers, calcium-channel blockers, and ACE inhibitors, especially in reducing 24-hour ambulatory BP.[33] The authors report that the drug is adequate for the daytime but loses its effectiveness during the night. In addition, they report that there are no data showing that it produces a reduction in morbidity and mortality. This is not true, however, for another thiazide diuretic, chlorthalidone.

The ADRs of thiazide diuretics are similar to those of the loop diuretics, except that thiazides may cause hypercalcemia. K^+ loss is also a significant problem in their use.

Potassium-Sparing Diuretics

Potassium-sparing diuretics act in the collecting tubule to inhibit Na^+ reabsorption and K^+ excretion. The Na^+ channel in the principal cell depolarizes the cell,

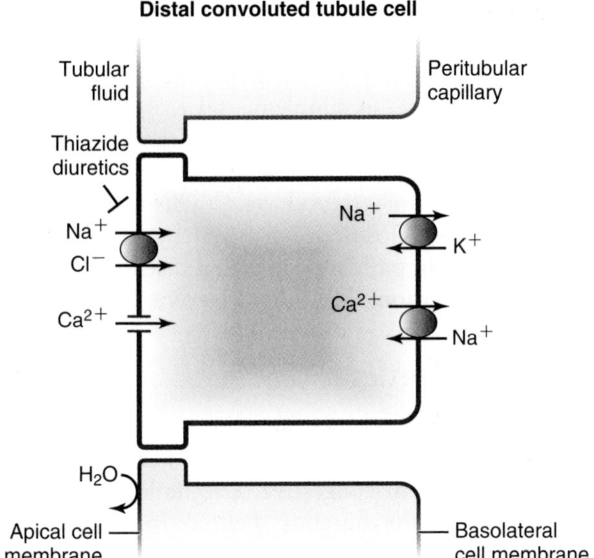

FIGURE 6-4 Cellular transport by distal convoluted tubule cells. Cell model for a distal convoluted tubule cell. As in the case of the thick ascending limb, this segment is relatively impermeable to water.

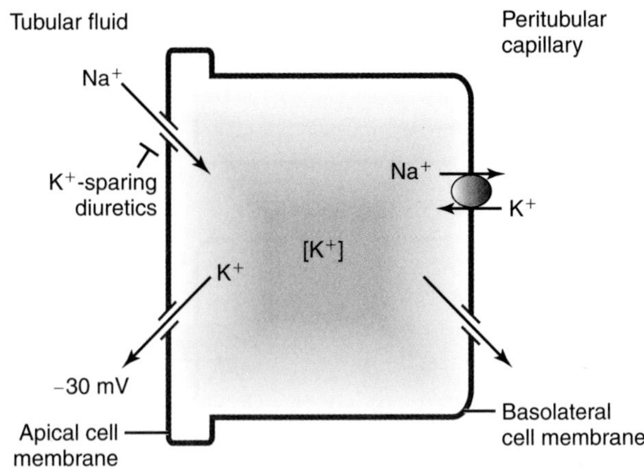

FIGURE 6-5 Cellular transport by principal cells of the collecting tubule. The principal cell contains both sodium (Na^+) and potassium (K^+) channels in the apical cell membrane. The Na^+ channel in the apical cell membrane depolarizes the cell membrane and thus provides an asymmetrical transepithelial voltage profile that favors K^+ secretion.

creating a positive charge that repels K^+.[29] Some of the K^+-sparing agents block this depolarization, so K^+ is not excreted into the tubular fluid (Figure 6-5). Other drugs that fall within this category block the aldosterone receptor; this explains their usefulness in patients with mineralocorticoid-producing tumors, adrenal hyperplasia, cirrhosis, and congestive heart failure, in which there is excessive aldosterone. However, because many of these drugs depend on the presence of excess aldosterone, they are not of significant use in the treatment of primary hypertension. In primary hypertension, they are used for their ability to prevent K^+ deficiency secondary to loss due to use of loop or thiazide diuretics. However, according to some authors, the rationale for using the K^+-sparing drugs along with thiazide drugs is not sound because only about 5% of patients taking thiazide diuretics lose too much K^+.[29]

Spironolactone blocks the receptor for aldosterone, but triamterene and amiloride block sodium channels on the lumenal side. They are all absorbed reasonably well from the gastrointestinal tract, but they have vastly different half-lives. Triamterene is short acting and must be administered two times per day.

Hyperkalemia is the most common ADR of spironolactone, but nausea, lethargy, and mental confusion may also occur. In addition, because this drug resembles adrenal sex steroids, it can produce gynecomastia in males and menstrual irregularities in females.

Therapeutic Concerns with Diuretics

In general, diuretics produce fluid depletion, hyponatremia, hypokalemia (except the K^+-sparing drugs), and orthostatic hypotension. Of particular concern is the K^+ level because a K^+ value that is too high or too low can trigger arrhythmias, particularly if the patient is also taking digitalis for heart failure.[30] Because many patients with hypertension also have cardiac disease, this is a special concern. Signs and symptoms of hypokalemia include an abnormal electrocardiogram (ECG) reading (flattened T waves), nausea, muscle weakness and fatigue, leg cramps, polyuria, hypotension, excessive sweating, and mental status changes. If hypokalemia is present, the patient may be given a K^+ supplement or encouraged to eat foods rich in K^+, such as apricots, bananas, raisins, and oranges. However, one concern is the need to consume a large number of calories to obtain a small amount of K^+. Hyperkalemia presents with ECG changes (elevated T waves); it also presents with nausea, diarrhea, and hyperreflexia progressing to weakness, numbness, and anuria. Syncope may be present in both the above scenarios if arrhythmias are present. Cardiac arrest can occur in both conditions. Frequent monitoring of K^+ levels is recommended for all new patients, and monthly monitoring is necessary for patients who have been taking the drug on a long-term basis.

Another issue with diuretics is that they produce hyperglycemia and abnormally affect lipids. This is of some concern because many patients who have hypertension also have diabetes and high cholesterol and triglyceride levels.[30] In terms of lipid levels, studies of less than 1-year duration show an increase in total cholesterol levels, especially LDL (15%) and triglyceride levels (23%). These percentages may significantly increase cardiovascular mortality. However, some longer-duration studies (1 year) indicate that lipoprotein levels are not significantly affected.[34] As with all studies, careful scrutiny of the data is imperative for accurate interpretation.

Interpretation of cholesterol levels must be analyzed in terms of the subgroup of patients showing the elevated levels, more specifically the subgroup responding with elevated lipid levels. Premenopausal women do not show elevated levels, but postmenopausal women seem to be prone to this increase in lipid levels. It has also been pointed out that successful adherence to a low-fat diet may negate the effects of thiazides on cholesterol. Because the findings have not been convincing, the controversy over whether the elevated cholesterol levels are significant across the population lingers.[35-37]

Treatment of hypertension, especially with thiazide diuretics, produces elevated glucose levels and glucose intolerance.[38] In 4736 patients treated with a thiazide diuretic for 1 year, there was a significant increase in fasting blood sugar levels. However, the percentage of patients newly diagnosed with diabetes during 3 years of drug administration was not significant. Because close control of glucose is imperative to decreasing the adverse effects of the disease, the use of diuretics in patients with diabetes remains controversial. In addition, a recent subanalysis of the Antihypertensive and Lipid-Lowering Treatment to Prevent Heart Attack Trial (ALLHAT) showed that there was no difference in cardiovascular event reduction between chlorthalidone (a thiazide diuretic) and amlodipine (a calcium channel blocker), doxazosin (an α-blocker), or lisinopril (an ACE inhibitor) in patients with metabolic syndrome.[39]

The adverse effects of diuretics have direct ramifications for therapy practice. Patients with diuretic-induced hypokalemia may experience muscle weakness or cramping. These drugs can also cause orthostatic hypotension, thus increasing the risk of falls.[40,41] The therapist must instruct the patient to perform leg extensions, ankle pumps, or other exercises before rising from a chair or bed. Avoiding sudden changes in position is also important. To monitor for dehydration, the therapist must check the patient for skin turgor, temperature, and moisture (including mucous membranes).[42] Any signs of dehydration must be reported immediately to the physician. The therapist should also monitor the patient for arrhythmias by checking the pulse for any irregularities. Older adults who are suffering from urinary incontinence may find this problem worsening when taking diuretics, and frequent urination may interrupt physical therapy.

Diuretics reduce exercise capacity, especially during periods of fluid loss. During exercise, patients with hypertension taking thiazide diuretics will show an attenuated increase in blood pressure and a reduced stroke volume.[43] Altered thermoregulation affecting heat dissipation, increased cardiovascular strain, reduced skeletal muscle blood flow, altered skeletal muscle metabolism, and increased perception of effort required to complete an exercise are also present.[44-46] Greater than 2% loss in body mass, due to fluid loss, produces exercise intolerance based on these mechanisms listed.[47] Electrolyte imbalance leads to dysrrhythmias, use arrhythmias, muscle weakness, and cramping, which also affect performance.

Because many patients taking diuretics may also be taking NSAIDs for arthritis, it is good medical practice to reduce patients' dependence on these drugs. NSAIDs cause Na^+ retention and decrease in renal perfusion, and this combination makes diuretics less effective.[48] Diuretics reduce blood pressure by preventing reabsorption of Na^+ through the kidney tubules, thus forcing diuresis.[29] These drugs have been prescribed to patients with hypertension more than any other agent, in part due to their low cost and relative effectiveness. However, they should not be the automatic first-choice agent for all patients. Diuretics can produce dehydration and orthostatic hypotension and negatively alter electrolyte balance, thus causing hypokalemia. These drugs are, without a doubt, useful as add-on drugs for difficult-to-control hypertension, but they are not indicated for healthy, physically active individuals. Thiazide diuretics are useful in the treatment of older adults with hypertension who are physically active but exercise only occasionally and in black patients who respond well to this treatment. The therapist can offer a variety of modalities, assistive devices, and intervention techniques to patients to reduce pain and inflammation associated with arthritis. The interventions by therapists can reduce the patient's dependence on potentially harmful pharmaceutical agents and this can be an incentive for physicians to employ or consult with therapists.

β-ADRENOCEPTOR BLOCKERS

β-Adrenoceptor blockers (antagonists) are primarily used to treat cardiovascular dysfunction. Specifically, they are used to reduce hypertension, angina, and arrhythmias and to increase survival after myocardial infarction. These drugs are also used for the treatment of glaucoma, thyrotoxicosis, anxiety, migraines, and benign essential tremors.

β-Blockers are competitive antagonists of β-adrenoceptors.[49] β-Blockers reduce heart rate and contractility, resulting in a reduction in cardiac output and blood pressure. These drugs also exert a central inhibitory effect on sympathetic activity, reducing peripheral vascular resistance. However, their most profound effect in terms of reducing blood pressure has to do with the blocking of renin release from the kidneys. The result is a reduction in circulating angiotensin II and aldosterone, which produces a vasodilatory effect.

β-Blockers are either selective or nonselective for β-adrenoceptors.[49] The nonselective antagonists will block β_1- and β_2-adrenoceptors. The selective agents will block only β_1-receptors, but this selectivity is lost at high doses. Propranolol is the prototypical nonselective agent.

Atenolol and metoprolol are selective β_1-adrenoceptor antagonists. The main difference between the two is that the nonselective agents will block the β_2-receptors in the bronchioles and will also block the β_2-receptors in skeletal muscle vasculature.

β-blockers have, for years, been recommended as first-line agents along with diuretics as monotherapy in the fight against uncomplicated hypertension. These drugs, especially atenolol, have recently been shown to be less effective than other antihypertensive agents, especially in the prevention of stroke.[50] Some guidelines (such as those from the British Hypertension Society, 2006) now list them as fourth-in-line treatment.[51,52]

β-Blockers with Intrinsic Sympathomimetic Activity

Pindolol is a partial agonist at the β_1-receptor and therefore is said to have intrinsic sympathomimetic activity. It inhibits excess β_1-receptor activity when the sympathetic system is stimulated, reducing blood pressure but with less reduction in resting heart rate than other β-blockers. Pindolol stimulates the β-receptor but at the same time blocks entrance of the more potent endogenous catecholamines. This is quite useful for the patient who tends to have bradycardia or for the patient who is receiving additional cardiac medications such as antiarrhythmic drugs, which slow heart rate by widening the QT interval. Pindolol should not be given to a patient who has already had a myocardial infarction or has angina.

Therapeutic Concerns with β-Blockers

The adverse effects of β-blockers are related to their receptor-blocking action. Blockade of β-receptors eliminates β_2-receptor–activated vasodilation. A reflex increase in peripheral vasoconstriction may also occur as a result of the hypotension induced by the drug. Both these factors may contribute to some peripheral vasoconstriction in certain susceptible persons, such as patients with Raynaud's disease.

Blocking β_2-receptors in the lungs also leads to bronchoconstriction. In patients with normal lung function, these drugs have little effect, but in patients with obstructive disease, they can produce fatal consequences. Bradycardia progressing to heart block is another adverse effect that may occur because the β-receptors on nodal tissue are blocked. At rest, these drugs may only produce small depressions in heart rate or cardiac output; however, during exercise these values are depressed enough to reduce exercise capacity. Excessive depression of heart rate and contractility will also exacerbate congestive heart failure. Abrupt withdrawal of a β-blocker will trigger dangerous arrhythmias, angina, and even myocardial infarction.

β-Blockers have several noncardiac-related adverse effects. Blocking β_2-receptors will decrease glycogenolysis and glucagon secretion. This is particularly worrisome in patients with diabetes because these drugs mask the symptoms of hypoglycemia and impair recovery from it. It has also been reported that the conventional β-blockers (nonselective and β_1-selective agents) may promote the development of type 2 diabetes in patients with hypertension.[48,53] Additional adverse effects include fatigue, dizziness, depression, sexual dysfunction, and an increase in LDL levels. In particular, an increase occurs in the number of smaller and denser LDL particles, which penetrate more easily into the vascular intima, causing damage.[54-56] Although β-blockers have been shown to reduce the mortality rate and incidence of reinfarction in patients recovering from myocardial infarction, their role in the prevention of primary infarcts has been a modest one.[57] Some speculate that the reason for this is the abnormality in lipid levels that occurs with these drugs. The significance of the increase in lipid levels with these drugs is currently being debated.[34]

Renal perfusion is also reduced with β-blockers because they block the prostaglandin-mediated vasodilation of the renal arteries. This does not appear to be a significant problem, except in cases of renal failure or when a patient is taking an NSAID along with the β-blocker.

In physical therapy, patients must be watched for signs of developing congestive heart failure. The allied health professional should note whether the patient is experiencing dyspnea, peripheral edema, increased weight, rales, jugular vein distension, or decreased urine output. Vital signs should be obtained frequently, particularly before the patient's next drug dose. The physician should be notified if systolic blood pressure falls below 90mm Hg or if the pulse is below 60 beats/min. Dosing would not typically be recommended in the presence of these values of vital signs.

α-ADRENOCEPTOR BLOCKERS

α-Blockers reduce the sympathetic tone of blood vessels, allowing vasodilation and a subsequent decrease in peripheral vascular resistance.[49] They are used in the treatment of pheochromocytoma (an epinephrine-secreting tumor), complex regional pain syndromes, and Raynaud's disease. In addition, these drugs are used to prevent autonomic hyperreflexia in patients with spinal cord injury and to improve urine flow in patients with benign prostatic hyperplasia.

Phenoxybenzamine is a nonselective α-blocker because it binds to both α_1- and α_2-receptors.[49] It irreversibly binds to the receptor, so it has a long duration of action, approximately 24 hours. The body must synthesize new receptors for the drug action to be terminated. It is used to induce vasodilation in some pain syndromes in which the vasculature is constricted. It is not useful in hypertension because norepinephrine can still act on the α_1-receptors of the heart to increase blood pressure. Also, blocking of α_2-receptors produces unrestricted norepinephrine release because the autoreceptors are blocked.

Prazosin, terazosin, and doxazosin are selective α_1-blockers (Figure 6-6). (Note the similar endings with -azosin.) These drugs are primarily used to lower peripheral vascular resistance, which, in turn, lowers blood pressure. They dilate both resistance and capacitance vessels. Unlike β-blockers, they have been shown to lower LDL and triglyceride levels, and they only minimally affect cardiac output and renal blood flow. Therefore, they do not produce any long-term tachycardia or increased renin release. However, in the short term, reflex tachycardia could be a problem.

α -Blockers are not used as monotherapy but only as add-on drugs to reduce blood pressure. This is, in part, due to findings from the ALLHAT study, in which the doxazosin arm of the study was discontinued early because of an increased incidence in heart failure caused by this drug.[58]

Therapeutic Concerns with α-Blockers

The adverse effects of α-blockers include postural hypotension, nasal stuffiness, reflex tachycardia, and arrhythmias. The increased heart rate and arrhythmias are the result of activation of the baroreceptor reflex, as well as

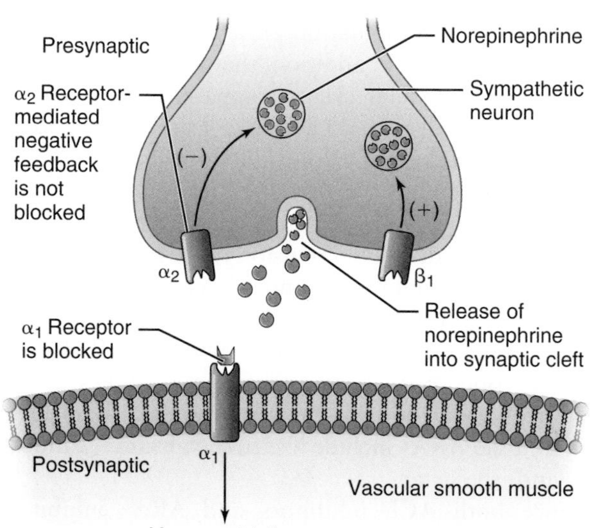

FIGURE 6-6 Antagonism at postsynaptic α_1-adrenoceptors. Prazosin (α_1-antagonist) prevents vasoconstriction by norepinephrine. Further effects of norepinephrine are reduced by a feedback mechanism, since presynaptic α_2-adrenoceptors are not blocked by prazosin; so the α_2-adrenoceptors can be occupied by norepinephrine, thereby activating a negative feedback pathway.

α_2-blockade, as explained previously. With a decrease in blood pressure, a reflex increase in heart rate occurs through the baroreceptors. This can produce angina in a patient who has poor cardiac perfusion and may be a reason for the increased incidence of heart failure during treatment with α-blockers compared with treatment with other antihypertensive agents.

The selective α_1-blockers may produce a significant drop in blood pressure, especially with the first dose. This is called first-dose syncope.[49] This effect may be minimized by starting with one half the usual dose and dosing at bedtime. Assisted ambulation may be necessary when this drug is first administered, especially when it is given to older adults.

DUAL α- AND β-BLOCKERS

Dual α- and β-blockers are helpful in reducing hypertension in patients who experience increased peripheral resistance while taking pure β-blockers. Labetalol and carvedilol are nonselective α_1- and β_1- receptor antagonists.[49] The ratio of β-blockade to α-blockade is 10:1 for carvedilol and 4:1 for labetalol. Labetalol also has some intrinsic sympathomimetic activity.[59] Adverse effects are similar to those of β-blockers and α-blockers.

CENTRAL ACTING α_2-AGONISTS

Centrally acting α_2-adrenoceptor agonists are primarily used to reduce blood pressure. Clonidine is the prototypical drug in this category, and it stimulates the autoinhibitory effects of norepinephrine on the sympathetic system.[49] Its action is particularly directed at the vasomotor center in the brain. This leads to a reduction of arteriolar tone and, with long-term use, a reduction in heart rate and cardiac output; however, there is less reduction in blood pressure than when the sympathetic system is blocked peripherally.[60]

The problem with these drugs is that they are highly sedating. They also produce dry mouth, orthostatic hypotension, erectile dysfunction, and galactorrhea. In addition, diffuse parenchymal injury to the liver and hemolytic anemia have been reported with some of these drugs. A rapid return of hypertension with tachycardia and restlessness is noted when the medication is withdrawn abruptly. Clonidine is now available as a transdermal preparation. The patch is changed every 7 days, providing good control of blood pressure with less sedation.[60] However, skin irritation has been reported.

VASODILATORS

Within the classification of vasodilators are calcium channel blockers and the direct vasodilators hydralazine, minoxidil, and nitroprusside.

Direct Vasodilators

Direct vasodilators dilate the arterioles by acting directly on the vascular smooth muscle as opposed to acting through adrenergic receptors. They were earlier used for the treatment of hypertensive emergencies with diastolic blood pressure over 120 mm Hg or in medical conditions such as hypertensive encephalopathy, dissecting aortic aneurysm, and pulmonary edema. They are rarely used today.[1]

Hydralazine and minoxidil are examples of direct vasodilators. Minoxidil is a more effective vasodilator and is useful in the patient who also has renal failure; however, it is rarely used because of its adverse effects. It works by opening an ion channel called the adenosine triphosphate (ATP)-sensitive K^+ channel. When this channel is opened, K^+ leaves the cell, leading to hyperpolarization. The more negative potential then reduces influx of Ca^{2+} through the L-type Ca^{2+} channel.

Calcium Channel Blockers

Like β-blockers, calcium channel blockers are used for many cardiovascular indications. They are used to treat angina, arrhythmias, and hypertension. They are particularly useful for patients with conditions that may contraindicate the use of β-blockers, for example, asthma, diabetes, and peripheral vascular disease. The mechanism of action in hypertension is blockade of calcium influx into arterial smooth muscle, producing vasodilation and decreased peripheral resistance.

Three classes of calcium channel blockers exist, each with different properties and indications.[60] Dihydropyridines have stronger affinity for vascular calcium channels than for the calcium channels in the heart. Therefore, they reduce arteriolar tone, with less effect on cardiac conduction. Examples include nifedipine, nicardipine, and amlodipine. These are the drugs primarily used for uncomplicated hypertension. The diphenyl alkylamine verapamil primarily affects the heart, and the benzodiazepine diltiazem affects both the vasculature and the heart. Both verapamil and diltiazem depress cardiac activity, produce conduction problems, and are negative inotropic agents. Verapamil can be especially problematic because it can produce atrioventricular nodal block and is contraindicated in congestive heart failure.

Therapeutic Concerns about Calcium Channel Blockers. Calcium channel blockers tend to produce a throbbing headache, dizziness, hypotension, bradycardia (verapamil and diltiazem), reflex tachycardia (nifedipine), sweating, tremor, flushing, and constipation. The combination of a β-blocker and verapamil is contraindicated because of the negative inotropic effects, and verapamil alone is contraindicated in congestive heart failure.

ACE INHIBITORS AND ACE RECEPTOR BLOCKERS (ACE RECEPTOR ANTAGONISTS)

ACE inhibitors and ACE receptor blockers are effective in reducing hypertension and reducing afterload in congestive heart failure; they are particularly recommended for patients who have diabetes along with cardiovascular disease.

ACE Inhibitors

ACE inhibitors block the action of ACE, reducing angiotensin II synthesis. Angiotensin II contributes to the development of hypertension by constricting arterioles and stimulating aldosterone release, which, in turn, stimulates Na^+ reabsorption from the kidney tubules. So, by blocking this synthesis, ACE inhibitors produce vasodilation and diuresis. These drugs also slow bradykinin inactivation, which, again, results in vasodilation. Long-term use of these drugs is associated with recovery of angiotensin II levels, even though blood pressure remains low. This suggests that some other mechanism might be partly responsible for their antihypertensive effects. ACE receptor antagonists (ARAs) interfere with the binding of angiotensin II to angiotensin receptors.

Both drug categories—ACE inhibitors and ARAs—are especially useful for patients with congestive heart failure because they do not depress cardiac function. In addition, they do not adversely affect lipid or glucose levels or heart rate. ACE inhibitors are as effective as diuretics or β-blockers; however, when an ACE inhibitor and a diuretic or β-blocker are used together, the effectiveness of the combination is better than when either drug is used alone. In addition, they have been shown to reduce cardiovascular events compared with placebo in high-risk patients who do not have heart failure and also to reduce cardiovascular mortality and morbidity compared with atenolol.[61-63]

ACE inhibitors are recommended as first-line drugs for the treatment of hypertension in diabetics.[63,64] However, both ACE inhibitors and ARAs have been shown to be renal protective by delaying the development of diabetic nephropathy in patients with type II diabetes, and to reduce proteinuria.[65,66] Some examples of ACE inhibitors are captopril, enalapril, ramipril, and lisinopril, and the ARAs include losartan, valsartan, candesartan, and irbesartan.

Since both ACE inhibitors and ARAs inhibit the renin–angiotensin system (RAS), it makes sense to ask whether one is more effective than the other and whether combination therapy is better than monotherapy. The majority of comparative effectiveness studies have shown that both types of drugs are about equally effective in most patients with uncomplicated hypertension.[67,68] When the two drugs were given together, they lowered

24-hour ambulatory BP by 4.7/3.9 mm Hg compared with an ACE inhibitor alone and by 3.8/2.9 mm Hg compared with monotherapy with an ARA.[69] The combination also reduced proteinuria by 30% and 39%, compared with an ACE inhibitor and ARA, respectively. However, what is not clear from these studies is whether monotherapy would be more efficacious if it was given at a higher-than-standard dose. What is clear, however, is that combination therapy is associated with greater adverse effects, particularly hyperkalemia (see below).

Therapeutic Concerns about ACE inhibitors and ACE Receptor Blockers. Common adverse effects of ACE inhibitors include dry cough, rashes, hypotension, hyperkalemia, and rarely, angioedema.[60] Cough occurs because the ACE inhibitors interfere with the metabolism of bradykinin in the lungs. At increased levels, this vasoactive peptide acts as a pulmonary irritant, although bradykinin also induces a beneficial vasodilation. In approximately 15% of patients, the resultant cough is so severe that the drug has to be withdrawn. Since NSAIDs block bradykinin-mediated vasodilation, they impair the hypertensive effects of the ACE inhibitors. Angiotensin receptor blockers (ARBs) have similar adverse effects, with the exception of the cough.

PLASMA RENIN INHIBITORS

Aliskiren (Tekturna) is the first drug in a new drug classification for the treatment of hypertension approved by the U.S. Food and Drug Administration (FDA) in 2007.[70,71] This drug directly blocks the activity of renin by inhibiting its catalytic activity. Plasma renin is reduced, which subsequently reduces angiotensin II and aldosterone. The ARA irbesartan shows similar reduction in blood pressure. In addition, with aliskiren, plasma renin concentration is markedly reduced, but this is not the case with either ACE inhibitors or ARAs, which researchers theorize could be responsible for persistent hypertension in some patients. Early reports of combination therapies with hydrochlorothiazide, amlodipine, ramipril, and valsartan showed greater reductions in blood pressure compared with any of these agents as monotherapy. Adverse effects include hypotension, hyperkalemia (especially when combined with an ACE inhibitor), rash, and gastrointestinal (GI) complaints, but these were not significantly different from those with placebo. However, the low incidence of adverse reactions may be reflective of the limited number of clinical trials and years of study rather than of the drug itself.

MANAGEMENT OF HYPERTENSIVE EMERGENCIES

Severe elevations (BP $\geq$180/110 mm Hg without visceral damage, or elevated BP with visceral damage) and sudden elevations in blood pressure represent medical emergencies. They pose substantial increases in the risks for heart failure, stroke, dissecting aneurysm, and death. Treatment of these severe episodes requires hospitalization and parenteral antihypertensive medications so that blood pressure can be lowered quickly within a few hours (25% in 2 hours). Close monitoring is necessary, however, to avoid cerebral hypoperfusion and brain injury.

One of the most commonly used drugs for severe hypertension is nitroprusside.[72] Sodium nitroprusside produces marked arterial and venous dilation, which reduces cardiac preload and afterload. It spontaneously breaks down to nitric oxide when entering smooth muscle cells. The nitric oxide activates guanylyl cyclase, which then increases cyclic guanosine monophosphate (cGMP) levels. Increased cGMP relaxes vascular smooth muscle. Nitroprusside is administered intravenously and produces a rapid reduction in blood pressure. Patients must be monitored carefully to ensure that hypoperfusion of organs does not occur while blood pressure is falling. Sodium nitroprusside is sensitive to light and degrades easily, so it must be prepared fresh before it is given to the patient. It also has a short duration of action and is metabolized in red blood cells liberating cyanide as a byproduct. Toxicity is related to the accumulation of cyanide from prolonged administration (1 week or more).

Fenoldopam is another drug for hypertensive emergencies; it primarily dilates peripheral arterioles and also acts as a diuretic in the kidneys by increasing renal blood flow.[73] It is a dopamine D_1 agonist. So far, it appears to be the ideal drug with wider applications because it does not cause bradycardia like parenteral β-blockers do and can therefore be used in the treatment of congestive heart failure.[74] The drug is also renal protective and does not trigger an increase in renin release. It is as effective as nitroprusside, but without the adverse effect of elevated cyanide levels.

Other parenteral medications that may be effective include labetalol (a β- & α-blocker), calcium channel blockers, esmolol (a β_1-blocker) and clonidine (an α_2-agonist).

GUIDELINES FOR THE TREATMENT OF HYPERTENSION

The first line of treatment for hypertension consists of lifestyle changes that include diet, exercise, and cessation of smoking.[75] If these changes are not effective, monotherapy is prescribed. Thiazide diuretics or β-blockers are usually the first drugs prescribed. Both have been shown to decrease coronary events in high-risk populations. ACE inhibitors are often more expensive alternatives, although some less expensive generics are available.

When deciding on the drug to be prescribed, some individual patient factors must be considered. ACE inhibitors are useful for patients with diabetes, for those who have abnormal lipid levels, and for those with heart failure. β-Blockers and calcium channel blockers are good for patients who have coexisting hypertension and angina. Race is also an important consideration. Black patients respond well to diuretics, and Asian patients are more sensitive to β-blockers. Older adults respond better to calcium channel blockers than to diuretics.

During the writing of the first edition of this book, diuretics were considered the best choice for the treatment of uncomplicated hypertension on the basis of their blood pressure lowering effect and their cost (cost–benefit analysis). The Antihypertensive and Lipid-Lowering Treatment to Prevent Heart Attack Trial (ALLHAT) compared the number of myocardial infarctions, strokes, and deaths in more than 33,000 subjects with hypertension who took chlorthalidone (a thiazide diuretic), amlodipine (a calcium channel blocker), or lisinopril (an ACE inhibitor) for 5 years.[76] Chlorthalidone was found to lower blood pressure slightly better than the other two drugs. However, as a result of increased blood glucose levels during treatment, patients receiving chlorthalidone had a risk of diabetes that was between 43% and 65% higher than had patients receiving an ACE inhibitor. Complications in terms of cardiac events associated with diabetes were not adequately studied during the 5-year study period.[77] Although diuretics have won some accolades with this study, it is still important to consider individual patient characteristics when a medication is chosen. The diuretic may be the cheapest and most effective in lowering blood pressure, but for the older adult who has mobility issues, the added trips to the bathroom may pose some hazards. In addition, hypokalemia may produce leg cramps or complicate the cardiovascular status. Thus, age, physical status, and the presence or absence of other medical conditions are important factors to consider while choosing a drug. The ALLHAT study did, however, show the clear superiority of diuretics over amlodipine and lisinopril in reducing blood pressure in black patients.[78]

The beneficial effects of calcium channel blockers have been supported in several large studies. Specifically, the Anglo-Scandinavian Cardiac Outcomes Trial (ASCOT) has demonstrated that amlodipine, with or without addition of an ACE inhibitor, reduced the risk of new-onset diabetes by 34% in 19,000 patients with hypertension.[79] This was compared with a β-blocker given with or without a thiazide diuretic. Calcium channel blockers also showed a reduction in stroke incidence.

Many studies have demonstrated the effectiveness of ACE inhibitors and ARAs in reducing hypertension and also in decreasing the incidence of new-onset type 2 diabetes. The Valsartan Antihypertensive Long-Term Use Evaluation (VALUE) trial compared treatment with amlodipine versus that with valsartan in over 15,000 high-risk patients with hypertension.[80] The results showed

BOX 6-1 First-Choice Drugs for Hypertension under the Following Conditions

Older adults with high systolic pressure	Diuretics, calcium channel blockers (dihydropyridines)
Diabetic nephropathy	Angiotensin-converting enzyme (ACE) inhibitors /ACE receptor antagonists with a calcium channel blockers
Post–myocardial infarction	β-Blockers, ACE inhibitors or ACE receptor antagonists
Heart failure	Diuretics, ACE inhibitors or ACE receptor antagonists
Hypertension in black Patients	Diuretics and calcium channel blockers

that no difference was found in cardiac endpoints, for example, strokes, myocardial infarctions, and all-cause deaths, between the two treatments. However, a clear reduction in heart failure and new-onset diabetes was seen in the valsartan group. The Appropriate Blood Pressure Control in Hypertensive and Normotensive Type 2 Diabetes Mellitus (ABCD trial) supported the use of an ACE inhibitor over a calcium channel blocker in patients who already had a confirmed diagnosis of diabetes.[81]

When one drug alone is not effective, combination therapy is the choice. By combining drugs with different mechanisms of action, the doses of each may be reduced, but the effects are usually additive. The β-blocker–diuretic combination has been the most commonly used, on the basis of the recommendations of the JNC 7 report, although this is expected to change in the future as β-blockers are moved to the positions of third- and fourth-line drugs.[51,52] Unless the patient has coexisting angina or an arrhythmia, either of these drugs is not recommended as monotherapy for hypertension.

ACE inhibitors or ARAs plus either a diuretic or a calcium channel blocker seems to be the most popular combination prescription at this time. In the ASCOT trial, mentioned above, the combination therapy arm of the trial demonstrated that the ACE inhibitor plus a calcium channel blocker was more effective than the β-blocker–diuretic combination.[79] This combination (amlodipine and valsartan) has recently been marketed as a single pill, Exforge.[82] The Avoiding Cardiovascular Events in Combination Therapy in Patients Living with Systolic Hypertension (ACCOMPLISH) trial further supports the combination of the ACE inhibitor benazepril plus the calcium channel blocker amlodipine.[83]

THERAPEUTIC CONCERNS ABOUT ANTIHYPERTENSIVE AGENTS

The allied health professional treating patients taking antihypertensive medications should be concerned about excessive lowering of blood pressure, orthostatic hypotension, and syncope. The physician should be notified if systolic blood pressure falls below 90mm Hg or if heart rate falls below 60 beats/min. Dosing should be stopped if this occurs, but this must always be the decision of the physician, not of the therapist. Patients should also be continuously monitored for reflex tachycardia. Slow rising and ankle pumping are useful techniques to prevent falls and syncope resulting from orthostatic hypotension. Patients are particularly vulnerable to falls because of urinary frequency and thus the need for many trips to the bathroom during the night. They should be instructed to stand holding on to a supporting object for at least 10 seconds before walking away. If a patient begins to feel lightheaded, he or she can cross one leg over the other and tighten the leg muscles. This has been shown to raise blood pressure.[84] Another helpful suggestion to the patient is to drink water throughout the day. Being dehydrated, even by a small amount, can cause blood pressure problems. A patient with orthostatic hypotension should drink a cup of water right before attempting to stand.[84]

Heat modalities should be avoided by those on antihypertensive medications that produce arterial vasodilation. The application of heat, especially from a whirlpool bath, will produce further vasodilation, will lower blood pressure, and may cause syncope.

β-Blockers, calcium channel blockers, vasodilators, and diuretics all decrease exercise performance and thus have ramifications for physical therapy. Exercise produces positive chronotropic and inotropic effects, but β-blockers produce negative chronotropic and inotropic effects. β-Blockers have been shown to decrease both resting and exercise heart rates in elite athletes and in patients with hypertension, but β-blockers that have intrinsic sympathomimetic action produce less reduction in these values. Lowering of maximum oxygen consumption per unit time (Vo_2 max) also occurs, regardless of whether the β-blocker is cardioselective or has intrinsic sympathomimetic action and regardless of whether the patients have normal or high blood pressure. One reason for these negative effects on exercise performance is that β-blockers reduce lipolysis and impair glycogenolysis, reducing fuels for exercise.[85,86] The masking of hypoglycemic symptoms can also be deleterious for a diabetic patient. Another important point with regard to β-blockers is that age-related equations to predict maximum heart rate do not apply because target heart rate is not attainable during administration of these drugs. A training rate that is 20 beats/min greater than the resting rate can be used as a maximum, provided the patient is free of symptoms at this level. β-Blockers should be reserved for those patients with coronary artery disease who are not engaged in endurance activities.

With regard to diuretics, exercise potentiates the fluid and potassium loss seen with the use of these drugs. Potassium depletion contributes to muscle fatigue, cramping, and possible arrhythmias; and fluid loss contributes to dehydration. Hypovolemia compromises venous return, so heart rate increases. Thermoregulation is also compromised because blood flow is shunted away from the skin to the muscles and because the peripheral arterioles undergo vasoconstriction. The results, including reduced sweating, translate into reduced exercise performance. Therefore, diuretics are not the best choice of drug for the serious endurance athlete.[87]

Additional information on the effects of α_1-blockers, calcium channel blockers, and ACE inhibitors on exercise performance is available from the literature. α_1-Blockers significantly reduce Vo_2 max, maximal workload, and duration of exercise on a bicycle ergometer in well-trained athletic men with hypertension.[88] Similar results have been reported for calcium channel blockers.[89] However, ACE inhibitors have been shown to cause less reduction in some of these values and may be better tolerated in terms of adverse effects.[90]

In addition to exercise counseling, physical therapists can play a significant role in helping patients reduce their blood pressure. Providing education on the physiology of blood pressure, encouraging patients to comply with their medication regimens, and carefully observing patients for any adverse reactions are forms of assistance that physical therapists can easily provide. Reducing blood pressure by even a small amount can be helpful in reducing morbidity and mortality. A recent meta-analysis of 61 long-term studies of initially healthy individuals showed that with every 20-point increase in systolic pressure or 10-point increase in diastolic pressure, the chance of having a fatal stroke or myocardial infarction doubles.[91] Reverse analysis demonstrates that reducing systolic pressure by 10 points or diastolic pressure by 5 points can produce a 30 to 40% decrease in the risk of fatal myocardial infarction and stroke.

TABLE 6-2 **Drugs for Hypertension**

Type	Drug	Main Action	Uses/Function	ADR
Adrenoceptor Antagonists	phenoxybenzamine	α-Antagonist (nonselective, irreversible)	Pheochromocytoma	Hypotension, flushing tachycardia, nasal congestion, erectile dysfunction
	phentolamine	α -Antagonist (nonselective), vasodilator	Rarely used	Same as phenoxybenzamine
	prazosin (Minipress)	α_1-Antagonist	Hypertension	Same as phenoxybenzamine
	tamsulosin (Flomax)	α_1-Antagonist (uroselective)	Prostatic hyperplasia	Failure of ejaculation
	propranolol (Inderal)	β -Antagonist (nonselective)	Angina, hypertension, cardiac arrhythmias, anxiety tremor, glaucoma	Bronchoconstriction, cardiac failure, cold extremities, fatigue and depression, hypoglycemia
	metoprolol (Lopressor)	β_1-Antagonist	Angina, hypertension, arrhythmias	Same as propranolol, less risk of bronchoconstriction
	Atenolol (Tenormin)	β_1-Antagonist	Angina, hypertension, arrhythmias	Same as propranolol, less risk of bronchoconstriction
	labetolol (Normodyne)	α/β -Antagonist	Hypertension in pregnancy	Postural hypotension, bronchoconstriction
	carvedilol (Coreg)	α/β -Antagonist	Heart failure	As for other β-blockers Exacerbation of heart failure Renal failure
Thiazide Diuretics	chlorothiazide (Diuril)	Block reabsorption of sodium, chloride, and water at the distal convoluted tubule	Management of edema and hypertension	Urinary loss of sodium, chloride, potassium Hyponatremia (low serum sodium) Hypokalemia (low serum potassium)
	chlorothalidone (Hygroton)	Same as chlorothiazide	Same as chlorothiazide	Same as chlorothiazide
	hydrocholorthiazide (Hydrodiuril)	Same as chlorothiazide	Same as chlorothiazide	Same as chlorothiazide
Loop Diuretics	furosemide (Lasix)	Inhibit sodium, chloride, and water absorption via the thick ascending limb of Henle's loop	Management of edema associated with congestive heart failure (CHF), cirrhosis of liver, and renal disease Used in treatment of hypertension	Urinary loss of sodium, chloride, potassium, and bicarbonate Hyponatremia and hypokalemia possible
	ethacrynic acid (Edecrin)	Same as furosemide	Same as furosemide	Same as furosemide
Potassium-Sparing Diuretics	spironoloactone (Aldactone)	Blocks aldosterone action on distal nephron causing potassium retention and sodium excretion	Used for treatment of CHF and hypertension	Urinary excretion of sodium, chloride, and bicarbonate Retention of potassium Hyperkalemia
	triamterene (Dyrenium)	Act on distal nephron decreasing sodium reuptake, reducing potassium secretion	Same as spironoloactone	Same as spironoloactone

TABLE 6-2 Drugs for Hypertension—cont'd

Type	Drug	Main Action	Uses/Function	ADR
β-Blockers	propranolol (Inderal)	β -Antagonist (nonselective)	Angina, hypertension, cardiac arrhythmias, anxiety tremor, glaucoma	Bronchoconstriction, cardiac failure, cold extremities, fatigue and depression, hypoglycemia
	metoprolol (Lopressor)	β_1-Antagonist	Angina, hypertension, arrhythmias	Same as propranolol, less risk of bronchoconstriction
	nadolol (Corgard)	β -Antagonist (nonselective)	Hypertension, angina, cardiac arrhythmias, hypertrophic cardiomyopathy, myocardial infarction (MI)	Drowsiness, tiredness or weakness Bradycardia, difficulty breathing, CHF, depression, diarrhea, constipation
	pindolol (Visken)	β -Antagonist (nonselective)	Hypertension	Lightheadedness, fatigue, weakness, reflex tachycardia
	atenolol (Tenormin)	β_1-Antagonist	Hypertension, angina, MI, anxiety tremors	Hypotension, dizziness, nausea, headache, fatigue, constipation, diarrhea
α-Blockers	doxazosin (Cardura)	α_1-Antagonist	Hypertension	Dizziness, asthenia, headache, edema
	prazosin (Minipress)	α_1-Antagonist	Hypertension	Hypotension, flushing tachycardia, nasal congestion, erectile dysfunction
	terazosin (Hytrin)	α_1-Antagonist	Hypertension	Dizziness, headache, unusually tired
α-Agonist	clonidine (Catapres)	α_2-Partial agonist	Hypertension, migraine	Drowsiness, orthostatic hypotension, edema and weight gain, rebound hypertension
Direct Vasodilators	hydralazine (Apresoline)	Relaxes vascular smooth muscle reducing blood pressure	Hypertension Treatment of CHF	Diarrhea, palpitations, tachycardia, headache, nausea, vomiting
	minoxidil (Loniten)	Direct action of vascular smooth muscle producing vasodilation of arterioles	Hypertension	Edema with concurrent weight gain
	fenoldopam (Corlopam)	Dopamine 1 (D_1) agonist	Severe hypertension	hypotension
Calcium Channel Blockers	amlodipine (Norvasc)	dihydropyridine	Hypertension	Hypotension Palpitations Tachycardia Peripheral edema Constipation
	Diltiazem (Cardizem)	Benzothiazepine	Hypertension, angina	Hypotension Palpitations Tachycardia or bradycardia Peripheral edema Constipation
	Nifedipine (Procardia)	dihydropyridine	Hypertension	Hypotension Palpitations Tachycardia Peripheral edema Constipation
	Verapamil (Calan)	Phenylalkylamine	Hypertension, angina, cardiac arrhythmias	Hypotension Heart failure/heart block

Continued

TABLE 6-2 **Drugs for Hypertension—cont'd**

Type	Drug	Main Action	Uses/Function	ADR
ACE Inhibitors	captopril (Capoten)	Suppresses renin-angiotensin-aldosterone system by preventing conversion to angiotensin II	Hypertension, CHF	Rash, headache, cough, insomnia, dizziness, fatigue, nausea, diarrhea/constipation
	enalapril (Vasotec)	Same as captopril	Hypertension, CHF	Hypotension, dizziness, headache, fatigue
ACE Receptor Blocker	candesartan (Atacand)	Angiotensin II receptor antagonist– blocking vasoconstrictor and aldosterone-secreting effects	Hypertension, CHF	Upper respiratory infection, dizziness, back and leg pain
	irbesartan (Avapro)	Same as candesartan	Hypertension, CHF	Upper respiratory infection, fatigue, diarrhea, cough
	valsartan (Diovan)	Same as candesartan	Hypertension, CHF	Insomnia, fatigue, heartburn, abdominal pain, dizziness, headache, diarrhea, nausea, vomiting, edema

ACTIVITIES 6

1. A.B. is a 46-year-old man who has a painful right wrist. He reports tripping over a rock while training for the New York City Marathon and landing on his outstretched arm. He has only 6 weeks left to train and does not want any lingering injuries while running the big race.

Medical History: A.B. has a history of hypertension for which he has been taking propranolol and hydrochlorothiazide, and over the last 2 days, he has been taking plenty of aspirin for the wrist pain. He denies having any other illness or musculoskeletal problem.

While performing your examination, you notice that the patient appears to be suffering from some cramping in his lower extremities. When you question him about this, he states that he just ran 8 miles to your clinic. You also notice that his clothes are dry, despite the high heat and humidity outside. You continue with the examination.

Vital Signs: Blood pressure, 90/60 mm Hg; resting pulse, 110 beats/min

Wrist Exam: Mild edema on the dorsum of the right hand with limited active and passive range of motion of the wrist. Strength testing demonstrates weakness caused by pain in the right hand but also a grade 4/5 for biceps, triceps, wrist flexors, and extensors. Grip strength measures only 25lb. Grip strength on the left measures 40lb. These results are not what you expected.

The patient continues to show evidence of mild cramping, and after further questioning, the patient reports feeling weak. You are very concerned and decide to call for an ambulance.

Labs: Results of tests on blood drawn from the patient 2 hours later are as follows: sodium concentration, 122mEq/L; potassium concentration, 2.5mEq/L; hemoglobin level, 16g/dL, creatinine clearance, 1.1mg/100mL; glucose level, 100mg/mL.

Arterial blood gases (ABGs): Metabolic alkalosis

Urinalysis: Positive for protein; a high specific gravity

Questions:

1. *Analyze the physical findings and lab work to determine what is abnormal.*
2. *What do you think is going on with this patient?*
3. *What type of medication changes should be made?*

2. A 54-year-old obese patient complains of dizziness and dyspnea while on the treadmill in your office. He reports that he fainted yesterday while he was walking briskly from his car to his office. He has been experiencing angina associated with exercise and stress for more than 2 years and is currently taking verapamil.

Medical History: Borderline type II diabetes; angina

Vital Signs: Blood pressure, 80/60 mm Hg; pulse, 48 beats/min

The patient is transported to the emergency department.

ECG: QRS is normal, but the PR interval is increased.

Labs: Blood urea nitrogen (BUN) level is slightly elevated. Blood glucose level is 70 mg/100 mL.

Chest: Scattered wheezes noted

Questions

1. *What do you think is going on with this patient? What is the immediate course of treatment?*

2. *What suggestions do you have for changing medications, and why?*
3. *What can you do in physical therapy to make sure that this does not happen again?*

3. *Research* the literature, and briefly review two articles that would help you decide on the best pharmacologic treatment for the following patient:
A 55-year-old man with mild hypertension (155/95mm Hg). The patient is slim and athletic (runs 3 miles, four times a week). Despite his low weight and dedication to exercise, he has high cholesterol (high-density lipoprotein level, 45mg/100mL; low-density lipoprotein, 270mg/100mL; triglyceride level, 300mg/100mL). What do you think might be prescribed for the hypertension? Note that he also had symptoms of diabetes 5 years ago when he was overweight.
4. Visit the supermarket or local general nutrition store and make a list of the most common ingredients in the so-called "energy drinks," and discuss what effects these drinks may have on blood pressure.
5. Search the literature for evidence that exercise lowers blood pressure.

REFERENCES

1. Elghozi JL, Azizi M, and Plouin PF: Hypertension. In S. A. Waldman and A. Terzic, editors: Pharmacology and therapeutics: Principles to practice, New York, 2009, Saunders.
2. Ostchega Y, Yoon SS, Hughes J, Louis T: Hypertension awareness, treatment, and control-continued disparities in adults: United States, 2005-2006. NCHS Data Brief No. 3. 2008. (website). http://www.cdc.gov/nchs/data/databriefs/db03.pdf. Accessed August 14, 2009.
3. Wong, ND, Lopez VA, L'Italien G: Inadequate control of hypertension in US adults with cardiovascular disease comorbidities in 2003-2004. Arch Intern Med 167:2431-2436, 2007.
4. Curtis MJ, Pugsley MK: Drugs and the cardiovascular system. In Page CP, Curtis M, Sutter MC, Walker M, editors: Integrated pharmacology, Philadelphia, 2002, Mosby.
5. Esler M, Rumantir M, Kaye D, et al: Sympathetic nerve biology in essential hypertension. Clin Exp Pharmacol Physiol 28(12):986-989, 2001.
6. Boulpaep EL: Organization of the cardiovascular system. In Boron WF, Boulpaep EL, editors: Medical physiology, Philadelphia, 2003, Saunders.
7. Boulpaep EL: Regulation of arterial Pressure and cardiac output. In Boron WF, Boulpaep EL, editors: Medical physiology, Philadelphia, 2003, Saunders.
8. Weems WA, Downey JM: Regulation of arterial pressure. In Johnson LR, editor: Essential medical physiology, New York, 1992, Raven Press.
9. Weems WA, Downey JM: The mechanical activity of the heart. In Johnson LR, editor: Essential medical physiology. 1992, Raven Press: New York.
10. Weisbrodt NW, Downey JM: Hemodynamics. In Johnson LR, editor: Essential medical physiology, New York, 1992, Raven Press.
11. Seeliger E, Safak E, Persson PB, Reinhardt HW: Contribution of pressure natriuresis to control of total body sodium: Balance studies in freely moving dogs. J Physiol 537(3):941-947, 2001.
12. Sonoyama K, Greenstein A, Price A, Khavandi K, Heagerty T: Vascular remodeling: Implications for small artery function and target organ damage. Ther Adv Cardiovasc Dis 1(2): 129-137, 2007.
13. Martinka P, Fielitz J, Patzak A, et al: Mechanisms of blood pressure variability-induced cardiac hypertrophy and dysfunction in mice with impaired baroreflex. Am J Physiol Regul Integr Comp Physiol 288(3):R767-R776, 2005.
14. Gericke A, Martinka P, Nazarenko I, Persson PB, Patzak A: Impact of α_1-adrenoceptor expression on contractile properties of vascular smooth muscle cells. Am J Physiol Regul Integr Comp Physiol 293(3):R1215-R1221, 2007.
15. Patzak A, Lai EY, Mrowka R, et al: AT1 receptors mediate angiotensin II-induced release of nitric oxide in afferent arterioles. Kidney Int 66(5):1949-1958, 2004.
16. Rahmouni K, Correia ML, Haynes WG, Mark AL: Obesity-associated hypertension: New insights into mechanisms. Hypertension 45(1):9-14, 2005.
17. Persson PB: Nitric oxide in the kidney. Am J Physiol Regul Integr Comp Physiol 283(5):R1005-R1007, 2002.
18. Busse R, Edwards G, Félétou M, et al: EDHF: Bringing the concepts together. Trends Pharmacol Sci 23(8):374-380, 2002.
19. Weber MA: Vasopeptidase inhibitors. Lancet 358:1525-1532, 2001.
20. Persson PB: Renin: Origin, secretion and synthesis. J Physiol 552(3):667-671, 2003.
21. Hao C-M, Breyer MD: Physiological regulation of prostaglandins in the kidney. Annu Rev Physiol 70(1):357-377, 2008.
22. Hao CM, Breyer MD: Physiological regulation of prostaglandins in the kidney. Annu Rev Physiol 70:357-377, 357-377 2008.
23. Brater DC: Effects of nonsteroidal antiinflammatory drug on renal function: Focus on cyclooxygenase-2 selective inhibition. Am J Med 107:65S-71S, 1999.
24. Chobanian AV, Bakris GL, Black HR, et al: The seventh report of the Joint National Committee on Prevention, Detection, Evaluation, and Treatment of High Blood Pressure (JNC 7). JAMA 289:2560-2572, 2003.
25. The Eighth Report of the Joint national Committtee on Prevention, Detection, Evaluation, and Treatment of High Blood Pressure (JNC 8) (website). http://www.nhlbi.nih.gov/guidelines/hypertension/jnc8/index.htm. Accessed August 14, 2009.
26. Cardiovascular Disease Risk Reduction, Adults Cholesterol Guidelines Update, ATP IV Hypertension Guidelines Update, JNC 8 Obesity Guidelines Update, Adults (website). http://www.nhlbi.nih.gov/guidelines/cvd_adult/background.htm. Accessed August 14, 2009.
27. Thune JJ, Signorovitch J, Kober L: Effect of antecendent hypertension and follow-up blood pressure on outcomes after high risk myocardial infarction. Hypertension 51:48-54, 2008.
28. Rang HP, et al: The kidney. In Rang HP, Dale MM, Ritter JM, Flower R, editors: Rang and Dale's pharmacology, Philadelphia, 2007, Churchill Livingstone.
29. Brater CD: Pharmacology of diuretics. Am J Med Sci 319(1):38-67, 2000.
30. Greenberg A: Diuretic complications. Am J Med Sci 319(1): 10-43, 2000.
31. Reid IR, Ames RW: Hydrochlorothiazide reduces loss of cortical bone in normal postmenopausal women: A randomized controlled trial. Am J Med 109:362-370, 2000.
32. Schoofs MW: Thiazide diuretics and the risk for hip fracture. Ann Intern Med (139):476-482, 2003.
33. Messerli FH, Makani H, Bangalore S: Hydrochlorothiazide is inappropriate for first-line antihypertensive therapy. In European Meeting on Hypertension, Milan, 2009.
34. Lakshman MR, et al: Diuretics and beta-blockers do not have adverse effects at 1 year on plasma lipid and lipoprotein profiles in men with hypertension. Arch Intern Med 159:551-558, 1999.
35. Moser M: Why are physicians not prescribing diuretics more frequently in the management of hypertension? JAMA. 279(22):1813-1816, 1998.

36. Golomb BA, Criqui MH: Antihypertensives. Arch Inten Med 159:535-537, 1999.
37. Peters AL, Hsueh W: Antihypertensive agents in diabetic patients. Arch Inten Med. 159:541-542, 1999.
38. Savage PJ, Pressel SL, Curb JD, et al: Influence of long-term, low-dose, diuretic-based, antihypertensive therapy on glucose, lipid, uric acid, and potassium levels in older men and women with isolated systolic hypertension. Arch Intern Med 158(7):741-751, 1998.
39. Wright JT, Harris-Haywood S, Pressel S: Clinical outcomes by race in hypertensive patients with and without the metabolic syndrome. Arch Intern Med 168:207-217, 2008.
40. Chutka DS, Evans JM, Fleming KC, Mikkelson KG: Symposium on Geriatrics—Part I: Drug prescribing for elderly patients. Mayo Clin Proc 70(7):685-693, 1995.
41. Evans JG: Drugs and falls in later life. Lancet 361: 448, 2003.
42. Goodman CC, Snyder TE: Problems affecting multiple systems. In Goodman CC, Boissonnault WG, Fuller KS, editors: Pathology implications for the physical therapist, Philadelphia, 2003, Saunders.
43. Lim PO, MacFadyen RJ, Clarkson PB, MacDonald TM: Impaired exercise tolerance in hypertensive patients. Ann Intern Med 124(1):41-55, 1996.
44. González-Alonso J, Mortensen SP, Jeppesen TD, et al: Haemodynamic responses to exercise, ATP infusion and thigh compression in humans: Insight into the role of muscle mechanisms on cardiovascular function. J Physiol 586(9):2405-2417, 2008.
45. Cheuvront, SN, et al: Daily body mass variability and stability in active men undergoing exercise-heat stress. Int J Sport Nutr Exerc Metab, 2004. 14(5):p. 532-540.
46. Montain SJ, Coyle EF: Thermal and cardiovascular strain from hypohydration: Influence of exercise intensity. J Appl Physiol 73:1340-1350, 1992.
47. Sawka MN, Noakes TD: Does dehydration impair exercise performance? Med Sci Sports Exerc 39(8):1209-1217, 2007.
48. Sarafidis PA, Bakris GL: Resistant hypertension: An overview of evaluation and treatment. J American Coll Cardiol 52(22):1749-1757, 2008.
49. Rang HP, Dale MM, Ritter JM, Flower R Noradrenergic transmission. In Rang HP, Dale MM, Ritter JM, Flower R, editors: Rang and Dale's pharmacology, Philadelphia, 2007, Churchill Livingstone.
50. Llindholm LH, Carlberg B, Samuelsson O: Should beta blockers remain first choice in the treatment of primary hypertension? A meta-analysis. Lancet 366:1545-1553, 2005.
51. Mancia G, De Backer G, Dominiczak A, et al: 2007 guidelines for the management of arterial hypertension: The Task Force for the Management of Arterial Hypertension of the European Society of Hypertension (ESH) and of the European Society of Cardiology (ESC). J Hypertens 25(6): 1105-1187, 2007.
52. Hypertension: Management of hypertension of adults in primary care (website). http://guidance.nice.org.uk/CG34. Accessed August 16, 2009.
53. Gress TW, Nieto FJ, Shahar E, Wofford MR, Brancati FL: Hypertension and antihypertensive therapy as risk factors for type 2 diabetes mellitus. Atherosclerosis Risk in Communities Study. N Engl J Med 342(13): 905-912, 2000.
54. Boquist S, Ruotolo G, Hellénius ML, Danell-Toverud K, Karpe F, Hamsten A: Effects of a cardioselective beta blocker on postprandial triglyceride-rich lipoproteins, low density lipoprotein particle size and glucose-insulin homeostasis in middle-aged men with modestly increased cardiovascular risk. Atherosclerosis 137:391-400, 1998.
55. Roberts W: Recent studies on the effects of beta-blockers on blood lipid levels. Am Heart J 117:709-714, 1989.
56. Superko HR, Haskell WL, Krauss RM: Association of lipoprotein subclass distribution with use of selective and nonselective beta-blocker medications in patients with coronary heart disease. Atherosclerosis 101:709-714, 1993.
57. Rochon PA, Tu JV, Anderson GM, et al: Rate of heart failure and 1-year survival for older people receiving low-dose beta-blocker therapy after myocardial infarction. Lancet 356(9230):639-644, 2000.
58. ALLHAT: Major cardiovascular events in hypertensive patients randomized to doxazosin vs chlorthalidone. JAMA 283:1967-1975, 2000.
59. Abramowicz M, editor: Treatment guidelines from the Medical Letter: Drugs for hypertension, Vol. 1(6), New Rochelle, NY, 2003, The Medical Letter.
60. Benowitz NL: Antihypertensive agents. In B. G. Katzung, editor: Basic and clinical pharmacology, New York, 2007, McGraw Hill.
61. Brenner BM, Cooper ME, de Zeeuw D, et al: Effects of losartan on renal and cardiovascular outcomes in patients with type 2 diabetes and neuropathy. N Engl J Med 345(12): 861-869, 2001.
62. Dahlöf B, Devereux RB, Kjeldsen SE, et al: Cardiovascular morbidity and mortality in the Losartan Intervention for Endpoint reduction in hypertension study (LIFE):A randomised trial against atenolol. Lancet 359:995-1003, 2002.
63. Yusuf S, Gerstein H, Hoogwerf B, et al: Ramipril and the development of diabetes. JAMA 286(15):1882-1885, 2001.
64. Yusuf S: Effects of an angiotensin-converting-enzyme inhibitor, ramipril, on cardiovascular events in high-risk patients. N Engl J Med 342(3):145-153, 2000.
65. Lewis EJ, Hunsicker LG, Clarke WR, et al: Renoprotective effect of the angiotensin-receptor anatgonist irbesartan in patients with neuropathy due to type 2 diabetes. N Engl J Med 345(12):851-860, 2001.
66. Kunz R, Friedrich C, Wolbers M, Mann JF. : Meta-analysis: Effect of monotherapy and combination therapy with inhibitors of the renin angiotensin system on proteinuria in renal disease. Ann Intern Med 148:30-48, 2008.
67. Smith DHG: Treatment of hypertension with an angiotensin II-receptor antagonist compared with an angiotensin-converting enzyme inhibitor: A review of clinical studies of telmisartan and enalapril, Clin Ther 24(10):1484-1501, 2002.
68. Izzo JL, Moser M: Clinical impact of renin-angiotensin system blockade: Angiotensin-converting enzyme inhibitors vs. angiotensin receptor antagonists. J Clin Hypertens 4(6 Suppl 2): 11-19, 2002.
69. Doulton TWR: ACE inhibitor-angiotensin receptor blocker combinations: A clinician's perspective. Mini Rev Med Chem 6(5):491-497, 2006.
70. Bomback AS, Toto R: Dual blockade of the renin-angiotensin-aldosterone system: Beyond the ACE inhibitor and angiotensin-II receptor blocker combination. Am J Hypertens, 2009.
71. Nussberger J, Gradman AH, Schmieder RE, et al: Plasma renin and the antihypertensive effect of the orally active renin inhibitor aliskiren in clinical hypertension. Int J Clin Prac 61(9):1461-1468, 2007.
72. Coons JC, Seidl E: Cardiovascular pharmacotherapy update for the intensive care unit. Crit Care Nurs 30(1):44-57, 2007.
73. Murphy MB, Murray C, Shorten GD: Drug therapy: Fenoldopam—a selective peripheral dopamine-receptor agonist for the treatment of severe hypertension. N Engl J Med 345(21):1548-1557, 2001.
74. Abramowicz M: Cardiovascular drugs in the ICU. Treat Guidelines Med Lett 1(4), 2002.
75. Appel LJ: Nonpharmacologic therapies that reduce blood pressure: A fresh perspective. Clin Cardiol 22(suppl 7):1-5, 1999.

76. The ALLHAT Officers and Coordinators for the ALLHAT Collaborative Group: Major outcomes in high-risk hypertensive patients randomized to angiotensin-converting enzyme inhibitor or calcium channel blocker vs diuretic. The Antihypertensive and Lipid-Lowering Treatment to Prevent Heart Attack Trial (ALLHAT). JAMA 288:1981-1997, 2002.
77. Messerli FH, Weber MA: ALLHAT—All hit or all miss? Key questions still remain. Am J Cardiol 92:280-281, 2003.
78. Wright JT Jr, Harris-Haywood S, Pressel S, et al: Clinical outcomes by race in hypertensive patients with and without the metabolic syndrome: Antihypertensive and Lipid-Lowering Treatment to Prevent Heart Attack Trial (ALLHAT). Arch Intern Med 168(2):207-217, 2008.
79. Dahlöf B, Sever PS, Poulter NR, et al: Prevention of cardiovascular events with an antihypertensive regimen of amlodipine adding perindopril as required versus atenolol adding bendroflumethiazide as required, in the Anglo-Scandinavian Cardiac Outcomes Trial-Blood Pressure Lowering Arm (ASCOT-BPLA):A multicentre randomised controlled trial. Lancet 366(9489):895-906, 2005.
80. Julius S, Weber MA, Kjeldsen SE, et al: The Valsartan Antihypertensive Long-Term Use Evaluation (VALUE) Trial: Outcomes in patients receiving monotherapy. Hypertension 48(3):385-391, 2006.
81. Schrier RW, Estacio RO, Mehler PS, Hiatt WR: Appropriate blood pressure control in hypertensive and normotensive type 2 diabetes mellitus: A summary of the ABCD trial. Nat Clin Pract Nephrol 3(8):428-438, 2007.
82. Allemann Y, Fraile B, Lambert M, Barbier M, Ferber P, Izzo JL Jr. : Efficacy of the combination of amlodipine and valsartan in patients with hypertension uncontrolled with previous monotherapy: The Exforge in Failure after Single Therapy (EX-FAST study). J Clin Hypertens 10(3):185-194, 2008.
83. Jamerson K, Weber MA, Bakris GL: Benazepril plus amlodipine or hydrochlorothiazide for hypertension in high-risk patients. N Engl J Med 359:2417-2428, 2008.
84. Skerrett PJ: Tricky forecast: Low pressure, In Lee TH, editor: Harvard Heart Letter, Vol. 14(3), Boston, 2003, Harvard Health Publications.
85. Lundborg P, Aström H, Bengtsson C, et al: Effect of beta-adrenoceptor blockade on exercise performance and metabolism. Clin Sci 61:299-305, 1981.
86. van Baak MA, Mooij JM, Schiffers PM: Exercise and the pharmacokinetics of propranolol, verapamil, and atenolol. Eur J Clin Pharmacol 43:547-550, 1992.
87. Swain R, Kaplan B: Treating hypertension in active patients. Physician Sportsmed 25(9):268-272, 1997.
88. Tomten SE, Kjeldsen SE, Nilsson S, Westheim AS. : Effect of alpha 1-adrenoceptor blockade on maximal VO_2 and endurance capacity in well-trained athletic hypertensive men. Am J Hypertens 7:603-608, 1994.
89. van Baak MA, Mooij JMV, Schiffers PMH: Exercise and the pharmacokinetics of propranolol, verapamil and atenolol. Eur J Clin Pharmacol 43:547-550, 1992.
90. Palatini P, Bongiovi S, Mario L, Mormino P, Raule G, Pessina AC. : Effects of ACE inhibition on endurance exercise haemodynamics in trained subjects with mild hypertension. Eur J Pharmacol 48:435-439, 1995.
91. Prospective Studies Collaboration: Age-specific relevance of usual blood pressure to vascular mortality: A meta-analysis of individual data for one million adults in 61 prospective studies. Lancet 360:1903-1913, 2002.

7

Drug Therapy for Coronary Atherosclerosis and Its Repercussions

Barbara Gladson

ISCHEMIC HEART DISEASE

Coronary blood flow is normally closely related to myocardial oxygen consumption, both at rest and during exercise. However, there are several factors that can alter coronary flow, creating a mismatch between perfusion (supply of oxygen) and demand. Ischemic heart disease or coronary artery disease (CAD) occurs when there is a lack of oxygen to the myocardium, usually resulting from coronary artery narrowing. This ischemic disease may present as unstable angina and acute myocardial infarction (MI) with specific electrocardiographic changes, chronic stable exertional angina, or ischemia caused by a vasospasm of the coronary vessels.

PATHOPHYSIOLOGY AND TREATMENT OF ISCHEMIC HEART DISEASE AND ANGINA

Heart rate, contractility, and wall stress (intraventricular pressure, ventricular volume, and wall thickness) during systole are the major determinants of myocardial oxygen demand (MVO_2).[1] Because the heart is continuously contracting, its oxygen needs are high; the heart uses 75% of the available oxygen, even at rest, leaving little reserve for other physical activities. Therefore, MVO_2 is a critical factor in producing ischemia because increased activity demands a greater oxygen supply (i. e. , perfusion); however, this value is usually fixed as a result of disease in the coronary arteries. Increased demand for oxygen in the normal heart is met by increasing coronary blood flow.

An indirect method for measuring MVO_2 is to calculate the "double product" (heart rate × systolic blood pressure).[2] Because coronary blood flows during the period of diastole, oxygen delivery is related to the duration of diastole. As heart rate increases and diastole shortens, the heart's demand for oxygen increases. Oxygen demand is also related to vascular tone. During systole, the heart must contract with a force that exceeds aortic pressure to eject blood. Therefore, the higher the blood pressure, the greater is the need for oxygen.

Coronary blood flow is inversely related to the diameter of the vessel to the fourth power.[1] Therefore, the diameter of the atherosclerotic lesion is a major determinant of resistance influencing coronary perfusion. A critical loss of perfusion occurs when the lesion extends across 70 to 80% of the diameter. At 80% or above, blood flow is so compromised that the nutrition needs of the myocardium are unmet even at rest and ischemia occurs.[3] However, lesions smaller than this may still cause problems if vasospasm is superimposed. In addition, little reserve exists for coronary flow, so problems begin to occur as activity and exercise increase the demand for blood flow.

Abnormalities in ventricular contraction impose further burdens on the remaining heart tissue, resulting in increased MVO_2, depletion of available oxygen, and, eventually, cardiac failure. Zones of reduced perfusion develop and are at risk for more ischemia, especially if the demand for oxygen is ongoing. The nonischemic areas of the heart attempt to compensate by developing more tension in an effort to maintain cardiac output, further increasing oxygen demand. In addition, the neurochemical and metabolic factors and the neural reflexes activated to reverse the diminished perfusion begin to fail. Severe coronary atherosclerosis increases the sensitivity of the coronary arteries to catecholamines and α_1-stimulation. The direct effect is vasoconstriction of the arteries both at rest and during activity, further increasing ischemia and pain. See Figure 7-1 for a summary of factors affecting the balance between oxygen supply and demand.

Within recent years there has been much focus directed on the role of oxidative stress and endothelial dysfunction.[4] Normal endothelial function depends on a balance between nitric oxide (NO), which reduces vascular tone, and reactive oxygen species such as hydrogen peroxide, which move the balance in the direction of vasoconstriction, inflammation, and thrombosis. NO is

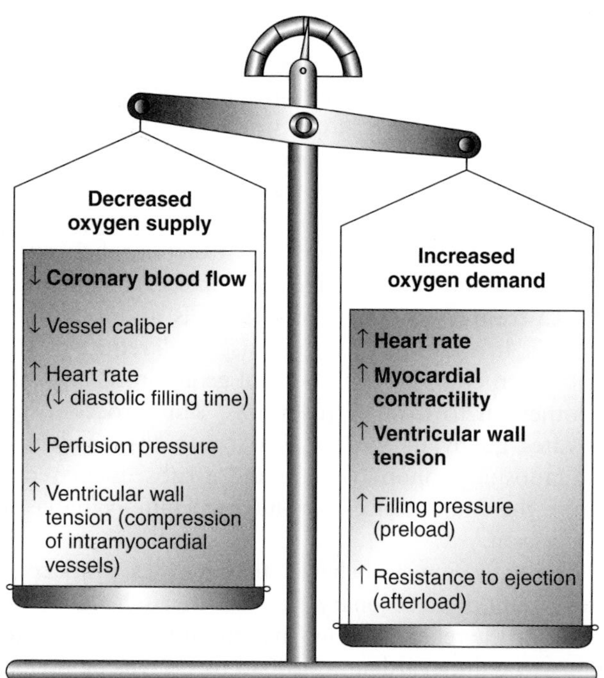

FIGURE 7-1 Factors affecting the balance of oxygen supply and demand in angina.

synthesized from L-arginine and molecular oxygen by the enzyme NO synthase. Endothelial NO synthesis appears to be released by "shear stress." Increased levels of oxidative stress lead to a reduction in NO activity. Much of the imbalance is the result of the common risk factors for cardiovascular disease, which include smoking, diabetes, dyslipidemia, and hypertension. Specifically, oxidized low-density lipoprotein (LDL) inactivates NO.

Small, dense LDL particles which contain a higher oxidized LDL in their lipid cores contribute to atherogenicity.[5,6] In particular, these particles can easily penetrate into the arterial wall and promote plaque instability. Further changes occur in the arterial wall (increased expression of matrix proteins, and growth factors), particularly when combined with elevated blood pressure, which results in structural changes such as decreased lumen diameter and thickened intimal media.

Endothelial dysfunction creates or at least adds to an inflammatory state.[7] The chemoattractant proteins (chemokines) that are released draw monocytes to the vessel wall; monocytes absorb oxidized LDL to become foam cells. These foam cells are the contributory factor for the formation of fatty streaks initially; then with further vascular remodeling and lipid uptake, these streaks become large plaques with necrotic centers, thin fibrous caps, and macrophages. Macrophages become activated by T cells into releasing metalloproteinases that break down the fibrous cap, and the plaque ruptures producing a sudden coronary event. Macrophage accumulation, which is associated with high levels of fibrinogen and cross-reactive (C-reactive) protein, has become a marker for predicting atherosclerotic cardiovascular disease.[8,9]

When plaque ruptures, the lipid core becomes exposed to blood, which then activates the coagulation pathway and initiates thrombus formation.[3] Platelets adhere to the area and assist in the formation of thrombin. Thrombin, in turn, converts fibrinogen into fibrin strands, which trap additional blood cells and platelets. What results is a large clot that may even completely block an artery. Thus what has been described here is a continuum of cardiovascular disease, starting with small changes in the diameter of the coronary arteries, which grow into a large plaque impairing coronary perfusion producing areas of ischemia and pain.[10] Ultimately, coronary perfusion may become so impaired that heart tissue becomes necrotic leading to a MI.

Even with some pharmaceutical agents that are designed to be potent arteriole dilators producing strong dilation of resistance vessels, ischemia may still continue. A fixed stenosis will greatly affect the collateral blood flow and the patient's response to activity and exercise in what has been labeled a *coronary steal*. Well-perfused tissue that is able to dilate will actually "steal" blood away from areas with fixed stenosis, which results in greater ischemia, especially if superimposed on vasospasm. Perfusion is compromised, and the vessels distal to the area of the fixed stenosis collapse. This makes treating angina a challenge.

Clinical Presentation of Angina

When demand for myocardial oxygen exceeds supply, ischemia develops and produces some typical signs and symptoms, including chest pain (angina) and ST-segment depression on an electrocardiogram. Patients often complain of pressure or the sensation of a heavy weight on their chests. They may also have a burning sensation or just a feeling of tightness in the chest. Shortness of breath along with a constrictive feeling around the larynx or upper trachea may occur. The location of the pain varies and may be limited to the sternum, left shoulder and arm, lower jaw, or lower cervical and upper thoracic spine. Radiation of pain to the left arm, and occasionally to the right arm, may occur. The typical anginal pain lasts from 30 seconds to 30 minutes and can be precipitated by exercise, a cold environment, emotional factors, walking against the wind, or walking after a large meal.

There are three major recognized forms of angina: exertional (stable), variant (Prinzmetal's), and unstable angina.[10,11] Exertional, or exercise-induced, angina is the most frequent type seen in patients with CAD. Usually, patients with exertional angina are free of pain at rest, but when a load is imposed on the heart, as with exercise, the supply of oxygen cannot meet the demand. Pain usually occurs at some predicted level of exertion, and there is a fixed narrowing of the coronary vessels.

Prinzmetal's angina results from a coronary spasm. Symptoms can occur at rest, usually during the night or in the early morning. In contrast to stable angina, ST-segment elevation may be seen during periods of pain. Pain is not usually experienced during exertion or emotional stress, and it is not typically relieved by rest.

Unstable angina is characterized by chest pain that increases in frequency, severity, and/or duration. Pain also occurs with less and less exertion and may even be present at rest. Unstable angina is often stratified into categories according to risk of impending nonfatal or fatal MI because it often occurs before an MI. Anginal episodes may occur with minimal activity, indicating a change from the predictable level of exertion that produces stable angina. Plaque rupture within the coronary artery may underlie this syndrome.

Treatment of Angina

Drug therapy for chest pain depends on the type of angina experienced. For the relief of acute anginal attacks, nitrates—particularly sublingual nitrate—are the drugs of choice.[3] Sublingual nitrate provides almost immediate relief of symptoms and may also be used to prevent an attack if administered just before any activity. Patients with stable angina may be treated with a variety of drugs used on a prophylactic basis to prevent anginal attacks (Table 7-1). These include long-acting nitrates, β-blockers, and calcium channel blockers. Nitrates, β-blockers, calcium channel blockers, aspirin, potassium channel openers, thrombin modulators, and some new agents called ranolazine and trimetazidine are part of the treatment regimen for unstable angina, in addition to surgical management such as coronary artery bypass graft or percutaneous transluminal coronary artery angioplasty. The goal in this case is to reduce pain and prevent progression to an MI. Variant angina is treated with drugs that dilate the coronary arteries, including nitrates, which may be used along with a calcium channel blocker.

Nitrates. Nitrates (nitroglycerin, isosorbide dinitrate, and isosorbide mononitrate) dilate the systemic veins and arterioles as well as the large and medium-sized coronary arteries.[12] Nitrates exert particular effects on the collateral vessels in the heart and thereby bypass the stiff and plaque-filled areas of the coronary arteries. Veins respond to the lowest dose of nitrates, and arteries respond to higher doses. Nitrates work directly on vascular smooth muscle as opposed to exerting action through a specific receptor. The exact mechanism of action is unknown, but evidence points to the liberation of NO from vascular endothelial cells and even from platelets. In addition, the nitrate itself will reduce to NO, which then combines with a thiol group in the vascular endothelium to form nitrosothiols. This process, then, activates guanylate cyclase, leading to the production of guanosine monophosphate and a subsequent reduction in the amount of intracellular calcium available for contraction.[13]

Originally, it was believed that nitrates produced a redistribution of coronary flow to the ischemic areas. However, the relief of angina may result from the nitrate's ability to reduce cardiac workload by decreasing preload and afterload.[11] Vasodilation of venous capacitance vessels, which causes a reduction in venous return and left ventricular filling pressure (preload), decreases ventricular wall tension and thus myocardial oxygen demand. Arterial resistance vessels (mainly the large arteries) dilate, producing a reduced resistance to ventricular emptying (afterload), which also decreases oxygen demand. Coronary artery dilation may occur as well, but to a limited extent. The specific beneficial effects of nitrates include decreases in ventricular volume, arterial pressure, ejection time, and ventricular diastolic pressure, as well as vasodilation of epicardial coronary arteries. Since the drug targets the collateral vessels, it does not produce the "coronary steal phenomenon."[11]

Nitrates come in a variety of forms, including intravenous (IV), sublingual, and topical preparations; a lingual

TABLE 7-1 Treatment for Stable Angina

Drug	Mechanism	⇧Time to Onset of ST Segment Depression	Anginal Episodes	Other Effects
β-blockers	Decreases O_2 consumption	+	+	
Calcium Blockers	Decreases O_2 consumption; Increases coronary blood flow	+	+	May prevent progression of atherosclerosis; Steal syndrome
Nitrates	Increases coronary blood flow	+	+	Antiplatelet effects
Ranolazine	Inhibits I_{Na} channel	+	+	
Ivabradine	Slows heart rate	+	+	
Nicorandil	Opens K+ channels and releases nitrates	+	+	

(Adapted from Ben-Dor I, Battler A: Treatment of stable angina, *Heart* 93:868–874, 2007.)

spray; chewable and oral tablets; and patches (Box 7-1). These preparations have different durations of action: the oral and transdermal forms are the long-acting versions for controlling the frequency of anginal attacks, and the sublingual, transmucosal, and chewable tablet preparations are the short-acting, quick responders. Most patients wear the transdermal patch for 12 hours during the day and carry sublingual nitroglycerin tablets for added exertional periods. Tolerance to nitrates develops quickly, so it is recommended that patients be free of the drug for at least 8 hours a day, preferably during sleep, to avoid this effect.[14] The patch must be placed above the elbow, preferably on the chest, for full effectiveness.

Sublingual nitroglycerin is kept in a tightly closed brown bottle that limits the drug's exposure to light.[12] It is kept in a glass container because it tends to adhere to plastic surfaces. It has a short shelf-life, maintaining potency for only 6 months, and 90 days after the bottle has been opened, any remaining tablets must be discarded. Patients are instructed to place a tablet under the tongue and let it dissolve, which takes 20 to 30 seconds. The drug will produce a gentle tingling or burning sensation if it is still active. If it does not produce this reaction, then the patient should obtain a prescription refill as soon as possible. Patients may also experience a vascular headache from meningeal artery vasodilation.[15]

Relief of angina should occur in 1 to 2 minutes. Drug action can be hastened by leaning forward in the sitting position and inhaling deeply. If at the end of 5 minutes, angina is still present, the patient may take a second dose. If another 5 minutes pass and the pain is still present, the patient may take a third sublingual dose. Up to three sublingual doses may be taken within 15 minutes. However, if pain is not relieved *after the first dose*, then the patient may be having an MI, and immediate transport to the hospital is warranted. Call 911 after first dose but patient can still take two additional doses.

Nitroglycerin is more effective when taken at the very beginning of chest discomfort or administered 5 to 10 minutes before an activity that might precipitate an acute attack, such as physical therapy. In practice, however, this is not usually done. Patients may reserve the medication for more severe episodes of pain that do not stop with cessation of activity. Some others have the notion that the less often they use nitroglycerin, the less serious is their cardiac condition. It is important for patients to understand that nitroglycerin is not addictive and that it is not a narcotic or a painkiller.

Therapeutic concerns with nitrates include monitoring for reflex tachycardia, dizziness, orthostatic hypotension, and weakness. Taking precautions against falls is warranted, especially with patients who are prone to orthostatic hypotension. Because nitrates cause vasodilation of arterioles and veins, thermal modalities that also cause vasodilation may exacerbate blood pooling in the lower extremities and lead to syncope. Long-term use of long-acting nitrates is associated with the development of abnormal hemoglobin, called *methemoglobin*, which compromises oxygen delivery. There exists a notion that long-term use of nitrates leads to the accumulation of oxygen-free radicals associated with further endothelial dysfunction.[16] This needs further study.

β-Blockers. β-Blockers are frequently used as initial therapy for stable angina along with short-acting nitrates in patients with no contraindications.[17] β-Blockers reduce myocardial oxygen demand by decreasing contractility and exertional tachycardia, which relieves angina. In patients with stable angina, the dose can be titrated to reduce resting heart rate to 55 to 60 beats/min. The dose should also be adjusted to limit exercise heart rate to within 75% of the rate that produces chest pain.[18] These drugs should be avoided in patients with bradycardia, asthma, hypotension, and heart block. Nebivolol is a new β-blocker that also enhances NO release to produce vasodilation and may be particularly useful in treating stable angina.[19]

β-blockers should not be used to treat angina due to coronary artery spasms (variant angina).[20] Since these drugs have no direct action on the coronary arteries and blocking of β-receptors may actually exacerbate β-adrenergic–mediated vasoconstriction of these vessels, vasospasm may worsen.

Calcium Channel Blockers. Because calcium in cardiac and smooth muscle is a key component for initiating contraction, blocking calcium channels reduces contractility and arteriole tone. Two types of calcium channels are known to exist in the heart: the L-type and the T-type.[21] The L-type channel produces a long, large, and high-threshold current, whereas the T-type channel produces a short, small, and low-threshold current. They are also active during different phases of the cardiac action potential. T-type channels may contribute to diastolic depolarization (phase 4), that is, they are involved in helping the sinoatrial node reach its threshold for depolarization. L-type channels are active during the upstrokes (phase 0) of the sinoatrial and atrioventricular nodal action potentials, and also during phases 1 and 2 of the ventricular and atrial muscle action potentials

BOX 7-1 Nitrate Preparations

Drug	Preparation
Nitrates & Nitrites	
Isosorbide dinitrate	Oral (Isordil), chewable tablets, sublingual
Isosorbide mononitrate	Oral (Ismo)
Nitroglycerin	Sublingual, buccal, metered-dose aerosol spray, oral (Nitro-Time), parenteral, transdermal (Nitro-Dur, Transderm-Nitro) patches, topical ointment (Nitro-Bid)

(see Chapter 8).[22] Therefore, the drugs that block calcium channels reduce cardiac contractility throughout the heart (reducing oxygen demand) and decrease sinoatrial and atrioventricular nodal activity. Smooth muscle contraction is also reduced, producing vasodilation (reducing preload and afterload). The calcium channel blockers in current clinical use block only the L-type channels.

As mentioned previously, there are three types of calcium channel blockers currently on the market. They differ in their vascular selectivity, with the dihydropyridines (e. g., nifedipine and amlodipine) having a greater ratio of vascular smooth muscle effects relative to the cardiac effects, compared with phenethyl alkylamines (e. g., verapamil and bepridil) and dibenzazepines (diltiazem). Verapamil and diltiazem reduce cardiac contractility and, in higher doses, slow conduction through nodal tissue.

Calcium channel blockers reduce and prevent the chest pain in stable angina associated with exercise as a result of a negative inotropic effect, which decreases myocardial oxygen demand. In addition, some of these drugs (diltiazem and nicardipine) have been shown to produce vasodilation in stenotic coronary arteries during exercise, preventing the coronary steal phenomenon.[23] However, some of the calcium channel blockers, particularly those in the dihydropyridine group, have induced this effect. The nondihydropyridine agents lower myocardial oxygen demand to a greater degree than do the dihydropyridines; however, if there is left ventricular function or a low heart rate, the dihydropyridine agents would be the preferred drug category.[14] Short-acting dihydropyridines have also been used to prevent variant angina, but there is evidence that these formulations increase the risk for MI.[24,25] They can produce reflex sympathetic stimulation in response to systemic vasodilation. In addition, the use of short-acting agents results in fluctuating drug levels, with reflex activity occurring during lower plasma levels of the drug. This sympathetic activity can produce a rather intense increase in heart rate and myocardial contractility that is not well tolerated by some patients. This effect can be avoided by giving the drug with a β-blocker or switching to longer-acting calcium channel blockers. A large meta-analysis completed in 1999 in which 143 studies were examined indicated that β-blockers produced outcomes similar to those achieved with calcium channel blockers but with fewer adverse effects.[20,26] However, in many of these studies the short-acting nifedipine was used, which is the formulation carrying greater risk. Calcium channel blockers are often used along with either β-blockers or nitrates. The combination of a dihydropyridine and a β-blocker produces only a small risk of heart block, but the use of verapamil or diltiazem along with a β-blocker is contraindicated because of the excessive depression of cardiac function caused by the combination.[3]

Many investigators have attempted to compare calcium channel blockers with both β-blockers and nitrates for the treatment of stable angina. In several randomized reports, with a combined total of approximately 2000 patients, calcium channel blockers were found to be as effective as β-blockers in reducing angina and increasing exercise time.[18] Other studies show that amlodipine is as effective as isosorbide dinitrate (a long-acting nitrate) in relieving exercise-induced angina. Several comparative studies have been performed, although not recently, that have shown little difference in these agents in reducing angina.[27] However, β-blockers continue to have a class I recommendation over calcium channel blockers.[14]

The adverse effects of these drugs are, in fact, extensions of their therapeutic effects.[2] The adverse effects associated with the dihydropyridines include dizziness, flushing of the skin, hypotension, reflex tachycardia, and peripheral edema. Verapamil and diltiazem can produce bradycardia, hypotension, congestive heart failure, heart block, and constipation.

Potassium Channel Openers. Nicorandil opens an adenosine triphosphate (ATP)–sensitive potassium channel, which allows the flow of potassium out of the cell, thus hyperpolarizing the cell membrane.[11] The more negative membrane potential inhibits the opening of the L-type calcium channels, producing vasodilation in the systemic and coronary arteries. Because of its relatively short half-life, this drug has not been widely used. It also produces a headache and significant reflex activation of the sympathetic nervous system, as well as dizziness, nausea, and vomiting.

Newer Antianginal Drugs. Ranolazine is a new antianginal drug that inhibits the late I_{Na} (sodium channel) and increases its action potential duration.[28,29] It is theorized that ischemia leads to the opening of this channel, thus increasing intracellular sodium accumulation. This elevated sodium level exchanges with calcium (three sodium ions exchange with one calcium ion per cycle) at the sarcolemma, bringing calicum back into the myocyte. This results in more intracellular calcium during diastole and activates contractile proteins, which increases energy consumption. The uniqueness of this drug is that it does not suppress systolic function. Adverse events include constipation, nausea, and dizziness. Studies are ongoing, but they do show the efficacy of these drugs in patients with stable angina and also an improvement in exercise performance in this patient group.

Ivabradine inhibits a channel in the sinus node producing bradycardia but without affecting contractility.[30] It increases exercise time and also reduces the number of anginal episodes. Early studies show that it might be as effective as atenolol.

Therapeutic Regimens

The choice of a drug or a combination of drugs for the treatment of stable angina depends on the presence of coexisting medical conditions and the patient's individual response. β-Blockers and nitrates are frequently used together because the combination seems to be more effective than when each drug is used alone. β-blockers reduce the reflex tachycardia caused by nitrates, and nitrates reduce the bradycardia produced by β-blockers. Nitrates are also more effective when given along with calcium channel blockers.

In patients who have both mild chronic stable angina and hypertension, monotherapy with a long-acting calcium channel blocker or β-blocker may adequately control symptoms. For more moderate symptoms, the β-blocker–calcium channel blocker combination is effective, but a patient may also respond well to two different calcium channel blockers, nifedipine and verapamil.

Nitrates and calcium channel blockers are effective in the treatment of variant angina. The mechanism for relief in this case is prevention of coronary artery spasm. Calcium channel blockers from all the categories can be effective in the treatment of this condition.

THROMBOSIS AND ANTITHROMBOTIC THERAPY

Platelet aggregation and vasoconstriction initiate the hemostatic process. When endothelial cells are damaged, platelets bind to the damaged vessel through the interaction of platelet glycoprotein (GP) receptors (GP Ib/IX and GP Ia/IIb) and exposed endothelial collagen.[3] The platelet becomes activated and releases thromboxane A_2 (TXA_2), adenosine diphosphate (ADP), epinephrine, von Willebrand's factor, fibrinogen, calcium, and serotonin. These substances activate and recruit other platelets into the growing thrombus. Similar substances are also released from the damaged vessel. Platelets furnish a surface on which clotting factors can bind and facilitate the conversion of prothrombin to thrombin (factor IIa). Thrombin converts fibrinogen to insoluble fibrin, assisting in the formation of a stable, insoluble clot. The activation of the platelet leads to a conformational change in the platelet glycoprotein receptors GP IIb/IIIa on the cell surface. These receptors then provide binding sites for fibrinogen molecules and adhesive molecules (von Willebrand's factor, fibronectin) and other platelets (Figure 7-2). TXA_2 is key in this cascade because not only does it promote platelet aggregation, but it also inhibits prostacyclin (a vasodilator) and neutralizes endogenous heparin produced by the vascular endothelium, all of which enhances coagulation.

The pathways that follow platelet aggregation involve a series of reactions leading to the generation of thrombin. This response to vascular injury involves many cells

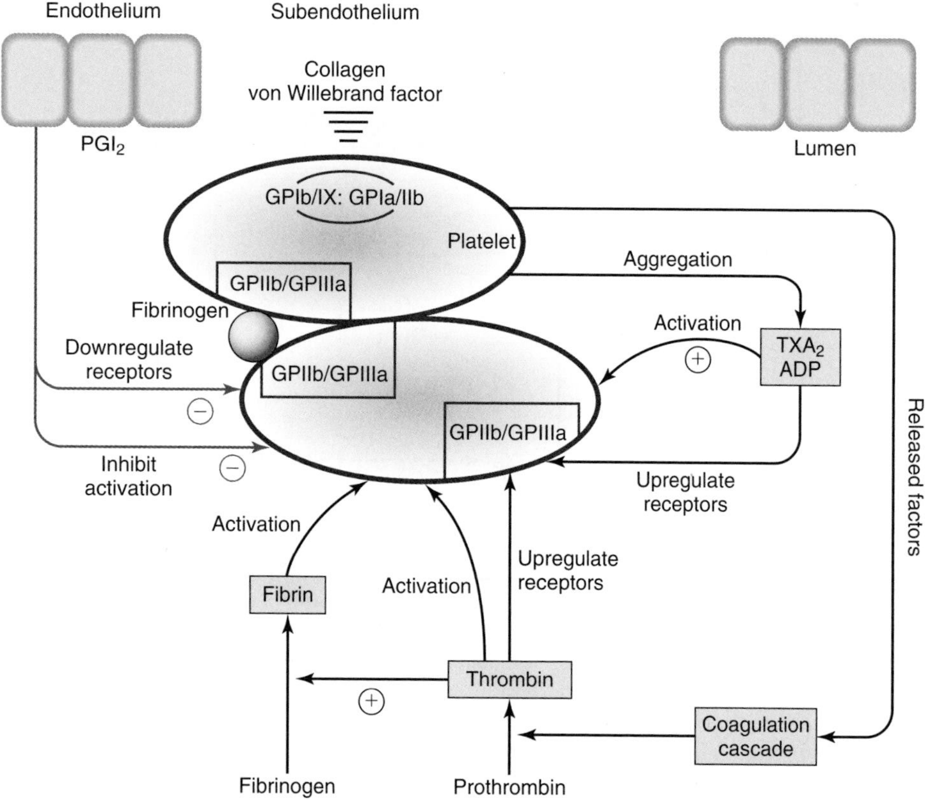

FIGURE 7-2 Platelets and platelet aggregation. Subendothelial macromolecules, such as collagen, interact with glycoprotein receptors (GP Ib/IX and GP Ia/IIb) on platelets, causing activation of platelets and upregulation of GP IIb/GP IIIa receptors, which are cross-linked by fibrinogen during aggregation. Synthesis of the proaggregatory thromboxane A_2 (TXA_2) and release of adenosine diphosphate (ADP) and 5-hydroxytryptamine occur. TXA_2 and thrombin cause further platelet activation and release of proaggregatory platelet contents. This leads to further upregulation of GP IIb/GP IIIa receptors. Prostacyclin (PGI_2) from endothelial cells inhibits activation and upregulation of GP IIb/GP IIIa receptors. Thrombin is generated by the action of factor Xa on prothrombin.

(platelets, leukocytes, and endothelial cells) along with the plasma blood-clotting proteins that ultimately form a fibrin clot and initiate inflammation and repair. The cascade of events leading to this final product is usually described as involving two distinct pathways, the extrinsic and intrinsic pathways (Figure 7-3). However, these pathways join forces to form the final common pathway, activation of factor X, and subsequent conversion of prothrombin (factor II) to thrombin (factor IIa) (Box 7-2).

The extrinsic system is initiated by the release of tissue thromboplastin (factor III) from damaged tissue.[31] A complex forms between this tissue factor and factor VIIa and calcium, followed by the sequential activation of factors VII, X, and prothrombin (factor II). The function of this pathway is measured by prothrombin time (PT) or by the international normalized ratio (INR).[32]

The intrinsic pathway begins when the exposed collagen acts in conjunction with kallikrein to activate factor XII to XIIa.[31] Several other factors become activated, and this pathway also joins the final common pathway. The function of this pathway is measured by the activated partial thromboplastin time (aPTT).[32]

The final common pathway involves the conversion of prothrombin into thrombin, which, in turn, converts fibrinogen to a stable clot. Thrombin also activates other coagulation factors to amplify its own production, as well as attracting platelets and white cells to the area of the clot. The intrinsic and extrinsic pathways are much slower than platelet aggregation and vasoconstriction.

Three categories of drugs are used to treat the various stages or conditions of thrombosis. The platelet aggregator inhibitors (aspirin, clopidogrel, ticlopidine) are used prophylactically to prevent formation of a platelet clot. Anticoagulants such as heparin and warfarin prevent the extension of a clot already present, and thrombolytics lyse a clot that has recently formed.

Antiplatelet Agents

Several agents are designed to prevent platelet plugs from forming and thus can be beneficial in preventing injury from stroke and MI. These agents include aspirin, ADP receptor antagonists, and glycoprotein IIb/IIIa receptor blockers.

Aspirin. Although aspirin has been primarily recommended for unstable angina (see below), it is also given to patients with cardiac disease to treat stable angina

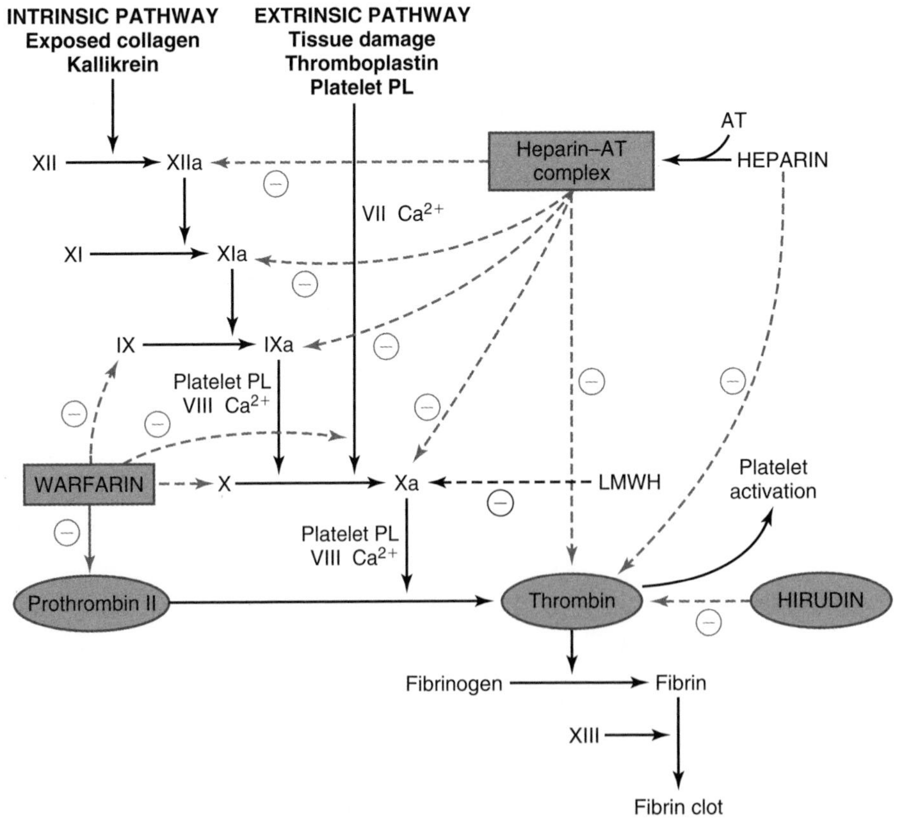

FIGURE 7-3 The coagulation cascade and action of anticoagulants. The complex cascade of clotting factor synthesis is initiated extrinsically by tissue damage. Activation of the clotting factors after damage requires platelet factors and calcium (Ca^{2+}). The provision of platelet products is further enhanced by the formation of thrombin, which then activates further platelets, as well as causing fibrin formation. Heparin acts at various sites in the cascade by activating the anticlotting factor antithrombin (AT) and inhibiting the activating protease clotting factors shown. Low-molecular-weight heparin (LMWH) acts on factor Xa. Hirudin inhibits thrombin (IIa) formation. Warfarin inhibits the synthesis of the vitamin K–dependent clotting factors VII, IX, X, and II (prothrombin). Roman numerals indicate the individual clotting factors. *PL*, Platelet phospholipid.

BOX 7-2 Blood Clotting Factors

Factor	Name	Target for:
I	Fibrinogen	
II	Prothrombin	Heparin, warfarin
III	Tissue thromboplastin	
IV	Calcium	
V	Proaccelerin	
VII	Proconvertin	Warfarin
VIII	Antihemophilic factor (AHF)	
IX	Christmas factor, plasma thromboplastin component	Warfarin
X	Stuart-Prower factor	Heparin, warfarin
XI	Plasma thromboplastin antecedent (PTA)	
XII	Hageman factor	
XIII	Fibrin-stabilizing factor	
Proteins C and S		Warfarin
Plasminogen		Thrombolytic enzymes

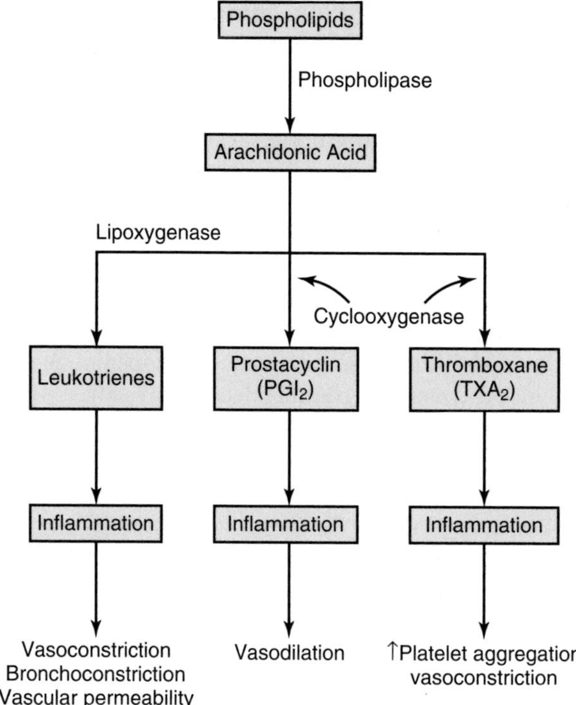

FIGURE 7-4 Mechanism of action of aspirin. Aspirin blocks the activity of cyclooxygenase and reduces the formation of prostacyclin and thromboxane A_2.

and for a generalized cardioprotective effect to lower the risk of an MI.[33] The goal in this case is to prevent a stable thrombosis from rupturing and producing unstable angina and a subsequent MI. Aspirin inhibits the action of the cyclooxygenase enzyme COX to block the conversion of arachidonic acid to prostaglandins and thromboxin (TXA_2) (Figure 7-4).[34] The aspirin achieves this by binding to the platelet irreversibly for the life of the platelet, thus inhibiting platelet aggregation for approximately 8 days. Thus platelet function is diminished for this period and results in prolonged bleeding time.

A loading dose of 325 mg of aspirin, followed by a daily dose of 80 mg, is recommended to reduce platelet aggregation and thus the incidence of angina and MI.[35] A higher dose is needed to produce an anti-inflammatory response. Chewable tablets are recommended for patients with chest pain and for those who might be having an MI. Chewed tablets will promote buccal rather than gastrointestinal (GI) absorption. Normal platelet function will return 36 hours after the last dose of the drug has been given because of the release of new platelets.[36] Aspirin reduces the incidence of death in acute MIs and also reduces the incidence of reinfarction, transient ischemic attacks, and stroke. This treatment reduces the risk of MI in patients with angina by 34%, by 46% in patients with unstable angina, and by 22 to 25% in patients with a previous MI, stroke, atrial fibrillation or peripheral arterial disease.[37] However, this does not completely reduce platelet activation because other pathways that enhance aggregation still exist. Women appear to benefit from a reduced risk of stroke but not of MI, whereas men may benefit by a reduction in both events.[38] Chewable aspirin at a dose of 162 mg to 325 mg can be given to patients presenting with acute coronary symptoms to achieve a reduction in mortality.[3] Aspirin may be combined with other antiplatelet agents such as ADP blockers, heparin, or warfarin for additive effects.

Adverse effects associated with aspirin include bleeding and GI irritation; however, there is still a positive benefit/risk ratio in patients who are taking aspirin for secondary prevention of cardiac events.[39] Tinnitus and central nervous system toxicity occur at higher doses, and bronchoconstriction may occur in susceptible patients. Taking a nonsteroidal anti-inflammatory agent (NSAID) concurrently with aspirin will reduce its cardioprotective effects unless the aspirin is administered at least 2 hours prior to the NSAID.[40,41] In physical therapy, deep tissue work, friction massage, and vigorous mobilization are contraindicated with the administration of aspirin. Patients receiving aspirin should be observed for bruising, joint swelling, blood in stools or urine, and bleeding from mucous membranes—all of which may mean that the dose is too high. See Chapter 11 for additional information on aspirin.

There is a growing group of physicians who suggest that low-dose aspirin be withdrawn from their patients. This is mostly in reaction to the growing number of gastritis cases, the development of anemia, and the need for renal dialysis in patients on this drug. In addition, aspirin interferes with the benefits achieved by an ACE inhibitor. It is argued that patients with a high risk of these complications have been excluded from studies, so the true benefit/risk ratio has not been determined.[42]

Adenosine Diphosphate Receptor Antagonists. Ticlopidine and clopidogrel block ADP-activated platelet aggregation, reducing the expression of GP IIb and IIIa receptors. Both are slightly more effective than aspirin in preventing recurrent stroke and transient ischemic attacks and are used separately or in combination with aspirin to prevent MI and in acute coronary syndromes without ST-segment elevation.[43,44] In addition, ticlopidine is used during stent placement to prevent thrombosis after percutaneous transluminal angioplasty. These drugs have an effect on bleeding similar to that of aspirin, but ticlopidine also produces neutropenia. A complete blood count is recommended 10 days after administration of the drug is started. As with aspirin, it takes 7 to 10 days for normal platelet function to return after these drugs have been discontinued.[45] It is important to monitor patients for excessive bleeding, since 10% of patients stop taking clopidogrel due to superficial or "nuisance" bleeding as defined by bleeding from small cuts, petechia, and bruising.[46]

Glycoprotein IIb/IIIa Receptor Blockers. Abciximab, eptifibatide, and tirofiban are given intravenously to patients undergoing angioplasty for the prevention of acute coronary events and to those undergoing fibrinolytic therapy.[47] These agents specifically inhibit the binding of fibrin and von Willebrand's factor to the glycoprotein receptors. Platelet inhibition occurs quickly (with maximum inhibition of platelet aggregation at 2 hours) but is reversed within 48 hours after the infusion is stopped. Adverse effects include bleeding, especially in older adults and patients with low body weight. The patients benefiting from this therapy are those who are in the acute phase of a coronary syndrome with ST segment changes on electrocardiogram (ECG) and those who are about to receive a percutaneous intervention.

Dipyridamole. Dipyridamole is used as a pharmacologic stressor to detect myocardial ischemia in patients who are unable to exercise.[48] It reduces the expression of GP IIb/IIIa platelet receptors but also inhibits the uptake of adenosine released by tissues when they are hypoxic. The excess adenosine produces vasodilation of the small resistance coronary arteries, which may already be maximally dilated. The net effect, therefore, is diversion of blood away from the ischemic area, which produces the coronary steal phenomenon. The heart is imaged before dipyridamole administration at rest and again after drug administration by using technetium-labeled thallium to view the ischemic areas. However, dobutamine, a β-agonist, used along with echocardiography, has been used increasingly for a preoperative risk assessment in patients with cardiac disease.[49,50]

Anticoagulant Agents

Anticoagulants are agents that prevent or delay blood coagulation by inhibiting certain clotting factors. They are available in intravenous (IV), injectable, and oral forms. Usually, patients receive heparin while in the hospital but are switched over to oral warfarin before discharge.

Heparin. Unfractionated heparin (UFH) is a glycosaminoglycan consisting of D-glucosamine and uronic acid. The standard preparation produces a large molecule, with molecular weights ranging from 3000 to 30,000 kd, with the larger molecule labeled *unfractionated heparin* and the smaller molecules labeled *fractionated* or *lower molecular weight heparin (LMWH)*.[51] The varying weights of the heparin molecule affect the pharmacokinetics of the drug and make parenteral administration necessary. The higher the molecular weight, the more rapidly the drug is cleared from the circulation.

Heparin acts by binding to the circulating endogenous protein antithrombin III to activate it. This complex then neutralizes activated clotting factors, particularly factors Xa, IXa, and IIa (thrombin). Inactivation of these factors prevents the conversion of prothrombin to thrombin through the intrinsic pathway. Without the presence of heparin, this inactivation of thrombin occurs very slowly; with heparin, the reaction is increased 1000-fold.[35] Heparin's major effect on hemostasis is direct inhibition of thrombin and, to a lesser degree, inhibition of other clotting factors. Only UFH, which has a greater effect on thrombin than do the LMWHs, can inhibit platelet aggregation.

Heparin is given either intravenously or by subcutaneous injection. IV administration is preferred in emergency situations because there is a 1- to 2-hour delay in action when heparin is given subcutaneously. When given intravenously, heparin is administered by repeated bolus injections or by continuous IV infusion. Its rate of elimination is dose dependent. The half-life is 30 minutes at low doses (25 units/kg) but increases many-fold at higher doses (100 to 400 units/kg).

Heparin treatment requires close monitoring because the therapeutic index of heparin is low. The degree of anticoagulation is monitored with aPTT, the lab test that measures the intrinsic coagulation pathway, particularly factors V, VIII, IX, X, XI, XII, fibrinogen, and prothrombin. An aPTT value that is 1.5 to 2.5 times the upper limit of normal (28 to 42 seconds) or 1.5 to 2.5 times the pretherapy value used to be recommended, but the American College of Chest Physicians has recommended different values depending on the condition being treated.[52] Additional tests may be used for monitoring and for measuring activated clotting time (ACT), antifactor Xa, or antifactor IIa.

Heparin is used for preventing and treating deep venous thromboembolism (DVT), pulmonary embolism (PE), and arterial thrombosis in selected cases of MI. In addition, it is used to prevent clotting in catheters and clotting that may occur after certain surgeries (e.g., hip and knee arthroplasties).

Bleeding is a common problem with heparin but can be reversed quickly by administration of protamine sulfate, which combines with heparin and inactivates it. Heparin-induced thrombocytopenia, a disorder that is paradoxically prothrombotic, may also occur.[53] This disorder is defined as a 50% drop in the platelet count with concurrent heparin use. This may occur within 4 to 10 days after heparin exposure or may be delayed with a mean of 9 days after the drug has been discontinued. Patients who are re-exposed to heparin will develop thrombocytopenia much more rapidly. The clinical presentation of this reaction is tachycardia, dyspnea, fever, hypertension, nausea, and cardiac arrest. Frequent platelet monitoring is necessary to detect thrombocytopenia, and if it occurs, all sources of heparin must be immediately discontinued. In addition, patients should not be exposed to the LMWHs while on heparin therapy, since there is some cross-reactivity. Actual treatment depends on the clinical manifestations of the patient, and if anticoagulation is still needed, the direct thrombin inhibitors argatroban and lepirudin are recommended. Osteoporosis is another adverse effect of long-term use (more than 3 months).

The risks associated with heparin were well publicized in the media when in 2007 it was reported that actor Dennis Quaid's twins had been exposed to 1000 times the normal dose of heparin.[54] An error had occurred in mixing the drug, in part due to different strengths of the drug being manufactured in "look-alike" packaging. The actor's children survived, but in another incident in 2006, three children had died. In addition, around the same time of these mishaps, 81 deaths had occurred because of a contaminant that had been added to heparin during the manufacturing process in a plant in China. As a result of these problems, new regulations and further safeguards have been put into place in many of the nation's hospital pharmacies to reduce the number of look-alike drugs.

Low Molecular Weight Heparins. LMWH, which are approximately one third of the molecular weight of the unfractionated heparin, is obtained by hydrolysis of the much larger heparin molecules.[3] They have high antifactor Xa activity compared with heparin, which has high antifactor IIa activity. This smaller molecule has several advantages over the unfractionated drug. The half-life is about 4 hours, much longer than that of the standard preparation. It also has greater bioavailability and a more predictable anticoagulant effect, which results in less bleeding. The LMWHs have a limited effect on platelets, which is another reason that there is less bleeding as compared with unfractionated heparin. The dose is based on the weight of the patient as opposed to laboratory monitoring, which makes home administration easier.[55] LMWHs are much more predictable than heparin, with less binding to plasma proteins, greater bioavailability, and peak plasma activity is obtained within 1 to 5 hours. Even though the half-life is 4 to 5 hours, their antifactor activity continues for 24 hours.

LMWHs are given subcutaneously every 12 hours for up to 6 weeks after orthopedic surgery for the prevention of deep vein thrombosis (DVT). However, protocols do vary, and some patients may only receive injections until they are mobile. LMWHs are currently under study to determine their effectiveness compared with that of heparin for the treatment of DVT, PE, and acute MIs. All indications show that they are equal in efficacy to heparin in the management of patients with acute coronary syndromes, and in some trials with enoxaparin, they showed superior efficacy.[56,57] In many of these trials, there was less bleeding with LMW heparins than with the UFHs, although exceptions include older adults; low body weight patients; patients who are taking clopidogrel, NSAIDs, or warfarin; and those with renal dysfunction. However, there was no difference in the rates of death or MI at 30 days when given to high-risk patients with acute coronary syndrome (ACS) receiving percutaneous intervention.[58] The anticoagulant effect of LMWH appears to be less easily reversed with protamine than with that of UFH.

Warfarin (Vitamin K Antagonist). Warfarin is an oral anticoagulant that inhibits the production of a reduced form of vitamin K that is a necessary cofactor for the synthesis of several coagulation factors (factors II, IX, and X, and especially factor VII) in the liver. It is indicated for the prevention and treatment of venous thromboembolism and acute MI and in the prevention of emboli resulting from atrial fibrillation and prosthetic heart valves.[59-61]

Warfarin is highly bound to albumin (99%) in the plasma, and therefore numerous drugs and conditions interact with warfarin (Box 7-3). Some drugs that increase the activity of warfarin and increase bleeding tendency include antibiotics, aspirin, NSAIDs, cimetidine, metronidazole, and phenytoin.[35] Drugs that reduce its activity and lead to increased clotting include barbiturates, carbamazepine, and rifampin. Ingestion of large amounts of vegetables that contain vitamin K, such as broccoli and cauliflower, will also decrease warfarin's effectiveness.

Warfarin is metabolized by the P450 enzymes, and it has a long half-life (36 to 40 hours). However, the plasma concentration of warfarin does not correlate directly with drug activity. Treatment with warfarin requires 4 to 5 days to be fully effective, partly because clotting factors are already present and active when administration is started. Therefore, administration of warfarin is usually started along with heparin so that almost immediate anticoagulation is attained. After treatment is stopped, the anticoagulant effect continues until new clotting factors are synthesized (Box 7-4).

In many patients who receive long-term warfarin therapy, warfarin is often combined with aspirin for a superior effect. Monitoring of prothrombin time is necessary to evaluate the activity of factors II, V, VII, and X (the extrinsic coagulation pathway). Factor VII is the

BOX 7-3 Drugs and Conditions Interacting with Warfarin Activity

Antibiotics	+
Amiodarone	+
Cimetidine	+
Clofibrate	+
Fluconazole	+
Metronidazole	+
Phenytoin	+
Barbiturates	−
Carbamazepine	−
Griseofulvin	−
Nafcillin	−
Rifampin	−
Sucralfate	−
Age	+
Biliary disease	+
Congestive heart failure	+
Hyperthyroidism	+
Hypothyroidism	−
Nephrotic syndrome	−

(From Page C, Curtis MJ, Sutter MC, Walker MJ, Hoffman BB, editors: *Integrated pharmacology* (2nd ed.). Philadelphia, 2002, Mosby.)
+, Increased activity; –, decreased activity.

clotting factor that is most sensitive to vitamin K deficiency. The international normalized ratio (INR), which compares the patient's prothrombin time with a controlled value, is becoming the more accepted mode of measurement.[62] Normally, this value is under 2.0. With warfarin therapy, an INR between 2.0 and 3.0 is considered acceptable, but any higher number indicates a much greater risk of bleeding. Specifically, 2.0 to 2.5 is the goal for prophylaxis of DVT; 2.0 to 3.0 is the goal for thromboprophylaxis in hip and femoral surgery and in the treatment of transient ischemic attacks and in the prevention of thromboembolism in atrial fibrillation; and 3.0 to 4.5 is the goal for prevention of recurrent DVT and thrombosis with mechanical heart valves. Since frequent monitoring of INR levels is imperative to the success of the treatment, home INR testing units have recently become available.[63]

The major adverse effect of warfarin is bleeding. It may be treated by withdrawal of the drug and IV administration of vitamin K. Bleeding can then be controlled within 6 hours. In addition, fresh frozen plasma or clotting factors can be infused intravenously for an immediate coagulant effect.

Warfarin crosses the placenta and is highly teratogenic, producing fetal central nervous system problems and bleeding. Pregnant women with thrombosis can be treated with standard heparin or LMWH, which do not produce fetal abnormalities.

Other Antithrombotic Drugs. Four direct thrombin inhibitors are available: hirudin, argatroban, lepirudin,

BOX 7-4 Coagulation Modifiers

Drug Category	Primary Indication
Antiplatelet Agents	
Aspirin	Pain Prevention of MI and stroke
ADP Receptor Antagonists	
Ticlopidine (Aggrastat)	Inhibition of platelet aggregation Prevention of recurrence of thrombotic strokes and TIAs
Clopidogrel (Plavix)	Inhibition of platelet aggregation Reduction of atherosclerotic events; NSTEMI
Glycoprotein IIb/IIIa Receptor Blockers	
Abciximab (ReoPro)	Percutaneous coronary procedures to prevent acute stent thrombosis, NSTEMI
Tirofiban (Aggrastat)	Percutaneous coronary procedures to prevent acute stent thrombosis, NSEMI
Eptifibatide (Integrilin)	Unstable angina, MI, percutaneous coronary procedures
Anticoagulant Agents	
Heparin	Thrombosis/embolism, DVT, PE
Warfarin (Coumadin)-Vitamin K antagonist	Thromboprevention and treatment of DVT, unstable angina, post-MI
Fondaparinux (Arixtra)	DVT prophylaxis, especially in orthopedic surgery
Enoxaparin (Lovenox)-LMWH	Thromboprevention and treatment of DVT, PE, atrial fibrillation, post-MI
Dalteparin (Fragmin)-LMWH	Thrombosis/embolism, DVT, PE
Tinazparin (Innohep)-LMWH	Thrombosis/embolism, DVT, PE
Lepirudin (Refludan)-thrombin inhibitor	Heparin-induced thrombocytopenia
Argatroban (Argatroban)-thrombin inhibitor	Heparin-induced thrombocytopenia
Thrombolytics	
Alteplase (Activase)	STEMI, cerebral thrombosis, PE
Streptokinase (Streptase)	STEMI, PE
Urokinase (Abbokinase)	STEMI, PE
Reversal Drugs	
Protamine sulfate	Heparin antagonist
Vitamin K	Warfarin antagonist

MI, myocardial infarction; *TIA*, transient ischemic attack; *NSTEMI*, non–ST segment elevation MI; *DVT*, deep venous thrombosis; *PE*, pulmonary embolism; *STEMI*, ST segment elevation MI.

and bivalirudin.[64] Hirudin, lepirudin, and argatroban may be used for the treatment of heparin-induced thrombocytopenia, but bivalirudin can be used instead of heparin in patients undergoing percutaneous intervention.[65]

Fondaparinux is a factor Xa inhibitor.[3] It is an analog of the antithrombin binding area found on heparin and LMWH. It is currently approved for patients undergoing major orthopedic surgery for the prevention of venous thromboembolism (VTE). It may also be used for the initial treatment of a VTE instead of heparin or LMWH. Early studies in ACS show that it is as effective as enoxaparin with less bleeding with non–ST-segment elevation.[66]

Thrombolytic Agents

Thrombolytic agents actively dissolve blood clots by promoting the conversion of plasminogen to plasmin, which, in turn, hydrolyzes fibrin.[35] However, high amounts of thrombin are released from the lysed clot, necessitating concurrent administration of aspirin or heparin. Examples of these drugs include streptokinase, urokinase, alteplase, and reteplase.

The thrombolytic agents are given intravenously or intra-arterially in the emergency department. Time is a critical factor, since ischemia for more than 30 minutes can produce permanent cell damage. Quick reperfusion may save some of the myocardium, but after 4 to 6 hours only minimal reversal can be obtained. The goal is a "door-to-needle time" of less than 30 minutes, especially for acute coronary events with ST segment elevation.[3] Even if time to needle stick is short, perfusion to the damaged area may be slow to return due to microvascular injury and reperfusion issues related to platelet activation, embolization, reactive oxygen, and edema. Therefore, other agents are also administered (see below).

Infusions generally last for 3 to 24 hours but in the case of streptokinase may continue for 72 hours. Infusions are indicated in the initial treatment of acute peripheral vascular occlusion, DVT, PE, and acute MI. Choice of agent depends on the patient's diagnosis and risk factors. Alteplase activates plasminogen bound to fibrin, which is thought to keep the fibrinolysis somewhat local. This is one reason why this drug is preferred over others for treating cerebral thrombosis. As with the other antithrombotic drugs, hemorrhage is a major adverse effect because the patient is placed in a general lytic state. These drugs are contraindicated in patients with internal bleeding, recent stroke, healing wounds, and metastatic cancer.

Therapeutic Concerns with Antithrombotic Drugs

Certain physical therapy interventions are contraindicated for patients who are taking anticoagulants. Débridement and rigorous manual techniques, such as deep tissue massage or chest percussions, are contraindicated. Dressing changes and wound care must be performed carefully to prevent bleeding. The patient should be observed for nosebleeds; bruising; and pain in the back, abdomen, or joints because these symptoms may indicate internal bleeding. The patient should also be asked to watch for blood in the urine or black, tarry stools, particularly after exercise.

PHARMACOLOGIC PREVENTION AND MANAGEMENT OF DEEP VEIN THROMBOSIS AND PULMONARY EMBOLISM

The balance between clot formation and lysis is intricately related to three factors that have been collectively labeled Virchow's triad.[67] The first is venous stasis, which is likely to develop from decreased velocity of blood flow, venous dilation and pooling, or venous obstruction. Venous stasis inhibits the blood's ability to dissipate locally activated clotting factors, leading to clot formation. Vessel wall injury is the second factor leading to DVT. Microtears in the vessel wall caused by distension or direct injury from a fracture, surgery, sepsis, or burn injury also damage the vessel's endothelial lining, further accelerating clotting. The lining becomes rough, causing platelet aggregation and adhesion. Even general anesthesia, by decreasing vascular tone, can disrupt the endothelial lining, increasing the patient's risk for DVT. The third factor that may be present in patients with DVT is a state of hypercoagulability. Certain medications (estrogens) and diseases (malignancies) are associated with hypercoagulability. Even surgery itself lowers fibrinolytic activity, which reaches its lowest point around the third postoperative day.[59]

Prevention of a DVT and subsequent PE begins by identifying patients at risk for these disorders. The eighth edition of *Antithrombotic and Thrombolytic Therapy: American College of Chest Physicians Evidence-Based Clinical Practice Guidelines* suggests assessing patients according to three levels of risk.[68] Low-risk patients include those receiving only minor surgery and patients who are fully ambulatory or mobile. Moderate-risk patients include those undergoing general surgery, gynecologic surgery, and those patients who will be at bed rest, and the high-risk group are those undergoing major orthopedic surgery, patients with spinal cord injury, or those who have sustained major trauma. No specific pharmacologic management is suggested for patients falling within the low-risk group. Those of moderate risk should receive LMWH, low-dose UFH, or fondaparinux for prevention. High-risk patients should receive LMWH, fondaparinux, and warfarin with an INR titrated to 2.0 to 3.0. Other recommendations include monitoring renal function to ensure that these agents do not accumulate in the body and to institute general prevention techniques, also known as *mechanical methods*. General prevention maneuvers have included mobilization, use of graduated compression elastic stockings and intermittent external compression devices, and insertion of a vena cava filter device.[67] This filter is recommended for patients when anticoagulant medications are contraindicated or for those who are at high risk for bleeding complications.[69] The filter is inserted into the femoral vein and threaded upward to the inferior vena cava. The filter will then trap the clots before they reach the heart or the lungs. Obviously, this device will prevent a PE but not a DVT. For the patient who requires bed rest, it is important to ensure that passive range-of-motion exercises are performed at least every 4 hours and that position is changed at least every 2 hours. The ACCP guidelines state that aspirin-alone should never be recommended for prophylaxis in any of the three groups.

The ACCP also recommends some more specific guidelines related to orthopedic surgery.[68] It recommends either LMWH, fondaparinux, or a vitamin K antagonist such as warfarin, aiming for a target INR of 2.5 for those patients undergoing hip or knee arthroplasty. Thromboprophylaxis continues for a minimum of 10 days for knee surgery but up to 35 days for hip surgery. For patients undergoing hip fracture surgery, the use of fondaparinux, LMWH, vitamin K antagonist, or low-dose UFH should be used with continued prophylaxis from 10 to 35 days after surgery. These guidelines are in contrast to those published by the American Association of Orthopedic Surgeons, which recommends 325 mg of aspirin for up to 6 weeks, LMWH for 7 to 12 days, fondaparinux for 7 to 12 days, or warfarin for 2 to 6 weeks for the patient with standard risk for both bleeding and pulmonary embolism (PE).[70] For patients at high risk for bleeding but not PE, aspirin or warfarin is recommended. If the patient is at high risk for PE, it recommends LMWH, fondaparinux, or warfarin. The key differences are the use of aspirin and the use of PE as an outcome as opposed to ACCP's recommendations which arose from using DVT as an outcome measure. Another reason for the discrepancy is that orthopedic surgeons are acutely aware of the extent of blood loss that occurs with their procedures and feel that additional loss due to pharmacologic prophylaxis will put their patients at greater risk than in patients undergoing general surgery or those at bed rest.

Before the use of LMWH, the traditional pharmacologic approach to treating newly diagnosed DVT was to hospitalize the patient for 5 to 7 days. The patient would receive intravenous heparin, followed by subcutaneous heparin during conversion to warfarin therapy. The patient would then continue to receive the oral anticoagulant for up to 6 months.[67] LMWHs have drastically changed this protocol, at least for patients with smaller thrombi. Instead of being hospitalized, many patients can be treated on an outpatient basis.[71-73] A multisite study enrolled 334 patients with DVT either with or without PE. It was an observational study utilizing once-daily dosing with a LMWH (tinzaparin) and warfarin therapy to treat patients at home. The study results demonstrated that home treatment with self-administered tinzaparin was safe and resulted in a low rate of adverse events. Although this and similar studies show low rates of recurrence and huge cost savings, patients recruited into these studies were carefully screened for their ability to follow through with the injections but also represented a varied patient population, one likely to be similar to those presently treated on an in-hospital basis, that is, of varied age ranges and varied diagnoses, with comorbidities, including cancer or diabetes, and at prolonged bed rest.

PHARMACOLOGIC MANAGEMENT OF PERIPHERAL ARTERIAL DISEASE

Systemic atherosclerosis is one of the major pathologic processes leading to atherosclerotic occlusion of the arteries to the legs, that is, peripheral arterial disease (PAD). Chronic ischemia of the legs and intermittent claudication result from atheromatous disease involving the iliac, femoral, and popliteal arteries. Clinical manifestations include claudication (pain in one or both legs, primarily in the calves, while walking but which is relieved by rest), an abnormal ankle-brachial index value, ischemic ulceration or gangrene, or leg ischemia at rest.[74] Patients with PAD have reduced walking ability that limits their activities of daily living (ADLs).

Treatment of chronic PAD begins with the modification of certain risk factors: cessation of smoking; and treatment of hyperlipidemia, diabetes, and hypertension—all of which negatively affect peripheral circulation. However, treatment of these conditions does not guarantee improvement in walking distance or relief of ischemic pain. Intensive therapy with insulin and oral hypoglycemic agents was associated with a reduction in MI but not a reduction in the number of amputations associated with PAD in diabetics.[75] However, several large clinical trials have shown that lowering cholesterol was associated with a reduction in disease progression.[76,77]

Antiplatelet drugs, particularly aspirin and clopidogrel, are considered the main drugs for preventing ischemic events in patients with PAD. This treatment is directed toward preventing further thrombosis and progression of the disease. The Antiplatelet Trialists' Collaboration demonstrated a reduction in MIs, strokes, and deaths from vascular causes in patients with claudication who received aspirin therapy.[74] This study also showed that aspirin improved vascular graft patency in those patients who were treated with bypass surgery for their arterial disease, and low-dose aspirin has been found to be as effective as high-dose aspirin in preventing graft occlusion.

Two other drugs may produce a small effect on maximal walking ability. Pentoxifylline is a drug that improves the ability of red and white blood cells to squeeze through small vessels. With treatment, erythrocytes can actually flow through capillaries that are smaller in diameter. In addition, the drug lowers plasma fibrinogen levels and has antiplatelet effects. Compared with placebo, it has been associated with a nonsignificant increase in walking distance.[74] Only one trial at a higher dose showed a significant increase in mean walking distance compared with placebo.[78] Cilostazol is another drug that has antiaggregation effects as well as some vasodilator effects on platelets. Its mechanism of action is not related to antiplatelet drugs because this drug appears to interact directly with vascular smooth muscle. It has been shown to significantly increase pain-free walking distances when compared with either placebo or pentoxifylline.[79] However, use of this drug is not yet widespread. Additional clinical trials specifically targeting patients with intermittent claudication are needed to determine the benefits of pentoxifylline and cilostazol, as well as the benefits of drugs that reduce the risk factors involved in the development of atherosclerosis, on the functional impairments produced by PAD. There are also some concerns with cilostazol, not because it is associated with adverse events but because some drugs that act similarly (milrinone and phosphodiesterase type 3 inhibitor) have been associated with increased mortality.[79]

There are several other agents that have been studied with respect to increasing walking distance, the supplements propionyl-L-carnitine, L-arginine, ginkgo biloba, vitamin E, and omega-3 fatty acids. The majority of these studies suffered from poor study design and were underpowered. Only propionyl-L-carnitine has received a class IIb recommendation from the American College of Cardiology, meaning that its usefulness has been established and its benefits outweigh the risks.[79]

PHARMACOLOGIC MANAGEMENT OF UNSTABLE ANGINA AND MYOCARDIAL INFARCTION

The major goal in treating MIs is to improve cardiac perfusion so that ischemia and myocyte cell death is reduced. As soon as a cardiac event is suspected, a patient should start receiving 325 mg non–enteric-coated aspirin, which should be chewed. In addition, patients should receive supplemental oxygen, which may limit the amount of ischemic damage. For ongoing ischemic pain, nitroglycerin can also be administered, up to three doses in 15 minutes, with the possibility of moving over to IV nitroglycerin in the emergency room. As soon as the type of cardiac event is determined by electrocardiography (ECG), decisions regarding the appropriate treatment can be made. The patient may be a candidate for reperfusion with fibrinolytics and percutaneous intervention with a stent if an ST-segment elevation MI is present, but this also depends on the patient's risk of bleeding, presence of shock, time since the beginning of symptoms, and time for transport to the location of the procedure.

In an ST segment elevation MI (STEMI), also known as a Q-wave MI, ruptured plaque with extensive thrombus and complete occlusion of the vessel occur. Treatment is begun with a thrombolytic agent, aspirin, nitrates, and a β-blocker (within the first 24 hours).[80,81] Clopidogrel, GP IIb/IIIa inhibitors, and LMWH may also be administered if needed. Morphine is given not only to reduce pain but also to reduce preload and afterload. Patients who are not candidates for fibrinolytic therapy may receive percutaneous coronary intervention or coronary bypass surgery.

In a non–ST segment elevation MI (NSTEMI), also known as a non-Q-wave MI (ruptured plaque with moderate thrombus), or in unstable angina, heparin is the drug of choice as opposed to thrombolytics.[3] Patients should also receive clopidogrel, β-blockers (within the first 24 hours), and aspirin. If unstable angina persists despite pharmacologic intervention, coronary artery revascularization with either coronary artery bypass graft surgery or percutaneous coronary artery angioplasty followed by insertion of a stent can be performed.

Immediately following recovery from an MI, the patient receives several pharmacologic interventions to promote survival and to prevent a secondary MI. Long-term management to prevent future MI should include aspirin, clopidogrel, β-blockers, angiotensin-converting enzyme (ACE) inhibitors, statins, revascularization with bypass or stent placement, or an implantable cardioverter-defibrillator.

ATHEROSCLEROSIS AND LIPID-LOWERING DRUGS

Reducing high levels of cholesterol has many positive implications for both short-term and long-term survival after an acute coronary syndrome. Specifically, lowering low-density lipoprotein (LDL) cholesterol levels has been shown to reduce the incidence of MI and stroke.[82]

Lipoproteins and the Atherogenesis Process

Lipids (triglycerides) and cholesterol are circulated in plasma as complexes consisting of lipid and proteins and are termed *lipoproteins*. They have been classified traditionally according to their density into chylomicrons, very-low-density lipoproteins (VLDLs), low-density lipoproteins (LDLs), and high-density lipoproteins (HDLs). Chylomicrons contain a very high concentration of triglycerides and basically transport dietary lipid to the liver, muscle, and adipose tissue. Lipoprotein lipase (located on the surface of the endothelial cells in the capillaries in muscle and adipose tissue) then splits the chylomicrons, releasing free fatty acids, which can be taken up in muscle and fat. Chylomicron remnants, consisting mainly of cholesterol, are then taken up by hepatocytes and stored, oxidized to bile acids, or released back into the plasma, along with newly synthesized triglycerides, as VLDL. This process is repeated as the VLDL transports the cholesterol and triglycerides back to the tissues; the triglyceride undergoes hydrolysis, and the VLDL now becomes LDL. The LDL with a large component of cholesterol is then either taken up in the tissues or liver via specific LDL receptors. However, if there is a deficiency in the LDL receptors or there is excess LDL, oxidation of LDL cholesterol takes place, leading to the formation of an atheromatous plaque in the arterial walls. HDL cholesterol is considered heart healthy. It takes up cholesterol from peripheral tissues and transfers it back to the liver as a reverse cholesterol transport. In general, a high HDL level or a low LDL cholesterol level is protective against heart disease.[83,84]

As discussed earlier in the chapter, the atherogenesis process begins with endothelial dysfunction occurring with an alteration in prostacyclin and nitric oxide synthesis, causing reduced vasodilator responses. Subsequent injury to this endothelium from hypertension or infection enhances monocyte attachment to the diseased endothelium. Monocytes and macrophages formed from monocytes then generate free radicals that oxidize the attached LDL, resulting in oxidatively modified LDL and also in the destruction of receptors needed for normal clearance of LDL. Macrophages bind to the oxidized LDL, becoming what are known as *foam cells*, and migrate subendothelially, forming fatty streaks in the lining of the vessel. The fatty streaks become an atheroma when platelets and endothelial cells release cytokines and growth factors, causing the deposit of connective tissue and a general fibroproliferative inflammatory reaction. Ultimately, this results in the formation of an atheromatous plaque that consists of a fibrous cap of connective tissue overlying a lipid center. This plaque can then rupture, thus providing surfacing for a thrombosis.

From this discussion, it would seem that a reduction in LDL levels would lower the risk of atherosclerosis, and this is partly true. However, as is true with most of medicine, the story is not so simple. Sophisticated laboratory methods involving analytical ultracentrifugation or polyacrylamide gradient gel electrophoresis have delineated seven subclasses of LDL cholesterol and three subclasses of HDL cholesterol.[85,86] The subclasses are based on the sizes of the LDL and HDL particles. The larger the LDL and HDL particles, the less likely a person is to experience CAD and hypertension.[87] Alternatively, persons with normal LDL levels but with a higher proportion of the LDL being small, dense particles (type IIIa+b) have a threefold higher risk for developing CAD.[6,85,86,88,89] In addition, those with this lipid profile have other health impairments, including insulin resistance, hypertension, impaired HDL cholesterol transport, increased platelet aggregability, and an increased postprandial lipid level. In fact, the frequent coexistence of small LDL particles with elevated triglyceride levels and low levels of HDL has been called the *lipid triad*, and patients who have this combination of risk factors are said to have an "atherogenic lipoprotein phenotype" or metabolic syndrome.

Leading cardiologists are proposing new standards for the measurement and diagnosis of lipoprotein disorders. The current method of delineating total, LDL, and HDL cholesterol levels along with fasting triglyceride levels is inadequate.[90] Research has shown that incorporating the LDL subclass distribution—as well as triglyceride, homocysteine, and lipoprotein (a) and (b) levels—provides the physician with more information to guide treatment toward the specific lipoprotein disorder.[91] All of these measures are considered independent risk factors for CAD, whereas high concentrations of apolipoprotein A-1, a major protein in HDL, are associated with a lower risk of disease. Unfortunately, few centers in the United States incorporate the scientific methodology needed to delineate the subclasses of LDL. However, patients can request their cardiologists to send a blood sample to the Berkeley HeartLab (in Berkeley, California) or LipoScience Inc. (in Raleigh, North Carolina) for evaluation of their LDL subclasses.

3-Hydroxy-3-Methylglutaryl Coenzyme A Reductase Inhibitors (Statins)

Statin drugs competitively inhibit the enzyme that catalyzes the rate-limiting step in synthesis of cholesterol by the liver (Figure 7-5). The reduction in cholesterol leads to a compensatory increase in LDL receptors and increased LDL clearance. Statins also reduce the production of VLDL and circulating triglycerides in the liver.[92] Statins only modestly raise HDL levels, but several large clinical trials have demonstrated that they reduce the risk of CAD in patients with low HDL and high LDL levels. Six statins are currently available: atorvastatin, fluvastatin, lovastatin, pravastatin, simvastatin, and rosuvastatin.

At least three very large 5- to 6-year clinical trials carried out with patients with CAD have shown that simvastatin or pravastatin can reduce cardiac mortality, lower the incidence of stroke, and decrease mortality from all causes.[93-95] Other studies have demonstrated the benefits of cholesterol-lowering drugs in the primary prevention of coronary disease in patients with average total cholesterol levels but low HDL levels and in patients with hypertension but average cholesterol readings.[96-99] The most compelling evidence for the use of statins comes from a large British trial.[100] The British Heart Protection Study enlisted more than 20,000 subjects between the ages of 40 and 80 years with some risk factors for CAD, diagnosed heart disease, or stroke; however, the subjects were not required to have high cholesterol levels. After 5 years, the results indicated that the subjects taking simvastatin had significantly fewer MIs, strokes, and cardiac procedures performed than subjects taking placebo. In addition, the study revealed that women benefited from the drug just as much as men, subjects older than 70 years benefited as much as younger subjects, and those with normal cholesterol levels also benefited from the drug. The results of this study suggested that the lower the LDL cholesterol achieved, the greater was the benefit, even when the LDL level was initially below the targeted value.[101] The study also showed that diabetic patients fared well with

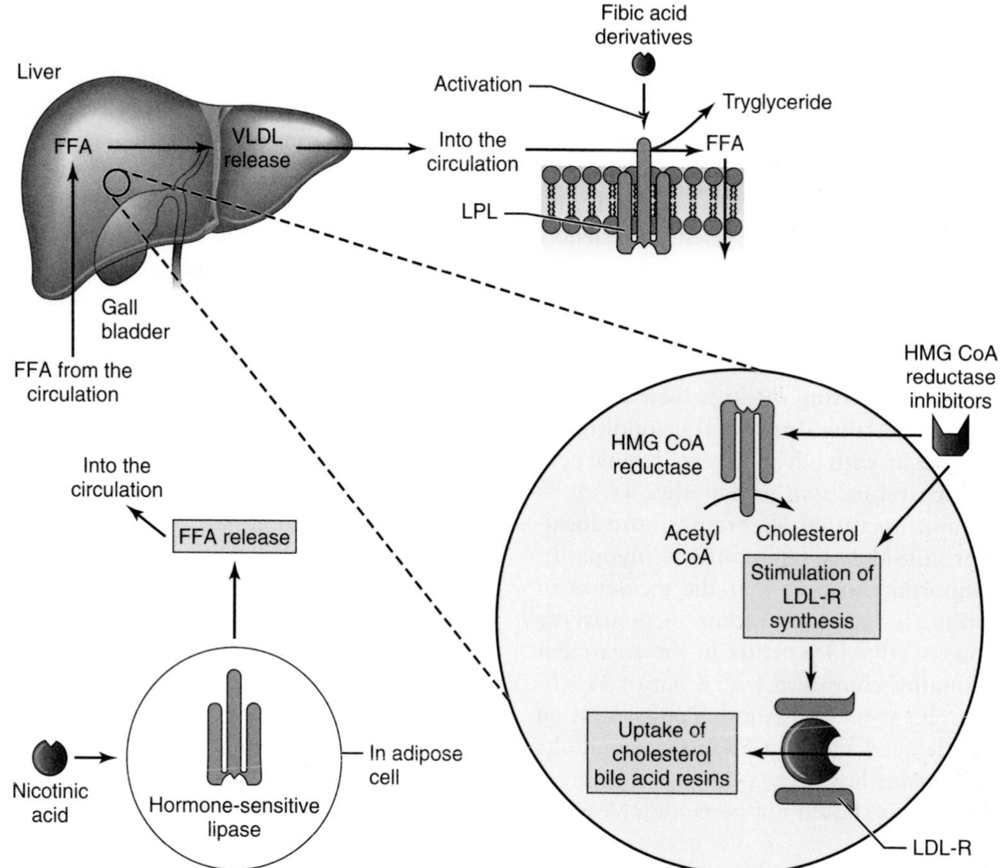

FIGURE 7-5 Sites of action of hypolipidemic agents. 3-Hydroxy-3-methylglutaryl coenzyme A (HMG CoA) reductase inhibitors lead to increased expression of low-density lipoprotein receptor (LDL-R) expression on hepatocytes and improved clearance of LDL from the plasma. Bile acid resins similarly lead to an increased LDL clearance, as well as increased cholesterol losses in bile. Fibric acid derivatives enhance lipoprotein lipase (LPL) action in peripheral tissues, which leads to improved clearance of triglyceride-rich particles. Nicotinic acid limits the flux of free fatty acids (FFA) from adipose tissue, which reduces the stimulus for hepatic very low-density lipoprotein (VLDL) production. When VLDL production is reduced, fewer remnant particles are available for LDL synthesis.

simvastatin in terms of cardiac events, even when LDL levels at baseline were low.

Even though all six statins have the same mechanism of action, their potency differs. A 20 mg tablet of pravastatin reduces LDL by 24%; the same dose of atorvastatin lowers cholesterol by 46%, and the newest drug rosuvastatin may be the most potent.[102] In terms of efficacy, atorvastatin used to be the top reducer of LDL, but rosuvastatin may lay claim to that position now.[103] This does not imply that all patients should take either of the two most potent or efficacious drugs because an individual may achieve his or her LDL target level with another drug that is less costly.

This discussion highlights the effectiveness of statins; however, they do have some limitations, and they are not well tolerated by all patients. Adverse effects fall into four main categories: (1) liver abnormalities, (2) muscle pain, (3) interactions with drugs and food, and (4) miscellaneous. Hepatic changes and muscle pain may occur fairly early during treatment. The liver utilizes one set of reactions to metabolize lovastatin, simvastatin, and atorvastatin and another set of reactions for fluvastatin. Still another group of reactions is used for pravastatin. Patients should have blood work done 6 weeks into treatment to monitor liver enzymes and every 6 months thereafter. An increase in the plasma aminotransferase level to more than three times normal is seen in only 1 to 2% of patients taking statins, and full-blown symptomatic hepatitis has been rare.[104] Patients who have elevated liver enzyme levels may do better by switching to another statin.

Myalgia and muscle weakness, though not always with elevated serum creatinine kinase (ck) levels, can also occur.[105,106] Reports of fatal myopathy linked to cerivastatin forced a recall of this drug from the market in August 2001. However, rarely has rhabdomyolysis or myoglobinemia been reported. The British Heart Protection Study put this problem into perspective.[100] Of more than 10,000 subjects who received simvastatin, only 49 had myopathy. This becomes even more insignificant when compared with the placebo group because 50 of these subjects had myopathy. Even though muscle weakness is rare during treatment with statins, it is more common when these drugs are combined with other lipid-lowering medications (e.g., fibrates or nicotinic acid). Safety concerns about these drugs surfaced when cerivastatin was withdrawn from the market after reports of fatal rhabdomyolysis. Rhabdomyolysis is a more severe form of muscle weakness resulting from sarcolemmal injury that causes release of myocyte contents (myoglobin, creatine kinase [CK], uric acid, and electrolytes) into the circulation. The patient experiences marked muscle damage and pain, dark-colored urine, and a CK level 40 times greater than normal (compared with 10 times the upper limit of normal in myositis) leading to acute renal failure.[107] Symptoms develop within a few months of starting therapy, increasing the dose, or adding an interacting drug.[108] The condition is also more likely to occur with advanced age, female gender, renal or hepatic dysfunction, or hypothyroidism.[109] Note that joint pain, nocturnal leg cramps, and localized pain are not considered symptoms of myopathy. However, it is important to note that the incidence of myopathy is extremely small. A recent meta-analysis showed that 9 out of 39,884 patients in the treatment arm reported myopathy, compared with 6 out of 39,817 patients in the placebo arm.[110,111] Another consideration is that many middle-aged individuals and older adults suffer from muscle pain; however, a diagnosis of myopathy or rhabdomyolysis should not be made unless the CK value is elevated.

The exact mechanism of statin-related myopathy is not really known. One theory is that the drug may lead to a ubiquinone (coenzyme Q10) deficiency. Ubiquinone is involved on a mitochondrial level altering cell signaling, differentiation, growth, and cell death, although how this specifically relates to muscle fibers is unknown. Coenzyme Q10 replacement has been proposed to lessen the likelihood of myopathy, but this remains controversial.

In addition to myopathy, tendonitis and tendon rupture with the use of statins have been reported.[112] During a 15-year period from 1990 to 2005, 96 cases of tendon complications were reported in France. The average age of the patient was 56 years old, with median time to onset after initiating statin therapy being 243 days. Many of those patients reporting symptoms had diabetes or hyperuricemia or participated in sports. As of March 2006, 247 cases of tendon rupture associated with statin therapy were reported in the U.S. Food and Drug Administration (FDA) adverse event data base. A case of biceps tendon rupture on one upper extremity with the administration of simvastatin/ezetimibe (Vytorin) and then a subsequent tendonitis in the contralateral biceps tendon when the patient underwent rechallenge with the drug has also been reported in a study by Pullatt et al.[113] Since statins inhibit metalloproteinase (MMP) expression, enzymes involved in the removal of denatured collagen from the extracellular matrix of tendons, these authors speculated that these drugs impair tendon repair and remodeling. They also promoted the idea that a certain segment of the population have a predisposition for tendinopathy.

Since myopathy and tendon lesions are rare, no guidance documents have been published for physical therapists treating patients on statins. There is no reason to withhold strengthening exercises for patients on these drugs, except when they report muscle pain. However, this decision is less clear if there are other conditions that may facilitate the risk of developing statin-related muscular abnormalities. In general, statins are metabolized in the liver by a group of enzymes known as CYP isoenzymes (CYP 3A4 enzyme). The activity of these enzymes can be either induced or inhibited by other drugs. If the CYP 3A4 enzyme is inhibited, patients will have higher plasma statin levels leading to toxicity. Also, certain ethnic and racial groups have a high incidence of a genetic polymorphism in this enzyme that also leads to high plasma statin levels. So if a patient develops unexplained muscle pain, a statin-related myopathy may be considered if the patient is consuming CYP 3A4 inhibitors, such as macrolide antibiotics; calcium channel blockers, such as diltiazem and nifedipine; and protease inhibitors. Statin-related myopathy should be considered if the patient is an older adult, experiences renal failure, or has several comorbidities. If any of these conditions exist, referral to a physician for further evaluation, particularly blood tests to measure CK, is necessary. The statin dose most likely would be lowered and the patient observed for reduction in symptoms. If symptoms dissipate, the patient may be rechallenged with another statin at a later date.

Statins interact with other drugs and with foods. Drugs or foods that affect the liver enzymes involved in metabolism will also affect plasma statin levels. Grapefruit juice will increase blood levels of lovastatin, simvastatin, and atorvastatin; but it does not usually affect the other drugs.[102] Other drugs that interact with the statins include antacids, some antibiotics, itraconazole, cyclosporine, and many human immunodeficiency virus (HIV) antiretrovirals. The remaining adverse effects that have been reported include constipation, dizziness, gastrointestinal (GI) problems, difficulty sleeping, rashes, and hair loss. There have also been some anecdotal reports of polyneuropathies with statin use.[104]

Statins are widely recommended and seem to be effective for anyone with a diagnosis of heart disease, a history of MI or stroke, high cholesterol levels, hypertension, diabetes, or PAD. Statins also have several nonlipid effects that are beneficial. Statins restore function to damaged vascular endothelium, although this may be a direct effect of lowered LDL cholesterol levels. Other benefits include the stabilization of atherosclerotic plaques, enhanced fibrinolysis, and reduction of inflammatory cell infiltration around atherosclerotic plaques.[114] There is also some evidence that statins may help prevent Alzheimer's disease and vascular dementia, but further study in this area is necessary.[115] These drugs come close to being miracle drugs for patients at high risk for developing heart disease, but some limitations to their use do exist. As mentioned earlier, the statins do not always lower LDL levels sufficiently, and increased doses of statins may not always continue to lower cholesterol levels. In addition, they have only a modest effect on HDL levels. For patients who do not reach their target cholesterol levels with these drugs, some alternatives are available (see the following sections). Some of these alternatives can be given safely along with a statin drug.

Bile Acid–Binding Resins

Cholestyramine, colesevelam, and colestipol are bile acid–binding resins that can successfully lower LDL levels by up to 20%.[104] These are insoluble agents that bind bile salts secreted into the duodenum, thus preventing enterohepatic circulation. Bile acids are synthesized from cholesterol in the liver and secreted into the gut to aid in the absorption of dietary fat. They are normally reabsorbed in the terminal ileum and sent back to the liver. Blocking bile acid reabsorption allows a compensatory increase in bile synthesis in the liver, leading to a further elimination of cholesterol. A lowered cholesterol level results in an upregulation of LDL receptors and a more rapid clearing of LDL particles.

The primary limitation to the widespread use of these drugs is GI intolerance—extreme diarrhea in some patients and constipation in others.[116] Another limitation is that the taste and texture are unacceptable to many individuals. These drugs come in a powder form and are mixed with food or drink. They may also interfere with the absorption of certain drugs (e.g., digoxin, warfarin, and thyroxine), and these drugs should be administered at least 1 hour before a bile acid–binding resin is taken.

Colesevelam is the newest bile acid sequestrant and appears to have some benefits over the older drugs. This drug has less potential to interfere with other medications, and therefore it can be given simultaneously with other drugs. In addition, when it is coadministered with the statins, an additive reduction in LDL cholesterol is seen. In fact, when colesevelam was given along with simvastatin, there was a greater reduction in the LDL level than when simvastatin was given alone with the dose doubled.[117] The primary disadvantage is that colesevelam attenuates the triglyceride reduction seen with the statins.

Fibrates

Bezafibrate, gemfibrozil, and ciprofibrate alter lipoprotein metabolism by activating gene transcription factors.[118] These factors are known as peroxisome proliferation activated receptors, and they increase lipoprotein lipase activity, thus enhancing the elimination of triglycerides from the lipoproteins in plasma. These drugs enhance free fatty acid uptake by the liver by inducing a fatty acid transport protein. Fibrates also convert small LDL particles to large LDL particles. In general, triglyceride levels are lowered by 25 to 50%, and the HDL level is increased 10 to 35%.

Adverse effects associated with fibrates include GI upset, increased risk of gallstones, and some drug–drug interactions with warfarin. Myositis has also been reported, but only when gemfibrozil was given along with a statin.

Nicotinic Acid/Niacin

Nicotinic acid is a B vitamin that at elevated levels increases HDL levels by 15 to 35%, reduces LDL levels by 5 to 25%, and decreases triglyceride levels by 20 to 35%.[116] This drug reduces free fatty acid mobilization from adipocytes and ultimately leads to a reduction in LDL cholesterol levels and even the proinflammatory lipoprotein (a).[119] In addition, the fact that it has a different mechanism of action from those of statins has provided a rationale for their concurrent use. Nicotinic acid plus lovastatin has been recommended for patients who continue to have high levels of triglycerides after monotherapy with a statin. A full-dose of niacin combined with a moderate dose of simvastatin is at least comparable with high-dose simvastatin. Adverse effects include flushing, pruritus, GI upset, blurred vision, fatigue, hyperuricemia, hepatic toxicity, and glucose intolerance. In general, this drug is poorly tolerated by patients.

BOX 7-5 Drugs for Dyslipidemias

HMG CoA Reductase Inhibitors	**% Reduction in LDL Based on 20 mg Dose**
Atorvastatin (Lipitor)	43
Fluvastatin (Lescol)	21
Lovastatin (Mevacor)	29
Pravastatin (Pravachol)	24
Rosuvastatin (Crestor)	48
Simvastatin (Zocor)	32
Bile Acid Sequestrants	**% Reduction in LDL Based on Recommended Dose Range**
Cholestyramine (Questran)	9–28
Colestipol(Colestid)	5–26
Colesevelam (Welchol)	15–19
Fibrates	
Fenofibrate (Tricor)	
Gemfibrozil (Lopid)	
Cholesterol Absorption Inhibitor	
Ezetimibe (Zetia)	
Combination Tablets	
Advicor (niacin plus lovastatin)	
Vytorin (eztimibe plus simvastatin)	

(Adapted from Jahangir A, Maria V: Coronary artery disease. In S. A. Waldman SA, Terzic A, Editors: *Pharmacology and therapeutics: Principles to practice*, Philadelphia, 2009, Saunders.)

Cholesterol Absorption Inhibitor

Ezetimibe is a new drug that inhibits the intestinal absorption of cholesterol. It also keeps the cholesterol in bile from recirculating back into the liver. According to Bruckert et al, it reduces LDL cholesterol levels by approximately 20% and produces modest but positive changes in other lipid markers.[120] The efficacy of ezetimibe when used alone is about equal to that of a high-dose statin. When ezetimibe was used in combination with a statin, a 21.45% greater reduction in LDL levels was achieved compared with statin plus placebo.[120]

The safety profile of ezetimibe is similar to that of placebo, and when it is given in combination with a statin, it is equal to that of the statin. The only warning that has been added to the ezetimibe label relates to a risk of angioedema, but at present, the absolute number of cases is not known because this adverse effect was not seen in clinical trials.[121]

Ezetimibe has been marketed as monotherapy for patients who are not able to tolerate statins and in combination with simvastatin (Vytorin) to help achieve LDL target levels. However, a recent study—Exetimibe and Simvastatin in Hypercholesterolemia Enhances Atherosclerosis Regression trial (ENHANCE)—comparing the Vytorin combination with simvastatin alone did not show a significant difference in carotid intima-media thickness, even though there were significantly greater reductions in LDL and cross reactive (C-reactive) protein levels.[122] However, it is important to realize that this is just one study, one that used surrogate markers, as opposed to firm outcomes such as cardiovascular events or death. These subtle points were, however, overshadowed by the feeling that the involved pharmaceutical companies, which in this case were Merck & Co and Schering-Plough, had been dishonest by delaying the release of this study data by many months. Other studies are ongoing with firmer endpoints.

Therapeutic Concerns with Lipid-Lowering Agents

In general, lipid-lowering drugs are safe with a low incidence of adverse effects. However, muscle soreness and rhabdomyolysis have occurred with some statins, particularly when used in combination with other lipid-lowering agents.[106] Rhabdomyolysis has also been reported when statins are used with erythromycin and some antifungal agents. Therapists should question their patients about the incidence of muscle soreness that appears greater than what would be expected from physical therapy.

ACTIVITIES 7

1. You are treating a 52-year-old man for chronic back pain related to a herniated disc in his lumbar area. His medical history is significant for an anterior myocardial infarction 2 years ago, and he is currently taking a β-blocker. His fasting plasma LDL level is 256, and his HDL level is 38. Both his orthopedic surgeon and cardiologist recommend exercise and weight loss to improve his functional abilities and medical status.

Questions

A. What advice would you give him?
B. What additional drugs would you recommend, and why?
C. What target cholesterol levels would you aim for?
D. What adverse effects should you stay alert for during therapy?

2. You are treating a 58-year-old man with adhesive capsulitis. The patient is receiving joint mobilization, passive stretching, and progressive resistive exercise. Shortly after he completes the weight lifting portion of his therapy session, he tells you that he has some chest pain. The patient has been lifting the same amount of weight for the past 2 weeks without problems. He reports that in the past he has been able to take one nitroglycerin tablet 5 minutes before activity but now he needs two tablets.

The patient has continued to smoke two packs of cigarettes each day and is concerned that his cardiac condition is worsening because of this increased need to take medication.

Vital Signs: Blood pressure, 135/80 mm Hg; pulse, 80 beats/min; respiratory rate, 18 breaths/min.

Physical Exam: Height, 5'8"; Weight, 220 lb; patient in no acute distress; no rales or crackles in the lungs; heart sounds are normal; no leg edema; and no jugular vein distention.

You decide to end the therapy session and refer the patient to an emergency clinic.

The patient returns to the clinic in the afternoon to report his test results.

The patient has an elevated glucose level (154 mg/dL), hypercholesterolemia, and hypertriglyceridemia. Blood urea nitrogen and creatinine levels are normal, and the electrocardiogram shows no signs of ischemia or infarction.

A chest X-ray film demonstrates left ventricular hypertrophy.

Questions

A. Why does the patient have increased chest pain despite the increased dose of nitroglycerin?
B. What is the patient's most likely diagnosis?
C. From a pharmacologic perspective, what changes need to be made?
D. Discuss why a patient may receive both warfarin and heparin at the same time.

3. Which type of patient should be monitored closely for deep vein thrombosis (DVT)?

4. Which complementary alternative agents increase the risk of bleeding when given with warfarin?

5. Grapefruit juice interacts with statin drugs and calcium channel blockers. Explain this interaction.

REFERENCES

1. Talbert RL: Ischemic heart disease. In DiPiro J, Talbert R, Yee G, Matzke G, Barbara W, Posey LM, editors: Pharmacotherapy: A pathophysiologic approach, Stamford, Connecticut, 1997, Appleton & Lange.
2. Katzung BG, Chatterjees MB: Vasodilators and the treatment of angina pectoris. In Katzung BG, editor: Basic and clinical pharmacology, New York, 2007, McGraw-Hill.
3. Jahangir A, Maria V: Coronary artery disease. In Waldman SA, Terzic A, editors: Pharmacology and therapeutics: Principles to practice, Philadelphia, 2009, Saunders.
4. Dzau VJ, Antman EM, Black HR, et al: The cardiovascular disease continuum validated: Clinical evidence of improved patient outcomes: Part I: Pathophysiology and clinical trial evidence (Risk factors through stable coronary artery disease). Circulation 114(25):2850-2870, 2006.
5. Mudd JO, Borlaug BA, Johnston PV , et al: Beyond low-density lipoprotein cholesterol: defining the role of low-density lipoprotein heterogeneity in coronary artery disease. J Am Coll Cardiol 50(18):1735-1741, 2007.
6. Zeller M, Masson D, Farnier M, et al: High serum cholesteryl ester transfer rates and small high-density lipoproteins are associated with young age in patients with acute myocardial infarction. J Am Coll Cardiol 50(20):1948-1955, 2007.
7. Libby P, Ridker PM:, Inflammation and atherosclerosis. Circulation 105:1135-1143, 2002.
8. Turk JR, Carroll JA, Laughlin MH, et al: C-reactive protein correlates with macrophage accumulation in coronary arteries of hypercholesterolemic pigs. J Appl Physiol 95:1301-1304, 2003.
9. Ridker PM: Clinical application of C-reactive protein for cardiovascular disease detection and prevention. Circulation 107:363-369, 2003.
10. Vitale JM, Hongyu Q, Depre C: Pre-emptive conditioning of the ischemic heart. In Cardiovascular and hematological agents in medicinal chemistry, Oak Park, IL, 2008, Bentham Science Publishers Ltd.
11. Rang, HP, et al: The heart. In Rang HP, Dale MM, Ritter JM, Flower R, editors: Rang and Dale's pharmacology, Philadelphia, 2007, Churchill Livingstone.
12. Graboys TB, Lown B: Nitroglycerin: The "mini" wonder drug. Circulation 108(11):e78-e79, 2003.
13. Waller DG, Renwick AG, Hillier K: Medical pharmacology and therapeutics. New York, 2001, W. B. Saunders.
14. Trujillo TC, Dobesh PP: Traditional management of chronic stable angina. Pharmacotherapy 27:1677-1692, 2008.
15. Peer CTH, Jacob TH: Nitroglycerin headache and nitroglycerin-induced primary headaches from 1846. and onwards: A historical overview and an update. Headache J Head Face Pain 49(3):445-456, 2009.
16. Gori T, ParkerJD: Nitrate-induced toxicity and preconditioning: A rationale for reconsidering the use of these drugs. J Am Coll Cardiol 52(4):251-254, 2008.
17. O'Rourke ST: Antianginal actions of beta-adrenoceptor antagonists. Am J Pharm Edu 71(5):1-6, 2007.
18. Fihn SD, Williams SV, Daley J, Gibbons RJ; American College of Cardiology; American Heart Association; American College of Physicians-American Society of Internal Medicine.: Guidelines for the management of patients with chronic stable angina: Treatment. Ann Intern Med 135(8 Part I):616-632, 2001.
19. Gielen W, Cleophas TJ, AgrawalR: Nebivolol: A review of its clinical and pharmacological characteristics. Int J Clin Pharmacol Ther 44(8):344-357, 2006.
20. Fraker TD Jr, Fihn SD, 2002 Chronic Stable Angina Writing Committee, American College of Cardiology, American Heart Association, et al: 2007 chronic angina focused update of the ACC/AHA 2002 guidelines for the management of patients with chronic stable angina: A report of the American College of Cardiology/American Heart Association Task Force on Practice Guidelines Writing Group to develop the focused update of the 2002 guidelines for the management of patients with chronic stable angina. J Am Coll Cardiol 50(23):2264-2274, 2007.
21. Moczydlowski EG: Electrical excitability and action potentials. In Boron WF, Boulpaep EL, editors: Medical physiology, Philadelphia, 2003, Saunders.
22. Lederer WJ: Cardiac electrophysiology and the electrocardiogram. In Boron WF, Boulpaep EL, editors: Medical physiology, Philadelphia, 2003, Saunders.
23. Kaufmann PA, Mandinov L, Seiler C, Hess OM. : Impact of exercise-induced coronary vasomotion on anti-ischemic therapy. Coron Artery Dis 11(4):363-369, 2000.
24. Epstein M: The calcium antagonist controversy: The emerging importance of drug formulation as a determinant of risk. Am J Cardiol 79(10A):9-19, 1997.
25. Frishman WH, Michaelson MD: Use of calcium antagonists in patients with ischemic heart disease and systematic hypertension. Am J Cardiol 79(10A):33-38, 1997.
26. Heidenreich PA, McDonald KM, Hastie T, et al: Meta-analysis of trials comparing beta-blockers, calcium, antagonists, and nitrates for stable angina. JAMA 281(20):1927-1936, 1999.
27. Dargie HJ, Ford I, Fox KM: Effects of ischaemia and treatment with atenolol, nifedipine SR and their combination on outcome in patients with chronic stable angina. Eur Heart J. 17:104-112, 1996.
28. Hassenfuss G, Maier LS: Mechanism of action of the new anti-ischemia drug ranolazine. Clin Res Cardiol 97:222-226, 2008.
29. Patel PD, Arora RR: Utility of ranolazine in chronic stable angina patients. Vasc Health Risk Manage 4(4):819-824, 2008.
30. Ben-Dor I, Battler A: Treatment of stable angina. Heart 93:868-874, 2007.
31. Furie B, Furie BC: Molecular and cellular biology of blood coagulation. N Engl J Med 326(12):800-806, 1992.
32. Vaughn G: Understanding and evaluating common laboratory tests. Upper Saddle River, NJ, 1999, Pearson Education.
33. Dentali F, Douketis JD, Lim W, Crowther M: Combined aspirin-oral anticoagulant therapy compared with oral anticoagulant therapy alone among patients at risk for cardiovascular disease: a meta-analysis of randomized trials. Arch Intern Med 167(2):117-124, 2007.
34. Curtis MJ, Pugsley MK: Drugs and the cardiovascular system. In Page C, Curtis M, Sutter M, Walker M, Hoffman BB, editors: Integrated pharmacology, Philadelphia, 2002, Mosby.
35. Zehnder JL: Drugs used in disorders of coagulation. In Katzung BG, editor: Basic and clinical pharmacology, New York, 2007, McGraw Hill.
36. Hu Z: Drugs and the blood, In Page C, Curtis M, Sutter M, Walker M, Hoffman BB, editors: Integrated pharmacology, Philadelphia, 2002, Mosby.
37. Collaboration meta-analysis of randomised trials of antiplatelet therapy for prevention of death, myocardial infarction, and stroke in high risk patients. Br Med J 324:71-86, 2002.
38. Ridker PM, Cook NR, Lee IM: A randomized trial of low-dose aspirin in the primary prevention of acardiovascular disease in women. N Engl J Med 352:1293-1304, 2005.
39. Hurlen M, Abdelnoor M, Smith P, Erikssen J, Arnesen H: Warfarin, aspirin, or both after myocardial infarction. N Engl J Med 347(13):969-974, 2002.
40. Catella-Lawson F, Reilly MP, Kapoor SC, et al: Cyclooxygenase inhibitors and the antiplatelet effects of aspirin. N Engl J Med 345(25):1809-1817, 2001.
41. MacDonald T, Wei L: Effect of ibuprofen on cardioprotective effect of aspirin. Lancet 361(9357):573-574, 2003.

42. Cleland JG: Chronic aspirin therapy for the prevention of cardiovascular events: A waste of time, or worse? Nat Clin Pract Cardiovasc Med 3(5):234-235, 2006.
43. The Clopidogrel in Unstable Angina to Prevent Recurrent Events Trial investigators Investigators: Effects of clopidogrel in addition to aspirin in patients with acute coronary syndromes without ST-segment elevation. N Engl J Med 345(7):494-502, 2001.
44. CAPRIE Steering Committee: A randomised, blinded, trial of clopidogrel versus aspirin in patients at risk of ischaemic events (CAPRIE). Lancet 348:329-1339, 1996.
45. Abramowicz M: Clopidogrel for reduction of atherosclerotic events. Med Lett Drugs Ther 40(1028):59-60, 1998.
46. Roy P, Bonello L, Torguson R: Impact of nuisance bleeding on clopidogrel compliance in patients undergoing intracoronary drug-eluting stent implantation. Am J Cardiol 102:1614-1617, 2008.
47. Tcheng JE, Kandzari DE, Grines CL, et al: Benefits and risks of abciximab use in primary angioplasty for acute myocardial infarction: The controlled abciximab and device investigation to lower late angioplasty complications (CADILLAC) trial. Circulation 108(11):1316-1323, 2003.
48. Elhendy A, Bax JJ, Poldermans D: Dobutamine stress myocardial perfusion imaging in coronary artery disease. J Nucl Med 43(12):1634-1646, 2001.
49. Sicari R, Nihoyannopoulos P, Evangelista A, et al: Stress echocardiography expert consensus statement: European Association of Echocardiography (EAE) (a registered branch of the ESC). Eur J Echocardiogr 9(4):415-437, 2008.
50. Fleisher LA, Beckman JA, Brown KA, et al: ACC/AHA 2007. Guidelines on peripoperative cardiovascular evaluation and care for noncardiac surgery: A report of the American College of Cardiology/American Heart Association Task Force on Practice Guidelines. Circulation 116:e418-e499, 2007.
51. Pangilinan JM: Current issues in heparin dosing. Medscape Pharmacists, 2007.
52. Hirsh J, Raschke R: Heparin and low-molecular-weight heparin: The seventh ACCP conference on antithrombotic and thrombolytic therapy. Chest 126:188S-203S, 2004.
53. Dager WE, Dougherty JA, Nguyen PH, Militello MA, Smythe MA: Heparin-induced thrombocytopenia: Treatment options and special considerations. Pharmacotherapy 27(4):564-587, 2007.
54. Heparin errors continue despite prior, high-profile, fatal events, 2008. (website). http://www.ismp.org/Newsletters/acutecare/articles/20080717.asp. Accessed August 20, 2009.
55. Blattler W, Kreis K, Blattler IK: Practicability and quality of outpatient management of acute deep venous thrombosis. J Vasc Surg 32:855-860, 2000.
56. Wong GC, Giugliano RP, Antman EM: Use of low-molecular-weight heparins in the management of acute coronary artery syndromes and percutaneous coronary intervention. JAMA 289(3):331-342, 2003.
57. Gibson CM, Murphy SA, Montalescot G, et al: Percutaneous coronary intervention in patients receiving enoxaparin or unfractionated heparin after fibrinolytic therapy for ST-segment elevation myocardial infarction in the ExTRACT-TIMI 25 trial. J Am Coll Cardiol 49(23):2238-2246, 2007.
58. Ferguson JJ, Califf RM, Antman EM: Enoxaparin vs unfractionated heparin in high-risk patients with non-ST-segment elevation acute coronary syndromes managed with an intended early invasive strategy: Primary results of the SYNERGY randomized trial. JAMA 292:45-54, 2004.
59. Salvati EA: Multimodal prophylaxis of venous thrombosis. Am J Orthoped 31(9S suppl):4-11, 2002.
60. Turpie AG, Gent M, Laupacis A, , et al: A comparison of aspirin with placebo in patients treated with warfarin after heart-valve replacement. N Engl J Med 329:524-529, 1993.
61. Coumadin Aspirin Reinfarction Study (CARS) Investigators: Randomised double-blind trial of fixed low-dose warfarin with aspirin after myocardial infarction. Lancet 350:389-396, 1997.
62. Turka J: Understanding international normalized ratio (INR). Nursing2005 35(8):2, 2005.
63. Heneghan C, Alonso-Coello P, Garcia-Alamino JM, Perera R, Meats E, Glasziou P: Self-monitoring of oral anticoagulation: a systematic review and meta-analysis. Lancet 367(9508): 404-411, 2006.
64. Weitz JI, Hirsh J, Samama MM: New antithrombotic drugs: American College of chest Physicians evidence-based clinical practice guidelines (8th edition). Chest 133:234S-256S, 2008.
65. Mureebe L: Direct thrombin inhibitors: Alternatives to heparin. Vascular 15(6):372-375, 2007.
66. Blick SK, Orman JS, Wagstaff AJ, Scott LJ: Spotlight on fondaparinux sodium in acute coronary syndromes. BioDrugs 22(6):413-415, 2008.
67. Church V: Staying on guard for DVT & PE. Nursing 30(2): 35-42, 2000.
68. Geerts WH, Bergqvist D, Pineo GF: Prevention of venous thromboembolism: American College of Chest Physicians evidence-based clinical practice guidelines. Chest 133(suppl 6): S381-S453, 2008.
69. Kaufman JM, Kinney TB, Streiff MB: Guidelines for the use of retrievable and convertible vena cava filters: Report from the Society of Interventional Radiology multidisciplinary consensus conference. Surg Obes Relate Dis 2:200-212, 2006.
70. Eikelboom JW, Karthikeyan G, Fagel N, Hirsh J: American Association of Orthopedic Surgeons and American College of Chest Physicians guidelines for venous thromboembolism prevention in hip and knee arthroplasty differ. Chest 135(2):513-520, 2008.
71. Partsch H: Bed rest versus ambulation in the initial treatment of patients with proximal deep vein thrombosis. Curr Opin Pulm Med 8:389-393, 2002.
72. Zidane M, van Hulsteijn LH, Brenninkmeijer BJ, Huisman MV: Out of hospital treatment with subcutaneous low molecular weight heparin in patients with acute deep-vein thrombosis: A prospective study in daily practice. Haematologica 91(8):1052-1058, 2006.
73. Hyers TM, Spyropoulos AC: Community-based treatment of venous thromboembolism with a low-molecular-weight heparin and warfarin. J Thromb Thrombolysis 24:225-232, 2007.
74. Hiatt WR: Drug therapy: Medical treatment of peripheral arterial disease and claudication. N Engl J Med 344(21): 1608-1621, 2001.
75. UK Prospective Diabetes Study (UKPDS) Group: Intensive blood-glucose control with sulphonylureas or insulin compared with conventional treatment and risk of complications in patients with type 2 diabetes. Lancet 352(9131):837-853, 1998.
76. Leng GC, Price JF, Jepson RG: Lipid-lowering for lower limb atherosclerosis. Cochrane Database Syst Rev 3, 2003.
77. Kroon AA, Van Asten W, Stalenhoef AF: Effect of apheresis of low-density lipoprotein on peripheral vascular disease in hypercholesterolemic patients with coronary artery disease. Ann Intern Med 125(12):945-954, 1996.
78. Dobesh PP, Stacy ZA, Persson EL: Pharmacologic therapy for intermittent claudication. Pharmacotherapy 29(5):526-553, 2009.
79. Dawson DL, Cutler BS, Hiatt WR, et al: A comparison of cilostazol and pentoxifylline for treating intermittent claudication. Am J Med 109(7):523-530, 2000.
80. Hilleman DE, Tsikouris JP, Seals AA, Marmur JD: Fibrinolytic agents for the management of ST-segment elevation myocardial infarction. Pharmacotherapy 27(11):1558-1570, 2007.

81. Antman EM, Hand M, Armstrong PW, et al: 2007 Focused Update of the ACC/AHA 2004. Guidelines for the Management of Patients With ST-Elevation Myocardial Infarction: a report of the American College of Cardiology/American Heart Association Task Force on Practice Guidelines: developed in collaboration With the Canadian Cardiovascular Society endorsed by the American Academy of Family Physicians: 2007. Writing Group to Review New Evidence and Update the ACC/AHA 2004. Guidelines for the Management of Patients With ST-Elevation Myocardial Infarction, Writing on Behalf of the 2004. Writing Committee. Circulation 117(2):296-329, 2008.
82. Aronow HD, Topol EJ, Roe MT, et al: Effect of lipid-lowering therapy on early mortality after acute coronary syndromes: An observational study. Lancet 357:1063-1068, 2001.
83. Francis GS, editor. Cholesterol size, not just levels, linked with cardiac health. The Cleveland Clinic heart advisor, Vol. 7(1), Greenwich, CT, 2004, Belvoir Publications.
84. Barter P, Gotto AM, LaRosa JC, et al: HDL cholesterol, very low levels of LDL cholesterol, and cardiovascular events. N Engl J Med 357(13):1301-1310, 2007.
85. Superko HR: Small, dense, low-density lipoprotein and atherosclerosis. Curr Atheroscler Rep 2(3):226-231, 2000.
86. Superko HR: Lipoprotein subclasses and atherosclerosis. Front Biosci 6:D355-D365, 2001.
87. Barzilai N, Atzmon G, Schechter C, et al: Unique lipoprotein phenotype and genotype associated with exceptional longevity. JAMA 290:2030-2040, 2003.
88. Superko HR, Hecht HS: Metabolic disorders contribute to subclinical coronary atherosclerosis in patients with coronary calcification. Am J Cardiol 88(3):260-264, 2001.
89. Kontush A, Chapman MJ: Antiatherogenic small, dense HDL—Guardian angel of the arterial wall? Nat Clin Pract Cardiovasc Med 3(3):44-153, 2006.
90. Superko HR: Hypercholesterolemia and dyslipidemia. Curr Treat Options Cardiovasc Med 2(2):173-187, 2000.
91. Benderly M, Boyko V, Goldbourt U: Apolipoproteins and long term prognosis in coronary heart disease patients. Am Heart J 157(1):103-110, 2009.
92. Law MR, Wald NJ, Rudnicka AR: Quantifying effect of statins on low density lipoprotein cholesterol, ischaemic heart disease, and stroke: Systematic review and meta-analysis. Br Med J 326:1-7, 2003.
93. Scandinavian Simvastatin Survival Study Group: Randomised trial of cholesterol lowering in 4444 patients with coronary heart disease: The Scandinavian simvastatin survival study. Lancet 344:1383-1389, 1994.
94. Sacks FM, Pfeffer MA, Moye LA, et al: The effect of pravastatin on coronary events after myocardial infarction in patients with average cholesterol levels. N Engl J Med 335:1001-1009, 1996.
95. The Long-term Intervention with Pravastatin in Ischaemic Disease (LIPID) Study Group: Prevention of cardiovascular events and death with pravastatin in patients with coronary heart disease and a broad range of initial cholesterol levels. N Engl J Med 339:1349-1357, 1998.
96. Downs JR, Clearfield M, Weis S, et al: Primary prevention of acute coronary events with lovastatin in men and women with average cholesterol levels: Results of AFCAPS/TexCAPS. JAMA 279:1615-1622, 1998.
97. Shepherd J, Cobbe SM, Ford I, et al: Prevention of coronary heart disease with pravastatin in men with hypercholesterolemia. N Engl J Med 333:1301-1307, 1995.
98. Ridker PM, Rifai N, Pfeffer MA, et al: Inflammation, pravastatin, and the risk of coronary events after myocardial infarction in patients with average cholesterol levels. Cholesterol and recurrent events (CARE) investigators. Circulation 98(9):839-844, 1998.
99. Sever PS, Dahlöf B, Poulter NR, et al: Prevention of coronary and stroke events with atorvastatin in hypertensive patients who have average or lower-than-average cholesterol concentrations, in the Anglo-Scandinavian Cardiac Outcomes Trial-Lipid Lowering Arm (ASCOT-LLA): A multicentre randomised controlled trial. Lancet 361:1149-1158, 2003.
100. Heart Protection Study Collaborative Group: MRC/BHF heart protection study of cholesterol lowering wiht simvastatin in 2053 high-risk individuals: A randomised placebo-controlled trial. Lancet 360:7-22, 2002.
101. Ballantyne CM: Current and future aims of lipid-lowering therapy: Changing paradigms and lessons from the heart protection study on standards of efficacy and safety. Am J Cardiol 92(4, suppl 2):3-9, 2003.
102. Lee TH, editor. Choose the statin that's right for you, Harvard Heart Letter, Vol. 14(4), Boston, MA, 2003, Harvard Health Publications.
103. Jones PH, Davidson MH, Stein EA, et al: Comparison of the efficacy and safety of rosuvastatin versus atorvastatin, simvastatin, and pravastatin across doses (STELLAR Trial). Am J Cardiol 92:152-160, 2003.
104. Abramowicz M, editor. Drugs for lipid disorders. Treatment Guidelines from the Medical Letter, Vol. 1(12), New Rochelle, NY, 2003, The Medical Letter Inc.
105. Wenisch C, Krause R, Fladerer P, El Menjawi I, Pohanka E: Acute rhabdomyolysis after atorvastatin and fusidic acid therapy. Am J Med 109(1):79, 2000.
106. Duell P, Connor W, Illingworth D: Rhabdomyolysis after taking atorvastatin with gemfibrozil. Am J Cardiol 81: 368-369, 1998.
107. Thompson, P, Clarkson P, Karas RH, Statin-Associated Myopathy. JAMA;289:1681-1690, 2003.
108. Armitage J: The safety of statins in clinical practice. Lancet 370(9601):1781-1790, 2007.
109. Harper CR, Jacobson TA, The broad spectrum of statin myopathy: from myalgia to rhabdomyolysis. Curr Opin Lipidol 18(4):401-408, 2007.
110. Baigent, C. , et al: Efficacy and safety of cholesterol-lowering treatment – Authors' reply. Lancet 367(9509):470-471, 2006.
111. Baigent C, Keech A, Kearney PM: Efficacy and safety of cholesterol-lowering treatment: prospective meta-analysis of data from 90, 056 participants in 14 randomized trials of statins. Lancet 366:1267-1278, 2005.
112. Marie I, Delafenetre H, Massy N: Tendinous disorders attributed to statins: A study on ninety-six spontaneous reports in the period 1990–2005 and review of literature. Arthritis Rheum 59:367-372, 2008.
113. Pullatt RC, Gadarla MR, Karas RH, Alsheikh-Ali AA, Thompson PD: Tendon rupture associated with simvastatin/ezetimibe therapy. Am J Cardiol 100:152-153, 2007.
114. Ridker PM, Rifai N, Clearfield M, et al: Measurement of C-reactive protein for the targeting of statin therapy in the primary prevention of acute coronary events. N Engl J Med 344(26):1959-1965, 2001.
115. Jick H, Zornberg GL, Jick SS, Seshadri S, Drachman DA. : Statins and the risk of dementia. Lancet 356:1627-1631, 2000.
116. Thompson PD: What's new in lipid management? Pharmacotherapy 23(9):34S-40S, 2003.
117. Knapp HH, Schrott H, Ma P: Effectiveness of colesevelam hydrocholoride in decreasing LDL cholesterol in patients with primary hypercholesterolemia. Am J Med 110:352-360, 2001.
118. Staels B, Dallongeville J, Auwerx J, Schoonjans K, Leitersdorf E, Fruchart JC: Mechanism of action of fibrates on lipid and lipoprotein metabolism. Circulation 98(19):2088-2093, 1998.

119. Scanu AM, Bamba R: Niacin and lipoprotein(a): Facts, uncertainties, and clinical considerations. Am J Cardiol 101(8, suppl 1):S44-S47, 2008.
120. Bruckert E, Giral P, Tellier P: Perspectives in cholesterol-lowering therapy: The role of ezetimibe, a new selective inhibitor of intestinal cholesterol absorption, Circulation. 107:3124-3128, 2003.
121. Neal RC, Jones PH: Lipid-lowering: Can ezetimibe help close the treatment gap? Cleve Clin J Med 70(9):777-783, 2003.
122. Kastelein JJ, Akdim F, Stroes ES, et al: Simvastatin with or without ezetimibe in familial hypercholesterolemia. N Engl J Med 358(14):1431–1443, 2008.

8

Drug Therapy for Congestive Heart Failure and Cardiac Arrhythmias

Barbara Gladson

DRUG TREATMENT FOR CONGESTIVE HEART DISEASE

Congestive heart failure (CHF) refers to the inability of the heart to pump sufficient cardiac output to maintain healthy tissue and to meet the body's physiologic needs. It is a progressive disorder, which in its severe form induces major physical limitations. There are over five million people in the United States who are living with heart failure, and there are over 550,000 new cases diagnosed each year.[1,2] The most common diseases or conditions that lead to the development of CHF include cardiomyopathy, myocardial ischemia and infarction, hypertension, valvular disease, congenital heart disease, and coronary artery disease.[3] Structural changes, either from the loss of cardiac myocytes in cardiomyopathy or from infarction, lead to reduced cardiac contractility. Excessive afterload from hypertension or aortic stenosis produces cardiac hypertrophy, and valvular defects (regurgitation) and tachycardia reduce stroke volume. Both cardiac hypertrophy and reduced stroke volume lead to the syndrome of heart failure.

In the early stages, the heart compensates for diminished cardiac output with tachycardia and increased contractility by means of myocardial hypertrophy. However, these compensations increase the cardiac workload, which further compromises pumping. The sympathetic system is activated to improve contractility, but the catecholamines produce vasoconstriction. The kidneys, sensing diminished perfusion begin to increase their secretion of renin, leading to release of angiotensin II and aldosterone. Water retention, increased blood pressure, and increased preload occur as a result. These neurohumoral compensations in response to the low blood pressure and diminished renal perfusion produce heart failure (Figure 8-1). As preload increases, more blood enters the heart, resulting in increased end-diastolic pressure, and cardiac dilation begins to occur. Angiotensin II also promotes arterial vasoconstriction and increased afterload. This cycle continues until the ventricles can no longer pump, and perfusion to the major organs is impaired.

CHF tends to develop from reduced left ventricular systolic contractility, also known as *systolic heart failure*. The hallmark of this condition is a reduced left ventricular ejection fraction (LVEF). Symptoms of left systolic heart failure include reduced cardiac output and blood pressure, which results in the backflow of fluid into the pulmonary system and pulmonary venous congestion. However, CHF can also result from impaired diastolic relaxation (diastolic heart failure).[4] In this case, the abnormality includes a slow or delayed relaxation of the ventricle with increased stiffness. Ventricular filling is incomplete (reduced preload), and therefore cardiac output is reduced; however, LVEF is normal or minimally reduced (≥45%). The tension in the ventricular muscle is thought to be maintained by calcium that is incompletely cleared from the actin–myosin cross-bridges. In time, ventricular geometry changes as a result of the myocardial stiffness, ischemia, and changes in wall thickness. The pathophysiology of the two conditions demonstrates that these are two separate conditions; however, the patient with systolic heart failure always has a mixture of systolic and diastolic pathologies, but the patient with diastolic heart failure can have a pure diastolic dysfunction. The pharmacologic management of the two conditions is similar, but some of the drugs used for systolic heart failure may have a negative effect on diastolic dysfunction.

In addition to systolic and diastolic heart failure, some patients may experience right ventricular heart failure. In this condition, fluid backflows into the venous circulation, which results in peripheral edema. The overall clinical presentation may include dyspnea, cyanosis, orthopnea, peripheral edema, ascites, and fatigue.

The American College of Cardiology (ACC) and the American Heart Association (AHA) have developed a classification scheme for heart failure that has replaced the New York Heart Association (NYHA) classification system.[5] First and foremost, it defines heart failure caused by systolic dysfunction as a left ventricular ejection fraction <40%. In addition, it presents CHF as a continuum based not only on symptoms but also on the

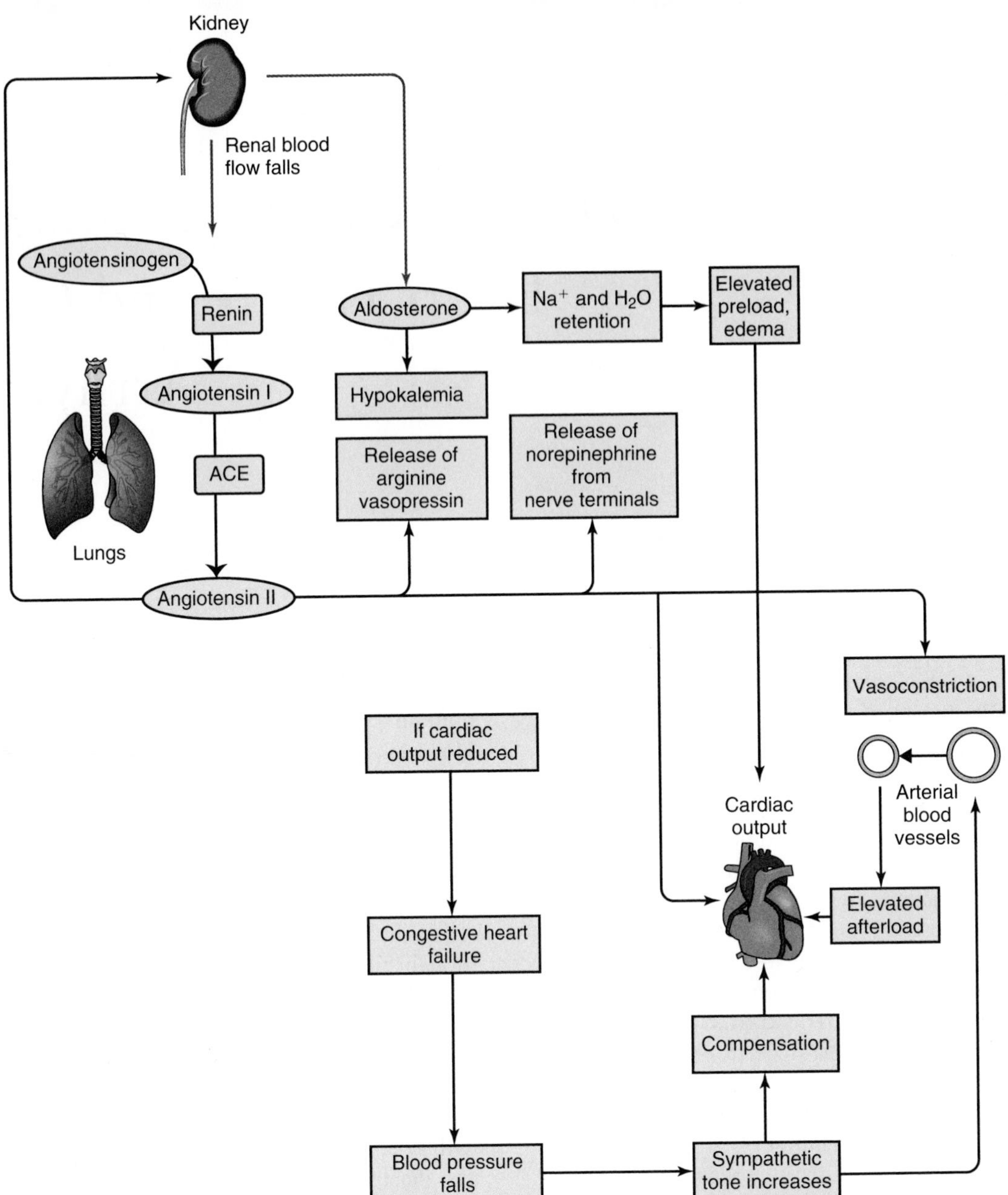

FIGURE 8-1 Neurohumeral compensation of Heart Failure. As blood pressure falls, sympathetic tone increases. This compensation results in elevated afterload. An elevation in preload results from renin release leading to formation of Angiotensin II. Angiotensin II stimulates release of Aldosterone causing Na^+ and H_2O retention. Angiotensin II is also a powerful arterial vasoconstrictor.

level of structural changes appearing in the heart and also takes into consideration risk factors. See Figure 8-2 for a more complete summary. However, since the NYHA system continues to be quoted in the literature, it has been provided as well in Box 8-1.[6]

Pharmacotherapeutic Goals in the Treatment of Congestive Heart Failure

The pharmacotherapeutic goals for treating heart failure include increasing contractility with positive inotropic drugs (cardiac glycosides and phosphodiesterase inhibitors), decreasing congestion and edema with diuretics, and decreasing preload and afterload with a vasodilator and/or an angiotensin-converting enzyme (ACE) inhibitor.

Cardiac Glycosides. Digitalis glycosides (digitalis, digoxin, and ouabain) are positive inotropic agents that enhance cardiac contractility by increasing the availability of free intracellular calcium (Ca^{2+}) to interact with contractile proteins. [3] Specifically, these drugs inhibit the sodium/potassium (Na^+/K^+)-ATPase pump on the cardiac cell membrane (Figure 8-3). This pump is normally responsible for maintaining low intracellular Na^+ and high intracellular K^+ concentrations. It pumps three

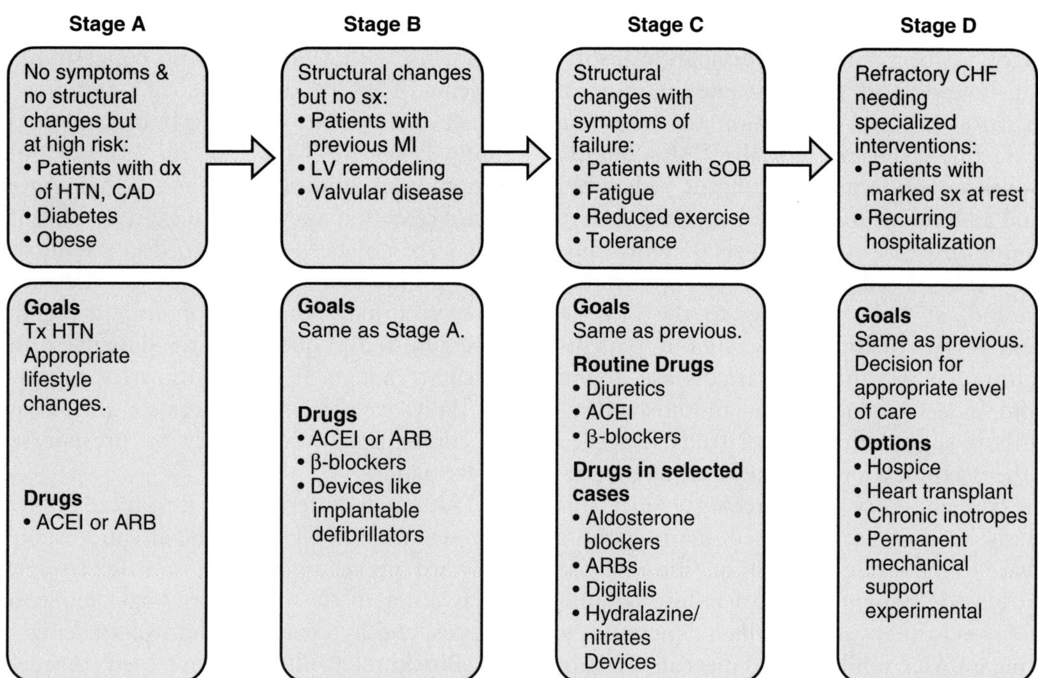

FIGURE 8-2 ACEI = angiotensin-converting enzyme inhibitor; ARB = ACE receptor blocker; HTN = hypertension; sx = symptoms. *(Hunt, SA et al: American College of Cardiology Foundation/American Heart Association Task Force on Practice Guidelines: 2009 Focused update incorporated into the ACC/AHA 2005 guidelines for the diagnosis and management of heart failure in adults.* Circulation *April 14; 119(14):e391–e479, 2009.)*

BOX 8-1 Classification System for Patients with Heart Failure

Class	Symptoms
I	No physical limitations
II	Slight limitation of physical activity; usual activity results in fatigue, palpitations, or dyspnea
III	Marked limitation of physical activity; less than usual activity produces fatigue, palpitation, or dyspnea
IV	Symptoms at rest and any activity increases discomfort

Adapted from the New York Heart Association Classification System for Patients with Heart Failure.[6]
http://www.abouthf.org/questions_stages.htm accessed on March 5, 2010.

Na^+ ions out of the cell in exchange for two K^+ ions into the cell against their concentration gradients. If the pump is inhibited, the high Na^+ concentration leads to inhibition of a membrane bound Na^+/Ca^{2+} exchange mechanism reducing the flow of calcium out of the cell. To summarize, the high Na^+ concentration intracellularly reduces the exchange function of the Na^+/Ca^{2+}, thus reducing the extrusion of calcium from the cell. The elevated level of Ca^{2+} is then pumped into the sarcoplasmic reticulum and now is available for subsequent depolarizations and enhanced excitation–contraction coupling. The result is greater contractility and therefore greater cardiac output and improved circulation. These changes reduce sympathetic activity and reduce angiotensin II and renin levels.

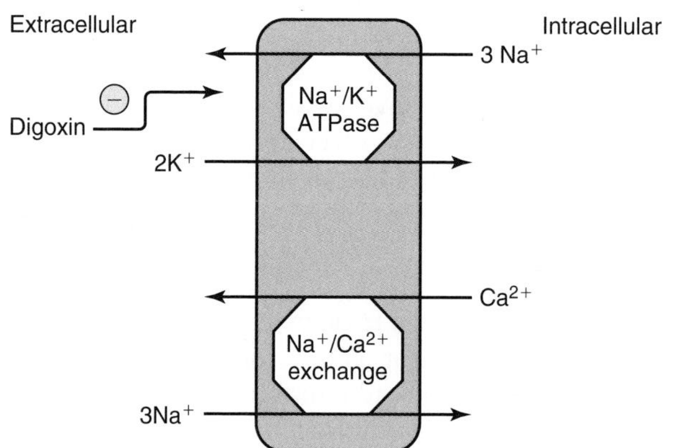

FIGURE 8-3 Digoxin blocks Na^+/K^+-ATPase which increases intracellular Na^+ and reduces Na^+ exchange with Ca^{2+}. Increased intracellular Ca^{2+} increases contractility.

Digitalis has effects on the kidneys and the parasympathetic system separate from its effects on the Na^+/K^+-ATPase pump. It enhances delivery of Na^+ to the distal tubules of the kidneys, producing diuresis, and it activates the parasympathetic system with resultant increased vagal tone, which produces an antidysrhythmic-effect.[7] When atrial fibrillation coexists with heart failure, digitalis use is clearly indicated because digitalis reduces ventricular response rates. However, because of its adverse effects, its use in heart failure in the absence of atrial fibrillation is becoming more difficult to justify.

The Digoxin Investigators Group studied more than 6800 patients without atrial fibrillation to determine whether digoxin reduced all-cause mortality.[8] After follow-up for 37 months, there was a significant reduction, 28% in hospital admissions for progressing heart failure but a reduction of only 6% in total hospital admissions. However, there were no reductions in all-cause mortality during this period, at least according to the original report. A recent review of the data, excluding patients with heart failure due to valvular heart disease, found that digoxin did, indeed, reduce deaths and hospitalizations.[9] The authors suggest that further study is needed to determine the usefulness of digoxin as adjunct treatment to more contemporary pharmacology. Since this post-hoc analysis has just been released, many authors are not yet aware of the results and still question the use of this drug at least in patients in heart failure without fibrillation.[10] However, in a study in which patients were already receiving an ACE inhibitor and digoxin, 28% of patients demonstrated a worsening of symptoms when the digoxin was withdrawn, compared with 6% in the group that was maintained on the two-drug regimen. Withdrawal resulted in a reduced exercise capacity and worsening of symptoms.[11]

The cardiac glycosides have a low therapeutic index because both therapeutic and toxic actions result from elevated cytoplasmic calcium levels. High intracellular Ca^{2+} precipitates arrhythmias. Arrhythmias may also result from cardiac K^+ loss and hypokalemia, especially when these drugs are given with diuretics, as they often are.[12] Additional adverse effects result from gastric irritation and stimulation of the chemoreceptor trigger zone, which results in nausea, vomiting, and diarrhea. Other effects include central nervous system (CNS) disturbances such as headaches, dizziness, visual disturbances, and hallucinations. Digitalis toxicity may occur and result in bradycardia. Treatment entails drug withdrawal, K^+ supplementation, and administration of atropine for sinus bradycardia. Careful monitoring of serum electrolyte and cardiac glycoside blood levels is needed.

Phosphodiesterase Inhibitors. Milrinone, amrinone, and vesnarinone are inhibitors of phosphodiesterase III found in cardiac and smooth muscles. [13] If this enzyme is blocked, there is an increase in intracellular cyclic adenosine monophosphate, which through a cascade of events, forces the release of Ca^{2+} stores. Cardiac contractility is improved, and elevated cyclic adenosine monophosphate levels in the arterial and venous smooth muscle result in marked vasodilation.

These drugs are not widely used because long-term administration with the oral formulation has been associated with increased mortality. However, they are still given intravenously for short periods. Adverse effects include nausea and vomiting, tachycardia, and serious arrhythmias.

Diuretics. Diuretics are essential in the treatment of patients with CHF and lung congestion or peripheral edema. They produce relief of symptoms more rapidly than do any other agent (in hours and days) and are the only drugs for CHF that can control fluid retention.[5] Short-term studies have shown that diuretics decrease fluid retention and improve exercise capacity, but diuretics have not been shown to decrease mortality or slow the progression of the disease.[14] Often, patients will receive a thiazide and a loop diuretic together, and doses are adjusted frequently as the patient's urine output and weight change. It is important for the patient to keep a daily weight record because this allows for more accurate dose adjustments to prevent severe volume overload.

Although diuretics are necessary to improve the clinical presentation in CHF, specific attention should be directed toward preventing hypotension, electrolyte imbalances, activation of the neurohormonal compensatory mechanisms, and hypokalemia and hyperkalemia.

β -Blockers. β-Blockers have been considered to be contraindicated for patients with CHF because they slow heart rate and decrease contractility.[14] However, several large clinical trials have shown that cardioselective β-blockers have some benefit for patients whose conditions have been stabilized with a diuretic and an ACE inhibitor.[6] The Cardiac Insufficiency Bisoprolol Study II evaluated 2647 symptomatic patients who had NYHA class III or IV CHF and who had an ejection fraction of less than 35%.[15,16] There was a 42% reduction in mortality and a significant reduction in hospital admissions in the bisoprolol group. Treatment effects were independent of the severity of heart failure. The OPTMIZE-HF (Organized Program to Initiate Lifesaving Treatment in Hospitalized Patients with Heart Failure) study showed that withdrawal of a β-blocker from standard therapy was associated with increased mortality at 60 to 90 days following hospitalization.[17]

Another study demonstrated that metoprolol improved the ejection fraction at rest and during exercise and decreased mortality among patients with mild-to-moderate heart failure (NYHA functional class II-III) who were taking ACE inhibitors.[18] These patients had CHF from either ischemic heart disease or idiopathic dilated cardiomyopathy, but both groups responded equally well to the β-blocker. Studies with carvedilol further substantiate a role for β-blockers in the treatment of CHF.[19] In fact, the beneficial effects of carvedilol, metoprolol, and bisoprolol on mortality and morbidity appear similar, regardless of the severity of CHF.[20]

Possible explanations for the usefulness of β-blockers in the treatment of CHF include the following: reduction in sympathetic nervous system activity, depression of the neurohumoral response to diminished cardiac output, antidysrhythmic properties of the drugs, and reduction of workload on the damaged myocardium. There are three β-blockers approved for use in CHF—bisoprolol and sustained release metoprolol which are both β1 selective blockers and carvedilol which blocks α1, β1, and β2 receptors. The updated 2009 guidelines for treatment of CHF suggest that all patients in stage C, or at the first sign of left ventricular dysfunction, receive one of the three β-blockers.[5] The dose should be titrated to make sure no adverse effects in terms of bradycardia or negative inotropy occur. Patients must also be selected carefully; those with edema are excluded from receiving a β-blocker, at least temporarily until fluid retention is under control. Even with careful selection, a patient may initially demonstrate some deterioration, followed frequently by an improvement. Adverse effects to watch for are hypotension, fluid retention, worsening heart failure, and bradyarrhythmias.

Angiotensin-Converting Enzyme Inhibitors. The beneficial effects of ACE inhibitors have been so convincing that these drugs are used not only in all stages of heart failure but also in patients with a high risk for CHF before symptoms and structural changes in heart tissue develop. These drugs reduce peripheral vascular resistance (afterload) and prevent aldosterone-mediated Na^+ and fluid retention. They have been shown to slow the progression of heart failure and prolong survival.[21,22] In the landmark Cooperative North Scandinavian Enalapril Survival Study (CONSENSUS-1), enalapril produced a reduction in mortality of 40% in patients with severe heart failure (NYHA class IV). In addition, there were reductions in heart size and in the need for diuretics in these patients.[23] ACE inhibitors have also been shown to protect against atherosclerosis through an antiproliferative effect and have an antimigratory effect on smooth muscle cells. At present, they are the first drugs prescribed for chronic CHF.

The major adverse effects of ACE inhibitors are infrequent but may include hypotension, cough, syncope, hyperkalemia, and angioedema. Several studies have shown that the beneficial effects of ACE inhibitors are diminished when concurrently given with aspirin but that they still outperformed other agents. In fact, there were no significant differences in outcomes when ACE inhibitors were administered with or without aspirin.[24,25]

Angiotensin-Converting Enzyme Receptor Blockers

These drugs were developed on the basis of the rationale that some angiotensin II remains despite inhibition of the angiotensin-converting enzyme. And since ACE inhibitors have proved to be beneficial in reducing mortality in patients with CHF, it was thought that ACE receptor blockers (ARBs) would be equally beneficial. In fact, several large clinical studies have shown this to be true. The Evaluation of Losartan In The Elderly (ELITE) trial compared losartan with captopril in 722 patients with CHF for 48 weeks.[26] The losartan group had fewer deaths and hospitalizations, as well as a 46% reduction in all-cause mortality. However, when the ELITE II trial, which was the ELITE trial extended for 2 additional years, was completed, no significant reduction in all-cause mortality was found.[27] The ELITE II trial, which enrolled more than 3000 subjects, did show, however, that ARBs were better tolerated than were ACE inhibitors.

The Optimal Trial in Myocardial Infarction with the Angiotensin II Antagonist Losartan (OPTIMAAL) demonstrated that losartan did not produce reduced mortality when compared with captopril, but the authors theorized that the poorer performance by losartan was due to the low dose used in the study.[28] The dose chosen for this study is the recommended starting dose for the treatment of hypertension and therefore is inadequate for patients with CHF. However, The Valsartan Heart Failure Trial demonstrated reduced mortality in patients who were either intolerant to or had never taken an ACE inhibitor, showing that these drugs are effective for patients with CHF.[29] Finally, in a recent meta-analysis, investigators attempted to determine whether ARBs reduced the number of deaths and hospitalizations among patients with CHF to a greater extent than ACE inhibitors.[30] This study failed to show any superiority of ACE blockers over ACE inhibitors but echoed the other studies in showing that an ACE blocker is better tolerated than an ACE inhibitor. However, the authors did discover that an ACE blocker given in combination with an ACE inhibitor was superior to use of the ACE inhibitor alone.[31] Currently, ACE inhibitors remain the first choice for patients with CHF over the ARBs.[5]

Nitrates. Nitrates reduce the myocardial oxygen requirement by dilating smooth muscle and increasing the volume of the venous vascular bed to reduce preload and ventricular filling pressure. Nitrates have been shown to reduce orthopnea and improve exercise tolerance in patients also taking ACE inhibitors.[32] For chronic heart failure, isosorbide dinitrate or mononitrate may be given orally, and isosorbide in either form is especially useful for patients who cannot tolerate ACE inhibitors because of hypotension or ensuing renal failure.

Aldosterone Receptor Blockers. Aldosterone release is elevated in CHF, promoting Na^+ retention, K^+ loss, sympathetic activation, myocardial and vascular fibrosis, and diminished vascular compliance. Spironolactone is a K^+-sparing diuretic that blocks the aldosterone receptor. It is currently being recommended for use in NYHA class IV CHF, but only if renal function is preserved. In the Randomized Aldactone Evaluation Study (RALES), roughly 1600 patients with moderate-to-severe heart failure were examined to determine whether spironolactone added to the regimen of an ACE inhibitor and a loop diuretic with or without digitalis prolongs life. This study was discontinued early after only 24 months because of the overwhelmingly significant benefit seen with spironolactone in terms of reducing the numbers of deaths and hospitalizations among patients with CHF.[33] Low-dose spironolactone, given along with an ACE inhibitor, has been shown to be beneficial for patients with CHF and moderate to severe impairment. It is theorized that the ACE inhibitors do not depress aldosterone levels, which are elevated in heart failure, so that the actions of spironolactone are needed to further alter the neurohumoral mechanism involved in this disease. Aldosterone antagonists are also believed to play a role in vessel wall and myocardial remodeling.[34] Additionally, aldosterone blockade has been shown to reduce vascular collagen turnover and significantly decrease the early morning rise in heart rate seen in heart failure.[35,36] However, because these drugs are K^+ sparing, the patients must be monitored for hyperkalemia and renal function. Another adverse effect is gynecomastia.

Eplerenone is the first aldosterone receptor blocker approved for administration following a myocardial infarction (MI). In one trial, when the drug was administered within 14 days of an MI, there was a 13.6% drop in mortality, compared with 11.8% with standard therapy. However, there was an unacceptable percentage of hyperkalemia.[37] A later study demonstrated a 15% drop in mortality at 30 days.[38]

Management of Decompensated CHF. Traditionally, β-agonists such as dobutamine have been used to treat decompensated CHF. Although these agents are effective in improving hemodynamics and decreasing some of the symptoms associated with CHF through β-receptor activation, improvement tends to be short term. Increasing β-activation leads to increased cardiac workload; and ultimately, symptomatic left ventricular dysfunction recurs.[39] In addition, frequent arrhythmias and tachycardia, which can be fatal, are adverse effects of this treatment. Dopamine may also be used in the emergency treatment of CHF. It is a β_1-agonist that also acts on the dopamine receptor. The advantage of this drug is that it produces renal arteriolar vasodilation which increases urinary output and a reduction in edema.

Many patients become dependent on intravenous inotropic infusions despite many weaning attempts.[10] Dependence is recognized by symptomatic hypotension, recurrent congestive symptoms, and worsening renal status shortly after the inotropic therapy is discontinued. When possible, the patient is sent home, and continuous inotropic therapy is used as a bridge to the use of a left ventricular assist device, to transplantation, or to the end of life.[40]

Human B-type natriuretic peptide (BNP) is a cardiac hormone that is secreted by the ventricular myocardium in response to fluid overload and ventricular wall stress.[41] BNP is thought to produce cardiac vasodilation and natriuresis. An elevated BNP level has now emerged as a marker for the diagnosis of CHF, helping to differentiate between heart failure and other causes of shortness of breath in the emergency department. ACE inhibitors, ARBs, and diuretics all reduce BNP levels. There is conflicting evidence regarding the effect of β-blocker on BNP level. It is now available as a member of a new drug classification—natriuretic peptides—and is named nesiritide.

Nesiritide is a BNP-like peptide that reduces preload and afterload and increases cardiac output without increasing heart rate.[5] In addition, this drug improves the glomerular filtration rate and has a sympatholytic cardiac effect. Its big advantage over β-agonists is that nesiritide reduces ventricular ectopy. It significantly reduced the number of ventricular tachycardic events and premature ventricular beats in a 24-hour period when compared with dobutamine. It is listed as a Drug Under Active Investigation in the 2009 guidelines for the treatment of CHF.[5]

Other drugs useful for decompensated heart failure include a loop diuretic such as intravenous furosemide, which produces rapid diuresis; sublingual nitroglycerin; and oxygen in high concentrations.[42] Morphine can also be used to help relieve shortness of breath, anxiety, and pain.[43] Morphine has a significant venodilator effect, which is helpful in reducing venous return. The patient's condition may improve once excess fluid is removed and the β-blocker and ACE inhibitor can be restarted. Figure 8-4 reviews the pharmacologic management of CHF and at what stage in the disease these drugs are introduced.

Treatment of Diastolic Heart Failure

Drug treatment for diastolic heart failure and systolic heart failure are similar except that there is greater emphasis on preventing tachycardia in diastolic heart failure.[4] Increased heart rate reduces diastolic filling time and coronary perfusion, so drugs that slow the heart rate, such as β-blockers and calcium channel blockers, can be useful. Digoxin can be tried with precautionary measures. It produces a lowering of heart rate via its vagal properties, but at the same time its inotropic effects may worsen this type of heart failure. Since this syndrome has only recently been recognized, studies on diastolic heart failure are at an infant stage.[5]

DRUG TREATMENT FOR CARDIAC ARRHYTHMIA

Technically, the term *arrhythmia* means no rhythm and the term *dysrhythmia* means an abnormal rhythm. In the literature and in clinical cardiology, particularly in the United States, they tend to be used interchangeably. Arrhythmias are a result of abnormal electrical events that occur in the heart as a result of ischemia, hypoxia, excessive myocardial fiber stretch, excessive discharge or sensitivity to catecholamines, scarred tissue, drug toxicity, or electrolyte imbalance.[3] Most arrhythmias result from disturbances in either impulse formation or impulse conduction. Heart rate may be faster or slower than normal but still maintain the appropriate shape on electrocardiogram (ECG; sinus tachycardia and sinus bradycardia). Impulse conduction may also be stopped,

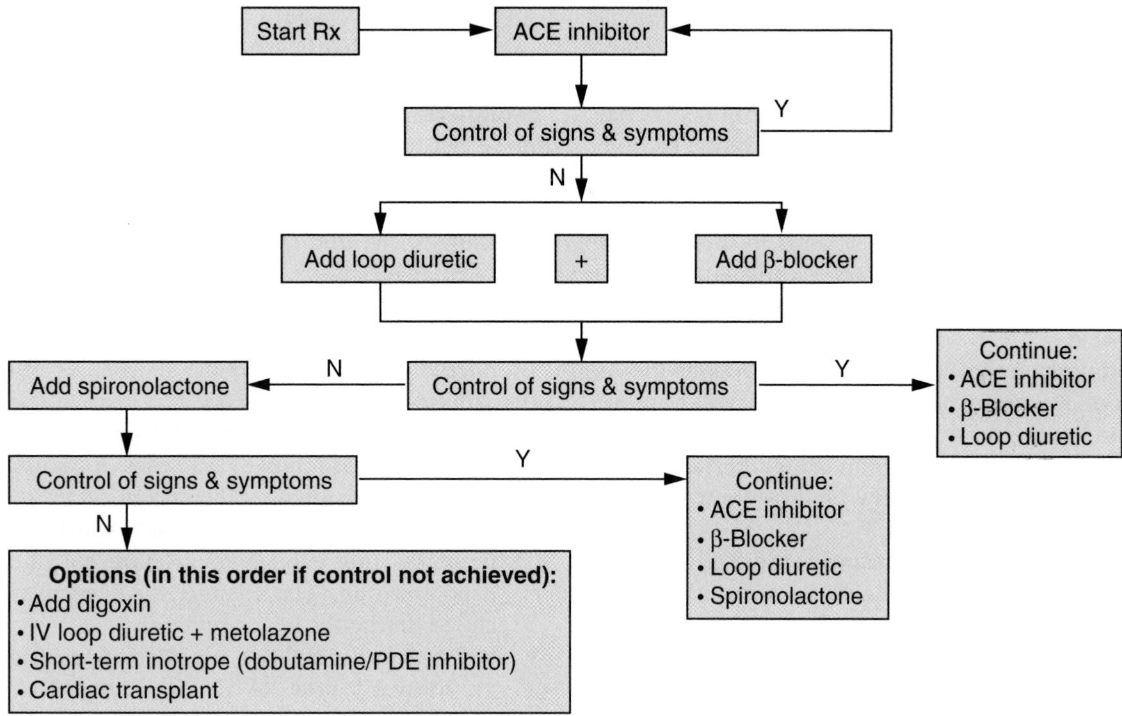

FIGURE 8-4 Management of chronic cardiac failure. *N*, no; *Y*, yes; *Rx*, treatment; *PDE*, phosphodiesterase. *(From Bennett PN, Brown MJ, editors.* Clinical pharmacology *(9th ed.). New York, 2003, Churchill Livingstone.)*

BOX 8-2 Drugs Used to Treat Heart Failure

Drug Category	Drug	Major Class Adverse Effects
β-blocker	Carvedilol (Coreg)	Fatigue, dizziness, hypotension, bradycardia, impaired recovery from hypoglycemia, increased risk of diabetes, increased LDL
	Metoprolol (Toprol XL)	
	Bisoprolol (Zebeta)	
ACE inhibitor	Lisinopril (Prinivil or Zestril)	Cough, hyperkalemia, hypotension, dizziness, weakness
	Fosinopril (Monopril)	
	Enalapril (Vasotec)	
	Benazepril (Lotensin)	
	Quinapril (Accupril)	
	Ramipril (Altace)	
ARBs	Losartan (Cozaar)	Hyperkalemia, hypotension, dizziness, weakness
	Candesartan (Atacand)	
	Valsartan (Diovan)	
	Ibesartan (Avapro)	
Aldosterone blocker	Spironolactone (Aldactone)	Hyperkalemia, gynecomastia in males (spironolactone), dizziness
	Eplerenone (Inspra)	
Inotropic agent	Digoxin	Nausea, vomiting, rhythm disturbances, especially bradycardia, electrolyte abnormalities, visual disturbances (colored vision)
	Milrinone	
Vasodilators	Isosorbide dinitrate	Dizziness, drowsiness, light-headedness, constipation, hypotension
	Hydralazine (Apresoline)	
Loop diuretics	Furosemide (Lasix)	Dizziness, hypokalemia, tinnitus, metabolic alkalosis, hypovolemia, hypotension, hyperuricemia, agranulocytosis
	Bumetanide (Bumex)	
	Ethacrynic acid (Edecrin)	
Thiazide diuretics	Hydrochlorothiazide (HydroDIURIL)	Dizziness, hypokalemia, hyponatremia, hypovolemia, hypotension, hyperglycemia, increased LDL
	Metolazone (Mykrox)	

LDL, low-density lipoprotein; *ACE*, angiotensin-converting enzyme, *ARB*, ACE receptor blocker.

commonly in or below the atrioventricular (AV) node producing a heart block or a bundle branch block. Arrhythmias also result from single or multiple beats originating from sites other than the pacemaker cell (sinoartial [SA] node), and these are noted as ectopic beats. Ectopic beats whose origin is in the atrium are called atrial premature contractions (APGs) and appear as abnormally timed P waves on ECG. If the origin is in the ventricle they are referred to as premature ventricular contractions (PVCs). Additional arrhythmic descriptions include the following:

- Atrial flutter occurs when atrial contractions are in excess of 300 beats/min. On ECG, there will be more than on P wave for every QRS complex.
- In atrial fibrillation, the atrium shows erratic twitching without distinct P waves with disruption of active pumping.
- Paroxysmal supraventricular tachycardia refers to an arrhythmia originating in the AV node resulting from retrograde travel through the node. Atrial tachycardia results.
- Ventricular fibrillation results in uncoordinated or asynchronous contractions causing the ventricles to remain partially contracted but unable to pump appropriately.

To understand these rhythm disturbances and how drug therapy suppresses them, we must review normal cardiac electrophysiology.

Contractility and its coordination throughout the heart are achieved by a specialized conduction system.[3] Sinus rhythm begins with impulses originating in the sinoatrial (SA) node and conducted through the atria, the AV node, bundle of His, Purkinje fibers, and finally to the ventricles. Cardiac cells and muscle are electrically sensitive because of various voltage-gated plasma membrane channels in which ions—including the Na^+, K^+, and Ca^{2+} ions—travel to control the electrical potential.

Ventricular and atrial cell membranes maintain a resting membrane potential between –85 and –90 mV as a result of an unequal distribution of electrolytes (high concentration of K^+ inside the cell compared with outside the cell).[44,45] This gradient is maintained by the Na^+/K^+-ATPase pump, which moves three Na^+ ions outward in exchange for two K^+ ions inward. An action potential is generated when voltage-gated Na^+ channels open and the entering ions depolarize the cell. This channel is referred to as the fast inward Na^+ current (I_{Na+}). If the Na^+ channel remains open for more than a few milliseconds, the channel will inactivate, and a second action potential cannot occur. This is called the *effective refractory period.* The hyperpolarizing phase of the action potential begins with the opening of different types of K^+ channels, which carry these ions in an outward direction. The slow inward Ca^{2+} current (ISI) is responsible for the plateau phase of the action potential. Calcium enters the cell, balancing an outward K^+ current.

At the SA and AV nodal tissue, the resting membrane potential is more positive and tends to be unstable.[44] This instability produces firing of the SA node at a rate that is faster than in any other region of the heart. The SA nodal action potential is conducted rapidly through the atria but then is delayed at the AV node because of dependence on a slow inward Ca^{2+} channel. Once the action potential enters the ventricle, it is conducted rapidly through the bundle of His, Purkinje fibers, and then ultimately through the entire ventricular mass.

Ventricular and SA node action potentials are different in shape owing to the different ion channels that produce them.[3] For the typical ventricular cell, the cardiac phases are as follows:

- Phase 0 is the period of rapid depolarization in which there is a rapid influx of Na^+ ions. It occurs when the membrane potential reaches its critical firing threshold (approximately –60 mV). The inward Na^+ current becomes large enough to produce an all-or-nothing depolarization. The channel then inactivates and is closed during the plateau phase.
- Phase 1 is early, brief repolarization, triggered by an outward flow of K^+ ions and Na^+ channel inactivation.
- Phase 2 is the plateau phase in which the K^+ current is balanced by a slow inward Ca^{2+} flux. This K^+ current is actually a specialized current known as an *inward rectifier*, which means that K^+ conductance falls as the membrane becomes more depolarized. Therefore, there is too little outward K^+ current to bring the potential down to resting. Thus, the inward Ca^{2+} current largely maintains the plateau at this point. Ca^{2+} channels behave like Na^+ channels, but in terms of activation and inactivation, they have a slower time course.
- Phase 3 is referred to as *repolarization.* At this point, the Ca^{2+} channels close, and the cell repolarizes as another K^+ channel opens and the ions flow out.
- Phase 4 is the resting phase, but for the SA node, this phase is called *diastolic depolarization.* In the SA node, several types of ion channels open to bring the membrane potential to threshold to trigger the full action potential.[46] This potential change is largely produced by increasing inward Ca^{2+} currents (from L-type and T-type calcium channels) during diastole. In addition, the SA node has greater susceptibility to Na^+ during this phase, even though it lacks the fast Na^+ current that characterizes phase 0 on the atrial or ventricular myocytes. Figure 8-5 shows the configuration of the action potential in different areas of the heart.

In the interval between phase 0 and the end of phase 2, the depolarizing channels become inactivated. This is also known as the *absolute refractory period* because the cell is unable to produce another action potential. However, during phase 3, a high amplitude stimulus may open enough Na^+ channels to produce another action potential, overcoming the K^+ outward current. Thus,

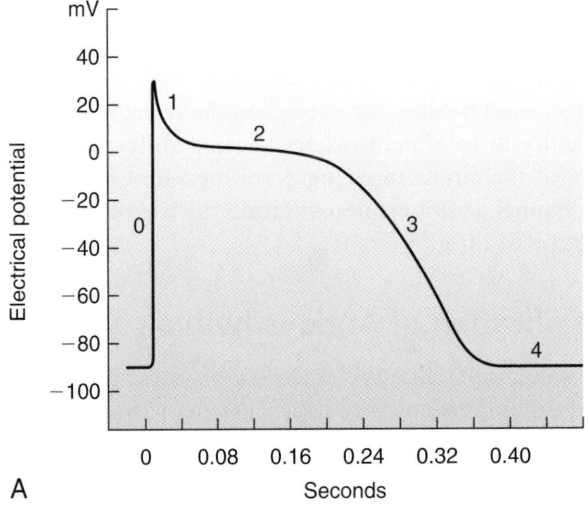

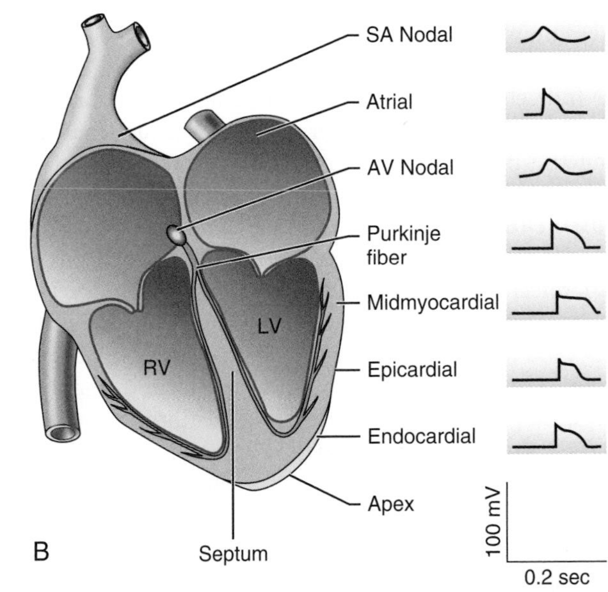

FIGURE 8-5 The cardiac action potential. **A**, Phases of the action potential: **0**, rapid depolarization; **1**, partial repolarization; **2**, plateau; **3**, repolarization; **4**, pacemaker depolarization. The *lower panel* shows the accompanying changes in membrane conductance for Na^+, K^+, and Ca^{2+}. **B**, Conduction of the impulse through the heart, with the corresponding electrocardiogram (ECG) trace. Note that the longest delay occurs at the atrioventricular (AV) node, where the action potential has a characteristically slow waveform.

this phase is known as the *relative refractory period*. The conduction of an electrical impulse is quite rapid but orderly, except in the case of disease. A localized ischemic area or tissue that has experienced a previous myocardial infarction may slow or interrupt a traveling impulse. For example, an impulse conducting down a Purkinje fiber may spread to an adjacent fiber that has failed to transmit and instead pass up it in a reverse direction. If this retrograde conduction should excite the original tissue that already transmitted the impulse, a re-entrant excitation occurs.

Mechanism for Arrhythmia

Abnormal impulse generation is responsible for many arrhythmias. This may be due to an enhanced normal automatic rhythm (nodal tachycardia) or an "abnormal automaticity." The pacemaker (SA) rate may be altered by shortening diastolic depolarization (increasing the slope of phase 4) through catecholamine stimulation. In addition, raising the resting diastolic potential (making it more positive) or making the threshold potential more negative will produce similar results, that is, trigger an action potential sooner. Likewise, slowing heart rate can be achieved by vagus nerve stimulation reversing the values just mentioned.

The SA node has the highest rate of spontaneous discharge (70 beats/min) and therefore controls the heart rate. If the SA node fails to initiate an electrical impulse, then the heart tissue with the next fastest rate takes over. This is often the AV node, which can initiate an impulse 45 times per minute. Next in line is the His–Purkinje system at 25 discharges per minute.

Abnormal automaticity occurs when an ectopic focus develops (usually in the Purkinje fibers) that presents with a faster rate than the SA node or other potential pacemaker. This is known as *ectopic pacemaker activity*. This type of activity can also lead to another phenomenon underlying many arrhythmias called *delayed after-depolarization*[47] (Figure 8-6). Delayed after-depolarizations occur in phase 4 in response to excess calcium release from the sarcoplasmic reticulum. They can also be induced by cardiac glycosides, norepinephrine, or phosphodiesterase inhibitors that increase intracellular Ca^{2+} levels. It is thought that excess calcium activates Na^+–Ca^{2+} exchange, which brings one Ca^{2+} ion out of the cell in exchange for transfer of three Na^+ ions into the cell, producing depolarization.

Abnormal automaticity may also be produced by early after-depolarizations. Early after-depolarizations occur during phase 3 and result from bradycardia or drugs that prolong the action potential. They may involve decreased conduction through one of the K^+ channels.

Abnormal impulse conduction refers to a heart block or circus re-entry movements.[47] The most common site for a heart block is the AV node. A first-degree block refers to slowing of the impulse through the node. A second-degree block occurs when not all the impulses from the SA node are transmitted to the ventricles, and a third-degree block occurs when there is complete blockage through the AV node. In a third-degree block, the atria and ventricles beat independently of each other, with the ventricles beating at their intrinsically slower rate or at a rate determined by whatever pacemaker activates distal to the block.

Re-entry rhythm underlies a variety of arrhythmias, and depending on the site of the re-entrant circuit, can affect the atria, ventricles, or nodal tissues.[47] Basically, the re-entry circuit describes a situation in which there is

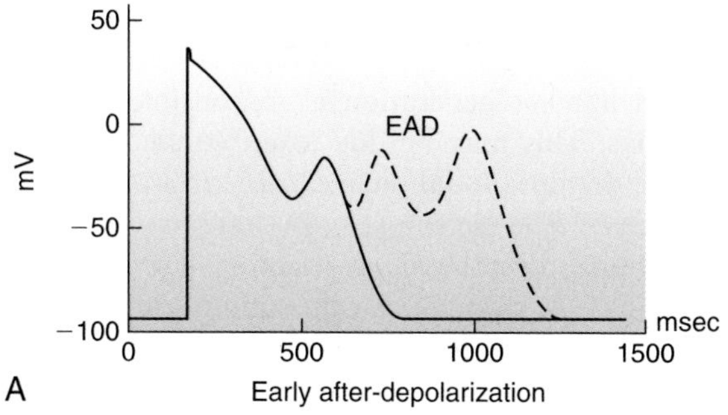

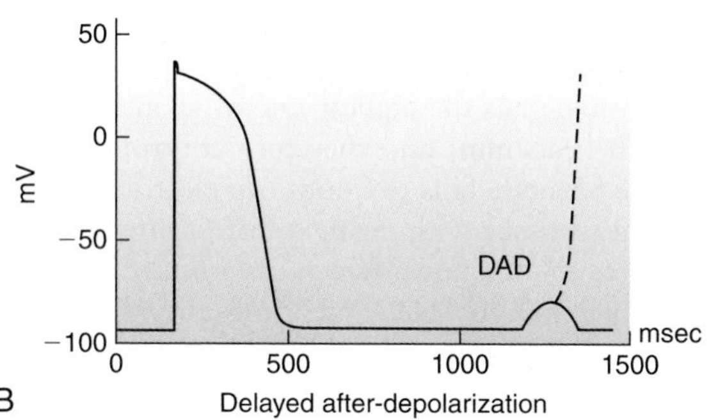

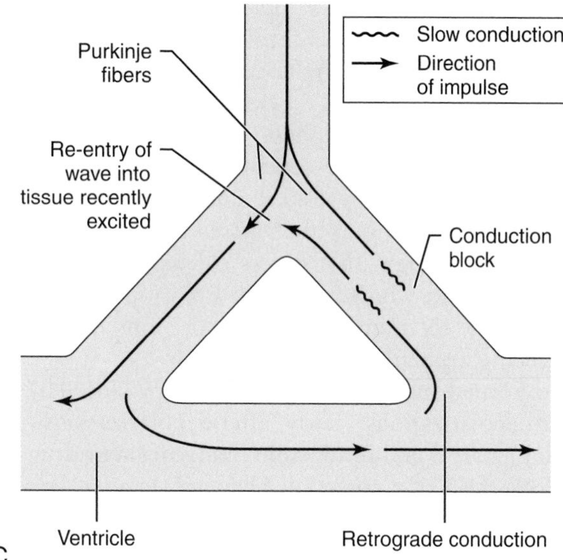

FIGURE 8-6 Main mechanism of arrhythmogenesis.

a partial conduction block. Normally, an impulse traveling around a ring of tissue will conduct in both directions, and the two impulses will extinguish themselves when they meet. However, if the area has ischemic damage, enough so that one impulse is blocked but the second can get through, a continuous circle of activity can occur. This is known as *circus movement* and occurs with a unidirectional block. Essentially, the impulse re-excites tissues that have just passed through their refractory period, but it does this over and over again (see Figure 8-6). Wolff-Parkinson-White syndrome is an anatomic anomaly that consists of a ring of tissue linking the atria and ventricles, which is often a location for circus re-entry arrhythmias. Treatment for this condition is directed at converting a unidirectional block into a bidirectional block or at extending the refractory period. Difficulty in treatment occurs because different components of the circus movement are mediated by different ion channel activities, necessitating the use of more than one type of drug.[48]

Classification of Antidysrhythmic Drugs

The Vaughan-Williams classification system proposed in 1970 offers a useful way to discuss the various antidysrhythmic drugs.[49,50] This system classifies drugs according to their major electrophysiologic effects and the phase of the cardiac cycle they affect. However, the student must realize that most of the drugs used for the treatment of arrythmias block multiple channels and have complex kinetics that limit the use of this classification scheme in clinical practice.[51] That being said, there are four classes of drugs: class I (drugs that block Na^+ channels); class II (β-blockers); class III (drugs that prolong the cardiac action potential); and class IV (Ca^{2+} blockers).

Class I Drugs. Class I drugs act by blocking Na^+ channels, slowing the rate of rise of phase 0. These drugs are also referred to as *membrane-stabilizing agents.* They are considered "use-dependent blockers," meaning that they bind more rapidly to open channels to block rapidly firing cells, rather than to fully repolarized channels. Thus, they do not affect the resting membrane potential. Class I drugs are further divided according to the duration of their effect on the action potential.[52] Class Ia

BOX 8-3 Vaughan–Williams Classification of Antidysrhythmic Drugs

Classification	Drug
Ia: Sodium channel blockers Moderate slowing of the action potential	Quinidine (Quinidex Extentabs) Procainamide (Pronestyl) Disopyramide (Norpace)
Ib Minimal slowing of the action potential	Lidocaine (Xylocaine) Mexiletine (Mexitil)
Ic Marked slowing of the action potential	Flecainide (Tambocor) Propafenone (Rythmol) Moricizine (Ethmozine)
II β-blockers	Propranolol (Inderal) Esmolol (Brevibloc)
III Prolongs the action potential	Amiodarone (Cordarone) Dronedarone (Multaq) Dofetilide (Tikosyn) Sotalol (Betapace)
IV Blocks calcium channels	Verapmil (Calan, Isoptin) Diltiazem (Cardizem, Dilacor)
Miscellaneous	Adenosine (Adenocard): opens K^+ channels

drugs produce a moderate slowing of the action potential (adjunctive class III action) by blocking K^+ currents, thus prolonging the effective refractory period. Examples of class Ia drugs include quinidine, disopyramide, and procainamide. Quinidine is the prototypical class Ia drug. In addition to its class Ia activity, quinidine has a positive inotropic effect (through a lengthening of ventricular systole) and an antimuscarinic effect. These agents are effective in suppressing premature ventricular beats, recurrent ventricular tachycardia, and re-entry arrhythmias. Because it slows conduction, quinidine can block re-entry by converting a unidirectional block to a bidirectional block. Adverse drug reactions include nausea, vomiting, and diarrhea. Larger doses may cause cinchonism (headache, vertigo, tinnitus, blurred vision, and disorientation). Perhaps most worrisome is that this drug and many other antiarrhythmics may exacerbate arrhythmias. Quinidine may cause not only SA and AV blocks but also sinus tachycardia. It is difficult to predict whether this drug will have a beneficial effect or a negative effect. Problems with this drug most definitely occur if hypokalemia is also present.

Class Ib drugs block Na^+ channels minimally, slowing depolarization but also decreasing the action potential duration by shortening the refractory period and suppressing conduction. Class Ib agents include lidocaine and the oral agents mexiletine and tocainide. As with class Ia drugs, use of these drugs is decreasing, although they are still used to inhibit ventricular tachycardia. Adverse effects occur primarily in the CNS and include drowsiness, slurred speech, paresthesias, confusion, and convulsions as the dose increases.

Class Ic drugs markedly slow phase 0 depolarization, even in healthy tissue, so conduction is slowed in all of the cardiac tissue, producing a prolonged depressant effect on conduction velocity and a wide QRS complex.[53] Flecainide and propafenone are class Ic agents. They are approved for treatment of refractory ventricular arrhythmias. Common adverse effects include dizziness, blurred vision, and headaches. Syncope can occur and is indicative of the proarrhythmic effects that these drugs have. Flecainide can induce life-threatening ventricular tachycardia and lead to death.[54]

To understand how these antidysrhythmic drugs may cause additional arrhythmias we need to further explore the concept of "use-dependent blocking." These class I drugs associate with open channels during systole and then dissociate during diastole. However, with tachycardia, there is less time for the drug to dissociate and blockage of the channel persists. For a drug like lidocaine that shows fast dissociation kinetics, little blockage remains in diastole, even at high heart rates. But the story is different for flecainide, which possesses slow dissociation kinetics. Therefore, the blockage remains even when heart rate returns to a normal range. This can be seen as a prolonged QRS segment on ECG. This overall slowing of conduction promotes re-entry impulses.

Class II Drugs. Class II antidysrhythmic drugs include the β-adrenergic antagonists. These drugs depress sinus node automaticity and prolong AV nodal conduction. They are useful in treating atrial flutter and fibrillation and can also prevent re-entry. These are excellent drugs for treating arrhythmias associated with exercise or any arrhythmia provoked by increased sympathetic activity.[55] The agents most commonly used for their antidysrhythmic effects include propranolol, acebutolol, and esmolol. Esmolol is a short-acting β_1-selective blocker used solely for the treatment of arrhythmias.[52] It is given intravenously and has a very short half-life (9 minutes), which allows it to be titrated rapidly against response.

Class III Drugs. Class III antidysrhythmic drugs prolong repolarization and the effective refractory period by blocking K^+ channels. They are considered to be the most effective antidysrhythmic leave agents. Amiodarone is one of the most commonly used drugs for ventricular arrhythmias.[56] It has some Na^+ and Ca^{2+} channel blocking abilities also and binds β-receptors noncompetitively. However, its usefulness is limited by its adverse effects. The list of adverse effects includes interstitial pulmonary fibrosis, gastrointestinal problems, thyroid dysfunction, blurred vision, ataxia, dizziness, liver toxicity, neuropathy, and bluish discoloration on exposed areas of the skin. Some of these may occur after only short-term use but will disappear when the drug is withdrawn. However, because of its long half-life (>50 days), several months may be needed for the drug to completely clear from the body. In terms of its cardiovascular adverse effects, amiodarone may cause bradycardia, heart block, and ventricular arrhythmias. The proarrhythmic effects of the class III drugs are particularly more prevalent in the hypertrophied heart.[57] In addition, the risk of developing life-threatening arrhythmias appears to be greater within the first few days of dosing. Some physicians propose 72-hour hospitalization when administration of these drugs is initiated to monitor patients for electrical changes.[58]

Dofetilide and sotalol are additional class III drugs.[47] Sotalol is actually a β-blocker, but it prolongs the action potential by delaying the outward K^+ current. It is not as effective as amiodarone in preventing ventricular arrhythmias but is free of some of its adverse effects. Other class III agents exist, but most have been withdrawn due to their adverse effects.

Class IV Drugs. Class IV drugs include the Ca^{2+} channel blockers.[47] These drugs inhibit Ca^{2+} transport through the membrane channels, resulting in depression of contractility there and also in suppression of automatic activity in the pacemaker cells. Verapamil and diltiazem are most commonly used for supraventricular tachycardia and atrial fibrillation. They decrease the SA nodal rate and AV nodal conduction.

Other Antiarrhythmics. Adenosine is another antidysrhythmic agent, but it does not fall within the Vaughan-Williams classification system. It stimulates adenosine receptors in the SA and AV nodes, which ultimately opens K^+ channels.[47,59] Re-entry movement is terminated by hyperpolarization and a decrease in action potential duration. Intravenous adenosine is used to stop supraventricular tachycardia. Adverse effects include bronchospasm and hypotension, which are usually not very serious because of adenosine's extremely short half-life (seconds) and the fact that this drug is not negatively inotropic like verapamil.

The last antidysrhythmic to discuss is digitalis.[47] This drug is primarily used in the treatment of CHF but is also used to control or slow ventricular rate in supraventricular tachycardia by prolonging the AV refractory period and also by producing a parasympathomimetic effect. It loses its effectiveness during exercise as the body shifts toward a more sympathetic control of heart function, so it is reserved for patients who are more sedentary.

Therapeutic Concerns with Antidysrhythmic Agents

The presence of adverse effects such as faintness, dizziness, or visual disturbances may indicate toxic drug effects from the antiarrhythmics or additional arrhythmias. All antidysrhythmic drugs can also produce arrhythmias, and efficacy in suppressing arrhythmias is only between 30% and 60%.[60] In addition, with the exception of amiodarone, no single antidysrhythmic agent shows superiority. Proarrhythmic effects are most likely to be seen with the drugs that prolong the QT interval (i.e., the action potential) on ECG.[61] Hypokalemia, in particular, increases the risk. Arrhythmias may only be detected by monitoring with electrocardiography. If ECG is not available, palpation of pulses for rate and regularity may detect rhythm disturbances.

Little information is available on how these drugs affect short- and long-term–duration exercise and how exercise affects arrhythmias.[55] Many antiarrhythmics have negative inotropic effects and therefore would impair exercise performance. Exercise may also increase rhythm disturbances as a result of an increase in circulating catecholamines and render the drugs ineffective during these periods.[52] Patients are cautioned to watch for signs of these disturbances and are also instructed not to stop exercising abruptly because this can cause an irregular rhythm.[62]

Treatment for Some Specific Arrhythmias

Although treatment of irregular rhythm is challenging, some effective protocols have been outlined for specific arrhythmias. Drugs, pacemakers, implantable defibrillators, and surgery may be used separately or in combination to treat a variety of arrhythmias.

Atrial Fibrillation. Atrial fibrillation is one of the most common cardiac arrhythmias.[63] It is defined as an "erratic quivering or twitching" of the atrial muscle caused by multiple ectopic atrial foci or a rapidly circulating circus movement.[64] There are no true P waves because the ectopic foci do not actually depolarize the atria. The AV node tends to control the impulses that produce a ventricular response; however, the ventricular rate can still be normal, slow, or very fast, and usually the QRS complex has an irregular rhythm.

There are pharmacologic and nonpharmacologic options for patients with atrial fibrillation. Despite unsatisfactory drug therapy, most patients are still treated with medications. However, a certain subset of patients will respond to various ablation procedures. These are individuals whose atrial fibrillation can be traced back to triggers in the pulmonary veins.[65] However, most individuals experience fibrillation sustained by "self-perpetuating macro–re-entrant circuits in the atria" and either need more widespread ablation or drug therapy.

In patients who have a ventricular response rate lower than 100 beats/min, cardiac output is not affected. However, if the patient exercises or if the ventricular rate is greater than 100 beats/min at rest, then cardiac output is diminished, and signs of heart failure may occur. Another problem with atrial fibrillation is the development of an atrial thrombus caused by coagulation of blood within the atria, leading to an embolus, and ultimately, a stroke.

There are several pharmacologic approaches to the management of atrial fibrillation. If the ventricular response rate is normal or slightly slowed, no pharmacologic management may be indicated. However, if the ventricular response rate is fast, treatment must be directed first toward control of this rate. Intravenous verapamil or diltiazem will produce a drop in ventricular rate within minutes. Diltiazem is preferred in patients with CHF but has also shown superiority over intravenous amiodarone and digoxin in achieving ventricular rate control.[66] β-Blockers can also be used to control ventricular rate. In fact, these are the drugs of choice when there are accessory electrical pathways that may become activated if the Ca^{2+} channel blockers produce a maximum slowing of AV nodal conduction.[52] In addition, they are very effective agents in thyrotoxicosis and in postoperative cardiac surgery. Esmolol is available for intravenous use, and oral β-blockers (atenolol and metoprolol) can be used for long-term rate control.

Until recently, there had been controversy over the primary initial approach to atrial fibrillation—rate control or rhythm control. However, two large studies have shown no difference in morbidity or symptoms between the two strategies.[67,68] This widens the treatment approach because trying to control rhythm with larger and larger doses of antidysrhythmic agents that have a poor benefit/risk ratio is not desirable if rate control can be achieved with a safer drug.[69]

If there is only a short history of atrial fibrillation and the heart is not enlarged, the patient may benefit from cardioversion and rhythm control. Electrical conversion is the choice if treatment is urgent, or the patient can be given amiodarone for conversion in hours to days.

For maintaining sinus rhythm over time, class Ia and Ic agents have been found to be helpful; however, amiodarone might still be the most effective drug.[70] However, it is still associated with a 30% recurrence rate after 1 year. For patients in whom sinus rhythm cannot be achieved with drugs, other therapies such as AV node ablation and pacemaker implantation or other implantable device–based therapy (implantable defibrillators with antitachycardia pacing) may be helpful.[71]

Atrial fibrillation promotes thrombus formation and an overall increased risk of stroke. If the patient is considered to be at low risk for a stroke, aspirin is recommended. For those who are at moderate to high risk of stroke (which is the majority of patients with atrial fibrillation), adequate anticoagulation with vitamin K antagonists is recommended.[72] New approaches with other antiplatelet drugs or anticoagulants are currently being explored for efficacy in reducing embolic events in these patients.

Ventricular Tachycardia. Ventricular tachycardia is a series of premature ventricular contractions that occur in a row.[73] It results from rapid firing by a single ventricular focus. P waves tend to be absent, and the QRS complexes are wide and bizarre. Ventricular rate is between 100 and 250 beats/min. This condition is often associated with ischemic heart disease but can also result from drugs that prolong the QT interval. Treatment consists of immediate injection with class I drugs, such as lidocaine or procainamide, or defibrillation. For recurrent ventricular tachycardia, amiodarone or sotalol may be chosen.

Ventricular Fibrillation. Ventricular fibrillation is the most prevalent arrhythmia in acute cardiac arrest. It presents as an irregular quivering of the ventricular muscle, resulting in severely diminished cardiac output. Treatment is defibrillation, followed by cardiopulmonary resuscitation (CPR). For recurrent fibrillation, suppression with sotalol or amiodarone with a β-blocker is suggested. An implantable cardioverter–defibrillator is also recommended.

Treatments for atrial and ventricular arrhythmias remain a challenge. The most significant problem with antidysrhythmic drugs is that they are proarrhythmic. Without an ECG, it is not always easy to recognize altered rate of rhythm in a patient. The therapist must pay particular attention to any reports of dizziness, light-headedness, palpations, chest pain, shortness of breath, or syncope. It is hoped that the new drugs that are more efficacious with reduced mortality than the ones currently available will be approved soon. It is also expected that nonpharmacologic treatments such as pacemakers, implantable cardioverter–defibrillators, and surgical ablation procedures will be improved and become more efficacious.

ACTIVITIES 8

1. AP is a 78-year-old woman who presents with a 1-week history of progressive shortness of breath (SOB). She reports the need to sleep on three pillows to breathe comfortably through the night. She also reports a 15-lb weight gain within the last month. The SOB has worsened considerably in the last 2 days so that she is unable to ambulate more than 10 feet without resting.

Medical History: Congestive heart failure (CHF) × 3 years, coronary artery disease (CAD) × 10 years, inferior wall myocardial infarction (MI) 1 year ago, type II diabetes × 20 years, degenerative joint disease (DJD) × 10 years

Social History: The patient lives alone. She uses a walker to ambulate throughout her house but requires a wheelchair for most outside excursions. Her daughter lives 1 hour away but visits her weekly to help with the shopping.

Medications: Lisinopril, furosemide, verapamil, warfarin, nitro patch, sublingual nitro, ibuprofen, glipizide (decreases blood glucose level in type II diabetics)

Physical Exam: Vital signs: blood pressure (BP), 135/88 mm Hg; pulse, 110 beats/min; respiratory rate (RR) 28 breaths/min; Weight, 190 lb

Neck: Mild jugular venous distension (JVD), no lymphadenopathy

Cardiac: Irregular rhythm, systolic murmur

Lungs: Crackles and wheezes noted

Extremities: Pedal edema, pedal pulses 1+ bilaterally, extremities cold to touch

Neurologic Findings: Within normal limits (WNL)

Labs: Na^+ 129 mEq/L; K^+ 4. 7 mEq/L; chloride 101 mEq/L; $PaCO^2$ 47 mm Hg; blood urea nitrogen (BUN) 53 mg/dL; serum creatinine 2. 3 mg/dL; glucose 130 mg/dL; hemoglobin 10. 0 g/dL; platelets 259, 000/mm^3; white blood cell (WBC) count 8800/mm^3; international normalized ratio (INR), 3.5

Chest X-Ray: Mild pulmonary edema and cardiomegaly

ECG: No acute ST or T wave changes

Questions

A. What signs and symptoms indicate the presence or severity of the patient's condition?
B. Could any of these problems have been caused by drug therapy?
C. What do you think is her diagnosis?
D. Would you recommend a medication change? If yes, what would you suggest, and what information should be provided to the patient about her new medications?
E. Are there any physical therapy interventions to reduce this patient's dependence on medications?

2. Interview a patient with CHF. Use the following questions to assess how much the patient understands about his/her condition, the medications, and his/her ability to determine when the condition is worsening.

Questions for Patient:

A. *Do you know when your heart failure began?*
B. *What medications are you taking, and what are they used for?*
C. *Do you know what adverse effects these drugs produce, and can you differentiate between the adverse drug effects and the symptoms of heart failure?*
D. *How do you monitor your symptoms of heart failure, and what do you do to manage them?*

Questions for Students

A. If you were seeing this patient in the home care setting, how would you determine whether this patient's medical condition is worsening?
B. What suggestions do you have regarding how to improve this patient's understanding of CHF, as well as his/her condition?

3. Heart failure is a major public health problem particularly among black men. Review the following article and discuss the reasons for the high prevalence among this population and what can be done to reverse this trend.
Bibbins-Domingo, K., et al., Racial differences in incident heart failure among young adults. *N Engl J Med* 360(12):1179–1190, 2009.

4. Since amiodarone is one of the most commonly used antidysrhythmic drugs, review its adverse effects and precautions that might influence therapy.

REFERENCES

1. Rosamond W, Flegal K, Furie K, et al: American Heart Association Statistical Update. Heart Disease and Stroke Statistics-2008 update. Circulation 115:e25-e146, 2007.
2. Djousse L, Driver JA, Gaziano JM: Relation between modifiable lifestyle factors and lifetime risk of heart failure. JAMA 302(4):394-400, 2009.
3. Page, C. , et al:, Drugs and the cardiovascular system. In Page C, Hoffman B, Curtis M, Walker M, editors: Integrated pharmacology, Philadelphia, 2006, Mosby.
4. Reddersen LA, Keen C, Nasir L, Berry D: Diastolic heart failure: State of the science on best treatment practices. J Am Acad Nurse Pract 20(10):506-514, 2008.
5. American College of Cardiology Foundation/American Heart Association Task Force on Practice Guidelines: 2009 Focused update incorporated into the ACC/AHA 2005 guidelines for the diagnosis and management of heart failure in adults. Circulation 119:e391-e479, 2009.
6. Klapholz M: β-Blocker use for the stages of heart failure. Mayo Clin Proc 84(8):718-729, 2009.
7. Lonn E, McKelvie R: Drug treatment in heart failure. Br Med J 320(7243):1188-1192, 2000.
8. The Digitalis Investigation Group: The effect of digoxin on mortality and morbidity in patients with heart failure. N Engl J Med 336:525-533, 1997.
9. Ahmed A, Waagstein F, Pitt B, et al: Effectiveness of digoxin in reducing one-year mortality in chronic heart failure in the Digitalis Investigation Group Trial. Am J Cardiol 103(1):82-87, 2009.
10. Stevenson LW: Clinical use of inotropic therapy for heart failure: Looking backward or forward? Part II: Chronic inotropic therapy. Circulation 108(4):492-497, 2003.
11. Adams KF Jr, Gheorghiade M, Uretsky BF, et al: Patients with mild heart failure worsen during withdrawal from digoxin therapy. J Am Coll Cardiol 30:42-48, 1993.
12. Dec GW: Digoxin remains useful in the management of chronic heart failure. Med Clin North Am 87(2):317-337, 2003.
13. Feldman AM: Heart failure. In Waldman SA, Terzic A: editors: Pharmacology and therapeutics principles to practice, Philadelphia, 2009, Saunders.
14. DiBianco R: Update on therapy for heart failure. Am J Med 115:480-488, 2003.
15. CIBIS-II Investigators: The Cardiac Insufficiency Bisoprolol Study II (CIBIS-II): A randomised trial. Lancet 353(9146): 9-13, 1999.
16. Simon T, Mary-Krause M, Funck-Brentano C, Lechat P, Jaillon P: Bisoprolol dose-response relationship in patients with congestive heart failure: A subgroup analysis in the cardiac insufficiency bisoprolol study (CIBIS II). Eur Heart J 24:552-559, 2003.
17. Fonarow GC, Abraham WT, Albert NM, et al: Influence of beta-blocker continuation or withdrawal on outcomes in patients hospitalized with heart failure, J Am Coll Cardiol 52(3). 190-199, 2008.
18. Waagstein F, Strömblad O, Andersson B, et al: Increased exercise ejection fraction and reversed remodeling after long-term treatment with metoprolol in congestive heart failure: A randomized, stratified, double-blind, placebo-controlled trial in mild to moderate heart failure due to ischemic or idiopathic dilated cardiomyopathy. Eur J Heart Fail 5(5):679-691, 2003.
19. Palazzuoli A, Bruni F, Puccetti L, et al: Effects of carvedilol on left ventricular remodeling and systolic function in elderly patients with heart failure. Eur J Heart Fail 4(6):765-770, 2002.
20. Bouzamondo A, Hulot JS, Sanchez P, Lechat P: Beta-blocker benefit according to severity of heart failure. Eur J Heart Fail 5(3):281-289, 2003.
21. Garg R, Yusuf S: Overview of randomized trials of angiotensin-converting enzyme inhibitors on mortality and morbidity in patients with heart failure. JAMA 273:1450-1456, 1995.
22. Flather MD, Yusuf S, Køber L, et al: Long-term ACE-inhibitor therapy in patients with heart failure or left-ventricular dysfunction: A systematic overview of data from individual patients. Lancet 355:1575-1581, 2000.
23. The CONSENSUS Trial Study Group: Effects of enalapril on mortality in severe congestive heart failure: Results of the cooperative north Scandinavian enalapril survival study (CONSENSUS). N Engl J Med 314:1547-1552, 1986.
24. Teo KK, Yusuf S, Pfeffer M: Effects of long-term treatment with angiotensin-converting enzyme inhibitors in the presence or absence of aspirin: A systematic review. Lancet 360:1037-1043, 2002.
25. Harjai KJ, Solis S, Prasad A: Use of aspirin in conjunction with angiotensin-converting enzyme inhibitors does not worsen long-term survival in heart failure. Int J Cardiol 88:207-214, 2003.
26. Pitt B, Segal R, Martinez FA, et al: Randomised trial of losartan versus captopril in patients over 65 with heart failure (Evaluation of Losartan in the Elderly Study, ELITE). Lancet 349:747-752, 1997.
27. Pitt B, Poole-Wilson PA, Segal R, et al: Effect of losartan compared with aptopril on mortality in patients with

symptomatic heart failure: randomised trial—The Losartan Heart Failure Survival Study ELITE II. Lancet 355:1582-1587, 2000.

28. Dickstein K, Kjekshus J: Effects of losartan and captopril on mortality and morbidity in high-risk patients after acute myocardial infarction: The OPTIMAAL randomised trial. Optimal Trial in Myocardial Infarction with Angiotensin II Antagonist Losartan. Lancet 360:752-760, 2002.
29. Maggioni AP, Anand I, Gottlieb SO, et al: Effects of valsartan on morbidity and mortality in patients with heart failure not receiving angiotensin-converting enzyme Inhibitors. J Am Coll Cardiol 40:1414-1421, 2002.
30. Jong P, Demers C, McKelvie RS, Liu PP: Angiotensin receptor blockers in heart failure: Meta-analysis of randomized controlled trials. J Am Coll Cardiol 39(3):463-470, 2002.
31. Blanchet M, Sheppard R, Racine N, et al: Effects of angiotensin-converting enzyme inhibitor plus irbesartan on maximal and submaximal exercise capacity and neurohumoral activation in patients with congestive heart failure. Am Heart J 149(5): 938-938, 2005.
32. Elkayam U, Hohnson JV, Shotan A: Double-blind, placebo controlled study to evaluate the effect of organic nitrates in patients with chronic heart failure treated with angiotensin-converting enzyme inhibition. Circulation 99:2652-2657, 1999.
33. The RALES Investigators: Effectiveness of spironolactone added to an angiotensin-converting enzyme inhibitor and a loop diuretic for severe chronic congestive heart failure (the Randomized Aldactone Evaluation Study [RALES]). Am J Cardiol 78:902-907, 1996.
34. Rajagopalan S, Pitt B: Aldosterone antagonists in the treatment of hypertension and target organ damage. Curr Hypertens Rep 3(3):240-248, 2001.
35. MacFadyen RJ, Barr CS, Struthers AD: Aldosterone blockade reduces vascular collagen turnover, improves heart rate variability and reduces early morning rise in heart rate in heart failure patients. Cardiovasc Res 35(1):30-34, 1997.
36. Pitt B: Do diuretics and aldosterone receptor antagonists improve ventricular remodeling? J Cardiac Fail 8(suppl 6):S491-493, 2002.
37. Pitt B, Williams G, Remme W: The EPHESUS trial: Eplerenone in patients with heart failure due to systolic dysfunction complicating acute myocardial infarction. Eplerenone Post-AMI Heart Failure Efficacy and Survival Study. Drugs Ther 15:79-87, 2001.
38. Pitt B, White H, Nicolau J: Eplerenone reduces mortality 30 days after randomization following acute myocardial infarction in patients with left ventricular systolic dysfunction and heart failure. J Am Coll Cardiol 46:425-431, 2005.
39. Burger AJ, Horton DP, LeJemtel T, et al: Effect of nesiritide (B-type natriuretic peptide) and dobutamine on ventricular arrhythmias in the treatment of patients with acutely decompensated congestive heart failure: The PRECEDENT study. Am Heart J 144:1102-1108, 2002.
40. Hon JK, Yacoub MH: Bridge to recovery with the use of left ventricular assist device and clenbuterol. Ann Thorac Surg 75:S36-S41, 2003.
41. Gallegos PJ, Maclaughlin EJ, Haase KK: Serial monitoring of brain natriuretic peptide concentrations for drug therapy management in patients with chronic heart failure. Pharmacotherapy 28(3):343-355, 2008.
42. Waller DG, Renwick AG, Hillier K: Medical pharmacology and therapeutics, New York, 2001, W.B. Saunders.
43. Johnson MJ, McDonagh TA, Harkness A, McKay SE, Dargie HJ: Morphine for the relief of breathlessness in patients with chronic heart failure-a pilot study. Eur J Heart Fail 4(6):753-756, 2002.
44. Guyton AC, Hall JE: Textbook of medical physiology (10th ed.), Philadelphia, 2000, W.B. Saunders Company.
45. Akar JG, Akar FG: Regulation of ion channels and arrhythmias in the ischemic heart, J Electrocardiol 40(6, suppl 1). S37-S41, 2007.
46. Baruscotti M, Robinson RB: Electrophysiology and pacemaker function of the developing sinoatrial node. Am J Physiol Heart Circ Physiol 293(5):H2613-H2623, 2007.
47. Darbar D, Roden DM: Rhythm disorders. In Waldman SA, Terzic A, editors: Pharmacology and therapeutics: Principles to practice, Philadelphia, 2009, Saunders.
48. Tsuchiya T, Okumura K, Honda T, Iwasa A, Ashikaga K: Effects of verapamil and lidocaine on two components of the re-entry circuit of verapamil-sensitive idiopathic left ventricular tachycardia. J Am Coll Cardiol 37(5):1415-1421, 2001.
49. Vaughan Williams EM: The relevance of cellular to clinical electrophysiology in classifying antidysrhythmic actions. J Cardiovasc Pharmacol 20(suppl 2):S1-S7, 1992.
50. Vaughan Williams . M: Classifying antidysrhythmic actions: By facts or speculation. J Clin Pharmacol 32(11):964-977, 1992.
51. Darbar D, Roden DM: Future of antidysrhythmic drugs. Curr Opin Cardiol 21(4):361-367, 2006.
52. Haugh KH: Antidysrhythmic agents at the turn of the twenty-first century. Crit Care Nurs Clin North Am 14(1):53-69, 2002.
53. Kawabata M, Hirao K, Horikawa T, et al: Syncope in patients with atrial flutter during treatment with class Ic antidysrhythmic drugs. J Electrocardiol 34(1):65-71, 2001.
54. Echt L: Mortality and morbidity in patients receiving encainide, flecainide, or placebo. N Engl J Med 324:781, 1991.
55. Belardinelli R: Arrhythmias during acute and chronic exercise in chronic heart failure. Int J Cardiol 90(2):213-218, 2003.
56. Siddoway LA: Amiodarone: guidelines for use and monitoring. Am Fam Physician 68(11):2189-2196, 2003.
57. El-Sherif N, Turitto G: Torsade de pointes. Curr Opinion in Cardiol 18(1):6-13, 2003.
58. Al-Khatib SM, LaPointe NM, Kramer JM, Califf RM: What clinicians should know about the QT interval. JAMA 289(16):2120-2127, 2003.
59. Pinter A, Dorian P: Intravenous antidysrhythmicagents. Curr Opin Cardiol 16:17-22, 2001.
60. Sanguinetti MC, Bennett PB: Antidysrhythmicdrug target choices and screening. Circ Res 93:491-499, 2003.
61. Wolbrette DL: Risk of proarrhythmia with class III antidysrhythmicagents: Sex-based differences and other issues. Am J Cardiol 91(6(suppl 1)):39-44, 2003.
62. Goodman CC: The cardiovascular system. In Goodman CC, Boissonnault WG, Fuller KS, editors: Pathology implications for the physical therapist, Philadelphia, 2003, Saunders.
63. Aronow WS: Atrial fibrillation. Heart Dis 4(2):91-101, 2002.
64. Summaries for patients. Management of newly detected atrial fibrillation: Recommendations from the American College of Physicians and the American Academy of Family Physicians. Ann Intern Med 139(12):I32-I35, 2003.
65. Haissaguerre M, Jais P, Shah DC: Spontaneous initiation of atrial fibrillation by ectopic beats originating in the pulmonary veins. N Engl J Med 339:659-666, 1998.
66. Siu CW, Lau CP, Lee WL, Lam KF, Tse HF: Intravenous diltiazem is superior to intravenous amiodarone or digoxin for achieving ventricular rate control in patients with acute uncomplicated atrial fibrillation. Crit Care Med 37(7):2174-2179, 2009.
67. Van Gelder IC, Hagens VE, Bosker HA, et al: A comparison of rate control and rhythm control in patients with recurrent persistent atrial fibrillation. N Engl J Med 347(23):1834-1840, 2002.
68. The Atrial Fibrillation Follow-up Investigation of Rhythm Management (AFFIRM) Investigators: A comparison of rate

control and rhythm control in patients with atrial fibrillation. N Engl J Med 347(23):1825-1833, 2002.

69. Connolly SJ: Preventing stroke in patients with atrial fibrillation: Current treatments and new concepts. Am Heart J 145:418-423, 2003.
70. Mazzini MJ, Monahan KM: Pharmacotherapy for atrial arrhythmias: Present and future. Heart Rhythm 5(6, suppl 1): S26-S31, 2008.
71. Maisel WH, Stevenson LW: Atrial fibrillation in heart failure: Epidemiology, pathophysiology, and rationale for therapy. Am J Cardiol 91(6 suppl 1):2-8, 2003.
72. Turpie AG: New oral anticoagulants in atrial fibrillation. Eur Heart J 29(2):155-165, 2008.
73. Hillegass E: Electrocardiography. In Hillegass E, Sadowsky HS, editors: Essentials of cardiopulmonary physical therapy, Philadelphia, 1994, Saunders.

9

Drug Therapy for Pulmonary Disorders

Barbara Gladson

REGULATION OF RESPIRATION AND AIRWAY SMOOTH MUSCLE TONE

The basic rhythm for respiration comes from the medullary rhythmicity center, which receives input from the pontine and higher central nervous system (CNS) centers, as well as vagal afferent input from the lungs.[1] Several chemical substances in the blood also affect the respiratory center. Peripheral control comes from carbon dioxide (CO_2) chemoreceptors in the medulla and oxygen chemoreceptors in the carotid bodies and aortic arch that respond to changes in the blood partial pressure of these substances. Respiratory rate is increased by elevated blood PCO_2 and lowered blood PO_2. There is also some degree of voluntary control that can be superimposed on automatic breathing, implying connections between the cortex and the muscles of respiration.

Airway smooth muscle tone is influenced by a balance maintained between the parasympathetic nervous system, sympathetic nervous system, circulating catecholamines, and a third nervous pathway called the *nonadrenergic–noncholinergic system* (Figure 9-1).[1] The parasympathetic nervous system, acting through the vagus nerve, releases acetylcholine to interact with muscarinic receptors. Of the five identified muscarinic receptors, three influence pulmonary ventilation: M_1 receptors exist in the parasympathetic ganglia in the airways, and mediate the transmission of acetylcholine to nicotinic receptors; M_2 receptors sit at the ends of cholinergic nerve terminals and are inhibitory autoreceptors in a feedback loop to modulate basal tone; and M_3 receptors are found on bronchial smooth muscle and glands and mediate the bronchoconstrictor response to cholinergic nerve stimulation or circulating cholinomimetics.[2] Stimulation of this system produces mainly bronchoconstriction in the larger airways and mucus secretion.

Sympathetic nerves directly innervate blood vessels and glands to produce constriction and inhibit secretion, but they do not innervate airway smooth muscle. Instead, the sympathetic effect on bronchial smooth muscle is produced by circulating catecholamines, specifically epinephrine from the adrenal glands, which primarily activates β_2-receptors.[3] Stimulation of these receptors relaxes smooth muscle, inhibits release of chemicals from mast cells, and increases mucociliary clearance. β_1-receptors are present but are localized to submucosal glands. α-Receptors also exist on the airways but appear to produce airway constriction only in diseased lungs. The nonadrenergic–noncholinergic mediators include nitric oxide (NO), which produces relaxation of the airways, and excitatory neuropeptides such as substance P and neurokinin A. These agents produce constriction, increase vascular permeability, and increase mucus secretion.

In addition to the efferent pathways, afferent pathways also contribute to airway regulation. Specialized irritant receptors and C fibers fire off in response to inflammatory mediators to produce coughing, bronchoconstriction, and mucus secretion.[1] Physical stimuli such as breathing in cold air can also stimulate these receptors and produce bronchoconstriction.

BRONCHIAL ASTHMA

Asthma is considered to be a chronic inflammatory disorder of the airways, which produces acute bronchoconstriction and shortness of breath.[3] The bronchi become hyper-reactive as a result of an inflammatory process involving a variety of stimulants, including allergens, environmental chemicals, exercise, cold air, aspirin-type drugs, and viruses. Cell types that participate in the inflammatory process include mast cells, T lymphocytes, immunoglobulin E (IgE) producing B lymphocytes, eosinophils, neutrophils, and macrophages. Eosinophils are particularly active in the inflammatory process in both acute and chronic asthma of mild to moderate severity, while neutrophils play a greater role in severe or steroid-resistant asthma. This is in contrast to chronic obstructive pulmonary disease (COPD), in which the neutrophil, macrophage, and $CD8^+$ T cells mediate inflammation.

In allergic asthma, also known as extrinsic asthma, inhaled allergens bind to IgE-bound mast cells and set off a cascade of events leading to destruction of the mast cell and liberation of a variety of chemical mediators that are damaging to the respiratory epithelium (Figure 9-2). Histamine is released preformed so that it produces an

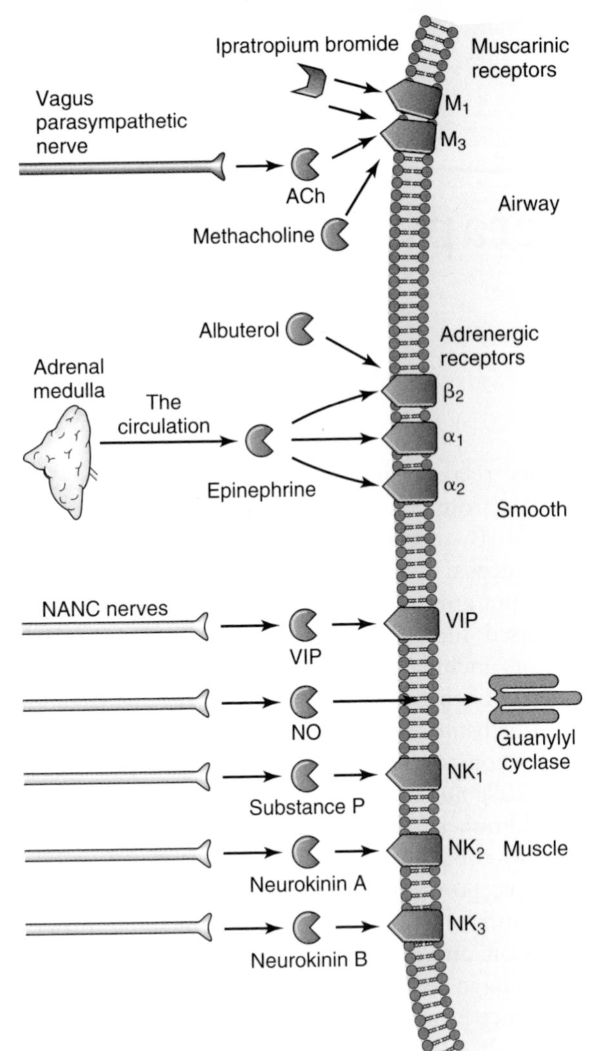

FIGURE 9-1 Airway smooth muscle tone and innervation. A constrictor tone is provided by the vagus nerve and release of acetylcholine (ACh). This is blocked by the mixed M_1/M_2 antagonist, ipratropium bromide. Methacholine challenge, to assess for asthma, activates these receptors. Epinephrine relaxes airway smooth muscle by activating β_2-receptors. This is mimicked by the therapeutic drug albuterol. The other features of the figure, including vasoactive intestinal polypeptide (VIP) activation of VIP receptors, nitrergic release of nitric oxide (NO), and activation of various neurokinin (NK) receptors, all part of the nonadrenergic noncholinergic (NANC) system, may represent targets for future drug development. *(From Page C, Curtis AB, Sutter MC, Walker MJ, Hoffman BB, editors:* Integrated pharmacology *(2nd ed.). Philadelphia, 2002, Mosby.)*

immediate bronchial reaction, which is responsible for the abrupt onset of symptoms. A later phase also produces a more sustained bronchial reaction, resulting from arachidonic acid release from damaged cell membranes and eosinophil accumulation. Metabolites of arachidonic acid from both the cyclooxygenase (prostaglandin D_2) pathway and lipoxygenase (cysteinyl-leukotrienes C4 and D4) pathways produce the second or late phase of bronchoconstriction (Figure 9-3).[4] Platelet activating factor is another mediator that is being increasingly recognized for its role in the production of asthma. These mediators interact to produce the typical signs of asthma, which include mucosal edema, mucus secretion, bronchoconstriction, and damage to the ciliated epithelium, resulting in wheezing, hyperventilation, cough, shortness of breath, and a reduction in the forced expiratory volume in 1 second (FEV_1).

Also, in allergic asthma, T helper cells (specifically Th2 cells as opposed to Th1 cells) are activated, and they release multiple proinflammatory cytokines, including Interleukin-4 (IL-4), IL-5, IL-5, IL-9, and IL-13.[4,5] Each of these cytokines has a particular role in maintaining the inflammatory process by increasing the production of IgE, esoinophils, mast cells, and Th2 cells and then being chemotactic for these cells. Again, the inflammatory mediators, histamines, leukotrienes, and prostaglandins become involved. A few hours later, eosinophil proteins, which cause tissue damage, become the ongoing stimulus for the asthma, producing the delayed phase.

Asthma not associated with a known allergy is considered intrinsic asthma. Two other categories of asthma are exercise-induced asthma (EIA) and asthma associated with COPD.[6] Exercise, especially when conducted in cold dry air, produces bronchoconstriction in some patients. This wheeze regularly occurs within just a few minutes of exercise. As described in the following section, preventive treatment with β_2-inhalers usually works well for this type of asthma. Asthma may coexist with COPD; if identified, treatment for this differs from treatment for COPD alone.

Inhalation Delivery Devices

Delivery of drug to the lungs by inhalation allows the medication to interact directly with the diseased tissue. This mode of administration reduces the risk of adverse effects, specifically systemic reactions, and allows for the reduction of dose compared with oral administration. Most of the inhaled drugs are administered through a pressurized metered-dose inhaler (pMDI). This is an aerosol delivery system that uses a chlorofluorocarbon propellant to spray the drug into the respiratory tract. The use of chlorofluorocarbons as a propellant is being phased out slowly and replaced with either no propellant or new, ozone-friendly propellants (hydrofluorocarbons).[7]

The pMDIs are convenient and inexpensive but require some coordination and practice for effective use. Correct use requires activation of the device and a simultaneous inhalation. Children and older adults seem to have problems maneuvering the device and coordinating the inhalation. The device containing the canister of drug is warmed to room temperature and then shaken well. The mouthpiece is held approximately 1 inch from the mouth, unless a spacer is used. The patient performs gentle exhalation to residual volume (RV) or functional residual capacity (FRC) and then presses down on the canister while breathing in slowly for 2 to 5 seconds.[8] The patient should hold the breath for up to 10 seconds, if

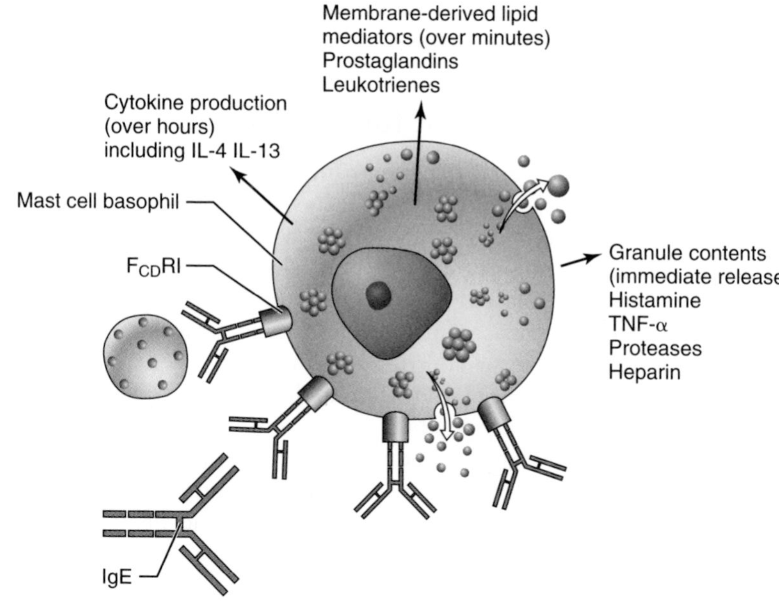

FIGURE 9-2 Mast cell mediator release. Tryptase is a serum marker of mast cell degranulation. *(Redrawn from Brody MJ, Larner J, Minneman KP, editors:.* Human pharmacology: Molecular to clinical *(3rd ed.). Philadelphia, 1998, Mosby.)*

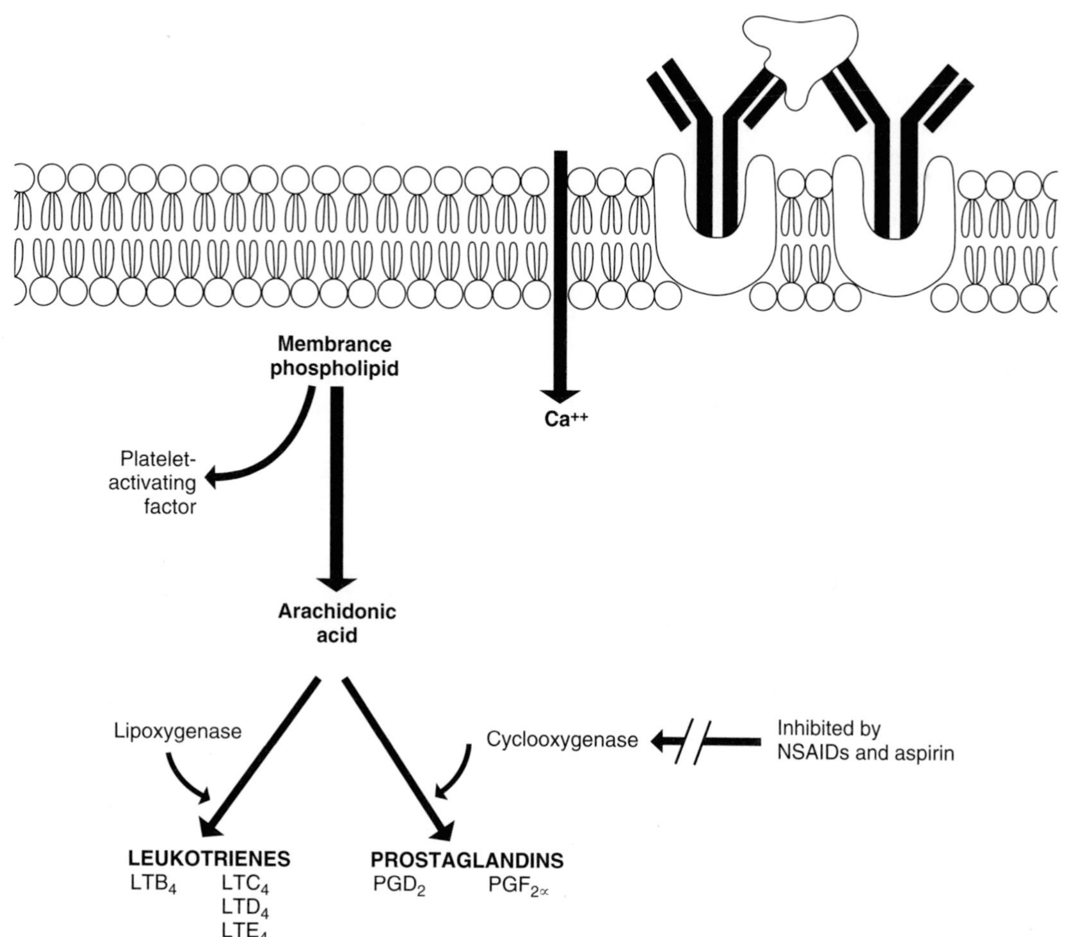

FIGURE 9-3 Newly generated lipid mast cell mediators. Specific leukotriene D_4-receptor antagonists are effective in the treatment of asthma. *NSAIDS*, nonsteroidal anti-inflammatory drugs. *(Redrawn from Brody MJ, Larner J, Minneman KP, editors:* Human pharmacology: Molecular to clinical *(3rd ed.). Philadelphia, 1998, Mosby.)*

possible, to allow the medicine to enter the lungs. If two puffs are prescribed, the patient should wait 5 minutes between inhalations. After the steroid has been inhaled, the mouth must be rinsed well with mouthwash. It has been found that many patients fail to exhale before the device is activated. A gentle exhalation appears to facilitate a deeper inhalation of the medication.

MDIs spray at high velocities, causing some of the drug particles to hit the back of the throat instead of being inhaled deeply into the lungs. A spacer is a cylinder that is attached to the MDI and helps capture the large high-velocity particles, allowing the slower, lower velocity drug particles to reach their target site deep in the lungs.[9] To reach and settle in the airways, particles must be between 2 and 6 microns in size.[10,11] The spacer also gives the patient some extra time to coordinate slow inspiration with the ejection of the drug from the canister. Even with the spacer, only about 20% of the drug inhaled reaches the lungs. Most of the drug is swallowed; some of it enters the systemic circulation through the gastrointestinal tract, and some is ejected with mouth rinsing. The addition of a spacer makes the device less portable, so one manufacturer has developed a collapsible spacer that can be used with the inhalation device.

Dry powder inhalers or breath-activated devices are delivery devices that scatter a fine powder into the lungs by means of a brisk inhalation.[7,12] These devices are easier to coordinate than MDIs, and some studies have shown that they are more effective. However, not all patients can inhale strongly enough to effectively use these devices, especially patients with severe airflow obstruction. Also, some patients find the dry powder irritating.

Another major drug delivery system for treating pulmonary problems is the nebulizer. This device dispenses liquid medication in oxygen or room air so that what is inhaled is a mist of extremely fine particles.[13] Use of the nebulizer simply requires the patient to breathe through a face mask or mouthpiece so that no coordination of inspiration is required.[14] Therefore it is often used by older adults and very young patients. These devices require an external gas source or an electronically powered compressor.

Drug Treatment for Asthma

The drugs used to treat asthma can be divided into two categories, short-term relievers and long-term controllers. The short-term relievers are those drugs that are used during acute asthma attacks. For this reason, they are also referred to as *rescue inhalers*. They include β_2-agonists, anticholinergics, and some sympathomimetics. The long-term controllers, which are used to prevent the occurrence of attacks, include steroids, leukotriene modifiers, theophylline, and cromolyn.

β_2-Adrenoceptor Agonists. β_2-Agonists are the most commonly prescribed drugs for the treatment of asthma.[3] These agents are delivered in MDIs and nebulizers, as well as in tablet and injectable forms. They produce relaxation of airway smooth muscle, resulting in bronchodilation, inhibit inflammatory mediator release from mast cells, and enhance mucociliary clearance.

Two categories of β_2-agonists are used in the treatment of asthma, short-acting agents and longer-acting agents (Table 9-1). After inhalation, the action of the short-acting agent is rapid, often within 5 to 10 minutes. Maximum effect usually occurs in 1 to 2 hours, and duration of action is 4 to 6 hours.[3] Examples of the short-acting agents include salbutamol, albuterol, and terbutaline.

Salmeterol and formoterol are longer-acting agents that produce bronchodilation for 12 hours.[3] These drugs contain a long lipophilic side chain on the molecule that binds to the membrane near the receptor, slowing the washout of the drug. These longer-acting agents are not appropriate for acute asthmatic episodes because of their delayed action, but they may be used to prevent nocturnal asthmatic attacks and provide protection for unanticipated or prolonged physical activity.

The usual dose for the short-acting β_2-agonists is two puffs every 4 to 6 hours or as needed.[6] If a patient uses more than two canisters per month, it probably means

TABLE 9-1 Commonly Used β_2-Agonists

Name	Dosing Interval (hr)	Onset of Action (min)	Peak Activity (hr)	Duration of Action (hr)	Comments
Short-Acting					
Albuterol (MDI or nebulization); Proventil, Ventolin	4–6	5	1–2	4–6	Most commonly used pMDI
Albuterol (oral); Volmax	6–8	30	2–3	6	Note that this is an oral dose
Pirbuterol; Maxair	4–6	5	0. 5–1	5	pMDI
Metaproterenol; Alupent	3–4	5	1	2–4	pMDI
Long-Acting					
Salmeterol; Serevent	12	30–50	2–4	12	Dry powder
Formoterol; Foradil	12	5	1	12	Dry powder

that he or she has inadequate control and that an adjustment on the long-term controller is needed. Regular use of the short-acting agents offers no advantage over as-needed use, and regular use may actually lead to tolerance.

Salmeterol and the other long-acting agents are given regularly, twice daily, and not on an as-needed basis.[6] As mentioned earlier, they are not indicated for acute asthma attacks because they have a slow onset of action and a prolonged effect. Patients taking these drugs regularly should use a short-acting bronchodilator as needed to control acute symptoms. Long-term daily use of salmeterol has been reported to lead to tolerance, at least in patients with exercise-induced asthma (EIA). Other studies have shown that the long-term agents can decrease responsiveness to the short-acting drugs, but this is still being debated. There also appears to be a subset of patients with asthma (African Americans with altered β_2-receptors) who have a small absolute increased risk of asthma-related death.[15] In addition, the Salmeterol Multicenter Asthma Research Trial (SMART) showed an increase in deaths due to respiratory complications with salmeterol; however, certain flaws in study design made this conclusion less convincing.[16] Nevertheless, efforts are being made to limit the use of these longer-acting agents, although they are recommended as an add-on therapy for patients taking an inhaled corticosteroid who need the next step in control of their symptoms.[17] This decision may be the preferred route as opposed to doubling the steroid dose.[18]

Oral β_2-agonists can also be given, but they are less effective, produce more adverse effects, and have a slower onset of action than the same drug given by inhalation. Oral syrup formulations are available and may be appropriate for small children with mild asthma who are unable to use an inhaler. Administering the drug through a nebulizer is also an option.

The adverse effects of β_2-agonists include tremor, tachycardia, hypokalemia, and hyperglycemia.[19] Increased mortality has been reported with the overuse of short-acting β_2-inhalers (greater than two canisters per month), but this was most likely due to worsening disease rather than the use of the drug. Less selective adrenergic agonists, such as epinephrine or isoproterenol, are more likely to produce adverse effects, particularly cardiac arrhythmias and rebound bronchospasm, than β_2-selective agents.

Anticholinergic Agents. Muscarinic receptor antagonists cause bronchodilation by blocking the action of acetylcholine on airway smooth muscle. These drugs do not prevent all types of bronchospasm but are effective against asthma produced by irritant stimuli. These drugs also decrease mucus secretion, which is why they are more effective in treating COPD than asthma.

The anticholinergic agents that may be used in asthma treatment include inhaled ipratropium and tiotropium (Table 9-2).[3] These synthetic compounds are permanently charged, preventing significant systemic absorption after inhalation, thus minimizing adverse effects. When inhaled, they produce maximum bronchodilation in 15 to 30 minutes, with duration of action up to 5 hours in COPD but a shorter onset of action in asthma. Both drugs have similar receptor-binding affinity but the tiotropium dissociates much more slowly, producing a longer duration of action and therefore needing only once-a-day inhalation. Ipratropium is available alone or in combination with the β_2-agonist albuterol. In general, dry mouth and pharyngeal irritation are the major adverse effects, but tachycardia may occur with excessive dosing. Although anticholinergic agents are primarily used in the treatment of COPD, they offer some additional efficacy in the treatment of asthma when combined with a β_2-agonist but are inferior to the β_2-agonists when used as monotherapy.[20]

Corticosteroids. Regular use of an inhaled corticosteroid can reduce bronchial inflammation and hyperresponsiveness in patients with persistent asthma.[21] Steroids block the release of arachidonic acid from airway epithelial cells, which, in turn, blocks the production of prostaglandins and leukotrienes. In addition, steroids inhibit transcription factors for the synthesis of interleukins and tumor necrosis factor, which are involved in stimulating the immune system. Related to this action, steroids decrease the number of mast cells and eosinophils that migrate into the area and also reduce edema formation by acting on the vascular endothelium. Specifically, they reduce the number of cytokines produced by the T2 helper cells that activate eosinophils and are responsible for facilitating the production of IgE.

Inhaled steroids have been the drugs of choice for reducing the number of asthma attacks in patients who have mild to moderate persistent asthma and for those who require β_2-inhalers more than once a day (Table 9-3).[18] Regular use of an inhaled steroid is

TABLE 9-2 Inhaled Anticholinergics

Name	Dosing Interval (hr)	Onset of Action (min)	Peak Activity (hr)	Duration of Action (hr)	Comments
Ipratropium (Atrovent)	6	5–15	1	3–6	MDI
Tiotropium (Spiriva)	12	15	4	36	Dry powder

TABLE 9-3 Classification of Asthma Severity and Treatment Recommendations

Severity	Symptoms	Nocturnal Symptoms	Lung Function	Medications
Mild Intermittent	Symptoms≤2×/wk	≤2×/month	FEV_1 ≥80% predicted between attacks	Short-acting β_2-agonists, as needed
Mild Persistent	Symptoms > 2×/wk but <1×/day	>2×/month	FEV_1 ≥80% predicted between attacks	Low-dose inhaled steroid; or leukotriene inhibitor; or mast cell stabilizer
Moderate Persistent	Daily symptoms with daily use of short-acting agents	>1×/week	FEV_1 >60% to <80%	Low-dose inhaled steroid + long-acting agent; or low-dose inhaled steroid + leukotriene inhibitor
Severe Persistent	Continual symptoms that limit activity; frequent exacerbations	Frequent	FEV_1<60% predicted	Medium-dose inhaled steroid + long-acting agent; if still not controlled, consider oral steroid or high-dose inhaled steroid + long-acting agent

FEV_1, forced expiratory volume in one minute.
(From Expert panel report 3: Guidelines for the diagnosis and management of asthma: NIH publication No. 08-4051. 2007.).[18]

BOX 9-1 Inhaled Steroids for Asthma

Beclomethasone (QVAR)
Budesonide (Pulmicort)
Flunisolide (AeroBid)
Fluticasone (Flovent)
Mometasone (Asmanex)
Triamcinolone (Azmacort)

associated with a reduced rate of deaths due to asthma. Examples of inhaled steroids include beclomethasone, budesonide, and fluticasone (Table 9-4). Fluticasone is also available in combination with salmeterol. In fact, the combination of the two drugs is more effective in improving lung function than doubling the dose of the inhaled steroid.[22] The combination of fluticasone and salmeterol is also more effective in improving FEV_1 than use of the inhaled fluticasone along with the oral leukotriene antagonist montelukast in patients with asthma not controlled by fluticasone alone.[23]

Although oral steroids are associated with some deleterious adverse effects, recommended use of inhaled steroids does not pose a risk of serious toxic effects. Dysphonia and oral candidiasis are the most common occurrences because of local deposition of the drug. Use of the spacer device and diligent rinsing of the mouth after inhalation can decrease these effects. Some other adverse effects include a dose-dependent slowing of growth in some children and adolescents but most likely with no effect on final adult height.[24,25] Decreased bone density, cataract formation, suppression of the hypothalamic–pituitary–adrenal axis, and glaucoma have also been reported.[26-29]

Oral or parenteral corticosteroids are the most effective treatments for acute exacerbations of asthma that do not respond well to β_2-agonists.[3] Even when patients do respond to short-term relievers, they may still receive a 10-day course of oral steroids to decrease symptoms and prevent relapses. Long-term daily use of oral steroids produces severe adverse effects, including hyperglycemia, weight gain, increased blood pressure, osteoporosis, cataracts, increased susceptibility to infection, muscle wasting, central fat deposition, moon facies, purple abdominal striae, atrophic skin, capillary fragility, and neuropsychiatric disorders. Because systemic use shuts down the hypothalamic–pituitary–adrenal axis, sudden withdrawal of steroids can be fatal, since the resumption of endogenous production of corticosteroids takes time. Corticosteroid adverse effects may be minimized by administering a single morning dose to correspond to the normal peak cortisol concentration that occurs in the early morning or by switching to alternate-day dosing. The benefits and adverse effects of steroids are more fully described in Chapter 13.

Leukotriene Antagonists and Leukotriene Receptor Blockers. Leukotrienes are inflammatory mediators released from mast cells, eosinophils, and basophils and are active during asthmatic attacks. They are a product of the lipoxygenase pathway (see Figure 9-3) and induce neutrophil and eosinophil chemotaxis as well as increasing vascular permeability, mucus production, and bronchocontriction.[30] Leukotriene antagonists and leukotriene receptor blockers block the actions of leukotrienes, decreasing the migration of eosinophils, production of mucus, and bronchoconstriction. Montelukast and zafirlukast are leukotriene receptor antagonists, and zileuton inhibits synthesis of leukotrienes. These drugs have been slightly less effective than the long-acting β-agonists and inhaled steroids, but the addition of these agents permits a reduction in corticosteroid dose. They can be used as primary monotherapy in mild persistent asthma with near-normal lung function, although a fast-acting inhaler may still be needed.[31] Montelukast is approved for children as young as 2 years old and, in spite of being inferior to inhaled steroids, has shown efficacy as monotherapy when assessing outcome measures of exacerbations.[32,33] In a cross-over study examining inhaled steroids versus montelukast, patients who had higher levels of eosinophilic/allergic inflammation were found to respond better to the steroids, and children who did not have these markers showed equal efficacy.[34] Occasionally, someone with moderate asthma (two or more bronchoconstrictive episodes per week) will do better with these drugs than with steroids.[30] One factor to consider may be cigarette smoking, which seems to impair the efficacy of the inhaled steroid in adults.[35]

Leukotriene blockers are given orally: montelukast is given once daily, and zafirlukast, twice daily. In several large clinical studies, they have demonstrated few adverse drug reactions.[36] The adverse-effect profile was similar to that of placebo with complaints of gastrointestinal upset and headache.[37] Montelukast is approved for use in children 6 to 12 years old and has a safety profile equal to that found for use in adults.

Cromolyn and Nedocromil. Cromolyn and nedocromil inhibit mast cell degranulation.[3] When stimulated, mast cells release granules containing histamine, leukotrienes, and prostaglandins—all of which produce an inflammatory response. These drugs block the release of these inflammatory mediators and thus decrease airway hyper-responsiveness, but they have no bronchodilating activity. They are used only for prophylaxis. The two compounds have equal efficacy, better than placebo in reducing the number of trips to the urgent care center, although nedocromil may be somewhat better in preventing exercise-induced asthma.[38] However, there may be little difference in some outcome measures, such as frequency of exacerbations, and they are far less effective than inhaled corticosteroids.

Cromolyn and nedocromil are not effective in all patients with asthma. A 4-week trial period may be necessary to determine their effectiveness. Children often respond better than adults to these drugs. A benefit of these drugs is that they have relatively few adverse effects, with the exception of their bitter taste.[39]

Theophylline. Theophylline is a methylxanthine, a substance found in coffee, tea, and chocolate. It was developed as a result of the observation that consuming great amounts of caffeine-containing beverages reduced the incidence of asthma. It acts as a phosphodiesterase inhibitor, which, in turn, increases intracellular cyclic adenosine monophosphate, which results in relaxation of smooth muscle. It also has some anti-inflammatory properties.[40] However, it has minimal effects on bronchoreactivity and offers significantly less control than do low-dose inhaled steroids.[41]

Theophylline was previously used as a long-term controller for asthma, but because of its low therapeutic index, it has largely been replaced by leukotriene antagonists.[42] The drug is still used in patients who do not respond to standard asthma agents. In addition, it may be used in the emergency department, along with oxygen, steroids, and bronchodilators, to treat acute and severe asthmatic attacks. It is occasionally used in the treatment of spinal cord injury because there is some evidence that it increases diaphragmatic strength and endurance.

Theophylline's adverse effects include nausea, vomiting, headache, insomnia, nervousness, tachycardia, and hypertension.[3] Arrhythmias may occur and signal that theophylline blood levels are too high. Frequent monitoring of blood levels is therefore essential. Factors that affect theophylline's clearance include enzyme inhibition by other drugs (cimetidine, erythromycin), congestive heart failure, liver disease, older age, viral infection, and a high-carbohydrate diet.

Acute Severe Asthma (Status Asthmaticus)

Status asthmaticus is a life-threatening condition requiring rapid and aggressive treatment. It may occur because the airways become refractory to the β_2-agonists, particularly when administered frequently within 36 to 38 hours to regain control over the airways. In addition, the mucus plugs that develop begin to impair the ability of the inhaled drugs to reach the distal airways.

Immediate treatment involves administering humidified oxygen by mask plus intravenous (IV) fluids for hydration to liquefy the mucus.[43] Additional treatment includes oral or IV steroids, followed by a β_2-agonist administered through a nebulizer. If cyanosis or bradycardia is observed or if breath sounds are absent, ipratropium and IV aminophylline (similar to theophylline) can be given.[44] If the patient's condition is still not improving, then the intensive care unit should be notified, and a decision regarding intubation and mechanical ventilation should be made. Monitoring the patient's response to treatment includes measurement of peak expiratory flow rate, oxygen saturation, and blood gases every 15 to 30 minutes.

Exercise-Induced Asthma

EIA, also known as *exercise-induced airway narrowing* or *exercise-induced bronchospasm*, involves acute airway constriction that occurs after exercise or strenuous exertion. Some patients with asthma exhibit symptoms only with exercise. EIA occurs in 40 to 90% of patients who experience bronchoconstriction and may have a prevalence of 11 to 50% in athletes overall.[45,46] In addition, it is not uncommon during cross-country skiing, swimming, and long-distance running, when ventilation is prolonged with subsequent mucosal evaporation of fluids through the nose or mouth. Chlorine from swimming pools and carbon dioxide emissions from indoor ice rinks act as allergic triggers, and outside allergens include cut grass and pollen.

There are two main theories regarding the pathogenesis of EIA. However, it is clear that neither one is sufficient to explain the hyperactive airways or full EIA.[45] One theory is that inhalation of cold and dry air leads to mucosal drying and increased osmolarity, stimulating mast cell degranulation. The fact that mast cell stabilizers (cromolyn and nedocromil) are effective in controlling EIA supports this hypothesis. However, EIA also occurs when hot, dry air is inspired during exercise. The other theory is that rapid airway rewarming after exercise produces vascular congestion, increased permeability, and edema, all of which can trigger the asthma attack. Proponents of this theory believe that the greater the difference in ambient temperature between the exercise and postexercise environments, the greater is the degree of bronchoconstriction.

There is a high incidence of EIA in elite athletes, so some clinicians have hypothesized that EIA in these cases may be due to airway injury from factors related to high-intensity exercises.[47] Repeated exposure of the airways to large amounts of plasma, particularly with airway injury from dehydration, may increase sensitivity to constriction. In addition, biopsies of the airways of elite athletes in cold-weather areas reveal a preponderance of neutrophils, which suggests microvascular leakage. Microvascular leakage and plasma exudation are responses seen following repetitive airway injury. Also, with intense exercising, smaller airways are recruited and may be subjected to damage as a result of dehydration not normally experienced at rest or with moderate exercise. Summer athletes show evidence of greater atopy or allergic asthma with elevated eosinophils and increased circulating levels of leukotrienes and prostaglandins, perhaps as a result of exposure to aeroallergens during training. Perhaps it is this difference in pathology that leads to differing responses to medications.

It is well recognized that repeated use of a β_2-agonist (daily administration) during training leads to the development of EIA.[48] In vitro mast cells incubated with β_2-agonists failed to release histamine after chemical challenge. Clinical studies have demonstrated increased tolerance to these agents, worsening of severity of EIA when exercise is performed 8 to 12 hours after drug administration, and longer time to recovery from EIA.

The clinical features of EIA include bronchospasm after at least 3 to 8 minutes of exercise and/or symptoms of cough, wheezing, dyspnea, and chest tightness. These symptoms reach their peak in about 15 minutes, and recovery generally occurs within 60 minutes. A late-phase response may also occur 4 to 6 hours after exercise. Although patients occasionally experience difficulty breathing during activity, EIA sometimes begins after the exercise has been completed, in about 5 to 10 minutes.[46] In addition, if a person who has EIA resumes exercising soon after the symptoms subside, he or she will experience less of a problem after the second bout of exercise than after the first. This is referred to as the *refractory period,* which generally lasts from 40 minutes to 4 hours.

The International Olympic Committee Medical Commission requires notification of the use of a β_2-agonist prior to a competitive event. Athletes must provide proof of their dependence on the drugs in the form of clinical and laboratory test results. Currently, an abnormal airway response from the eucapnic voluntary hyperpnoea (EVH) test confirms that the participant indeed has EIA.[49] The test requires the individual to breathe in air that is dry and contains 21% oxygen, 4.9 to 5.1% carbon dioxide, and nitrogen making up the balance. The subject hyperventilates this mixture for $30 \times FEV_1$ which is equivalent to 85% the maximum voluntary ventilation for 6 minutes. However, the duration, temperature, and ventilation level can be altered to mimic the specific conditions for a given sport. The FEV_1 is measured three times before the test and then twice immediately after the challenge and then at 5, 10, 15, and 20 minutes after the test. The rapid breathing simulates an exercise response. Generally, a fall of 10% in post-test FEV_1 is considered positive for EIA.[50] Other bronchial provocation tests for EIA include administration of methacholine (a cholinergic agonist) or histamine, both of which produce airway constriction in susceptible individuals, and hyperosmolar aerosols such as 4.5% saline and mannitol.[50,51] Field testing involving the specific sport can also be used as a challenge (see Chapter 29).

EIA may be treated with or without drugs. A high level of fitness is important in decreasing EIA because patients who exercise regularly do not demonstrate the abrupt increases in ventilation experienced by their more sedentary counterparts; abrupt increases are more likely to stimulate bronchoconstriction. Swimming is often recommended over outdoor running because warm humidified air does not seem to trigger EIA. Other recommendations include warming up before exercise, covering the mouth and nose with a scarf during cold weather, and incorporating a cool-down period before ending exercise.[46]

Pharmacologic agents can be used just before exercise to reduce the incidence of EIA.[52] Inhaled short-acting β_2-agonists are the most commonly used agents for this purpose. They are effective in preventing symptoms if they are administered between 15 minutes and 1 hour before exercise. Duration of the drug's action is up to 4 hours. The patient is instructed to use two puffs of the short-acting agent 30 to 60 minutes before exercise. Patients who exercise for a prolonged period generally use a long-acting β_2-agonist such as formoterol. Formoterol has a more rapid onset of action (15 minutes) than salmeterol and is effective for up to 12 hours. It has been shown to decrease EIA after as-needed single doses as well as with regular use.

Other agents commonly used to decrease EIA are inhaled cromolyn and nedocromil.[45] They are used 10 to 20 minutes before exercise, and although they attenuate the symptoms, they are less effective than the

β_2-agonists.[53] The leukotriene antagonists, which have been shown to reduce bronchoconstriction during exercise challenges, are some other choices.[54] Single doses of montelukast and zafirlukast are protective for 1 hour to 24 hours after administration, and some studies show equal effectiveness when compared with salmeterol early in the course of treatment, but after dosing for several weeks, the leukotriene antagonists demonstrate superiority.[55] Additionally, montelukast shows greater efficacy over salmeterol at 24 hours in adults.[56] In 6- to 14-year-old children with asthma, montelukast has also been shown to reduce EIA more effectively compared with placebo.[57] Other pharmacologic agents including anticholinergic drugs, theophylline, and antihistamines have been shown to offer some protection against EIA when added to a daily regimen of asthma control medications.[45] However, only certain drugs are approved by the U. S. and International Olympic Committees for use in those engaging in athletic competition because β-agonists have the potential to be anabolic when taken in the oral form.[58-60] Although the use of these agents for increasing voluntary muscle strength holds some promise in the treatment of weakened skeletal musculature, it is doubtful that someone would want to compete against an athlete taking these agents. All inhaled corticosteroids, leukotriene antagonists, cromolyn/nedocromil, theophylline, and ipratropium are approved; but of the list of β_2-agonists, only albuterol, terbutaline, and salmeterol are approved agents. Athletes who require the use of these agents must submit clinical and laboratory values that prove their need for these drugs to the International Olympic Committee Medical Commission.[61]

New Alternatives

Targeting the cytokines and other immune components in asthma with specific monoclonal antibodies is a new approach to treatment. Since IgE is implicated in producing mast cell degranulation, the anti-IgE drug omalizumab has been developed.[62] Omalizumab is a recombinant humanized monoclonal antibody that acts against circulating IgE. It is used in patients with moderate-to-severe asthma whose disease has not been controlled well on inhaled steroids. It is administered by subcutaneous injection every 2 to 4 weeks. The dosing schedule and the amount of drug administered are dependent on serum IgE levels. Omalizumab has been shown to reduce exacerbations of the disease. Anti–IL-5 targeting eosinophils and anti–TNF-α α drugs are other therapies currently under study.

OTHER DRUGS USEFUL IN RESPIRATORY DISORDERS

Cough, nasal congestion, and thick mucus are symptoms of respiratory disorders. For each of these indications, specific drugs for symptom reduction are available.

Antitussives

These drugs are used to treat recurrent or persistent cough.[63] Nonspecific cough, not resulting from asthma or as an adverse effect of angiotensin-converting enzyme (ACE) inhibitors, may be triggered by mechanical or chemical stimulation of the upper respiratory tract. This stimulus is relayed to the cough center in the medulla and then to the respiratory muscles. The efferent pathway for cough involves the phrenic nerve and the abrupt contraction of the intercostals muscles. Cough is necessary as a protective mechanism to expel foreign bodies or to help produce and expel mucus, but a nonproductive cough can be bothersome. Peripheral cough receptors are sensitive to local anesthetics, so topical application of lidocaine is used to inhibit cough during bronchoscopy.

Drugs that suppress cough act by decreasing the activity of the afferent nerves or by decreasing the sensitivity of the cough center. Menthol vapor inhalation is effective in reducing the sensitivity of the peripheral cough receptors. Inhalation of menthol vapors or sucking on lozenges containing menthol will lessen the urge to cough. Topical anesthetics such as lidocaine, benzocaine, and bupivacaine will also reduce the sensitivity of the peripheral receptors. Opioids reduce the sensitivity of the central cough center. Codeine and hydrocodone are common ingredients in cough medicines. Narcotic preparations must be used with caution in patients with head trauma or renal or liver disease. These drugs produce sedation, drowsiness, and constipation, as well as nausea and vomiting. Because the overdose effects include hypotension, bradycardia, and respiratory depression, narcotics must be used with caution in patients with COPD. In addition, codeine decreases secretions in the bronchioles, thickening the sputum and producing a reduction in clearance. Dextromethorphan is similar in structure and just as effective as codeine but without its analgesic properties.

Drugs for Rhinitis and Rhinorrhea

Rhinitis is an acute or chronic inflammation of the nasal mucosa, and *rhinorrhea* is the production of watery nasal secretions. Both these conditions may result from a viral infection of the nasal mucosa or an IgE-type allergy. Essentially, blood flow and vascular permeability to the mucosa are increased, resulting in fluid buildup in the nasal passages and difficulty breathing. Sympathomimetic drugs or better alpha agonists drugs that constrict the blood vessels are the major ingredients in nasal sprays. However, the major adverse effects of these drugs are vasoconstriction and elevated blood pressure. They can also aggravate hyperthyroidism, diabetes, glaucoma, and benign prostatic hyperplasia. This is particularly true with the oral mixtures that contain phenylephrine. Patients will develop tolerance to topical agents, if used repeatedly, but will not usually develop tolerance to oral decongestants.

Other treatments for rhinitis and rhinorrhea take an immunologic approach. Autocoids such as histamine are released as a result of an immunologic reaction. Antihistamines and the local administration of glucocorticosteroids are useful in controlling disease associated with these reactions. Histamine acts on the nasal mucosa, largely on H_1 receptors. The antihistamines, or H_1 receptor blockers, reduce nasal congestion, mucosal irritation, and cough by reducing secretions. The first-generation H_1 antagonists, such as diphenhydramine and chlorpheniramine, were effective; however, they interfered with learning and motor performance and posed a safety hazard because of the excessive somnolence they caused.[63] The newer antihistamines, such as loratadine, cetirizine, and fexofenadine, do not cross the blood–brain barrier and therefore produce less sedation than their older counterparts did. Glucocorticosteroids that are applied topically to the nasal mucosa include triamcinolone, beclomethasone, fluticasone, and over-the-counter (OTC) cromolyn—all of which are sprayed directly into the nasal passages.

The leukotriene receptor antagonist montelukast has also been approved for the treatment of seasonal allergic rhinitis in adults and children.[64] It has been found to decrease symptoms better than placebo, and in one study of 460 patients, the combination of montelukast and loratadine was more effective than either drug alone. However, in a larger study of 907 subjects, the combination was found to be no better than each drug taken individually.[65] Montelukast is less effective than intranasal corticosteroids.

Mucolytics

Respiratory mucus consists of water and glycoproteins that are cross-linked by disulfide bonds. Normally, only about 100 mL of fluid is produced in the respiratory tract per day, and most of this is swallowed. In disease states, more mucus is produced, and it tends to be more viscous. The purpose of mucolytics is to liquefy mucus so that it can be cleared from the airway by coughing. Carbocysteine and mecysteine open disulfide bonds and reduce the viscosity of mucus. They can be given orally or by inhalation and are particularly useful in treating cystic fibrosis (CF). Water inhalation (breathing over a bowl of hot water) and the use of a humidifier or vaporizer are also considered mucolytic treatments because hydration can lower viscosity.

Dornase alfa is a phosphorylated glycosylated recombinant human deoxyribonuclease that hydrolyzes DNA and is effective for airway clearance in CF.[66,67] Copious amounts of neutrophil-derived DNA accumulate in the airways of patients with CF, and DNA accumulates as a result of degenerating neutrophils. Recombinant human deoxyribonuclease I also breaks down DNA to reduce the viscosity of sputum. The most common adverse reactions associated with this treatment are upper airway irritations, including pharyngitis and laryngitis.

Respiratory Stimulants

Drugs that are used to stimulate the respiratory system are called *analeptics*. They are CNS stimulants with very low therapeutic indexes. Doxapram increases both the rate and depth of respiration. It acts on the medullary respiratory center. Nasal intermittent positive pressure ventilation has largely replaced its use. However, it may still be used to treat postoperative respiratory depression and opiate overdose. Aminophylline may also be used as a respiratory stimulant when given slowly by IV infusion.

Oxygen Therapy

Oxygen therapy should be initiated whenever there is moderate or new-onset hypoxia, with $PaO_2 < 50$ mm Hg. Patients with chronic hypoxia may be able to maintain adequate oxygenation with a PaO_2 less than this by such compensations as increasing red blood cell mass. However, low concentrations of oxygen may still be indicated, particularly when $PaCO_2$ is increased, which is usually seen in COPD. The stimulus to breathe is the elevated CO_2, but this can be diminished in patients with chronically high CO_2 and replaced instead by a drive connected to a low oxygen level. Elevating the oxygen level therefore might remove the stimulus to breathe. High-concentration oxygen therapy is indicated when both oxygen and CO_2 levels are low, as might be seen in a patient with a pulmonary embolism, pneumonia, or myocardial infarction and early in an acute severe asthma attack. Long-term continuous oxygen therapy is given to patients with severe hypoxia and cor pulmonale caused by COPD.

CHRONIC OBSTRUCTIVE PULMONARY DISEASE

Clinical signs and symptoms of COPD include excessive production of sputum with mucus plugging, cough, increased respiratory rate, hypoventilation, hypercapnia, and hypoxia.[68] Anatomic changes that occur include glandular hypertrophy, goblet cell metaplasia, and inflammation and fibrosis of the airways (greater in smaller airways than in larger airways), leading to a narrowing of the lumen and obstructive flow. Many of these changes are irreversible, which is the feature that separates this illness from asthma. In addition, biopsies of the bronchial airways and lung parenchyma show a preponderance of neutrophils and T cells but absent mast cell activation as opposed to the eosinophils seen in asthma.[4] Drugs are used to improve functional abilities, to turn around the reversible component of the disease, and to improve the quality of life.

The therapeutic approach to COPD needs to be flexible enough to keep up with the progression of the disease. The American Thoracic Society recommends spirometry measurements to determine the presence and severity of COPD. The ratio of FEV_1 to forced vital capacity (FVC) is used to determine airflow obstruction. An FEV_1/FVC ratio <70% or <88% and <89% of predicted value for men and women, respectively, along with X-ray evidence and clinical symptoms are positive for a diagnosis. Mild COPD is defined by a postbronchodilator FEV_1 of 70 to 80% or greater of predicted value; moderate COPD, as an FEV_1 of 50 to 80% of predicted value; severe COPD, as an FEV_1 of 30 to 49% of predicted value; and very severe COPD, as an FEV_1 <30% of predicted value.[69,70] Note that FEV_1 is the best predictor of mortality and an FEV_1 less than 50% of predicted value has a risk of higher mortality.

During the early, largely asymptomatic phase, the therapeutic goal is to slow the loss of lung function. At this point, patients may show reversible bronchoconstriction and eosinophils in their sputum and respond to steroid treatments in the same way as patients with asthma.[4] Inhaled corticosteroids, with and without long-acting β_2-agonists, can be used, and some patients will respond with improved FEV_1 and a reduction in symptoms. However, this response is individually determined. Patients who are likely to respond are those with a history of asthma, sputum eosinophilia, and a good response to β_2-agonists. The best way to determine responsiveness to steroids is with a trial. It is recommended that the patient receive oral prednisone for 2 to 3 weeks. If the patient responds to the prednisone, then weaning to inhaled steroids can be initiated. However, failure to respond to steroids in a baseline state does not necessarily mean that the patient will not respond during an exacerbation. Given the adverse effects associated with steroid use and the fact that several studies show that steroids have no effect on the decline of lung function, they must be used with caution.[71] However, a study showed that the combination of fluticasone and salmeterol improved lung function and reduced the severity of shortness of breath in patients receiving this combination over a 1-year period.[72] The combination was superior to use of each drug alone.

One of the best treatment options for early stage COPD is, of course, the cessation of cigarette smoking. Behavioral approaches and nicotine replacement therapy can thus be helpful.[73] Patients should also be administered the pneumococcal vaccine and the appropriate influenza vaccine yearly and be careful to limit exposure to upper respiratory tract infections, as these can all lead to acute exacerbations.[74] As the disease progresses, patients with COPD become less responsive to either inhaled or oral high-dose steroids.

Bronchodilators are almost universally used to provide relief in all stages of the disease. Traditionally, patients have used a combination of short-acting β_2-agonists and inhaled anticholinergic drugs. Short acting β_2-agonists are useful in treating intermittant dyspnea. However, combination therapy appears to be slightly better than monotherapy with short-acting β_2-agonists in reducing exacerbations but is not superior to monotherapy with ipratropium. Salbutamol and ipratropium given four times daily is the most common combination. They are packaged together in a single inhaler for patient convenience. The anticholinergic compounds reduce neurogenic control of mucus, which is probably why monotherapy with ipratropium is efficacious. However, there is little evidence that either monotherapy or combination therapy slows the decline in lung function or improves survival.[3]

Longer-acting agents, such as the β_2-agonists formoterol and salmeterol, and the anticholinergic agent tiotropium have also been used as treatment for COPD (Table 9-4).[75] These medications should be utilized in patients with less than 60% of FEV_1. A few clinical trials that examined FEV_1 changes over a 1-year period, exacerbation rates, and quality-of-life issues have demonstrated the efficacy of these agents over placebo as well as the correspondingly shorter-acting agents. No studies have shown that the β_2-agonists or anticholinergic agents are either superior or inferior to each other. But combining a longer-acting β_2-agonist with ipratropium is more effective than combining a short-acting agent with ipratropium. Hence, the practice of combining the longer-acting agent of each type of drug is catching on. However, patients must carry around two inhalers because the available long-acting β_2-agonists are given twice daily, but tiotropium is given only once, which makes combining them into a single inhaler not feasible at this time. Tiotropium has shown improved clinical outcomes, improved exercise capacity, and reduced exacerbations compared with ipratropium, since it has action at the M_1 and M_3 receptors but not at the M_2 autoreceptor.[76-78] The once-a-day dosing also improves compliance.

Other treatments for COPD include antibiotics and mucolytic agents. Antibiotics are often needed because the presence of copious amounts of sputum provides a fertile ground for bacterial growth. Mucolytics, such as N-acetylcysteine, reduce the viscosity of the mucus, but because the most effective means for mobilizing mucus from the airways is a strong cough, these patients should also receive chest physical therapy and learn how to bring up secretions to the tracheal level so that they can be expelled.[79]

As COPD progresses, oxygen therapy becomes necessary to relieve hypoxemia and prolong survival.[60] Long-term administration of oxygen for at least 15 hours per day to maintain a PaO_2 of 60 mm Hg has resulted in a reduction of deaths in patients with severe disease (resting hypoxemia PaO_2 ≤55 mm Hg, FEV_1 <30%).[70] Less favorable results were noted when patients were treated with oxygen for 9 to 13 hours per day.[80] Routine use of oxygen is contraindicated in less severe hypoxemia, unless the patient has end-organ dysfunction or mental status changes, because in COPD the respiratory drive is diminished and may be reduced even further if the hypoxemic drive to breathe is removed.

TABLE 9-4 Inhaled Anticholinergics

Name	Dosing Interval (hr)	Onset of Action (min)	Peak Activity (hr)	Duration of Action (hr)	Comments
Ipratropium (Atrovent)	6	5–15	1	3–6	MDI
Tiotropium (Spiriva)	12	15	4	36	Dry Powder

CYSTIC FIBROSIS

Cystic fibrosis (CF) is a multisystem disease, in which there is a defect in a gene on chromosome 7 that encodes a chloride channel common to epithelial cells (CFTR, cystic fibrosis transmembrane conductance regulator).[81] Failure to develop this channel affects the epithelial cells lining the airways, intestines, biliary and pancreatic ducts, vas deferens, and sweat ducts. The result is that fluid secretion is diminished, and what is secreted becomes more viscous, leading to plugging of ducts. There is also an upregulation of sodium channels, particularly in the airways, leading to reabsorption of sodium. Proinflammatory pathways are also upregulated in the airways, and bacterial killing is diminished.

Malnutrition and failure to thrive are common presentations of CF. Failure of the pancreas to produce digestive enzymes leads to the inability to absorb fats and protein. Specifically, the fat-soluble vitamins A, D, E, and K cannot be absorbed.[82] The deficiency of vitamin K may lead to bleeding. Supplementation with water-miscible forms of these vitamins is therefore necessary for patients with CF. In addition, pancreatic enzymes are given in a microencapsulated form to improve their survival in an acid environment. Drugs that inhibit acid secretion may also be administered to enhance the survival of the pancreatic enzymes.

The pathophysiology of the lungs appears to be due to two mechanisms: (1) impaired secretion of chloride (Cl^-) in serous cells of airway submucosal glands and (2) enhanced absorption of sodium (Na^+) with subsequent hyperabsorption of electrolytes and fluids at the airway surface epithelium, leading to mucus plugging and impaired mucociliary clearance.[68] This removal of salt and water from the lining of the airways results in loss of lubrication and the collapse of cilia. Mucus is produced in the glands but has difficulty getting out, which leads to hypertrophy of the gland. Several drugs to correct these defective ion channels are under study. Some Na^+ channel blockers can block the specific type of Na^+ channel involved in CF (ENaC, amiloride-sensitive epithelial Na^+ channel). Amiloride is a potassium (K^+)-sparing diuretic, which blocks Na^+ absorption in the kidney collecting duct. An aerosolized form is available to patients with CF. Benzamil is a related drug that has a longer effect on the Na^+ channels. Other drugs that attempt to activate an alternative calcium-activated chloride channel or activate mutant CFTRs (cystic fibrosis transport regulator) are being tested. Additionally, rehydrating agents such as hypertonic saline and inhaled mannitol are also being explored.[83]

Because of mucus plugging, an intense regimen for airway clearance is necessary. In addition to the mucus plugging, the lungs in CF tend to harbor bacteria. Three organisms predominate: *Haemophilus influenzae*, *Staphylococcus aureus*, and *Pseudomonas aeruginosa*.[82-84] *P. aeruginosa* will establish itself in the lungs of approximately 80% of patients by young adulthood. *P. aeruginosa* forms "protective biofilms" over microcolonies to guard them against immune attack and antibiotic action. Antibiotics with sensitivities for these infections are frequently given to patients with CF. The antibiotic should be chosen after culture of a specimen obtained from sputum or a deep throat swab. Sensitivity testing is paramount in preventing antibiotic resistance. Depending on the severity of infection, oral, inhaled, or IV antibiotics may be used. Inhaled tobramycin is sometimes used every other month to help control *Pseudomonas* infections. Beta lactam antibiotics (penicillins, cephalosporins, carbapenems) or a quinolone (ciprofloxacin, levofloxacin) may be added. Typically, higher doses are needed in CF due to the influence the disease process has on drug pharmacokinetics and because drug metabolism and elimination tend to be accelerated. Due to the need for frequent IV antibiotics, many patients will require establishment of central catheters for drug administration.

Many patients with CF are also prescribed a β_2-agonist.[85] However, there is little evidence that these drugs are effective, and some patients may even show deterioration in lung function while taking these drugs. If the patient experiences symptomatic relief with these drugs, they can be prescribed. Theophyllines act as bronchodilators, but they also directly affect mucociliary function.[86] Despite this effect, these drugs are used only on a limited basis because of their low safety index.

Two other categories of drugs that are frequently used in the treatment of pulmonary problems are leukotriene antagonists and steroids. Several studies have shown the presence of leukotrienes in CF, but no large study has demonstrated that leukotriene antagonists are helpful in treating this disease. Oral steroids are being prescribed, even on a long-term basis, to many patients with CF. Given their rather extensive list of adverse effects, this practice is not considered acceptable.

A surprise candidate for further consideration in the treatment of CF is the non-steroidal anti-inflammatory agent ibuprofen.[87] A 4-year trial from 1995 to 2002 and another 2-year trial in reported in 2007—with a total of 232 children—demonstrated a reduction in pulmonary function decline (a 29% reduction in FEV_1 deterioration) and in the number of hospitalizations in the ibuprofen-treated group versus the untreated group. In general, the treated group received a dose of 20 to 30 mg/kg twice daily, which was carefully controlled on the basis of the individual patient reaching a specific peak plasma concentration of the drug known to be safe. Gastrointestinal (GI) symptoms, including an occasional bleed, were reported, but given the intestinal manifestations of CF, it is difficult to attribute that effect entirely to ibuprofen. On the basis of results in this small number of patients, ibuprofen therapy is recommended in patients age 6 to 17 years with an FEV_1 above 60% predicted value. However, a much larger study is needed to verify these results.

THERAPEUTIC CONCERNS WITH DRUGS FOR RESPIRATORY DISORDERS

Patients with respiratory illnesses will commonly receive drugs from any of the following categories: steroids, β_2-agonists, and anticholinergic agents. The therapeutic concerns are largely related to their adverse effects. Patients receiving anticholinergic agents must be monitored for tachycardia, hypertension, and urinary retention. In addition, although dry mouth is seemingly a mild adverse effect associated with anticholinergic drugs, this reaction becomes magnified with drug inhalation and pursed lip breathing. Dry mouth can produce swallowing difficulty and over the long term, lead to an increased risk of dental caries. Caution should be exercised when working with patients taking inhaled or oral steroids. Thrush and oral candidiasis are often seen with use of inhaled steroids; and bruising, osteoporosis, increased risk of infection, hypertension, hyperglycemia, and atrophy of skin and muscle are adverse effects of both formulations. Therapists must pay special attention to the strength and force of any manipulations and perform integumentary evaluations before and after the use of modalities.

The adverse effects associated with β_2-agonists include tremor, tachycardia, hypokalemia, and hyperglycemia. Monitoring for angina is particularly important when patients are receiving these drugs. Adequate hydration is necessary in all patients with thickened and copious amounts of mucus.

Patients with respiratory illnesses may experience significant dyspnea and diminished exercise tolerance related to muscle weakness, cardiac impairment, and hypoxemia. Pulmonary rehabilitation programs have been developed to address some of these impairments. Although these programs vary, they usually consist of exercise training, education, and behavior modifications. Aerobic training, emphasizing endurance training, and inspiratory respiratory muscle strengthening form the core of these programs.[88] Several clinical trials have shown that these programs improve health status and increase exercise tolerance but may have little effect on mortality.

In addition to demonstrating the merits of regular exercise, a few centers have started collecting data on how the bronchodilators affect exercise hemodynamics and performance.[89] β_2-agonists as well as anticholinergic drugs are expected to raise heart rate during both rest and exercise. However, studies have shown that only the β_2-agonist fenoterol, and not the anticholinergic drug oxitropium, produces increases in heart rate and a decrease in PaO_2 at rest. During exercise, these differences were not observed, and both drugs were equally effective in attenuating exercise-induced elevations in right heart afterloads (pulmonary artery pressure, pulmonary capillary wedge pressure, and right atrial pressure). Normally, in COPD, these values increase during exercise, even in the absence of cardiac disease, because trapped air in the peripheral airways leads to end-expiratory positive airway pressure. Improvement in pulmonary mechanics with the bronchodilators leads to a fall of intrathoracic pressure, followed by a fall in capillary wedge pressure. A similar study also indicated that there was no difference in dyspnea scoring after walking and no difference in the distance walked in 12 minutes with either albuterol or ipratropium.[90]

Although anticholinergics and β_2-agonists appear equally effective during exercise, there is one drug that may improve performance beyond the individual's standard drug therapy.[91] The unlikely candidate is the opiate morphine. Patients with COPD are often limited by breathlessness because of the increased work of breathing. It is thought that morphine reduces the ventilatory drive in response to elevated CO_2, hypoxia, and exercise. The reduced respiratory effort may reduce shortness of breath. In addition, morphine produces a sedating effect that reduces anxiety. When a low dose of morphine is administered along with prochlorperazine for relief of nausea, there is a significant reduction in breathlessness along with an increase in walking distance and an increase in maximum oxygen consumption of 20%. It is significant that in addition to being used for nausea, prochlorperazine is also a "stimulant of the hypoxic response." Similar results have been reported with another opiate, dihydrocodeine.[92] However, other studies have not demonstrated an opiate's effect on exercise, and given the concerns regarding respiratory depression, reduced arterial oxygen saturation, and the potential for producing addiction and altering mental function with opiates, more work in this area is needed before these agents can be recommended for improving exercise tolerance or functional abilities.

ACTIVITIES 9

1. A 50-year-old woman with a history of asthma reports increasing shortness of breath (SOB) and wheezing over the past few days. She has increased the use of her inhalers to approximately six times per day. She reports disposing of her prednisone last month because she was "gaining weight."

   Medical History: Asthma × 10 years, Heart burn, HTN × 2 years

   Social History: EtOH: Two beers/day; tobacco use: one pack/day; divorced mother of two teenagers

   Employed in the Housekeeping Department of a large city-managed hospital

   Medications: Albuterol metered-dose inhaler (MDI) two puffs q4-6h prn; lisinopril (started 2 weeks ago); cimetidine; prednisone

   Vital Signs: Blood pressure (BP) 160/90; pulse (P) 120; respiratory rate (RR) 30; temperature (T) 98.7°F; weight (Wt) 150 lbs

   Chest: Bilateral expiratory wheezes; X-ray shows hyperinflated lungs with air trapping

   Labs: Sodium 140 mEq/L, potassium 3.2 mEq/L, Chloride 105 mEq/L, blood urea nitrogen (BUN) 17 mg/dL, serum creatinine 1.0 mg/dL, glucose 110 mg/dL

   Hemoglobin 14.6 g/dL, platelets 200, 000/mm^3, white blood cells (WBC) 7000/mm^3

   FEV_1: 40%

   Arterial Blood Gases: PaO_2, 60; $PaCO_2$ 50 mm Hg; pH 7.30; HCO_3 25 mEq/L

   Questions:

   A. What could have caused the patient's increased wheezing?

   B. What are the immediate pharmacologic goals for this patient, and how should they be achieved?

   C. What pharmacologic interventions would you recommend for the patient after this acute exacerbation is controlled?

   D. How will you monitor the efficacy and adverse effects of your treatment plan (after the acute attack subsides), and how will you address compliance issues with this patient? Why should you monitor the heart rate in this patient, and what response would warrant a call to the physician?

   E. This patient desires to make major lifestyle changes, that is, lose weight, stop smoking, and start exercising. What advice do you have for her on how to avoid exercise-induced asthma?

2. A 72-year-old male has had severe COPD for the last 10 years. His FEV_1 is approximately 35% of predicted value. He is taking ipratropium, albuterol, and an inhaled corticosteroid through inhalers. This patient stopped smoking 1 year ago, but his illness has progressed, and he is now having dyspnea even at rest. On clinical examination, he is found to have some peripheral lower extremity edema and elevated jugular venous pressure. Lung fields are clear at this time. Blood gases show a PaO_2 of 52 mm Hg, $PaCO_2$ of 52 mm Hg, SaO_2 of 89%, and a pH of 7.32. Would oxygen therapy be recommended for this patient? What other advice should the patient receive regarding use of the three inhalers?
3. A 15-year-old boy with cystic fibrosis (CF) has been referred to your clinic for deconditioning. He has just recovered from a severe bacterial infection and needs help developing an exercise program. Discuss what category of medications he might be on, and also prepare some general exercise guidelines for him, keeping in mind his medical status.
4. Compare and contrast the procedure for inhaling drugs using a metered-dose inhaler (MDI) versus a dry powder inhaler.
5. Research the literature to determine what nutritional interventions are available that will help reduce the number of asthmatic exacerbations in a patient.

REFERENCES

1. Brashers VL, Huether SE: Structure and function of the pulmonary system. In Huether SE, McCance KL, editors: Understanding pathophysiology, St. Louis, 2008, Mosby.
2. Eglen RM: Muscarinic receptor subtypes in neuronal and non-neuronal cholinergic function. Auton Autacoid Pharmacol 26(3):219-233, 2006.
3. Kraft WK, Leone FT: Asthma and chronic obstructive pulmonary disease. In Waldman SA, Terzic A, editors: Pharmacology and therapeutics: Principles to practice, St Louis, 2009, Saunders.
4. Barnes PJ: Immunology of asthma and chronic obstructive pulmonary disease. Nat Rev Immunol 8(3):183-192, 2008.
5. Barnes PJ: The cytokine network in asthma and chronic obstructive pulmonary disease. J Clin Invest 118(11):3546-3556, 2008.
6. Busse, WW, Boushey, HA, Camargo, CA, et al: Guidelines for the Diagnosis and Management of Asthma—part 4: Managing Special Situations and Exacerbations 2007 (website). http://cme.medscape.com/viewarticle/564675. Accessed July 6, 2009.
7. Berger W: Aerosol devices and asthma therapy. Curr Drug Deliv 6(1):38-49, 2009.
8. Self TH, Pinner NA, Sowell RS, Headley AS: Does it really matter what volume to exhale before using asthma inhalation devices? J Asthma 46(3):212-216, 2009.
9. Lavorini F, Fontana GA: Targeting drugs to the airways: The role of spacer devices. Expert Opin Drug Delivery 6(1): 91-102, 2009.
10. Kelly HW, Ahrens RC, Holmes M, et al: Evaluation of particle size distribution of salmeterol administered via metered-dose inhaler with and without valved holding chambers. Ann Allergy Asthma Immunol 87(6):482-487, 2001.
11. Usmani OS, Biddiscombe MF, Nightingale JA, Underwood SR, Barnes PJ: Effects of bronchodilator particle size in asthmatic patients using monodisperse aerosols. J Appl Physiol 95(5):2106-2112, 2003.
12. Epstein S, Maidenberg A, Hallett D, Khan K, Chapman KR: Patient handling of a dry-powder inhaler in clinical practice. Chest 120(5):1480-1484, 2001.

13. Kelly HW: Comparison of two methods of delivering continuously nebulized albuterol. Ann Parmacother 37(1):23-26, 2003.
14. Melani AS: Inhalatory therapy training: A priority challenge for the physician. Acta Biomed 78(3):233-245, 2007.
15. Wechsler ME, Lehman E, Lazarus SC, et al: Beta-adrenergic receptor polymorphisms and response to salmeterol. Am J Respir Critical Care Med 173:519-526, 2006.
16. Nelson HS, Weiss ST, Bleecker ER, et al: The Salmeterol Multicenter Asthma Research Trial: A comparison of usual pharmacotherapy for asthma or usual pharmacotherapy plus salmeterol. Chest. 129:15-26, 2006.
17. Wijesinghe M, Perrin K, Harwood M, Weatherall M, Beasley R: The risk of asthma mortality with inhaled long acting beta-agonists. Postgrad Med J 84(995):467-472, 2008.
18. Expert panel report 3: Guidelines for the diagnosis and management of asthma: NIH publication No. 08-4051. 2007.
19. Murray JJ: Cardiovascular risks associated with beta-agonist therapy. Chest 127:2283-2285, 2005.
20. Qureshi F, Pestian J, Davis P, Zaritsky A: Effect of nebulized ipratropium on the hospitalization rates of children with asthma. N Engl J Med 339(15):1030-1035, 1998.
21. Suissa S, Ernst P, Benayoun S, Baltzan M, Cai B: Low-dose inhaled corticosteriods and the prevention of death from asthma. N Engl J Med 343(5):332-336, 2000.
22. Postma DS, Kerstjens HAM, ten Hacken NHT: Inhaled corticosteroids and long-acting beta-agonists in adult asthma: A winning combination in all? Naunyn-Schmiedeberg's Arch Pharmacol 378:203-215, 2008.
23. Shrewsbury S, Pyke S, Britton M: Meta-analysis of increased dose of inhaled steroid or addition of salmeterol in symptomatic asthma (MIASMA). Br Med J 320(7246):1368-1373, 2000.
24. Silverstein MD, Yunginger JW, Reed CE, et al: Attained adult height after childhood asthma: Effect of glucocorticoid therapy. J Allergy Clin Immunol 99(4):466-474, 1997.
25. Guilbert TW, Morgan WJ, Zeiger RS, et al: Long-term inhaled corticosteroids in preschool children at high risk for asthma. N Engl J Med 354(19):1985-1997, 2006.
26. Barnes PJ, Pedersen S, Busse WW: Efficacy and safety of inhaled corticosteroids. Am J Respir Crit Care Med 157(3): S1-S53, 1998.
27. Wong CA, Walsh LJ, Smith CJ, et al: Inhaled corticosteroid use and bone-mineral density in patients with asthma. Lancet 355(9213):1399-1403, 2000.
28. Casale TB, Nelson HS, Stricker WE, Raff H, Newman KB: Suppression of hypothalamic-pituitary-adrenal axis activity with inhaled flunisolide and fluticasone propionate in adult asthma patients. Ann Allergy Asthma Immunol 87(5):379-385, 2001.
29. Roland NJ, Bhalla RK, Earis J: The local side effects of inhaled corticosteroids: Current understanding and review of the literature. Chest 126:213-219, 2004.
30. Barnes PJ: Anti-leukotrienes: Here to stay? Curr Opin Pharmacol 3(3):257-263, 2003.
31. Barnes N, Wei LX, Reiss TF, et al: Analysis of montelukast in mild persistent asthmatic patients with near-normal lung function. Respir Med 95(5):379-386, 2001.
32. Garcia Garcia ML, Wahn U, et al: Montelukast, compared with fluticasone, for control of asthma among 6- to 14-year-old patients with mild asthma: The MOSAIC study. Pediatrics 116(2):360-369, 2005.
33. Sorkness CA, Lemanske RF Jr, Mauger DT, et al: Long-term comparison of 3 controller regimens for mild-moderate persistent childhood asthma: The Pediatric Asthma Controller Trial. J Allergy Clin Immunol 119(1):64-72, 2007.
34. Zeiger RS, Szefler SJ, Phillips BR, et al: Response profiles to fluticasone and montelukast in mild-to-moderate persistent childhood asthma. J Allergy Clin Immunol 117(1):45-52, 2006.
35. Chalmers GW, Macleod KJ, Little SA, Thomson LJ, McSharry CP, Thomson NC: Influence of cigarette smoking on inhaled corticosteroid treatment in mild asthma. Thorax 57(3):226-230, 2002.
36. Lipworth BJ: Leukotriene-receptor antagonists. Lancet 353: 57-62, 1999.
37. Reiss TF: Montelukast, a once daily leukotriene receptor antagonist in the treatment of chronic asthma: A multicenter randomized, double blind trial. Arch Intern Med 158:1213-1220, 1998.
38. Tasche MJ, Uijen JH, Bernsen RM, de Jongste JC, van der Wouden JC: Inhaled disodium cromoglycate (DSCG) as maintenance therapy in children with asthma: A systematic review. Thorax 55(11):913-920, 2000.
39. van der Wouden JC, Uijen JH, Bernsen RM, Tasche MJ, de Jongste JC, Ducharme F: Inhaled sodium cromoglycate for asthma in children. Cochrane Database Syst Rev, (3) (CD002173), 2003.
40. Jaffar ZH, Sullivan P, Page C, Costello J: Low-dose theophylline modulates T-lymphocyte activation in allergen-challenged asthmatics. Eur Respir J 9(3):456-462, 1996.
41. Dahl R, Larsen BB, Venge P: Effect of long-term treatment with inhaled budesonide or theophylline on lung function, airway reactivity and asthma symptoms. Respir Med 96(6):432-438, 2002.
42. Weinberger M, Hendeles L: Drug therapy: Theophylline in asthma. N Engl J Med 334(21):1380-1388, 1996.
43. Rang HP, et al: The Respiratory system. In Rang JP, Dale MM, Ritter JM, Flower R, editors: Rang and Dale's pharmacology, St. Louis, 2007, Churchill Livingstone.
44. Boushey HA: Drugs used in asthma. In Katzung BG, editor: Basic and clinical pharmacology, New York, 2007, McGraw Hill.
45. Tan RA, Spector SL: Exercise-induced asthma: Diagnosis and management. Ann Allergy Asthma Immunol 89:226-236, 2002.
46. Parsons JP, Mastronarde JG: Exercise-induced bronchoconstriction in athletes. Chest 128:3966-3974, 2005.
47. Andersen SD, Kippelen P: Exercise-induced bronchoconstriction: Pathogenesis. Curr Allergy Asthma Rep 5:116-122, 2005.
48. Anderson SD, Brannan JD: Long acting beta$_2$-adrenoceptor agonists and exercise-induced asthma: Lessons to guide us in the future. Paediatr Drugs 6:161-175, 2004.
49. Anderson SD, Argyros GJ, Holzer MK: Provocation by eucapnic voluntary hyperpnoea to identify exercise induced bronchoconstriction. Br J Sports Med 35:344-347, 2001.
50. Fitch KD, Sue-Chu M, Anderson SD, et al: Asthma and the elite athlete: Summary of the International Olympic Committee's Consensus Conference, Lausanne, Switzerland, January 22-24, 2008. J Allergy Clin Immunol 122(2):254-260. e7, 2008.
51. Joos GF, O'Connor B: Indirect airway challenges. Eur Respir J 21(6):1050-1068, 2003.
52. Raissy HH, Harkins M, Kelly F, Kelly HW: Pretreatment with albuterol versus montelukast for exercise-induced bronchospasm in children. Pharmacotherapy 28(3):287-294, 2008.
53. Kelly KD, Spooner CH, Rowe BH: Nedocromil sodium versus sodium cromoglycate in treatment of exercise-induced bronchoconstriction: A systematic review. Eur Respir J 17:39-45, 2001.
54. Leff JA, Busse WW, Pearlman D, et al: Montelukast, a leukotriene-receptor antagonist, for the treatment of mild asthma and exercise-induced bronchoconstriction. N Engl J Med 339(3):147-152, 1998.
55. Villaran C, O'Neill SJ, Helbling A, et al: Montelukast versus salmeterol in patients with asthma and exercise-induced bronchoconstriction. Montelukast/Salmeterol Exercise Study Group. J Allergy Clin Immunol 104(1):547-553, 1999.

56. Philip G, Pearlman DS, Villarán C, et al: Single-dose montelukast or salmeterol as protection against exercise-induced bronchoconstriction. Chest 132:875-883, 2007.
57. Kemp JP, Dockhorn RJ, Shapiro GG, et al: Montelukast once daily inhibits exercise-induced bronchoconstriction in 6- to 14- year old children with asthma. J Pediatr 133(3):424-428, 1998.
58. Martineau L, Horan MA, Rothwell NJ, Little RA: Salbutamol, a β_2-adrenoceptor agonist, increases skeletal muscle strength in young men. Clin Sci 83:615-621, 1992.
59. van Baak MA, Mayer LH, Kempinski RE, Hartgens F: Effect of salbutamol on muscle strength and endurance performance in nonasthmatic men. Med Sci Sports Exer 32(7):1300-1306, 2000.
60. Goubault C, Perault MC, Leleu E, et al: Effects of inhaled salbutamol in exercising non-asthmatic athletes. Thorax 56:675-679, 2001.
61. McKenzie DC, Stewart IB, Fitch KD: The asthmatic athlete, inhaled beta agonists, and performance. Clin J Sport Med 12(4):225-228, 2002.
62. Bhowmick B, Singh D: Novel anti-inflammatory treatments for asthma. Expert Rev Resp Med 2(5):617-629, 2008.
63. Abramowicz M, editor: Over-the-counter (OTC) cough remedies. In The Medical Letter, Vol. 43(1100). New Rochelle, NY, 2001, The Medical Letter, Inc.
64. Abramowicz M, editor: Montelukast (Singulair) for allergic rhinitis. In The Medical Letter, Vol. 45(1152). New Rochelle, NY, 2003, The Medical Letter, Inc.
65. Nayak AS, Philip G, Lu S, Malice MP, Reiss TF; Montelukast Fall Rhinitis Investigator Group: Efficacy and tolerability of montelukast alone or in combination with loratadine in seasonal allergic rhinitis: A multicenter, randomized, double-blind, placebo-controlled trial performed in the fall. Ann Allergy Asthma Immunol 88(6):592-600, 2002.
66. Harms HK, Matouk E, Tournier G, et al: Multicenter, open-label study of recombinant human DNase in cystic fibrosis patients with moderate lung disease. Pediatr Pulminol 26: 155-161, 1998.
67. Johnson CA, Butler SM, Konstan MW, Breen TJ, Morgan WJ: Estimating effectiveness in an observational study: A case study of dornase alfa in cystic fibrosis. J Pediatr 134(6):734-739, 1999.
68. Brashers VL: Alterations of pulmonary function. In Huether SE, McCance KL, editors: Understanding pathophysiology, St. Louis, 2008, Mosby.
69. Man SF, McAlister FA, Anthonisen NR, Sin DD: Contemporary management of chronic obstructive pulmonary disease. JAMA 290:2313-2316, 2003.
70. Qaseem A, Snow V, Shekelle P, et al: Diagnosis and management of stable chronic obstructive pulmonary disease: A clinical practice guideline from the American College of Physicians. Ann Intern Med 147(9):633-638, 2007.
71. Lung Health Study Research Group: Effect of inhaled triamcinolone on the decline in pulmonary function in chronic obstructive pulmonary disease. N Engl J Med 343:1902-1909, 2000.
72. Calverley P, Pauwels R, Vestbo J, et al: Combined salmeterol and fluticasone in the treatment of chronic obstructive pulmonary disease: A randomised controlled trial. Lancet, 2003. 361: p. 449-456.
73. Jorenby DE, Smith SS, Fiore MC, et al: Varying nicotine patch dose and type of smoking cessation counseling. JAMA 274(17):1347-1352, 1995.
74. Sin DD, McAlister FA, Man SF, Anthonisen NR: Contemporary management of chronic obstructive pulmonary disease. JAMA 290(17):2301-2312, 2003.
75. Scullion JE: The development of anticholinergics in the management of COPD. Int J COPD 2(1):33-40, 2007.
76. Barr RG, Bourbeau J, Camargo CA, Ram FS: Tiotropium for stable chronic obstructive pulmonary disease: A meta-analysis. Thorax 61:854-862, 2006.
77. Vincken W, Van Noord JA, Greefhorst APM: Improved health outcomes in patients with COPD during 1 year's treatment with tiotropium. Eur Respir J 19:209-216, 2006.
78. Travers J, Laveneziana P, Webb KA, Kesten S, O'Donnell DE: Effect of tiotropium bromide on the cardiovascular response to exercise in COPD. Respir Med 101(9):2017-2024, 2007.
79. Grimes GC: Pharmacologic management of stable COPD reviewed. Am Fam Physician 76:1141-1148, 2007.
80. Chaouat A, Weitzenblum E, Kessler R, et al: A randomized trial of nocturnal oxygen therapy in chronic obstructive pulmonary disease patients. Eur Respir J 14:1002-1008, 1999.
81. Kunzelmann K, Mall M: Pharmacotherapy of the ion transport defect in cystic fibrosis. Clin Exper Pharmacol Physiol 28:857-867, 2001.
82. Davis PB: Cystic fibrosis. Pediatr Rev 22(8):257-264, 2001.
83. Clunes MT, Boucher RC: Front runners for pharmacotherapeutic correction of the airway ion transport defect in cystic fibrosis. Curr opin Pharmacol 8(3):292-299, 2008.
84. Elpern EH, Patel G, Balk RA: Antibiotic therapy for pulmonary exacerbations in adults with cystic fibrosis (Cover story). MEDSURG Nursing 16(5):293-297, 2007.
85. Bennett WD: Effect of beta-adrenergic agonists on mucociliary clearance. J Allergy Clin Immunol 110(suppl 6):S291-S297, 2002.
86. Jaffe A, Balfour-Lynn IM: Treatment of severe small airways disease in children with cystic fibrosis: Alternatives to corticosteroids. Paediatr Drugs 4(6):381-389, 2002.
87. Konstan MW: Ibuprofen therapy for cystic fibrosis lung disease: Revisited. Curr Opin Pulm Med 14:567-573, 2008.
88. Ries AL: New guidelines highlight benefits of pulmonary rehabilitation. Chest 131:4s-42s, 2007.
89. Saito S, Miyamoto K, Nishimura M, et al: Effects of inhaled bronchodilators on pulmonary hemodynamics at rest and during exercise in patients with COPD. Chest 115(2):376-382, 1999.
90. Blosser SA, Maxwell SL, Reeves-Hoche MK, Localio AR, Zwillich CW: Is an anticholinergic agent superior to a beta$_2$-agonist in improving dyspnea and exercise limitation in COPD? Chest 108:730-735, 1995.
91. Light RW, Stansbury DW, Webster JS: Effect of 30 mg of morphine alone or with promethazine or prochlorperazine on the exercise capacity of patients with COPD. Chest 109(4):975– 981, 1996.
92. Woodcock AA, Gross ER, Gellert A, Shah S, Johnson M, Geddes DM: Effects of dihydrocodeine, alcohol, and caffeine on breathlessness and exercise tolerance in patients with chronic obstructive lung disease and normal blood gases. N Engl J Med 305(27):1611-1616, 1981.

SECTION III

Pain Control

10

Anesthetic Agents

Barbara Gladson

TYPES OF ANESTHESIA

There are three basic categories of anesthetics: general, local, and regional. Within each category, there are different modes of administration. General anesthesia may be given by the inhaled or intravenous (IV) mode. Local anesthesia can be administered through an injection or by topical application, and regional anesthesia involves numbing a large area of the body, as in spinal anesthesia.

GENERAL ANESTHESIA

General anesthesia produces a progressive and reversible central nervous system (CNS) depression. Many different drugs are used to induce anesthesia, each with individual characteristics and different adverse effects. The ideal agent must produce a loss of consciousness, analgesia, amnesia, skeletal muscle relaxation, and inhibition of sensory and autonomic reflexes and must have a rapid onset.[1] In addition, it must be nontoxic and achieve the desired effect without producing hypoxia, laryngospasm, excessive tracheobronchial secretions, or respiratory depression. However, none of the anesthetic agents available today meet these criteria. Therefore, it is common practice to administer several different medications in small amounts to produce the desired effects while minimizing toxic effects. This practice is called *balanced anesthesia*, and it involves administering a combination of inhaled and IV anesthetics along with narcotics and neuromuscular blocking agents.

Induction of anesthesia involves the patient passing through different levels of CNS depression.[1] The first stage is *analgesia*, followed by the second stage, *delirium*. In this stage, consciousness is lost, and excitement and muscle activity may be marked. Rapid respirations and vomiting may occur, and breathing is irregular. The third stage is referred to as *surgical anesthesia*. It is marked by rhythmic breathing with deep respirations. The fourth stage is *medullary paralysis*, characterized by respiratory and cardiovascular collapse. Blood pressure falls, pupils dilate, and spontaneous breathing ceases. Anesthesia is irreversible at this point.

In today's practice of anesthesia, these phases, as described previously, are somewhat unrecognizable. Drug-induced rapid loss of consciousness, premedication, and assisted ventilation produce a blurring of these stages. Basically, the adequacy of anesthesia is now assessed by certain respiratory and cardiovascular responses.

Premedication

Premedication, that is, drug administration before anesthesia is induced, is done for a variety of reasons, including sedation, analgesia, antiemesis, infection control, and minimization of anesthetic adverse effects; disease-modifying agents may also be given to control for any adverse effects on a patient's underlying medical condition.[2] Preoperative sedation with a benzodiazepine or a barbiturate may be given 1 to 2 hours before surgery. These drugs are not only effective at reducing anxiety but also provide a certain baseline sedation that facilitates a loss of consciousness with reduced anesthesia.

The patient might receive promethazine to combat the nausea and vomiting produced by the anesthetics. This drug is an antihistamine with antiemetic, anticholinergic, and sedative properties. Recent food in the stomach poses a risk of aspiration because the normal protective airway responses are diminished in the absence of consciousness.[2] Preoperative fasting and postponement of the surgery are options, but these strategies will not always guarantee an empty stomach because opioids reduce gastric mobility; nor is this practical in an emergency. Intubation along with neuromuscular paralysis can be instituted as soon as the IV anesthesia takes effect as a means of guarding against aspiration when surgery must be performed on an emergency basis.

Antimicrobial prophylaxis (usually a single intramuscular injection within an hour of the start of surgery) can decrease the incidence of infection, particularly wound infection after certain procedures, but this benefit must be weighed against the risk of allergic reactions and the development of resistant bacteria.[3] It is recommended for procedures associated with high infection rates such as those involving implantation of prosthetic material, those involving the gastrointestinal tract, and those involving trauma in which the wound is already dirty. Host factors such as immunosuppression or the presence of valvular and other cardiac diseases also warrant prophylaxis. Patients who have had long preoperative hospitalization also need prophylaxis because they may have been exposed to hospital-based resistant organisms.

Patients with pre-existing chronic obstructive pulmonary disease (COPD) or respiratory limitations are predisposed to atelectasis, pneumonia, hypoxia, and respiratory failure after surgery, particularly abdominal or thoracic surgery. Pretreatment with bronchodilators and antibiotics and chest physical therapy should be standard treatment for several days before the surgery.[1] General anesthetics decrease myocardial performance, so patients with congestive heart failure (CHF) should also receive premedication to control cardiac symptoms.

Certain medications should be discontinued before surgery (Table 10-1).[2] Diuretics can create hypovolemia and hypokalemia, which must be corrected over several days to decrease the risk of arrhythmias during surgery. In addition, diabetic patients should have their oral diabetic drugs withheld on the morning of the procedure to prevent hypoglycemia, and patients who receive insulin will be asked to reduce their dose and quite possibly will receive IV glucose. Anesthetic agents can also interact with pre-existing drug therapy (Table 10-2).

Inhaled Anesthesia

Commonly used inhalation agents include nitrous oxide, halothane, methoxyflurane, isoflurane, desflurane, and sevoflurane. Nitrous oxide is used primarily during dental surgery.[4] Inhalation agents are vaporized and mixed with oxygen and then given through a mask or endotracheal tube. Once gas exchange occurs in the lungs, these drugs are circulated to the brain and other organs. From there, these drugs diffuse into fats because of their great lipid solubility. Over time, these drugs diffuse back out into the general circulation and then again into the brain. This phenomenon is responsible for the "hangover" that many patients experience the day after surgery.

The degree of anesthesia is determined by a drug's concentration in the CNS. The rate at which an effective concentration of drug reaches the brain (the rate of anesthetic induction) is related to a variety of factors, including the solubility of the drug, concentration of drug in the inspired air, respiratory rate and depth, blood flow to the lungs, and the loss of drug through expired air. The anesthetic agent must first transfer from the alveolar air to the blood and then to the brain. The rate at which this occurs depends on the solubility of the agent in the blood. The "blood:gas partition coefficient" is an index explaining the relative affinity of the drug to blood versus air. For desflurane, sevoflurane, and nitrous oxide, this index is quite low, indicating their low solubility in blood (range of 0.47 to 0.69).[2] Methoxyflurane is extremely soluble and has a much higher index of 12.[5] There is an inverse relationship between solubility in blood and the rate of increase in a drug's partial pressure

TABLE 10-1 Drugs to Be Stopped, Continued, or Started Preoperatively

	Drugs	Perioperative Aims
Stop	Oral hypoglycemics	Avoid hypoglycemia and cerebral damage
	Monoamine oxidase inhibitors (MAOIs)	Avoid hypertensive crisis and hyperpyrexia
	Warfarin (e.g., for atrial defibrillation or prosthetic valve; convert to heparin, and discontinue shortly before surgery)	Avoid excessive bleeding intraoperatively (with minimal increase in risk for cerebral embolism and stroke)
	Diuretics	Avoid hypovolemia and hypokalemia
Continue	Opioids	Avoid preoperative pain
	Anticonvulsants	Avoid seizure
	Bronchodilators	Avoid bronchoconstriction
	Antihypertensive and cardiac drugs, with exception of diuretics	Avoid hypertension, angina, congestive heart failure, arrhythmia
	Adrenocorticosteroids (increase dose)	Avoid adrenal insufficiency
	Insulin (decrease dose)	Avoid ketoacidosis
Start	Histamine H_1- and H_2-receptor antagonists	Allergy prophylaxis in atopic patients
	Benzodiazepine	Provide anxiolysis and anterograde amnesia in frightened patients
	Bronchodilators (inhaled)	Avoid bronchoconstriction in patients with stable asthma
	Anticholinergics	Avoid bradycardia in young children (cardiac output depends on the heart rate)
	Adrenocorticosteroids (increase dose)	Avoid adrenal insufficiency if drug history positive in the last year
	Antacids, histamine H_1-receptor antagonists, gastric motility agents	Increase gastric pH and decrease gastric residual volume
	Antiemetics	Reduce risk of nausea and vomiting
	Heparin	Prevent deep vein thrombosis and pulmonary embolism
	Antibiotics	Prevent wound infection and subacute bacterial endocarditis

From Page C, Curtis MJ, Sutter MC, Walker MJ, Hoffman BB, editors: *Integrated pharmacology* (2nd ed.). Philadelphia, 2002, Mosby.

TABLE 10-2 Anesthetic Interactions with Pre-existing Therapy

Body Location	Drug	Anesthetic Interaction
Brain	Acute alcohol intoxication	Potentiates general anesthetics
	Long-term alcohol abuse	Increases general anesthetic requirements
	Clonidine	Potentiates general anesthetics (but continue preoperatively to avoid intraoperative "rebound" hypertension because of its short half-life)
Lung	Smoking	Pulmonary injury decreases oxygen transfer, and carbon monoxide decreases blood oxygen capacity
	Past use of bleomycin	High FiO_2 can precipitate adult respiratory distress syndrome
Circulation	Diuretics	Hypovolemia increases risk of hypotension and acute hypokalemia; increases risk of arrhythmias during general anesthesia
	β-Adrenoceptor agonists, bronchodilators	Potentiate arrhythmias from volatile inhaled anesthetics
	β-Adrenoceptor antagonists	Potentiate myocardial depression from general anesthetics
	Ca^{2+} antagonists	Potentiate myocardial depression from general anesthetics
	Monoamine oxidase inhibitors (MAOIs)	Sympathetic stimulants or meperidine may precipitate hypertension and hyperpyrexia
	Past use of doxorubicin	Cardiomyopathy increases risk of heart failure from anesthesia
	Aminoglycosides	Potentiate nondepolarizing neuromuscular blockers

FiO_2, fractional concentration of oxygen in inspired gas.
From Page C, Curtis MJ, Sutter MC, Walker MJ, Hoffman BB, editors: *Integrated pharmacology* (2nd ed.). Philadelphia, 2002, Mosby.

or tension. When a drug of low solubility is inhaled and diffuses into arterial blood, only a few molecules are required to raise its partial pressure, and arterial tension rises quickly. However, when the drug has high solubility, more molecules dissolve in the blood before there is a significant change in the partial pressure, causing the arterial tension of the gas to rise slowly. Raising the minute ventilation and increasing the concentration of the drug in the inspired air also enhance the uptake and distribution of the inhaled agent. Cardiac output or blood flow to the lungs slows the induction of anesthesia because more blood going to the lungs reduces the relative concentration of the drug and necessitates a greater partial pressure to achieve anesthesia.[1]

The major route of elimination of inhaled agents is through expired air, although some agents are metabolized by the liver enzymes.[1] How quickly elimination occurs is related to the drug's solubility. Agents that have a low solubility in the blood will be the most quickly eliminated. Therefore, rapid recovery from anesthesia occurs with nitrous oxide and slow recovery with methoxyflurane. The speed of onset and recovery mimic each other.

The potency of an inhaled anesthetic agent is not expressed by the kd or median effective dose (ED50), but rather by the minimum alveolar concentration (MAC) that suppresses movement in response to a surgical incision in 50% of subjects.[5,6] It is estimated that 1.3 times the MAC will prevent movement in 95% of subjects.

The mechanism of action of inhaled drugs is not completely understood. One theory is that the molecules of gas dissolve in the phospholipid bilayer of the neuronal membrane, causing the membrane to expand and impeding the opening of sodium channels.[7] However, it has been pointed out that anesthetics cause only a slight upset in the lipid membrane.[8] Another theory is that these agents block the sodium channels in neurons.[9] However, it is more likely that inhaled agents act differently in different neural tissues and affect a variety of specific membrane proteins and ion channels, particularly enhancing the inhibitory effects of gamma (γ)-aminobutyric acid (GABA) receptors. Anesthetics also inhibit the function of excitatory receptors, including glutamate, acetylcholine (ACh), and 5-hydroxytryptamine. Currently, researchers are investigating an anesthetic-sensitive potassium (K^+) channel labeled TREK.[10,11] When the inhaled drug activates this channel, neural membrane excitability becomes depressed. Anesthetics affect all parts of the nervous system, but it is thought that most of the influence takes place at the thalamus, cortex, and hippocampus, producing a lack of interest in sensory input and memory loss.

Most inhaled anesthetics have a profound effect on the cardiovascular system.[5] Most decrease arterial pressure and depress contractility, producing reflex tachycardia. The heart may also become sensitized to epinephrine, resulting in arrhythmias. However, some argue that inhaled agents are, in fact, cardioprotective if heart rate does not become elevated extensively. Myocardial depression reduces myocardial oxygen demand on an ischemic heart.[12] A recent meta-analysis specifically showed a reduction in the incidence of myocardial infarction (MI) following cardiac surgery with desflurane, but this has not been seen in other types of surgeries. Inhaled anesthetics also reduce the responsiveness of the chemoreceptors to carbon dioxide and oxygen; This reduced response is confounded by the administration of opioids, these drugs should not be used in patients with CHF. In the case of the pulmonary system, a reduction in respiratory rate and mucociliary function occurs. Inhaled agents also have the potential to produce hepatotoxicity and nephrotoxicity and an increase in cerebral blood flow, so they are not recommended for use in patients with increased intracranial pressure caused by head trauma or a brain tumor.

Another complication of inhaled anesthetics is malignant hyperthermia.[5] This is a genetically related condition characterized by extreme muscular rigidity, hypertension, tachycardia, and fatal hyperthermia resulting from exposure to certain anesthetic agents, particularly halothane and methoxyflurane.[13] The pathologic condition involves excessive calcium release from the sarcoplasmic reticulum. Quick administration of dantrolene (a drug that inhibits calcium release from the sarcoplasmic reticulum) may prevent death.

Despite their adverse effects, not all inhaled agents produce the same level of risk. Isoflurane and desflurane have limited effects on the cardiovascular system, and because inhaled agents are never used in isolation, the addition of another type of drug may work synergistically so that the concentration of the inhaled agent may be reduced, thus diminishing the risks. A thorough assessment by the anesthesiologist is always necessary in determining the appropriate drugs for anesthesia.

Intravenous Anesthetic Agents

In recent years, the use of IV drugs in anesthesia has increased. Anesthetic agents that comprise the IV category are a diverse group of drugs that include barbiturates, short-acting hypnotics, opioids, benzodiazepines, and neuroleptics.[1] IV anesthetics act as adjuncts to inhaled drugs or may be given on their own. They require no specialized equipment such as a face mask for administration and induce anesthesia very rapidly. Induction occurs as soon as the drug reaches the brain and may be faster than that achieved with some of the newer inhaled agents. IV anesthetics—particularly thiopental, etomidate, and propofol—are the drugs of choice for the induction of anesthesia. The recovery rate with many of these agents is fast enough that they may be used in short, outpatient procedures; propofol, in particular, matches the recovery time of the fastest inhaled drug.

Ultra-Short-Acting Barbiturates: Thiopental. Thiopental is a short-acting barbiturate and is one of the most commonly used agents for the induction of anesthesia. Its mechanism of action is its binding to the GABA-gated chloride channel, which enhances the inhibitory effect of GABA. This drug produces a more satisfactory rapid induction than any of the inhaled anesthetics. After IV injection, the drug is rapidly distributed to the brain as a result of its extensive blood flow and high lipid solubility. Loss of consciousness occurs within 10 to 30 seconds.[5] However, the blood concentration drops off rapidly by about 80% in the first 1 to 2 minutes after injection as equilibration with the brain occurs. After a short period, the concentration in the brain decreases as the drug is redistributed to other tissues. This redistribution, rather than the drug's metabolism, accounts for the short duration of action. Recovery occurs within about 5 to 10 minutes, unless more drug is injected, and after several hours, much of the thiopental in the body will have been redistributed into the body fat. Redistribution back into the brain occurs again and is responsible for the hangover effect. Hepatic metabolism occurs quite slowly, so with repeated administration, the drug accumulates in the body which causes delayed awakening. Therefore, thiopental is not used to maintain surgical anesthesia but only for induction.

The disadvantages of thiopental include poor analgesic action and inadequate skeletal muscle relaxation; so, frequently, pain medication and muscle relaxants must also be administered. In addition, as the dose increases, thiopental produces decreases in arterial blood pressure (caused by venodilation), stroke volume, heart rate, and cardiac output. There is actually a narrow margin between the anesthetic dose and the dose that produces cardiovascular depression.[14] Other adverse effects include respiratory depression, bronchospasm, laryngospasm, and reflex tachycardia if the patient experiences excessive hypotension.

Methohexital is another ultra-short-acting barbiturate. It is stronger than thiopental and shorter acting. It is often used in oral surgery and fracture reduction and during electroconvulsive therapy. This drug is less likely to produce bronchospasm, so it may be used in patients with asthma.

Etomidate. Etomidate is used for induction of anesthesia and along with other agents for balanced sedation.[15] It has a larger margin of safety compared with thiopental and is associated with minimal cardiovascular and respiratory depression.[16] Loss of consciousness occurs in seconds, and recovery occurs within 3 to 5 minutes. It is also metabolized more rapidly than the barbiturates and therefore does not produce a hangover effect. The negative aspects of this drug include lack of analgesic effect, production of involuntary movements during induction, pain on injection, and significant postoperative nausea and vomiting.

Ketamine. Ketamine is a short-acting hypnotic, nonbarbiturate agent that is related to phencyclidine, an anesthetic agent used in veterinary medicine.[5] It binds to N-methyl-D-aspartate (NMDA) receptors, inhibiting the excitatory effects of glutamate. This drug preserves muscle tone and the protective airway reflexes, and limits its respiratory depression. It is often used in burn units where patients are frequently anesthetized for dressing changes, since it also possesses analgesic properties.[17] Induction occurs in 2 to 4 minutes, and anesthesia lasts for approximately 20 minutes.[1]

Ketamine produces dissociative anesthesia characterized by catatonia, amnesia, and analgesia without loss of consciousness. Its mechanism of action is not fully understood, but ketamine produces a generalized sensory blockade in the higher brain centers. The patient's eyes remain open and are characterized by nystagmus and an appearance of staring into space.[18] Although the patient is not completely unconscious, responses to questions tend to be minimal. It produces a rapid induction with good pain control and has a higher therapeutic index than other IV anesthetics.

Ketamine increases the tone of skeletal, cardiac, and respiratory muscles, which results in raising blood pressure, heart rate, and respiratory rate. Ketamine also increases secretions from the salivary and bronchial glands, produces vomiting, and increases intracranial pressure. Because of these adverse effects, this drug is not recommended for patients with ischemic heart disease or COPD or for those who have sustained head trauma. Another major drawback of this drug is the occurrence of "emergence reactions." Some patients will experience hallucinations or disturbing dreams as the drug wears off. Diazepam, a benzodiazepine, administered with ketamine will reduce these reactions.

Propofol. Propofol is one of the most popular IV anesthetics because it has few adverse effects. Induction of anesthesia is smooth and occurs within 40 seconds after administration. It lowers blood pressure without myocardial depression and also lowers intracranial pressure. It acts as an antiemetic agent and is safe to use in patients with a previous history of malignant hyperthermia.[19-21] Propofol is the ideal agent for ambulatory anesthesia because it has a short duration of action without a hangover effect or significant postoperative drowsiness. It is used not only to induce anesthesia but also for maintenance of anesthesia during surgery. At lower doses, it can be used to attain a state of conscious sedation, a drug-induced reduction in anxiety that allows the patient to maintain an airway and respond to verbal commands. It is also administered as a sedative to critically ill patients.[22]

The major drawback to using propofol is that it offers little pain control, so the addition of an analgesic is required. Propofol can cause lethal metabolic acidosis and skeletal myopathy, a condition called *propofol infusion syndrome*, and it is occasionally associated with dystonic movements and seizure-like activity.[23-25]

At the time of this writing, the world was awaiting the autopsy report on the pop star Michael Jackson. The news media reported that his body was found hooked up to an IV, and propofol was the suspected cause of death. Propofol addiction has recently been recognized; during the period between 1992 and 2007, 38 cases of abuse have been reported in the literature.[26] The most probable cause of death was apnea, hypoxia, and hypotension. Not surprisingly, several of the reported fatalities were among medical professionals themselves.

Benzodiazepines. A few members of the class of drugs known as benzodiazepines—diazepam and midazolam—are used in anesthesia practice. Midazolam is more potent than diazepam, and its onset of action when given intravenously is usually less than 2 minutes.[15] Complete recovery takes approximately 90 minutes after a single dose, so it is not used to induce or maintain anesthesia but rather as premedication. Used intravenously, it prolongs the postanesthetic recovery period but also produces anterograde amnesia, which is usually desirable. Cardiovascular adverse effects are uncommon at the doses used for sedation, and the associated respiratory depression is usually tolerable.

Opioid Use in Anesthesia. Optimal treatment with opioids should provide a rapid onset of analgesia and rapid recovery without postoperative pain. With large doses, general anesthesia can be achieved. At lower doses, opioids help maintain anesthesia produced by other agents. Commonly used agents include IV morphine, fentanyl, remifentanil, and sufentanil.[15]

IV opioids are not good amnesic agents and cause respiratory depression and chest wall rigidity, which may impair ventilation.[1] They also are responsible for the postoperative nausea and vomiting. Naloxone is a narcotic antagonist that can rapidly reverse the respiratory depression associated with opioids.

Neuroleptanesthesia. Neuroleptanesthesia is general anesthesia produced by a combination of a neuroleptic agent (dopamine antagonist, antipsychotic) and an opioid analgesic.[1] Commonly used drugs are fentanyl and droperidol. Patients are neither asleep nor fully awake but are in a profound state of analgesia and will experience retrograde amnesia. Neuroleptanesthesia is used for short procedures requiring some patient cooperation. The combination of fentanyl and droperidol is given as an adjunct to other anesthetic drugs for maintenance of anesthesia. Adverse effects include bradycardia, bronchospasm, and muscle rigidity.

Adjuvants to Anesthesia

In addition to the anesthetic agents already discussed, several other types of drugs may be given during the perioperative period to augment the anesthesia process. Atropine is administered to prevent bradycardia and the excessive respiratory secretions associated with many of the anesthetic agents, but this may delay voiding after surgery. There are also reports that dextromethorphan, an NMDA antagonist, can block receptor sites in the spinal cord and CNS, leading to a reduction in the amount of postoperative pain medication required.[27] Clonidine, an α_2-agonist, also lessens the need for pain medication after surgery and reduces nausea and shivering as well.

Other intraoperative agents include neuromuscular blocking agents.[2] These are required for intubation, as laryngeal spasms can cause reflex closure of the vocal cords and subsequent hypoxemia. Neuromuscular blockers are also needed in abdominal and thoracic surgery to prevent reflex muscle contractions and in delicate surgeries such as microsurgery. There are two types of neuromuscular blockers: nondepolarizing blockers and depolarizing blockers. Nondepolarizing blockers are competitive antagonists of ACh at the neuromuscular junction. Examples of these are tubocurarine, pancuronium, and rocuronium. These drugs block the access of ACh to its binding site without activating the receptor. Rocuronium produces its effect in 90 seconds. Partial recovery occurs in about 30 minutes. After surgery, neostigmine, an anticholinesterase agent, can be used to reverse the effects of these drugs if recovery time needs to be shortened.

Depolarizing blockers bind and depolarize the motor end plate.[2] The end plate remains depolarized throughout the procedure because the drug is only broken down by the cholinesterase in the plasma. Initially, muscle fasciculations and unsynchronized contractions occur, followed by flaccid paralysis. Succinylcholine is the only drug of this kind available, and it is very useful in facilitating endotracheal intubation. It takes effect rapidly (similar to rocuronium) and has a short plasma half-life of about 5 minutes.

Drug Selection Process for General Anesthesia

The crucial goal for all anesthesiologists is to maintain proper pain control, amnesia, and sedation in patients undergoing surgical procedures. Current guidelines recommend propofol for short-term, same-day surgery procedures when rapid awakening is needed.[28] This may be combined with midazolam for sedation in an anxious patient and with fentanyl for pain relief. For longer procedures and for procedures which require hospitalization, induction of anesthesia is usually achieved with a barbiturate, followed by administration of an inhaled anesthetic for maintenance. Lorazepam is recommended for achieving amnesia in longer procedures, and morphine or hydromorphone is recommended for pain control and sedation. As the dose of any these types of drugs is increased, the dose of the true anesthetic can be minimized. Reversal agents are also kept on hand to correct any mishaps or lingering effects of the opioids and neuromuscular blockers.

Therapeutic Concerns with Anesthesia

When a patient returns to therapy after surgery, he or she may not have completely recovered from the effects of anesthesia. If the therapist is treating a patient the day after surgery, the patient may still be confused or "woozy" and may show signs of neuromuscular weakness. General anesthetics depress mucociliary clearance in the airways, leading to pooling of mucus and secretions. The patient should be encouraged to cough and to breathe deeply. This will help expel some of the anesthetic gases and also mobilize the pooled secretions. Proper guarding during ambulation is necessary because of lingering weakness from the anesthesia. Despite the hangover effect, patients should be encouraged to move so that abdominal distention caused by the anesthetic and muscle relaxant drugs can be reduced.

Another more recent concern with general anesthesia is anesthesia-induced neuroapoptosis.[29] Animal studies have shown that anesthesia in a dose-dependent manner can cause neuronal cell death. This recognition has led to some epidemiologic studies that suggest an association between the number of surgical procedures performed in children and the development of learning disabilities. Future studies are needed to establish a cause-and-effect relationship.

REGIONAL AND LOCAL ANESTHESIA

Regional anesthesia is an alternative to general anesthesia for surgery performed on the extremities or even the lower abdomen.[30] Regional anesthesia involves the administration of a local anesthetic agent by a variety of methods, including topical anesthesia, infiltration anesthesia, peripheral nerve block, IV regional block, and epidural or spinal administration. Essentially, regional anesthesia can be divided into three categories based on the site of injection: (1) A *central neuraxial* block is the injection of a drug into the epidural or intrathecal space; (2) a *peripheral nerve* block refers to an injection near a nerve or the plexus innervating the area undergoing surgery; and (3) a *field* block is the injection of the anesthetic into adjoining tissues for the expressed purpose of drug diffusion to the surgical area for minor procedures in the hand or foot. The choice of regional versus general anesthesia is related to the patient's medical status and type of surgery and also the anesthesiologist's experiences and preferences. Both types of anesthesia may be given together to reduce the need for high doses of general anesthetics. In some cases, regional anesthesia may be unsuccessful, and general anesthesia will then be necessary.

Local Anesthetic Agents

Local anesthetic agents have a similar structure consisting of a lipophilic aromatic ring and a hydrophilic tertiary amine separated by a carbon chain. This link can be either an amide or an ester bond (Figure 10-1).[30] The structural–functional way of looking at these compounds is important because this is how they are classified. Esters, including cocaine, procaine, tetracaine, and benzocaine, are rapidly metabolized by blood pseudocholinesterase,

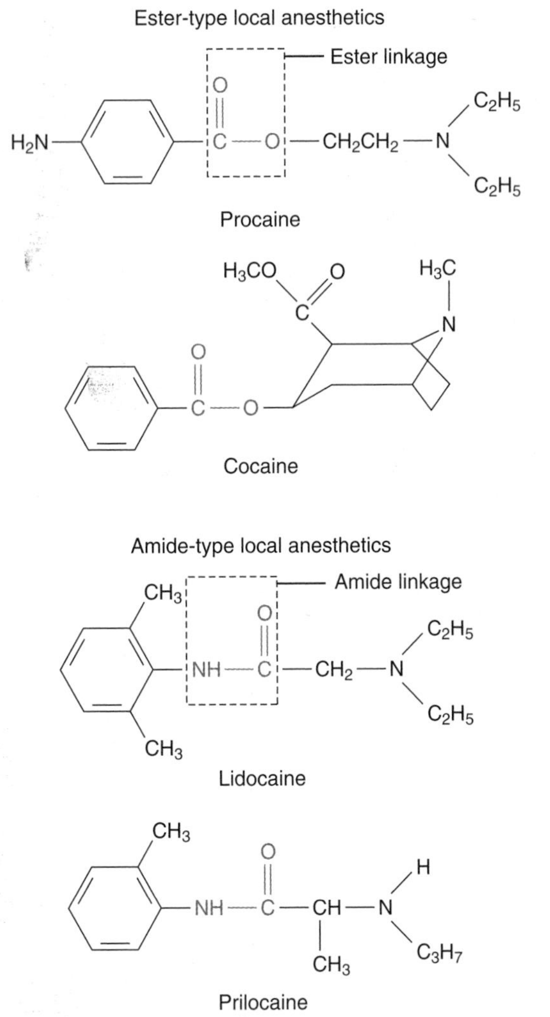

Ester-type local anesthetics

Ester linkage

Procaine

Cocaine

Amide-type local anesthetics

Amide linkage

Lidocaine

Prilocaine

FIGURE 10-1 Structures of local anesthetics. The general structure of local anesthetic molecules consists of the aromatic group (*left*), the ester or amide group (*shaded*), and the amine group (*right*). Benzocaine is an exception, lacking a side-chain amino group.

ending in the formation of para-aminobenzoic acid, a possible allergen. Amides, such as lidocaine, mepivacaine, bupivacaine, and prilocaine, are metabolized more slowly in the liver and rarely produce an allergic reaction. Procaine has a short (20 to 45 minutes) duration of action; lidocaine has an intermediate (1 to 2 hours) duration; and bupivacaine has a long (3 to 6 hours) duration. Most local anesthetics, with the exception of cocaine, cause vasodilation. Epinephrine increases the duration of action by vasoconstricting the area receiving the injection and decreasing the rate of absorption. Epinephrine is added in a ratio of 1 to 200,000 of lidocaine, which doubles the anesthetic's duration of action. Repeated injection will also prolong the anesthesia.[18] A vasoconstrictor should not be used for nerve block of a finger, toe, or nose because the entire blood supply to these areas may be stopped due to intense vasoconstriction. Other additives that help extend the duration of action include clonidine (an α_2 agonist) and sodium bicarbonate.[18] Clonidine may inhibit the release of substance P and reduce sensory neuron firing when used to block peripheral nerves. Sodium bicarbonate is often added to lidocaine to alkalize the area receiving the injection. The lidocaine then exists in its uncharged form and can easily traverse the nerve cell membrane (see below).

Local anesthetic agents are weak bases and tend to remain ionized at physiologic pH and acidic pH. They become neutral at high pH. Thus a local anesthetic agent needs a more basic environment to penetrate the nerve sheath and axon membrane and to reach the sodium channel where it binds. Once inside the axon, it becomes ionized again and binds to the channel. This is significant because during inflammation, the environment tends to be acidic and therefore resistant to local anesthetic agents.

Local anesthetics selectively block conduction of the small myelinated axons (A delta and C fibers) more readily than do the larger fibers.[31] The mechanism of action is blockade of sodium channels. Because nociceptive input is carried on these smaller fibers, pain sensation is blocked more than other sensations such as touch and proprioception. Because they are quite large, motor axons tend to be unaffected by these agents, unless the dose injected is excessive. However, exceptions occur when the motor nerves in the large nerve trunks are located circumferentially and therefore exposed to the drug first. In this case, motor paralysis occurs before sensory loss. Local anesthetics also exhibit use-dependent blockade. They block nerves that have a high firing rate as seen when A delta and C fibers transmit pain impulses.

Adverse reactions to local anesthetic drugs may occur but are rare. They can result from excess drug entering the systemic circulation. Adverse effects tend to be a mixture of CNS stimulation and depressant effects. Restlessness, tremors, and confusion may progress to convulsions, then finally to CNS depression.[31] Cardiac adverse reactions include arrhythmias, followed by bradycardia, hypotension, and cardiac arrest. Respiratory depression can also occur. Resuscitative drugs and equipment should be kept nearby. Any tissue that depends on conduction or transmission of impulses may be affected.

The advantages of local anesthesia include quick recovery, low systemic toxicity, and action confined largely to nerve tissue. The disadvantages may include incomplete analgesia and the longer time to achieve anesthesia.

Clinical Uses for Local Anesthetics and Their Modes of Administration

A variety of nerve blocks are used in rehabilitation medicine. Differential nerve blocks are particularly useful to identify the nerves that may be involved in the production of pain. In addition, this type of administration can provide pain relief for certain nonsurgical procedures, such as therapy for musculoskeletal injuries. Injection of a local anesthetic near the sympathetic stellate ganglion is a specialized type of nerve block that is used to reduce pain in chronic regional pain syndrome. The presence of analgesia, increases in skin surface temperature, and/or the appearance of Horner's syndrome have been considered by some clinicians as being diagnostic of chronic regional pain syndrome. However, others argue that to use this block diagnostically, the results need to be compared with the results of injection of saline solution in the same region.[32]

Infiltration anesthesia is produced by injecting the drug throughout the area to be numbed.[27] It is performed by injecting the drug along a prospective incision line or along the edges of a laceration to be sutured. It has been used as the primary form of pain control for several procedures, including removal of skin lesions, foreign body removal, and breast biopsies. Infiltration of the local anesthetic also reduces the need for supplemental analgesics after surgery.

Local anesthetics are administered during laparoscopic procedures by continuous infusion and are given intra-articularly during arthroscopic knee surgery.[27] Continuous infusion has also been used after digital tenolysis surgery to facilitate immediate postoperative movement without pain.[33] Use of indwelling brachial plexus catheters filled with ropivacaine for pain relief after shoulder arthroscopy has also been reported.[34] In some instances, these catheters are attached to patient-controlled anesthesia (PCA) pumps.[35]

Topical anesthesia is the application of drug to the skin or mucous membranes. It is often used in eye treatments; ear, nose, and throat procedures; and rectal surgery.[30] When used in this mode, drugs should be capable of rapidly penetrating the skin or mucosa with diminished ability to flow away from the local site of pain. Cocaine penetrates well through the nasal mucosa, so it has been used for nose and throat procedures. It also has the ability to vasoconstrict, which is partly why it has a medium duration of action as opposed to a short duration.

Drugs can also be administered by iontophoresis or phonophoresis to produce analgesia for minor surgery (specifically dermatologic procedures).[36-38] Technically, this is transdermal administration of local anesthetics.

Intravenous regional block, also known as the *Bier block*, is the injection of drug into a vein that has been previously exsanguinated with a tourniquet.[39] After cuff inflation, the limb is raised to drain the venous system. The veins are then filled with the local anesthetic, and the cuff is kept tight for at least 20 minutes. This procedure may be used to numb an entire distal part of an extremity and is frequently used in hand surgery for procedures lasting less than 45 minutes.

Epidural and intrathecal injections of local anesthetics are other modes of administration. Epidural anesthesia, used in the thoracic, lumbar, and sacral regions of the spinal column, requires the drug being injected into the space between the dura and bony canal where it can act on nerve roots. Lumbar epidurals achieve excellent pain relief in a laparotomy and are also used extensively in obstetrics. The catheter can be left in place safely for up to 7 to 10 days.[40] Hypotension is an adverse effect; there is also a risk of developing a hematoma if the patient has been receiving lower-molecular-weight heparins (LMWHs). Permanent neurologic injury has occurred during this procedure in patients who had been taking anticoagulants. Intrathecal migration of the catheter and intraneural injection are other risks.

Subarachnoid or intrathecal block is the injection of the drug into the subarachnoid space, usually between the third and fourth lumbar vertebrae.[41] The anesthetic solution subsequently spreads, but where it actually ends up depends on the density of the solution and the posture of the patient. For low spinal anesthesia, the patient is placed either flat or in Fowler's position. The anesthetic is mixed with a solution denser than the cerebrospinal fluid (CSF), and the solution tends to diffuse downward. If a higher level of anesthesia is desired, the patient can be placed in the Trendelenburg position with the head sharply flexed. In this case, the anesthetic agent is mixed with a solution that has a lower specific gravity than that of the CSF, so it will diffuse upward. If the solution is equal to the CSF in specific gravity, the anesthesia will act at the site of injection.

Intrathecal injections are indicated for lower abdominal procedures and for procedures in the inguinal area or lower extremities.[42] Onset of action occurs within 1 to 2 minutes, and the duration is between 1 and 3 hours, depending on the choice of drug. Headache appears to be the most common complaint associated with spinal blocks. This results from actual puncture of the dura, which may remain open for days to weeks after the procedure, facilitating the loss of CSF. The headache lessens as CSF pressure returns to normal. Hypotension may also occur.

Caudal anesthesia results from the injection of the anesthetic agent into the sacral part of the vertebral canal so that the drug infuses around the cauda equina.[42] This type of anesthesia is used in obstetrics and in genital surgery. The advantages of this block are decreased headaches and less hypotension.

Therapeutic Concerns with Local Anesthetic Agents

Local anesthetic agents offer several benefits over general anesthetics. Patients experience rapid recovery without the hangover effect, and there usually is no interference with cardiovascular, respiratory, or renal function. However, therapists should be aware that if they are seeing patients immediately after a block, as often occurs in patients with chronic regional pain syndrome, sensation and strength will be diminished.[42] Sensory and strength testing will therefore be necessary before applying modalities or attempting motor activities. In addition, the force of any manipulation will also need to be carefully controlled because the patient will not be able to provide accurate feedback.

ACTIVITIES 10

1. Many disease states can alter a patient's response to general anesthesia. List some interactions that might occur in relation to the following illnesses or conditions:
   a. Alcoholism
   b. Obesity
   c. Pediatric surgery
   d. Older age
   e. Smoking
   f. Recent head trauma
2. Research how each of the following drug groups affects anesthesia:
   a. Steroids
   b. Antibiotics
   c. Antiepilepsy drugs
   d. Antihypertensives
   e. Psychotropic drugs
   f. Oral contraceptives
   g. Anticoagulants
3. Discuss the following local anesthetics in terms of the tissue affected and therapeutic use:
   a. Topical
   b. Infiltration
   c. Block
   d. Spinal
4. Discuss the differences between conscious sedation and general anesthesia.

REFERENCES

1. Trevor AJ, Miller RD: General anesthetics. In Katzung BG, editor: Basic and clinical pharmacology, New York, 2007, McGraw Hill.
2. Ries CR, Quastel DMJ: Drug use in anesthesia and critical care. In Page C, Curtis MJ, Sutter MC, Walker MJ, Hoffman BB, editors: Integrated pharmacology (2nd ed.), Philadelphia, 2002, Mosby.
3. Lampiris HW, Maddix DS: Clinical use of antimicrobial agents. In Katzung BG, editor: Basic and clinical pharmacology, New York, 2007, McGraw Hill.
4. Becker DE, Rosenberg M: Nitrous oxide and the inhalation anesthetics. Anesth Prog 55:124-131, 2008.
5. Foss JF, Martua MA: General anesthesia and sedation. In Waldman SA, Terzic A, editors: Pharmacology and therapeutics: Principles to practice, Philadelphia, 2009, Saunders.
6. Eger E: Age, minimum alveolar anesthetic concentration, and minimum alveolar anesthetic concentration-awake. Anesth Analg 93(4):947-953, 2001.
7. Carmody JJ: Some scientific reflections on possible mechanisms of general anaesthesia.(Clinical report). Anaesth Intensive Care 37(2):175(15), 2009.
8. Campagna JA, Miller KW, Forman SA: Mechanisms of actions of inhaled anesthetics. N Engl J Med 348(21):2110-2124, 2003.
9. Hemmings HC: Sodium channels and the synaptic mechanisms of inhaled anaesthetics. Br J Anaesth 103(1):61-69, 2009.
10. Franks NP, Honore E: The Trek K2P channels and their role in general anaesthesia and neuroprotection. Trends Pharmacol Sci 25(11):601-608, 2004.
11. Westphalen RI, Krivitski M, Amarosa A, Guy N, Hemmings HC Jr: Reduced inhibition of cortical glutamate and GABA release by halothane in mice lacking the K+ channel, TREK-1. Br J Pharmacol 152:939-945, 2007.
12. Landoni G, Fochi O, Tritapepe L, et al: Cardiac protection by volatile anesthetics. A review. Minerva Anesthesiol 75: 269-273, 2009.
13. Parness J: You're "hot" from pumping iron? Anesth Analg 108(3):711-713, 2009.
14. Huynh F, Mabasa VH, Ensom MH: A critical review: Does thiopental continuous infusion warrant therapeutic drug monitoring in the critical care population? Ther Drug Monit 31(2):153-169, 2009.
15. Tesniere A, Servin F: Intravenous techniques in ambulatory anesthesia. Anesthesiol Clin North Am 21(2):273-288, 2003.
16. Nestor NB, Burton JH: ED use of etomidate for rapid sequence induction. Am J Emerg Med 26(8):946-950, 2008.
17. Strayer RJ, Nelson LS: Adverse events associated with ketamine for procedural sedation in adults. Am J Emerg Med 26(9):985-1028, 2008.
18. Khushal Latifzai BA, Sites BD, Koval K: Orthopaedic anesthesia. Bull NYU Hosp Joint Dis 66(4):297-305, 2008.
19. Visser K, Hassink EA, Bonsel GJ, Moen J, Kalkman CJ: Randomized controlled trial of total intravenous anesthesia with propofol versus inhalation anesthesia with isoflurane-nitrous oxide. Anesthesiology 95(3):616-626, 2001.
20. Gare M, Parail A, Milosavljevic D, Kersten JR, Warltier DC, Pagel PS: Conscious sedation with midazolam or propofol does not alter left ventricular diastolic performance in patients with preexisting diastolic dysfunction: A transmitral and tissue Doppler transthoracic echocardiography study. Anesth Analg 93(4):865-871, 2001.
21. Migita T, Mukaida K, Hamada H, et al: Effects of propofol on calcium homeostasis in human skeletal muscle. Anaesth Intensive Care 37:415-425, 2009.
22. Angelini G, Ketzler JT, Coursin DB: Use of propofol and other nonbenzodiazepine sedatives in the intensive care unit. Crit Care Clin 17(4):863-880, 2001.
23. Short TG, Young Y: Toxicity of intravenous anaesthetics. Best Pract Res Clin Anaesthesiol 17(1):77-89, 2003.
24. Schramm BM, Orser BA: Dystonic reaction to propofol attenuated by benztropine (cogentin). Anesth Analg 94(5):1237-1240, 2002.
25. Orsini J, Nadkarni A, Chen J, Cohen N: Propofol infusion syndrome: Case report and literature review. Am J Health Syst Pharm 66(10):908-915, 2009.
26. Kirby RR, Colaw JM, Douglas MM: Death from propofol: Accident, suicide, or murder? Anesth Analg 108:1182-1184, 2009.
27. Redmond M, Florence B, Glass P: Effective analgesic modalities for ambulatory patients. Anesthesiol Clin North Am 21(2):329-346, 2003.
28. Liu LL, Gropper MA: Postoperative analgesia and sedation in the adult intensive care unit: A guide to drug selection. In Drugs, 2003:63-755-767, ADIS International Limited.
29. Istaphanous GK, Loepke AW: General anesthetics and the developing brain. Curr Opin Anaesthesiol 22:368-373, 2009.
30. White PF, Katzung BG: Local anesthetics. In Katzung BG, editor: Basic and clinical pharmacology, New York, 2007, McGraw Hill.

31. Tezlaff JE: Local anesthesia. In Waldman SA, Terzic A, editors: Pharmacology and therapeutics: Principles to practice, Philadelphia, 2009, Saunders.
32. Price DD, Long S, Wilsey B, Rafii A: Analysis of peak magnitude and duration of analgesia produced by local anesthetics injected into sympathetic ganglia of complex regional pain syndrome. ClinJ Pain 14(3):216-226, 1998.
33. Schneider LH, Berger-Feldscher S: Tenolysis: Dynamic Approach to surgery and Therapy. In Hunter JM, Mackin EJ, Callahan AD, editors: Rehabilitation of the hand: Surgery and therapy, Philadelphia, 1995, Mosby.
34. Klein SM, Nielsen KC, Martin A, et al: Interscalene brachial plexus block with continuous intra-articular infusion of ropivacaine. Anesth Analg 93(3):601-605, 2001.
35. Corda .M, Enneking FK: A unique approach to postoperative analgesia for ambulatory surgery. J Clin Anesthesiol 12(8):595-599, 2000.
36. Byl NN: The use of ultrasound as an enhancer for transcutaneous drug delivery: Phonophoresis. Phys Ther 75(6): 539-553, 1995.
37. Núñez M, Miralles ES, Boixeda P, et al: Iontophoresis for anesthesia during pulsed dye laser treatment of port-wine stains. Pediatr Dermatol 14(5):397-400, 1997.
38. Tachibana K, Tachibana S: Use of ultrasound to enhance the local anesthetic effect of topically applied aqueous lidocaine. Anesthesiology 78(6):1091-1096, 1993.
39. Latifzai K, Sites BD, Koval K: Orthopaedic anesthesia Part 2. Common techniques of regional anesthesia in orthopaedics. Bull NYU Hosp Joint Dis 66(4):306-316, 2008.
40. Mandabach MG: Perspectives in pain management: Intrathecal and epidural analgesia. Crit Care Clin 15(1):105-123, 1999.
41. Lilley LL, Harrington RA, Snyder JS: General and local anesthetics. In Lilley LL, Harrington RA, Snyder JS, editors: Pharmacology and the nursing process. St. Louis, 2007, Mosby.
42. Linchitz RM, Raheb JC: Subcutaneous infusion of lidocaine provides effective pain relief for CRPS patients. Clin J Pain 15(1):67-72, 1999.

11

Drugs for the Treatment of Pain and Inflammation

Barbara Gladson

PHYSIOLOGY OF PAIN

Pain is usually a direct response to some event that produces tissue damage. The cause may be injury, inflammation, or cancer. However, it also may arise from an unrecognized event or cause (e.g., trigeminal neuralgia) and continue long after the precipitating injury has healed (e.g., phantom limb pain). Pain is also a subjective experience, difficult to see, difficult to quantify, and difficult to treat—especially if there is no known physical or anatomic reason for discomfort. Pain can be described as any unpleasant sensation that can range from mild discomfort to severe and debilitating pain. This is quite a simplistic definition that does not help in identifying the mechanism of pain, which remains quite complex. Despite this, however, we have divided pain into three major categories: (1) nociceptive, (2) neuropathic, and (3) psychogenic.

Nociceptive pain is produced by an injury and may be described as a stabbing or aching sensation. It tends to be well localized when it comes from soft tissue, bone, or muscle but less identified when is originates from the viscera. *Neuropathic pain* is described as a burning or tingling sensation and indicates nerve involvement. Examples include peripheral neuropathies, postherpetic neuralgia, and chronic regional pain syndrome, formerly called reflex sympathetic dystrophy. *Psychogenic pain* assumes an origin or relationship to a psychological disorder. None of these types are mutually exclusive, and patients may begin with one type of pain and end up with another. Also, the presence of pain increases sensitivity to further noxious stimulation and pain and leads to central sensitization.

The study of pain is complex because pain is often related to an affective component that cannot be easily reproduced in an animal model. Commonly used procedures to test analgesic drugs involve applying a noxious stimulus to an animal and then watching the animal's response. Measuring the time it takes for a rodent to withdraw its tail when exposed to heat and measuring the threshold force that results in withdrawal of an inflamed paw when it is pinched repetitively with greater strength are two research methods commonly used. Similar tests are also conducted on human subjects, but they still lack the affective component that is intertwined with patients' pain.

Neural Mechanisms of Pain and Their Modulation

Two mechanisms may be involved with pain production: (1) nociceptive afferent neurons and (2) abnormal central control over the afferent input. One or both may be present with a pain syndrome. The nociceptive afferent neurons are unmyelinated C fibers and finely myelinated A delta fibers that have sensory endings in the peripheral tissue, which activate in response to noxious input from mechanical, thermal, or chemical stimuli. Stimulation of the A delta fibers produces sharp, intense, and well-localized discomfort; whereas stimulation of the unmyelinated C fibers produces a dull, burning, diffuse type of pain.[1]

Tissue injury results in the local release of several chemicals that stimulate the afferent receptors and neurons. The cell bodies of these neurons lie in the dorsal root ganglia. The fibers enter the spinal cord via the dorsal root and terminate in the laminae. The A delta nociceptor fibers synapse in laminae I and V (Figure 11-1).[1] C fibers synapse in laminae I and II (the substantia gelatinosa). They synapse with neurons containing excitatory amino acids and neuropeptides that act as neurotransmitters between the primary afferents and spinal cord nociresponsive neurons.

In the dorsal horn, nociceptive block is attained by N-methyl-D-aspartate (NMDA) blockers, by substance P antagonists, and by inhibitors of nitric oxide (NO) synthesis.[2] Substance P is an excitatory transmitter released by the nociceptive afferent neurons, and this produces a slow depolarizing response in the postsynaptic cell that increases in amplitude with repetitive stimulation. Substance P also enhances NMDA receptor transmission resulting in calcium (Ca^{2+}) influx and activation of NO synthesis. The released NO enhances pain perception and transmission in ways that have not yet been

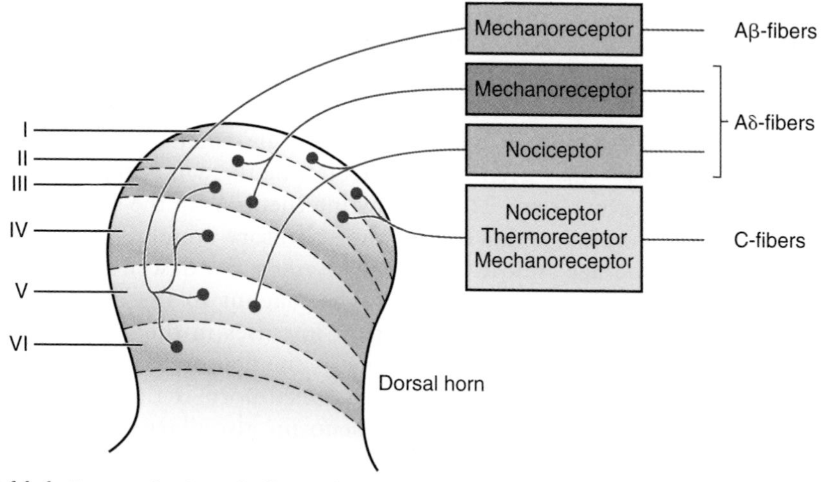

FIGURE 11-1 The termination of afferent fibers in the six laminae of the dorsal horn of the spinal cord.

fully explained. Substance P also acts in the periphery to produce inflammation, as does the calcitonin gene-related peptide released along with substance P.

The substantia gelatinosa consists mainly of short inhibitory interneurons that project to laminae I and V.[1] These interneurons modulate transmission at the first synapse in this pain pathway, between the primary afferents and the spinothalamic tract. It is often given the gatekeeper function allowing impulses from one group of afferent fibers to regulate the transmission of nociceptive fibers. The substantia gelatinosa is rich in opioid peptides and opioid receptors and is the site of action for morphine-like drugs. From laminae I and V, sensory information is then projected upward to the thalamus.

Some descending pathways make up another gating mechanism that controls pain transmission in the dorsal horn.[3] This descending portion originates in the periaqueductal gray area of the midbrain. These fibers project downward first to the nucleus raphe magnus and then back down to lamina I, where they synapse on enkephalinergic and serotoninergic interneurons. These neurotransmitters then diminish pain by blocking the release of substance P and inhibiting the spinothalamic neurons (Figure 11-2). There is also a similar pathway from the locus ceruleus; this pathway inhibits transmission in the dorsal horn, which contains norepinephrine.

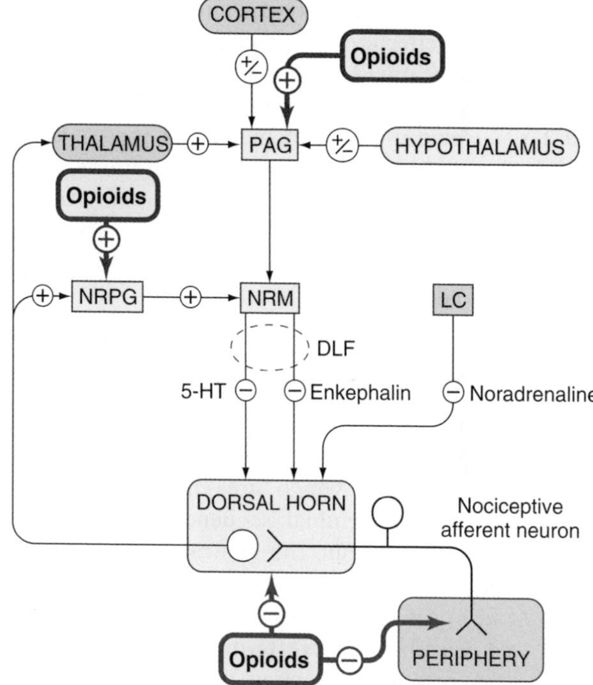

FIGURE 11-2 The descending control system, showing the main sites of action of opioids on pain transmission. Opioids excite neurons in the periaqueductal gray matter (PAG) and in the nucleus reticularis paragigantocellularis (NRPG), which, in turn, project to the rostroventral medulla, which includes the nucleus raphe magnus (NRM). From the NRM, 5-HT- and enkephalin-containing neurons run to the substantia gelatinosa of the dorsal horn, and exert an inhibitory influence on transmission. Opioids also act directly on the dorsal horn as well as on the peripheral terminals of nociceptive afferent neurons. The locus ceruleus (LC) sends noradrenergic neurons to the dorsal horn, which also inhibit transmission. The pathways shown in this diagram represent a considerable oversimplification but depict the general organization of the supraspinal control mechanisms. Shaded boxes represent areas rich in opioid peptides. *DLF*, dorsolateral funiculus; *5-HT*, 5-hydroxytryptamine. *(From Rang HP, Dale MM, Ritter JM, Moore JL.* Pharmacology *(5th ed.). New York, 2003, Churchill Livingstone.)*

Chemical Mediators of Pain

Stimulation of nociceptive endings in the periphery is often chemical in nature. These chemicals are released as a result of inflammatory or ischemic changes in tissues. Better understanding of these chemicals and receptors may provide strategies for treatment.

The vanilloid receptor was recognized after it was observed that capsaicin, the chemical in chili peppers, caused intense pain when injected into the skin or applied on sensitive tissues.[4] Capsaicin binds to the receptor, opening up an ion channel permeable to several cations, which initiates a depolarization and an action potential. Other substances including hydrogen (H^+) and even heat produce a similar response on these receptors. Essentially, a large influx of Ca^{2+} occurs in the nerve terminal, producing release of substance P and calcitonin gene-related peptide. This Ca^{2+} may even be enough to produce nerve terminal degeneration. This has been the premise behind the use of topical capsaicin, but the initial painful response has discouraged researchers from pursuing further study of this treatment.

Bradykinin is another pain-producing substance that becomes more potent in the presence of prostaglandins.[4] Bradykinin receptors are coupled in some ways to the activation of the vanilloid receptor channel. Pain research is directed toward finding safe bradykinin antagonists that have analgesic and anti-inflammatory properties.

Prostaglandins of the E and F series are released during inflammatory states and also during ischemia.[5] They do not produce pain themselves, but they enhance the pain-producing effects of other chemicals such as serotonin and bradykinin. Aspirin-type drugs inhibit prostaglandin synthesis and, in turn, reduce pain.

Other peripheral chemical mediators that initiate a painful response include serotonin, histamine, lactic acid, adenosine triphosphate, and potassium.[4] Antagonists to some of these mediators have been experimentally studied but have been shown to produce only limited pain reduction.

Neurotransmitters Involved in the Nociceptive Pathway

Substance P and neurokinin A (NKA) are members of the tachykinin family, which are characterized by a specific amino acid terminal sequence. They are dispersed widely throughout the central nervous system (CNS), especially in the nociceptive primary afferent neurons and in the dorsal horn. They are released from central and peripheral nerve terminals and trigger an inflammatory response known as *neurogenic inflammation*. The response of smooth muscle to tachykinins, including that in the gastrointestinal (GI) tract and bronchial airways, tends to be constriction. On blood vessels, there is a mix of constriction and dilation along with increased permeability, which leads to edema. Substance P and NKA act on NK1 and NK2 receptors, respectively, creating a slow excitatory synaptic potential in the dorsal horn neurons. This synaptic potential builds to become a burst of action potentials that continues even after the stimulus stops, which is called *wind-up*. Several tachykinin antagonists have been developed; unfortunately, they have not been very effective in decreasing pain in humans but have been somewhat useful in the treatment of depression.

Other centrally acting neurotransmitters involved in pain production include glutamate, gamma (γ)-aminobutyric acid (GABA), serotonin, norepinephrine, and adenosine.[6] Glutamate is an excitatory amino acid that is involved in fast synaptic transmission at the first synapse in the dorsal horn by acting on γ-amino-3-hydroxy-5-methylisoxazole-4-propionate (AMPA) receptors. Glutamate also acts on NMDA receptors, facilitating the wind-up phenomenon. GABA is released by interneurons in the spinal cord and inhibits some of the excitatory impulses in the dorsal horn. Serotonin is involved in the descending pathway from the nucleus raphe magnus to the dorsal horn, acting to interrupt pain impulses in the ascending pathway. Norepinephrine is the neurotransmitter from the locus ceruleus to the dorsal horn, acting as an antinociceptive pathway. Adenosine also plays a role in regulating the pain pathways by producing analgesia when acting on the purine A_1-receptors but causes the reverse when acting on the purine A_2-receptors.

Theoretically, any compound that acts on the neurotransmitters and chemical mediators listed previously should have an impact on the pain pathways. However, in practice, coming up with an effective drug for pain has been quite challenging.

Opiate Peptides and Their Receptors

The term *opioid* refers to any substance, whether endogenous or synthetic, that produces morphine-like effects that are blocked by the morphine antagonist naloxone.

Naturally occurring opioids in plants are called *opiates*, and those found in humans are called *opioid peptides*. They originate from three protein precursors—proopiomelanocortin, prodynorphin, and proenkephalin—which produce β-endorphin, met-enkephalin, leu-enkephalin, and dynorphin.[7] A fifth opioid peptide that has been discovered recently is called *nociceptin;* in contrast to endorphins and enkephalins, this opioid peptide *produces* pain. These five peptides are widespread in the brain but are also found in more localized areas of the spinal cord. Dynorphin is found mainly in the interneurons of the spinal cord; enkephalins are detected in the long descending pathways from the midbrain to the dorsal horn and are involved in modulating ascending pain impulses.

There are three main types of opioid receptors—μ (mu), δ (delta), and κ (kappa)—which mediate the pharmacologic actions of opiates.[8] Each type has distinctive subtypes, and all are located in the central regions involved with nociception as well as in the periphery.[9] In addition, peripheral inflammation or chronic arthritis has been shown to increase the expression of opioid receptor genes, resulting in receptor manifestation in inflamed synovia.[7] Interaction with the μ-receptor produces analgesia and euphoria but is also associated with respiratory depression, bradycardia, emesis, a slowing of GI motility, pruritus, and a high abuse potential. The respiratory depression appears to be due to the μ_2-receptor as are the pruritus and the dependence. The

BOX 11-1 Functional Effects Associated with the Main Types of Opioid Receptors

	μ	δ	κ
Analgesia			
• Supraspinal	+++	−	−
• Spinal	++	++	+
• Peripheral	++	−	++
• Respiratory depression	+++	++	−
• Pupil constriction	++	−	+
• Reduced GI motility	++	++	+
• Euphoria	+++	−	−
• Dysphoria	−	−	+++
• Sedation	++	−	++
• Physical dependence	+++	−	+

GI, gastrointestinal.
From Rang HP, Dale MM, Ritter JM, Moore JL: *Pharmacology* (5th ed.). New York, 2003, Churchill Livingstone.

δ-receptors produce spinal analgesia and respiratory depression and have a low abuse potential. The κ-receptor produces spinal analgesia, miosis, constipation, and sedation and is associated with a low abuse potential. A fourth receptor, σ (sigma), was thought to be responsible for some of the dysphoric effects of opiates, namely, anxiety, hallucinations, and nightmares; but at present, it is unclear whether these are true opioid receptors. They may be a target site for phencyclidine (PCP, phenylcyclohexylpiperidine) instead.[1,8] See Box 11-1 for a list of the main pharmacologic effects produced by drug interaction with opiate receptors. All of the opioid receptors are G-protein linked and facilitate the opening of potassium (K^+) channels, producing hyperpolarization. The result is inhibition Ca^{2+} influx and blocking of neurotransmitter release.

MORPHINE AND SIMILAR OPIOID ANALGESICS

Opium is derived from the juice of the seed pod of the poppy (*Papaver somniferum*) plant. It has been used for centuries to reduce pain and produce analgesia and sleep and also as an anti-diarrheal agent.[10] It was primarily used in the Middle East by citizens of all means but was used only by the elite in Europe and the United States. In the 1800s, use of morphine-containing tinctures became more common and widely available from doctors and pharmacists. However, with the invention of the hypodermic syringe in the 1900s, street use of opioids in the form of heroin escalated. By the end of the 1940s when the nature of opiate addiction became known, opioid use became tightly restricted by government regulation. Legal use of opioids is now controlled solely by health care providers (e.g., physicians, dentists, nurses). However, this presents certain problems because health care providers could face criminal charges if they prescribe these drugs inappropriately. This has led to reluctance on the part of physicians to prescribe opioids, often leaving chronic pain that is not related to a terminal illness untreated. Consensus statements put out by the American Academy of Pain Medicine and American Pain Society support the use of opioids after nonopioid therapy has failed and after a comprehensive medical examination has been conducted, along with mutually-agreed-on goals for treatment and specific follow-up.

Opioid drugs are the first choice for treatment of severe pain. On a basic science level, these drugs decrease the influx of Ca^{2+} in the presynaptic terminal of the nociceptive C fibers and A delta fibers, preventing the release of substance P and glutamate.[9] They also increase K^+ influx, which results in hyperpolarization and a decrease in nerve transmission. A third area of action is the inhibition of GABAergic transmission in the brainstem, where GABA inhibits a pain inhibitory neuron. There is also evidence that these drugs are involved in the mesolimbic dopamine system to produce euphoria, which is separate from their action on the pain pathways. The last suspected mechanism of action is to block NMDA receptors, activating the descending serotonin and noradrenaline pain pathways from the brain stem. Stimulation of these same NMDA receptors is involved in the perpetuation of neuropathic pain.

Analgesics That Are Strong μ-Agonists

Opiates may be divided according to how strongly they interact with their receptors, on their chemical composition, and also based on the drug Enforcement Agency (DEA) classification (Table 11-1). Opioids can be further subdivided based on their actions at the receptors, that is, as pure agonist, agonist/antagonist, and partial agonist (Table 11-2 and Box 11-2) For the purposes of this book, opioids will be classified on the basis of their relative affinity for the μ-receptor. Drugs that fall within the "strong agonist" category include morphine, fentanyl, hydromorphone, meperidine, methadone, and oxycodone. They have a strong affinity for the μ-receptor and less affinity for the δ- and κ-receptors. They have similar pharmacodynamic effects, but they differ in terms of analgesic potency and elimination half-life. Some of the strong agonists metabolize into active metabolites, extending the duration of action. Morphine, in particular, metabolizes into morphine-6-glucuronide, extending its analgesic activity. Morphine-6-glucuronide is 20 to 40 times more potent than morphine.[11] It is eliminated by the kidneys, so it will quickly accumulate in patients with renal failure. Accumulating metabolites present problems even in patients with healthy kidneys when therapy is continued for more than 1 to 2 days.

Oxycodone is often marketed with either aspirin (Percodan) or acetaminophen (Percocet) for an additive effect. The rationale behind combining drugs in pain management is based on the fact that one drug is not always capable of controlling pain.[12] If only one drug

TABLE 11-1 Drug Enforcement Administration (DEA) Classification of Opioids

Schedule	Criteria	Example
I	No medical use, high abuse potential	Heroin, benzylmorphine, dihydromorphinone
II	Used medically, high abuse potential	Morphine, oxycodone, methadone, fentanyl, meperidine, oxymorphone, hydromorphone
III	Used medically, potential for addiction	Hydrocodone, codeine compounds, buprenorphine
IV	Used medically, low abuse potential	Butorphanol, pentazocine, propoxyphene
V	Used medically, low abuse potential	Buprenex, phenergan with codeine

Modified from Trescot AM, Datta S, Lee M, Hansen H: Opioid pharmacology. *Pain Physician* 11(2 Suppl):S133–S153, 2008.

TABLE 11-2 Opioid Analgesics and Equianalgesic Doses Compared with Morphine

Drug	Pharmacologic Class	IM/SQ/IV (mg)	PO (mg)
Morphine (Astramorph, Duramorph, Roxanol, MS-Contin–continuous release)	Opiate analgesic, full agonist	10 (standard)	30 (standard)
Fentanyl (Duragesic–patch; Actiq–buccal; Sublimaze–parenteral)	Opiate analgesic, full agonist	0.1	Not available
Methadone (Dolophine)	Opiate analgesic, full agonist	10	20
Codeine (generic)	Full agonist but less effective	75–100	300
Oxycodone (OxyContin–continuous release)	Full agonist	Not available in injection	15–20
Oxymorphone (Numorphan)	Full agonist	1.0	10 (rectal)

IM, intramuscular; *SQ*, subcutaneous; *PO*, oral.

were administered, a higher dose might be required to control the pain than if two different drugs were used at lower doses. Therefore, combining drugs may be a useful way to reduce adverse effects. However, since 1996, the manufacturer has released oxycodone as a single entity and in the controlled-release tablet form (OxyContin) in doses ranging from 10 to 160 mg.[13] The tablets are intended for use every 12 hours, but they have become a popular drug for abuse. OxyContin tablets are being crushed to make the entire dose immediately available and are then snorted or dissolved in water and injected intravenously. When taken in this manner by people who have not built up tolerance to the drug, a single 80-mg dose can be fatal. For this reason, the 160-mg tablets were withdrawn from the market shortly after their introduction.

Meperidine has a higher rate of adverse drug reactions (ADRs) and is no longer recommended for acute or chronic pain. The American Pain Society recommends that it not be used for more than 48 hours and that it should be avoided especially in patients with reduced liver or kidney function. As the blood levels increase, neurotoxic metabolites (normeperidine) accumulate and can produce anxiety, hyper-reflexia, myoclonus, and seizures.[14] This drug should only be used if the patient cannot tolerate other opioids.

Most opioids, including strong agonists, are available in a variety of different dose forms and modes of administration, including oral, transdermal, intramuscular, intravenous (bolus, continuous infusion, patient-controlled), subcutaneous infusion, rectal, epidural, intrathecal, intranasal, and transmucosal (lollipop). Proper dosing can be complicated, especially during a switch from one mode of administration to another, and therefore should be conducted by a skilled, experienced clinician. For example, the relative potency of intramuscular to oral morphine is 1:6, but this ratio changes with repeated administration or when patients receive the drug on a regular schedule. In these circumstances, the intramuscular to oral ratio is reduced to 1:2 or 1:3.[9] Delayed-release preparations are

BOX 11-2 Other Opioid Drugs

Drug	Pharmacologic Class
Hydromorphone (Dilaudid)	Opiate analgesic, full agonist
Meperidine (Demerol)	Opiate analgesic, full agonist
Pentazocine (Talwin)	Considered both partial agonist and agonist–antagonist
Buprenorphine (Buprenex)	Considered both partial agonist and agonist–antagonist
Nalbuphine (Nubain)	Considered both partial agonist and agonist–antagonist
Tramadol (Ultram)	Miscellaneous agonist
Buprenorphine (Buprenex)	Partial agonist
Codeine/acetaminophen (Tylenol with codeine)	Opioid combination
Codeine/aspirin (Empirin compound)	Opioid combination
Hydrocodone/acetaminophen (Vicodin, Lortab)	Opioid combination
Hydrocodone/ibuprofen (Vicoprofen)	Opioid combination
Oxycodone/acetaminophen (Percocet)	Opioid combination

also available for some opioids. MS-Contin is an oral morphine that provides pain relief for 8 to 12 hours. This provides for better compliance and longer-lasting pain relief before repeated dosing. For management of "breakthrough" pain, the immediate-release morphine IR-Contin can be used.

Transdermal fentanyl is also a useful drug for improving compliance and for providing longer pain relief. It has a long half-life, only needing to be replaced every 72 hours.[15] This drug is indicated for patients who could benefit from continuous infusion of an opioid and also for those patients who are unable to swallow or who have GI problems. However, physical activity and exposure to heat and humidity result in increased drug delivery. Ashburn and colleagues used "controlled heat," delivering approximately 107.6°F (42°C) for a duration of up to 240 minutes, to determine if reaching a serum therapeutic level could be hastened.[16] The heat source was placed over a portion of a 25 mcg/h patch. Higher fentanyl concentrations were obtained during the heating periods, but the overall "area under the concentration curve" was similar to that in the sessions without heat. The authors concluded that the controlled application of heat to the patch is one method to hasten the onset of the drug's effect. However, out of the 10 subjects participating in this study, 5 developed respiratory depression and needed to be treated with verbal stimulation and nasal oxygen. Several deaths and cases of severe toxicity have been reported with this patch; In 1998, a 44-year-old male with a painful human immunodeficiency virus (HIV)-related neuropathy was treated with a 75-ug patch along with two oxycodone doses for breakthrough pain.[17] He attended a camp with his family and was participating in outdoor activities (hiking and playing ball) in warm weather. On the third day, the patient reported feeling tired and was later found unresponsive with pinpoint pupils. Naloxone IV was administered, and the patient became responsive again. In 2005, the U.S. Food and Drug Administration (FDA) issued a Public Health Advisory on the fentanyl patch when a woman was prescribed a 50-mcg patch for sciatic pain.[18] The patch was placed on her buttocks, the site of pain, along with a heating pad, and she was found dead two days later..[19]

In 2006, a fentanyl iontophoretic transdermal delivery system was approved by the FDA.[14] A low-intensity electric current is used to deliver a preprogrammed dose of fentanyl across the skin without a needle. This technique provides rapid absorption of the drug, 40% in the first hour but 100% by the tenth hour. The device is activated by the patient, but the number of doses is limited to six per hour. The system locks after 80 doses have been delivered or after 24 hours. This system is comparable with standard morphine IV through patient-controlled analgesia (PCA).

Care must be taken when patients are switched from immediate-release formulations to other modes of administration because ADRs can become exaggerated.[20] In addition, switching from one opioid to another also presents certain challenges. Even though fentanyl and sufentanil are in the same category as morphine, their potencies differ vastly.[11] Sufentanil is 625 times more potent than morphine and 12 times more potent than fentanyl. When sufentanil is injected intravenously, analgesia is achieved instantaneously, but with morphine, it takes several minutes for pain relief to occur. Conversion charts have been developed but are not always accurate. Methadone has a potency equal to that of morphine but a much longer duration of action. However, because methadone is converted to two inactive metabolites, in terms of pain control, its analgesic effects often wear off before the signs of physical withdrawal develop. Patients with opioid addiction may be given methadone to assist with the withdrawal process.[21,22] It is given in two to three daily doses and then tapered over time, producing a much gentler withdrawal. In addition, when injected in the presence of methadone, morphine does not cause the same euphoria as it does when administered alone.[8]

Diamorphine (heroin) is rapidly converted to morphine, so diamorphine's effects should be similar to those of morphine.[1] However, diamorphine has greater lipid solubility, so it crosses the blood–brain barrier more rapidly than does morphine, giving the patient a greater "rush." It also has a shorter duration of action than morphine's.

When pain relief with strong opioids is inadequate, a common quandary for the physician is whether to change the drug or keep the drug but change its mode of administration.[23] When the physician desires to change the drug and not the mode of administration, comparisons regarding equianalgesic doses must be made. When changing the mode of administration, the dose must be adjusted. This is especially true when switching from the oral route to the parenteral route. Debate regarding the best course of action continues.

Weak Opioids

Drugs that fall within the mild to moderate agonist category include codeine, codeine combinations, and propoxyphene. Some authors have included oxycodone in this category as well. This class of opioids is considered to comprise the "weaker opioids," although they are effective in treating pain of moderate intensity. However, withdrawal from these drugs may not be any easier than withdrawal from stronger opioids.

Codeine is 50% less potent than morphine, but it is absorbed well when given orally, which makes it the preferred opioid in some cases.[8] It has almost no pain-relieving action on its own, but it converts to morphine and then to morphine-6-glucuronide. It also has a marked antitussive effect, so it is often formulated as a cough medicine.

Opioid Agonist–Antagonists (Partial Mixed Agonists)

The opiate agonist–antagonist drugs are agonists at the κ- and δ-receptors but show partial and weak agonist activity at the μ-receptor.[9] Included in this category are pentazocine, butorphanol, nalbuphine, and buprenorphine. These drugs produce an analgesic effect in patients who cannot tolerate morphine, but they precipitate a withdrawal reaction in patients who had previously been receiving strong agonist drugs. The reason for this is that a strong agonist is displaced off the receptor by the partial mixed agonist drug, thereby triggering withdrawal.

Nalbuphine is a strong κ-agonist and a μ-antagonist. It is used for decreasing mild to moderate pain; however, it can exacerbate psychiatric conditions, and can produce dysphoria, nightmares, and hallucinations. Its real advantage over some of the other opioids is that there is less potential for abuse.

Buprenorphine is a new opioid that shows high affinity for the μ-receptor but has lower efficacy than the other opioids. The maximal effect (E_{max}) on the dose–response curve is less than the E_{max} produced by a full agonist, so it cannot control pain as well as can strong agonists.[11] However, it appears to be quite effective as an alternative to methadone in preventing withdrawal symptoms in patients who are physically dependent on morphine or heroin. it is often given in combination with a small amount of naloxone to reduce its potential for abuse.[24,25] A systematic review revealed that sublingual buprenorphine given three times a week was just as effective as methadone for maintenance.[26] Buprenorphine is available in tablet forms for sublingual and oral administration. The major limitation of this drug is that the E_{max} dose of buprenorphine is equivalent to only 70 mg of oral methadone, lower than what is needed to combat heroin addiction.

Miscellaneous Analgesics

Tramadol is another weak μ- and κ-receptor agonist. It is an oral opioid that also blocks the reuptake of norepinephrine and serotonin and is marketed for moderate pain relief. It is about one tenth as potent as morphine but is available in combination with acetaminophen for better efficacy.[27] It is not widely known as an opioid, and some physicians have actually prescribed it as an anti-inflammatory agent. The assumption has been that it does not produce dependence, but some opioid-type dependence has been reported.

Adverse Effects of Opioids

The adverse effects of opioids can be divided into CNS effects and peripheral effects (Box 11-3). Major CNS effects include sedation, respiratory depression, cough suppression, miosis, truncal rigidity, and vomiting. The sedative effect is one of drowsiness with depressed mentation and impaired reasoning.[28] Cognitive impairment appears to be worse during the first few days of use and in the first few hours after a dose is given. Patients also score poorly on timed performance tests in psychomotor function when taking these drugs.

Respiratory depression, which is produced by a depressed response to carbon dioxide at the respiratory centers in the pons and medulla, occurs even at usual doses. Therefore, opiates should be avoided in patients with respiratory diseases because rate and depth of respiration will be reduced. Opioid-induced respiratory depression remains one of the most significant challenges for pain management physicians.

BOX 11-3 Adverse Effects of Opioids

Euphoria or dysphoria in some
Sedation
Depressed cognition
Respiratory depression
Cough suppression
Miosis
Truncal rigidity
Nausea and vomiting
μ receptor agonists produce hyperthermia; κ receptor agonists produce hypothermia
Constipation
Biliary colic
Neuroendocrine: stimulates the release of ADH and prolactin, but inhibits luteinizing hormone
Pruritus
Little effect on cardiovascular system except hypotension

Cough suppression may be considered a desirable effect or an adverse effect depending on the indication for opioid use. Obviously, cough suppression is the desired effect as adjunctive treatment for an upper respiratory infection. However, cough suppression can cause harm in older adults recovering from surgery who are at risk for pneumonia.

Pupillary constriction is caused by stimulation of the oculomotor center. The patient may also have reddened eyes from cerebral vessel dilation. This dilation is a result of respiratory depression and hypoxia. It is an important diagnostic finding because most other causes of coma and respiratory depression produce papillary dilation. Nausea and vomiting result from stimulation of the chemoreceptor trigger zone located in the medulla. Lastly, increased tone, particularly truncal rigidity, is another adverse effect of opioids. In patients with normal tone, this increased rigidity is of little consequence, but in a patient with spasiticity, this tone may alter function significantly. In addition, the rigidity reduces thoracic mobility, further impairing ventilation. Most of these adverse effects, with the exception of miosis, diminish after prolonged administration.

Peripheral adverse effects include constipation, urinary retention, and bronchospasm. These occur as a result of the activation of the opiate receptors in the perspective areas. Delayed gastric emptying can retard the absorption of other drugs. Biliary tract irritability may also occur because opioids produce contraction of the gall bladder but at the same time cause constriction of the sphincter. Therefore, opioids should be avoided in patients with gall bladder disease. Some opiates also cause histamine release from mast cells, which is responsible for pruritus, or frictopathia, as well as bronchoconstriction.

Opioids have the potential to produce complex immunosuppressant and hormonal effects. Animal studies and in vitro assays have shown that opioids can depress immune function.[10,29] They have been shown to increase immunosuppression in patients with acquired immune deficiency syndrome (AIDS), and they may actually increase the viral load.[30] Along with the obvious risk of sharing needles, this fact also helps explain the prevalence of AIDS in opioid-addicted individuals. In terms of hormonal effects, opioids influence the hypothalamic–pituitary–adrenal axis and the hypothalamic–pituitary–gonadal axis. Morphine reduces plasma cortisol levels and also causes a decrease in luteinizing hormone, follicle-stimulating hormone, testosterone, and estrogen.[10] In combination, these effects lead to decreased libido, aggression, and amenorrhea. However, prolactin levels are noticeably increased and may result in galactorrhea.

Tolerance and Treatment for Dependence

There is no doubt that opioids have helped many people with severe pain. However, more people could be helped by these drugs than those who actually receive them. Patients may fear addiction and refuse to take these medications. Physicians are also reluctant to prescribe opioids. Many stories of celebrity drug addictions reinforce the notion that addiction is a real concern. However, several studies have shown that addiction problems related to these drugs are unusual in older patients.[31,32] In addition, rarely do patients with cancer pain become addicted. Proponents of opioid therapy for relief of pain believe that it is unlikely that a patient who does not have a history of addiction or alcoholism will experience such problems with these drugs.[33]

The CNS-mediated effects of opioids, which are the most likely to lead to misuse after long-term administration, include psychological and physical dependence.[9] The development of physical dependence and tolerance is predictable, but these are separate entities from psychological dependence (addiction). Unfortunately, tolerance to opioids develops quickly, and the patient must continually administer a higher dose to get the same effect. Tolerance begins after the first administration, and often an increase in dose is needed in just 2 to 3 weeks. Tolerance may be minimized by switching to another opioid (known as *opioid rotation*).[34] When given regularly over time, withdrawal symptoms begin within 6 to 10 hours after a dose is missed. This onset of withdrawal is usually accompanied by feelings of anxiety, irritability, and alternating chills and hot flashes. Other signs include body aches, runny nose, diarrhea, shivering, gooseflesh, stomach cramps, insomnia, sweating, tachycardia, yawning, nausea, and vomiting.[35] Symptoms reach their peak at 24 to 72 hours. These are physical impairments indicating that the patient is physically dependent, but not necessarily psychologically dependent, on the drug.

Addiction refers to deliberately seeking out a drug for its mood-altering abilities.[35] This tends to occur when opioids are used in excessive doses after the need for pain relief has passed. Opioids mediate this effect by increasing synaptic dopamine levels in the limbic system in susceptible patients. It is believed that the drug triggers biologic changes that lead to compulsive craving. Addiction can be treated with pharmaceuticals, but treatment is not always successful.

Whether treatment is with methadone or buprenorphine, all patients undergo a health screening prior to medication-assisted withdrawal; Patients undergo testing for hepatitis, HIV infection, and other infectious diseases, including sexually transmitted infections (STIs). Screening is also performed to rule out any acute or life-threatening condition that may be masked by opioids and the presence of other drugs such as benzodiazepines. Induction with drug therapy usually begins when there are no signs of opioid intoxication or sedation, although some patients may start receiving their medication at the onset of withdrawal. Observed therapy is required as patients swallow oral doses of methadone or utilize a sublingual tablet of buprenorphine. After the first dose, patients are asked to stay for an observation period of about 1 hour. Federal regulations require that methadone be given daily under observation for 6 or 7 days. If the clinic is closed on a Sunday, patients are allowed a take-home dose.

Initial dosing of methadone is between 20 and 30 mg. If withdrawal symptoms persist after 2 to 4 hours, the initial dose can be increased by 5 to 10 mg. Patients who become sick during the peak period of maximum blood concentration of methadone (2 to 4 hours after taking a dose) tend to ask for an additional dose.[36] However, due to the drug's long half-life, they may need more time for the blood level to increase (reach steady state) rather than a dose increase. In inpatient settings, split doses can be given, which may improve the comfort level.

The maintenance phase of withdrawal begins when a patient is responding to the current dose of methadone and no longer needs dose adjustments.[36] This is the dose that will minimize withdrawal and reduce cravings. Hopefully, at this point, the patient has stopped abusing opioids and has resumed some normalcy in his or her life. Patients may stay on the maintenance dose for months; however, during periods of increased stress or physical activity or when in an environment that encourages reverting to illicit use, an increase in methadone may be warranted.

For many patients, the therapeutic range of methadone is between 80 to 120 mg/day but can be much higher. Studies show that patients receiving the higher dose tend to relapse less.

Once the patient has been stabilized on a maintenance dose, medically supervised withdrawal may begin. Usually, there is a reduction of 5 to 10% every 1 to 2 weeks. Withdrawal is done slowly, and at times the dose may need to be increased rather than decreased. However, at some point, as the number of occupied receptors increase, patients may start to feel discomfort and craving for the drug may reappear. Those patients who have a good support system and have received psychological counseling tend to manage without relapsing during this time.

Another way to withdraw from opioid abuse is to detoxify first and then be maintained on methadone, buprenorphine, or even naloxone (see below). Success of methadone treatment for addiction has been uncertain in recent years. Part of the problem is that many patients have multidrug addictions. In addition, the number of comorbidities remains high and necessitate the use of other medications that may impair the effectiveness of the withdrawal treatment.

Opioid Antagonists

Naloxone in repeated doses is used to reverse respiratory depression and coma in opioid overdose. It is a competitive antagonist at the μ-, κ-, and δ-receptors but has the highest affinity for the μ-receptor. This explains why it rapidly reverses respiratory insufficiency but has little effect on analgesia. It is given intravenously, and its actions are almost immediate. It also precipitates withdrawal in physically dependent patients but produces no effect in healthy subjects. Naloxone is used during labor to reverse the effect of an opioid on a newborn baby.

Naltrexone is similar to naloxone but has a longer duration of action. It is can be used after detox to help quell the patient's drug cravings, and it does not create any euphoria.[36] It is usually administered either daily (at 50 mg/day) or three times a week (e.g., 100 mg/day on Monday and Wednesday and 150 mg on Friday).

Patient-Controlled Analgesia

Patient-controlled analgesia (PCA) allows the patient to self-administer the analgesic medication on an as-needed basis, usually on top of a preprogrammed continuous infusion. This method consists of an infusion pump that is electronically controlled and connected to a timing device. PCA devices may be small pumps that are worn by the patient, implantable delivery devices, or larger pumps that are attached to a pole or rest on a bedside table. The catheter delivering the medication may be placed intrathecally, intravenously, or in the epidural space.[37] The patient presses on a thumb button whenever he or she feels pain. The pump then releases a preset amount of drug through the indwelling intravenous catheter. The timer is programmed to lock out additional doses until the first dose has had a chance to reach peak effect. The "lock out" interval can be changed as necessary. Typically, patients receive 1.0 to 1.5 mg of morphine with a 4 hour limit of 30 to 40 mg and a lockout interval of 7 to 10 min.[38] However, fentanyl and hydromorphone are also used. Meperidine has been used previously, but due to its high rate of ADRs, it is rarely used now.

PCA has grown in popularity since the development of infusion pumps.[39] Patients seem to like the fact that they can give themselves medication without having to rely on a nurse. A background of continuous analgesia prevents the peaks and troughs associated with drug administration every 4 hours. Supporters of PCA also report that recovery from surgery is accelerated because factors such as muscle guarding, poor chest expansion, and immobility caused by pain are avoided. However, this mode of administration is not without problems.

Programming errors, mechanical problems, adverse reactions associated with the medication, and infections such as epidural abscesses and meningitis can occur.[40] Simple kinking of the tube may cause changes in the dose the patient receives, although there is a pump occlusion alarm to alert the patient if it occurs. The catheter can move from the epidural space into the subarachnoid space or from the subarachnoid space into the vascular system. In addition, the catheter may press on neural tissue, nerve roots, or the spinal cord. Signs of catheter migration include aspiration of cerebrospinal fluid as indicated by a wet catheter dressing and the patient complaining of a throbbing, continuous occipital headache. If the catheter has migrated into the vascular system, blood will be apparent in the catheter. The therapist should also be on the alert for any sudden nausea and vomiting, hypotension, and respiratory depression. Compression of nerve tissue is indicated by motor weakness and bowel and bladder dysfunction. There has also been a case report of a delayed diagnosis of a myocardial infarction in a patient who received PCA after a radical cystoprostatectomy.[41]

The Medical Device Reporting Regulations require that manufacturers, distributors, and facilities that use the devices report deaths or serious injuries associated with these pumps to the FDA.[42] In addition, health care providers are encouraged to voluntarily report adverse events to the FDA through MedWatch. Errors that have been reported include those related to product packaging, drug concentration programming errors, and improper installation of tubing. In several cases, patients experienced respiratory depression related to overdose of morphine when part of the shipping package was left in place, allowing a free flow of drug into the patient. Narcotic overdose can also result when the pump is programmed with a lower concentration of drug than what is actually filled in the drug reservoir. The pump's calculation of the rate of infusion is based on the drug concentration in the reservoir. A higher infusion rate occurs if the concentration is underestimated.[40] One study confirmed that operator errors led to a greater number of adverse events than did mechanical problems, and another study cited "PCA by proxy" indicating that someone other than the patient (often a family member) was pressing on the delivery button.[43] Another study reported that even though operator-related events were less frequent than device-related issues, they were more devastating in terms of outcomes for patients.[44] The use of computerized order sets is being explored to reduce programming errors.[45] Another problem is faulty installation of tubing, resulting in continuous drug infusion. Ideally, the pumps should be designed so that parts fit together only in one way.

Some new types of infusion pumps are undergoing extensive testing and are expected to cut down on drug programming errors.[46] To program these devices, a health care provider can scan a bar-coded label on a drug package or intravenous fluid container. This will automatically program the pump to the correct infusion rate. A patient-controlled transdermal fentanyl patch that uses iontophoresis to deliver the drug as described above is also being used and has shown to be as effective as PCA with IV morphine in terms of pain relief and equal in safety.[43] Some advantages to this system include no required tubing and improved mobility for patients, as they are not tied to an IV pole. Regardless of the system used, therapists must be alert for excessive sedation and respiratory depression.

Therapeutic Concerns with Opioids

Rehabilitative therapists working with patients who have recently started using opioids need to be prepared for adverse effects. The patient may experience drowsiness or dizziness, and dulled cognitive function may be seen. In many cases, the patient will develop tolerance for the adverse effects, with the exception of miosis and constipation. Until these symptoms disappear, patients should take commonsense precautions such as not driving, avoiding fall hazards (such as throw rugs), holding onto the stair railings, and not making any important decisions while on opioid medication.[13] An important concern for patients wearing patches is to avoid heat, pressure, and exercise in the area of the patch, since all of these may increase the rate of drug absorption. In addition, some patches need to be removed prior to certain medical procedures such as magnetic resonance imaging (MRI), since the radiofrequency pulses in these procedures generate electrical currents that can overheat the metallic component of the patch. Several patches used for pain control, for example, Duragesic (fentanyl), LidoSite (lidocaine/epinephrine), and Synera (lidocaine/tetracaine), contain this component.[47]

Therapy should be scheduled when the opioid has nearly reached its peak action so that the patient can fully cooperate with the program. However, this also means that the patient will not be able to accurately report when a technique is painful. In addition, the therapist must take into consideration the possibility of respiratory depression when planning an exercise program.

ANTI-INFLAMMATORY AGENTS

Nonsteroidal anti-inflammatory drugs (NSAIDs) are quite possibly the most widely used group of drugs in the world (Box 11-4).[48] They are often self-administered or prescribed by a physician for musculoskeletal pain and injury or to treat an inflammatory condition such as

BOX 11-4 Commonly Used NSAIDs

Celecoxib (Celebrex)
Diclofenac (Voltaren)
Diflunisal (Dolobid)
Fenoprofen (Nalfon)
Flurbiprofen (Ansaid)
Ibuprofen (Motrin, Rufen, Advil, Nuprin)
Indomethacin (Indocin)
Ketoprofen (Orudis)
Ketorolac (Toradol)
Meloxicam (Mobic)
Nabumetone (Relafen)
Naproxen (Naprosyn, Aleve)
Piroxicam (Feldene)
Sulindac (Clinoril)
Tolmetin (Tolectin)

rheumatoid arthritis. At least 20 different NSAIDs are available in the United States, but none is perfect in eliminating symptoms or benign in terms of adverse effects. Many of them work by primarily blocking prostaglandin synthesis.

Prostaglandins and Their Role in Inflammation

Prostaglandins have been detected in almost every tissue of the body in response to cell damage. They are not stored but rather released when an injury, inflammation, or tumor is present. There are several types of prostaglandins delineated by a letter (A, B, C, D, E, F, H, I) and nonprostaglandins (thromboxanes).[49] Subscript numbers are added to indicate that a prostaglandin exists in a series (e.g., PGH_2). PGI_2 is also known as prostacyclin. All prostaglandins are derived from arachidonic acid, which is a fatty acid that is ingested through diet and stored as phospholipids in the cell membrane. Arachidonic acid is cleaved by the enzyme phospholipase A_2 and is then acted on by two enzyme systems, cyclooxygenase (COX) and lipoxygenase. Prostaglandins, prostacyclins, and thromboxanes come from the cyclooxygenase pathway, and leukotrienes come from the lipoxygenase pathway (Figure 11-3).

Prostaglandins have many diverse actions: PGAs, PGEs, and prostacyclin produce vasodilation; PGF_2 and thromboxanes produce vasoconstriction and make platelets sticky; other actions include increased cardiac output, increased capillary permeability, stimulation of uterine contractions, either vasodilation or constriction of bronchioles (PGE_1 and PGE_2 dilate; PGF_2 constricts), pain production, platelet aggregation, inhibition of gastric acid secretion and stabilization of the gastric mucosa, elevation of body temperature, and vascular dilation in the kidneys which helps regulate renal vascular resistance. Some of these effects, particularly those on the kidneys and GI mucosa, are quite helpful; whereas other effects produce pain and discomfort.[50,51] Along with prostaglandins, kinins also play a role in inflammation. Kinins, including bradykinin, are formed as a result of injury and are strong vasodilators. Vasodilation is accompanied by increased permeability of capillaries, resulting in redness, edema, and pain. Leukotrienes, histamines, and serotonin have similar roles.

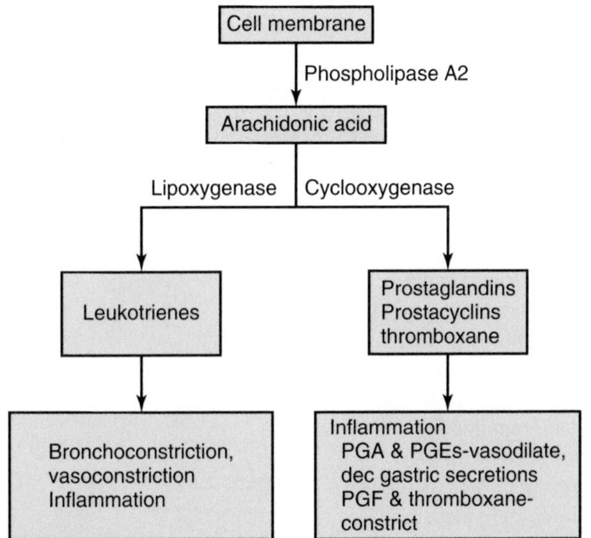

FIGURE 11-3 The cyclooxygenase (COX) and lipoxygenase pathway. *NSAIDs*, Nonsteroidal antiinflammatory drugs; *PG*, prostaglandin.

Cyclooxygenase Enzyme

There are two different isoforms of the COX enzyme, but they are incompletely understood.[52] COX-1 is found in the platelets, kidneys, and stomach. COX-2 is induced and found in synoviocytes, endothelial cells, and macrophages and catalyzes the conversion of arachidonic acid to PGF_2. However, there is some evidence that COX-2 may also exist in the kidney expressed in the cortical thick ascending limb and macular densa.[53,54] Both forms are found in the synovial fluid of patients with rheumatoid arthritis. Drugs that act largely on the COX-2 form of the enzyme have been developed and are called COX-2 inhibitors.

Both COX-1 and COX-2 are long channels associated with the cell membrane, with COX-2 being wider than COX-1. Each has a bend toward the terminal end of the channel. Arachidonic acid enters the channel and becomes twisted around the bend. At this point, two oxygen molecules are inserted, and a free radical is extracted. The result is the five-carbon ring recognized as a prostaglandin.

A third form of the enzyme, COX-3, has recently been identified in the human brain, spinal cord, and heart and in canine and murine species.[55] This enzyme is inhibited by acetaminophen but is relatively insensitive to aspirin and shows reduced sensitivity to diclofenac and indomethacin (nonselective NSAIDs).[55,56] This may explain acetaminophen's role in fever reduction.

Aspirin

Aspirin (acetylsalicylic acid) is one of the most widely used analgesic, antipyretic, and anti-inflammatory drugs. A national survey conducted in American households between 1998 and 1999 showed that 17% of subjects reported taking an aspirin in the preceding week, 23% reported using acetaminophen, and another 17% reported using ibuprofen. Given the wide prevalence of these agents, it is prudent to thoroughly review their pros and cons. Aspirin blocks prostaglandin synthesis by blocking the action of both forms of COX. It binds irreversibly to a specific serine molecule (serine 530 for COX-1 and serine 516 for COX-2) toward the end of the tubular channel, inactivating the enzyme.[49]

Beneficial Effects of Aspirin. Aspirin has major beneficial effects, including an antipyretic effect, an analgesic effect, an anti-inflammatory effect, and an antithrombotic effect.[57] The antipyretic action results from blockade of prostaglandins in the hypothalamus. Bacterial endotoxins produce the release of pyrogens from macrophages, which stimulate PGEs. These PGEs raise the set point for body temperature. COX-2 and COX-3 have a role in inducing pyrogen release, causing fever. The analgesic effect of aspirin results from decreased production of prostaglandins that sensitize nociceptors, and the anti-inflammatory response comes from blockade of prostaglandin-induced increased vascular permeability. As previously described, aspirin is also used in vascular disorders to inhibit platelet-induced thrombus formation by irreversibly inhibiting thromboxane production (80 mg/day). However, this positive effect of aspirin can cause serious bleeding. Bleeding time is increased, and bruising is more common. The inhibition of platelet aggregation is a desirable effect for some patients, but the therapist must always be alert to excessive bleeding and bruising, especially if it occurs with a minor injury.

Higher doses are needed for analgesic activity (two 300-mg tablets administered four times per day) and even higher doses (12 to 20 tablets) are needed for anti-inflammatory effects. Other beneficial effects include reducing the incidence of colon and rectal cancers. Aspirin appears to have proapoptotic properties.[58] There is also early evidence that aspirin delays the onset of Alzheimer's disease by inhibiting aggregation of amyloid-beta and by scavenging for radicals.[59,60] However, other studies indicate that aspirin and NSAIDs fail to produce changes in cognitive function in these patients.[61]

Adverse Effects of Aspirin. Regular aspirin use produces GI problems ranging from minor stomach discomfort to hemorrhage and ulceration. Even at normal doses, between 3 and 8 mL of blood may be lost in the feces per day, which may cause anemia. Normally, PGI_2 inhibits gastric acid secretion, and PGE_2 stimulates mucus production in both the stomach and small intestine. Both these prostaglandins are the result of COX-1 action. If these functions are blocked by aspirin, the epithelial membrane of the stomach will be damaged.[50] Common GI adverse effects include dyspepsia, diarrhea, nausea, vomiting, and gastric bleeding and ulceration. It is estimated that one in five aspirin and NSAID users will experience some gastric injury. This damage may grow silently for years eventually leading to hemorrhage, perforation, or both. Therefore, it is suggested that aspirin be taken with food and a large volume of fluid to diminish the GI problems. Misoprostol (a PGE_1 analog) or omeprazole (a proton pump inhibitor) is sometimes given along with aspirin or NSAIDs to decrease the incidence of GI problems.[62]

One of the other major adverse effects of aspirin is renal dysfunction.[51] PGE_2 and PGI_2 are important for maintaining renal blood flow by helping dilate the renal artery, particularly in individuals who have angiotensin-mediated vasoconstriction. Loss of this mechanism results in decreased sodium, potassium, and water excretion and facilitates hypertension. High doses can also produce acute renal failure.

Another problem with aspirin is that it readily binds to plasma proteins, producing several drug-drug interactions. Examples include raising unbound methotrexate levels, enhancing the hypoglycemic affect of sulfonylurea drugs used for diabetes, and increasing the anticoagulant effect of warfarin.

Salicylates produce metabolic changes that increase with the dose.[63] Large but normal doses can alter the acid–base balance. The increase in acidity leads to higher levels of carbon dioxide production, which stimulates respiration. Hyperventilation produces a respiratory alkalosis, which, in turn, is compensated for by renal excretion of bicarbonate. However, as the plasma aspirin level increases, respiration is suppressed, leading to retention of carbon dioxide on an already low bicarbonate level and metabolic acidosis. Fever is likely to be present because of an increased metabolic rate, and dehydration caused by vomiting may follow. Salicylate poisoning is also associated with headache, nausea, tinnitus, and confusion. It is more serious in children in whom the primary disturbance tends to be metabolic acidosis, whereas in adults, it results primarily in respiratory alkalosis.

Less common adverse effects of aspirin include skin rashes and photosensitivity, bronchospasm in patients with aspirin-sensitive asthma, liver dysfunction, and bone marrow depression. Aspirin has also been epidemiologically linked with encephalitis (Reye's syndrome) when given to children with viral infections.

Nonsteroidal Anti-inflammatory Drugs (Nonselective Cyclooxygenase Inhibitors)

NSAIDs act by reversibly inhibiting the COX enzyme, with varying effects on COX-1 versus COX-2 (Figure 11-4). In contrast, aspirin displays irreversible binding to the COX enzyme. NSAIDs are also more potent than aspirin at equal doses, and they have just about identical beneficial and adverse effects, with the exception that they are not used for cardiac protection as will be explained later. Among older adults, they are responsible for 10 to 20 of 1000 hospitalizations per year for peptic ulcer disease and for a fourfold increased risk of death from GI bleeding.[64] Data collected between 1998 and 2008 show that mortality in cases of upper GI bleed or perforation with concurrent NSAID use was 20.9%, but the authors caution against using this number, since differences in study design, patient characteristics, risk factors, and recording outcomes reduce the validity of this number.[65] Nevertheless, GI bleeds and other related conditions are associated with NSAID use. GI toxicity can be reduced with the addition of proton pump inhibitors (omeprazole and lansoprazole), prostaglandin

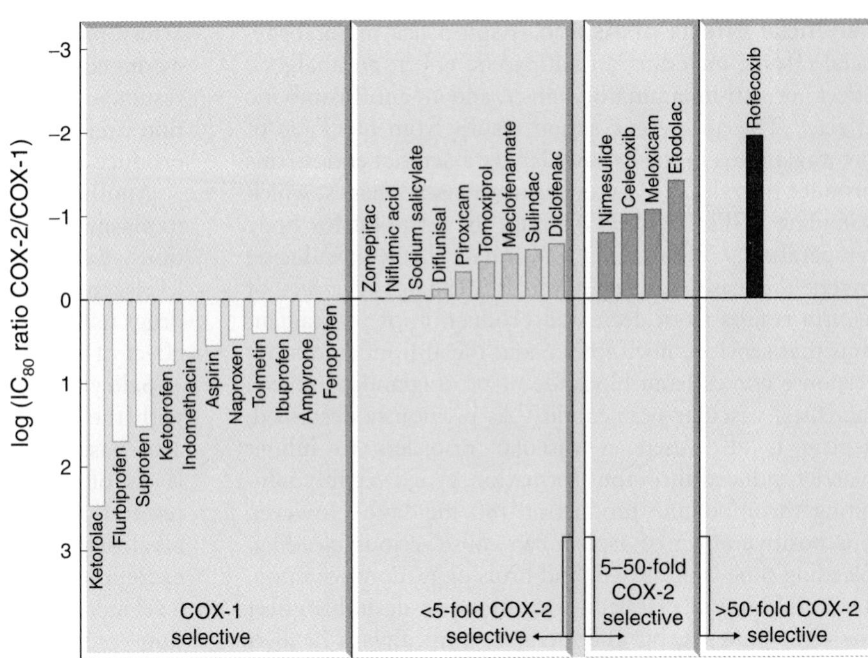

FIGURE 11-4 A comparison of cyclooxygenase (COX) isozyme selectivity of nonsteroidal anti-inflammatory drugs (NSAIDs). The graph shows the effect of various NSAIDs on COX-1 at a dose that gives an 80% inhibition of COX-2. The *zero line* indicates equal potency. Those below the line have selectivity for COX-1. Some above the line have a less than fivefold selectivity for COX-2. The next group (containing meloxicam, etodolac, celecoxib, and nimuselide) has a 50-fold selectivity for COX-2; but note that all can produce full inhibition of COX-1. Only rofecoxib has a greater than 50-fold selectivity for COX-2. Activity measured in whole blood assay. *(From Rang HP, Dale MM, Ritter JM, Moore JL.* Pharmacology *(5th ed.). New York, 2003, Churchill Livingstone. Modified from Warner, et al:* Proc Natl Acad USA *96:7563–7568, 1999, as adapted by Vane SJ: Aspirin and other anti-inflammatory drugs,* Thorax *55 (Suppl):S3–S9, 2000.)*

analog (misoprostol), and double doses of histamine-2 (H_2) receptor blockers (equivalent to 300 mg of ranitidine twice daily).[66]

The individual NSAIDs have differences in potency, toxicity, patient tolerance, and relative selectivity for COX-1 and COX-2. For example, diclofenac is said to be more GI sparing, and sulindac is safer on the kidneys (Figure 11-5). NSAIDs associated with a shorter half-life produce less injury to the GI system than those with longer half-lives as measured by the degree of fecal blood loss. The theory is that the gastric mucosa has a chance to repair itself between doses of short-acting drugs but not with a longer-acting agent.[67] Indomethacin and ketoprofen produce greater degrees of GI toxicity and have longer half-lives.[68] Sulindac is somewhat renal sparing because it is converted to an inactive drug in the kidneys and thus may inhibit renal COX to a lesser extent than the other NSAIDs. However, both these drugs have the tendency to produce liver damage. Effects on the CNS also vary among the NSAIDs. Indomethacin, naproxen, and ibuprofen have been reported to produce occasional cognitive dysfunction, confusion, behavioral disturbances, and dizziness.[69] In general, if a patient has a negative reaction to one NSAID, it does not automatically imply that he or she will react in the same manner to other agents in this class.

Cyclooxygenase-2 Inhibitors

As mentioned previously, two different isoforms of the COX enzyme are well known. COX-1 is found in various locations in the body, whereas COX-2 is more prevalent when induced by inflammation or surgery. The development of COX-2 inhibitors is a more recent approach to preventing some of the traditional renal and GI complications of aspirin and NSAIDs while exploiting their anti-inflammatory action.[49] Celecoxib and rofecoxib (now withdrawn) are the oldest and most studied of the group. They have been found to produce less GI toxicity than the nonselective NSAIDs, particularly up through the first 6 months of treatment.[70] After that, the difference between the selective and nonselective agents in terms of their effects on the GI system is less clear.[71] This study, however, was confounded by the concurrent use of low-dose aspirin for cardiac protection. When subjects who did not take the aspirin were examined, there was clear superiority of the COX-2 inhibitor.[72] However, the hypertensive effects and nephrotoxic potential may remain.[73,74] Animal studies have revealed that the COX-2 isoform is important for renal PGE_2 synthesis, and in human studies in which celecoxib was compared with naproxen, both drugs showed similar decreases in sodium excretion. However, in another study in which rofecoxib was compared with indomethacin, only indomethacin caused a decrease in glomerular filtration rate.[75] The authors hypothesized that the COX-1 enzyme is important in maintaining renal perfusion and the COX-2 enzyme in sodium regulation.

Several single-dose, randomized, double-blind studies have shown that COX-2 inhibitors are as effective as ibuprofen or naproxen in reducing postsurgical pain as well as pain due to osteoarthritis.[71,76,77]

Besides their effects on the GI and renal systems, the nonselective COX inhibitors and the COX-2 inhibitors have a few other differences.[78] These selective inhibitors do not inhibit platelet aggregation or increase bleeding time, so they are of no value in decreasing thrombotic effects. However, the fact that they do not influence bleeding time makes them useful as pain medication after surgery.[79] The exception to this is cardiovascular

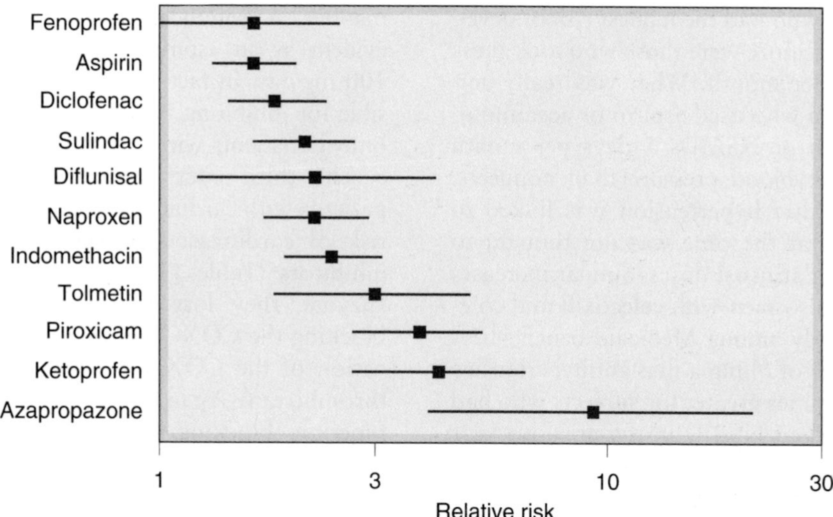

FIGURE 11-5 The risk of gastrointestinal complications with various nonsteroidal anti-inflammatory drugs (NSAIDs), relative to the risk with ibuprofen (relative risk = 1). Ibuprofen, given in a dose of 1200 mg daily, itself carries a risk of double that of placebo. The lines represent 95% confidence intervals. *(From Hawkey CJ: Gastrointestinal toxicity of non-steroid anti-inflammatory drugs. In: Vane JR, Botting RH, editors:* Therapeutic roles of selective COX-2 inhibitors, *London, 2001, William Harvey Press.)*

surgery (see below). NSAID use after surgery has been previously limited because of concerns about blood loss. In addition, postoperative use of these drugs has been shown to reduce opioid use, pain, vomiting, and sleep disturbances and to improve range of motion in patients who have had orthopedic surgery.[80]

Nonsteroidal Anti-inflammatory Drugs and Muscle

NSAIDs are widely used by patients of physical therapy as well as by competitive and elite athletes to prevent delayed muscle soreness.[81] There are many legitimate reasons to administer NSAIDs; however, there are several reports of professional and amateur athletes consuming excessive amounts of these agents to minimize pain during intense training. This self-prescribed and excessive use of NSAIDs is under scrutiny due to mounting evidence that they negatively affect satellite cells that are crucial for muscle hypertrophy and hence strengthening.

In normal adult skeletal muscle, there are two populations of satellite cells.[82-84] One group resides underneath the basal lamina of the muscle fiber, and the other group sits outside the laminal layer in the connective tissue. Following an injury, these cells differentiate into myoblasts and then myotubes. These myotubes then fuse together with each other and also with the injured myofiber. Satellite cells are stimulated to proliferate in response to exercise and also after a mild or more severe injury. Eccentric contractions appear to produce a stronger response from these cells than do concentric strengthening activities. But cessation of training results in both decreased differentiation and in actual numbers of satellite cells.

Several studies suggest that the COX enzyme is necessary for satellite cell proliferation, differentiation, and fusion to muscle fibers during healing. And both selective and nonselective COX inhibitors have been shown to suppress muscle regeneration and repair in both animal and human models, with the inhibition of COX-2 producing a greater impairment in the function of satellite cells.[85-87] The clinical implication of these studies is huge for patients of physical therapy and suggests that these anti-inflammatory agents impair muscle healing as well as the normal hypertrophy that occurs with resistive exercise training. However, current research does not offer guidelines regarding which NSAID produces the least deleterious effect and at what time, if any, it would be safe to take the drugs during the healing process. It is thought that NSAIDs could be administered safely a few days after an injury (after the initial stages of inflammation) but should be avoided in the subacute and chronic stages of healing.[88] However, further study about this is necessary.

Nonsteroidal Anti-inflammatory Drugs and Heart Disease

Some short- and long-term studies indicate that NSAIDs can produce elevations in blood pressure, leading to a diagnosis of hypertension.[89,90] This includes aspirin, but at anti-inflammatory doses and not at the lower doses used to prevent thrombotic events. In 1990, questions were added to the Nurses' Health Study survey regarding the frequency of use of aspirin, acetaminophen, and other NSAIDs and the onset of hypertension. Follow-up questions were mailed every 2 years for 8 years. The study was completed in 51,630 women between the ages of 44 and 69 years who had no history of high blood pressure at the beginning of the study. However, by the end of the study, 10,579 new cases of hypertension were identified. The women who had the highest risk of developing elevated blood pressure were those who took these drugs 15 to 22 days per month. What was really surprising was that women who used aspirin or acetaminophen 1 day per month or NSAIDs 5 days per month had significantly higher blood pressure than nonusers. Another surprise was that hypertension was linked to acetaminophen, which at the time was not thought to influence renal function at usual doses. Similar increases in blood pressure are also seen with celecoxib and rofecoxib.[91] In another study among Medicaid beneficiaries in New Jersey, the odds of filling a first antihypertensive prescription were two times greater for subjects who had filled a prescription for an NSAID in the previous year than for those who had not.[90] In addition, the Joint National Committees Sixth Report on Hypertension states that NSAIDs adversely affect blood pressure.[92]

The mechanism of action for this link is probably interference with the synthesis of the renal vasodilator prostaglandins and sodium excretion from the kidney tubules. However, it was surprising that acetaminophen was associated with hypertension because it was believed at that time that this drug blocks prostaglandin synthesis in the CNS and not in the peripheral tissue.[92] Perhaps the COX-3 isoform exists in the kidneys, or acetaminophen acts on a CNS site for blood pressure regulation.

Another observation regarding NSAIDs and high blood pressure is that these drugs actually make antihypertensive medication less effective.[93,94] Older adults who were taking hydrochlorothiazide to lower blood pressure found that their supine systolic and standing systolic pressures were significantly increased when they were taking ibuprofen compared with placebo. Other studies that examined the combination of aspirin and angiotensin-converting enzyme (ACE) inhibitors in patients with heart failure also showed a dose-mediated conflict between the two drugs.[95,96] Aspirin alters arterial properties by blocking the synthesis of certain vasodilating prostaglandins. Therefore, the vasodilating goal of an ACE inhibitor is attenuated by the use of aspirin in a dose-dependent manner. A significant effect on arterial properties is evident at an aspirin dose of 325 mg/day, but not at 100 mg/day. In fact, this dose of aspirin may be responsible for inhibiting half the effectiveness of an ACE inhibitor in patients with difficult-to-treat heart failure.[97]

The third issue regarding the use of NSAIDs in patients with cardiac disease has to do with the increased risk of cardiovascular events associated with COX-2 inhibitors (Table 11-3). By targeting only the COX-2 enzyme, they lose the cardioprotection afforded by blocking the COX-1 enzyme. As mentioned earlier, activation of the COX-1 enzyme induces the synthesis of thromboxane-A_2 in the platelet, enhancing its clotting function. Blocking this enzyme is the principle behind using low-dose aspirin for cardiac protection. Four major studies, in which 16,000 subjects were enrolled, compared the number of cardiac events among patients who took a COX-2 inhibitor with those among patients who received a traditional NSAID. COX-2 inhibitors, specifically rofecoxib, increased the absolute risk of cardiovascular events by 1% compared with an increase in risk of 0.47% with naproxen.[98] Those patients who took 50 mg of rofecoxib (higher than the recommended 25-mg dose) were five times more likely to have a myocardial infarction than those who were given 1000 mg of naproxen. At the time of this finding, it was not known whether this result was due to a reduction in cardiovascular events with the nonselective agent, an increase in cardiovascular events with the COX-2 inhibitor, or coincidence.[99] Continued study revealed that patients taking rofecoxib at a dose of 50 mg were almost two times more likely to have a coronary event than patients taking nonselective NSAIDs, but there was no increased risk associated with a dose of 25 mg or lower.[100] Some confounding factors in this study were that 17% of the rofecoxib users were taking 50 mg for 30 days, whereas only a 5-day regimen is recommended at this dose, and the study included some subjects with the diagnosis of rheumatoid arthritis, which is also associated with an increased cardiovascular risk.[101,102] Comparisons of

TABLE 11-3 Cardiovascular Safety of NSAIDs

Drug	High COX-2 Selectivity	Cardiovascular Effects	Hypertension	Interaction with Aspirin
Naproxen	–	–	–	+
Ibuprofen	–	++	+++	+++
Diclofenac	+	++	+++	–
Rofecoxib	+++	+++	–	–
Celecoxib	+	+++	+++	–
Lumiracoxib	+++	++	–	–
Valdecoxib	++	++	–	–
Etoricoxib	+++	+++	+++	–

Adapted from Farkouh ME, Greenberg BP: An evidence-based review of the cardiovascular risks of nonsteroidal anti-inflammatory drugs, *Am J Cardiol* 103(9):1227–1237, 2009.

COX-2 inhibitors also demonstrated that rofecoxib was associated with an increased risk of cardiac events, whereas an increased risk was not seen with celecoxib.[103] Finally, on September 30, 2004, Merck & Company announced a worldwide withdrawal of rofecoxib.[104] This decision was based on a 4-year study designed to assess the drug's effectiveness in treating colon polyps. Analysis of data from 2600 patients revealed that in the group of patients taking rofecoxib, there were twice as many cardiovascular events, including strokes, compared with the placebo group. A similar trial with celecoxib (Adenoma Prevention with Celecoxib trial) was terminated early due to the rofecoxib recall, but analysis revealed an increase in cardiovascular events, although the numbers were comparatively lower in the celecoxib study.[105] The current speculation is that the drug's increased risk of cardiovascular disease is due to its inhibition of prostacyclin formation and lack of a positive effect on platelet aggregation.[106] In addition, several systematic reviews and meta-analyses of the cardiovascular safety of nonselective NSAIDs have shown similar safety concerns as those for the COX-2 inhibitors, with the exception of naproxen.[107] Current American Heart Association guidelines recommend these drugs only when other alternatives have been exhausted in patients at high risk for cardiac disease.[14]

The last issue to discuss regarding the use of NSAIDs and heart disease is the fact that NSAIDs reduce the cardioprotective effects of low-dose aspirin.[108,109] The original study that sounded the alarm regarding this issue included 80 healthy volunteers. These subjects were given low-dose aspirin (81 mg) each morning, followed by 400 mg of ibuprofen 2 hours later, for 6 days. Another group of subjects followed the same procedure with the aspirin, but 2 hours later they were given acetaminophen, rofecoxib, or diclofenac. The next week the order of drug administration was reversed so that the NSAID was given first, followed 2 hours later by the low-dose aspirin. The investigators found that taking the aspirin a few hours before ibuprofen irreversibly inhibited platelet aggregation. However, when ibuprofen was taken before the aspirin, platelet aggregation was reversibly inhibited, thus eliminating the cardioprotective effects. The reason for this is that aspirin binds to the COX enzyme in the platelet for the life of the platelet. When taken first, aspirin will block access to the binding site for the NSAID. However, if the NSAID binds to the COX first, it will keep the aspirin from entering its binding site, but only temporarily. Reversible binding implies that the NSAID disengages from the platelet so that its antithrombotic action does not persist throughout the dosing interval. The other drugs examined did not influence the beneficial effect of aspirin, regardless of timing of administration. In another study, 7000 men with heart disease who took low-dose aspirin were followed up for an 8-year period and tracked regarding their NSAID use. Those who took ibuprofen and aspirin together were almost twice as likely to have died from a cardiovascular problem than those who took only aspirin.[108] However, naproxen and diclofenac appeared to preserve aspirin's ability to prevent blood clots. The present recommendation for concurrent use of low-dose aspirin and an NSAID is to administer the aspirin 2 hours prior to the anti-inflammatory drug.

Acetaminophen

Acetaminophen (also known as *paracetamol* in Europe) is a common non-narcotic analgesic and antipyretic agent. It is believed to inhibit prostaglandin synthesis in the CNS, and new research has demonstrated its ability to block the COX-3 enzyme.[56] It has only weak peripheral anti-inflammatory properties.

Acetaminophen is primarily used to reduce pain and fever. Although not quite as effective as NSAIDs, it has become the standard treatment for osteoarthritis when NSAIDs can no longer be tolerated.[110,111] Trends in medication use show a decline in NSAID use and, instead, an increased acetaminophen use for osteoarthritis.[112] Acetaminophen is also used in combination with NSAIDs to reduce the NSAID dose needed for symptom relief. This, in turn, reduces the adverse effects associated with the anti-inflammatory agents.

The advantage of acetaminophen over aspirin is that at a normal therapeutic dose, it is free of adverse effects and can also be used for prolonged periods without problems.[113] However, at high doses (two to three times the maximum therapeutic dose), especially when combined with alcohol, acetaminophen may produce significant liver and kidney damage. The initial signs of acetaminophen toxicity are nausea and vomiting. The hepatotoxicity may be delayed for 24 to 48 hours. Antidotes given within 12 hours of acute ingestion reduce liver damage.

Therapeutic Concerns with Nonsteroidal Anti-inflammatory Drugs

The main therapeutic concerns with NSAIDs have to do with bruising and increased risk of bleeding. If GI adverse effects are present, the therapist should be alert for any diarrhea or vomiting that may interfere with therapy services. Last, because so many patients are taking aspirin for its cardioprotective effects and also taking NSAIDs for their musculoskeletal aches and pains, patients should be questioned regarding dosage timings for these medications and referred to their physicians for counseling if the drugs are not being administered properly. Because many patients take over-the-counter NSAIDs, the drugs are often viewed as being insignificant and thus never discussed with the physician. Also, some patients may be taking a prescription NSAID as well as an over-the-counter NSAID without the physician's knowledge.

NEUROPATHIC PAIN

Neuropathic pain is pain that is associated with disease or injury to the peripheral or central nervous system.[114] Diabetes, immune deficiencies, shingles, trauma, multiple sclerosis, ischemic issues, and cancer can all produce neuropathic pain. It is thought that sustained noxious input leads to altered processing of noxious information and that this plasticity can occur at several neural levels from the spinal cord on up to the cortex.

Mediators of inflammation that may be involved in neuropathic pain syndromes include neuropeptides (bradykinin, calcitonin gene-related peptide, substance P, vasoactive intestinal peptide), cytokines (interleukins 1-β, 6, and 8 and tumor necrosis factor-α), and eicosanoids ($PGF_2\alpha$ and PGE_2 and leukotriene B_4).[115]

Clinical signs of neuropathic pain include a variety of stimulus-independent and stimulus-dependent pains. Stimulus-independent pain can be shooting, shock-like, aching, crushing, burning, or electric-shock-like. These types of pain may be related to nerve compression or entrapment syndromes. The underlying mechanism may be increased sensitization of C fibers and A delta fibers. Stimulus-dependent pains result from mechanical, thermal, or chemical stimuli. Patients may experience hyperalgesia (including cold or heat hyperalgesia), mechanical allodynia, dysesthesias, paresthesias, and paroxysms. Paroxysms involve shooting, electric-shock-like or shock-like pain that results from a benign tactile stimulus. Referred pain, sympathetic hyperactivity, and a loss of some afferent sensory function are also common in neuropathic pain conditions.

Drugs in monotherapy are usually insufficient to treat neuropathic pain. In fact, even though neuropathic pain can be diminished with traditional analgesics, this syndrome is unfairly represented among patients who respond poorly to opioids. The reason for combining drugs in pain management is that one drug does not always eliminate pain and use of two or more drugs with different mechanisms of action enhances pain relief. Antidepressants and anticonvulsants are frequently used as adjuncts in the treatment of these pain syndromes.[116] Antidepressants such as amitriptyline and imipramine have been used to treat pain associated with diabetic neuropathy, postherpetic neuralgia, polyneuropathy, and nerve injury associated with cancer. The mechanism of action for decreasing pain has not been identified, but it appears to be separate from their antidepressive effect. The assistance with analgesia occurs at lower doses than those used to treat depression. In addition, these medications can relieve symptoms such as sleeping problems commonly seen in patients with chronic pain.[117] The older tricyclic antidepressants have a sedating effect that helps the patient ease into a more restful sleep. The newer serotonin reuptake inhibitors are less sedating but have also been effective in decreasing chronic pain.

Anticonvulsants such as carbamazepine, phenytoin, lamotrigine, and gabapentin are also effective in the treatment of neuropathic pain.[118-121] Although the pathogenesis of neuropathy is not directly known and in many cases the exact mechanism of action of the antiseizure drugs is not known, there is speculation that relief of pain with these drugs is due to blockade of sodium channels.[122]

Other medications for neuropathic pain include clonidine and oral cannabinoids.[123,124] Epidural clonidine is indicated for neuropathic pain and is effective in approximately 50% of patients who do not respond to epidural opioids. Clonidine may decrease pain by its action on α_2-adrenergic receptors. Oral cannabinoids (dronabinol) have demonstrated pain-relieving effects in animal models of nerve injury but may not offer significant relief in refractory neuropathic pain. Investigations on the use of these drugs in pain syndromes are ongoing and may provide some new forms of pain relief for difficult cases.

In an effort to improve pharmacologic effectiveness in the treatment of neuropathic pain, there has been a push toward pairing individual symptoms to treatment with specific drugs.[125] For patients whose primary complaints are static hyperalgesia (pain in response to gentle pressure caused by sensitized C-fiber nociceptors), the drugs of choice are systemic and topical lidocaine and opioids. When there is hyperalgesia in response to light stroking of the skin, NMDA antagonists such as ketamine and dextromethorphan (a low-affinity NMDA channel blocker) may be indicated. The pain-producing mechanism in this case may be "central sensitization" from increased input. In cases in which the symptoms are related to sympathetic hyperactivity, norepinephrine blockade is recommended with either clonidine or a stellate ganglion block with lidocaine. In summary, the recommended protocols are as follows: opioids or lidocaine for sensitized C-nociceptors, adrenergic blockers for sympathetic maintained pain, lidocaine for pain and itching associated with vasodilation, and NMDA antagonists for centrally mediated pain produced by excess activity at these receptors.

PAIN RELATED TO CANCER

Cancer-related pain may result from primary tumor growth, metastatic disease, or the toxic effects of chemotherapy and radiation.[126] Invasion of bone, joint, or muscle can cause continuous pain. Bone pain appears to be common, but not all bone metastases become painful. The spine is the most common site for bone metastases. Extension of the tumor from the vertebra may produce spinal cord or cauda equina compression and result in neurologic compromise. The pain complaints tend to be variable; patients may complain of aching pains or dysesthesias anywhere in the dermatomal area innervated by the compressed neural tissue. However, many studies report undertreatment of pain in cancer patients.[127]

Treatment-related pain syndromes are also common and can result from chemotherapy, radiation, or surgery. Necrosis of bone may result from treatment with steroids or radiation. Visceral pain may result from intraperitoneal chemotherapy, scar tissue from surgery, or radiation-induced fibrosis.

Regular administration of NSAIDs is the usual starting point for mild pain associated with cancer. However, the beneficial response of pain control needs to be balanced with the risks (GI problems, bleeding tendencies, and masking of fever that indicates infection). When these drugs are no longer effective, a weak opioid may be added to or substituted for the NSAID. Codeine and hydrocodone preparations are recommended. When combinations of codeine-like drugs and NSAIDs are not sufficient and pain is severe, strong opioids are recommended. Morphine, hydromorphone, transdermal fentanyl, and oxycodone are appropriate. Sequential opioid trials (opioid rotations) are used to identify the drug that strikes the best balance between pain relief and adverse effects. During a switch to a stronger opioid, the dose of the new drug is reduced by approximately 30 to 50%.[126] Fixed schedule dosing appears to be preferred over dosing on an as-needed basis. Patients with limited opioid exposure are started on a low dose, equivalent to 5 to 10 mg of parenteral morphine every 4 hours. Rescue medication is supplied for breakthrough pain. Patients with bone cancer pain generally require significantly higher doses of morphine than those with postoperative pain.[128]

When the opioid regimen fails to control pain, the adjuvant pain medications discussed earlier (antidepressants, NMDA antagonists, antiseizure medications, and local anesthetics) can be added, or the mode of administration (e.g., PCA or patches) can be changed.[126] The oral mode of administration is preferred but may need to be avoided if the patient has dysphagia or is vomiting. Corticosteroids can be administered after full opioid effectiveness has been exploited. Steroids are considered multipurpose drugs to relieve pain, anorexia, and nausea. They can also reduce tumor size in certain types of cancers (lymphomas). Drugs for bone pain include bisphosphonates (see Chapter 14) and calcitonin, which can be added to the opioid regimen.[128] Even the Ca^{2+} channel blocker nifedipine has been used to decrease bone pain. Aggressive management of opioid and chemotherapy adverse effects also reduces discomfort. Anticholinergics can be used to reduce vomiting, and laxatives can be used for relief of opioid-induced constipation.

ACTIVITIES 11

1. You are treating a 62-year-old woman with metastatic breast cancer in her home. This patient is currently receiving intravenous morphine through a PCA device. When you arrive at the patient's house, you find the front door open and a note from the patient's caregiver saying that she had a family emergency and had to leave. You suspect that the caregiver had left several hours ago, which means that the patient had not been checked or repositioned during that time. When you arrive at the patient's bedside, she is difficult to awake. She responds to stimuli but falls back to sleep. Blood pressure is 120/70 mm Hg, pulse is 86 beats/min, and respirations are 6 breaths/min. On your last visit, the patient was weak but fully responsive and cooperative with therapy.

Questions

A. What is your immediate course of action?
B. What factors could have contributed to the patient's change in condition?
C. What drug might be prescribed for this patient?
D. What did this case teach you about working with patients who are receiving opiates?
E. If this patient were receiving morphine through an epidural catheter, what signs would indicate catheter malposition?

2. A 63-year-old man presents with severe, unrelenting midthoracic pain. The patient reports an insidious increase in pain over the past 2 months. He denies any falls or injuries to his back. He also reports a loss of 15 lb in the same period and constipation. Medical history includes squamous cell carcinoma of the lung 2 years ago, treated with chemotherapy until remission 6 months ago and hypertension, benign prostatic hypertrophy, and hyperlipidemia. Current medications include finasteride, simvastatin, and enalapril.

Labs: Alanine aminotransferase level, 40 IU/L; aspartate aminotransferase level, 45 IU/L; γ-glutamyl transferase level, 100 IU/L; alkaline phosphatase level, 350 IU/L; blood urea nitrogen level, 20 mg/dL; total calcium concentration, 30 mEq/L; total cholesterol level, 260 mg/dL; sodium concentration, 140 mEq/L; chloride concentration, 105 mEq/L; potassium concentration, 3.0 mEq/L; serum creatinine level, 1.0 mg/dL, red blood cell count, $5.0 \times 106/mm^3$, white blood cell count, $7000/mm^3$; platelets, $80{,}000/mm^3$

X-Ray: Compression fracture of T9-T12

Bone Scan: Metastatic disease localized in areas of ribs and spine

Questions:

A. Analyze the patient's lab values and physical findings, and list his medical problems.
B. How would you manage the patient's pain, both from a pharmacologic perspective and a physical therapy perspective?
C. Discuss the issue of psychological dependence and addiction associated with opiate use in patients with cancer.
D. How should the patient be monitored in terms of efficacy, tolerance, and adverse effects?

3. A 62-year-old female fell on her right knee 2 years ago. She treated her injury with ice, elevation, and compression. The acute pain and swelling resolved within 2 weeks. However, over the past year she has experienced increasing pain and stiffness in this knee. She reports morning stiffness and additional discomfort with activity. She is a retired elementary school teacher. She lives alone in a second floor walkup.

Past Medical History: HTN × 5 years

Meds: Ibuprofen, hydrochlorothiazide

X-Ray: Knee: narrowed joint spaces bilaterally; right more than left; consistent with osteoarthritis

Questions

A. What information would the physician need to know about this patient before prescribing medications?

B. Would you change her existing medications? If yes, what would you prescribe?

C. How would you monitor this patient for adverse effects and efficacy of the medications?

D. If conservative therapy does not help, should this patient receive a COX-2 inhibitor?

4. Pain medication is administered through a variety of methods. Describe the delivery methods best used for the patients below:

A. Patient with metastatic bone cancer

B. Patient with multiple herniated discs that has produced chronic debilitating pain for the past 5 years.

C. Severe postoperative pain following cardiac bypass surgery

5. Physicians prescribing opioids use a Patient Reassessment Model called the "four A's of Pain." This stands for Analgesia, Activities of daily living, Adverse effects, and Aberrant drug-taking behavior. Describe how you might monitor your patient on the basis of this model.

REFERENCES

1. Rang, HP, et al: Analgesic Drugs. In Rang HP, Dale MM, Ritter JM, Flower R, editors: Rang and Dale's Pharmacology, New York, 2007, Churchill Livingstone.
2. Parsons CG: NMDA receptors as targets for drug action in neuropathic pain. Eur J Pharmacol 429:71-78, 2001.
3. Millan MJ: Descending control of pain. Prog Neurobiol 66(6):355-474, 2002.
4. Julius D, Basbaum AI: Molecular mechanisms of nociception. Nature 413:203-210, 2001.
5. Wang H, Woolf CJ: Pain TRPs. Neuron 46(1):9-12, 2005.
6. Yaksh TL: Spinal systems and pain processing: Development of novel analgesic drugs with mechanistically defined models. Trends Pharmacol Sci 20(8):329-337, 1999.
7. Przewlocki R, Przewlocki B: Opioids in chronic pain. Eur J Pharmacol 429:79-91, 2001.
8. Trescot AM, Datta S, Lee M, Hansen H: Opioid pharmacology. Pain Physician 11(2 suppl):S133-S153, 2008.
9. Inturrisi CE: Clinical pharmacology of opioids for pain. Clin J Pain 18(suppl 4):S3-S13, 2002.
10. Ballantyne CM, Mao J: Opioid therapy for chronic pain. N Engl J Med 349(20):1943-1953, 2003.
11. Camu F, Vanlersberghe C: Pharmacology of systemic analgesics. Best Pract Res Clin Anaesthesiol 16(4):475-488, 2002.
12. Curatolo M, Sveticic G: Drug combinations in pain treatment: A review of the published evidence and a method for finding the optimal combination. Best Pract Res Clin Anaesthesiol 16(4):507-519, 2002.
13. Abramowicz M: Oxycodone and OxyContin, The medical letter, Vol. 43(1113), New Rochelle, NY, 2001, The Medical Letter, Inc.
14. Gandhi K, Heitz JW, Viscusi E: Treatment of pain. In Waldman SA, Terzic A, editors: Pharmacology and therapeutics: Principles to practice, Philadelphia, 2009, Saunders.
15. Vallerand AH: The use of long-acting opioids in chronic pain management. Nurs Clin North Am 38(3):435-445, 2003.
16. Ashburn MA, Ogden LL, Zhang J, Love G, Basta SV: The pharmacokinetics of transdermal fentanyl delivered with and without controlled heat. J Pain 4(6):291-297, 2003.
17. Newshan G, Newshan G: Heat-related toxicity with the fentanyl transdermal patch. J Pain Symptom Manage 16(5):277-278, 1998.
18. Safety warnings regarding use of fentanyl transdermal (skin) patches (website). http://www.fda.gov/cder/drug/advisory/fentanyl.htm. Accessed February 16, 2009.
19. ISMP calls for more action to safeguard pain patches (website). http://www.ismp.org/pressroom/PR20050818.pdf. Accessed February 16, 2009.
20. Kornick CA, Santiago-Palma J, Moryl N, Payne R, Obbens EA: Benefit-risk assessment of transdermal fentanyl for the treatment of chronic pain. Drug Saf 26(13):951-973, 2003.
21. Amato L, Davoli M, Minozzi S, Ali R, Ferri M: Methadone at tapered doses for the management of opioid withdrawal. Cochrane Database Syst Rev 2(CD003409), 2003.
22. Layson-Wolf C, Goode JV, Small RE: Clinical use of methadone. J Pain Palliat Care Pharmacother 16(1):29-59, 2002.
23. McQuay H: Opioids in pain management. Lancet 353: 2229-2232, 1999.
24. Mintzer IL, Eisenberg M, Terra M, MacVane C, Himmelstein DU, Woolhandler S: Treating opioid addiction with buprenorphine-naloxone in community-based primary care settings. Ann Fam Med 5(2):146-150, 2007.
25. Boothby LA, Doering PL: Buprenorphine for the treatment of opioid dependence. Am J Health Syst Pharm 64(3):266-272, 2007.
26. Abramowicz M: Buprenorphine: An alternative to methadone. In The medical letter, Vol. 45(1150), New Rochelle, NY, 2003, The Medical Letter, Inc.
27. Schnitzer T: The new analgesic combination tramadol/acetaminophen. Eur J Anaesthesiol 20(Suppl 28):13-17, 2003.
28. Chapman SL, Byas-Smith MG, Reed BA: Effects of intermediate- and long-term use of opioids on cognition in patients with chronic pain. Clin J Pain 18(4):S83-S90, 2002.
29. Shavit Y, Ben-Eliyahu S, Zeidel A, Beilin B: Effects of fentanyl on natural killer cell activity and on resistance to tumor metastasis in rats: Dose and timing study. Neuroimmunomodulation 11:255-260, 2004.
30. Peterson PK, Sharp BM, Gekker G, Portoghese PS, Sannerud K, Balfour HH Jr: Morphine promotes the growth of HIV-1 in human peripheral blood mononuclear cell cocultures. AIDS 4(9):869-873, 1990.
31. Potent Painkillers: Addictive? Johns Hopkins Med Lett Health After 50 16(1), 2004.
32. Pergolizzi J, Böger RH, Budd K, et al: Opioids and the management of chronic severe pain in the elderly: Consensus statement of an international expert panel with focus on the six clinically most often used World Health Organization step III opioids (buprenorphine, fentanyl, hydromorphone, methadone, morphine, oxycodone). Pain Pract 8(4):287-313, 2008.

33. Strain EC: Assessment and treatment of comorbid psychiatric disorders in opioid-dependent patients. Clin J Pain 18(4): S14-S27, 2002.
34. Estfan B, LeGrand SB, Walsh D, Lagman RL, Davis MP: Opioid rotation in cancer patients: Pros and Cons. Oncology 19(4):511-516, 2005.
35. Savage SR, Joranson DE, Covington EC, Schnoll SH, Heit HA, Gilson AM: Definitions related to the medical use of opioids: Evolution towards universal agreement. J Pain Symptom Manage 26(1):655-667, 2003.
36. Medication-assisted treatment for opioid addiction in opioid treatment programs (website). http://download.ncadi.samhsa.gov/Prevline/pdfs/bkd524.pdf. Accessed September 2, 2009.
37. Jones TF, Feler CA, Simmons BP, et al: Neurologic complications including paralysis after a medication error involving implanted intrathecal catheters. Am J Med 112(1):31-36, 2002.
38. Kissin IMD.P: Patient-controlled-analgesia: Analgesimetry and its problems. Anesth Analg 108(6):1945-1949, 2009.
39. Shang AB, Gan TJ: Optimising postoperative pain management in the ambulatory patient. Drugs 63(9):855-867, 2003.
40. Vicente KJ, Kada-Bekhaled K, Hillel G, Cassano A, Orser BA: Programming errors contribute to death from patient-controlled analgesia: Case report and estimate of probability. Can J Anaesthesiol 50(4):328-332, 2003.
41. Finger MJ, McLeod DG: Postoperative myocardial infarction after radical cystoprostatectomy masked by patient-controlled analgesia. Urology 45(1):155-157, 1995.
42. Brown SL, Bogner MS, Parmentier CM, Taylor JB: Human error and patient-controlled analgesia pumps. J Intraven Nurs 20(6):311-316, 1997.
43. Viscusi ER, Siccardi M, Damaraju CV, Hewitt DJ, Kershaw P: The safety and efficacy of fentanyl iontophoretic transdermal system compared with morphine intravenous patient-controlled analgesia for postoperative pain management: An analysis of pooled data from three randomized, active-controlled clinical studies. Anesth Analg 105(5):1428-1436, 2007.
44. Hankin CS, Schein J, Clark JA, Panchal S: Adverse events involving intravenous patient-controlled analgesia. Am J Health Syst Pharm 64(14):1492-1499, 2007.
45. Weber LM, Ghafoor VL, Phelps P: Implementation of standard order sets for patient-controlled analgesia. Am J Health Syst Pharm 65(12:1184-1191, 2008.
46. General-purpose infusion pumps: Evaluating the B. Braun Outlook Safety Infusion System. Health Devices 32(10):382-395, 2003.
47. ISMP Medication Safety Alert! Burns in MRI patients wearing transdermal patches: (website). http://www.ismp.org/Newletters/acutecare/articles/20040408.asp. Accessed April 8, 2004.
48. Van Thuyne W, Delbeke FT: Declared use of medication in sports. Clin J Sport Med 18(2):143-147, 2008.
49. Bjorkman DJ: The effect of aspirin and nonsteroidal anti-inflammatory drugs on prostaglandins. Am J Med 105 (1, suppl 2):8S-12S, 1998.
50. Eberhart CE, Du Bois RN: Eicosanoids and the gastrointestinal tract. Gastroenterology 109:285-301, 1995.
51. Brater DC: Effects of nonsteroidal antiinflammatory drug on renal function: Focus on cyclooxygenase-2 selective inhibition. Am J Med 107:65S-71S, 1999.
52. Vane J: Towards a better aspirin. Nature 367:215-216, 1994.
53. Matzdorf C, Kurtz A, Hocherl K: COX-2 activity determines the level of renin expression but is dispensable for acute upregulation of renin expression in rat kidneys. Am J Physiol Renal Physiol 292(6):F1782-F1790, 2007.
54. Hao CM, Breyer MD: Physiological regulation of prostaglandins in the kidney. Ann Rev Physiol 70(1):357-377, 2008.
55. Schwab JM, Beiter T, Linder JU, et al: COX-3—A virtual pain target in humans? FASEB J 17(15):2174-2175, 2003.
56. Warner TD, Mitchell JA: Cyclooxygenase-3 (COX-3): Filling in the gaps toward COX continuum? Proc Nat Acad Sci USA 99(21):13371-13373, 2002.
57. Lilley LL, Harrington RA, Snyder JS: Anti-inflammatory, antirheumatic, and related drugs. In Lilley LL, Harrington RA, Snyder JS, editors: Pharmacology and the nursing process, St. Louis, 2007, Mosby.
58. Elwood PC, Gallagher AM, Duthie GG, Mur LA, Morgan G: Aspirin, salicylates, and cancer. Lancet 373(9671):1301-1309, 2009.
59. Asanuma M, Nishibayashi-Asanuma S, Miyazaki I, Kohno M, Ogawa N: Neuroprotective effects of non-steroidal anti-inflammatory drugs by direct scavenging of nitric oxide radicals. J Neurochem 76(6):1895-1904, 2001.
60. Thomas T, Nadackal TG, Thomas K: Aspirin and non-steroidal anti-inflammatory drugs inhibit amyloid-beta aggregation. Neuroreport 12(15):3261-3267, 2001.
61. Aisen PS, Schafer KA, Grundman M, et al: Effects of rofecoxib or naproxen vs placebo on Alzheimer disease progression: A randomized controlled trial. JAMA 289(21):2819-2826, 2003.
62. Chan FK, Hung LC, Suen BY, et al: Celecoxib versus diclofenac and omeprazole in reducing the risk of recurrent ulcer bleeding in patients with arthritis. N Engl J Med 347(26): 2104-2110, 2002.
63. Lilley LL, Harrington RA, Snyder JS: Anti-inflammatory, Antirheumatic, and Related Drugs. In Lilley LL, Harrington RA, Snyder JS, editors: Pharmacology and the Nursing Process, Philadelphia, 2007, Mosby.
64. Ray WA, Stein CM, Byrd V, et al: Educational program for physicians to reduce use of non-steroidal anti-inflammatory drugs among community-dwelling elderly persons: A randomized controlled trial. Med Care 39(5):425-435, 2001.
65. Straube, S, et al: Mortality with upper gastrointestinal bleeding and perforation: Effects of time and NSAID use. BMC Gastroenterol 9:1-7, 2009.
66. Rostom A, Dubé C, Jolicoeur E, Boucher M, Joyce J: Gastroduodenal ulcers associated with the use of non-steroidal anti-inflammatory drugs: A systematic review of preventive pharmacological interventions. Ottawa, Ontario, 2003, Canadian Coordinating Office for Health Technology Assessment.
67. Scharf S, Kwiatek R, Ugoni A, Christophidis N: NSAIDs and faecal blood loss in elderly patients with osteoarthritis: Is plasma half-life relevant? Aust N Z J Med 28:436-439, 1998.
68. Furst DE, Munster T: Nonsteroidal anti-inflammatory drugs, disease-modifying antirheumatic drugs, nonopioid analgesics, and drugs used in gout. In Katzung BG, editor: Basic and clinical pharmacology, New York, 2002, McGraw-Hill.
69. St Lawrence KS, Ye FQ, Lewis BK, Weinberger DR, Frank JA, McLaughlin AC: Effects of indomethacin on cerebral blood flow at rest and during hypercapnia: An arterial spin tagging study in humans. J Magnet Reson Imag 15(6):628-635, 2002.
70. Goldstein B: Gastrointestinal event rates in the CLASS study: 6 month vs longer-term follow-up analysis. Gastroenterology 122(Suppl 1):A469-A483, 2002.
71. Singh G, Fort JG, Goldstein JL, Levy RA, et al: Celecoxib versus naproxen and diclofenac in osteoarthritis patients: SUCCESS-I Study. Am J Med 119(3):255-266, 2006.
72. Singh G, Goldstein J, Bello AE: The effect of low dose aspirin on the incidence of UGI symptoms among patients receiving celecoxib or conventional NSAIDs: Analysis of the SUCCESS-1 and CLASS trials. J Clin Rheum 8(Suppl):S62-S71, 2002.
73. Perazella MA: COX-2 selective inhibitors: Analysis of the renal effects. Expert Opin Drug Saf 1(1):53-64, 2002.
74. Gambaro G, Perazella MA: Adverse renal effects of anti-inflammatory agents: Evaluation of selective and nonselective

cyclooxygenase inhibitors. J Intern Med 253(6):643-652, 2003.
75. Catella-Lawson F, McAdam B, Morrison BW, et al: Effects of specific inhibition of cyclooxygenase-2 on sodium balance, hemodynamics, and vasoactive eicosanoids. J Pharmacol Exper Therapy, 289:735-741, 1999.
76. Abramowicz M, editor: Valdecoxib (Bextra)—A new cox-2 inhibitor (Vol. 44[1129]), New Rochelle, NY, 2002, The Medical Letter, Inc.
77. Martin-Mola E, Munoz-Gomez J, Sanchez-Burson J: Celecoxib is as effective as ibuprofen in treating pain associated with osteoarthritis of the knee. Ann Rheum Dis 64(Suppl III): 495-496, 2005.
78. Abramowicz M: Drugs for pain. Med Lett Drugs Ther 42(1085):73-78, 2000. .
79. Gajraj NM: COX-2 inhibitors celecoxib and parecoxib: Valuable options for postoperative pain management. Curr Top Med Chem 7(3):235-249, 2007.
80. Buvanendran A, Kroin JS, Tuman KJ, et al: Effects of perioperative administration of a selective cyclooxygenase 2 inhibitor on pain management and recovery of function after knee replacement. JAMA 290(18):2411-2418, 2003.
81. Alaranta A, Alaranta H, Heliövaara M, Airaksinen M, Helenius I: Ample use of physician-prescribed medications in Finnish elite athletes. Int J Sports Med 27(11):919-925, 2006.
82. Järvinen TA, Järvinen TL, Kääriäinen M, Kalimo H, Järvinen M: Muscle injuries: Biology and treatment. Am J Sports Med 33(5):745-764, 2005.
83. Hawke TJ, Garry DJ: Myogenic satellite cells: Physiology to molecular biology. J Appl Physiol 91(2):534-551, 2001.
84. Hawke TJ: Muscle stem cells and exercise training. Exerc Sport Sci Rev 33(2):63-68, 2005.
85. Mendias CL, Tatsumi R, Allen RE: Role of cyclooxygenase-1 and -2 in satellite cell proliferation, differentiation, and fusion. Muscle Nerve 30(4):497-500, 2004.
86. Bondesen BA, Mills ST, Kegley KM, Pavlath GK: The COX-2 pathway is essential during early stages of skeletal muscle regeneration. Am J Physiol Cell Physiol 287(2):C475-C483, 2004.
87. Mackey AL, Kjaer M, Dandanell S, et al: The influence of anti-inflammatory medication on exercise-induced myogenic precursor cell responses in humans. [see comment]. J Appl Physiol 103(2):425-431, 2007.
88. Chazaud B, Brigitte M, Yacoub-Youssef H, et al: Dual and beneficial roles of macrophages during skeletal muscle regeneration. Exerc Sport Sci Rev 37(1):18-22, 2008.
89. Dedier J, Stampfer MJ, Hankinson SE, Willett WC, Speizer FE, Curhan GC: Nonnarcotic analgesic use and the risk of hypertension in US women. Hypertension 40:604-608, 2002.
90. Gurwitz JH, Avorn J, Bohn RL, Glynn RJ, Monane M, Mogun H: Initiation of antihypertensive treatment during nonsteroidal anti-inflammatory drug therapy. JAMA 272(10):781-786, 1994.
91. Whelton A, White WB, Bello AE, Puma JA, Fort JG; SUCCESS-VII Investigators: Effects of celecoxib and rofecoxib on blood pressure and edema in patients >65 years of age with systemic hypertension and osteoarthritis. Am J Cardiol 90:959-963, 2002.
92. Egan B: Nonnarcotic analgesis use and the risk of hypertension in US women. Hypertension 40(5):601-603, 2002.
93. Gurwitz JH, Everitt DE, Monane M, et al: The impact of ibuprofen on the efficacy of antihypertensive treatment with hydrochlorothiazide in elderly persons. J Gerontol A Biol Sci Med Sci 51(2):M74-M79, 1996.
94. Meune C, Mourad JJ, Bergmann JF, Spaulding C: Interaction between cyclooxygenase and the renin-angiotensin-aldosterone system: Rationale and clinical relevance. J Renin Angiotensin Aldosterone Syst 4(3):149-154, 2003.
95. Meune C, Mahé I, Mourad JJ, et al: Aspirin alters arterial function in patients with chronic heart failure treated with ACE inhibitors: A dose-mediated deleterious effect. Eur Journal of Heart Fail 5(3):271-279, 2003.
96. Park MH: Should aspirin be used with angiotensin-converting enzyme inhibitors in patients with chronic heart failure? Congest Heart Fail 9:206-213, 2003.
97. Hall D: The aspirin-angiotensin-converting enzyme inhibitor tradeoff: To halve and halve not. J Am Coll Cardiol 35: 1808-1812, 2000.
98. Mukherjee D, Nissen SE, Topol EJ: Risk of cardiovascular events associated with selective COX-2 inhibitors. JAMA 286(8):954-959, 2001.
99. Cleland JGF: No reduction in cardiovascular risk with NSAIDs-including aspirin? Lancet 359(9301):92-93, 2002.
100. Ray WA, Stein CM, Daugherty JR, Hall K, Arbogast PG, Griffin MR: COX-2 selective non-steroidal anti-inflammatory drugs and risk of serious coronary heart disease. Lancet 360(9339):1071-1073, 2002.
101. DeMaria AN: Relative risk of cardiovascular events in patients with rheumatoid arthritis. Am J Cardiol 89(suppl):33D-38D, 2002.
102. Griffin MR, Stein CM, Graham DJ, Daugherty JR, Arbogast PG, Ray WA: High frequency of use of rofecoxib at greater than recommended doses: Cause for concern. Pharmacoepidemiol Drug Saf 13(6):339-343, 2004.
103. Solomon DH, Schneeweiss S, Glynn RJ, et al: Relationship between selective cyclooxygenase-2 inhibitors and acute myocardial infarction in older adults. Circulation 109(17): 2068-2073, 2004.
104. Cohen R, Silverman E: FDA blasted for how it handled Vioxx after studies raised flags, Newark, NJ, 2004, The Sunday Star-Ledger.
105. Solomon SD, McMurray JJ, Pfeffer MA, et al: Cardiovascular risk associated with celecoxib in a clinical trial for colorectal adenoma prevention. N Engl J Med 352:1071-1080, 2005.
106. Ray WA, Stein CM, Hall K, Daugherty JR, Griffin MR: Nonsteroidal anti-inflammatory drugs and risk of serious coronary heart disease: An observational cohort study. Lancet 359(9301):118-123, 2002.
107. Farkouh ME, Greenberg BP: An evidence-based review of the cardiovascular risks of nonsteroidal anti-inflammatory drugs. Am J Cardiol 103(9):1227-1237, 2009.
108. MacDonald T, Wei L: Effect of ibuprofen on cardioprotective effect of aspirin. Lancet 361, 2003.
109. Catella-Lawson F, Reilly MP, Kapoor SC, et al: Cyclooxygenase inhibitors and the antiplatelet effects of aspirin. N Engl J Med 345(25):1809-1817, 2001.
110. Acetaminophen for osteoarthritis. Cochrane Database Syst Rev 2(CD004257), 2003.
111. Case JP, Baliunas AJ, Block JA: Lack of efficacy of acetaminophen in treating symptomatic knee osteoarthritis: A randomized, double-blind, placebo-controlled comparison trial with diclofenac sodium. Arch Intern Med 163(2): 169-178, 2003.
112. Ausiello JC, Stafford RS: Trends in medication use for osteoarthritis treatment. J Rheumatol 29(5):999-1005, 2002.
113. Abramowicz M, editor: Acetaminophen safety. In The Medical Letter (Vol. 44[1142]), New Rochelle, NY, 2002, The Medical Letter, Inc.
114. Jensen J: Nutritional concerns in the diabetic athlete. Curr Sports Med Rep 3:192-197, 2004.
115. Boddeke E: Involvement of chemokines in pain. Eur J Pharmacol 429:115-119, 2001.
116. Jensen TS, Gottrup H, Sindrup SH, Bach FW: The clinical picture of neuropathic pain. Eur J Pharmacol 429:1-11, 2001.

117. Asburn MA, Staats PS: Management of chronic pain. Lancet 353:1865-1869, 1999.
118. Eisenberg E, Damunni G, Hoffer E, Baum Y, Krivoy N: Lamotrigine for intractable sciatica: Correlation between dose, plasma concentration and analgesia. Eur J Pain 7(6):485-491, 2003.
119. Serpell MG: Gabapentin in neuropathic pain syndromes: A randomised, double-blind, placebo-controlled trial. Pain 99(3):557-566, 2002.
120. Wermeling DP, Berger JR: Ziconotide infusion for severe chronic pain: Case series of patients with neuropathic pain. Pharmacotherapy 26(3):395-402, 2006.
121. Finnerup NB, Otto M, Jensen TS, Sindrup SH: An evidence-based algorithm for the treatment of neuropathic pain. MedGenMed 9(2):36, 2007.
122. Fields HL: Multiple mechanisms of neuropathic pain: Evolving concepts and treatments, Medscape Medical News 2008. (website). http://www.medscape.com/viewarticle/508718_1. Accessed March 5, 2010.
123. Attal N, Brasseur L, Guirimand D, Clermond-Gnamien S, Atlami S, Bouhassira D: Are oral cannabinoids safe and effective in refractory neuropathic pain? Eur J Pain 8(2): 173-177, 2004.
124. Ackerman LL, Follett KA, Rosenquist RW: Long-term outcomes during treatment of chronic pain with intrathecal clonidine or clonidine/opioid combinations. J Pain Symptom Manage 26(1):668-677, 2003.
125. Sindrup SH, Jensen TS: Efficacy of pharmacological treatments of neuropathic pain: An update and effect related to mechanism of drug action. Pain 83:389-400, 1999.
126. Portenoy RK, Lesage P: Management of cancer pain. Lancet 353:1695-1700, 1999.
127. Shi Q, Wang XS, Mendoza TR, Pandya KJ, Cleeland CS: Assessing persistent cancer pain: A comparison of current pain ratings and pain recalled from the past week. J Pain Symptom Manage 37(2):168-174, 2009.
128. Luger NM, Sabino MA, Schwei MJ, et al: Efficacy of systemic morphine suggests a fundamental difference in the mechanisms that generate bone cancer vs inflammatory pain. Pain 99(3):397-406, 2002.

12

Drug Treatment for Arthritis-Related Conditions

Barbara Gladson

DRUG TREATMENT OF RHEUMATOID ARTHRITIS

Rheumatoid arthritis (RA) is a chronic and progressive inflammatory disorder, primarily affecting the synovium of the joints and leading to pain, stiffness, joint damage, and disability. The progression and general virulence of the disease may vary, but the course of disease is generally downward. In addition, patients with RA experience earlier mortality than do their healthy counterparts and experience a greater incidence of cardiac concerns.[1,2] Despite years of study, the cause and mechanism of disease in RA remain unknown. Even the diagnostic process of using a set of clinical criteria is unrefined by today's standards of biologic markers for disease. Treatment of RA has not been sensibly based on a thorough understanding of its pathogenesis but has instead been borrowed from that of other diseases. Treatment has consisted of an array of anti-inflammatory and immunosuppressive drugs with their weak justification following some clinical efficacy. However, certain strides in treatment have been made and consist of extensive use of methotrexate (a chemotherapy agent), aggressive early treatment, biologic response modifiers, and the development of effective combination treatments.[3]

Clinical Presentation

RA typically develops slowly over weeks to months, and symptoms include fatigue, weakness, low-grade fevers, and joint pain.[4] Stiffness, particularly of the hands, and myalgias precede the onset of inflammation. Joint involvement is commonly symmetrical and tends to affect the small joints of the hands, wrist, and feet; but some larger joints such as the elbows, shoulders, hips, knees, and ankles may also be involved. Symptoms of inflammation and joint swelling may be visible or palpable. The soft tissue around the joints feels soft, spongy, and warm and appears erythematous. Over time, slow destruction of ligaments and tendons leads to joint deformities, including metacarpophalangeal subluxations and other deformities involving the proximal interphalangeal joints, such as swan-neck deformity, boutonniere deformity, and ulnar deviation. Extra-articular systemic involvement, including vasculitis, pleural effusion, pericarditis, and lymphadenopathy, is also prevalent.

Diagnosis is based on the American Rheumatism Association's criteria for classification of RA.[5,6] These criteria include the presence of morning stiffness, symmetric arthritis, rheumatoid nodules, radiographic changes, and some laboratory values. Laboratory tests may show anemia, depressed bone marrow, elevated erythrocyte sedimentation rate (ESR), positive rheumatoid factor (60 to 70% of patients), and a positive antinuclear antibody (ANA) titer (25% of patients). There is a new serologic test for RA, anticyclic citrullinated peptide (CCP) antibody.[7] This marker is more specific for the disease compared with rheumatoid factor.

Pathogenesis of Rheumatoid Arthritis

RA has typically been considered an autoimmune disease; however, none of the laboratory markers strictly support this notion. In addition, a "unique autoantigen" has not been found, proving that this is strictly an autoimmune disorder.[3] At present, much of the attention regarding the pathogenesis of RA centers on the role of the T lymphocytes in the inflamed joint and proinflammatory cytokines.

RA is genetically linked to the histocompatibility antigens human leukocyte antigen (HLA) DR-1 and DR-4.[8] This genetic connection is related to the presentation of antigen to the T lymphocytes that signal inflammation with synovial lining cell hyperplasia, T-lymphocyte infiltration, and the secretion of toxic proteases into the joint (collagenases, stromelysin, and free radicals). Activation of the cellular and humoral immune responses (B cell and cell-mediated) begins with involvement of chemokines, cell adhesion molecules, and cytokines, resulting in loss of cartilage and bony erosions.

Because T lymphocytes are abundant in inflamed synovial tissue, researchers have spent time developing T-cell–depleting agents (novel monoclonal antibodies), but this approach has been largely ineffective.[3] Researchers' disappointment with this approach has led to a new focus on the other cellular components of the inflamed synovium—macrophage-like synoviocytes and fibroblastic synoviocytes—and on a new model of RA as a "chronic tissue-specific inflammatory process," with a variety of immune mediators playing a role.

Analysis of the inflamed synovium has shown that it contains principally two types of synoviocytes in abundance: type A and type B.[9] Type A synoviocytes are members of the monocyte–macrophage family, which secretes large amounts of proinflammatory cytokines. This family is also known for its phagocytic ability. Type B synoviocytes are the specialized fibroblasts that produce hyaluronic acid and collagen, but under inflammatory conditions, these cells may also secrete cytokines and proteases into the joints. Neutrophils in the synovial fluid and chondrocytes in the cartilage also contribute inflammatory mediators. Early in the disease, the synovium begins to invade the cartilage.

The focus of research has become even more narrowed as new information about cytokines has been discovered. Cytokines are proteins that work as intercellular messengers for the immune system. Some cytokines have been classified as interleukins, but others have been named according to their function, such as tumor necrosis factor-α (TNF-α). Cytokines are produced in response to other cytokines (sort of a chain reaction) and are also activated in response to specific stimuli such as microbial products. They bind to specific cell receptors which ultimately signal transduction systems that regulate transcription of specific genes. They tend to act locally but can have significant systemic effects. Cytokines have been shown to induce metabolic effects, including alterations in lipids and peripheral insulin resistance that promote atherogenesis, and they may be responsible for early death caused by coronary heart disease in patients with RA.[10,11]

In RA, cytokines are involved extensively in all aspects of inflammation and joint destruction. Table 12-1 lists the cytokines that are seen in inflamed synovial tissue, with TNF and interleukin-1 (IL-1) the most abundant.[3,12] TNF was originally discovered as a factor that can induce regression and cell death in some tumors, but it may also be responsible for cachexia in cancer. Its level in RA coincides with the extent of inflammation and bone erosion, as well as with the expression of adhesion molecules, synthesis and release of proteases, and synovial neoangiogenesis (production of blood vessels in the synovium). IL-1 has many of the same properties as TNF. With all this new understanding of RA, research has been directed toward neutralizing or blocking TNF and IL-1.

Monoclonal antibodies to TNF are being used clinically. These drugs block TNF expression and also cause decreases in IL-1, IL-6, and some other adhesion molecules, thus reducing inflammatory infiltration. Another new approach is the administration of soluble TNF receptors that bind TNF, reducing its biologic activity. TNF blockers and soluble receptors show great promise for patients with RA. However, research on these agents is new, and it is still unknown whether they are more effective than the traditional drugs used in the treatment of RA. Many of the initial studies have been placebo-controlled trials, and only recently have these drugs been compared with methotrexate, the gold standard treatment. Another concern is that these new drugs have still not elucidated a clear cause of RA, but the research has

TABLE 12-1 Cytokines Detected in Rheumatoid Arthritis Synovial Tissue or Fluid

Cytokine	Quantity	Level of Tissue Damage
TNF	+++	+++
IL-1β	+++	+++
IL-6	++	++
IL-8	++	++
IL-10	++	–
IL-12	+	++
IL-15	+	++
IL-2	+/–	+
IL-17	+	++
IFN-γ	+	++
TGF-β	++	–
GM-CSF	++	++

TNF, tumor necrosis factor; *IL*, interleukin; *IFN*, interferon; *TGF*, transforming growth factor; *GM-CSF*, granulocyte-macrophage colony-stimulating factor; *M*, monocyte/macrophage; *F*, fibroblast; *T*, T lymphocyte; –, inhibitory effect; +, low abundance/mild effect; ++, moderate abundance/moderate effect; +++, high abundance/high effect.

From Fox DA: Cytokine blockade as a new strategy to treat rheumatoid arthritis: Inhibition of tumor necrosis factor, adapted from *Arch Intern Med* 160:437–444, 2000.

helped explain why some of the older agents such as antimalarials, gold, sulfasalazine, and steroids have been useful because all of them inhibit cytokine production to some extent.

Antirheumatoid Drugs

Three primary categories of drugs are used to treat RA: (1) nonsteroidal anti-inflammatory drugs (NSAIDs), including aspirin and other salicylates for their anti-inflammatory actions; (2) disease-modifying antirheumatic drugs (DMARDs) that attempt to alter the disease; and (3) corticosteroids, which bridge the gap between the above two. NSAIDs and cyclooxygenase 2 (COX-2) inhibitors, which are used early in the course of the disease, only provide symptomatic relief but do not prevent joint destruction. Because these drugs have been extensively reviewed in Chapter 11, they will not be discussed in this section, but they are very important for the patient with RA. The DMARDs that are currently in use include methotrexate, leflunomide, sulfasalazine, and hydroxychloroquine. These are more effective than some older drugs and have fewer adverse effects, but the time it takes to see clinical improvement (3 to 6 months) has not changed. Older agents such as injectable gold, penicillamine, cyclosporine, and cyclophosphamide are no longer used due to their high risk/benefit ratio and therefore will not be reviewed in this text.

Corticosteroids. The corticosteroid drug prednisone can produce quick and significant symptomatic improvement in inflammation. Prednisone is the synthetic version of cortisol, the natural endogenous corticosteroid found in humans. Cortisol is secreted from the adrenal cortex in response to the adrenocorticotropic hormone (ACTH) coming from the anterior pituitary gland. The major physiologic effects of cortisol include increase in gluconeogenesis and lipolysis to provide fuel for activity and for brain function. Cortisol also enhances epinephrine synthesis and sensitizes tissues to the effect of catecholamines. It is considered to be the "stress hormone," meaning that physical, emotional, or chemical stress triggers its release.

Prednisone is used in the treatment of RA because it reduces inflammation and suppresses the immune system. When given exogenously, prednisone interferes with inflammatory cell adhesion and migration through the vascular endothelium, impairs leukotriene and prostaglandin synthesis by blocking phospholipase A_2, impairs transport of immune complexes, makes antigens susceptible to phagocytosis, and inhibits the release of immune cytokines through the inhibition of their transcription factors.[13] Additionally, steroids have a direct effect on depressing bone marrow cells, which results in neutropenia, leukopenia, and eosinopenia. The result is immune system depression.

Excess glucocorticosteroids, given for extended periods, are associated with a variety of adverse effects, which has led to reluctance to prescribe them on a long-term basis. Steroids have a catabolic effect on all types of supportive joint tissue, producing osteoporosis, increased incidence of fracture, tendon rupture, thinned skin, and muscle wasting. Exogenous steroid use leads to Cushing's syndrome, which is characterized by muscle weakness, truncal obesity, "moon faces," fragile skin and capillaries, easy bruising, hypertension, diabetes, and neuropsychiatric disorders.[14] Poor wound healing, increased risk of infection, stomach ulcers, acne, and cataracts can also occur.

Because osteoporosis occurs in about 50% of patients with RA, the American College of Rheumatology has developed some guidelines to prevent loss of bone density. The recommendations include administering the lowest effective dose. In addition, patients should adhere to certain lifestyle principles that have been shown to slow bone reabsorption. Avoidance of smoking, limiting alcohol intake, and maintaining a healthy weight are suggested. A baseline bone scan should be performed before steroid treatment is started, and follow-up scans should be done every 6 months to 1 year. Patients must also take 1500 mg of calcium and 400 to 800 international units (IU) of vitamin D daily. Administration of growth hormone is useful in children receiving steroids to prevent slowing of linear bone growth.[15] Treatment with the anti-osteoporosis drugs alendronate, risedronate, and calcitonin is also recommended (see Chapter 14).

The adverse effects of steroids may be minimized by alternate-day dosing or by using an alternative route of administration such as inhalation or topical application. Alternate-day dosing only works with prednisone and only if it is given at precisely the correct time. Another problem with using prednisone for chronic conditions is that patients must be convinced to withdraw the drug when the time is appropriate. Steroids produce a therapeutic effect but also create some euphoria and energizing effects, and therefore some patients may be reluctant to discontinue using them.

Because the adrenal glands stop producing steroids during exogenous administration (negative feedback), these drugs are withdrawn slowly over time. The purpose of the weaning process is to give the adrenal glands time to resume the production of steroids and also to help prevent a recurrence of the arthritis, which often occurs.

There has been renewed interest in the use of low doses of prednisone as a treatment for RA, given the belief that many of the adverse effects are dose related. A dose of prednisone may range anywhere from 5 to 150 mg/day. A low dose of prednisone is considered to be around 10 mg/day and is usually given in divided doses (5 mg twice a day). Several studies have shown that this level of prednisone to be more effective in limiting the number of tender and swollen joints, improving grip strength, and retarding the progression of bony erosions when used as monotherapy in patients with a recent diagnosis of RA, compared with placebo.[13,16] Prednisone can slow the course of RA, but this effect is limited.

Therefore, it is not recommended as monotherapy but should be combined with some other DMARDs for added benefit. Low-dose prednisone is well tolerated, although some adverse effects, including high blood sugar levels, weight gain, bruising, and osteopenia, are still documented.[17] Tapering is usually started at 6 months and is performed slowly with 1-mg decreases every couple of weeks to a month.

Sulfasalazine. Sulfasalazine suppresses the immune system by reducing natural killer cell activity and alters lymphocyte function. It may inhibit TNF-α in macrophages as well.[18] It also has some antimicrobial action and has been used for the treatment of ulcerative colitis.

Nausea and rash are fairly common adverse effects, but serious reactions such as hepatitis, pneumonitis, and bone marrow suppression occur. Dose-related symptoms include headache, gastrointestinal (GI) upset, leukopenia, and megaloblastic anemia. A lupus-like reaction has been reported in some patients. Monitoring of blood counts is advised once a month for the first 3 months and at monthly intervals thereafter. The efficacy of sulfasalazine may be equal to that of hydroxychloroquine, but the former may act more quickly.[19]

Hydroxychloroquine. This drug has been used to treat malaria, but since it appears to suppress T lymphocytes, it has been used in the treatment of RA as well.[20] This drug improves symptoms but does not seem to delay the bony lesions seen in RA. Adverse effects include dyspepsia, nausea, abdominal pain, rashes, nightmares, and visual disturbances.

Methotrexate. Methotrexate is a folic acid antagonist that impairs deoxyribonucleic acid (DNA) synthesis by inhibiting purine biosynthesis.[8] It inhibits leukotriene synthesis and decreases TNF-α levels. It is also known to decrease IL-1 levels and inhibit the proliferation of rapidly replicating monocytes and lymphocytes. It basically acts as an immunosuppressant but was originally and still is used as a chemotherapy agent at a higher dose. It is now the drug of choice for patients with RA and often produces improvement within 1 month, more quickly than many of the other DMARDs can.

Methotrexate administration is started at a dose of 7.5 to 10 mg once a week, which can be taken as a single dose or over a 24-hour period.[21] Intramuscular or subcutaneous injections are also available. Methotrexate is generally well tolerated at this low dose. However, it is most frequently associated with stomatitis, anorexia, and abdominal cramping and rarely with alopecia. Administration of folic acid is an effective way to reduce methotrexate's adverse effects. The more severe adverse effects include bone marrow suppression and pulmonary and hepatic toxic effects. Measurements of the liver transaminases must be performed regularly. Also, herpes zoster and *Pneumocystis carinii* infection are more common among patients taking this drug. There is even a link to lymphoma, which spontaneously resolves when the drug is discontinued. Methotrexate is teratogenic and therefore has found use as an abortifacient in ectopic pregnancy. Concurrent use with NSAIDs increases the toxic effects of methotrexate, especially in older adults with diminished renal function.

Research on methotrexate has led to some major changes in rheumatology practice. Several clinical trials have indicated that aggressive pharmacologic treatment of RA should occur early in the disease.[19] The beneficial effect of methotrexate is greater in patients during the first 2 years of the disease than in those who have had RA for 2 to 5 years.[22] Longitudinal radiographic studies have shown that the drug can retard the progression of the disease. Additionally, methotrexate has been found to lower mortality risk in RA by protecting against cardiovascular events.[23] It is the standard against which all new DMARDs are evaluated. Additional studies have shown that methotrexate is even more effective when combined with some of the other DMARDs.[24]

Leflunomide. Leflunomide is a prodrug, whose active metabolite inhibits the enzyme ribonucleotide uridine monophosphate, which is required for pyrimidine nucleotide synthesis.[25] In regard to RA, this drug interferes with the synthesis of activated lymphocytes by interfering with their cell cycle progression because of inadequate stores of uridine monophosphate (see Chapter 22). Cells undergoing division need an adequate supply of pyrimidine nucleotides, but in the presence of leflunomide, this supply is dramatically reduced.

Patients with RA used to begin a leflunomide regimen with 100 mg a day for 3 days and then switch over to a maintenance dose of 10 to 20 mg/day.[26] The reason for the loading dose is that the drug is almost completely protein bound. It has a long half-life, 15 days, which indicates that the effectiveness of the drug lasts for a while even after its discontinuation. However, at present, clinicians start with the usual dose of 10 mg, since the time to reach steady state is not much different from when a loading dose is given. Leflunomide undergoes repeated enterohepatic recirculation, so patients can take the resin cholestyramine, which will bind the drug in the GI tract with final elimination in the stool.

In a clinical trial that included 482 patients with active disease, there was more than 20% improvement in swollen joints, and in general, more than 40% of subjects experienced a reduction in symptoms.[27] This was compared with 35% improvement in the methotrexate-treated group and 19% improvement in the placebo group. In addition, the Sharp X-ray score (a measure of disease progression) showed the least progression in subjects taking leflunomide. In another year-long study of 402 patients, researchers found that this drug was as effective as methotrexate (50% success rate in both groups).[28] Leflunomide may also be given along with methotrexate. Adverse effects reported included diarrhea, alopecia, rash, and increases in aminotransferase activity, indicating some liver damage. Leflunomide is also carcinogenic and teratogenic in animals.

Tumor Necrosis Factor Inhibitors. TNF represents a new target for inhibition in patients with RA. Etanercept, adalimumab, and infliximab are three new drugs that can bind and inactivate TNF. Etanercept is an artificial bioengineered molecule that consists of two TNF receptors attached to a human immunoglobulin molecule.[29] This drug is administered subcutaneously two times per week, and long-term self-administration is required. This is significant in terms of patient compliance because some patients with RA will not have the dexterity to self-administer the injections.

Etanercept has been shown to be effective when compared with placebo and in some cases has been shown to be more effective than methotrexate.[30,31] Adverse effects reported have been mainly injection-site reactions, which do not necessitate removal of the drug. Repeated dosing is associated with the development of antinuclear antibodies, and a few patients have experienced a lupus-like syndrome. Demyelinating disorders, including multiple sclerosis and myelitis, have rarely been associated with etanercept.[32]

Infliximab is an antibody that targets TNF. It is administered intravenously at 0, 2, and 6 weeks and then every 8 weeks. Repeated administration has been associated with the development of antibodies to the drug. For this reason, infliximab has only been studied with simultaneous administration of methotrexate. The combination of infliximab plus methotrexate has been shown to be as effective as etanercept plus methotrexate and more effective than methotrexate plus placebo.[33] Adverse effects have included headache, infusion reactions (fever, urticaria, dyspnea, and hypotension), aseptic meningitis, and worsening congestive heart failure (CHF).[21] In some patients, anti-infliximab antibodies have developed, but combining this drug with methotrexate may decrease the development of these antibodies.

Serious infections, including reactivation of tuberculosis and sepsis, have been reported with both etanercept and infliximab.[21] These usually occur within the first 2 to 7 months of treatment. Lupus-like symptoms have also been reported. Skin testing for *Mycobacterium tuberculosis* and a chest X-ray are now recommended before therapy with these drugs is started. These drugs should not be given to patients with recently developed malignancy.

Adalimumab is the newest TNF inhibitor that is administered by weekly subcutaneous injection.[34] This drug may be effective in the treatment of severe RA that is refractory to other drugs, such as methotrexate, when given either as a single agent or in combination with methotrexate. Adverse effects are similar to those of the other two drugs in this category.

There is consensus that all three TNF-α inhibitors work similarly with similar efficacy, so no comparison studies have been released. Etanercept and adalimumab are approved for monotherapy but they are usually given along with methotrexate for added efficacy.

All three TNF-α inhibitors have the potential for disseminated infections.[35] The most common infection seen is a reactivation of latent tuberculosis, which usually occurs within the first few months of treatment. Other infections include listeriosis, *Pneumocystis carinii* infection, and fungal infections. There also is a risk of malignancy with these drugs, although this remains controversial, since patients with RA already have an elevated risk for lymphoma.[36]

Abatacept. Abatacept is an analog of cytotoxic T-lymphocyte–associated antigen 4 ($CTLA_4$), a molecule that reduces the activation of T cells. It has high affinity for the cell surface receptors on the surface of antigen-presenting cells that bind to T cells. This drug is approved for severe disease that has not responded to other DMARDs. When given in combination with methrotrexate to patients who were nonresponders to methotrexate, the combination slowed joint destruction and improved symptoms.[37] Adverse effects include increased upper respiratory tract infections and infusion reactions.

Rituximab. Rituximab is a monoclonal antibody that targets CD20 marked B lymphocytes developed to treat B-cell non-Hodgkin's lymphoma.[38] These B cells play a role in facilitating synovitis. It is given intravenously (IV); it may result in infusion reactions, including rigors, fever, nausea, cough dyspnea, and vacillating blood pressure.

Anakinra. Anakinra is another new drug that is a genetically engineered IL-1 receptor antagonist.[21] Compared with placebo, this drug has produced only modest improvements in the signs and symptoms of RA, and therefore it will probably be used only in combination with methotrexate. Adverse effects include injection-site reactions and infections similar to those caused by TNF inhibitors, but there has been no report of reactivation of tuberculosis with anakinra alone. Complications appear to occur more often when it is combined with TNF inhibitors.

Rehabilitation Concerns with Disease-Modifying Antirheumatic Drugs

DMARDs have not been studied with respect to how they affect exercise performance or how exercise affects their efficacy or pharmacokinetics. Most of these drugs can produce renal and liver toxic effects, immunosuppression, and fatigue. Frequent laboratory tests are necessary to evaluate liver function and to monitor for bone marrow suppression which is indicated by anemia, thrombocytopenia, and neutropenia. The therapist should also watch for clinical signs of bone marrow suppression, such as easy bruising and lowered exercise tolerance; and patients must be monitored for any infections, particularly if they are taking TNF inhibitors. Many of these drugs also produce skin rashes, which are often a sign of drug toxicity. Skin inspection should be a regular part of the therapy appointment. In addition,

BOX 12-1 Disease-Modifying Antirheumatic Drugs

Drug	Comments
Methotrexate (Rheumatrex)	Monitor CBC, albumin, and liver enzymes every 4–8 wk; May cause myelosuppression, hepatotoxicity, pulmonary fibrosis, oral ulcers, GI problems
Leflunomide (Arava)	Monitor CBC, albumin, and liver enzymes every 4–8 wk; May cause hepatotoxicity and GI problems
Sulfasalazine (Azulfidine)	Monitor CBC and liver enzymes q mo for 3 mo then q 3 mo; may cause myelosuppression, hepatotoxicity, rash
Hydroxychloroquine (Plaquenil)	Perform ophthalmologic exam every 6–12 mo; may cause macular damage
Biologic Response Modifiers	
Abatacept (Orencia)	Blocks stimulation of T cells by binding to CD80/86 on antigen-presenting cells, preventing interaction with the T-cell molecule CD28
Etanercept (Enbrel)	Binds to TNF-α to prevent its binding to its receptor
Infliximab (Remicade)	Monoclonal antibody to TNF α
Adalimumab (Humira)	Monoclonal antibody to TNF α
Rituximab (Rituxan)	Monoclonal antibody to CD20, which is a cell-surface molecule found on mature B cells; produces depletion of B cells
Anakinra (Kineret)	IL-1 inhibitor

CBC, complete blood count; *GI*, gastrointestinal; *TNF*, tumor necrosis factor; *IL*, interleukin.

patients should remain hydrated to protect renal function. Some of these drugs produce toxic metabolites that undergo renal elimination; keeping fluids moving through the kidneys can help decrease the accumulation of these metabolites. Last, for patients also receiving steroids, the catabolic effects of DMARDs should be considered, especially when strengthening, stretching, or deep tissue work is performed, so that tissue injury and rupture may be avoided (Box 12-1).

Rational Dosing and Combination Therapy for Rheumatoid Arthritis

The current approach for treating RA is to start DMARD therapy as soon as the disease is suspected. This differs from the older approach that withheld these drugs until there was damage to the joint surfaces. In addition, combination therapy is utilized, since it has definitely been shown to be more effective than the use of individual drugs. The typical regimen prior to the use of biologic response modifiers consisted of methotrexate, hydroxychloroquine, and sulfasalzine.[39] Low-dose prednisone was also added to this treatment and was later tapered as the DMARDs began to work.

Most rheumatologists begin treatment with methotrexate at 7.5 to 10.0 mg/wk and increase the dose by 2.5 to 5.0 mg/wk each month. An incomplete response will require that additional drugs be added. This may be a biologic response agent or hydroxychloroquine, sulfasalazine, or leflunomide. A study published in 2005 revealed that combination therapy started early was the best approach rather than switching sequentially from one drug to another or even starting with methotrexate and then combining it with other agents as necessary. The best approach—starting right at the outset with combination of methotrexate and sulfasalazine or of methotrexate with infliximab—was demonstrated by radiographic assessment 2 years later.

New Drugs in Clinical Trials

There are several monoclonal antibodies that are in various phases of clinical trials.[9] Certolizumab pegal and golimumab are close to full regulatory approval as of this writing. Both are administered every 4 weeks and demonstrate similar efficacy to the other TNF inhibitors. Tocilizumab is a humanized monoclonal antibody to the IL-6 receptor, and ocrelizumab is a monoclonal antibody to the CD_{20} on B cells. It is hoped that this last agent will reduce the number of infusion reactions compared with rituximab.

DRUG TREATMENT OF GOUT

Gout is a metabolic disorder in which the plasma urate concentration is elevated because of overproduction (hyperuricemia), deficient elimination, or a combination of the two.[40] Uric acid is produced by the degradation of purine-containing compounds such as nucleic acids, and the level tends to increase with age. Hyperuricemia is defined as a plasma level of more than 7.0 mg/dL in men and more than 6.0 mg/dL in women.[41] Hyperuricemia by itself does not always lead to gout; however, hyperuricemia is a necessary factor in the development of gout.

Gout tends to be more common in men in their thirties and forties and also in postmenopausal women. It is associated with cardiovascular disease, alcoholism, obesity, hypertriglyceridemia, and insulin resistance; and it is also seen in patients with renal insufficiency. Elevated uric acid production is responsible for approximately 10% of cases of gout, which can be associated with an inherited enzyme deficiency or a myeloproliferative disorder. In the remaining 90% of cases, patients appear to have diminished urinary excretion of uric acid. Treatment with some drugs—including the thiazide diuretics, angiotensin receptor blockers, and cyclosporine (used to prevent transplant rejection)—is also associated with a greater risk of developing gout because these drugs are thought to interfere with the kidneys' ability to excrete urate.[42,43] High doses of aspirin appear to be uricosuric, but low doses cause uric acid retention. In fact, low-dose aspirin produces significant changes in renal function in patients with no known renal disease. Given the widespread use of low-dose aspirin for cardiac protection, it is recommended that health care providers become alert to the signs and symptoms of gout.

The clinical manifestations of gout include intermittent bouts of acute monoarthritis produced by the deposition of crystals of sodium urate in the joint synovial fluid or a tophus (a nodular or needle-shaped bundle of urate crystals in the soft tissue).[41] The classic presentation is arthritis of the first metatarsophalangeal joint, but it can occur at the knee and even inside the carpal canal, producing carpal tunnel syndrome.[44] The onset of the arthritis is often rapid; and the affected joint becomes warm, erythematous, painful, and swollen. Monoarthritis is the most common form, but a patient, especially an older adult, may present with involvement of several of the proximal interphalangeal and distal interphalangeal joints of the hand. The result is an inflammatory response involving the synthesis and activation of lipoxygenase products and the migration of neutrophils to the area. The crystals become engulfed by phagocytosis, producing tissue damage and release of proteolytic enzymes. Patients may also have systemic involvement such as symptoms associated with uric acid kidney stones (urolithiasis).

Management of gout involves treating the arthritic inflammation and urolithiasis, if present, and also lowering uric acid levels to prevent exacerbations.[45] Drugs used are those that inhibit uric acid synthesis, increase uric acid excretion, inhibit migration of white cells into the joints, and reduce inflammation (Box 12-2).

Treatment of Acute Gout

NSAIDs can be very effective in reducing the symptoms of acute gout. Indomethacin is the most common drug used, but there is little evidence that one NSAID is better than another.[41] Because gout is related to worsening renal function, caution should be used when these drugs are prescribed, particularly for older adults. Cyclooxygenase-2 (COX-2) inhibitors might be quite effective in this disorder because COX-2 has also been implicated in crystal formation.[45,46] Opioids are frequently prescribed for pain relief. Corticosteroids are also effective in acute gout, especially if patients do not respond to the NSAIDs or to colchicine (see below).

BOX 12-2 Drugs for the Treatment of Gout

Treatment of Acute Gout
NSAIDS (indomethacin)
Colchicine
Corticosteroids

Treatment of Chronic Gout
Allopurinal (Zyloprim)
Probenecid
Sulfinpyrasone (Anturane)

Colchicine is an old drug but one that is still found to be quite effective in reducing the symptoms of gout. In a placebo-controlled trial, two thirds of patients in the colchicine group experienced improvement within 48 hours, compared with only one third in the placebo group.[47] The drug prevents migration of neutrophils by binding to tubulin (a major protein that helps form the intracellular skeleton of the mitotic spindle), impairing the cells' ability to achieve chemotaxis and thus decrease phagocytosis. Colchicine may also inhibit crystal-induced COX-2 expression. It is administered by the oral route every 1 to 2 hours until pain subsides or a specific maximal dose is reached. Its use is primarily limited by GI adverse effects, including severe diarrhea, nausea, and vomiting, which begin before the acute gouty symptoms are relieved. Large doses may also produce GI hemorrhage and kidney damage. After an acute bout of gout, colchicine may be used at low doses along with some of the other preventive agents to prevent flare-ups. However, long-term use has been associated with bone marrow depression, renal failure, and even rhabdomyolysis and polyneuropathy.[48] In cases in which patients do not respond to NSAIDs or colchicine or the adverse effects of this therapy cannot be tolerated, good alternatives include oral prednisone and intravenous or intra-articular steroids.[49]

Long-Term Treatment of Gout

Drugs used to treat chronic gout or to prevent recurrence include medications that lower blood uric acid levels. The uricosuric agents (probenecid and sulfinpyrazone) increase excretion of uric acid by the kidneys. They block the reabsorption of filtered uric acid in the renal tubules, leading to increased clearance. They are most effective in patients whose urine contains only small amounts of uric acid and in those who have good renal function. They are not helpful for the treatment of acute gout attacks and should not be administered until the acute attack subsides. The most common adverse effects of these drugs are rash and GI discomfort. Another limitation of these drugs is that they should not be taken concurrently with doses of aspirin greater than 325 mg/day because salicylates interfere with their uricosuric effects. However, low-dose aspirin is acceptable as long as patients are counseled to stay away from other aspirin-containing products.[50] Lastly, sufficient hydration is imperative, particularly during intensive exercise sessions.

Allopurinol represents another approach to the long-term management of gout.[40] This drug inhibits uric acid synthesis by blocking the enzyme xanthine oxidase, which controls the last two steps in purine metabolism (conversion of adenine or guanine to uric acid). This drug tends to be more effective in patients whose urine contains large amounts of uric acid, indicating excessive production.[51] Like the uricosuric agents, allopurinol is not helpful during acute attacks, and if administration is started during this time, it may actually prolong the attack. However, allopurinol is quite helpful in preventing future attacks and kidney stones. Adverse effects are usually minor and include headaches, heartburn, and diarrhea. However, it can produce a number of drug interactions, most significantly inactivation of oral anticoagulants. Patients taking allopurinol must undergo frequent monitoring of their blood coagulability with international normalized ratio (INR).

The uricosuric agents sulfinpyrazone and probenecid are drugs that block reabsorption of uric acid.[52] They are used in patients who underexcrete uric acid but who have normal renal function. Frequent monitoring of renal function is necessary, and the drugs should be stopped if nephrolithiasis occurs. In addition, surprisingly the angiotensin-converting enzyme (ACE) inhibitor losartan, vitamin C, and fenofibrate all act as uricosuric agents.

Although the choice of drugs for the treatment of gout is clear, the correct time to start administration of urate-lowering drugs is controversial.[42] Some physicians recommend starting therapy only in patients who experience more than four flare-ups per year. Others recommend earlier treatment, believing that it is more cost-effective to treat patients who have only had two attacks per year. Complicating the decision is the fact that gout is not always a progressive problem and patients with hyperuricemia do not always have gout. Instead, a trial of nonpharmacologic management, reducing alcohol, meat, and seafood (anchovies, herring) consumption, as well as reducing weight may be useful.[53] Many unanswered questions regarding the treatment of this disease remain, for example, how low plasma urate levels should be, how long patients should be treated with urate-lowering drugs, and whether intermittent use of the drugs is equal in effectiveness to continuous use.

DRUG TREATMENT OF SYSTEMIC LUPUS ERYTHEMATOSUS

Systemic lupus erythematosus (SLE) is an autoimmune disease affecting a variety of organs.[54] Constitutional symptoms such as fever, weight loss, and fatigue are common, as are a number of other clinical manifestations affecting the skin, joints, kidneys, heart, and vascular and nervous systems (Box 12-3).

The immunologic dysfunction includes the development of antinuclear antibodies to components of the cell nucleus, particularly to double-stranded DNA.[55] This disorder promotes B-cell activity to both self-antigens and foreign antigens. Normally, B lymphocytes provide help to T cells, produce cytokines, trigger antigen-induced production of immunoglobulin antibodies, and act as memory cells awaiting antigen re-exposure.[56] However, in SLE, B lymphocytes provide help to the autoreactive T cells; induce production of autoantibodies, creating destructive immune complexes; and undergo clonal proliferation. The direct infiltration of these immune complexes into the kidneys, joints, liver, and other organs leads to the destruction of tissue and the development of clinical symptoms.

BOX 12-3 Clinical Presentation of Systemic Lupus Erythematosus by System

System	Presentation
Musculoskeletal	Arthritis of small joint of the hand and wrist but without joint erosions
Skin and mucosal surfaces	Photosensitivity
	Malar or butterfly rash (30%)
	Discoid lesions (raised, erythematous plaques on face, scalp, and neck)
	Papulosquamous rash on trunk
	Diffuse alopecia
	Oral ulcers (40%)
	Raynaud's phenomenon
Neuropsychiatric	Cognitive dysfunction
	Mood disorder
	Headaches
	Cerebrovascular accident
	Autonomic neuropathy
	Peripheral neuropathy
Renal	Glomerulonephritis
	Interstitial nephritis
Cardiovascular	Valvular heart disease
	Coronary artery disease
	Vasculitis
	Pericarditis
Pulmonary	Pleuritis
	Acute pneumonitis
Gastrointestinal	Peritonitis
	Hepatitis
	Pancreatitis
Hematologic	Anemia
	Leukopenia
	Thrombocytopenia

Treatment of SLE involves a combination of anti-inflammatory and immunosuppressive drugs, and even some chemotherapy agents. The appropriate medication depends on the particular array of symptoms, organ involvement, and severity of disease (Table 12-2).

Treatment of Mild to Moderate Systemic Lupus Erythematosus

In patients with mild to moderate SLE without major organ involvement, treatment tends to be a combination of NSAIDs, corticosteroids, and the antimalarial agent

TABLE 12-2 Drugs Utilized for Specific Symptoms of Systemic Lupus Erythematosus

Drug	Constitutional Symptoms	Cutaneous Symptoms	Musculoskeletal Symptoms	Organ Damage
NSAIDs	X		X	
Corticosteroids				
Topical		X		
Low dose	X	X	X	
High dose				X
Antimalarials	X	X	X	
Dapsone		X		
Hydroxychloroquine		X		
Retinoids		X		
Immunosuppressive				
Azathioprine	X	X	X	X
Cyclophosphamide				X
MMF (Cellcept)				X
Methotrexate			X	X
TNF-α agents		X		
Rituximab	X		X	X
Danazol (Danocrine)				X

NSAIDs, nonsteroidal anti-inflammatory drugs; *MMF*, Mycophenolate mofetil; *TNF*, tumor necrosis factor.

hydroxychloroquine.[54] NSAIDS are quite helpful in reducing the pain and inflammation associated with arthritis and arthralgias, and they are useful in combating SLE-induced fevers.

Acute inflammation in the skin and joints may be treated with steroids. Options include topical creams for inflammatory rashes and low-dose oral steroids for immune modulation. Prednisone is the preferred oral agent because it is available in small doses that allow for convenient titration if symptoms progress.

Hydroxychloroquine has also been shown to be effective for the skin lesions and arthritis.[57] This drug can also reduce fatigue and prevent more serious flare-ups of the disease. A placebo-controlled trial that examined the effect of discontinuing hydroxychloroquine in stable SLE demonstrated that flare-ups were 2.5 times more frequent in the group that discontinued the drug.[58] Methotrexate and leflunomide are two other drugs that can be used to treat moderate SLE.

Treatment of Severe Systemic Lupus Erythematosus

Patients with major organ involvement such as glomerulonephritis, pneumonitis, neurologic disease, or hematologic disorders are considered to have severe disease. Prompt treatment is necessary to prevent death or long-term organ damage. Initial therapy involves high-dose corticosteroids, usually administered intravenously. Other immunosuppressive medications—including cyclophosphamide, methotrexate, azathioprine, and mycophenolate mofetil—can be added.

Cyclophosphamide might be the most effective agent at this time for treating severe SLE, particularly when there is coexisting lupus nephritis.[59] It is a chemotherapy agent that covalently binds to nucleic acids with an alkyl group (saturated carbon atoms). The drug may bind to one or both strands of DNA, producing cross-linkages between the strands. Essentially, this inhibits the activation of inflammatory cell division. High-dose cyclophosphamide induces maximal immunosuppression. It is also quite useful to treat lupus nephritis. In a small study of 14 patients with refractory SLE, high-dose cyclophosphamide was shown to achieve a complete response in five patients and a partial response in six patients.[60] Outcomes were defined by using the Responder Index for Lupus Erythematosus (RIFLE). At follow-up 32 months later, the five complete responders continued to be free of disease, and the partial responders had their symptoms controlled with drugs that were previously ineffective for them. Although the authors of this study reported that the treatment was well tolerated, cyclophosphamide has some very serious adverse effects. In addition to alopecia, nausea, vomiting, diarrhea, and bone marrow depression, it produces hemorrhagic cystitis, which leads to bladder fibrosis. The toxic metabolite acrolein is eliminated in the urine, but not before it has done damage. In this study, the patients were well hydrated, and they also received intravenous (IV) injections of MESNA (sodium 2-mercaptoethane sulfonate) to help inactivate these toxic compounds. MESNA binds to the irritant metabolites in the bladder to prevent cystitis. It was given intravenously 30 minutes before cyclophosphamide and again at 3, 6, and 8 hours after the alkylating agent was administered. In addition, patients received IV ondansetron to prevent nausea and antibiotics, antivirals, and antifungal agents to prevent infection until their white blood cell counts returned to safe levels, aided by granulocyte cell-stimulating factors (see Chapter 23). In another study in which high-dose treatment with cyclophosphamide was compared with a low-dose regimen, little difference in the percentage of responders was found, but the high-dose group experienced a significantly greater number of severe infections.[61]

In addition to these adverse effects, there are also concerns of effects on fertility, mutagenesis and carcinogeneis, and wound healing. Treatment with this agent is quite involved and requires tremendous cooperation from the patient. A complete blood count (CBC) should be performed every 1 to 2 weeks until the patient is stable on the drug and then at monthly intervals thereafter. Patients remain on the drug for extended periods, although the dose is "pulsed," that is, given first at monthly intervals and then quarterly.

Other immunosuppressive agents are currently available for the treatment of SLE. Mycophenolate mofetil (MMF) was found to be as effective for SLE nephritis as prednisone combined with cyclophosphamide.[62] It has been reserved for use in cyclophosphamide-resistant patients. Common adverse effects include constipation or diarrhea, nausea, vomiting, and headaches. More serious reactions include hypertension, GI hemorrhage, leukopenia, myelosuppression, infections, lymphoma, mental status changes, and peripheral edema. In milder degrees of organ involvements, azathioprine may be used. Again, it is an immunosuppressive agent that is much safer in low doses for mild disease than is cyclophosphamide. This drug is often used as maintenance therapy. Recent studies evaluating the effectiveness of cyclophosphamide, mycophenolate mofetil, and azathioprine show equal effectiveness in the maintenance phase after acute treatment with cyclophosphamide.[63] A hope for the future may lie with the newly synthesized biologic agents. Rituximab is engineered to target activated mature B lymphocytes.[56] Because these B cells are implicated in the pathogenesis of SLE, anti–B-cell therapy may hold some promise for this disease. Currently, this drug has been studied on patients who have failed conventional immunosuppressive treatment. The studies are small, but nevertheless these patients have shown considerable improvement in both laboratory results and symptomotology.[64,65]

Danazol is a steroid that is derived from ethisterone. It decreases the hypothalamic–pituitary response to decreased estrogen production and has been used in the treatment of endometriosis and fibrocystic breast disease. It also is used in SLE to treat hemolytic anemia. Compared with corticosteroids and immunosuppressive agents, when used for hemolytic problems, it is least likely to be abandoned due to adverse effects.[66] Adverse effects include edema, acne, hirsutism, weight gain, and abnormal menstruation.

Drug Treatment for the Cutaneous Signs of Systemic Lupus Erythematosus

Approximately 80% of patients with SLE experience skin and mucous membrane involvement. SLE is associated with many types of skin conditions, including alopecia, urticaria, Raynaud's phenomenon, and vasculitis as well as the more common discoid and malar rash. The goal of therapy is to prevent pigment changes and scarring. Some of these rashes may be treated or at least avoided with some preventive measures such as limiting sun exposure, use of sun block, and wearing light sun-blocking clothes. Once the rashes develop, treatment with topical corticosteroids is beneficial.[66] Application of 1% hydrocortisone twice a day is effective and safe. More potent topical steroids such as 0.1% triamcinolone may also be indicated, especially for discoid lesions. Hydroxychloroquine has been used for cutaneous lesions, although few studies support this use. For severe skin lesions, either systemic corticosteroids or immunosuppressive agents are indicated.

Therapeutic Concerns about Drugs for Systemic Lupus Erythematosus

Because disease-modifying therapy for SLE consists largely of immunosuppressive agents, treatment for SLE carries significant risks of infection.[67] Patients with SLE appear to have a propensity for infection, so special concern is warranted when this factor is combined with treatment with cyclophosphamide and high-dose steroids. Bacterial infections account for the majority of infections in SLE, greater than 80%. The most common infections are with *Staphylococcus aureus*, *S. pyogenes*, *S. pneumoniae*, and *Escherichia coli*. Clinical presentations vary from full-blown sepsis to soft-tissue infection. Tissues most affected include lung, sinus, skin, and bone tissues. The most common viral infection is herpes zoster, and fungal infections are most commonly caused by the *Candida* species.

Therapists should regularly monitor the skin and soft tissue of their patients who are receiving immunosuppressive therapy and should look for reddened and warm areas. In addition, patients should be instructed to report low-grade fever. Equipment should be kept clean, and patients should be isolated from anyone who might be infectious.

Another concern for patients with SLE is exposure to ultraviolet A (UV-A) and UV-B sun rays.[59,68] It has been determined that both forms of sunlight are harmful to patients with SLE because these rays induce inflammatory events in which local lymphocyte activation occurs. Other drugs such as the thiazide diuretics, neuroleptics, and tetracyclines also cause photosensitivity that may compound this problem in patients with SLE. Patients should wear sun-protective clothing and use broad-spectrum sunscreens frequently, as mentioned above. The optimal sunscreen should contain titanium dioxide or zinc oxide and UV-A absorbers such as Parsol 1789 or Mexoryl-SX. Common sense dictates that UV light therapy is contraindicated for these patients. However, studies have indicated that phototherapy has some benefit for both cutaneous and systemic lupus erythematosus.[69] The underlying mechanism of action is unknown, but studies to determine it are ongoing. For now, UV therapy should be avoided in patients with SLE.

Drug-Induced Rheumatic Syndromes

Many new and older drugs have resulted in a drug-induced rheumatic syndrome.[70] For a diagnosis of a drug-related syndrome, a patient must have been exposed to the drug, exhibit clinical and laboratory evidence of the syndrome without having a history of the syndrome, and demonstrate rapid improvement in symptoms and laboratory values after discontinuation of the drug. Specifically, drug-induced rheumatic syndromes include SLE, vasculitis, scleroderma, and myositis.

Currently, more than 80 drugs are associated with development of SLE.[70] One of the more recently implicated drugs is minocycline, a tetracycline antibiotic used to treat acne. A recent prospective study included 20 patients with minocycline-induced SLE with arthritis, a positive antinuclear antibody titer, and at least one other symptom of SLE.[71] By the sixteenth week after drug discontinuation, all symptoms resolved. Similar situations have occurred with etanercept and sulfasalazine, both used in the treatment of rheumatoid arthritis (RA).[72]

Other commonly used drugs implicated in SLE include lisinopril, an ACE inhibitor, and simvastatin, a cholesterol-lowering drug.[70] Fosinopril, another ACE inhibitor, has also been implicated in drug-induced scleroderma, and the statin drugs are associated with drug-induced myositis.

DRUG TREATMENT OF OSTEOARTHRITIS

Osteoarthritis is the most frequently diagnosed chronic medical condition.[73,74] It is responsible for 40 to 60% of degenerative states of the musculoskeletal system. It is characterized by cartilage degeneration, subchondral bone thickening, osteophytes, and bone cysts. Usually, the weight-bearing joints of the legs are affected, but osteoarthritis can also occur in the smaller joints of the hands and in the spine. These anatomic changes result in gradual development of joint pain, stiffness, and loss of range of motion (ROM).

Pathophysiology of Osteoarthritis

The common prevailing theory on osteoarthritis is that this disease reflects the aging process, meaning that repetitive use of joints results in cartilage erosion.[75] However, recent studies have introduced another explanation for this condition, describing osteoarthritis as a complex interaction of genetic, mechanical, and biologic factors.[76] In addition, it is no longer thought to just involve the cartilage but also involves the subchondral bone, menisci, ligaments, periarticular muscle, capsule, and synovium.

Normal articular cartilage can absorb shock and reduce friction at the joint surfaces.[74] Collagen fibers provide the strength to counter the shear forces during movement. Within this network of fibers are proteoglycans made of glycosaminoglycans (GAGs) attached to protein chains. The principal GAGs of cartilage are chondroitin sulfate and keratin sulfate. These give the cartilage its elasticity and ability to resist compression through their fluid-absorbing abilities. Under pressure, the fluid is squeezed out, providing hydrostatic lubrication. As the cartilage ages, it loses fluid; the proteins become fragmented; and the levels of chondroitin sulfate, keratin sulfate, and hyaluronic acid change, but the cartilage retains most of its functions. It is important to realize that articular cartilage lacks blood supply and therefore gains it nutrients from the synovial fluid. It is also devoid of nerve innervations and lymphatic drainage.

In contrast, in osteoarthritis, the cartilage has an increase in fluid content and normal proteins; but the levels of GAGs, hyaluronic acid, and keratin sulfate decrease. The balance between cartilage synthesis and degradation is disrupted, and the structural properties of the collagen change. The chondrocytes, which are initially stimulated to repair the damage, also produce cytokines such as IL-1β and TNF-α, which are proinflammatory. The chondrocytes themselves produce abnormal types of collagen and increase their synthesis of proteinases, specifically matrix metalloproteinases (MMPs), causing the breakdown of proteoglycans.

Another area of study is the role of bone, especially subchondral bone in the development of osteoarthritis.[77,78] The progression of cartilage degeneration is associated with intensive remodeling of the subchondral bone. New bone synthesis—as evidenced by higher osteopontin (a bone-specific matrix protein) levels and elevated alkaline phosphatase levels—occurs. Both osteopontin and alkaline phosphatase are produced by the osteoblast. Proinflammatory cytokines (IL-1β, IL-6, prostaglandin E_2, and leukotriene B_4) are also products of the dysfunctional osteoblast.[79] IL-1β and IL-6 promote matrix degradation as a result of their activation of the MMPs. Prostaglandin E_2 stimulates bone formation at low concentrations but inhibits it as the concentration increases. Leukotrienes activate the osteoclasts. It is theorized that these cytokines run through the bone–cartilage interface to activate cartilage breakdown through channels and fissures. Thus the subchondral bone changes and cartilage destruction mirror each other, with the cytokines being the go-between. It is unclear, however, whether the changes in the subchondral bone precede the changes in the cartilage. There is evidence of thickening of the subchondral cortical plate prior to changes in the cartilage. Increased thickness and stiffening of this area reduce its ability to absorb energy, thus placing more strain on the articular cartilage. Eventually, the cartilage erodes, and the bones directly contact each other.

Therapeutics for Osteoarthritis

Aspirin, NSAIDs, and acetaminophen are the main treatments offered to reduce pain in osteoarthritis. However, given the fact that these drugs neither actually alter pathogenesis nor repair the damage already present, there is new interest in viscosupplementation as well as in drugs that may repair damaged cartilage.

Aspirin and Acetaminophen. The primary treatments for osteoarthritic pain are acetaminophen and NSAIDs. Acetaminophen has been the drug preferred by physicians, as evidenced by a decline in NSAID use from 1989 to 1998.[80] The reason for this decline has been the recognition by physicians of the adverse cardiac and renal effects of the NSAIDs, particularly in older adults. This decline has been met with an increase in acetaminophen use, although to reach the same level of effective pain relief as the NSAIDs, regular dosing of up to 4 g/day may be necessary.[74] However, several studies have shown that acetaminophen is not as effective in reducing pain as are the NSAIDs, even at a dosage of 4 g/day.[81,82] In a small study of seven patients with osteoarthritis, in which a crossover design was used, NSAIDs and acetaminophen were each favored by one patient, whereas five patients reported experiencing no difference between the two treatments. These five subjects went on to take acetaminophen, but 3 months later, they had all switched to an NSAID for greater effectiveness.

Hyaluronan. Viscosupplementation is a relatively new treatment option for patients with osteoarthritis of the knee. This procedure involves injecting into the knee joint a derivative of hyaluronan, a component of the synovial fluid responsible for its lubrication properties. Animal studies have suggested that hyaluronic acid may promote bovine cartilage growth, and although they may alleviate pain in humans, there is no evidence that they alter disease progression.[83] The U.S. Food and Drug Administration (FDA) has approved three hyaluronan derivatives: two containing sodium hyaluronate (Hyalgan and Supartz), which are injected once a week for 5 weeks; and Hylan G-F 20 (Synvisc), which is injected three times with 1 week between injections. This is a costly treatment resulting in only modest improvements.[84,85] Some patients experience only a slight reduction in pain compared with placebo injections or use of oral naproxen. In addition, there is no overall effect on joint space width.[86,87] Adverse effects include pain at the injection site, swelling, and a rash that dissipates in time.

Glucosamine and Chondroitin Sulfates. More than 250 years ago, a British naval surgeon designed the first controlled, prospective, clinical experiment in which lemons and oranges were used to cure scurvy.[88] This led to the recognition that dietary deficiencies can cause disease. Out of this research was born the belief that eating cartilage or its component molecules rebuilds joints and prevents arthritis. However, for years, knowledgeable scientists have refuted claims made by the dietary food industry that glucosamine and chondroitin can relieve the pain of osteoarthritis, stimulate proteoglycan synthesis in articular cartilage and hyaluronan synthesis in synovial tissue, and also decrease cartilage degradation. Neither glucosamine nor chondroitin is approved by the FDA; rather, both are considered dietary supplements. This has led to their widespread use by the public in spite of lack of rigorous scientific documentation of their effectiveness. However, recently, several well-conducted studies have demonstrated that glucosamine and chondroitin might be effective not just in terms of reducing pain but also in preventing the progression of the disease.[89]

Glucosamine is an aminosaccharide that acts as a basic constituent and building block for the synthesis of the glycosaminoglycans and proteoglycans in the cartilage matrix and synovial fluid, particularly the proteoglycan aggrecans, a matrix structural protein.[90,91] Aggrecans plays an essential role in maintaining the health of cartilage by regulating its fluid content.[92] In vitro studies show that glucosamine appears to stimulate cartilage cells to synthesize aggrecans and to reduce MMPs.[92,93] In has been shown in animal studies that oral glucosamine has a beneficial effect on immune-mediated arthritis. Chondroitin is a glycosaminoglycan that is found in articular cartilage, bone, skin, ligaments, and tendons. Along with aggrecans, it plays a role in creating an osmotic pressure that expands the cartilage matrix. In animal studies, chondroitin has been reported to maintain joint viscosity, stimulate cartilage repair, and inhibit the enzymes involved in cartilage degradation. However, some sources indicate that the chondroitin molecule is too large to enter the synovium.

Human studies, of varying lengths from 4 weeks to 3 years, in which glucosamine was primarily used, with chondroitin added for some of the trials, demonstrated beneficial effects for patients with mild to moderate osteoarthritis, primarily of the knee.[94] Outcome measures used in many of the studies included measures of pain (visual analog scale during walking), joint space narrowing shown on plain radiographs, and the Western Ontario and McMaster Universities (WOMAC) Osteoarthritis Index Pain Subscale. One study, in particular, was a double-blind trial, in which 212 patients were treated with either 1500 mg of glucosamine or placebo, once daily for 3 years.[95] The treated group demonstrated a 20 to 25% reduction in symptoms on the WOMAC Osteoarthritis Index Pain Subscale, whereas the placebo group showed a slight worsening of symptoms. Careful measurements of joint space narrowing with fluoroscopy to correct lower limb positioning and X-ray beam alignment showed no average loss of joint space in the patients receiving glucosamine, but those receiving placebo had significant changes detected on X-ray films. Similar numbers of patients in the two groups took at least one dose of a "rescue drug," either acetaminophen or an NSAID. Consumption of these drugs was inconsistent between the groups and also within each group. Adverse effects were similar in both groups and were no more serious than GI complaints of abdominal pain and diarrhea. Routine laboratory tests did not show any abnormalities in either group, and there was no change in glucose tolerance.

Perhaps the most definitive trial on glucosamine was the Glucosamine/Chondroitin Arthritis Intervention Trial (GAIT) sponsored by the National Institutes of Health (NIH).[96] This was a 2-year, double-blind, placebo-controlled trial conducted at multiple sites. Patients received either glucosamine 500 mg three times per day, chondroitin sulfate 400 mg three times per day, celecoxib 200 mg daily, or placebo. The main outcome measure was medial tibiofemoral joint space width (JSW), which was measured at baseline, at 12 months, and at 24 months. The supplements were manufactured specifically for this study, since the researchers were unable to locate a consistent amount of the active ingredient. This guaranteed that all subjects received the same amount of active drug. The results were disappointing to the proponents of this therapy. At 2 years, none of the treatment groups were significantly different from the placebo group. However, all the groups lost less JSW than predicted. The study authors recommended that future studies include a more structural knee evaluation, longer duration, and stratification by severity of arthritis to determine if mild or moderate osteoarthritis might respond better.

Intra-articular Corticosteroids. Triamcinolone acetonide (kenalog) and methylprednisolone acetate (Depo-Medrol) are the two most common injectable corticosteroids.[97] Often they are mixed with lidocaine or bupivacaine to reduce pain immediately, especially since the steroid takes 24 to 48 hours to work. Adverse effects include post-injection flare-up of pain—induced by the crystalline composition of the solution—that may last 48 hours, as well as atrophy of tissues, including those of the skin and tendons. Typically, these injections are used only on patients with very painful and edematous joints, and no more than four injections are given per year per joint. Depending on the severity of the joint problem, relief of pain and improved function may last for 1 week or more.

Topical Agents. Topical NSAIDs, particularly diclofenac (Voltaren Gel), has been shown to reduce pain for the short term. Since there is less systemic absorption with topical agents, there is less GI and renal toxicity.[98] However, there has been little interest in the study of topical NSAIDs, so further studies are necessary, especially comparison trials with oral NSAIDs. This drug may be a good alternative to the oral agents in patients with a history of acid reflux, GI bleed, and ulcer.

Capsaicin is derived from the hot chili pepper plant.[97] It appears to decrease pain by the depletion of substance P from local neurons. It is applied to the skin in small amounts following the application of topical anesthetic agents, since it produces a burning sensation and if too much of it is applied, it may cause skin irritation. Great care must be taken to avoid contact with eyes, nose, mouth, as severe burning may result.

Future Agents to Control the Osteoarthritic Process

As discussed previously, the pharmacologic management of osteoarthritis has been mainly symptomatic, with little emphasis placed on the biologic factors that lead to joint degradation. In part, this has been due to inadequate outcome measures that make it difficult to document efficacy. Pain and functional assessment have been used for symptom-modifying drugs, but JSW assessed by plain radiographs has been used for structure-modifying agents. This standard measurement for joint space does not give us any information on the cartilage itself because it is not imaged. Newer techniques in magnetic resonance imaging (MRI) now allow adequate visualization of the joint structures, particularly the cartilage and its pathologic progress.[64] Some new quantitative measurements (assessment of cartilage volume) may be obtained, allowing specific, sensitive, and valid assessment of the progression of the disease. Incorporation of these outcome measurements into the research is the key to identifying possible structure-modifying agents for osteoarthritis.

Other advances in pharmacotherapy for osteoarthritis include the discovery of an IL-1β receptor antagonist and an IL-1β–converting enzyme blocker, both of which can be used to reduce several different cartilage breakdown processes.[74] The IL-1β–converting enzyme inhibitor is in clinical trials and is responsible for blocking the conversion of IL-1β into its mature form. Research is also being conducted on finding agents to block the activity of MMPs. Efforts are directed toward inhibiting their synthesis or blocking the conversion of the pro-MMPs into active MMPs. In addition, inhibition of the intracellular signaling pathways that signal the cell to produce MMPs is another attractive target. Another interesting route under study in osteoarthritis has to do with the activation of inflammation by nitric oxide (NO).[99,100] NO and its byproducts are capable of inducing tissue damage and may cause chondrocyte death. NO is also capable of increasing the activity of COX-2. In fact, a selective inhibitor of NO synthase showed a significant reduction in the severity of cartilage lesions in dogs. The mechanism of action appears to be the ability of the inhibitor to reduce IL-1β and MMP levels and also to reduce chondrocyte death. Lastly, licofelone, a new COX and lipoxygenase inhibitor, has been found to block the production of leukotriene B_4 and prostaglandin E_2, as well as several biomarkers seen in osteoarthritis.[97,101]

ACTIVITIES 12

1. Review some of the literature presented in this chapter for outcome measures that are used to determine drug efficacy in rheumatoid arthritis (RA). Indicate which ones might be useful in determining the effectiveness of a rehabilitative intervention.
2. Interview a patient with RA regarding drugs he or she has taken since the diagnosis was made. List the drugs, and indicate the length of time they were administered, adverse effects, and the impact the drugs had on disease progression. In addition, indicate the reason for discontinuing the drugs.
3. What steps can be taken to minimize the deleterious effects of corticosteroids?

REFERENCES

1. Gabriel SE, Crowson SC, Kremers HM: Survival in rheumatoid arthritis: a population based analysis of trends over 40 years. Arthritis Rheum 48:54-58, 2003.
2. Nicolo PJ, Maradit-Kremers H, Roger VL: The risk of congestive heart failure in rheumatoid arthritis: a population based study over 46 years. Arthritis Rheum 52:412-420, 2005.
3. Fox DA: Cytokine blockade as a new strategy to treat rheumatoid arthritis: Inhibition of tumor necrosis factor. Arch Intern Med 160:437-444, 2000.
4. Pincus T, Callahan LF: The 'side effects' of rheumatoid arthritis: joint destruction, disability and early mortality. Br J Rheumatol 32([suppl 1]):28-37, 1993.
5. Wells BG, DiPiro JT, Schwinghammer TL: Pharmacotherapy handbook (5th ed.), New York, 2003, McGraw Hill.
6. Arnett FC, Edworthy SM, Bloch DA, et al: The American Rheumatism Association 1987 revised criteria for the classification of rheumatoid arthritis Arthritis Rheum 31(3): 315-324, 1988.
7. van der Helm-van Mil AH, Verpoort KN, Breedveld FC, Toes RE, Huizinga TW: Antibodies to citrullinated proteins and differences in clinical progression of rheumatoid arthritis. Arthritis Res Ther 7(5):R949-R958, 2005.
8. Day, R, et al:, Connective tissue and bone disorders. In Carruthers SG, Hoffman B, Melmon K, Nierenberg DW, editors: Melmon and Morrelli's clinical pharmacology, New York, 2000, McGraw Hill.
9. Keating, RM, Rheumatoid arthritis. In Waldman SA, Terzic A, editors: Pharmacology and therapeutics: Principles to practice, Philadelphia, 2009, Saunders.
10. Sattar N, McCarey DW, Capell H, McInnes IB: Explaining how "high-grade" systemic inflammation accelerates vascular risk in rheumatoid arthritis. Circulation 108(24):2957-2963, 2003.
11. del Rincon I, Escalante A: Atherosclerotic cardiovascular disease in rheumatoid arthritis. Curr Rheumatol Rep 5(4): 278-286, 2003.
12. Redlich K, Schett G, Steiner G, Hayer S, Wagner EF, Smolen JS: Rheumatoid arthritis therapy after tumor necrosis factor and interleukin-1 blockade. Arthritis Rheum 48(12):3308-3319, 2003.
13. Gotzsche PC, Johansen HK: Short-term low-dose corticosteroids vs placebo and nonsteroidal antiinflammatory drugs in rheumatoid arthritis. Cochrane Database Syst Rev 2 (CD000189), 2001.
14. Buckbinder L, Robinson RP: The glucocorticoid receptor: molecular mechanism and new therapeutic opportunities. Curr Drug Targets Inflamm Allergy 1(2):127-136, 2002.
15. Mauras N: Growth hormone therapy in the glucocorticosteroid-dependent child: Metabolic and linear growth effects. Horm Res 56(suppl 1):13-18, 2001.
16. van Everdingen AA, Jacobs JW, Siewertsz Van Reesema DR, Bijlsma JW: Low-dose prednisone therapy for patients with early active rheumatoid arthritis: Clinical efficacy, disease-modifying properties, and side effects: A randomized, double-blind, placebo-controlled clinical trial. Ann Intern Med 136(1):1-12, 2002.
17. Conn, DL, Lim SS: New role for an old friend: prednisone is a disease-modifying agent in early rheumatoid arthritis. Curr Opin Rheumatol 15(3):193-196, 2003.
18. Rodenburg RJ, Ganga A, Van Lent PL: The anti-inflammatory drug sulfasalazine inhibits tumor necrosis factor alpha expression in macrophages by inducing apoptosis. Arthritis Rheum 43:1941-1950, 2000.
19. American College of Rheumatology Subcommittee on Rheumatoid Arthritis Guidelines: Guidelines for the management of rheumatoid arthritis: 2002. update. Arthritis Rheum 46(2):328-346, 2002.
20. Furst DE, Ulrich RW: Nonsteroidal anti-inflammatory drugs, disease-modifying antirheumatic drugs, nonopioid analgesics, & drugs used in gout. In Katzung BG, editor: Basic and clinical pharmacology, New York, 2007, McGraw-Hill.
21. Abramowicz M, editor: Drugs for rheumatoid arthritis. In Treatment guidelines from the medical letter (Vol. 1[5]), New Rochelle, NY, 2003, The Medical Letter, Inc.
22. Weinblatt ME: Rheumatoid arthritis: Treat now, not later. Ann Intern Med 124:773-774, 1996.
23. Choi HK, Hernán MA, Seeger JD, Robins JM, Wolfe F: Methotrexate and mortality in patients with rheumatoid arthritis: A prospective study. Lancet 359(9313):1173-1177, 2002.
24. Landewé RB, Boers M, Verhoeven AC, et al: COBRA combination therapy in patients with early rheumatoid arthritis: Long-term structural benefits of a brief intervention. Arthritis Rheum 46(2):347-356, 2002.
25. Fox RI, Herrmann ML, Frangou CG, et al: Mechanism of action for leflunomide in rheumatoid arthritis. Clin Immunol 93(3):198-208, 1999.
26. Kremer JM: Rational use of new and existing disease-modifying agents in rheumatoid arthritis. Ann Intern Med 134(8): 695-706, 2001.
27. Abramowicz M, editor: New drugs for rheumatoid arthritis. In The medical letter (Vol. 40[1040]), New Rochelle, NY, 1998, The Medical Letter, Inc.
28. Strand V, Cohen S, Schiff M, et al: Treatment of active rheumatoid arthritis with lefulunomide compared with placebo and methotrexate. Arch Intern Med 159:2542-2550, 1999.
29. Moreland LW, Baumgartner SW, Schiff MH, et al: Treatment of rheumatoid arthritis with a recombinant human tumor necrosis factor receptor (p75)-Fc fusion protein. N Engl J Med 337(3):141-147, 1997.
30. Genovese MC, Bathon JM, Martin RW, et al: Etanercept versus methotrexate in patients with early rheumatoid arthritis: two-year radiographic and clinical outcomes. Arthritis Rheum 46(6): p. 1443. 1450, 2002.
31. Bathon JM, Martin RW, Fleischmann RM, et al: A comparison of etanercept and methotrexate in patients with early rheumatoid arthritis. N Engl J Med 343(22):1586-1593, 2000.
32. Robinson WH, Genovese MC, Moreland LW: Demyelinating and neurologic events reported in association with tumor necrosis factor alpha antagonism: by what mechanisms could tumor necrosis factor alpha antagonists improve rheumatoid arthritis but exacerbate multiple sclerosis? Arthritis Rheum 44(9):1977-1983, 2001.
33. Maini R, St Clair EW, Breedveld F, et al: Infliximab (chimeric anti-tumour necrosis factor alpha monoclonal antibody)

versus placebo in rheumatoid arthritis patients receiving concomitant methotrexate: a randomised phase III trial. ATTRACT Study Group. Lancet 354(9194):1932-1939, 1999.

34. Abramowicz M, editor: Adalimumab (Humira) for rheumatoid arthritis. In The medical letter (Vol. 45[1153]), New Rochelle, NY, 2003, The Medical Letter, Inc.
35. Hamilton CD: Infectious complications of treatment with biologic agents. Curr Opin Rheumatol 16:393-398, 2004.
36. Wolfe E, Michaud K: Lymphoma in rheumatoid arthritis the effect of methotrexate and anti-tumor necrosis factor therapy in 18, 572 patients. Arthritis Rheum 50:1740-1751, 2004.
37. Kremer JM, Genant HK, Moreland LW: Effects of abatacept in patients with methotrexate-resistant active rheumatoid arthritis. Ann Intern Med 144:865-876, 2006.
38. Cohen S, Emery P, Greenwald M: Prolonged efficacy of rituximab in rheumatoid arthritis patients with inadequate response to one or more TNF inhibitors: 1 year follow-up of a subset of patients receiving a single course in a controlled trial (REFLEX study). Ann Rheum Dis 65(Suppl2):183, 2006.
39. O'Dell JR, Leff R, Paulsen G: Treatment of Rheumatoid arthritis with methotrexate and hydroxychloroquine, methotrexate and sulfasalazine, or a combination of the three medications: results of a two year, randomized, double-blind placebo-controlled trial. Arthritis Rheum 46:1164-1170, 2002.
40. Wortmann R: Gout and hyperuricemia. Curr Opin Rheumatol 14(3):281-286, 2002.
41. Rott KT, Agudelo CA: Gout. JAMA 289(21):2857-2860, 2003.
42. Schlesinger N, Schumacher HR: Gout: Can management be improved? Curr Opin Rheumatol 13(3):240-244, 2001.
43. Schlesinger N, Schumacher HR: Update on gout. Arthritis Care Res 47(5):563-565, 2002.
44. Mockford BJ, Kincaid RJ, Mackay I: Carpal tunnel syndrome secondary to intratendinous infiltration by tophaceous gout. Scand J Plast Reconstr Surg Hand Surg 37(3):186-187, 2003.
45. Terkeltaub RA: Gout. N Engl J Med 349(17):1647-1655, 2003.
46. Agudelo CA, Wise C: Gout: diagnosis, pathogenesis, and clinical manifestations. Curr Opin Rheumatol 13(3):234-239, 2001.
47. Ahern MJ, Reid C, Gordon TP, McCredie M, Brooks PM, Jones M: Does colchicine work? The results of the first controlled study in acute gout. Aust N Z J Med 17(3):301-304, 1987.
48. Hsu WC, Chen WH, Chang MT, Chiu HC: Colchicine-induced acute myopathy in a patient with concomitant use of simvastatin. Clin Neuropharmacol 25(5):266-268, 2002.
49. Groff GD, Franck WA, Raddatz DA: Systemic steroid therapy for acute gout: A clinical trial and review of the literature. Semin Arthritis Rheum 19(6):329-336, 1990.
50. Harris M, Bryant LR, Danaher P, Alloway J: Effect of low dose daily aspirin on serum urate levels and urinary excretion in patients receiving probenecid for gouty arthritis. J Rheumatol 27:2873-2876, 2000.
51. Perez-Ruiz F, Calabozo M, Pijoan JI, Herrero-Beites AM, Ruibal A: Effect of urate-lowering therapy on the velocity of size reduction of tophi in chronic gout. Arthritis Care Res 47(4):356-360, 2002.
52. Keith MP, Gilliland WR, Uhl K: Gout. In Waldman SA, Terzic A, editors: Pharmacology and therapeutics: Principles to practice, Philadelphia, 2009, Saunders.
53. Lee SJ, Terkeltaub RA, Kavanaugh A: Recent developments in diet and gout. Curr Opin Rheumatol 18:193-198, 2006.
54. Dall'Era M, Davis JC: Systemic lupus erythematosus. Postgrad Med 114(5):31-40, 2003.
55. Rekvig OP, Nossent JC: Anti-double-stranded DNA antibodies, nucleosomes, and systemic lupus erythematosus: A time for new paradigms? Arthritis Rheum 48(2):300-312, 2003.
56. Silverman GJ, Weisman S: Rituximab therapy and autoimmune disorders: Prospects for anti-B cell therapy. Arthritis Rheum 48(6):1484-1492, 2003.
57. Fabbri P, Cardinali C, Giomi B, Caproni M: Cutaneous lupus erythematosus: Diagnosis and management. Am J Clin Dermatol 4(7):449-465, 2003.
58. The Canadian Hydroxychloroquine Study Group: A randomized study of the effect of withdrawing hydroxychloroquine sulfate in systemic lupus erythematosus. N Engl J Med 324(3):150-154, 1991.
59. Wallace DJ: Management of lupus erythematosus: Recent insights. Curr Opin Rheumatol 14(3):212-219, 2002.
60. Petri M, Jones RJ, Brodsky RA: High-dose cyclophosphamide without stem cell transplantation in systemic lupus erythematosus. Arthritis Rheum 48(1):166-173, 2003.
61. Houssiau FA, Vasconcelos C, D'Cruz D, et al: Immunosuppressive therapy in lupus nephritis: The Euro-Lupus Nephritis Trial, a randomized trial of low-dose versus high-dose intravenous cyclophosphamide. Arthritis Rheum 46(8):2121-2131, 2002.
62. Chan TM, Li FK, Tang CS, Wong RW, et al: Efficacy of mycophenolate mofetil in patients with diffuse proliferative lupus nephritis. N Engl J Med 343(16):1156-1162, 2000.
63. Contreras G, Tozman E, Nahar N: Main therapies for proliferative lupus nephritis: mycophenolate mofetil, azathioprine and intravenous cyclophosphamide. Lupus 14(suppl 1):s33-s38, 2005.
64. Leandro MJ, Cambridge G, Edwards JC: B cell depletion in the treatment of patients with systemic lupus erythematosus: a longitudinal analysis of 24 patients. Rheumatology 44:1542-1545, 2005.
65. Willems M, Haddad E, Njaader P: Rituximab therapy for childhood-onset systemic lupus erythematosus. J Paedr 148: 623-627, 2006.
66. Gilliland WR, Keith MP, Uhl K: Systemic lupus erythematosus. In Waldman SA, Terzic A, editors: Pharmacology and therapeutics: Principles to practice, Philadelphia, 2009, Saunders.
67. Kang I, Park SH: Infectious complications in SLE after immunosuppressive therapies. Curr Opin Rheumatol 15(5):528-534, 2003.
68. Millard TP, Hawk JL, McGregor JM: Photosensitivity in lupus. Lupus 9(1):3-10, 2000.
69. Millard TP, Hawk JL: Ultraviolet therapy in lupus. Lupus 10(3):185-187, 2001.
70. Brogan BL, Olsen N: Drug-induced rheumatic syndromes. Curr Opin Rheumatol 15(1):76-80, 2003.
71. Gordon MM, Porter D: Minocycline induced lupus: Case series in the west of Scotland. J Rheumatol 28:1004-1006, 2001.
72. Shakoor N, Michalska M, Harris CA, Block JA: Drug-induced systemic lupus erythematosus associated with etanercept therapy. Lancet 359(9306):579-580, 2002.
73. Martel-Pelletier J, Pelletier JP: Osteoarthritis: Recent developments. Curr Opin Rheumatol 15(5):613-615, 2003.
74. Morehead K, Sack KE: Osteoarthritis. Postgrad Med 114(5):11-17, 2003.
75. Verzijl N, Bank RA, TeKoppele JM, DeGroot J: AGEing and osteoarthritis: A different perspective. Curr Opin Rheumatol 15(5):616-622, 2003.
76. Aigner T, Dudhia J: Genomics of osteoarthritis. Curr Opin Rheumatol 15(5):634-640, 2003.
77. Laufer S: Role of eicosanoids in structural degradation in osteoarthritis. Curr Opin Rheumatol 15(5):623-627, 2003.
78. Burr DB: The importance of subchondral bone in the progression of osteoarthritis. J Rheumatol 70(suppl):77-80, 2004.
79. Lajeunesse D, Reboul P: Subchondral bone in osteoarthritis: A biologic link with articular cartilage leading to abnormal remodeling. Curr Opin Rheumatol 15(5):628-633, 2003.

80. Ausiello JC, Staffore RS: Trends in medication use for osteoarthritis treatment. J Rheumatol 29(5):999-1005, 2002.
81. Case JP, Baliunas AJ, Block JA: Lack of efficacy of acetaminophen in treating symptomatic knee osteoarthritis: A randomized, double-blind, placebo-controlled comparison trial with diclofenac sodium. Arch Intern Med 163(2):169-178, 2003.
82. Towheed TE, Maxwell L, Judd MG, Catton M, Hochberg MC, Wells G: Acetaminophen for osteoarthritis. Cochrane Database Syst Rev 2(CD004257), 2003.
83. Akmal M, Singh A, Anand A: The effects of hyaluronic acid on articular chondrocytes. J Bone Joint Surg 87:1143-1149, 2005.
84. Lo GH, LaValley M, McAlindon T, Felson DT: Intra-articular hyaluronic acid in treatment of knee osteoarthritis: A meta-analysis. JJAMA 290(23):3115-3121, 2003.
85. Felson DT, Anderson J: Hyaluronate `sodium injections for Osteoarthritis: Hope, hype, and hard truths. Arch Intern Med 162:245-247, 2002.
86. Jubb RW, Piva S, Beinat L, Dacre J, Gishen P: A one-year, randomised, placebo (saline) controlled clinical trial of 500-730 kDa sodium hyaluronate (Hyalgan) on the radiological change in osteoarthritis of the knee. Int J Clin Prac 57(6):467-474, 2003.
87. Cubbage K: Does intra-articular hyaluronate decrease symptoms of osteoarthritis of the knee? J Fam Pract 51(5):411, 2002.
88. Buckwalter JA, Callaghan JJ, Rosier RN: From oranges and lemons to glucosamine and chondroitin sulfate: Clinical observations stimulate basic research. J Bone Joint Surg 83 (A-8):1266-1268, 2001.
89. Abramovicz D: Update on glucosamine for osteoarthritis. Med Lett 43(1120), 2001.
90. Towheed TE, Anastassiades TP: Glucosamine and chondroitin for treating symptoms of osteoarthritis. JAMA 283(11):1483-1485, 2000.
91. Richy F, Bruyere O, Ethgen O, Cucherat M, Henrotin Y, Reginster JY: Structural and symptomatic efficacy of glucosamine and chondroitin in knee osteoarthritis. Arch Intern Med 163:1514-1522, 2003.
92. Reginster JY, Deroisy R, Rovati LC, et al: Long-term effects of glucosamine sulphate on osteoarthritis progression: A randomised, placebo-controlled clinical trial. Lancet 357:251-256, 2001.
93. Deal CL, Moskowitz RW: Nutraceuticals as therapeutic agents in osteoarthritis. Rheum Dis Clin North Am 25:778-799, 1999.
94. McAlindon TE, LaValley MP, Gulin JP, Felson DT: Glucosamine and chondroitin for treatment of osteoarthritis: A systematic quality assessment and meta-analysis. JAMA 283(11):1469-1475, 2000.
95. Reginster JY: Long term effects of glucosamine sulphate on osteoarthritis progression: A randomized placebo-controlled clinical trial. Lancet 357:251-256, 2001.
96. Sawitzke AD, Shi H, Finco MF, et al: The effect of glucosamine and/or chondroitin sulfate on the progression of knee osteoarthritis: A report from the glucosamine/chondroitin arthritis intervention trial. Arthritis Rheum 58(10):3183-3191, 2008.
97. Harvey WF, Hunter DJ: Osteoarthritis. In Waldman SA, Terzic A, editors: Pharmacology and therapeutics: Principles to practice, Philadelphia, 2009, Saunders.
98. Lin J, et al: Efficacy of topical non-steroid antiinflammatory drugs in the treatment of osteoarthritis: meta analysis of randomized controlled trials. Br Med J 329:324, 2004.
99. Pelletier JP, Martel-Pelletier J: Therapeutic targets in osteoarthritis: from today to tomorrow with new imaging technology. Ann Allergy Asthma Immunol, 2003.
100. Pelletier JP, Jovanovic DV, Lascau-Coman V, et al: Selective inhibition of inducible nitric oxide synthase reduces progression of experimental osteoarthritis in vivo. Arthritis Rheum 43(6):1290-1299, 2000.
101. Paredes Y, Massicotte F, Pelletier JP, Martel-Pelletier J, Laufer S, Lajeunesse D: Study of the role of leukotriene B4 in abnormal function of human subchondral osteoarthritis osteoblasts: Effects of cyclooxygenase and/or 5-lipoxygenase inhibition. Arthritis Rheum 46(7):1804-1812, 2002.

SECTION IV

Endocrine Pharmacology

13

Selective Topics in Endocrine Pharmacology

Barbara Gladson

OVERVIEW OF THE ENDOCRINE SYSTEM

The endocrine system consists of a group of ductless glands that release hormones into the circulation for transport to their target organs. In most instances, the release of hormones is controlled through a negative feedback mechanism in which the stimulus initiates a response that reduces the original stimulus; or more simply stated, hormones inhibit their own release. The glands involved in this system include the hypothalamus, pituitary gland, thyroid gland, adrenal glands, gonads, pancreatic islets, and the parathyroid glands. See Table 13-1 for a review of the functional anatomy of the endocrine system.

Hypothalamic–Pituitary Axis

The hypothalamus and pituitary glands integrate physiologic signals to produce the release of hormones that regulate the function of other glands. The hypothalamus produces releasing or inhibiting hormones that travel to the anterior pituitary gland via a portal venous system in the pituitary stalk (Figure 13-1).[1] These include growth hormone (GH)–releasing hormone, growth hormone–inhibitory hormone (also known as *somatostatin*), prolactin-releasing factor, thyrotropin-releasing hormone, corticotrophin-releasing hormone, gonadotropin-releasing hormone (GnRH), melanocyte-stimulating hormone, and prolactin-inhibiting factor (Table 13-2). This portal venous system provides a delivery route for the hypothalamic hormones that regulate anterior pituitary function. The hypothalamus also synthesizes antidiuretic hormone (ADH) and oxytocin, which undergoes neurosecretory release into the posterior pituitary gland for storage and future systemic secretion.

In response to the hypothalamic releasing hormones, the anterior pituitary gland secretes GH, thyroid-stimulating hormone (TSH), adrenocorticotropic hormone (ACTH), follicle-stimulating hormone (FSH), luteinizing hormone (LH), and prolactin, which then bind to specific receptors in a variety of target tissues.[1]

An example of how the hypothalamic–pituitary axis integrates with a target tissue, such as the adrenal glands, is as follows. If a low concentration of circulating cortisol is sensed by the hypothalamic receptors sensitive to this hormone, there is a resultant release of corticotrophin-releasing hormone from the hypothalamus. This hormone is then released into the portal veins to act on receptors in the anterior pituitary gland. Stimulation of receptors in the anterior pituitary gland leads to the release of ACTH into the systemic venous system. The adrenal glands are then directed to synthesize and release cortisol into the general circulation. As the level of cortisol is increased, the hypothalamus reduces the amount of corticotrophin-releasing hormone released, forming a negative feedback loop. Similar types of feedback loops exist for the release of thyroid and sex hormones.

Drugs have many clinical uses in endocrinology, and one of the most common is replacement therapy.[2] In diabetes, exogenous insulin is given if the body can no longer produce its own. GH is also administered when there is a deficiency. Another use of endocrine drugs is to help diagnose an endocrine disorder. The dexamethasone suppression test will suppress cortisol release when the dysfunction is at the pituitary gland but will not in the presence of a cortisol-secreting tumor in the adrenal gland. Birth control pills alter normal endocrine function by providing low doses of estrogen and progestin to suppress ovulation because the estrogen causes a negative feedback effect on the release of LH and FSH.

PATHOPHYSIOLOGY AND PHARMACOLOGY RELATED TO THE PITUITARY GLAND

Hypothalamic and pituitary diseases may affect either single or multiple hormonal systems, leading to symptoms that appear similar to deficiencies of the target organs. Given the critical role of the hypothalamic and pituitary glands in the regulation of the endocrine system, dysfunction at this level affects many organ functions.

Pituitary Hypofunction (Hypopituitarism)

Pituitary hypofunction may be caused by neoplasms, trauma, infection, or vascular infarction.[3] There might be hypofunction of several hormones or diminished

TABLE 13-1 Functional Anatomy of the Endocrine and Metabolic Systems*

Endocrine Function	Regulatory Factors	Endocrine Organ/Hormone	Target Tissues
Availability of fuel	Serum glucose, amino acids, enteric hormones (somatostatin, cholecystokinin, gastrin, secretin), vagal reflex, sympathetic nervous system	Pancreatic islets of Langerhans/ insulin, glucagon	All tissues, especially liver, skeletal muscle, adipose tissue, indirect effects on brain and red blood cells
Metabolic rate	Hypothalamic thyrotropin-releasing hormone (TRH), pituitary thyrotropin (TSH)	Thyroid gland/ triiodothyronine (T_3)	All tissues
Circulatory volume	Renin, angiotensin II, hypothalamic osmoreceptor	Adrenals/aldosterone Pituitary/vasopressin	Kidney, blood vessels, central nervous system (CNS)
Somatic growth	Hypothalamic growth hormone–releasing hormone (GHRH), somatostatin, sleep, exercise, stress, hypoglycemia	Pituitary/growth hormone Liver/insulin-like growth factors (IGFs)	All tissues
Calcium homeostasis	Serum Ca^{2+} and Mg^{2+} concentration	Parathyroid glands/parathyroid hormone, calcitonin, vitamin D	Kidneys, intestines, bone
Reproductive function	Hypothalamic gonadotropin-releasing hormone (GnRH), pituitary follicle-stimulating hormone (FSH), and luteinizing hormone (LH), inhibins	Gonads/sex steroids Adrenals/androgens	Reproductive organs, CNS, various tissues
Adaptation to stress	Hypothalamic corticotrophin-releasing hormone (CRH), pituitary adrenocorticotropic hormone (ACTH), hypoglycemia, stress	Adrenals/glucocortico-steroids, epinephrine	Many tissues: CNS, liver, skeletal muscle, adipose tissue, lymphocytes, fibroblasts, cardiovascular system

From Page C, Curtis AB, Sutter MC, Walker L, Hoffman BB, editors: *Integrated pharmacology*. Philadelphia, 2002, Mosby.

*The endocrine and metabolic systems regulate seven major bodily functions. For each target tissue effect, endocrine glands release hormones in response to regulating factors, which include physiologic (e.g., sleep and stress), biochemical (e.g., glucose and calcium), and hormonal (e.g., hypothalamic and enteric hormones) stimuli.

levels of a single hormone. Multiple endocrine deficits such as hypogonadism (decreased FSH and LH levels), secondary adrenal insufficiency (decreased ACTH), altered fluid regulation (decreased ADH), hypothyroidism (decreased TSH), and diminished growth (decreased GH) may all occur. The treatment is to replace the hormones that are deficient (Table 13-3).

Adrenocorticotropic Hormone. The primary use of ACTH (Acthar) is diagnostic for differentiating primary adrenal insufficiency (Addison's disease) from secondary adrenal insufficiency caused by poor secretion of ACTH by the pituitary gland.[4] In Addison's disease, the addition of ACTH will have no effect on cortisol production, but in secondary adrenal insufficiency, the added ACTH will cause the adrenals to produce the glucocorticosteroid. ACTH stimulates the adrenocorticosteroid pathway, converting cholesterol to cortisol in the adrenal cortex (Figure 13-2). Cortisol is then responsible for providing the necessary glucose for brain function and fuel.

Antidiuretic Hormone. ADH (also known as *arginine vasopressin*, AVP) has a critical role in maintaining proper fluid balance in the body. An increase in plasma osmolality is one of the main stimuli for ADH release. A decrease in blood volume is also responsible for hormone release. Baroreceptors in the cardiovascular system sense a decrease in blood pressure, which results in release of hormone from the posterior pituitary gland. ADH has two main target tissues: (1) vascular smooth muscle via stimulating V_1 and V_3 receptors, leading to an influx of calcium into the cell; and (2) the kidney distal tubule and collecting duct via a V_2 receptor. Renal actions include increasing the number and rate of water channels in the luminal membrane, thus increasing water reabsorption, which results in concentrated urine. Nonrenal effects include contraction of smooth muscle, particularly in the cardiovascular system, although this is only seen when the levels of ADH are elevated.

Various analogs of ADH are offered for replacement therapy. Vasopressin (Pitressin), which is actually ADH itself, has a short duration of action and must be given by subcutaneous or intramuscular injection.[5] It is not highly selective for the V_2 receptors, so its use will result in nonrenal effects. Desmopressin (DDAVP, Stimate) is more selective for V_2 and also has a longer duration of action. It is usually administered in the form of a metered-dose nasal spray.

ADH and its analogs are used to treat diabetes insipidus and also to stop bleeding of esophageal varices through their action on smooth muscle. In addition,

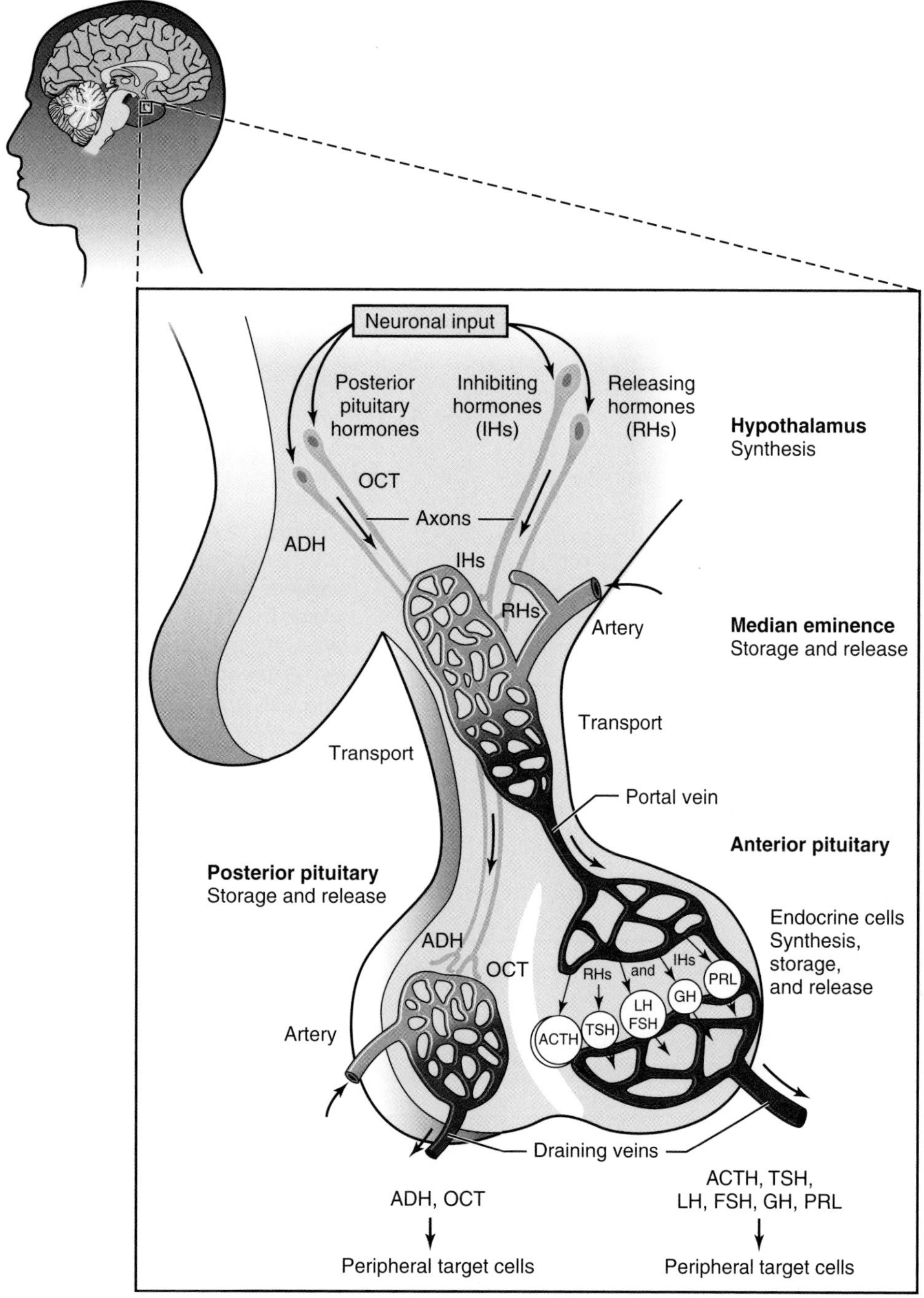

FIGURE 13-1 Schematic diagram of vascular and neural relationships among the hypothalamus, the posterior pituitary, and the anterior pituitary. The main portal vessels to the anterior pituitary lie in the pituitary stalks and arise from the primary plexus in the hypothalamus, but some (*the short portal vessels*) arise from the vascular bed in the posterior pituitary (*not shown*).

desmopressin is used for nocturnal enuresis in older children and adults and in patients with mild to moderate hemophilia to prevent bleeding. Parenteral desmopressin increases the concentration of factor VIII in the blood. Adverse effects of these drugs are related to water intoxication and hyponatremia and include headache and tremors.

Growth Hormone Deficiency. GH originates in the somatotroph cells in the anterior pituitary. This gland contains more GH than any of the other pituitary hormones. Secretion is high in the newborn, decreasing to an intermediate level by the age of 4 years, and declining further after puberty. Secretion is pulsatile, varying throughout the day, with higher levels during deep sleep and in the early morning hours. The plasma concentration may fluctuate from 10-fold to 100-fold during the day.

GH has anabolic effects on several tissues, including skeletal muscle and epiphyseal cartilage.[6] It stimulates protein synthesis and the uptake of amino acids into cells. It stimulates the production of insulin-like growth

TABLE 13-2 Hormones Secreted by the Hypothalamus and the Anterior Pituitary

Hypothalamic Factor/ Hormone (and Related Drugs)	Hormone Affected in Anterior Pituitary (and Related Drugs)	Main Effects of Anterior Pituitary Hormone
Corticotrophin-releasing factor (CRF)	Adrenocorticotropic hormone (ACTH; corticotropin, tetracosactide)	Stimulates secretion of adrenal cortical hormones (mainly glucocorticoids); maintains integrity of adrenal cortex
Thyrotropin-releasing hormone (TRH; protirelin)	Thyroid-stimulating hormone (TSH; thyrotropin)	Stimulates synthesis and secretion of thyroid hormones, thyroxine and triiodothyronine; maintains integrity of thyroid gland
Growth hormone–releasing factor (GHRF)	Growth hormone (GH; somatotropin)	Regulates growth, partly directly, partly through evoking the release of somatomedins from the liver and elsewhere; increases blood glucose; stimulates lipolysis
Growth hormone–releasing inhibiting factor (GHRIF; somatostatin, octreotide)	Growth hormone	As above
Gonadotropin-releasing hormone (GnRH; somatorelin, sermorelin)	Follicle-stimulating hormone (FSH) Luteinizing hormone (LH) or interstitial-cell-stimulating hormone (ICSH)	Stimulates the growth of the ovum and the Graafian follicle in the female and gametogenesis in the male; with LH, stimulates the secretion of estrogen throughout the menstrual cycle and progesterone in the second half; stimulates ovulation and the development of the corpus luteum; with FSH, stimulates secretion of estrogen and progesterone in menstrual cycle; in males, regulates testosterone secretion
Prolactin release-inhibiting factor (PRIF, probably dopamine)	Prolactin	Together with other hormones, prolactin promotes development of mammary tissue during pregnancy; stimulates milk production in the postpartum period
Prolactin-releasing factor (PRF)	Prolactin	As above
Melanocyte-stimulating hormone (MSH) releasing factor (MSH-RF)	α-, β-, and γ-MSH	Promotes formation of melanin, which causes darkening of skin; MSH is anti-inflammatory and helps regulate feeding
MSH release-inhibiting factor (MSH-RIF)	α-, β-, and γ-MSH	As above

From Rang HP, Dale MM, Ritter JM, Moore JL, editors: *Pharmacology* (5th ed.). New York, 2003, Churchill Livingstone.

TABLE 13-3 Selected Pituitary Drugs

Drug Class	Drug	Indications
Adrenal cortex stimulating hormone	Corticotropin (Acthar, ACTH, Acthar Gel)	Diagnosis of adrenocortical insufficiency
ADH	Desmopressin (DDAVP, Stimate), Vasopressin (Pitressin)	Nocturnal enuresis; diabetes insipidus; DDAVP is also an antihemophilic hormone
GH inhibitor (somatostatin analog)	Octreotide (Sandostatin, Sandostatin LAR Depot)	Acromegaly
GH analog	Sometrem (Protropin), somatropin (Genotropin, Humatrope, Serostim)	Growth failure; AIDS-related wasting syndrome (Serostimony)

ADH, antidiuretic hormone; *ACTH*, adrenocorticotropic hormone; *GH*, growth hormone; *AIDS*, acquired immune deficiency syndrome.

factor–1 (IGF-1) and insulin-like growth factor–binding protein 3 from the liver, which mediates the anabolic effect of GH, activating receptors on bone and muscle to promote growth. IGFs are also called *somatomedins*. Somatomedin receptors exist on many other cell types as well, including liver and fat cells. The result of IGF production is stimulation of bone and muscle growth.

A deficiency in GH results in pituitary dwarfism. This condition may be produced by a lack of GH-releasing hormone or a diminished production of IGF. The pharmacologic treatment is replacement with recombinant human GH, somatropin, or an analog called somatrem. Both of these are marketed for pediatric GH deficiency, short stature related to Turner's syndrome, and idiopathic,

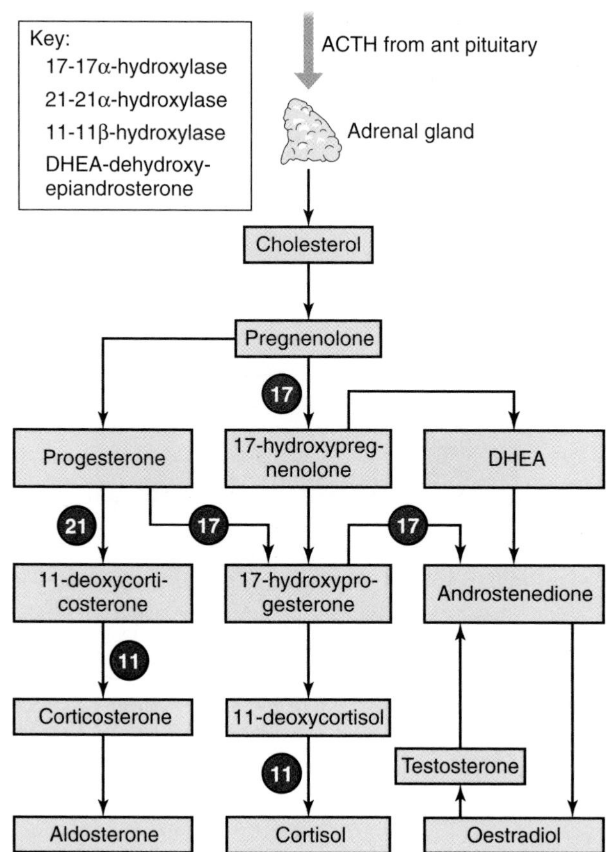

FIGURE 13-2 Main pathways in the biosynthesis of corticosteroids and adrenal androgens. Glucocorticoids synthesis is stimulated by ACTH; aldosterone synthesis is stimulated by angiotensin II. *ACTH*, adrenocorticotropic hormone.

non–GH-deficient short stature in children more than 2.25 standard deviations below the mean height for their age.[7,8] Administration of the hormone results in linear skeletal growth and anabolic effects on organs and soft tissue. Children, ages 9 to 15 years who received somatropin three times per week over a 4-year period, had a final height measurement of 3.3 cm more than children who received placebo. In another study in which a high dose and a low dose of somatropin were compared, children who received the higher dose were 3.3 cm taller than those who had received the lower dose. Eighty-two percent of the subjects in the higher-dose group who were followed up into adulthood were found to have achieved an adult height greater than the fifth percentile compared with 47% in the lower dose group. A meta-analysis of 10 controlled studies of children with short stature showed that GH injections for 5 years resulted in a gain of 4 to 6 cm.[9]

GH is usually administered as intramuscular injections three times per week until epiphyseal closure occurs. The total dose per week is determined by the weight of the child, but GH may be given in divided doses as often as six times per week.[8] This resembles the pulsatile release of endogenous GH. It is usually given in the evening. Patients with idiopathic GH deficiency might later develop normal GH secretion, so the dose may be tapered as the child ages. Adverse effects are minimal, with none on pubertal development, but may include insulin resistance or glucose intolerance. Some cases of intracranial hypertension, probably related to increased sodium retention, have been reported. There have also been some reports of gynecomastia, pancreatitis, and increased growth of pre-existing nevi. Children should be monitored for these effects if they have an appropriate risk profile. For example, obese children should be screened periodically for diabetes. Occasionally, children may develop coarsening of facial features due to GH overdosing. There is also the concern that GH injections may promote tumorgenesis.[10]

In 1989, the results of two placebo-controlled studies of GH replacement in GH-deficient adults were published. GH administered to individuals in these studies was found to be beneficial in terms of body composition and lipid levels.[11] Since then, more published evidence has indicated beneficial but inconsistent effects of GH for adults with hypopituitarism, patients with human immunodeficiency virus (HIV) infection, patients with fibromyalgia, children with cystic fibrosis, and even frail older adults.[12-15] In general, GH given to adults reduces central obesity, improves lipid levels, and increases bone density and lean body mass. When given along with resistive training to healthy older adult men for 12 weeks, GH was found to increase isokinetic muscle strength compared with exercise alone, exercise with placebo injection, or placebo alone.[16] Exercise alone produced a significant increase in muscle strength, but the GH-only group did not show any improvement. The investigators concluded that in healthy older adult men, GH can augment the strengthening effect of exercise, but not when it is the only therapy. Subjects who took GH did, however, show positive changes in body composition consisting of decreased fat mass. A similar study performed with frail older adults for 6 months demonstrated that GH combined with exercise as well as exercise alone did increase muscle strength significantly.[13] Treatment with GH alone resulted in a nonsignificant trend toward increased quadriceps strength. Musculoskeletal adverse effects reported among the adults included carpal tunnel syndrome, arthralgias, and lower extremity edema. Although further study is needed to determine the benefits of GH administration in adults, the current guidelines indicate that if a patient perceives no benefit after 6 months of treatment, withdrawal should begin.[3]

Another indication for GH administration is to offset some of the adverse effects associated with long-term use of steroids for certain disease processes.[17] Steroids suppress linear growth and become GH antagonists, particularly when given to children. However, because both therapies are associated with insulin resistance and hyperglycemia, children receiving this regimen must be monitored frequently for type 2 diabetes.

Insulin-like growth factor-I (IGF-1) is another treatment for growth hormone deficiency that is resistant to replacement therapy.[5,18] Recombinant human IGF-1 (rhIGF-1) and rhIGF-1/IGFBP3 (insulin growth factor binding protein 3) complex offers an alternative treatment. Children around the age of 6 years at the start of therapy grew from a velocity of 2.8 cm/yr before treatment to 8.0 cm/yr during the initial year of treatment. Adverse effects included mild hypoglycemia and lipohypertrophy at the injection sites.[19]

Therapeutic Concerns with Hypopituitarism. As reviewed previously, hypopituitarism can entail the partial or complete loss of anterior pituitary hormone secretion. Once it occurs, it is generally permanent and requires multiple hormone replacement therapies. In patients who have panhypopituitarism (multiple deficiencies), cortisol should be replaced first, followed by thyroxine (T_4) (see discussion of thyroid deficiency and corticosteroid deficiency).[3] Sex steroids may be replaced when the patient's medical condition has stabilized. The last to be replaced is GH.

Hypopituitarism requires complicated treatment regimens that are often imprecise, with levels sometimes exceeding the normal range.[3] Achieving the optimum dose is a trial-and-error process. The therapist treating patients who are receiving hormone replacement must be alert to the adverse effects of excessive hormone levels. Unexpected interactions between hormones may also occur; therefore any ailment not usually seen should be reported to the patient's endocrinologist. Children and adults who have low GH levels have decreased bone mineral density and therefore are at increased risk for fractures. Slipped capital femoral epiphyses have been associated with GH deficiency.[8] It might be prudent to suggest that these children have GH levels determined, especially if they have any other metabolic bone disease or renal insufficiency. Likewise, children with known GH deficiency who have hip pain should be thoroughly evaluated.

Acromegaly

Acromegaly results from excessive production of GH caused by a pituitary adenoma in adults.[6] Clinical features include excessive growth of bone and soft tissue with their resultant musculoskeletal problems, as well as some complex metabolic abnormalities (hyperglycemia, insulin resistance, elevated IGF-1 levels). Patients with this disorder display skin thickening; thyroid enlargement; excessive sweating; enlarged hearts; and enlargement of the hands, feet, and facial features (Figure 13-3). Severe arthritis, carpal tunnel syndrome, sleep apnea, and impaired cardiovascular function with hypertension are also seen. When this disorder occurs in children, it is labeled as *gigantism*; this disorder results in linear bone growth because the growth plates are still active.

Treatment of GH-secreting tumors usually involves surgery and radiation. However, if the patient is not a candidate for surgery or the tumor >1 cm, drug intervention can be used.[5] The dopamine agonist bromocriptine can block GH release in a certain percentage of patients. In healthy individuals, bromocriptine will increase secretion of GH; however, in patients with acromegaly, the drug appears to have a paradoxical effect. Because bromocriptine is not always effective, somatostatin analogs have become the drugs of choice.

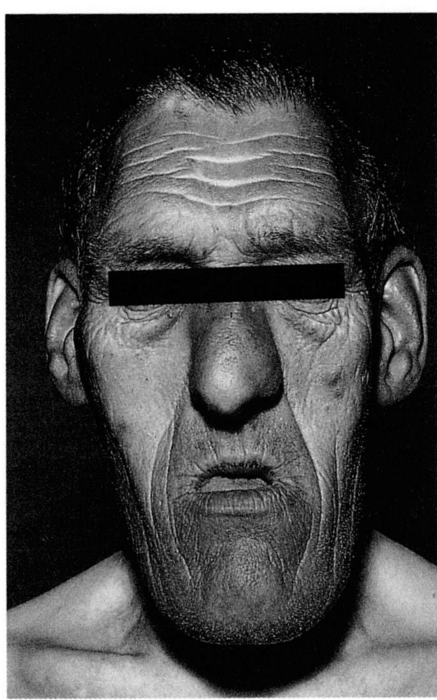

FIGURE 13-3 Characteristic facial features of acromegaly. *(Courtesy Dr. C. D. Forbes and Dr. W. F. Jackson. From Rang HP, Dale MM, Ritter JM, Moore JL:* Pharmacology *(5th ed.), New York, 2003, Churchill Livingstone.)*

Somatostatin diminishes GH concentration in both healthy subjects and patients with acromegaly. Somatostatin has multiple functions, acting as a neurotransmitter, regulating the release of GH—and when secreted by the pancreatic delta cells—acting to inhibit both insulin and glucagon release.[20] During the initial studies, this hormone showed promise in the treatment of diabetes. However, its benefit is limited by its extremely short half-life (1 to 3 minutes).

Octreotide is a longer-acting synthetic somatostatin analog. Its half-life is 80 to 100 minutes, and it is effective in reducing GH levels in 94% of patients and can help lower IGF-1 to normal levels in about 70% of patients.[21] The initial dosage of octreotide is three subcutaneous injections daily. The dose and number of injections may be increased if needed. Some newer depot preparations of octreotide (octreotide LAR) have improved compliance by reducing the need for injections to only once or twice a month. Octreotide used preoperatively also improves postoperative results. Adverse effects of octreotide include nausea, abdominal cramps, diarrhea, flatulence, and gallbladder dysfunction. Tolerance for these adverse effects develops quickly. Lanreotide acetate is another long-acting somatostatin analog that is given once a month subcutaneously.

Pegvisomant is a GH receptor antagonist used as parenteral treatment for acromegaly.[22] This treatment is reserved for patients who are not candidates for surgery or in cases in which surgery has failed. This drug binds to the GH receptors and blocks attachment by endogenous GH.

The patient is initially given a 40-mg subcutaneous loading dose, followed by daily doses starting at 10 mg. In a 12-week trial, reported adverse effects included injection-site reactions, nausea, diarrhea, chest pain, and flu-like symptoms. Increased hepatic enzyme levels have also been seen in a few patients.

THYROID DISEASES

Thyroid hormone (TH) controls the basal metabolic activity of all tissues by regulating genes that increase cell metabolism and protein synthesis.[23] In addition, these hormones stimulate tissue oxygen consumption, complement the sympathetic nervous system, and enhance gluconeogenesis; however, all this occurs at the expense of wasting tissue in order to supply glycogen. TH increases the metabolism of carbohydrates, fats, and proteins by influencing insulin, glucagon, glucocorticoids, and the catecholamines—either directly or indirectly—by regulating the activity of some enzymes involved in carbohydrate metabolism. Other important physiologic effects of TH include regulating body temperature, increasing cardiac rate and contractility, and enhancing red blood cell mass and circulatory volume. An adequate TH level is critical for normal bone growth, and there is evidence that TH stimulates both osteoblasts and osteoclasts, but in patients with hyperthyroidism, the net effect on bone cells is bone reabsorption, leading to osteoporosis and increased risk of fracture.[24]

The thyroid gland secretes three main hormones: T_4, triiodothyronine (T_3), and calcitonin.[25] Calcitonin is involved in regulating the plasma calcium level and will be discussed in Chapter 14. T_3 and T_4 are formed by the iodination of tyrosine residues on a large peptide (thyroglobulin), which is synthesized and secreted into the lumen of the follicle (the functional unit of the thyroid gland). The follicles are surrounded by a rich capillary network, which produces a high rate of blood flow into the gland.

The first step in producing TH is the uptake of iodide by the follicle cells.[25] Iodide is taken up by a sodium/iodine (Na^+/I^-) co-transporter, which receives energy from the Na^+/K^+–ATPase (adenosine triphosphatase) pump. Next, the iodide is oxidized by the enzyme thyroperoxidase, and attaches to the tyrosine residue on thyroglobulin (Figure 13-4). The coupling of two iodinated tyrosines forms diiodotyrosine. When two diiodotyrosines are coupled, they form T_4 (Figure 13-5). Hormone secretion occurs when endocytotic vesicles fuse with the wall of the follicle cell. Thyroglobulin is reabsorbed into the follicle cells, and T_4 and T_3 are secreted into the circulation. Most of T_3 is formed by the deiodination of T_4 in extrathyroidal tissues, generating about 80% of the circulating T_3.[26] T_3 is the more active hormone with a higher affinity for thyroid receptors.

The regulation of thyroid function comes from the release of TSH by the hypothalamus and the subsequent release of thyrotropin-releasing hormone from the anterior pituitary gland.[26] The production of TSH is regulated by a negative feedback effect from T_3 and T_4 as well. The plasma iodide concentration also influences hormone

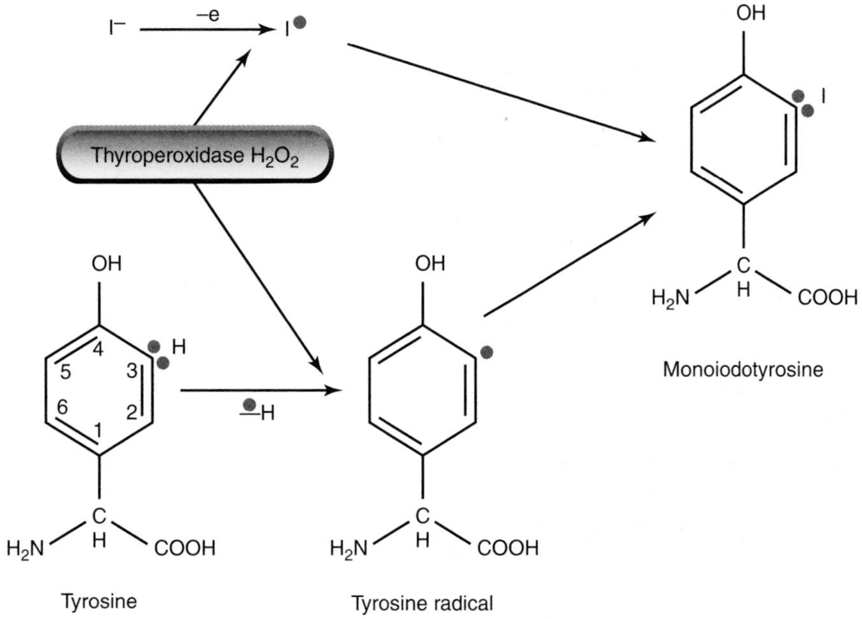

FIGURE 13-4 Iodination of tyrosine residues by thyroperoxidase *(From Rang HP, Dale MM, Ritter JM, Moore JL: Pharmacology (6th ed.), New York, 2007, Churchill Livingstone.)*

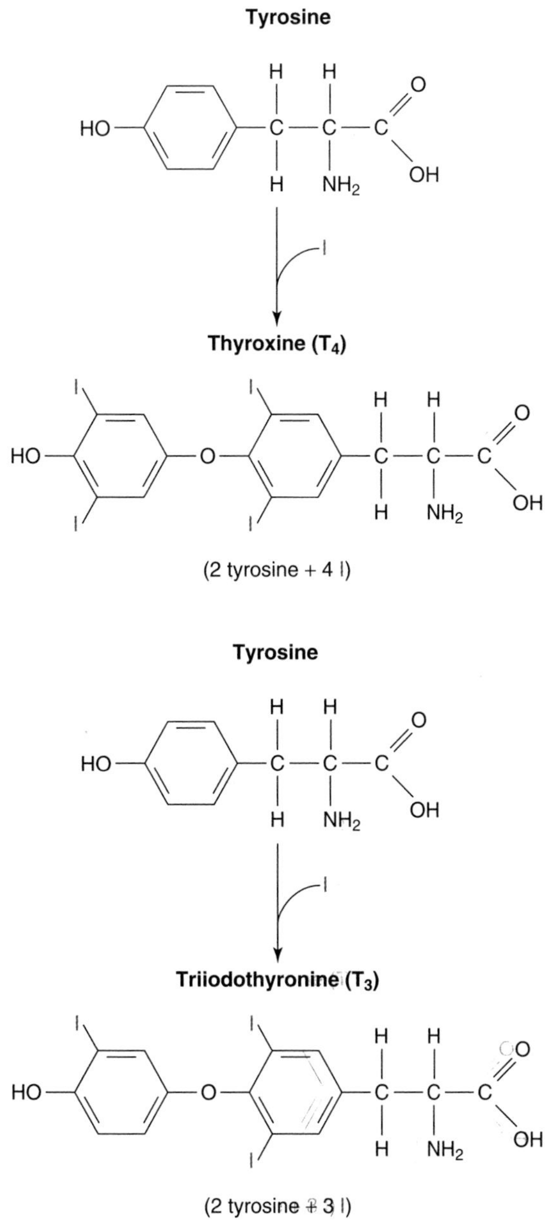

Tyrosine

Thyroxine (T_4)

(2 tyrosine + 4 I)

Tyrosine

Triiodothyronine (T_3)

(2 tyrosine + 3 I)

FIGURE 13-5 Iodinated tyrosine residues. Monoiodotyrosine and diiodotyrosine are shown in peptide linkage, as in thyroglobulin. When thyroxine (T_4) is used as a drug, it is given as the salt of the amino acid.

production. The thyroid gland requires the uptake of at least 500 nmol of iodide daily (equal to 70 mg of iodine). If the plasma level of iodide is reduced, there will be a reduction in hormone production and an increase in TSH secretion. An elevated level of plasma iodide has the opposite effect—a reduction in hormone production.

Hyperthyroidism (Thyrotoxicosis)

Hyperthyroidism occurs due to an overproduction of the endogenous hormone or excessive ingestion of exogenous hormone.[27] Symptoms include nervousness, weight loss, heat intolerance, tremor, tachycardia, hyperhidrosis, exophthalmos, and enhanced reflexes (Figure 13-6). The most common cause for hyperthyroidism is Graves' disease, an autoimmune disease, in which circulating immunoglobulins stimulate the TSH receptor. The result is sustained overproduction of TH. The diagnosis is made by elevated serum T_4 and or T_3 levels and a diminished TSH level.

Thionamides (Propylthiouracil, Methimazole). Treatment for hyperthyroidism includes antithyroid drugs, surgical removal, and radioactive iodine.[27] Propylthiouracil and methimazole inhibit iodine coupling to thyroglobulin by binding to the peroxidase enzyme. Propylthiouracil also inhibits deiodination of T_4 to T_3. Skin rashes, fever, arthralgias, abnormal taste sensation, liver dysfunction, and bone marrow depression may occur as adverse effects; therefore, close monitoring is important. These drugs require 6 weeks of administration before success is realized, as they do not affect the thyroglobulin already stored in the gland. These drugs require longer for those patients with very large goiters. Thionamides are frequently administered as long-term therapy for Graves' disease or prior to radioactive iodine (see below).

Iodide and Radioactive Iodine. Another treatment for hyperthyroidism is the administration of iodide, which, if administered in excess, will inhibit the iodination of tyrosines. It is often used during a "thyroid storm" or to reduce TH levels until surgery can be performed. It is called *Lugol's solution* and consists of liquid drops added to fruit juice taken three times a day. Adverse effects include diarrhea, nausea, burning of the mouth, and a metallic taste in the mouth.

Destruction of the thyroid gland can be achieved with radioactive iodine (^{131}I).[27] The radioisotope, which is taken up into the thyroid follicular cells, slowly destroys the gland. Onset of action is within 2 to 4 weeks and peaks between 2 and 4 months. Treatment with the thionamides should precede this treatment to achieve euthyroidism, since administering radioiodine to an overactive thyroid gland can precipitate a thyroid crisis. Patients will remain radioactive for a period of time after treatment has ceased. Passing security checkpoints or other devices that measure radioactivity will most likely trigger an investigation by law enforcement, so when traveling patients should carry with them some documentation from their physician. Once the thyroid gland is destroyed, supplemental TH is required.

β-Adrenoceptor Antagonists. β-Blockers are considered adjuncts in the treatment of hyperthyroidism.[25] They are usually given to reduce some of the symptoms of excess TH levels until the radioisotope treatment becomes effective. These drugs are effective in reducing symptoms related to adrenergic hyperstimulation, such as tachycardia and tremor. Use of a β-blocker continues until the patient achieves euthyroidism.

Treatment of Thyroid Storm. A *thyroid storm* represents a severe form of thyrotoxicosis and is considered a medical emergency.[25] Symptoms include fever, delirium, excessive tachycardia, hypotension, vomiting, and

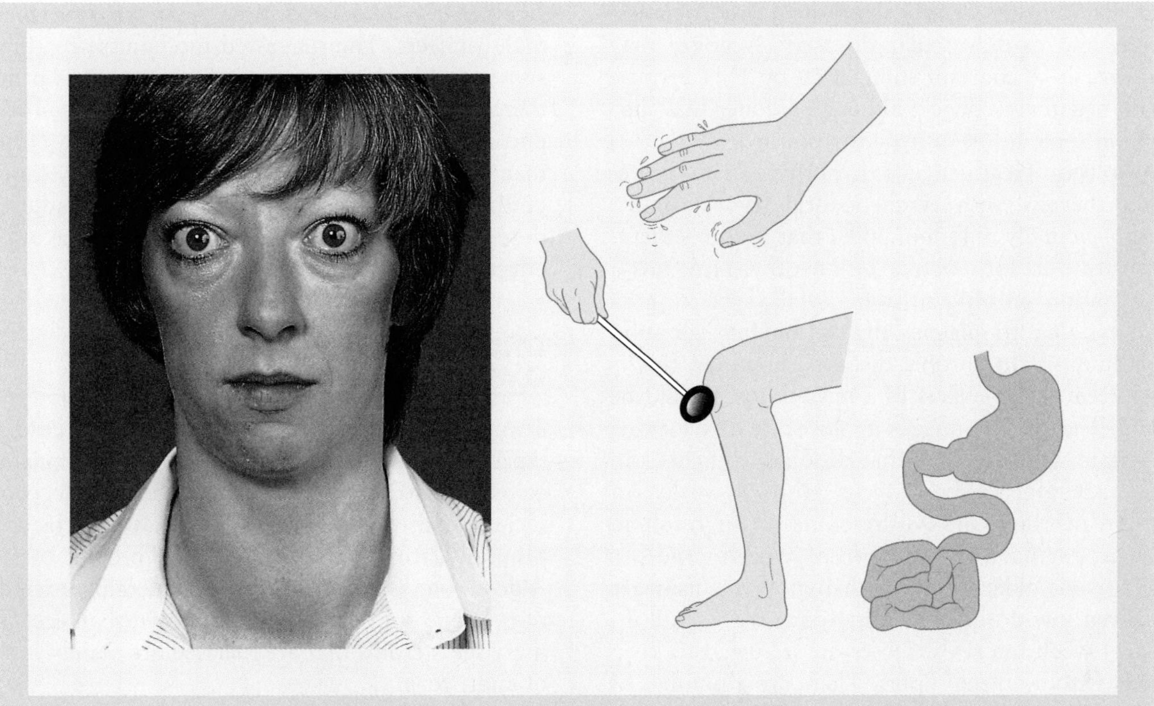

FIGURE 13-6 Signs and symptoms of hyperthyroidism. Hyperthyroidism leads to characteristic symptoms of nervousness, weight loss, heat intolerance, and fatigue. Signs such as tachycardia, tremor, accelerated reflexes, smooth skin, hyperhidrosis, and ocular stare are common to hyperthyroidism of any cause. Proptosis, diplopia, and corneal inflammation are specific findings in Graves' disease. *(Photograph courtesy Dr. C. D. Forbes and Dr. W. F. Jackson. From Page C, Curtis AB, Sutter MC, Walker L, Hoffman BB, editors:* Integrated pharmacology, *Philadelphia, 2002, Mosby.)*

TABLE 13-4 Treatment for Thyroid Storm

Drug Class	Drug	Indication
Antithyroid agents	Propylthiouracil (PTU)	Prevents production of T_4 and T_3 in the gland; blocks conversion of T_4 to T_3 outside the thyroid
	Methimazole (Tapazole)	Prevents production of thyroid hormone
Iodides	Lugol's solution	Blocks release of stored thyroid hormone
	Saturated solution of potassium iodide (Pima)	Blocks release of stored thyroid hormone
Glucocorticoids	Dexamethasone (Decadron) Hydrocortisone	Blocks conversion of T_4 to T_3
β-Blockers	Propranolol (Inderal) Esmolol (Brevibloc Injection)	Reduces tachycardia, tremor, and restlessness

diarrhea. Supportive treatments such as intravenous hydration, cortisol, and large doses of propylthiouracil are needed. Oral potassium iodide to block TH release and β-blockers to lower heart rate are also needed (Table 13-4).

Hypothyroidism

TH deficiency is usually caused by autoimmune destruction of the gland or directed destruction as a result of treatment for hyperthyroidism.[28] The most common cause of primary hypothyroidism when there is available dietary iodine is Hashimoto's thyroiditis and results from antibody-mediated destruction of the thyroid gland. Secondary hypothyroidism results from reduced secretion of either TSH from the pituitary gland or reduced TRH from the hypothalamus. Patients can have a subclinical condition with normal T_3 and T_4 levels but elevated TSH or overt hypothyroidism with low thyroid hormone levels. Symptoms include bradycardia, anemia, lethargy, weight gain, cold intolerance, menstrual irregularities, generalized muscle weakness, and myxedema (generalized nonpitting edema, including the periorbital area). Hypothyroidism is also associated with altered lipoprotein metabolism, which results in elevated low-density lipoprotein (LDL) cholesterol levels and cardiovascular disease.[29] A goiter may form as a result of constant stimulation by TSH because there is no negative feedback, although a goiter may also be present in some forms of hyperthyroidism.

Levothyroxine. Treatment of hypothyroidism is replacement therapy with synthetic oral levothyroxine. This drug is actually a T_4 look-alike that requires metabolic activation to form active T_3. Levothyroxine has a long elimination half-life of about 6 days because of extensive binding to plasma thyroid-binding globulin and to albumin.[25] In chronic diseases, however, this is preferred because the effects of a missed dose would be minimized. The disadvantage is its slow rate of achieving a steady state, which means that dose adjustments can only be made after several weeks (4 to 8 weeks) of therapy. An overdose of levothyroxine might result in arrhythmias, angina, and symptoms of hyperthyroidism. For this reason, older adults with hypothyroidism are initially given low doses of levothyroxine with small increases at 4-week intervals. Doses are adjusted to keep TSH levels within normal limits. There are a number of generic T_4 preparations that have varying degrees of bioavailability, so when a patient is switched to a new brand, serum TSH should be checked at 6 weeks to make sure that the dose is correct. In addition, ingestion of iron or calcium along with T_4 may affect its absorption. Therefore, these supplements should be taken at least 4 hours apart from the T_4. Combination generics consisting of T_3 and T_4 are available as well, but they have not shown any superiority over monotherapy with T_4, and the combination may affect pharmacokinetics (Box 13-1).[30,31]

Therapeutic Concerns for Patients Receiving Therapy for Hypothyroidism. It is well known that hyperthyroidism increases bone reabsorption, leading to osteoporosis and increased risk of fractures.[32] Some studies have demonstrated a similar risk for patients receiving long-term levothyroxine therapy. In a recent large study[32] of 23,183 subjects receiving TH, fracture of the femur was significantly associated with levothyroxine therapy in male subjects. The suggested mechanism for this risk is subclinical hyperthyroidism. Therefore, it is prudent for therapists to take this fracture risk into consideration, particularly when treating older men with TH replacement. Therapists should also watch for any signs of hyperthyroidism in their older clients, so that adjustment in dose can be made as quickly as possible to avoid adverse effects.

BOX 13-1 Thyroid Hormone Preparations

T_4 (levothyroxine) Preparations
- Synthroid
- Levoxyl
- Thyro-Tab
- Unithroid
- Levothroid
- L-thyroxine

T_3 (Liothyronine) Preparations
- Cytmel

Combination Preparations
- Thyrolar
- Thyroid USP
- Armour Thyroid

DRUG THERAPY FOR ADRENAL DYSFUNCTION

The adrenal cortex is responsible for the secretion of three types of steroid hormones: glucocorticoids, mineralocorticoids, and sex steroids. The endogenous glucocorticoids include hydrocortisone (cortisol) and corticosterone and primarily affect carbohydrate and protein metabolism. Aldosterone is the endogenous mineralocorticoid and is responsible for water and electrolyte balance. The primary sex steroids that are released are mainly in the form of androgens.

Glucocorticoids

The glucocorticoids are secreted from the adrenal cortex in response to ACTH from the anterior pituitary gland.[33] The initial step in cortisol synthesis is the conversion of cholesterol to pregnenolone (see Figure 13-2). Basal release follows a diurnal variation with a marked elevation in the predawn hours of the morning and a marked reduction during the late evening hours. Replacement therapy attempts to mimic this normal cycle (Figure 13-7). Psychological factors and physical stimuli such as excessive heat or cold, injury, surgery, illness, or infection will

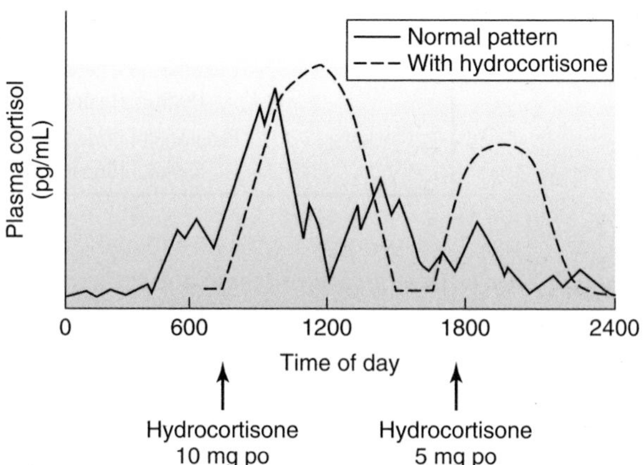

FIGURE 13-7 Glucocorticosteroid replacement therapy. An average adult produces approximately 10 mg of cortisol per day. Cortisol production shows marked diurnal variation, with an initial elevation in the pre-waking hours. Physiologic replacement with oral hydrocortisone attempts to mimic this endogenous pattern. *(From Page C, Curtis AB, Sutter MC, Walker L, Hoffman BB, editors:* Integrated pharmacology, *Philadelphia, 2002, Mosby.)*

increase secretion, which is why cortisol is called the *stress response hormone*.[3]

Cortisol activates the GR-α and GR-β receptors located in the cell cytoplasm in almost every tissue of the body.[34] This steroid–receptor complex then moves to the nucleus of the cell and binds to steroid-responsive elements in the DNA. The net effect is to turn off transcription of genes for the cyclooxygenase-2 (COX-2) enzyme, various cytokines and adhesion factors, the vitamin D_3 induction of the osteocalcin gene in osteoblasts, and nitric oxide (NO) synthase. Another effect of this steroid–receptor complex is to induce the formation of annexin-1 (previously known as *lipocortin-1*).[35] Annexin-1 has strong anti-inflammatory action, as well as negative feedback action, on the hypothalamus and anterior pituitary gland.

The major metabolic effects of cortisol include increasing gluconeogenesis and lipolysis to provide fuel for physical activity and brain function.[36] Cortisol also produces a decrease in the uptake of glucose, resulting in a trend toward hyperglycemia. The effect on proteins is an increase in catabolism, and the effect on fat is redistribution to the trunk. Cortisol also decreases calcium absorption from the gastrointestinal tract and increases its excretion in the kidney tubules.

The anti-inflammatory and immune suppressive actions of cortisol are the pharmacologic reasons for its use. In the area of inflammation, influx and activity of leukocytes, eicosanoids, and fibroblasts are decreased. In chronic inflammation, proliferation of blood vessels is decreased. In the lymphoid areas production of T and B cells, cytokines, tumor necrosis factor (TNF), and immunoglobulin G (IgG) is decreased.

Excess Glucocorticoids (Cushing's Syndrome). Excessive amounts of glucocorticoids lead to Cushing's syndrome, characterized by muscle weakness, osteoporosis, central obesity, moon facies, fragile skin and capillaries, hypertension, diabetes, and neuropsychiatric disorders (Figure 13-8). This syndrome resembles the unwanted effects of cortisol and the adverse drug effects of exogenous steroid administration. Cushing's syndrome may result from an ACTH-secreting adenoma, a cortisol-secreting adrenal tumor, or ectopic ACTH production from certain tumors in the lungs or gastrointestinal tract. Treatment for Cushing's syndrome is usually surgical, but drug treatment with ketoconazole or metyrapone is advocated for several weeks before surgery or in cases where surgery has failed in order to reverse some of the catabolic and metabolic effects (Table 13-5).[36] Metyrapone blocks the enzyme 11β-hydroxylase, inhibiting the terminal step in cortisol synthesis (see Figure 13-2). The precursors of these pathways, such as 17-hydroxyprogesterone, are funneled into the mineralocorticoid and sex hormone pathways, leading to adrenal androgen formation and hirsutism, salt formation, and hypertension. Ketoconazole is an antifungal drug that inhibits the first step in cholesterol synthesis and also ACTH secretion. An alternative drug

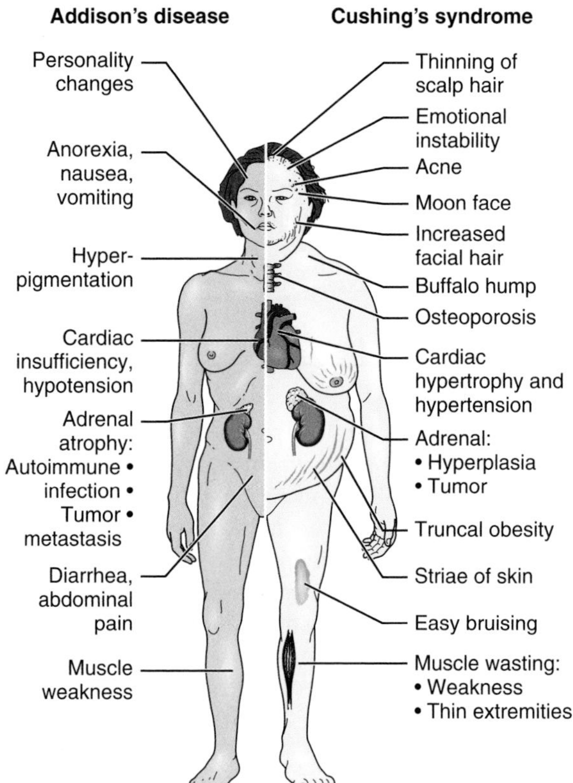

FIGURE 13-8 Glucocorticoid excess and deficiency.

is trilostane, which inhibits an earlier enzymatic step in cortisol formation. Mitotane represents another approach to treating this condition.[37] This drug is an active ingredient in dichlorodiphenyltrichloroethane, commonly known as the insecticide DDT. It acts on the mitochondria in the cells of the adrenal cortex and has an active metabolite that produces a necrosis of the adrenocortical cells. It takes up to 6 to 9 months to be effective; and since the drug has many adverse effects, only a low dose should be administered. These adverse effects include nausea, vomiting, anorexia, rash, ataxia, confusion, leukopenia, and gynecomastia. Hypercholesterolemia, hypouricemia and hepatotoxicity can occur. Patients will also develop cortisol deficiency, but this is expected as the adrenal cells die. However, when the deficiency will occur cannot always be predicted, so replacement therapy with glucocorticoids is also indicated.

Glucocorticoid Deficiency. Diminished levels of cortisol lead to devastating effects, even in nonstressful situations. This deficiency can result from hypothalamic–pituitary disease, autoimmune destruction of the adrenal cortex (Addison's disease), or suppression of the hypothalamic–pituitary–adrenal axis after steroid withdrawal. Symptoms include weight loss, fatigue, arthralgias, and reduced cardiovascular function. If the insult is at the adrenal gland, additional symptoms such as low blood pressure and hyperkalemia are present as a result

TABLE 13-5 Drugs Used to Treat Cushing's Syndrome

Drug	Mechanism of Action	ADRs
Mitotane	Inhibits 11β-hydroxylase	Nausea/vomiting, anorexia, rash, diarrhea, gynecomastia, leukopenia
Metyrapone	Inhibits 11β-hydroxylase	Hypertension, acne, hirsutism
Aminoglutethimide	Inhibits conversion of cholesterol to pregnenolone	Sedation, rash, bone marrow suppression, hypothyroidism, cholestasis
Ketoconazole	Blocks conversion of cholesterol to pregnenolone; inhibits 11β-hydroxylase	Headache, sedation, amenorrhea, gynecomastia, erectile dysfunction

of the loss of aldosterone. Treatment for this deficiency is hormone replacement. Previously, there was an attempt to simulate physiologic secretion by giving 10 mg of cortisone or hydrocortisone in the morning and 5 mg in the evening. However, now patients are administered the longer-acting agents such as prednisone once a day.[38] Adverse effects of treatment include symptoms resembling Cushing's syndrome. Therapeutic concerns with steroids have been reviewed previously.

Mineralocorticoids

Aldosterone is the primary mineralocorticoid as described previously. Its secretion is regulated by a variety of factors, with angiotensin II, hyponatremia, and hyperkalemia being the primary factors. The actions of aldosterone include increasing the permeability of the kidney distal tubules (luminal side) to sodium by increasing the number of sodium channels. Water is then passively reabsorbed following the osmotic pressure gradient. Aldosterone also stimulates the Na+/K+–ATPase pump in the basolateral membrane, leading to sodium reabsorption and excretion of potassium and hydrogen.

Mineralocorticoid Deficiency. Mineralocorticoid deficiency is characterized by reduced extracellular volume, resulting in orthostatic hypotension, dehydration, oliguria, and poor skin turgor. Fludrocortisone is the synthetic version of aldosterone used for replacement therapy.[39] Adverse effects include sodium retention, hypokalemia, and hypertension.

Mineralocorticoid Excess. Excess aldosterone is usually produced by an adenoma in the zona glomerulosa of the adrenal cortex (Conn's syndrome).[39] The primary treatment for this tumor is surgical resection, but drug therapy is recommended for patients who are not candidates for surgery. The drug of choice for this problem is the potassium-sparing diuretic spironolactone.

DRUG TREATMENT FOR THE REPRODUCTIVE SYSTEM

The hypothalamic–pituitary–gonadal axis regulates short-term control over events such as spermatogenesis, follicular development, and the menstrual cycle but is also involved in long-term control to maintain the secondary sex characteristics and initiate puberty and then menopause. Hypothalamic gonadotropin-releasing hormone (GnRH) is the master hormone that interacts in a complex way with the anterior pituitary gland to release LH and FSH. LH stimulates sex steroid production in the gonads and also converts the adrenal androgens to testosterone and estrogens. Estrogens are also produced by the aromatase enzyme in the gonads and adipocytes, which then become the sole source of estrogen in postmenopausal woman after ovarian failure. FSH is the major regulator of gamete production.

Androgens and the Male Reproductive System

Dihydrotestosterone (DHT) and its precursor testosterone are androgens that produce anabolic and masculinizing effects in both sexes. They are produced in the testes by the androgenic precursors dehydroepiandrosterone and androstenedione coming from the adrenal glands, and in small amounts by the ovaries in response to LH. Testosterone is an active ligand in muscle and liver, but in other tissues (prostate, seminal vesicles, epididymis, and skin) it is converted to the more powerful DHT by the enzyme 5α-reductase (Figure 13-9). The aromatase enzyme in the gonads and adipose tissue converts the testosterone precursors to estrogens.

The mechanism of action of testosterone really occurs through its active metabolite DHT. Testosterone itself causes masculization of the male embryo's genital tract and later on regulates LH production from the anterior pituitary cells, also known as ICSH (interstitial cell-stimulating hormone) in the male. Both testosterone and DHT increase gene transcription. Actions of testosterone and DHT include development of the male testes, penis, epididymis, seminal vesicles, and prostate at puberty, along with growth of axillary, pubic, facial, and chest hair and maintenance of these tissues throughout adulthood. These hormones are also responsible for the stimulation of sexual function and behavior and, of course, spermatogenesis in the adult. In terms of their metabolic actions, they are anabolic agents, increasing the size of muscles and bone. Testosterone stimulates the

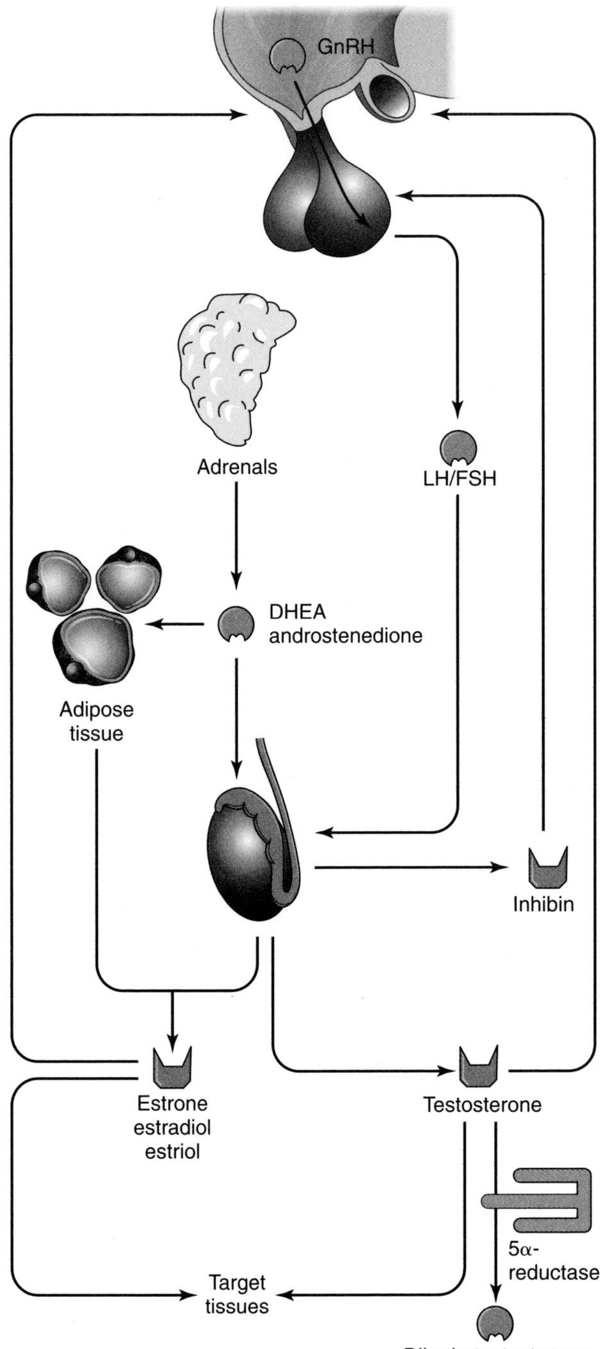

FIGURE 13-9 Regulation of sex steroids. Hypothalamic gonadotropin-releasing hormone (GnRH) stimulates the release of luteinizing hormone (LH) and follicle-stimulating hormone (FSH) from the gonadotrophs of the anterior pituitary. LH and FSH stimulate sex steroid production in the gonads. Adrenal androgens are further metabolized to more potent androgens in the gonads. The aromatase enzyme in both the gonads and adipose tissue converts androgens to estrogens. In certain target tissues, the enzyme 5α-reductase converts testosterone to the more potent androgen dihydrotestosterone. In postpubertal males, sex steroid production is constant. In females, gonadotropins and sex steroids are released in a complex pattern during the menstrual cycle. *ACTH*, adrenocorticotropic hormone; *DHEA*, dehydroepiandrosterone.

synthesis of clotting factors in the liver and also stimulates the production of erythropoietin by the kidneys, giving men a higher hemoglobin concentration than in women.

Androgen Deficiency. Diminished androgen levels in prepubertal boys will cause a delay in puberty, especially in the development of secondary sex characteristics. Failure of the testes to produce enough testosterone in adults leads to low energy, decreased libido, erectile dysfunction, decreased growth of axillary and pubic hair, anemia, osteoporosis, and atrophy of muscle. Testosterone serum levels normally decrease with age, 1 to 2% per year after the age of 30 years.[40,41] Hypogonadism can be primary from testicular failure or secondary from decreased GnRH secretion. Other causes of hypogonadism include Klinefelter's syndrome, mumps, orchiectomy, alcoholism, chemotherapy, and radiation therapy for pituitary or hypothalamic tumors. Treatment with testosterone will stimulate spermatogenesis and cause male sex characteristics to appear, regardless of whether the condition is due to primary testicular failure with elevated FSH and LH levels or secondary failure caused by decreased gonadotropin secretion.

Because testosterone has poor bioavailability, oral synthetic analogs, transdermal applications, intramuscular injections, and topical gels have been developed.[42] Some commonly used intramuscular preparations (testosterone enanthate, testosterone cypionate) have an oil-based solution to slow the absorption from the site of injection. This allows dosing intervals of 2 to 4 weeks compared with an aqueous solution that only lasts 3 days. However, this mode of administration produces great peaks and troughs in concentrations.[43] Oral synthetic agents (methyltestosterone, oxandrolone) can produce a more evenly controlled serum level but have been associated with hepatic tumors. Testosterone patches are applied once daily and are also capable of producing a stable concentration; however, a patch worn on the scrotum has a tendency to fall off with exercise and sweating and requires that the scrotum be shaved frequently. A patch formulated to be worn on the upper arm, thigh, back, or abdomen is available, but it frequently produces skin reactions. It is estimated that 10% of the testosterone dose is absorbed through the skin from the patch. This then serves as a reservoir, slowly releasing the hormone into the body over a 24-hour period. A buccal tablet is also available; it is placed inside the cheek or just above the incisor tooth and held there for 30 seconds.[44] The tablet remains in place by forming a gel that slowly releases the hormone across the oral mucosa. Twice-a-day dosing is necessary, and each tablet stays in place for 12 hours. Adverse effects have included gum and mouth irritation, as well as a bitter taste, but apparently, oral activities, such as eating and brushing the teeth, are not affected. Testosterone can also be rubbed onto the skin, but topical application requires 30 minutes to 4 hours to reach a normal concentration, and vigorous skin-to-skin contact 2 to 12 hours after application did result in a doubling of testosterone levels in female partners.[45] A long-acting testosterone undecanoate formulation has shown efficacy and safety comparable with those of the intramuscular androgen formulation testosterone enanthate and requires dosing at 12-week intervals.[46]

Testosterone replacement therapy is associated with some potential risks and adverse events.[47] When administered to boys at puberty who are deficient in the hormone, secondary sex characteristics develop rapidly with an increase in muscular strength. Height increases at a slower rate. However, if administered to prepubertal males, full predicted height is never reached due to premature closure of the epiphyses of the long bones. Other effects include retention of salt and water, darkening of the skin, growth of facial and pubic hair and a lowering or deepening of the voice. Lipid levels in patients taking testosterone are inconsistent but suggest a neutral effect when the hormone is administered as replacement; however, a significant reduction in high-density lipoprotein (HDL) levels is seen at supraphysiologic doses. Other areas of concern are the potential for developing benign prostatic hyperplasia and prostate cancer. However, multiple studies have not demonstrated a worsening of voiding symptoms, which is an indication of increased prostate size, with replacement therapy. But there is a lowered risk of prostate cancer in men treated with finasteride, a 5α-reductase inhibitor that reduces the DHT level.[48] Monitoring of prostate-specific antigen (PSA) levels and digital rectal examinations are recommended. Other potential adverse events include hepatic neoplasms, seen only with the use of oral preparations, and sleep apnea. Some rather benign adverse effects include breast tenderness and reduced testicular size (from downregulation of gonadal receptors).

Supraphysiologic Use of Testosterone. Studies assessing muscle size and strength in healthy eugonadal men given high doses of testosterone have shown significant increases in bench-press and squat exercise capacity, as well as increases in fat-free mass, particularly when treatment was combined with exercise.[49] However, physiologic doses of testosterone given to older men, not all of whom had hypogonadism, have shown inconsistent gains in strength and physical function. This explains why athletes abusing androgens not only use supraphysiologic doses but also use several different androgen preparations simultaneously. The typical physiologic dose is 100 mg of testosterone enanthate, given weekly as intramuscular injections. The typical supraphysiologic dose may be 1 g or more.[40] Therapists should be aware that although many people associate the term *steroid* with androgens, the term actually describes the basic chemical structure of many endogenous substances, including cholesterol, estrogen, progesterone, and cortisol.

The testosterone precursors dehydroepiandrosterone (DHEA), androstenedione, and androstenediol are considered dietary supplements, believed to enhance muscle strength.[50,51] However, when they were given according to manufacturers' directions to men 35 to 65 years old with normal testosterone levels, no greater strength was detected with the drugs compared with resistance training alone. However, older women but not men showed an increase in bone mineral density probably because supplementation does result in increases in estrogen level. DHEA also abnormally affects the lipid profile.[52,53] However, it is important to recognize that many athletes who take these supplements consume much greater doses than recommended and that the adverse effects cannot always be anticipated.

Additional Uses for Testosterone. From the previous discussion, it is clear that testosterone is useful in physiologic doses for men with hypogonadism, especially when given together with GH in terms of producing an increase in lean mass, muscle strength and endurance.[54] However, when administered in large amounts to eugonadal men, its adverse effects may outweigh the benefits. Despite this risk/benefit ratio, research is being conducted on the use of testosterone and its precursors in various states of illness. Synthetic testosterone analogs have been studied in men with wasting associated with acquired immune deficiency syndrome (AIDS).[55,56] Wasting is defined as a loss of more than 10% of body weight. In several placebo-controlled studies, the testosterone group gained a significant amount of weight and lean body mass compared with the placebo group; some actually experienced increased muscle strength, although this was variable.[57,58] Additional uses for testosterone in older men may include treatments for osteoporosis, Alzheimer's disease, diabetes, and congestive heart failure.[59]

Another area in which testosterone and its analogs are used is treatment of androgen insufficiency in women.[60] Low levels of androgens in women produce depression, fatigue, and decreased libido. Androgen replacement in these women improves their sex drive, increases bone density, reduces menopausal symptoms, and in general creates a feeling of well-being.[61,62] Adverse effects in this population may include acne, hoarse voice, virilization, and hirsutism, although these signs are much more prevalent at supraphysiologic doses than at doses used for treating loss of libido.

Androgen Excess. Androgen excess in women is manifested as hirsutism and acne, which are common symptoms of polycystic ovary syndrome.[62] This syndrome presents as a hormone imbalance, high LH and low FSH (the reverse of normal) levels, and is associated with infertility, obesity, diabetes, and high estrogen and androgen levels. Danazol is an androgen analog used for the treatment of androgen excess and polycystic ovary syndrome.[63] It has few androgenic effects on peripheral tissues and is not converted to estrogen. However, it is able to provide feedback inhibition to the hypothalamus, reducing the release of GnRH. It is also used to reduce gonadal activity in endometriosis, precocious puberty, and fibrocystic breast disease. Adverse effects include nausea, fluid retention, mild hirsutism, reduction in breast size, hepatic dysfunction, and symptoms associated with menopause. Other agents that can be used for treating excess testosterone in women include spironolactone, which has potent antiandrogen properties, and some insulin-sensitizing agents such as metformin, which is used in diabetes.[64] Metformin was originally used in the treatment of polycystic ovary syndrome to help obese women lose weight. It was later discovered that these patients had lowered androgen levels and improved menstrual cycle regularity when on the drug. The mechanism of action is not clear, but there seems to be a connection between insulin resistance and a high androgen level, so that if one is reduced, the other could be expected to follow.

Androgen excess in men may also be treated with spironolactone, but when androgen excess is combined with prostatic growth and male pattern baldness, the drug of choice is finasteride. Finasteride is a 5α-reductase inhibitor that is used for treating benign prostatic hypertrophy.[65] This results in a decrease in the formation of DHT by the prostate, a subsequent decrease in prostate size, and improvement in urinary flow. It is mildly effective, reducing prostate size by about 20%. Adverse effects include decreased libido and erectile dysfunction. This drug and the newer dutasteride must not be touched by pregnant women because they can be absorbed through the skin and may cause birth defects in their offspring (Table 13-6).[66]

Anabolic Steroid Use

Anabolic steroids, also referred to as *anabolic-androgenic steroids* (AASs) are used as doping agents to increase muscle hypertrophy and strength. Some athletes use them to increase physical capabilities in their sports, but it is especially prevalent among body builders.[67] The drugs are often manufactured clandestinely, and the individuals taking these agents have little regard for the impurities that might be present or even the physiologic and psychological consequences associated with the use of these drugs.

AASs are synthetic compounds that have a similar chemical structure to testosterone. They bind to an androgen receptor and produce amplification of testosterone and DHT.[68] They have both androgenic (hormone-induced maleness) and anabolic functions (muscle building). They were originally developed by pharmaceutical companies for the treatment of aplastic anemia, disseminated carcinoma of the breast, and osteoporosis. Researchers intended to make a drug that retained the anabolic properties of testosterone but not its androgenic or virilizing effects. However, all products labeled as AASs still possess significant androgenic adverse effects.

There are three classes of AASs based on their route of administration and the fluid carrier.[69] Oral AASs are acidic preparations that undergo little degradation. They are absorbed through the stomach or the proximal small intestines. These drugs have a short half-life, so frequent dosing throughout the day is necessary. Oil-based injectable preparations have a longer half-life (1 to 4 weeks) but cause pain at the injection site. Because they are slowly absorbed into the systemic circulation, the dose reaching the liver at any one time is low, so there is less of a compromise on the metabolizing enzymes than with the oral drugs. The last category comprises injectables that are dissolved in a water-based solution. They have a shorter half-life (1 to 2 weeks) compared with the drug dissolved in oil, so more frequent injections are needed, but they also cause less discomfort at the injection site due to the lower viscosity of the carrier agent.

AASs are typically used during training as opposed to during competition so that traces of the drugs are not detected during drug tests. The transdermal, sublingual, and oral doses can be cleared from the body quickly in 2 to 14 days, but the water-soluble drugs take about 4 weeks to clear. Athletes have learned about the half-lives of the agents administered and usually can time the administration so that the drug becomes untraceable by the time of competition. However, increased "out-of-competition" testing has identified more athletes who abuse these agents. In 1993, after the collapse of East Germany, records from a seized pharmaceutical company revealed that an

TABLE 13-6 Selected Drugs used in Men's Health

Drug Class	Drug	Indications
5α-reductase inhibitor	Finasteride (Propecia, Proscar), dutasteride (Avodart)	Male androgenetic alopecia (baldness), benign prostatic hyperplasia (BPH)
Phosphodiesterase inhibitor	Sildenafil (Viagra), vardenafil (Levitra),	Erectile dysfunction
Synthetic androgen	Methyltestosterone (Methitest, Virilon, Android)	Delayed puberty or hypogonadism in males; inoperable breast cancer in women
Androgenic hormone	Testosterone, transdermal (Testoderm, Androderm, AndroGel)	Male hypogonadism

injectable form of epitestosterone propionate had been produced primarily for a government-sponsored doping program.[69] This agent is a steroid devoid of any anabolic activity; however, when administered with testosterone, it prevents superphysiologic levels of testosterone from appearing in the urine. However, epitestosterone can be detected in the urine. As a result, the World Anti-Doping Agency (WADA) has now set a urinary threshold for this drug. However, a few years back, the Bay Area Laboratory Cooperative (BALCO) in California was found to produce a transdermal preparation called "The Cream" that contained both testosterone and epitestosterone. The WADA laboratory and a lab at the University of California, Los Angeles (UCLA) have developed tests for these agents.

Athletes using these agents have developed some complex methods of administration. The terms *stacking*, *blending*, and *shot gunning* refer to using more than one drug simultaneously in an attempt to augment the effect of each drug.[69] *Cycling* is another mode of administration, in which the athlete uses different drugs for a finite period, perhaps 6 to 12 weeks, followed by a period of abstinence for the same length of time before the drugs are resumed. *Pyramiding* refers to taking the maximum dose within a certain period, followed by a much smaller dose for the same length of time.

Two examples of anabolic steroids are nandrolone and stanozolol. Nandrolone is given by intramuscular injections, and stanozolol is taken orally. There are few medical indications for the use of these steroids; nandrolone has been used to promote erythropoiesis in aplastic anemia. Adverse effects that might be expected with these drugs in order of greatest number of reports to lesser incidences include water retention, testicular atrophy, insomnia, loss of libido, hair loss, acne, and nose bleeds. Congestive heart failure (CHF) has also been reported as an adverse effect.[70] Psychological adverse effects reported include increased libido, a sense of being more powerful and more confident, mood changes, aggression, and the urge to harm others.[71] Other effects that have been reported are priapism, oligospermia, increased LDL (low-density lipoprotein) levels, weight gain from muscle hypertrophy and fluid retention, and hepatotoxicity.[72] In addition, gynecomastia may occur as a result of the transformation of androgens to estrogens. Further investigations are needed to assess the risk for prostate or testicular cancer with these elevated levels of hormones (Box 13-2).

Erectile Dysfunction

Erectile dysfunction, previously referred to as *impotence*, is defined as the inability to achieve or maintain an erection for sexual intercourse. Among the many contributing factors to this disorder are aging, smoking, hypertension, diabetes, hyperlipidemia, arterial disease, psychological issues, as well as the certain drugs (Box 13-3).[73,74] An erection is achieved by a complex integration of neuronal and hormonal mechanisms that lead to blood accumulating under pressure in the penis.[75] This process can occur only if the smooth muscle of the arteries and sinusoids have vasodilated and relaxed. The erectile tissue then fills with blood and the resultant pressure expands the trabecular walls against the tunica albuginea compressing venous outflow. This results in a rigid penis (Figure 13-10).

The nervous systems involved in attaining an erection are the sympathetic and the nonadrenergic noncholinergic (NANC) nitric oxide (NO) systems. With sexual stimulation, nitric oxide is released and acts to increase production of cyclic guanosine monophasphate (cGMP) within the cavernosal smooth muscle cells. cGMP then decreases intracellular calcium concentration, which, in turn, leads to smooth muscle relaxation. cGMP is degraded by an enzyme called *phosphodiesterase type 5* (PDE5).

Several drugs are now available for the treatment of erectile dysfunction. Papaverine and phenoxybenzamine are vasorelaxant agents that must be injected into the intracavernosal tissue. For obvious reasons, as well as penile fibrosis that occurs as an adverse effect, this therapy has largely been abandoned and replaced by the PDE5 inhibitors sildenafil (Viagra), vardenafil (Levitra), and tadalafil (Cialis).

Sildenafil is only effective when combined with sexual stimulation. It is absorbed within an hour after administration and has a half-life of 4 to 6 hours; the effect can be longer, with some men reporting an erection lasting up to 36 hours after the dose. Tadalafil is longer acting

BOX 13-2 Anabolic Steroids

Oral AAS	Injectable AAS
Methyltestosterone (Android)	Nandrolone decancate (Androlone-D, Hybolin)
Fluoxymesterone (Android-F, Halotestin)	Nandrolone phenylpropionate (Anabolin, Androlone)
Stanozolol (Winstrol)	Stanozolol (Winstrol-V)
Ethylestrenol (Maxibolin)	Testosterone enanthate (Andro LA 200)
Norethandrolone (Nilevar)	Testosterone propionate (Androlan)

BOX 13-3 Drugs That Can Cause Erectile Dysfunction

Drug Class	Specific Drugs
Antihypertensives	Clonidine, methyldopa, hydrochlorothiazide, β-blockers, spironolactone, digoxin
Psychotropic agents	MAO inhibitors, tricyclic antidepressants, benzodiazepines, risperidone
CNS Depressants	Benzodiazepines, opioids, alcohol
Miscellaneous	Estrogens, chemotherapy drugs, histamine-2 blockers, indomethacin, levodopa, fibrates, phenytoin

CNS, central nervous system; *MAO*, monoamine oxidase.

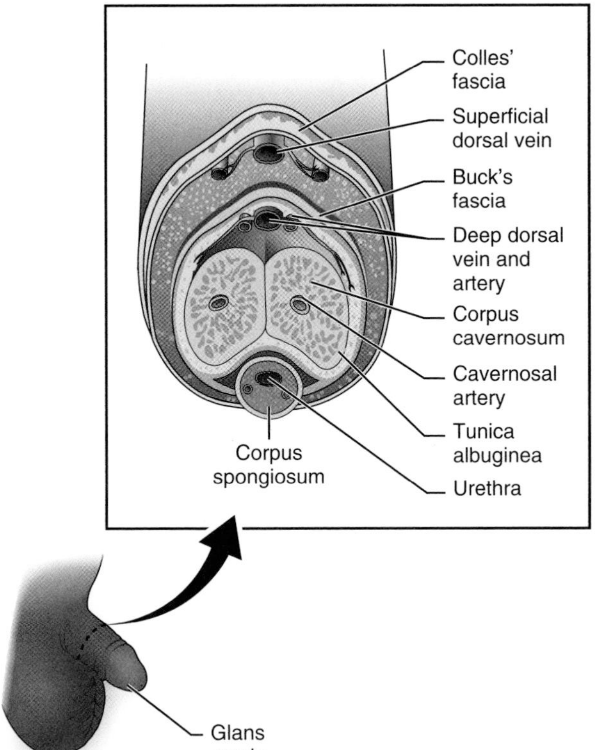

FIGURE 13-10 Structure of the penis. The procreative function of the penis depends upon erection, which results from dilation of the cavernosal artery and filling of the corpora cavernosa and corpus spongiosum with arterial blood. The various fascias, particularly the tunica albuginea, prevent excessive dilation of the penis and limit venous drainage. Both arterial dilation, which increases flow, and reduction of venous outflow are important for maintaining erection.

than sildenafil and therefore can be taken more than an hour before sexual activity. Adverse effects include headache, flushing, and nasal stuffiness. PDE5 inhibitors may also produce visual disturbances (changes in color perception, blurred vision, flashing lights, and a blue haze) and occasionally priapism.[76] However, one of the main concerns with these drugs include the enhanced effect of nitrates on blood pressure that may result in a dangerous life-threatening hypotension.

Estrogen, Progesterone, and the Female Reproductive System

Each ovary contains about seven million ova (eggs) at birth, but most of the ova die during childhood, leaving about 400,000 at puberty; of these, only about 400 are actually ovulated.[1] GnRH, FSH, and LH maintain an intimate balance to ensure that one egg matures and undergoes ovulation each month from puberty to menopause. The menstrual cycle begins with shedding of the uterine endometrium, which lasts approximately 5 days. This is followed by the follicular or proliferative phase in which GnRH induces release of FSH and LH, which, in turn, stimulate follicles to develop. The prolonged low-level release of gonadotropic hormones results in continued maturation of one Graafian follicle. The remaining follicles undergo regression, but the developing follicle continues to mature and converts the androgens produced by the thecal cells of the follicle into estradiol (Figure 13-11). Estradiol, in turn, causes the uterine endometrium to proliferate. In the late follicular phase, the granulosa cells of the maturing follicle start to express LH receptors. These granulosa cells are then stimulated by LH to secrete progesterone. A higher estradiol concentration at midcycle then promotes LH secretion and the LH surge, a reverse of the usual negative feedback mechanism. The LH surge begins to stop androgen and estrogen synthesis and induces the release of ovarian cytokines, prostaglandins, and histamine, causing a rupture of the ovary wall and ovulation. Ovulation starts the luteal phase when the ruptured follicle becomes a corpus luteum, producing progesterone. The progesterone readies the uterine endometrium for implantation. Plasma LH levels fall and remain low for the remainder of the cycle. The progesterone produced by the corpus luteum suppresses LH and FSH production by negative feedback on the hypothalamus and pituitary. If fertilization does not occur, the corpus luteum decreases its progesterone secretion, and the endometrium starts to slough off. When fertilization does occur, progesterone secretion is maintained by human chorionic gonadotropin (hCG) secreted from the fertilized egg until the placental hormones take over in about 6 to 8 weeks (Box 13-4).

Estrogens. Endogenous estrogens have many actions but the primary one is pubertal development in girls and preparation of the endometrium for follicular implantation. The most potent of the naturally existing estrogens is 17β-estradiol with estrone and estriol, second and third.[77] Estrogens come from either androstenedione or testosterone in the ovarian granulosa cell, testicular Sertoli and Leydig cells, adipose cells, adrenal cortex, the placenta, and even in regions of the brain. In premenopausal women, the primary source is the ovary, but after menopause, fat tissue and the adrenal glands become the primary sources. Synthetic estrogens are available, as are external compounds that are estrogenic, including flavones and isoflavones found in plants and even chemicals found in pesticides and some plastics.

Estrogens bind to the ERα and the ERβ receptors, which appear to have different functions.[78] ERαs are located in the reproductive tract, mammary gland, hypothalamus, and vascular smooth muscle. ERβs are expressed in the prostate, ovaries, lung, brain, and bone. Since estrogen is lipophilic, oral formulations are well absorbed. There are also transdermal preparations and creams. The creams are administered to the upper thigh and calf and also to the vaginal area. A 3-month vaginal ring is also available.

Exogenous estrogens have a variety of indications, including stimulating secondary sexual characteristics in girls with primary hypogonadism, and are given along with progesterone to women with primary amenorrhea to induce a menstrual cycle. In addition,

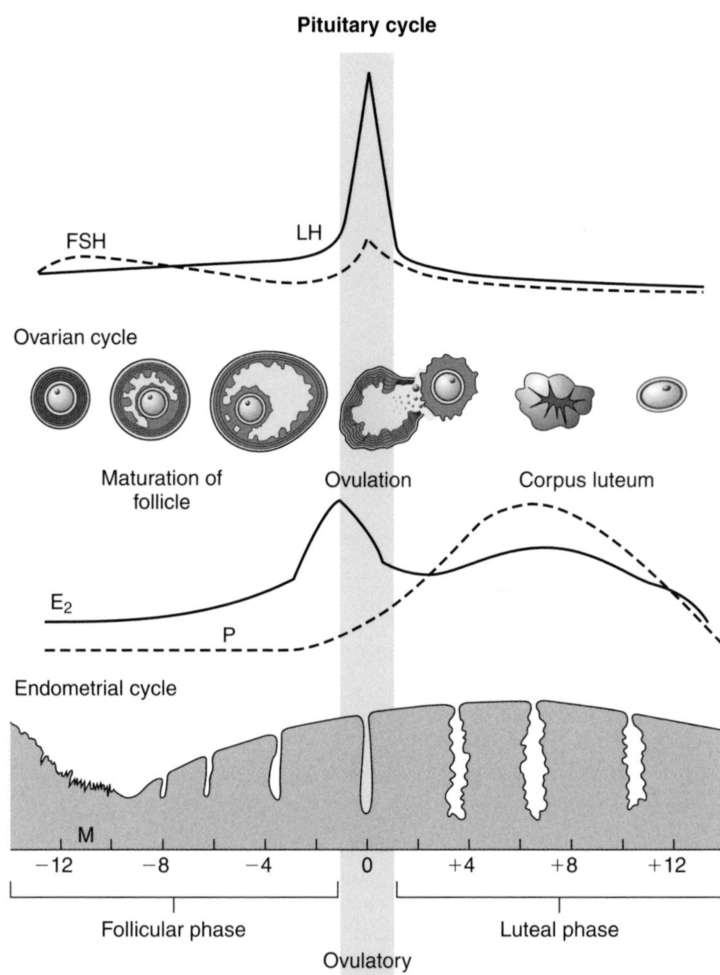

FIGURE 13-11 Menstrual Cycle

BOX 13-4 Hormonal Control of Female Reproduction

- The menstrual cycle begins on Day 1 of menstruation.
- GnRH from the hypothalamus acts on the anterior pituitary to release FSH and LH.
- FSH stimulates follicular development in the ovary and stimulates the release of estrogen.
- Estrogen is released by granulosa cells in the follicle and is responsible for endometrial proliferation and increases its thickness and vascularity.
- LH surge at midcycle stimulates ovulation.
- Cells of the ruptured follicle form the corpus luteum, which secretes progesterone.
- Progesterone acts on the endometrium to prepare it for implantation.
- If fertilization does not occur, the corpus luteum dies, and progesterone secretion stops.
- Low levels of estrogen and progesterones cause endometrial shedding and the beginning of menstruation.

estrogen–progesterone combination pills are used for contraception and also postmenopausally to reduce bone loss and menopausal symptoms such as atrophic vaginitis and vasomotor symptoms. Other beneficial effects of estrogen include increased HDL levels and bone formation. However, estrogen produces a variety of cardiovascular and carcinogenic effects (Boxes 13-5 and 13-6).

Progestins. Among the natural and synthetic progestins, the most active is progesterone. The other two major natural agents are 17-hydroxyprogesterone, which is an inactive metabolite of progesterone, and pregnenolone, which is the precursor to all steroid hormones that is synthesized from cholesterol. Since natural progesterone is inactive when administered orally, synthetic progesterone is used in contraceptive agents to decrease the frequency of GnRH pulses. The synthetic progestin is also known as *progestogen*. Progestins are also used to treat uterine bleeding caused by a hormonal imbalance or fibroids, and along with estrogen after menopause. Some synthetic progestins include medroxyprogesterone, hydroxyprogesterone, megestrol, noretindrone, and norgestrel (Box 13-7).

BOX 13-5 Beneficial and Negative Effects of Estrogen

- Cardiovascular: increased high-density lipoproteins, hypertension, thrombophlebitis, edema, increased risk of stroke
- Gastrointestinal: nausea, vomiting, diarrhea, constipation
- Genitourinary: prevents atropic vaginitis; unopposed estrogen produces amenorrhea with breakthrough uterine bleeding and endometrial hyperplasia; enlarged uterine fibromyomas
- Dermatologic: facial skin discoloration, hirsutism, alopecia
- Breast Health: tender breasts; increased risk of breast cancer
- Bone Health: increased bone mineral density
- Other: fluid retention, decreased carbohydrate tolerance, headaches; replacement therapy decreases hot flashes

BOX 13-6 Estrogenic Drugs

- Conjugated estrogens (Cenestin, Premarin)
- Estradiol (Estrace)
- Estradiol transdermal (Estraderm, FemPatch, Vivelle, Climara, Menostar)

BOX 13-7 Progestins

- Hydroxyprogesterone (Hylutin)
- Medroxyprogesterone, MPA (Amen, Cycrin, Provera, Depo-Provera)
- Megestrol (Megace)
- Norethindrone acetate (Aygestin)
- Norgestrel (Ovrette, Ovral)
- Progesterone (Prometrium, Crinone)

Contraceptive Agents. Oral contraceptives contain either a combination of a synthetic estrogen and a progestogen or progestogen alone (Table 13-7).[79] The estrogen component is usually ethinyl estradiol, but occasionally it is mestranol. These synthetic estrogens closely resemble the natural estradiol produced in the body. Ethinyl estradiol differs by only one substitution, making it more resistant to metabolism. Over the years, the dose of estrogen has been reduced, and the so-called *second-generation pills* produced now have only 20 to 30 mcg of ethinyl estradiol compared with the 50 mcg in the older preparations. Several different progesterones have also been used for many years. The first-generation progestogens had significant androgenic activity, causing acne and reduced HDL cholesterol levels. The newer third-generation progestogens lack androgenic effects and allow for greater expression of estrogen on lipoproteins, which increases HDL levels. Examples of the progestogens currently in use in the combination pill include desogestrel, gestodene, and norgestimate. A combined oral contraceptive that contains a new progestogen, drospirenone (Yaz), is also available. This progestogen has some antimineralocorticoid activity that has been shown to decrease water retention; however, it is associated with a tendency to retain potassium. Other progestogens include the 17-hydroxyprogesterone acetate derivatives, which are devoid of androgenic activity and are mainly used in intramuscular preparations for dysfunctional bleeding or for depot forms of contraception. Medroxyprogesterone (MPA) is also a derivative of the 17-hydroxyprogesterone acetate but is mainly used in hormone replacement therapy (HRT).

The mechanism of action of oral contraceptives is mainly the disruption of the precise hormonal balance that controls the menstrual cycle.[78] The estrogen component suppresses LH and FSH secretion and follicular development by providing negative feedback to the hypothalamus and pituitary. The progestogen component also inhibits production of gonadotropins and makes the cervical mucus thick and unfriendly to sperm. Both components affect fallopian tube motility in opposite ways, thus altering the rate of ovum transport.

Oral combined contraceptives are available in three different combinations. (1) The monophasic pill contains fixed amounts of estrogen and progestogen that are taken together for 21 days before drug administration is stopped to allow 1 week of withdrawal bleeding. (2) Some newer contraceptives are given consecutively for 3 months allowing menstruation to occur only four times a year. (3) The multiphasic combinations (biphasic and triphasic) have a stepwise increase in both hormones and some that just provide increases in the progesterone concentration.

The progestogen-only pill is useful for women who should not take estrogen (especially those who have a history of thromboembolic disorders). It is considered just a little less effective than the combined pills but must be taken within 3 hours of the usual time every day without any breaks. In addition, more irregular bleeding and breakthrough bleeding are associated with this type of pill. The intramuscular injection of progestogen can provide contraception for up to 8 to 12 weeks. Ovulation is more reliably inhibited than with the oral progestogen pill.

The oral contraceptive pills have several benefits in addition to preventing pregnancy. These pills reduce premenstrual tension, dysmenorrhea, and irregular bleeding and thus reduce anemia, ovarian cysts, and endometriosis. There is also strong evidence that they reduce the risk of ovarian cancer by simply limiting the explosive effect of ovulation on the ovary.[80]

Because noncompliance can be a problem with daily contraceptive regimens, there has been new emphasis on development of drugs for women who have trouble remembering to take a daily pill.[81] The norelgestromin–ethinyl estradiol patch and the etonogestrel–ethinyl estradiol vaginal ring are now available. The patch inhibits ovulation in the same manner as the daily pill, but the patch is applied once a week for 3 weeks, followed by a patch-free week for withdrawal bleeding. Application sites include the upper arm, buttocks, lower abdomen, and upper torso. The vaginal ring requires even less patient compliance. It releases ethinyl estradiol and etonogestrel;

TABLE 13-7 Contraceptive Agents

Drug Class	Drug	Indications
Oral contraceptives (OCs)	Norethindrone/ethinyl estradiol (Ortho-Novum, Necon, Jenest) Norethindrone/ethinyl estradiol (Loestrin, Modicon, Necon) Norethindrone/ethinyl estradiol (Ortho-Novum 7/7/7, Estrostep, Tri-Norinyl	Biphasic OCs used to prevent pregnancy Monophasic OCs used to prevent pregnancy Triphasic OCs used to prevent pregnancy
Injectable contraceptives (Depot)—Progestin only	Medroxyprogesterone (Depo-Provera)	Prevention of pregnancy
Transdermal contraceptives	Norelgestromin/ethinyl estradiol	Fixed-combination estrogen-progestin transdermal contraceptive
Intravaginal contraceptives	Etonogestrel-ethinyl estradiol vaginal ring (NuvaRing)	Fixed-combination estrogen-progestin intravaginal contraceptive

it is placed in the vagina for 3 weeks and then removed for 1 week. Menstrual bleeding occurs during the ring-free week. A new combined hormonal injection of MPA acetate and estradiol cypionate can be given monthly. Lastly, a long-acting progestin-only contraceptive consisting of six Silastic capsules containing 36 mg of levonorgestrel is available; it is implanted under the skin and remains in place for 5 years. The progestin is released at a constant rate. Because a surgical incision is required for insertion of the implants, complications such as pain, edema, and bruising may occur. There have also been reports of nerve injury with placement or removal, cellulitis, ulceration, and excessive scarring at the insertion site.

Some annoying adverse effects associated with birth control pills include breakthrough bleeding, nausea, headaches, and breast tenderness; but in time, most women learn to tolerate these.[82] Adverse drug reactions that are more worrisome include increased risk of deep vein thrombosis (DVT), ischemic stroke, myocardial infarction (MI), and pulmonary embolism (PE). However, since the doses of estrogen and progestin were reduced in the 1970s, the safety profile has improved. In addition, estrogens alone are associated with an increase in plasma HDL cholesterol levels, although this factor may be negated by the tendency to increase clotting factors, retain fluid, and produce more renin. Another problem is that some of the newer progestogens, especially norethisterone and MPA, oppose some of the beneficial effects of estrogens on lipid profiles; gestodene and desogestrel may be associated with a slightly higher risk of DVT.[83] Critics speculate that the newer oral contraceptives pose no risk at all, if patients with other cardiovascular risk factors such as smoking, advanced age, and diabetes are excluded.

Despite years of study, the effect of oral contraceptive use on breast cancer continues to be controversial. Data from a pooled analysis of 54 studies published in 1996 showed a small increase in the risk of breast cancer, and a more recent meta-analysis corroborates this finding.[84] But there also have been reports that show no increased risk among women who were currently using oral contraceptives.[85] The study also demonstrated no added risk for women who had ever used the pill or for those who had used the pill on a long-term basis. However, it has been determined that use of oral contraceptives increases breast proliferation significantly in the first week of use compared with placebo.[86] This plus the fact that estrogen has neoplastic influences on the mammary gland as evidenced by the reduction in breast cancer recurrence with estrogen receptor blockers, suggests that contraceptives increase the risk of cancer. In 2005, the International Agency for Research in Cancer reported that there is enough evidence to suggest that contraceptives increase the risk of breast, cervical, and liver cancers. They also reported a protective effect against endometrial and ovarian cancers.[87] Although this subject remains controversial, it is clear that women who have a *BRCA1* or *BRCA2* gene mutation for breast cancer and those with a strong family history of the disease should not take oral contraceptives.

Postcoital Pill. High-dose estrogen and progestogen combinations have traditionally been administered within 72 hours of insemination to prevent pregnancy.[77] Although this approach is 75% successful, it is associated with a high degree of nausea and vomiting. Mifepristone (RU 486) is an antiprogestin that has been approved for the termination of a pregnancy of 49 days or less.[88] This drug has a high affinity for progesterone receptors. Removal of progesterone's influence on the pregnancy produces uterine contractions. In addition, the drug increases prostaglandins, which also stimulate uterine contractility. The recommended dose is three 200-mcg mifepristone tablets taken as a single dose. If abortion does not occur within 3 days, then two more

200-mcg misoprostol tablets (given as a single dose) may be administered. Misoprostol also acts to stimulate uterine contractions. This drug combination terminates early pregnancy in approximately 95% of women. Adverse effects include vaginal bleeding and cramping abdominal pain. Recently, a dose as low as 10 mg has been shown to be effective.[89]

Treatment for Infertility. Infertility may be due to problems with ovulation, an anatomic abnormality of the fallopian tubes such as scarring or endometriosis, or male factors; or it may be unexplained.[90] Unexplained infertility is probably caused by poor quality or quantity of eggs. Ovulation induction or controlled ovarian hyperstimulation is the hallmark of assisted reproduction techniques and is used to treat most cases of infertility. Stimulating the maturation of multiple follicles improves the odds of becoming pregnant in combination with intrauterine insemination or in vitro fertilization. For these procedures to be successful, a complex protocol with several different drugs is needed.

Women undergoing these techniques begin with injections of GnRH agonists. Three are currently available in the United States: leuprolide acetate, nafarelin acetate, and goserelin.[91] Administration of any of these agents initially increases the pituitary release of FSH and LH, but after 7 to 10 days, gonadal secretions are diminished. The goal of this part of the protocol is to prevent premature ovulation. Adverse effects include those associated with menopause, such as hot flashes. These drugs may also be used to treat precocious puberty, endometriosis, uterine fibroids, breast and uterine neoplasms, prostate cancer, and other hormone-sensitive cancers.

Once the reproductive system is turned off, patients are given injectable FSH and LH agonists in an attempt to stimulate growth of multiple follicles.[90] Daily injections over a period of 8 to 12 days will cause the maturation of many follicles in preparation for egg retrieval. The patient is monitored by means of ultrasonography and measurement of serum estradiol levels to determine when the follicles are ready to be harvested. When the follicles reach 18 to 20 mm in diameter, the patient will receive an injection of hCG to induce final egg maturation and ovulation by simulating an LH surge. The eggs are then subsequently retrieved and mixed with sperm to achieve fertilization.

While the egg and sperm are mixing, the mother-to-be receives supplemental progesterone.[91] Most commonly, this entails daily intramuscular injections of progesterone in oil to prepare the uterine lining for implantation. Any time between day 3 and day 6 of fertilization, the embryos are transferred to the mother for implantation. Progesterone injections continue until the placenta begins its own progesterone support at approximately 8 weeks. If pregnancy is not achieved, administration of progesterone is discontinued, and shedding of the uterine lining begins.

Clomiphene is another drug used to treat infertility by promoting follicular maturation, although at much lower numbers than the FSH/LH combinations. Clomiphene is not a gonadotropin but rather an antiestrogen. It antagonizes the normal negative feedback of estrogen on the hypothalamus and pituitary and results in an increased FSH level.Two major adverse effects are associated with induced ovulation.[90] Ovarian hyperstimulation syndrome is a serious complication, in which fluid collects in the abdomen, leading to weight gain, severe pelvic pain, vomiting, and dyspnea. Fatalities are rare but have been reported. Another adverse effect of these drugs is enlargement of the ovaries in all women. This occurs because multiple eggs are maturing, which causes the ovaries to expand. Aerobic activity and activities that include jumping and running are contraindicated. Overheating may affect egg maturity, and jumping activities are contraindicated because an ovary may twist on itself, cutting off its blood supply.

Hormone Replacement Therapy. Hormone replacement therapy (HRT) has been used extensively in postmenopausal women experiencing symptoms resulting from decreasing estrogen levels. Estrogen therapy is useful in reducing vasomotor symptoms (hot flashes), atrophic vaginitis, osteoporosis, mood swings, and insomnia associated with menopause. In addition, for years, physicians were convinced that HRT was cardioprotective because it produces a decrease in LDL and an increase in HDL cholesterol levels. However, in some recent well-conducted and large-scale studies, investigators have expressed serious doubt as to the cardioprotection offered by HRT. These studies have given women more reason to worry about the risk of breast cancer as well.

HRT has been supplied most commonly in tablet form. Estrogen is taken daily with the addition of a progestin tablet for 10 to 14 days a month. This regimen leads to predictable monthly vaginal bleeding at least in the initial years of use. Another alternative has been to take an estrogen tablet daily and a progestin tablet for 10 to 14 days every 3 months. The typical regimen for women who have undergone a hysterectomy is estrogen alone (unopposed estrogen). The reason for this is that estrogen stimulates growth of the endometrial lining, which if left unchecked, can develop into endometrial cancer. However, women who no longer have a uterus do not need to be concerned about endometrial carcinoma.

The most popular form of HRT had been a pill containing 0.625 mg of conjugated equine estrogen and 2.5 mg of MPA acetate, known by the trade name Prempro (manufactured by Wyeth-Ayerst). However, in 1998, studies began to be published in the literature that questioned the benefit-versus-risk of this form of HRT.[92] In the first published study, known as the HERS trial (Heart and Estrogen-Progestin Replacement Study), 2700 women between the ages of 44 and 79 years with known heart disease were examined. These women were randomly assigned to take conjugated estrogen plus progestin or placebo. The study showed that adding HRT did not reduce the incidence of heart attack. There was actually an increase in the number of deaths caused by coronary heart disease (CHD) in the first year of the study, followed by a decrease over the next 3 years, but without an overall reduction in events. A later report in which the same subjects were examined revealed no reduction in the risk of stroke.[93] The next study, released in August 2000 and called the Estrogen Replacement and Atherosclerosis (ERA) trial, indicated that the use of HRT did not slow the progression of coronary artery blockages.[94] The follow-up to the HERS trial, the HERS II trial, which extended observation of the original subjects, showed that after 6.8 years, HRT did not reduce the risk of CHD.[95] The most disturbing study released in July 2002, called the Women's Health Initiative (WHI) Randomized Controlled Trial, indicated that the risks of HRT exceeded the benefits in healthy postmenopausal women.[96] In this study, 16,608 women between the ages of 50 and 79 years were followed up for 5.2 years. They received either placebo or the same estrogen and progesterone combination used in the previous studies. The trial was stopped early because of an increased risk of coronary events, stroke, DVT, gallbladder disease, and invasive breast cancers. The incidence of breast cancer, which appeared to be greater among women who took HRT for more than 5 years, was also greater among women receiving the combination of estrogen and progesterone when compared with other studies of women taking estrogen alone. Absolute risks of taking the hormone combination per 1000 women per year were as follows: for breast cancer, 3.8 with HRT versus 3.0 with placebo; for strokes, 2.9 with HRT versus 2.1 with placebo; for MI, 3.0 with HRT versus 2.3 with placebo; and for blood clots, 3.4 with HRT versus 1.6 with placebo. Positive outcomes included a reduction in hip fractures (33%) and colorectal cancers (37%).[97]

The important point is that these studies were performed with a specific type of HRT, conjugated equine estrogen plus MPA acetate, so these results cannot be generalized to all kinds of HRT (e.g., estrogen ring or estrogen patch). In addition, the type of breast cancer exhibited in the WHI study was more invasive than the tumor that has been typically associated with estrogen. This has led to speculation that the culprit for the breast cancer is the MPA, and not the estrogen.

To determine which hormone is responsible for the increases seen in breast cancer and to more definitively determine the cardiovascular risk associated with estrogen, investigators allowed one arm of the WHI study to continue. The WHI investigators continued to study 10,739 healthy women who had previously had a hysterectomy in the WHI Estrogen-Alone Trial. These women were randomly assigned to receive unopposed estrogen or placebo. This study was also recently stopped prematurely, almost a year before its scheduled end.[98] This was a difficult decision made by the National Institutes of Health (NIH) with the aid of extra advisors because the safety monitoring board could not reach a consensus. The hypothesis of this study was that hormone therapy would reduce the risk of CHD, which did not occur, although early CHD was reduced in the estrogen-alone group. The risk of stroke was still present and was, in fact, a commonality for all three major studies—the HERS study, the WHI study, and the WHI-Estrogen-Alone Trial. However, in the estrogen-alone trial, only 0.12% additional cases of stroke were seen per year. A pattern of increased PE was observed in all the studies, but it was not statistically significant in the estrogen-alone trial.

The major finding of the estrogen-alone trial was the effect of hormones on breast cancer. In the HERS and WHI studies, the risk of breast cancer was seen to have increased by about 25%. In the WHI Estrogen-Alone Trial, the risk of breast cancer was seen to have reduced by 23%. Therefore combining the results of all three studies demonstrates that estrogen plus progestin, particularly MPA, is associated with a higher risk of breast cancer. In fact, some animal and human studies demonstrated that progestins are mitogenic on the human breast but that this risk varies among the different progestins.[99-101] In addition, the synthetic progestins acting through the androgen receptor, which normally confers protection against breast cancer, disrupts the balance between estrogen and progesterone on breast tissue.[102] Furthermore, studies conducted in Europe, where the HRT consists of oral micronized progesterone rather than the synthetic progestin, have not shown the same increase in breast cancer risk.[103]

So who should be receiving HRT? It is clear that HRT has its benefits, such as reducing menopausal symptoms, osteoporosis, and colorectal cancers.[104] However, estrogen therapy is associated with stroke, venous thromboembolism, gallbladder disease, and breast cancer. MPA is associated with a different form of breast cancer, one that is more invasive. Women must carefully weigh the risks versus the benefits of this therapy. They must be adequately informed regarding the cardiovascular events that may occur within the first 1 to 2 years of therapy, and these should be balanced against the severity of menopausal symptoms. Perhaps HRT may be prescribed for a short time, 6 months, and only for women who do not have cardiovascular risk factors. Other forms of HRT such as skin patches, vaginal creams, and vaginal rings might not present the same risks; but further study of these products is warranted.[105]

ACTIVITIES 13

1. You are evaluating a 52-year-old female for difficulty with fine motor skills secondary to a fine tremor of her hands. As part of your evaluation, you attempt to take a detailed medical history. The patient does not remember when the tremors started or what makes them better or worse. She only knows that activities such as buttoning up a shirt and writing are becoming more difficult. The only other piece of information she offers is that she has felt very nervous and is

hoping a massage could be part of her treatment program. You proceed with the evaluation.

This patient is a thin, active woman who states she has trouble keeping weight on. She has prominent eyes and presents with hot, moist skin despite the fact that she has been sitting in your waiting area for at least 45 minutes. Upper extremity range of motion is within normal limits, and strength is normal, although the patient reports some proximal weakness in her legs when she goes from sit-to-stand. Likewise, the cervical range is normal but you found a lump on palpation of the neck, probably representing an enlarged thyroid gland.

Questions

A. Discuss the most likely diagnosis for this patient, and list some other symptoms associated with this condition. Which signs and symptoms might negatively affect rehabilitative interventions?

B. You are alarmed about your findings, and refer the patient to her doctor. The patient's physician prescribes propylthiouracil. Why was this drug chosen?

C. Following surgical removal of the thyroid gland, the patient will receive thyroid replacement therapy. What signs or symptoms should you look out for, and what should the patient know about replacement therapy?

2. You are treating a 13-year-old boy for impairments related to cerebral palsy. The child also has a growth hormone deficiency and is currently taking somatrem. He has recently demonstrated more limitations in function, and you have noticed additional tightness in the hamstrings and heel cords bilaterally. You also notice that his clothes seem too short for his body. Review of the patient's chart reveals that he has grown at least 3 cm in the last 4 months. What are your recommendations?

3. Discuss the use of growth hormone, including recommended uses as well as off-label uses. What risks are involved with the off-label uses?

4. You are asked to evaluate a patient admitted to the hospital following an automobile accident. He has absent sensation below the waist and lower extremity paralysis consistent with a spinal cord injury. The patient is receiving high-dose IV steroids. What is the purpose of using a steroid in this situation, and what are some things the therapist needs to take into consideration when planning treatment?

5. What are some alternative treatments for hormone replacement therapy (HRT) in menopausal women?

6. Research the literature for recent articles on the use of testosterone for the treatment of the following illnesses: diabetes, metabolic syndrome, congestive heart failure, cardiovascular disease, Alzheimer's disease, and mood disturbances. How strong is the evidence for its use in these conditions?

REFERENCES

1. Guyton AC, Hall JE: Textbook of medical physiology (10th ed.), Philadelphia, 2000, W.B. Saunders Company.
2. Miller JW: Drugs and the endocrine and metabolic systems. In Page CP, Curtis MJ, Sutter MC, editors: Integrated pharmacology, Philadelphia. 2002, Mosby.
3. Lamberts SW, de Herder WW, van der Lely AJ: Pituitary insufficiency. Lancet 352:127-134, 1998.
4. Lilley LL, Harrington RA, Snyder JS: Pituitary drugs. In Lilley LL, Harrington RA, Snyder JS, editors: Pharmacology and the nursing process, Philadelphia, 2007, Mosby.
5. Yu R, Braunstein GD: Disorders of the hypothalamic-pituitary axis. In Waldman SA, Terzic A, editors: Pharmacology and therapeutics: Principles to practice, Philadelphia, 2009, Saunders.
6. Okada S, Kopchick JJ: Biological effects of growth hormone and its antagonist. Trends Mol Med 7(3):126-132, 2001.
7. Abramowicz, M, Growth Hormone for Normal Short Children. In The Medical Letter, New Rochelle, NY, 2003, The Medical Letter Inc.
8. Vance ML, Mauras N: Growth hormone therapy in adults and children. N Engl J Med 341(16):1206-1216, 1999.
9. Finkelstein BS, Imperiale TF, Speroff T, Marrero U, Radcliffe DJ, Cuttler L: Effect of growth hormone therapy on height in children with idiopathic short stature. Arch Pediatr Adolesc Med 156(3):230-240, 2002.
10. Ergun-Longmire B, Mertens AC, Mitby P: Growth hormone treatment and risk of second neoplasms in the childhood cancer survivor. J Clin Endocrinol Metab 91:3494-3498, 2006.
11. Murray RD, Shalet SM: Adult growth hormone replacement: Lessons learned and future direction. J Clin Endocrinol Metab 87(10):4427-4428, 2002.
12. Hütler M, Schnabel D, Staab D, et al: Effect of growth hormone on exercise tolerance in children with cystic fibrosis. Med Sci Sports Exerc 34(4):567-572, 2002.
13. Hennessey JV, Chromiak JA, DellaVentura S, et al: Growth hormone administration and exercise effects on muscle fiber type and diameter in moderately frail older people. J Am Geriat Soc 49(7):852-858, 2001.
14. Paiva ES, Deodhar A, Jones KD, Bennett R: Impaired growth secretion in fibromyalgia patients: Evidence for augmented hypothalamic somatostatin tone. Arthritis Rheum 46(5):1344-1350, 2002.
15. Burgess E, Wanke C: Use of recombinant human growth hormone in HIV-associated lipodystrophy. Curr Opin Infect Dis 18:17-24, 2005.
16. Lange KH, Andersen JL, Beyer N, et al: GH administration changes myosin heavy chain isoforms in skeletal muscle but does not augment muscle strength or hypertrophy, either alone or combined with resistance exercise training in healthy elderly men. J Clin Endocrinol Metab 87(2):513-523, 2002.
17. Mauras N: Growth hormone therapy in the glucocorticosteroid-dependent child: Metabolic and linear growth effects. Hormone Res 56(suppl 1):13-18, 2001.
18. Laron Z: Insulin-like growth factor-1 (IGF-1): Safety and efficacy. Pediatr Endocrinol Rev 2(suppl 1):78-85, 2004.
19. Chernausek SD, Backeljauw PF, Frame J, Kuntze J, Underwood LE: Long-term treatment with recombinant insulin like growth factor (IGF)-1 in children with severe IGF-1 deficiency due to growth hormone insensitivity. The J Clin Endocrinol Metab 92(3):902-910, 2007.
20. Lamberts SW, van der Lely AJ, de Herder WW, Hofland LJ: Octreotide. N Engl J Med 334:246-254, 1996.
21. Colao A, et al: Extensive personal experience: Acromegaly. J Clinical Endocrinol Metabol 82:3395-3402, 1997.
22. Abramowicz M: Pegvisomant (Somavert) for acromegaly. In The Medical Letter, New Rochelle, NY, 2003, The Medical Letter, Inc.

23. Zhang J, Lazar MA: The mechanism of action of thyroid hormones. Annu Rev Physiol 62:439-466, 2000.
24. Yen PM: Physiological and molecular basis of thyroid hormone action. Physiol Rev 81(3):1097-1142, 2001.
25. Baron HL, Singer PA: Disorders of the thyroid. In Waldman SA, Terzic A, editors: Pharmacology and therapeutics: Principles to practice, Philadelphia, 2009, Mosby.
26. Wood AJ: Drugs and thyroid function. N Engl J Med 333(25):1688-1694, 1995.
27. Gittoes N, Franklyn JA: Hyperthyroidism. Drugs 55(4): 543-553, 1998.
28. Lindsay RS, Toft AD: Hypothyroidism. Lancet 349:413-417, 1997.
29. Brent GA: The molecular basis of thyroid hormone action. N Engl J Med 331(13):847-853, 1994.
30. Walsh JP, Shiels L, Lim EM: Combined thyroxin/liothyronine treatment does not improve well-being, quality of life, or cognitive function compared to thyroxine alone: A randomized controlled trial in patients with primary hypothyroidism. J Clin Endocrinol Metab 88:4543-4550, 2003.
31. Escobar-Morreale HF, Botella-Carretero JI, Gomez-bueno M: Thyroid hormone replacement therapy in primary hypothyroidism: A randomized trial comparing L-thyroxine plus liothyronine with L-thyroxine alone. Ann Intern Med 142:412-424, 2005.
32. Sheppard MC, Holder R, Franklyn JA: Levothyroxine treatment and occurrence of fracture of the hip. Arch Intern Med 162:338-343, 2002.
33. Bakheit AM, Thilmann AF, Ward AB, et al: A randomized, double-blind, placebo-controlled, dose-ranging study to compare the efficacy and safety of three doses of botulinum toxin type A (Dysport) with placebo in upper limb spasticity after stroke. Stroke 31:2402-2406, 2000.
34. Funder JW: Glucocorticoid and mineralocorticoid receptors: Biology and clinical relevance. Annu Rev Med 48:231-240, 1997.
35. Buckingham JC, Flower RJ: Lipocortin 1: A second messenger of glucocorticoid action in the hypothalamo-pituitary-adrenocortical axis. Mol Med Today July:296-302, 1997.
36. Rang HP, et al: The pituitary and the adrenal cortex. In Rang HP, Dale MM, Ritter JM, Flower R, editors: Rang and Dale's pharmacology, New York, 2007, Churchill Livingstone.
37. Terzolo M, Pia A, Berruti A, et al: Low-dose monitored itotane treatment achieves the therapeutic range with manageable side effects in patients with adrenocortical cancer. J Clin Endocrinol Metab 85:2234-2238, 2000.
38. Coursin DB, Wood KI: Corticosteroid supplementation for adrenal insufficiency. JAMA 287:236-240, 2002.
39. Hamaker L, Jabbour S: Adrenal disorders. in Waldman SA, Terzic A, editors: Pharmacology and therapeutics: Principles to practice, Philadelphia, 2009, Saunders.
40. Bhasin S, Woodhouse L, Storer TW: Proof of the effect of testosterone on skeletal muscle. J Endocrinol 170:27-38, 2001.
41. Travison TG, Araujo AB, Hall SA, McKinlay JB: Temporal trends in testosterone levels and treatment in older men. Curr Opin Endocrinol Diabet Obesity 16(3):211-217, 2009.
42. Testim and Striant—Two new testosterone products. Med Lett 45:1164, 2003.
43. Dobs AS, Meikle AW, Arver S, Sanders SW, Caramelli KE, Mazer NA: Pharmacokinetics, efficacy, and safety of permeation-enhanced testosterone transdermal system in comparison with bi-weekly injections of testosterone enanthate for the treatment of hypogonadal men. J Clin Endocrinol Metab 84(10):3469-3478, 1999.
44. Dobs AS, Hoover DR, Chen MC, Allen R: Pharmacokinetic characteristics, efficacy, and safety of buccal testosterone in hypogonadal males: A pilot study. J Clin Endocrinol Metab 83(1):33-39, 1998.
45. Androgel. Med Lett 42:1080, 2000.
46. Minnemann T, Schubert M, Freude S, et al: Comparison of a new long-acting testosterone undecanoate formulation vs testosterone enanthate for intramuscular androgen therapy in male hypogonadism. J Endocrinol Invest 31(8):718-723, 2008.
47. Rhoden EL, Morgentaler A: Risks of testosterone-replacement therapy and recommendations for monitoring. N Engl J Med 350(5):482-492, 2004.
48. Wirén S, Stattin P: Androgens and prostate cancer risk. Best Pract Res Clin Endocrinol Metab 22(4):601-613, 2008.
49. Bhasin S, Storer TW, Berman N, et al: The effects of supraphysiologic doses of testosterone on muscle size and strength in men. N Engl J Med 335:1-7, 1996.
50. Broeder CE, Quindry J, Brittingham K, et al: The Andro Project: Physiological and hormonal influences of androstenedione supplementation in men 35 to 65 years old participating in a high-intensity resistance training program. Arch Intern Med 160:3093-3104, 2000.
51. Brown GA, Vukovich MD, Sharp RL, Reifenrath TA, Parsons KA, King DS: Effect of oral DHEA on serum testosterone and adaptations to resistance training in young men. J Appl Physiol 87(6):2274-2283, 1999.
52. King DS, Sharp RL, Vukovich MD, et al: Effect of oral androstenedione on serum testosterone and adaptations to resistance training in young men: A randomized controlled trial. JJAMA 281(21):2020-2028, 1999.
53. Weiss EP, Shah K, Fontana L, Lambert CP, Holloszy JO, Villareal DT: Dehydroepiandrosterone replacement therapy in older adults: 1- and 2-y effects on bone. Am J Clin Nutr 89(5):1459-1467, 2009.
54. Sattler FR, Castaneda-Sceppa C, Binder EF, et al: Testosterone and growth Hormone Improve body composition and muscle performance in older men. J Clin Endocrinol Metab 94(6):1991-2001, 2009.
55. Corcoran C, Grinspoon S: Drug therapy: Treatments for wasting in patients with the acquired immunodeficiency syndrome. N Engl J Med 340(22):1740-1750, 1999.
56. Bhasin S, Storer TW, Javanbakht M, et al: Testosterone replacement and resistance exercise in HIV-infected men with weight loss and low testosterone levels. JAMA 283(6):763-770, 2000.
57. Knapp PE, Storer TW, Herbst KL, et al: Effects of a supraphysiological dose of testosterone on physical function, muscle performance, mood, and fatigue in men with HIV-associated weight loss. Am J Physiol Endocrinol Metab294(6):E1135-E1143, 2008.
58. Miller K, Corcoran C, Armstrong C, et al: Transdermal testosterone administration in women with acquired immunodeficiency wasting: A pilot study. J Clin Endocrinol Metab 83:2717-2725, 1998.
59. Stanworth RD, Jones TH: Testosterone for the aging male; Current evidence and recommended practice. Clin Interven Aging 3(1):25-44, 2008.
60. Chi MC, Lobo RA: Formulations and use of androgens in women. Mayo Clin Proc 79(4):S3-S7, 2004.
61. Shifren JL: The role of androgens in female sexual dysfunction. Mayo Clin Proc 79(4):S19-S24, 2004.
62. Guzick DS: Polycystic ovary syndrome. Obstet Gynecol 103(1):181-193, 2004.
63. Nissen D: Mosby's drug consult, St. Louis, 2004, Mosby.
64. Tsilchorozidou T, Prelevic GM: The role of metformin in the management of polycystic ovary syndrome. Curr Opin Obstet Gynecol 15(6):483-488, 2003.
65. McConnell JD, Bruskewitz R, Walsh P, et al: The effect of finasteride on the risk of acute urinary retention and the need for surgical treatment among men with benign prostatic hyperplasia. N Engl J Med 338(9):557-563, 1998.

66. Abramowicz M: Dutasteride (Avodart) for benign prostatic hyperplasia. In The Medical Letter, New Rochelle, NY, 2002, The Medical Letter, Inc.
67. Baker JS, Graham MR, Davies B: Steroid and prescription medicine abuse in the health and fitness community: A regional study. Euro J Int Med 17:479-484, 2006.
68. Shadidi NT: A review of the chemistry, biological action, and clinical applications of anabolic-androgenic steroids. Clin Ther 23:1355-1390, 2001.
69. Graham MR, Davies B, Grace FM, Kicman A, Baker JS: Anabolic steroid use: patterns of use and detection of doping. Sports Med 38(6):505-525, 2008.
70. Ahlgrim C, Guglin M: Anabolics and cardiomyopathy in a bodybuilder: Case report and literature review. J Cardiac Fail 15(6):496-500, 2009.
71. Graham MR, Davies B, Kicman A, Cowan D, Hullin D, Baker JS: Recombinant human growth hormone in abstinent androgenic-anabolic steroid use: psychological, endocrine, and trophic factor effects. Curr Neurovasc Res 4:9-18, 2007.
72. Christiansen K: Behavioural effects of androgen in men and women. J Endocrinol 170:39-48, 2001.
73. Uçok A, Incesu C, Aker T, Erkoç S: Sexual dysfunction in patients with schizophrenia on antipsychotic medication. Eur Psychiatry 22(5):328-333, 2007.
74. Reffelmann T, Kloner RA: Sexual function in hypertensive patients receiving treatment. Vasc Health Risk Manag 2(4):447-455, 2006.
75. Lue TF: Drug therapy: Erectile dysfunction. N Engl J Med 342:1802-1813, 2000.
76. Hatzimouratidis K: Sildenafil in the treatment of erectile dysfunction: An overview of the clinical evidence. Clin Interv Aging 1(4):403-414, 2006.
77. Lilley LL, Harrington RA, Snyder JS: Women's health drugs. In Lilley LL, Harrington RA, Snyder JS, editors: Pharmacology and the nursing process, St. Louis, 2007, Mosby.
78. Stovall DW, Strauss JF: Reproductive health. In Waldman SA, Terzic A, editors: Pharmacology and therapeutics: Principles to practice, Philadelphia, 2009, Saunders.
79. Waller DG, Renwick AG, Hillier K: Medical pharmacology and therapeutics, New York, 2001, W.B. Saunders.
80. Ness RB, Grisso JA, Klapper J, et al: Risk of ovarian cancer in relation to estrogen and progestin dose and use characteristics of oral contraceptives. Am J Epidemiol 152(3):233-241, 2000.
81. Herndon E: New contraceptive options. Am Fam Phys 69:853-860, 2004.
82. Petitti DB: Clinical practice: Combination estrogen-progestin oral contraceptives. N Engl J Med 349(15):1443-1450, 2003.
83. Rosing J, Tans G, Nicolaes GA, et al: Oral contraceptives and venous thrombosis: Different sensitivities to activated protein C in women using second- and third-generation oral contraceptives. Br J Haematol 97(1):233-238, 1997.
84. Kahlenborn C, Modugno F, Potter DM: Oral contraceptive use as a risk factor for premenopausal breast cancer: A meta-analysis. Mayo Clin Proc 81(10):1290-1302, 2006.
84. Marchbanks PA, McDonald JA, Wilson HG, et al: Oral contraceptives and the risk of breast cancer. N Engl J Med 346(26):2025-2032, 2002.
86. Garcia y Narvaiza D, Navarrete MA, Falzoni R, Maier CM, Nazário AC: Effect of combined oral contraceptives on breast epithelial proliferation in young women. Breast J 14(5):450-455, 2008.
87. Casey PM, Cerhan JR, Pruthi S: Oral contraceptive use and the risk of breast cancer. Mayo Clin Proc 83(1):86-91, 2008.
88. Abramowicz M: Mifepristone (RU 486). In The Medical Letter, New Rochelle, NY, 2000, The Medical Letter, Inc.
89. Gemzell-Danielsson K, Mandl I, Marions L: Mechanisms of action of mifepristone when used for emergency contraception. Contraception 68(6):471-476, 2003.
90. Abramowicz M: Drugs for assisted reproduction. In Treatment guidelines from the medical letter, New Rochelle, NY, 2003, The Medical Letter, Inc.
91. Huirne JA, Lambalk CB: Gonadotropin-releasing-hormone-receptor antagonists. Lancet 358:1793-1803, 2001.
92. Hulley S, Grady D, Bush T, et al: Randomized trial of estrogen plus progestin for secondary prevention of coronary heart disease in postmenopausal women. JAMA 280(7):605-613, 1998.
93. Simon JA, Hsia J, Cauley JA, et al: Postmenopausal hormone therapy and risk of stroke: The Heart and Estrogen-progestin Replacement study. Circulation 103(5):638-642, 2001.
94. Herrington DM, Reboussin DM, Brosnihan KB, et al: Effects of estrogen replacement on the progression of coronary-artery atherosclerosis. N Engl J Med 343(8):522-529, 2000.
95. Grady D, Herrington D, Bittner V, et al: Cardiovascular disease outcomes during 6.8 years of hormone therapy: Heart and Estrogen-progestin Replacement study follow up. JAMA 288(1):49-57, 2002.
96. Investigators: Writing group for the Women's Health Initiative: Principal results from the Women's Health Initiative randomized controlled trial. JAMA 288(3):321-333, 2002.
97. Chlebowski RT, Wactawski-Wende J, Ritenbaugh C, et al: Estrogen plus progestin and colorectal cancer in postmenopausal women. N Engl J Med 350(10):991-1004, 2004.
98. Hulley S, Grady D: The WHI estrogen-alone trial—Do things look any better? JAMA 291(14):1769-1771, 2004.
99. Santen RJ: Risk of breast cancer with progestins: Critical assessment of current data. Steroids 68(10-13):953-964, 2003.
100. Nilsen J, Brinton RD: Divergent impact of progesterone and medroxyprogesterone acetate (Provera) on nuclear mitogen-activated protein kinase signaling. Proc Nat Acad Sci USA 100(18):10506-10511, 2003.
101. Brinton LA, Schairer C: Postmenopausal hormone-replacement therapy—Time for a reappraisal? N Engl J Med 336(25):1821-1822, 1997.
102. Birrell SN, Butler LM, Harris JM, Buchanan G, Tilley WD: Disruption of androgen receptor signaling by synthetic progestins may increase risk of developing breast cancer. FASEB J 21(10):2285-2293, 2007.
103. Fournier A, Berrino F, Riboli E, Avenel V, Clavel-Chapelon F: Breast cancer risk in relation to different types of hormone replacement therapy in the E3N-EPIC cohort. Int J Cancer 114:448-454, 2005.
104. Kocjan T, Gordana M: Hormone replacement therapy update: Who should we be prescribing this to now? Curr Opin Obstet Gynecol 15(6):459-464, 2003.
105. Stevenson JC, Oladipo A, Manassiev N, Whitehead MI, Guilford S, Proudler AJ: Randomized trial of effect of transdermal continuous combined hormone replacement therapy on cardiovascular risk markers. Br J Haematol 124(6):802-808, 2004.

14

Drug Treatment for Osteoporosis and Diabetes

Barbara Gladson

DRUG TREATMENT FOR OSTEOPOROSIS

Osteoporosis is the loss of bone mass caused by a loss of mineral content, which reduces the strength of bone. All individuals lose bone mass as they age, but for women, there is a marked increase in bone loss after menopause that corresponds to the loss of estrogen. Other factors that influence the loss of bone include smoking, significant alcohol use, hereditary factors, immobility, and age. Age-related bone loss results from increased bone reabsorption and increased apoptosis of osteocytes, decreasing the repair response. In addition, fracture risk is increased because of comorbid conditions, cognitive impairment, medications, deconditioning, and inadequate calcium and vitamin D intake. There is a lower incidence of osteoporosis among men, probably resulting from higher peak bone mass to begin with, shorter life expectancy, and a more gradual cessation of hormone production. Bone loss in the younger group of older adults is associated with trabecular loss and may predispose these individuals to spontaneous vertebral fractures. Osteoporosis in older patients is associated with loss of cortical bone, increasing the risk of traumatic fracture, particularly at the neck of the femur. However, the development of osteoporosis is viewed on a continuum with multiple processes occurring at once. Many drugs are marketed for the prevention and treatment of osteoporosis, particularly postmenopausal osteoporosis. However, drug intervention for this disorder has become much more complicated by the news that hormone replacement therapy (HRT) increases the incidence of cardiovascular diseases and breast cancer.

Bone Remodeling

Bone is specialized connective tissue designed as a load-bearing structure. It is formed by a combination of dense compact (cortical) bone and cancellous (trabecular) bone. Trabecular bone is a honeycomb of vertical and horizontal bars filled with marrow and fat. Trabecular bone is located in the vertebral bodies, pelvis, and proximal femur.[1] The mineral components of bone are calcium and phosphorus, and the organic matrix is type I collagen. Two major cell types that are found in bone include (1) the osteoclast, responsible for removing the mineralized matrix, and (2) the osteoblast, responsible for producing the matrix. These cell types are the commanders of the bone remodeling process.

Bone is constantly undergoing remodeling with a delicate balance between reabsorption by osteoclasts and bone formation by osteoblasts. Bone remodeling occurs in small packets of cells called basic multicellular units (BMUs).[2] The BMU is approximately 1 to 2 mm long and 0.2 to 0.4 mm wide and is composed of a group of osteoclasts in the front, osteoblasts in the back, a central vascular capillary, and a nerve supply. Each BMU begins at a particular place and advances toward a target, which is the area that needs replacement. The BMU travels through bone across a surface, excavating and then replacing. Osteoclasts adhere to bone and remove it by proteolytic digestion and acidification. Osteoblasts move to cover the excavated area and begin forming new bone. The lifespan of the BMU is 6 to 9 months, and at any one time there are one million active BMUs.

The precursors of osteoblasts are mesenchymal stem cells, which also give rise to bone marrow stromal cells, chondrocytes, muscle cells, and adipocytes, whereas the precursors of osteoclasts are hematopoietic cells of the monocytes/macrophage lineage.[3] The development and differentiation of these cells are controlled by growth factors and cytokines produced in the bone marrow environment. Several cytokines are involved in the early stages of hematopoiesis and in osteoclastogenesis. Interleukin-6 (IL-6), in particular, is involved in both pathways but alone is able to stimulate osteoclastogenesis and promotes bone reabsorption.

The regulation of cell numbers and alterations in the functional activity of the osteoclasts and osteoblasts, termed *cell vigor*, contributes to changes in the rate of reabsorption and formation. Several molecules have been proposed to coordinate this function. Three proteins that are involved in this signaling pathway have been identified.[4] Two of these proteins are membrane-bound cytokine-like molecules called *receptor activator of nuclear factor* (RANK) and the *RANK ligand* (RANKL). RANK is present on osteoclast precursor cells and when activated promotes osteoclast maturation by increasing the expression of specific genes. RANKL is produced by and exists on the surface of osteoblasts. Thus, if an osteoclast precursor encounters an osteoblast, the resulting interaction between RANK and RANKL stimulates the osteoclast precursor to mature into the bone-reabsorbing osteoclast. Activation of RANK by RANKL induces the expression of interferon-β (IF- β) in osteoclast precursor cells, which ultimately leads to a decrease in osteoclast differentiation by means of negative feedback.[5] Osteoblasts also produce osteoprotegerin (OPG), which binds to RANKL and prevents it from binding to RANK. This inhibits RANKL-mediated osteoclast maturation. It is believed that these chemical factors are involved in modulating the strength of the osteoclast response and in stimulating more frequent cycles of reabsorption.

The mature osteoblast secretes the bone matrix whose major product is type I collagen.[3] Extracellular processing of this collagen results in three-chained type I collagen molecules, which then form a collagen fibril. The osteoblasts also synthesize other proteins that are incorporated into the bone matrix, including osteocalcin and osteonectin (noncollagenous proteins), as well as glycosaminoglycans, biglycan, and decorin; osteoblasts help regulate the local concentrations of calcium and phosphate in a way that promotes the formation of hydroxyapatite. Osteoblasts express large amounts of alkaline phosphatase, which is thought to play a role in the mineralization of bone. Bone mineralization lags behind matrix production, and matrix synthesis determines the volume of bone, but mineralization of the matrix increases the density of bone by displacing water. Osteoblasts become osteocytes as they are buried within the mineralized matrix. They are regularly spaced throughout the matrix and communicate with each other and with other cells on the bone surface via multiple extensions of their plasma membrane. Osteoblasts communicate with the cells of the bone marrow stroma. Communication actually extends from the osteocytes to the osteoblasts to bone marrow and finally to the endothelial cells of the vascular supply. Thus, the location of the osteocytes can indicate the need for repair and transmit this need to the bone marrow to stimulate differentiation of additional osteoblasts. Osteocytes can also detect changes in the levels of hormones that circulate through the blood vessel, such as estrogen and glucocorticoids, which influence their function.

Osteoclasts are large multinucleated cells that have a ruffled border, described as a complex system of finger-shaped projections of membrane.[5] This structure is surrounded by a specialized area called the *clear zone*, which attaches the osteoclast to bone and seals off the area to be excavated. Here, the osteoclast secretes the matrix metalloproteinases to degrade the matrix.

Systemic hormones, primarily parathyroid hormone (PTH) and 1,25-dihydroxyvitamin D_3, are strong stimulators of osteoclast formation and regulate calcium absorption and excretion from the intestine and kidneys, maintaining calcium homeostasis.[6] Specifically, PTH increases calcium reabsorption from bone, increases calcium reabsorption from the kidneys, increases intestinal absorption of calcium, and promotes the formation of 1,25-dihydroxyvitamin D_3. At the same time, PTH decreases phosphate reabsorption from the kidneys. The result is an increase in the serum calcium level and a decrease in the serum phosphate level.

Vitamin D is produced in the skin by UV light (D_3) or ingested in the diet (D_3 and D_2).[7] Because vitamins D_2 and D_3 have identical biologic actions, they are referred to as vitamin D. However, vitamin D must undergo successive hydroxylations to act as a hormone. In the liver, it is hydroxylated to 25-hydroxyvitamin D_3, and then in the kidneys, it is further activated to 1,25-dihydroxyvitamin D_3. At physiologic levels, vitamin D increases bone formation. It stimulates absorption of calcium, phosphate, and magnesium from the intestines and plays a significant role in bone formation. Vitamin D is responsible for mineralization of newly formed osteoid along the calcification front. The mechanism of action may be the synthesis of osteocalcin and fibronectin. In addition, it increases calcium and phosphorus reabsorption from the kidneys. At high levels, however, the action of vitamin D mimics the action of PTH.

Calcitonin inhibits osteoclast development and promotes osteoclast apoptosis.[6] It decreases reabsorption and enhances bone formation. Other hormones including estrogen, androgen, glucocorticoids, and thyroid hormone have strong influences over the development of osteoblasts and osteoclasts by producing different cytokines.

Pathogenesis of Osteoporosis

The rate of differentiation of osteoblasts and osteoclasts, their relative vigor, and the timing of their death—all influence the bone repair process.[3] The lifespan of the osteoclast is about 2 weeks, whereas the osteoblast exists for 3 months. Normally, estrogen and androgens suppress IL-6 and also directly act on osteoclasts to promote their cell death. The sex steroids also have an antiapoptotic effect on osteoblasts. Therefore, the loss of sex steroids, particularly after menopause, leads to a shortened lifespan for osteoblasts. In addition, a delay in the cell death of osteoclasts leads to the formation of deeper reabsorptive cavities and perforation of the trabeculae.

All of the cells involved in bone remodeling possess estrogen receptors; osteoblasts, osteocytes, and osteoclasts. In addition, estrogen affects bones via its effects on cytokines and growth factors. In estrogen deficiency, T cells are found to encourage osteoclast recruitment and differentiation and extend longevity with the help of IL-1, IL-6, and tumor necrosis factor–α (TNF-α). T cells may also prevent osteoblast maturation and promote its cell death. Lastly, an estrogen-deficient state enhances bone sensitivity to parathyroid hormone (PTH), which is responsible for maintaining serum calcium levels and can promote calcium release from bone. Other mechanisms which may be active in the pathogensis of osteoporosis include an increase in RANKL production, increased cytokine production, or changes in the osteoclast themselves. Estrogen therapy was found to rapidly (3 weeks) lower the percentage of cells expressing RANKL and to reduce the "osteoclastogenic response" to RANKL.[8]

The amount of bone formed during each remodeling phase decreases with age, regardless of sex. Specifically, there is a decrease in wall thickness, and this has become a marker for reduced remodeling. Changes in the production of bone cells, that is, a reduction in progenitor cells, provide an explanation for osteoporosis caused by senescence independent from sex steroid loss. Decreased osteoblastogenesis as a result of aging is associated with an increase in adipogenesis and myelopoiesis, suggesting a change in the expression of the genes toward differentiation of multipotent mesenchymal stem cells to adipocytes instead of osteoblasts.[9,10] There is strong evidence for an association of dietary fat and lipoproteins with bone marrow differentiation, osteoporosis, and atherogenesis. In fact, mice fed a high-fat diet for 4 months showed decreases in osteogenic cell differentiation.[10,11]

Another cause of osteoporosis is drug-induced loss of bone mineral density (BMD) (Box 14-1). Glucocorticoids, in particular, have been shown to inhibit osteoblastogenesis and increase osteoblast cell death, making decreased bone formation the cardinal feature.[11] However, an early loss of BMD occurs, which suggests that steroid use increases osteoclast numbers, despite decreasing osteoclast production, by decreasing osteoclast cell death. BMD can decrease by 2 to 4% after just 6 months of steroid use in healthy men, after which the rate of loss declines. In one short-term study, 10 days of steroid administration to mice increased osteoclast numbers. Thus, the adverse effect of steroids on bone occurs in two phases, (1) an early phase characterized by excessive bone reabsorption and (2) a slower, later phase in which the loss is due to decreased formation.[12] Another feature of glucocorticoid-induced osteoporosis is osteonecrosis, which results in the collapse of the large joints.[13] This osteonecrosis is explained by still another mechanism, increasing osteocyte apoptosis.

Prevention and Treatment of Osteoporosis

For patients at risk for developing osteoporosis, the goals of treatment include obtaining optimal peak bone mass and minimizing further bone loss. Ideally, prevention begins in childhood with a healthy diet and adequate intake of calcium and vitamin D (see discussion of calcium and vitamin D). It is estimated that the highest rate of calcium accumulation occurs at a mean age of 12.5 years in girls and at 14 years in boys.[14] After this period of rapid accumulation, a period of bone consolidation occurs, during which calcium levels change little but periosteal expansion takes place. The actual age of peak bone mass is unknown because of its variability, but it may be the twenties at the proximal femur and near age 30 for the spine in healthy women. Multiple factors affect attainment of peak bone mass, including nutrition, eating disorders, genetics, weight cycling, and conditions that lead to hypoestrogenism such as heavy exercise, low body fat, and premature menopause. Although current data are insufficient to set specific recommendations for premenopausal women, it is clear that some interventions to prevent this disease must be instituted early. However, often women do not direct their attention toward preventing osteoporosis until later in life after fracture or loss of height has been noted (Box 14-2)

Typically, the need for drug therapy is determined by bone densitometry.[15] Measurement of hip and spine BMD with dual-energy X-ray absorptiometry is the gold standard for an osteoporosis diagnosis. The test is based on the fact that calcium absorbs much more radiation than does protein or soft tissue. The amount of energy that is absorbed by the calcium in a section of bone represents the bone mineral content. This is a noninvasive

BOX 14-1 Medications That Cause Osteoporosis

- Corticosteroids: Prednisone (≥5 mg/day for ≥3 months
- Anticonvulsants: Phenytoin, barbiturates, carbamazepine (associated with vitamin D deficiency)
- Heparin (long-term)
- Chemotherapeutic/transplant drugs: Cyclosporine, tacrolimus, cyclophosphamide, ifosfamide, methotrexate
- Hormonal/endocrine therapies: Gonadotropin-releasing hormone agonists, luteinizing hormone-releasing hormone analogs, depomedroxyprogesterone, excessive thyroid supplementation
- Lithium
- Aromatase inhibitors: Exemestane, anastrozole

BOX 14-2 Risk Factors for Osteoporosis

- Endocrine disorders: Hyperparathyroidism, hypogonadism, hyperthyroidism, diabetes, Cushing's syndrome, prolactinoma, acromegaly, adrenal insufficiency
- Gastrointestinal or nutritional conditions: Inflammatory bowel disease, celiac disease, malnutrition, gastric bypass, chronic liver disease, anorexia nervosa, vitamin D or calcium deficiency
- Renal diseases
- Rheumatologic diseases
- Hematologic diseases: Multiple myeloma, thalassemia, leukemia, lymphoma, hemophilia, sickle cell disease
- Genetic disorders: Cystic fibrosis, osteogenesis imperfecta, Marfan syndrome, hemochromatosis

and painless test that is used to identify osteoporosis, determine the risk of fracture, and monitor the patient's response to treatment. This test measures the patient's BMD and compares it with "young normal" (30-year-old healthy adult) and age-matched norms. The comparisons with the young normal norms are listed as T-scores, and the aged-matched comparisons are listed as Z-scores (Box 14-3).[16,17] The World Health Organization (WHO) defines osteoporosis on the basis of bone density levels. Individuals with a T-score within 1 standard deviation (SD) of the norm (+1 or −1) are considered to have normal bone density. Scores below the norm are indicated by negative numbers. Low bone mass or osteopenia is bone density 1 to 2.5 SDs below the young adult mean (−1 to −2.5 SDs). Osteoporosis is 2.5 SDs or more below the young adult mean (<−2.5 SDs). For this test, −1 SD equals approximately a 10 to 12% decrease in bone density. The guidelines by the National Osteoporosis Foundation (NOF) recommend that all women aged 65 years or older and men aged 70 or older, be offered a screening test. In addition, patients who are younger than 65 years old but who have strong risk factors for a fracture or another condition linked to osteoporosis should also be tested. This list includes a smoking history, body weight less than 56.3 kg, history of fracture after age 50, long-term (>3 months) oral steroid therapy, rheumatoid arthritis or conditions that cause osteoporosis, and the need to brace oneself with the arms when rising from a chair.

BMD is usually measured every 1 to 2 years during drug therapy to determine whether the patient is responding to therapy.[16] However, determining a response is not always easy. Patients may lose BMD even if they are responding to medication; they may just be losing bone at a slower rate. In addition, some women lose bone with treatment, only to regain it, even if therapy is unaltered. There is variability within the test, but this is less than 5%.

When to start therapy is also not always easy to determine. At initial screening, many patients have BMD too high to require treatment, but BMD may decline rapidly, especially within 5 years of menopause.[16] After about 60 years of age, bone loss declines so that women tend to lose less than 1% of hip bone density a year, reducing the T-score 1 point over 10 years. The general recommendation is that therapy should be started when T-scores fall below –2.5 for the femoral neck in patients without previous fracture or secondary causes (Box 14-4). Patients with T-scores between –1.0 and –2.5 (osteopenia) should be considered for therapy if they have other risk factors. However, treatment for patients with only osteopenia has been controversial. The Fracture Intervention Study, in which the effects of alendronate on the risk of hip and nonspine fractures were examined, demonstrated clear benefits of treatment for women with T-scores less than –2.5 but not for women with higher scores.[18]

BOX 14-3 Diagnostic Criteria by the National Osteoporosis Foundation*

- T-score of −1 to −2.5 SD = osteopenia
- T-score of less than −2.5 SD = osteoporosis
- T-score of less than −2.5 SD with fragility fracture = severe osteoporosis

From National Osteoporosis Foundation: *What the numbers mean?*: http://www.nof.org/osteoporosis/bmdtest.htm: Accessed September 22, 2009.

*This criteria should not be applied to premenopausal women, pediatric patients, or men younger than 50 years of age.

Currently, several effective treatments for osteoporosis can slow the rate of bone reabsorption. The decision about which drug to administer and the duration of therapy is based on careful consideration of the risks versus the benefits and the patient's individual risk factors for fractures, coronary events, and breast cancer.[19]

Estrogens. Until recently, estrogen had been the number one drug used to prevent osteoporosis in postmenopausal women. A recent study in older women indicated that 0.625 mg of estrogen per day with or without progesterone increased both spine and hip BMD, and even lower doses of estrogen (0.3 or 0.45 mg/day) increased bone density.[20,21] The Women's Health Initiative (WHI) study discussed in Chapter 13, showed a significant reduction in the number of hip and vertebral fractures in women receiving HRT compared with placebo.[22] However, as discussed previously, estrogen therapy was found to produce an increased risk of coronary heart disease, and when combined with medroxyprogesterone, it was associated with a virulent form of breast cancer. Because long-term estrogen use had been recommended to prevent bone loss, the women who were taking it for this purpose must now consider their individual risk-versus-benefit ratio and decide to either continue with this approach or choose an alternative therapy. Low-dose Premarin is available and approved for a limited period with frequent monitoring.

Calcium and Vitamin D. Dietary and supplemental calcium are effective in reducing the rate of bone loss in older women and in those with very low calcium intake.[23,24] It was initially thought that supplementation with calcium would have an early positive effect but that this effect would not last despite continued dosing. However, one study demonstrated that the positive effects of calcium were at least sustained over a 4-year period. At present, all regimens approved for the treatment and prevention of osteoporosis include supplemental calcium and vitamin D. Current recommendations include an elemental calcium intake of 1000 mg for all adults between the ages of 19 and 50 years and 1200 mg for everyone older than 50 years.[17] Calcium salts (calcium carbonate, calcium gluconate, calcium lactate, and calcium phosphate) are used for nutritional supplementation. One of the most commonly used calcium salts is calcium carbonate, but it requires an acid medium to

BOX 14-4 National Osteoporosis Foundation Criteria for Phamacologic Treatment of Postmenopausal Women and Men age 50 or older

- Hip or vertebral fracture
- Other prior fractures and low bone mass (T-score between −1.0 and −2.5 SD at the femoral neck, total hip, or spine
- T-score less than −2.5 SD at the femoral neck, total hip, or spine, without secondary cause
- Low bone mass (T-score between −1.0 and −2.5 SD at the femoral neck, hip, or spine) and secondary causes associated with high risk of fracture (steroid use or immobilization)
- Low bone mass (T-score between −1.0 and −2.5 SD at the femoral neck, hip, or spine and a 10-year probability of hip fracture of 3% or more using the WHO Fracture Risk Assessment Tool*

* WHO Fracture Risk Assessment Tool: http://www.shef.ac.uk/FRAX/tool.jsp?locationValue=9: Accessed September 22, 2009.

form a soluble compound; however, calcium citrate, calcium gluconate, and calcium lactate are pH independent and therefore are better absorbed.

The minimum daily requirement for vitamin D in adults younger than 50 years is 400 to 800 IU (international unit), but this increases to 800 to 1000 IU for those over 50. Vitamin D is recommended along with calcium because it improves calcium absorption from the gastrointestinal (GI) tract, decreases calcium renal excretion, and is responsible for bone mineralization. This combination has been especially recommended for nursing home residents who have low sunshine exposure.[25]

Supplementation with calcium and vitamin D is generally safe.[26] GI problems such as constipation and excess gas may occur. Some of the adverse effects may be lessened when supplements are taken with a meal; this also improves bioavailability because acid secretion is greatest at mealtime. Supplements should be used with caution by persons who are prone to kidney stones.

Bisphosphonates. Bisphosphonates inhibit bone reabsorption by reducing recruitment of osteoclasts and by inducing their cell death. They have a strong affinity for calcium phosphate and therefore are absorbed directly into bone.[6] Bisphosphonates have different anti-reabsorptive potential, with the potencies of etidronate, pamidronate, alendronate, risedronate, and ibandronate being 1, 100, 1000, 5000, and 10,000, respectively. Their oral bioavailability is very low, since they are highly negatively charged with only 1 to 3% bioavailability, and their bioavailability is further impaired by food, calcium, iron, coffee, tea, and orange juice. They must be taken with a full glass of water, and patients must maintain an upright position for 30 to 60 minutes after intake to avoid heartburn. The safety profile of these drugs is good, but as many as 30% of patients report mild to moderate GI discomfort consisting of esophagitis, nausea, and abdominal pain. Osteonecrosis of the jaw has been reported in patients with cancer when given intravenous (IV) bisphosphonates.[27] The risk is enhanced with concomitant glucocorticoid therapy and in patients who have had recent dental extractions. Bone pain and musculoskeletal pain have also been reported, but establishing a cause-and-effect relationship has been difficult, since patients who have osteoporosis also experience these problems.

Studies of alendronate in approximately 4000 postmenopausal women (the Fracture Intervention Trial, FIT) with an existing vertebral fracture or osteoporosis, as defined by a T-score less than −2.5 at the femoral neck, but without vertebral fracture showed a significant reduction in fracture rate during a 3- to 4-year period when compared with placebo.[28] BMD at the spine increased by 8% and by 3.5% at the hip. Other studies in which alendronate was used have also had positive outcomes. Alendronate given for 2 years to 1174 postmenopausal women younger than 60 years without osteoporosis increased BMD at the lumbar spine (3.5%) and at the hip (1.9%), and when the original FIT study performed on patients with osteoporosis was extended, it was found that the drug was effective and well tolerated over a 10-year period.[29] This study, known as the Fracture Intervention Trial Long-term Extension (FLEX) study, took the women who were enrolled in the treatment arm of the FIT study and randomized them to either continued use of alendronate for an additional 5 years or placebo.[30] Those subjects who were switched to placebo had a decrease in BMD at the total hip and spine; however, levels remained above the pretreatment levels obtained 10 years earlier. In addition, the placebo group did not have any higher fracture risk, other than vertebral fractures, than did the treatment group. The women in the treatment group continued to show increases in BMD, and their vertebral fracture risk was significantly lowered. The conclusion of this study is that continuation of alendronate after a 5-year period is associated with a reduction in vertebral fractures but no difference in the number of other fractures. Therefore, patients who are at high risk for vertebral fractures should consider additional dosing beyond 5 years. The half-life of alendronate is extremely long (nearly 10 years), and it is credited with helping to maintain BMD above pretreatment levels even when patients are on placebo.

Studies performed with risedronate have also shown positive outcomes. In 5 years, BMD at the lumbar spine increased by 9.2%, whereas there were no significant changes in the placebo group.[31] This drug also demonstrated an increase in BMD in patients with normal BMD in the spine and hip. Both alendronate and risedronate are available in a once-a-week formulation. This type of administration is just as effective as daily dosing but is associated with improved compliance.[32]

Oral alendronate, risedronate, and ibandronate are approved for the prevention and treatment of osteoporosis. IV zoledronic acid and pamidronate are used to treat skeletal metastases from breast and prostate cancers, and IV etidronate and pamidromate are used for the treatment of hypercalcemia secondary to cancer. Some are also used to treat Paget's disease.

Selective Estrogen Receptor Modulators. Tamoxifen and raloxifene are estrogen agonists in some tissues and antagonists in other tissues. Tamoxifen has been used for the treatment of estrogen-sensitive breast cancer because it blocks estrogen receptors in breast tissue. It is a partial agonist in bone but also in the endometrium and may cause endometrial cancer. Raloxifene is a related drug that has been found to be an agonist in bone but an antagonist in both breast tissue and endometrium, which favors its use in the treatment of osteoporosis.[33]

In a double-blind, placebo-controlled, 2-year study of more than 600 postmenopausal women, raloxifene was shown to increase BMD in the lumbar spine, hip, and femoral neck.[34] Three different doses of raloxifene were administered, and the results showed greater BMD with a greater dose. Concentrations of total cholesterol and low-density lipoprotein (LDL) cholesterol decreased in the treatment group, whereas these measures did not change in the placebo group. No change in endometrial thickness was detected. In terms of cardiovascular events, a 4-year study in which raloxifene was compared with placebo showed that the drug did not affect the overall risk of cardiac events but did significantly reduce the number of events in women who had cardiac risk factors at the beginning of the study.[35] In addition, raloxifene was associated with a reduction in estrogen-sensitive breast cancer but not in estrogen-receptor–negative cancers over a 4-year period.[36] Although these studies have shown positive outcomes, raloxifene is assumed to be less effective than estrogen or the bisphosphonates.[37]

Adverse effects of raloxifene are similar to those of estrogen and include hot flashes, leg cramps, and an increased risk of thromboembolic events.[38] Long-term studies are needed to more fully assess these adverse effects and also to study the possible occurrence of endometrial hyperplasia.

Tibolone is an oral steroid derived from norethynodrel, but it is not exactly considered a selective estrogen receptor modulator. However, this drug has estrogenic, progestogenic, and weak androgenic activity. The Long-Term Intervention on Fractures with Tibolone (LIFT) was a randomized, double-blind, placebo-controlled study that examined the effect of tibolone on reducing vertebral fractures in women with osteoporosis. Patients in the treatment group had a 46% reduction in relative risk for vertebral fracture and a reduced risk of nonvertebral fracture of 26%. However, the study was halted at 3 years due to an increased risk of stroke, particularly in women over the age of 70.[39] There were also some cases of endometrial cancer in the treatment group compared with none in the placebo group. Several other studies have shown that tibolone has beneficial effects on the vasculature and cholesterol levels.[40,41] However, there is some indication that this drug may promote tumor cell growth in breast cells.[42]

Calcitonin. Calcitonin is a peptide produced by thyroid cells that binds to receptors on osteoclasts to inhibit their function.[6] It is approved for the treatment, but not the prevention, of osteoporosis. It is available as a subcutaneous injection or a nasal spray. A tablet form is not available because when calcitonin is taken orally, much of the drug is broken down in the GI tract. A 5-year study with salmon calcitonin showed a reduction in vertebral fractures, but not in peripheral fractures.[43] Salmon calcitonin is preferred, since it is approximately 20 times more potent than human calcitonin and takes longer to clear from the body. Injected calcitonin produces an increase in trabecular bone in the spine but not cortical bone by 2% over 2 years, and the nasal spray is associated with a greater reduction in vertebral fractures than what is expected based on BMD.[6] Subcutaneous injection may produce nausea and flushing, and rhinitis is associated with the nasal preparation, but no other adverse effects have been reported. This drug is usually reserved for women who cannot take other more effective options.

Denosumab. Denosumab is a monoclonal antibody to RANKL that is currently being investigated. In studies it has been administrated by injection subcutaneously at 3-month and 6-month intervals for a year, and has demonstrated increased BMD compared with placebo.[44]

Anabolic Therapies. All the osteoporotic treatments discussed previously are considered anti-reabsorptive agents that generally work on osteoclasts to reduce bone loss. They do increase BMD but by only a few percentage points. These treatments are not curative, and if medication is stopped, bone loss resumes. However, a new class of drugs called anabolic agents, capable of stimulating significant increases in BMD, is under development.[45] The goal of these agents is to increase bone mass and mechanical strength over a short time to replace the bone lost. The agents currently under study include the statin drugs, (PTH) and related peptides, growth hormone (GH), fluoride, and insulin-like growth factor-1 (IGF-1). Of these agents, the statins and PTH-related peptides look most promising. Fluoride stimulates new bone formation but interferes with bone mineralization, so the new bone is not resistant to fractures. Studies of GH demonstrate increases in bone mass; however, this effect is inconsistently sustained after treatment.[46-48] IGF-1 stimulates the proliferation of osteoblasts, but this therapy has been associated with edema, hypotension, and tachycardia.[49,50] Further studies on all of these agents are continuing.

Native PTH (hPTH-[1-84]) is the principal regulator of serum calcium, and as discussed earlier, an increase in PTH leads to excessive bone reabsorption and bone loss.[49] However, there is evidence that intermittent PTH injections improve bone strength by stimulating new bone formation. The primary target with this type of administration is the osteoblast. Osteoblasts are stimulated to express genes for factors such as IGF-1, vascular endothelial growth factor, and transforming growth factor-β (TGF-β) which stimulate the proliferation of osteoblast precursor cells. PTH works by increasing the number of osteoblasts and by extending their lifespan. The results are an increase in the size of remaining trabeculae and increased cortical thickness from bone added at the endocortical surfaces. However, PTH also produces bone reabsorption, and this becomes more evident with prolonged continuous dosing.

Animal and human studies with teriparatide have shown favorable outcomes. Many of the animal studies have used the sexually mature oophorectomized rat model required by the U.S. Food and Drug Administration (FDA) for evaluation of new therapies for osteoporosis. Oophorectomized rats experience tremendous loss of trabecular bone during the initial weeks after removal of the ovaries. Daily injections of small amounts of PTH simulate new cortical and trabecular bone in these animals.[51] PTH has also been noted to greatly increase callus volume of a fractured rat tibia by 175% over control values.[52] Similar to the animal studies, compared with placebo, daily doses of 15 to 50 mg of PTH given to 1600 postmenopausal women significantly increased BMD at the spine and hip.[53] In fact, this was the study that convinced the FDA to approve teriparatide despite some reservations regarding the development of osteosarcomas in PTH-treated rats.

In a study comparing PTH administered daily for 15 months versus cyclic PTH (3 months on followed by 3 months off for 15 months) versus placebo, the two groups treated with PTH demonstrated similar increases in spinal BMD. Given the fact that both PTH regimens were equally effective but that one group received a much greater amount of drug, the conclusion may be that the intermittant treatment produced anabolic changes in bone but continuous treatment produced some catabolic changes, that is, bone reabsorption.[54]

Because PTH receptors are found throughout the body, it might be assumed that PTH and PTH analogs would have many adverse effects.[49] However, other than hypercalcemia, there have been no serious adverse effects. There are some reports of hypotension and tachycardia but no fatalities. Since the safety and efficacy of PTH has not been studied beyond a 2-year period, in practice it is used for only 2 years and must be followed with another agent, usually a bisphosphonate.

Besides PTH, the other big news regarding anabolic agents for osteoporosis is the use of statins. This is an exciting development because these drugs have already been shown to offer many positive benefits. It was originally noted that statins induced a bone protein involved in osteoblastogenesis, and when lovastatin or simvastatin was injected into the calvariae of mice, a significant increase in bone formation was seen.[45] Clinical studies have supported the findings of these animal studies by showing a reduction in fracture risk in postmenopausal women; however, the exact manner in which the statins get into bone remains unknown.[55,56]

Combination Therapy. Because there are several different types of drugs now available for the treatment of osteoporosis, combination therapy may be an option for patients with severe osteoporosis (Table 14-1).[57] Combinations of alendronate with HRT, and alendronate and raloxifene, have already been shown to increase BMD more than each agent independently.[58,59] Even sequential treatment with PTH and alendronate resulted in an increase in spinal bone density compared with treatment with each agent separately.[60] This treatment regimen might offer the best hope for preserving the anabolic effects of PTH, particularly because the long-term effects of PTH injections are not known yet.

Therapeutic Concerns Regarding Antiosteoporosis Agents. In general, antiosteoporosis agents do not have direct therapy concerns. The action of these drugs appears to have limited effects on rehabilitative interventions. However, a few guidelines should be remembered when patients receiving these drugs are treated. First, many of these agents are administered by daily injections. Patients should be asked where their injection sites are located, and use of modalities or exercise in these areas should be avoided. In the case of patients receiving the bisphosphonates, exercises that increase intra-abdominal pressure as well as those performed in the supine position should be avoided. The reason for this is that many patients taking these drugs have esophagitis or esophageal reflux, so the supine position or increased abdominal pressure will exacerbate this condition.

DRUG TREATMENT FOR DIABETES

Diabetes is a chronic metabolic disorder characterized by hyperglycemia associated with either insulin insufficiency (type 1) or combined insulin insufficiency with insulin resistance (type 2). Published data from 2001 have shown that the incidence of diabetes in the United States has tripled since the late 1950s, turning what was once considered only a minor disease into a major threat worldwide.[61] Worldwide, 220 million people are expected to have the disease by 2010 and 300 million by 2025. The Centers for Disease Control and Prevention (CDC) Diabetes Data and Trends reported in 2006 that 16.8 million

TABLE 14-1 Approved Drugs for Osteoporosis

Drug Class	Drug	Dosing Form	Adverse Drug Reactions
Vitamin/mineral	Calcium	Tablet; 1200–1500 mg daily for postmenopausal women	Constipation
	Vitamin D	Tablet: 800–1000 IU daily for postmenopausal women	Constipation
Bisphosphonate	Alendronate (Fosamax; Fosamax plus D)	*Treatment*: 70 mg PO qwk or 10 mg PO qd; *Prevention*: 35 mg PO qwk or 5 mg PO qd; 70 mg liquid suspension also available	GI irritation ranging from minor to esophageal abnormalities, especially when taken with aspirin or NSAIDs; coadministration with calcium decreases absorption—separate dosing by 30 min; osteonecrosis of the jaw in cancer patients
	Risedronate (Actonel; Actonel with calcium)	*Treatment or prevention*: 5 mg PO qs; 35 mg PO qwk; 75 mg tablet PO on two consecutive days monthly; or 150 mg tablet PO qmo	Same as for alendronate
	Ibandronate (Boniva)	*Treatment or prevention*: Oral: 150 mg PO qmo; or 2.5 mg PO qd IV: 3 mg IV q3mo	Same as for alendronate
	Zoledronic acid (Reclast)	5 mg IV over 15 min once yearly	Same as for alendronate
Hormone	Parathyroid (Teriparatide-Forteo)	Given intermittently; used also for Paget's disease 20 mcg SC qd	Increased risk for osteosarcoma; hypercalcemia
	Raloxifene (Evista)	60 mg PO qd	Thrombophlebitis; may antagonize warfarin; caution with drugs that are highly protein bound (e.g., diazepam, diazoxide, lidocaine); not for premenopausal women; discontinue 72 h before prolonged immobilization or surgery
	Calcitonin (Miacalcin, Calcimar, Cibacalcin)	200 IU (1 puff) qd in alternating nostrils 100 IU IM/SC qod	Nasal irritation, monitor for hypocalcemia
	Conjugated estrogens (from natural sources); low-dose Premarin or low-dose Prempro)	0.3 mg PO qd given continuously or in cyclical regimens (25 days on, 5 days off); adjust to lowest level while still maintaining effective control	Abnormal or excessive bleeding; thrombophlebitis; DVT; breast and endometrial cancers

IU, international unit; *PO*, orally; *GI*, gastrointestinal; *NSAIDs*, nonsteroidal anti-inflammatory drugs; *IV*, intravenous; *SC*, subcutaneous; *IM*, intramuscular; *DVT*, deep venous thromboembolism.

individuals in the United States were positive for diabetes, and the 2008 Behavioral Risk Factor Surveillance System (BRFSS) reported that 8.3% of individuals living in this country have the disease.[62,63] To make matters worse, there are approximately 6.3 million adults in the United States that have undiagnosed disease.[64] Environmental and lifestyle changes have resulted in escalating obesity, which is linked to diabetes.

Pathophysiology and Classification of Diabetes

The normal response to eating a meal is that carbohydrates from food are converted to glucose, which then enters the plasma. Glucose also enters the blood from the breakdown of stored glycogen in the liver, which is caused by the hormone glucagon and other hormones (Table 14-2). In response to the rise in blood sugar, the pancreas produces insulin from its beta cells; the insulin is then secreted into the bloodstream and interacts with its receptors on cell surfaces, enhancing glucose entry into the cell for fuel. Leftover glucose is converted to glycogen in the liver and muscles and stored for future use. As a result, the blood glucose level drops, reducing the need for insulin.

Type 1 diabetes is considered an autoimmune disease in which the body produces antibodies that attack the beta cells.[65] Patients with type 1 diabetes tend to be young (children or adolescents) and not obese. There is a strong inherited predisposition, and associations with

TABLE 14-2 Effect of Hormones on Blood Glucose Levels

Hormone	Main Actions	Main Stimulus for Secretion	Main Effect
Main regulatory hormone			
Insulin	↑ Glucose uptake ↑ Glycogen synthesis ↓ Glycogenolysis ↓ Gluconeogenesis	Acute rise in blood glucose	↓ Blood glucose
Main counter-regulatory hormones			
Glucagon	↑ Glycogenolysis ↑ Gluconeogenesis	Hypoglycemia (i.e., blood glucose <3 mmol/L), e.g., with exercise, stress, high-protein meals, etc.	↓ Blood glucose
Adrenaline	↑ Glycogenolysis ↓ Glucose uptake		
Glucocorticosteroids	↑ Gluconeogenesis ↓ Glucose uptake and utilization		
Growth hormone	↓ Glucose uptake		

From Rang HP, Dale MM, Ritter JM, Moore JL, editors: *Pharmacology* (5th ed.). New York, 2003, Churchill Livingstone.

some specific histocompatibility antigens exist, but it is believed that exposure to a virus is the precipitating event. Initially, the ability of the beta cells to produce insulin is just impaired, but as time goes on (usually less than a year), the pancreas ceases to produce the hormone. Because little or no insulin is being produced, the blood sugar level rises in response to a meal,. The pancreas tries to compensate by producing more insulin, but eventually it cannot keep up with demand.

In type 2 diabetes, insulin is plentiful, at least in the beginning of the illness, but resistance to the hormone is present. The liver and muscles become less sensitive to the action of insulin. Sensing an elevated blood glucose level, the pancreas attempts to increase production of insulin, but eventually the pancreas "burns out." At that point, the patient with type 2 diabetes will need supplemental insulin. Unlike type 1 diabetes, this form of the disease is associated with obesity.[66] Obesity itself can cause some degree of insulin resistance. Patients who are not considered obese may have an increased percentage of body fat distributed in the abdominal area. Type 2 diabetes usually develops during adult life, although the growing number of children with this disease is emerging as a major public health problem.[67]

Heredity also plays a role in type 2 diabetes.[68] A polygenic basis for type 2 diabetes has been discussed because many patients with this disease have a relative with diabetes. It has been shown that first-degree relatives without diabetes are insulin resistant. Parental history of hypertension and diabetes has also been associated with diabetic nephropathy in offspring with type 1 diabetes.[69]

Other specific types and causes of diabetes have been identified.[66] Genetic defects may be present in the beta cell. In fact, this is associated with the onset of hyperglycemia before the age of 25 years and is referred to as maturity-onset diabetes of the young. It is characterized by impaired insulin secretion but with minimal or no insulin resistance. Some genetic defects prevent the conversion of proinsulin to insulin, resulting in mild glucose intolerance, as well as defects that alter the structure of the insulin receptor. Acquired processes are also involved in the development of diabetes. Any injury to the pancreas caused by infection, carcinoma, or trauma and endocrinopathies such as acromegaly, Cushing's syndrome, pheochromocytoma, and glucagonomas can also produce diabetes. Several drugs, such as steroids, thiazide diuretics, and protease inhibitors (used for the treatment of acquired immune deficiency syndrome, AIDS), raise the blood glucose level and trigger diabetes in susceptible patients. Gestational diabetes mellitus (GDM) is an acquired glucose intolerance seen during pregnancy. This may disappear after delivery but can also predict future problems of impaired glucose tolerance.

The terms *impaired glucose tolerance* and *impaired fasting glucose* refer to a metabolic state intermediate between normal carbohydrate metabolism and diabetes. The exact name depends on the screening test used—fasting plasma glucose (FPG) or oral glucose tolerance test (OGTT)—although these terms have recently been given the diagnostic category of prediabetes.[66] A diagnosis of prediabetes automatically puts one at greater risk for developing diabetes. Prediabetes is associated with insulin resistance syndrome (formerly known as *metabolic syndrome*). Insulin resistance syndrome includes decreased sensitivity to insulin, compensatory hyperinsulinemia, abdominal obesity, dyslipidemia (high triglyceride and/or low high-density lipoprotein [HDL] cholesterol levels), and hypertension.[70] A body mass index greater than 25, family history of type 2 diabetes, GDM, and PCOS are associated with this disorder.

Diabetes is a multifactorial problem. Fasting glucose level is elevated when it should be low, and insulin secretion is reduced or delayed after a meal when it should be elevated. Hyperglycemia occurs in both types of diabetes as a result of uncontrolled hepatic glucose production and reduced uptake by cells, as well as the inability of the α cells to sense glucose level and reduce glucagon release. There is also a defect at the level of the insulin receptor. Either the receptor no longer recognizes insulin, or the cascade of events that must occur to mobilize glucose transporters has gone awry.

Several events lead up to type 2 diabetes. Lipotoxicity and its associated obesity and glucotoxicity appear to be one of the main causes of type 2 diabetes.[71] An excess of free fatty acids (FFAs) leads to dysregulation at the level of the adipocyte. There is deficient differentiation of preadipocytes to adipocytes and then a reduced number of mature, insulin sensitive cells that store fat. This leaves large amounts of hypertrophic adipocytes that secret excessive amounts of proinflammatory cytokines. Excessive fat accumulates within the liver, skeletal muscle, and also the β-cells. Visceral fat appears to be the major source of these cytokines. This results in a preferential use of FFAs instead of glucose as fuel, leading to underutilization of glucose and elevated levels causing increased insulin secretion. Ultimately, the pancreas cannot keep up with the demand for insulin and begins to fail.

Symptoms of Diabetes

The initial symptoms of diabetes are related to hyperglycemia.[72] Diabetic ketoacidosis may appear suddenly in type 1 diabetes when there is nearly a complete absence of insulin and the body is forced to utilize other sources for energy. In an effort to produce fuel, fatty acids are released from adipose tissue and broken down in the liver into ketone bodies. These strong acids accumulate in the blood, leading to metabolic acidosis. In addition, the excess blood glucose is filtered through the kidney glomerulus, taking with it large quantities of water, causing polyuria and severe dehydration. Other symptoms of ketoacidosis include a fruity breath, nausea, slowing respirations, changes in mental state, and finally a collapse of the cardiovascular system.

In contrast to type 1 diabetes, type 2 diabetes may develop very slowly, so some patients may not notice symptoms for years. The classic symptoms include polyuria, polydipsia, weight loss despite increased food intake, and weakness. Other symptoms that may occur include blurred vision caused by changing levels of glucose in the eye, recurrent vaginal yeast infections, and frequent skin infections.

Long-term complications are also common with this disease, especially if a patient has had difficulty controlling his or her glucose level. Several prospective studies have demonstrated greater degrees of microvascular and macrovascular disease with long-term poor control of glucose level.[73-75] Retinopathy, nephropathy, neuropathy, autonomic neuropathy, glaucoma, cataracts, skin infections, coronary heart disease, stroke, and peripheral vascular disease are more likely to occur when glycemic control is not maintained. Advanced glycation end products have been implicated in the development of dysfunction of the vascular endothelium. These are nonenzymatic products of glucose and albumin. Oxygen-derived free radicals and increased activation of the diacylglycerol–protein kinase C signal transduction pathway have also been identified in diabetic animals.[76] Protein kinase C activation leads to deposition of extracellular matrix, resulting in a thickening of the capillary basement membrane. This change is associated with increased vascular permeability, impaired regulation of vascular tone, endothelial cell proliferation, and microaneurysm formation, leading to many of the ischemic events seen in diabetes. Specific diacylglycerol–protein kinase C pathway inhibitors are being explored as adjunct treatments for diabetes.

Diagnostic Testing for Diabetes

In an effort to promote early detection, the American Diabetes Association (ADA) recommends that persons of any age be tested for diabetes if they have a BMI ≥25 kg/m^2 and an additional risk factor such as inactivity, have a first-degree relative with diabetes, are a member of a high-risk ethnic population, or have hypertension or high cholesterol and triglycerides.[77] Other risk factors include PCOS, previous GDM, and a history of cardiovascular disease. High-risk racial and ethnic groups include black, Hispanic, and Native American. If no risk factors are present, then testing begins at age 45 and every 3 years thereafter. Children should be tested starting at age 10 if they are overweight (BMI>85th percentile for age and sex) and have two risk factors such as ethnicity, family history, signs of insulin resistance, and maternal history of GDM. Testing should be initiated sooner if symptoms appear. Signs of insulin resistance include acanthosis nigricans, hypertension, dyslipidemia, and PCOS.

A diagnosis of diabetes can be made in three ways.[77] A diagnosis can be made when the blood glucose level climbs above 200 mg/dL (11.1 mmol/L) in a blood sample obtained at any time of the day and under any circumstances, along with the classic symptoms of thirst, frequent urination, and weight loss. A diagnosis can also be made with an FBG test or an OGTT. The FBG test requires that the patient abstain from eating or drinking for 8 hours before a blood sample is obtained. A normal FBG test result is less than 100 mg/dL. A positive result for the disease is an FBG value greater than or equal to 126 mg/dL (7.0 mmol/L). FBG values between 100 and 125 mg/dL indicate impaired glucose tolerance and identify patients who may need counseling regarding diet and exercise and also those who must be regularly screened in the future. The third test is the OGTT, which is performed by having the patient drink a solution containing 75 g of glucose, followed by sampling the blood every half hour for 2 hours. Glucose levels of 140 mg/dL and lower obtained at 2 hours after glucose administration are considered normal. Impaired glucose tolerance is defined by a level between 140 and 200 mg/dL 2 hours after administration, and any value of 200 mg/dL or greater is considered positive for diabetes (Table 14-3).

The normal and diagnostic values cited previously are values adopted by the American Diabetes Association in 1998.[78] This diagnostic "cut point" for diabetes and impaired glucose tolerance results from collection of clinical and epidemiologic data that correlate glucose levels with the onset of microvascular and macrovascular disease, indicating that measurements above these values are associated with a significant increase in morbidity.

Another test called the hemoglobin A_{1C} (HbA_{1C}) test, also known as the *glycohemoglobin test* or the *glycated hemoglobin test*, is not used for diagnostic purposes but is used to assess blood glucose control over the previous 3 months in persons known to have the disease.[78] The test is based on the fact that some glucose absorbed from the intestine attaches to hemoglobin and remains there for the life of the red blood cell, which is approximately 120 days. This combination of glucose and hemoglobin is called *glycosylated hemoglobin*. When glucose levels are consistently high, the amount of glycosylated hemoglobin increases. A normal HbA_{1C} value in persons without the disease is between 4% and 6% (Table 14-4). The ADA recommends an HbA_{1C} value under 7% for people with diabetes. This test is given twice a year to people who successfully manage their glucose level and is recommended every 3 months for those patients who have inconsistent levels or for those who might not be as interested in managing their blood glucose level as they should be. The factors contributing to the A_{1C} level include glucose released by the liver overnight and postprandial glucose level, with the second factor having much more influence, hence the emphasis on reducing post-meal rises in glucose level through drug therapy.

Other laboratory tests important to perform for patients with diabetes include tests of blood urea nitrogen (BUN), blood creatinine, and protein (albumin) in the urine, which provide useful data for evaluating kidney damage. Measurements of triglyceride, total, LDL, and HDL cholesterol levels are also needed on a regular basis to assess for cardiac risk factors.

Common sense tells us that maintaining tight control over blood glucose level will reduce the complications of diabetes. Several recent trials have tried to determine the target A_{1C} level that will safely reduce the risk of cardiovascular disease (CVD) in patients with diabetes. The Action to Control Cardiovascular Risk in Diabetes (ACCORD) randomized patients to receive intensive glycemic control to a A_{1C} target of <6% or to enough glycemic control to reach the standard target of 7%. Multiple antidiabetic drugs were administered to reduce the A_{1C} levels, which went from 8.1% to 6.4% in a year. The control group reached an A_{1C} of 7.5%. This study was stopped in 2008 due to an increased rate of death in the intensive control group. Two similar studies were conducted, the Action in Diabetes and Vascular Disease (ADVANCE) study and the Veterans Affairs Diabetes Trial (VADT) study. The ADVANCE study showed no increase in mortality in the treatment group; however, the VADT trial showed an increase in mortality, but this was not significant.[79] Intense analysis of these studies have led to the conclusion that the greater the number and severity of hypoglycemic events, the

TABLE 14-3 Criteria for Diagnosis of Diabetes and Prediabetes

Prediabetes (Impaired Glucose Tolerance)	Diabetes
• FBG≥100 mg/dL (5.6 mmol/L but <126 (7.0 mmol/L)	• FBG≥126 mg/dL (7.0 mmol/L) with no caloric intake for at least 8 hr
OR	OR
• 2-hr values in the OGTT ≥140 mg/dL (7.8 mmol/L but <200 mg/dL (11.1 mmol/L)	• Symptoms of hyperglycemia and a casual plasma glucose ≥200 mg/dL (11.1 mmol/L). *Casual* is defined as any time of the day. Symptoms include polyuria, polydipsia, and unexplained weight loss
	OR
	• 2-hr plasma glucose≥200 mg/dL during an OGTT using 75 g glucose dissolved in water

OGTT, oral glucose tolerance test; FPG, fasting plasma glucose test.
Adapted from Diagnosis and classification of diabetes mellitus, *Diabetes Care* 32(suppl 1):S62–S67, 2009.

TABLE 14-4 Correlation of A_{1C} with Plasma Glucose Level

A_{1C} %	Plasma Glucose (mg/dL)	Plasma Glucose (mmol/L)
6	126	7.0
7	154	8.6
8	183	10.2
9	212	11.8
10	240	13.4
11	269	14.9
12	298	16.5

Data taken from Standards of medical care in diabetes, *Diabet Care* 32 (suppl 1):S13–S61, 2009.

greater is the mortality. In addition, an older patient who has had diabetes for greater than 12 years may not be able to tolerate lower levels of A_{1C}.[80] Therefore, the ideal A_{1C} level of patients with diabetes still needs to be determined.

Self-Monitoring of Blood Glucose Level

Self-monitoring of blood glucose level is essential for patients with diabetes. Regular measurement and keeping a log of the values, food intake, and activity level are recommended. Not only is monitoring useful for indicating when a patient needs to be more aggressive in management, it also allows the patient to make rapid changes in diet, medication, or activity level to keep glucose levels within an acceptable range. High or low levels at the same time of the day suggest the need for a medication change. Although unexpected alterations in glucose readings may simply be traced to eating unusually large or small amounts of food, they may also be caused by variation in activity level or even psychological stress that the patient might be experiencing on a particular day. The log is helpful for identifying these anomalies. Patients are encouraged to check glucose levels frequently; before meals, 2 hours after meals, and before bedtime (Box 14-5). Glucose monitoring requires only a single drop of blood, which can be withdrawn from a fingertip by a lancet or by the meter itself. The blood is placed on a reagent strip containing an enzyme called *glucose oxidase*. The strip is inserted into a meter, which provides a digital readout of the blood glucose level. If the patient is only willing to test blood glucose once a day, then "block testing" is recommended. This means that the fasting glucose should be measured one day, the postprandial glucose the next day, then perhaps 2 hours after breakfast the following day, and 2 hours after lunch the day after. Obviously, for improved patient compliance, the testing schedule needs to take into consideration the patient's activity level, work and lifestyle influences, and desire for tight control of diabetes.

Many different types of monitors with variable features are available. Factors to consider when choosing a monitor include how large the numbers are on the readout, how difficult the meter is to use, and whether it has memory features that could make record keeping easy. Some models can download meter results to a computer and print out summaries. The type of test strips required by the monitor should also be considered. These strips have a shelf life and therefore are packaged either in a vial or individually wrapped in foil. A patient with arthritis might have difficulty opening the individually wrapped strips. Some monitors have a roll of test strips inserted inside so the patient does not have to handle them directly. Older patients should be informed that Medicare pays for the meters and testing supplies.

In the past few years, the FDA has approved several new methods for testing glucose levels.[81] The Freestyle blood glucose monitoring system (TheraSense, Alameda, California), the One Touch FastTake system (LifeScan, Milpitas, California), and the Sof-Tac Diabetes Management System (Abbott Laboratories, MediSense Products, Bedford, Massachusetts) all allow blood to be drawn from the forearm, which is less sensitive than the fingertip. Studies have shown that blood glucose measurements obtained from the arm with the automated devices are just as accurate as those obtained by the fingerstick method. The Sof-Tac device, in particular, is easy to use as well, since it combines the two steps of lancing the skin and transferring the blood to the test strip. The patient places the device on either the forearm or the upper arm. When the device is engaged, it creates a vacuum seal against the skin, releasing the lancet and drawing blood onto the strip. Strips can be loaded up to 8 hours before testing. Blood glucose results are provided in 40 seconds from the time the device is engaged. There also are several noninvasive devices in development, including a skin patch to monitor blood glucose levels in interstitial fluid, contact lenses that sense the level of glucose in tears, and infrared devices.[82]

The GlucoWatch Biographer (Animas Corporation, West Chester, Penn.) and the mimiMed CGMS represents another innovation in testing.[83] This is an automatic, noninvasive glucose monitoring device. It is worn on the wrist like a watch and consists of a disposable

BOX 14-5 Glycemic Recommendations for Adults with Diabetes

A_{1C}	<7.0%*
Preprandial capillary plasma glucose	70–130 mg/dL (3.9–7.2 mmol/L)*
Peak postprandial capillary plasma glucose	<180 mg/dL (<10.0 mmol/L)*
Postprandial capillary plasma glucose at 2 hours	<160 mg/dL
Fasting capillary plasma glucose (FPG)	70–94 mg/dL**
Bedtime capillary plasma glucose	110–130 mg/dL**
3 AM capillary plasma glucose	>80 and <120 mg/dL

*Data from Standards of medical care in diabetes. *Diabet Care* 32(suppl 1):S13–S61, 2009.

**Data from Bergenstal RM, Johnson M, Powers MA, et al: Adjust to target in type 2 diabetes: Comparison of a simple algorithm with carbohydrate counting for adjustment of mealtime insulin glulisine, *Diabet Care* 31:1305–1310, 2008.

Values vary depending on reference.

single-use electrochemical sensor that contains two glucose oxidase–containing gel discs and two electrodes. A small electric current is emitted through the skin, which measures glucose-containing interstitial fluid from adjacent cells by means of reverse iontophoresis. Glucose measurements may be obtained as often as once every 20 minutes within a 12-hour period. Each reading is the average of two 10-minute periods and lags behind blood glucose readings because of processing and the 5-minute delay between blood and tissue sugar levels. This device demonstrates good correlation with the glucose measurements obtained by the fingerstick method, but the manufacturer states that it is not meant to replace regular blood monitoring. However, it is not accurate in low ranges of blood glucose and may cause persisting edema and redness of the skin under the device. Another problem is that it must be recalibrated with the fingerstick readings every 12 hours before use.

The MimiMed Continuous Glucose Monitoring System (CGMS) is connected to a subcutaneous sensor via a wire.[82] The sensor is inserted into the abdominal wall and then taped securely to the skin. The patient can wear the device for up to 72 hours while recordings are made every 10 seconds. Average glucose measurements are made every 5 minutes for a total of 288 recordings in a 24-hour period. Patients still need to calibrate the device with at least four capillary glucose tests and record this information on the device. In addition, the data must be downloaded into a computer for viewing. A newer model is the Guardian Real-Time Continuous Glucose Monitoring System, which provides real-time data and sends alarms when the glucose level is outside the preset range. The DexCom STS System (DexCom, San Diego, California) is an even more revolutionary device that uses a disposable sensor placed just below the skin. The sensor can stay in place for a week and is comfortable for the patient to wear. The device is about the size of a cell phone and worn at the waist. Although these devices appear to be a step toward reducing the burden of this disease, they are not meant to replace traditional fingertip/forearm testing. In addition, studies on these devices have shown that they do not help improve clinical outcomes, particularly in patients with poorly controlled diabetes.

Insulin and the Other Pancreatic Islet Hormones

The pancreatic islets of Langerhans contain at least three main types of cells: beta cells that secrete insulin, alpha cells that secrete glucagon, and delta cells that secrete somatostatin.[84] Each islet contains mainly the beta cells surrounded by the alpha cells interspersed with delta cells.

The main action of insulin is to preserve energy stores by stimulating the uptake and storage of glucose, amino acids, and fats after a meal. It responds quickly to reduce the blood glucose level by acting on the liver, muscle, and fat. In the liver, insulin inhibits glycogenolysis (glycogen breakdown) and gluconeogenesis (synthesis of glucose from amino acids) while enhancing glycogen synthesis and increasing glucose utilization (Table 14-5). In addition, insulin stimulates carrier-mediated transport of glucose into several tissues. These carriers are called *glut carriers* and range in number from 1 to 5. Glut 4 carriers are responsible for glucose entry into muscle and adipose tissue (Figure 14-1). In adipose tissue, insulin enhances glucose metabolism, which results in the formation of glycerol, a precursor to triglycerides, and also inhibits lipolysis. In terms of protein metabolism, insulin stimulates the uptake of amino acids into muscle and increases protein synthesis.

Insulin is initially synthesized as one long peptide chain called *preproinsulin* in the rough endoplasmic reticulum. Preproinsulin is then transported to the Golgi apparatus, where it is cleaved into a smaller peptide called *proinsulin* and then finally to insulin and a fragment called *C-peptide*. The exact function of C-peptide is unknown, but it is stored in granules in the beta cells

TABLE 14-5 Summary of the Effects of Insulin on Carbohydrate, Fat, and Protein Metabolism in Liver, Muscle, and Adipose Tissue

Type of Metabolism	Liver Cells	Fat Cell	Muscle
Carbohydrate metabolism	↑↓ Gluconeogenesis ↓ Glycogenolysis ↑ Glycolysis ↑ Glycogenesis	↑ Glucose uptake ↑ Glycerol synthesis	↑ Glucose uptake ↑ Glycolysis ↑ Glycogenesis
Fat metabolism	↑ Lipogenesis ↓ Lipolysis	↑ Synthesis of triglycerides ↑ Fatty acid synthesis ↓ Lipolysis	—
Protein metabolism	↓ Protein breakdown	—	↑ Amino acid uptake ↑ Protein synthesis

From Rang HP, Dale MM, Ritter JM, Moore JL, editors: *Pharmacology* (5th ed.). New York, 2003, Churchill Livingstone.

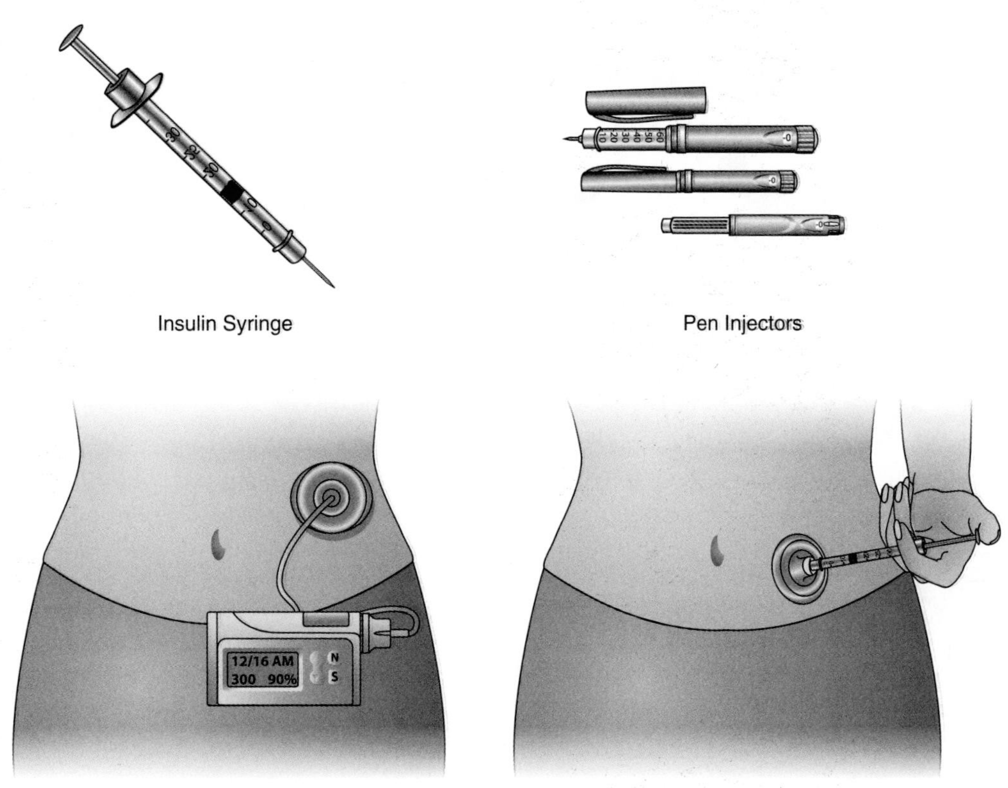

FIGURE 14-1 Self-monitoring tools for measuring glucose level.

along with insulin and released by exocytosis in equimolar amounts. Some proinsulin may be released as well.

Beta cells respond to an absolute glucose concentration in the blood and also to a change in concentration. Glucose enters the beta cell via a Glut 2 transporter. There it undergoes metabolism, producing intracellular adenosine triphosphate (ATP). This ATP blocks a specialized ion channel called an *ATP-sensitive potassium (K+) channel* (Figure 14-2). The channel closes, blocking the outflow of K+ ions from the cell and producing a membrane depolarization. The positive change in membrane potential opens the voltage-gated calcium channels, leading to calcium (Ca^{2+}) influx. Calcium entry triggers exocytosis and insulin release.

The beta cell responds to glucose in two phases—an initial rapid secretion of insulin, followed by a slower delayed release.[85] In addition, a low-level basal release of insulin occurs (Figure 14-3). Many factors other than just glucose control the release of insulin. GI hormones (e.g., gastrin, secretin, cholecystokinin) trigger the release of insulin. These hormones are released by both the visual and physical activities of eating, and this explains why there is a greater release of insulin in response to food than when the same amount of glucose is given intravenously. Other stimuli for insulin release include amino acids, fatty acids, and the parasympathetic nervous system (Figure 14-4). The sympathetic system exerts an inhibitory effect on insulin release.

Once released, insulin binds to a specialized membrane-bound receptor linked to a tyrosine kinase (Figure 14-5). This is a large receptor consisting of two α- and two β-subunits. The α-subunits are extracellular, and each contains an insulin-binding site. The β-subunits exist both outside and inside cells and have tyrosine kinase activity. Tyrosine kinase activity allows autophosphorylation of the receptor, leading to a signal cascade that ultimately turns on several genes involved in cell growth and metabolism. The development of insulin resistance is thought to be related to the loss of this tyrosine kinase activity.

Glucagon acts in opposition to insulin, increasing the blood glucose level and stimulating protein and fat breakdown.[85] Its secretion is stimulated by low levels of glucose and fatty acids in the plasma and a high-protein meal but is inhibited by high levels of glucose and fats. Sympathetic nervous activity and circulating epinephrine also stimulate glucagon release. Essentially, glucagon guarantees available plasma glucose to fuel the brain and muscles for activity and stimulates glycogen breakdown and gluconeogenesis.

Somatostatin opposes the action of both insulin and glucagon because it inhibits their secretion.[85] It is widely found outside the pancreas, secreted by the hypothalamus, which then inhibits the release of GH from the anterior pituitary. Hence, somatostatin lowers the blood glucose level by several mechanisms.

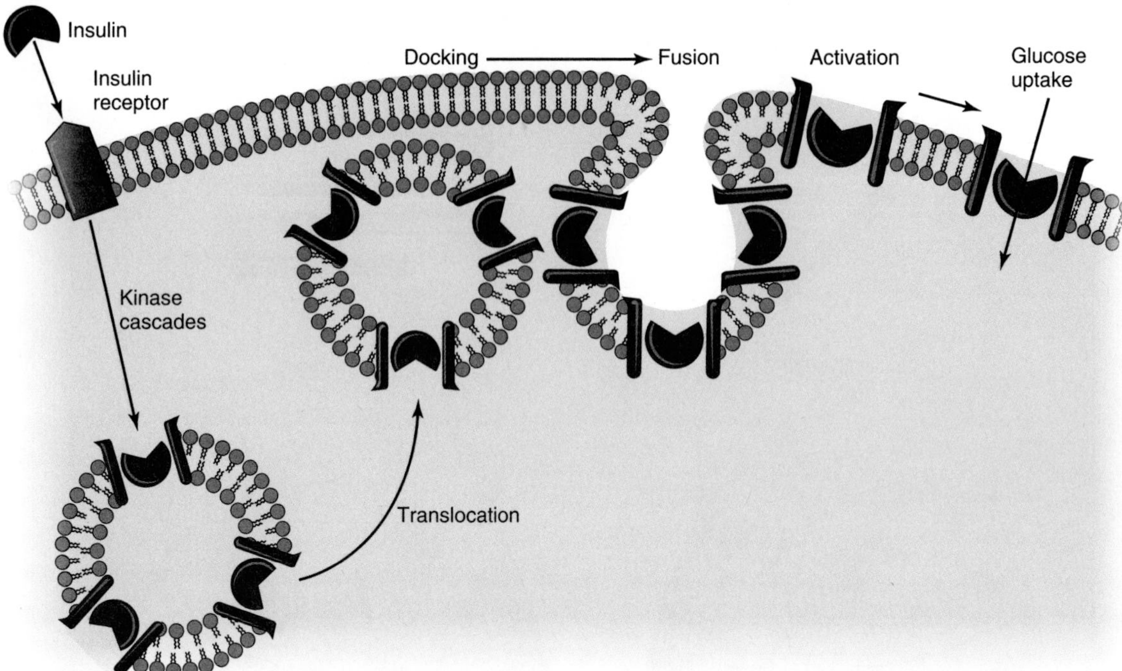

FIGURE 14-2 Intracellular kinase cascades cause translocation of glucose transporters from an endosomal compartment to the plasma membrane, where they increase glucose uptake.

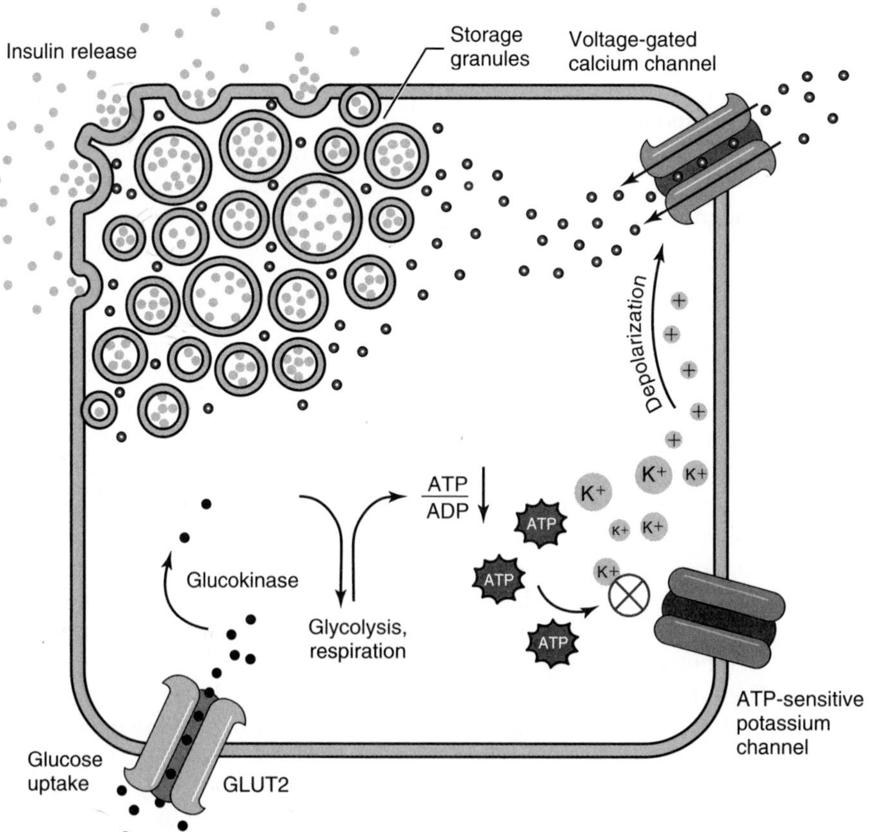

FIGURE 14-3 Insulin secretion. Insulin release from pancreatic beta cells is stimulated by the release of calcium (Ca^{2+}) from the endoplasmic compartment by voltage-sensitive channels and by the influx of extracellular Ca^{2+}. The adenosine triphosphate (ATP)–dependent potassium (K^+) channel on the plasma membrane maintains the intracellular resting potential. Inhibition of this K^+ channel by sulfonylurea or meglitinide agents results in depolarization and activation of the Ca^{2+} channels, resulting in enhanced insulin secretion.

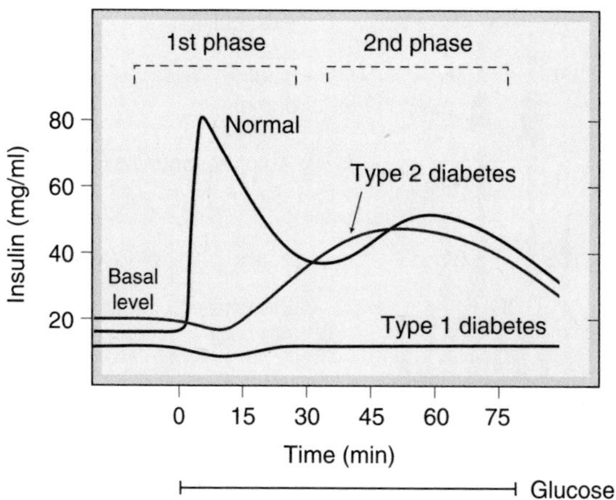

FIGURE 14-4 Schematic diagram of the two-phase release of insulin in response to constant glucose infusion. The first phase is missing in type 2 (non–insulin-dependent) diabetes mellitus, and both phases are missing in type 1 (insulin-dependent) diabetes mellitus. The first phase is also produced by amino acids, sulfonylureas, glucagons, and gastrointestinal tract hormones. *(Data from Pfeifer MA, Halter JB, Porte D Jr: Insulin secretion in diabetes mellitus,* Am J Med *70:579–588, 1981.) (From Rang HP, Dale MM, Ritter JM, Moore JL, editors:* Pharmacology *(5th ed.). New York, 2003, Churchill Livingstone.)*

Insulin Treatment

All insulins were originally isolated from beef or pork pancreases until 1982 when genetically engineered human insulin became available.[86] This innovation has led to a number of insulin analogs that have improved pharmacokinetic properties; however, replacement of physiologic insulin and return of glycemic control remain difficult goals to achieve.

The goal of insulin therapy is to match plasma insulin level to food intake and exercise.[87] In healthy individuals, the concentration of glucose in the plasma remains within a narrow range throughout the day, despite the amount of food consumed and activity level. After a meal, the glucose level rises to a peak in 30 to 60 minutes and then returns to baseline concentrations within 2 to 3 hours. The lowest glucose level occurs around 2:00 to 3:00 A.M., but basal secretion rises again before breakfast, probably in response to GH secretion. Insulin must be secreted or provided in appropriate amounts to match this level of glucose. This includes meal-related secretion, a low-level basal release, and the morning rise.

Insulin Formulations. Four types of insulin are available: ultra-short-acting, short-acting or regular, intermediate, and long-acting insulin (Figure 14-6). Ultra-short-acting insulins (lispro and aspart) can be taken 5 minutes before a meal, peak at 1 hour, and have a duration of

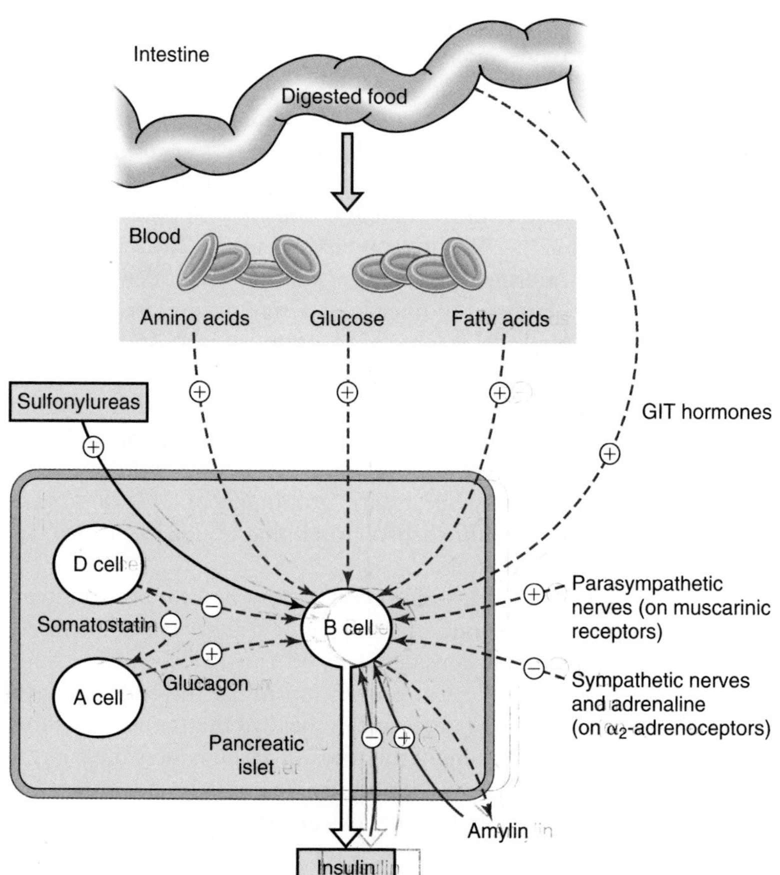

FIGURE 14-5 Factors regulating insulin secretion. Plasma glucose level is the most important factor. Drugs used to stimulate insulin secretion are shown in boxes. Glucagon potentiates insulin release but opposes some of its peripheral actions and increases the plasma glucose level. *GIT*, gastrointestinal tract.

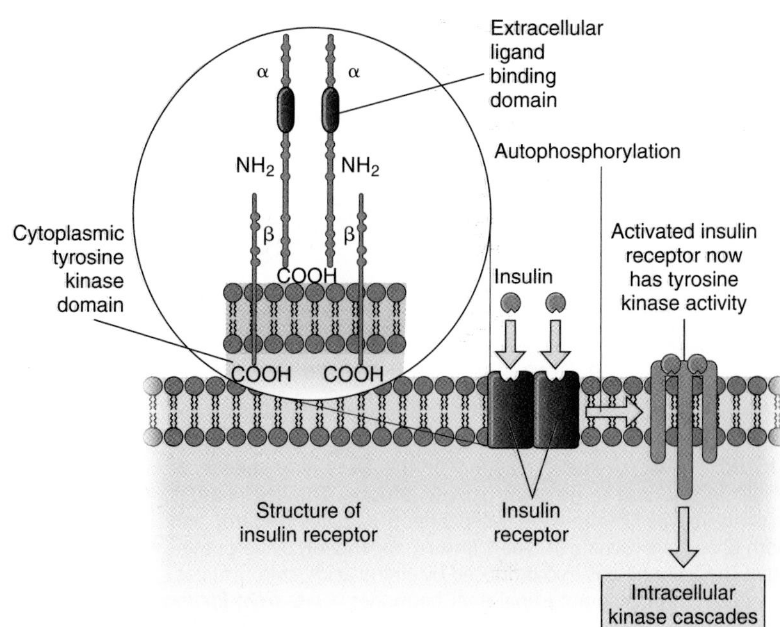

FIGURE 14-6 Insulin action. The insulin receptor is a heterodimeric transmembrane receptor consisting of two α- and two β-subunits. The intracellular portions of the β-subunits contain tyrosine kinase activity. Insulin receptor stimulation leads to phosphorylation of multiple intracellular signaling molecules. Phosphorylation of tyrosine kinase residues on intracellular kinases leads to activation of serine/threonine kinase cascades.

3 to 5 hours.[88-90] An ultra-short-acting insulin acts more rapidly but for a shorter time than does regular insulin. Regular insulin has an onset of action within 30 minutes, peaks in about 2 hours, and has a duration of action of 6 to 8 hours.[91] Regular insulin has no additives to delay absorption. The ultra-short-acting insulins offer slightly better control of postprandial rise in glucose level, but there may be a more rapid onset of hypoglycemia and less time for symptom recognition. In addition, the use of the ultra-short-acting agents alters the glucose monitoring schedule. It is customary for the patient to measure premeal glucose levels to determine the amount of regular insulin needed.[90] However, if the patient uses lispro or aspart at noon with the anticipation that the next dose will be at 6:00 P.M. before dinner, the predinner glucose measurement would be inaccurate. This is because the rapid-acting analogs might only be effective for 4 hours compared with the 6 hours with regular insulin. By dinner time, premeal glucose levels will be quite high, and the patient will then have the tendency to increase the next insulin dose, possibly triggering a hypoglycemic event.

Intermediate-acting insulin has a more gradual onset. It begins working after about 1 to 4 hours, and peak action occurs after about 6 to 12 hours. Effects may continue for 14 to 24 hours. A cationic protein, protamine (neutral protamine Hagedorn, or NPH), is added to regular insulin zinc suspensions to slow absorption. The intermediate-acting insulins have the advantage of longer duration but slower onset than the short-acting agents.

Long-acting insulin (Ultralente) contains zinc and a buffer to delay absorption, postponing onset for 4 to 6 hours with duration lasting up to 36 hours.[92] Ultralente peaks in 8 to 20 hours. This insulin has now been withdrawn from the market and has been replaced by the long-acting agents glargine and detemir. Insulin glargine is a new long-acting insulin that has recently been approved.[93,94] The mean onset of action is within 1 hour of injection, but the duration of action is similar to that of Ultralente. It has no peak and instead mimics continuous infusion of rapid-acting regular insulin from a subcutaneous pump. Long-acting insulins are intended to provide adequate basal insulin concentrations in a single daily dose.[95]

All insulins are available in concentrations of 100 units/mL.[91] There is one regular insulin formulation available in a 20-mL vial containing 500 units/mL for patients who require more than 200 units/day. Regular and ultra-short-acting insulins can be combined in the same syringe with intermediate-acting insulin and Ultralente but not with glargine (another long-acting insulin) because glargine will delay the absorption of the shorter-acting agent.[96] Patients can identify an insulin by checking its appearance. Regular and ultra-short-acting insulins and glargine are clear; the other insulins appear cloudy. Premixed insulins containing 70% NPH and 30% regular, 70% insulin aspart protamine and 30% aspart, or 75% insulin lispro protamine and 25% lispro are available.

Unopened insulin products may be kept at room temperature, but once the stopper or seal has been punctured, the insulin is considered to be "in use."[91] In-use insulin vials can be kept at room temperature for up to 28 days. However, it has been recommended that in-use measured syringes containing mixtures of insulins be stored in the refrigerator. Any unused insulin must be discarded if it freezes. Insulin travel packs are also available.

Insulin Regimens for Type 1 Diabetes. Combinations of insulin types are used to control glucose. This strategy of mixing types is known as the *basal/bolus regimen*.[97] Low levels of insulin are required from bedtime until early morning, and higher levels are required during the daytime hours with significant increases at meal times. One regimen is called *split and mixed* and consists of a mixture of rapid-onset insulin (regular or ultra-short-acting) and intermediate or Ultralente insulin, with the first injection given before breakfast and a second given before supper (Figure 14-7). The supper dose of the NPH may be adjusted to achieve euglycemia before breakfast the next morning without producing hypoglycemia in the middle of the night. When the desired fasting morning level of glucose is achieved, the morning dose of the intermediate-acting insulin may be adjusted to attain euglycemia before supper. This regimen requires two injections per day. A disadvantage to this regimen is that there might not be enough active insulin available to cover lunch. Also, nocturnal hypoglycemia may occur around midnight, especially if the patient did not eat a snack after dinner. In addition, and perhaps more important, patients rarely achieve adequate control with this program.[97]

For the purpose of improving night-time control, the second intermediate-acting insulin can be held until bedtime (9:00 P.M.). This regimen is called *split and mixed with bedtime intermediate*. Three injections are required: (1) one at breakfast consisting of regular or ultra-short-acting insulin mixed with NPH, (2) short-acting insulin at dinner, and (3) an injection of intermediate-acting insulin before bed. Nocturnal hypoglycemia is delayed and the level instead corresponds to early morning hyperglycemia.

The "multiple dosing" regimen includes preprandial regular insulin and bedtime intermediate insulin for a total of four injections (Figure 14-8). This system covers each meal as well as the slow climb toward hyperglycemia in the 5:00 to 8:00 A.M. period. The longer-acting insulins (detimir and glargine) may be substituted for the intermediate-acting insulin at bedtime, depending on the patient's caloric intake and activity level[97] (Figure 14-9). This regimen offers the most flexibility in terms of meal size and timing in that each meal is covered with regular insulin and the longer-acting agents cover the basal

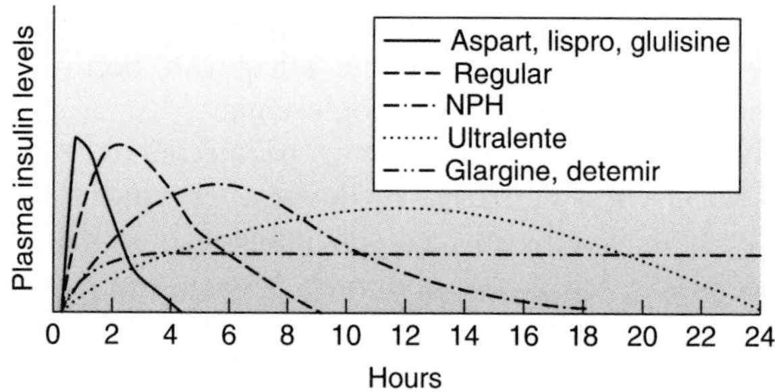

FIGURE 14-7 Types of insulin and their times of onset and duration of action.

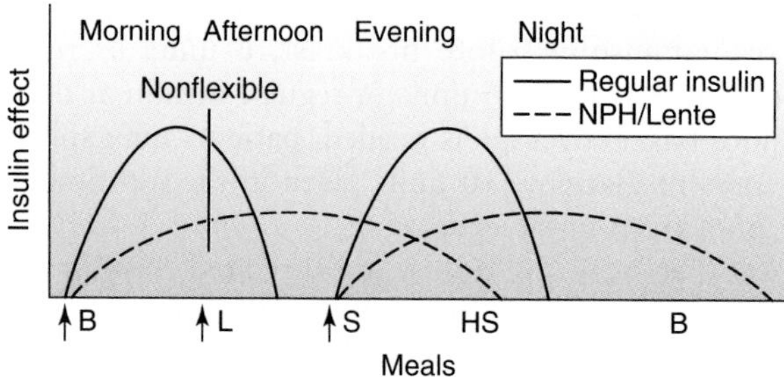

FIGURE 14-8 Split and mixed insulin regime. Patient receives an injection of ultra-short-acting insulin along with intermediate-acting insulin before breakfast and again before dinner.

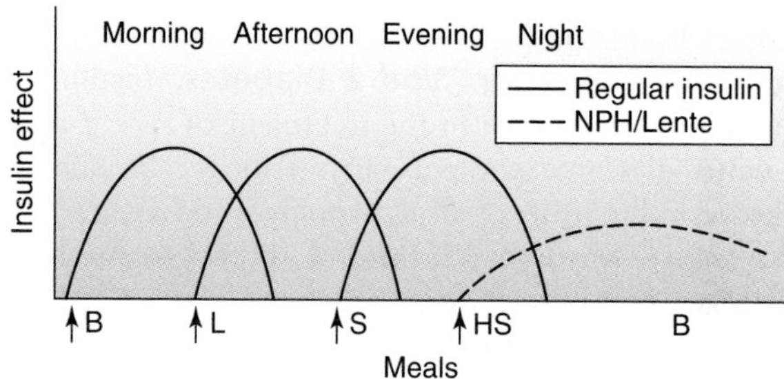

FIGURE 14-9 Premeal regular or ultra-short-acting insulin with bedtime intermediate insulin.

insulin release during the night. However, any large depot of insulin can easily lead to hypoglycemia (see the following section).

Dosing Guidelines. Insulin doses are expressed in units instead of milliliters. For the initial insulin dose, most patients are started with an average dose of intermediate-acting insulin or long-acting insulin. This dose may range from 10 to 30 units per day. The obese patient will require a greater amount. The dose is then adjusted to meet the patient's diet and activity level. Patients are asked to coordinate increases in dose with their FPG test. For example, an FPG value of 120 to 140 requires an increase of 2 units/day and 140 to 180 requires an increase of 4 to 6 units/day. If the FPG value is over 180, the dose is adjusted by 8 units/day. Insulin level is increased weekly as long as there are no severe hypoglycemic events (plasma glucose <72 mg/dL).

After dosing with the intermediate- or long-acting insulins, the meal-related dose must be configured. Short-acting insulins administered with each meal should achieve a peak postprandial blood glucose level of less than 160 mg/dL.[98] Blood glucose at bedtime should be between 110 and 135 mg/dL. Patients are encouraged to check glucose levels frequently, especially after a change in regimen, and also around 2:00 A.M. to check for hypoglycemia. Nightmares may be a signal that the patient is hypoglycemic during sleep. A sample insulin program might include 20 units of glargine in the evening, 8 units of regular insulin before breakfast, 6 units of regular insulin at lunch, and 6 units of regular insulin at dinner. If more basal coverage is needed, patients may split the 20 units of glargine, 10 units given in the morning and 10 units given in the evening.

Another way to adjust meal-related insulin dose is through counting carbohydrates. In this method, the insulin dose is adjusted on the basis of the number of grams of carbohydrate expected to be consumed. The greater the amount of carbohydrates ingested, the greater is the amount of insulin that must be administered. The general rule is for every 10 g of carbohydrate, patients should receive 1 unit of insulin. Determining the correct dose of insulin to administer and the most effective regimen for a patient is complicated, and therefore patients should be encouraged to see a nutritionist certified as a Diabetes Educator.

Insulin Regimens for Type 2 Diabetes. Insulin is a very important adjunct in the treatment of type 2 diabetes when glycemic control can no longer be achieved with a combination of oral hypoglycemic agents, diet, and exercise. More than a third of all patients with type 2 diabetes will require treatment with insulin.[72] Therefore, early insulin replacement in type 2 diabetes is becoming a new strategy to achieve optimal metabolic control. It is believed that this strategy improves insulin sensitivity by reducing "glucotoxicity" and may reduce cardiovascular risk.[97]

In general, patients with type 2 diabetes begin therapy with an oral insulin sensitizer or insulin secretagogue (see discussion of oral hypoglycemic agents).[97] As insulin resistance develops, the patient begins receiving an evening basal insulin replacement in addition to the oral agents. This requires only one daily injection without the need to mix different preparations. Insulin-naïve patients start with an average dose of 15 units of glargine at night and then make adjustments according to the FBG test result the next morning. If patients are switching to glargine from once-daily NPH or Ultralente, the initial dose should be the same. However, if they are switching from twice-daily NPH, the initial dose of glargine must be reduced by 20%. Comparison studies of NPH insulin and glargine at bedtime showed equivalent glycemic control and similar weight gain. However, patients who took glargine had less symptomatic hypoglycemia and better glycemic control in the late afternoon.[99] Patients may also end up needing twice-daily injections of basal insulin, one at bedtime and the other at breakfast, and the total dose may not be increased but rather split between a bedtime dose and a morning dose.

Adverse Effects of Insulin. The main adverse effect of insulin is hypoglycemia, which may occur as a result of a delayed or missed meal, excess insulin, decreased carbohydrate content of a meal, increased insulin absorption rates, or exercising without first eating a snack.[96] Symptoms include sweating, tachycardia, nervousness, headache, faintness, weakness, and numbness in the fingers and around the mouth. Neurologic manifestations include coma, convulsions, transient hemiparesis, stroke, and cognitive dysfunction. Cardiac events such as arrhythmias and myocardial ischemia may also occur. Many of these manifestations can lead to accidents and injuries, particularly if the patient is behind the wheel of a car. The annual prevalence of severe hypoglycemia is about 1.0 to 1.7 episodes per patient per year.[100] Severe hypoglycemia is classified as needing assistance for recovery. These responses occur as a result of epinephrine release and are considered to provide a warning to the patient to eat something with sugar, usually fruit juice (4 to 6 oz) or hard candy (5 to 7 pieces).[72] Glucose tablets are also available for this purpose. Other signs include double vision, confusion, and finally seizures, coma, and death. Once the confusion begins, the patient may not be able to get to food or help.

Patients using insulin should carry at least 15 g of carbohydrate to be administered orally in the event of a hypoglycemic event.[72] The glucose level can be stabilized in about 15 minutes with 10 to 15 g of carbohydrate in cases of mild hypoglycemia. Family members and friends should receive instruction on how to use glucagon when the patient cannot be given sugar orally. Quick fixes that can be administered by the patient include 4 oz of orange juice, 6 oz of regular soda, 6 to 8 oz of 2% or skim milk, three graham crackers, six jelly beans, and 2 tablespoons of raisins.[101] Patients can use the "Hypoglycemia Protocol" to raise their glucose level.[102] This protocol is also known as the *Rule of 15*. If blood glucose is 70 mg/dL or below, the patient needs to eat 15 g of carbohydrate and recheck the glucose level in 15 minutes. If the reading is still not above 70 mg/dL, then the patient is instructed to eat another 15 g and test again in 15 minutes. If the level is still not above the 70 mg/dL mark, another 15 g of carbohydrate should be consumed and the physician should be contacted. Patients who take β-blockers or who have had nerve damage from their diabetes may not be able to recognize the signs of hypoglycemia and must be quite vigilant about measuring their glucose levels.

Other adverse effects of insulin include lipoatrophy, a benign condition in which a loss of subcutaneous fat occurs at the injection site; lipohypertrophy; local injection site reactions; and the Somogyi effect or rebound hyperglycemia.[72] The Somogyi effect can occur 6 to 12 hours after periods of hypoglycemia.

Delivery of Insulin. Insulin must be injected to be effective because it is destroyed by digestive enzymes if taken orally. It is usually injected subcutaneously in different areas of the body: the abdomen (except for 2 inches around the navel), the front and outer side of the thigh, the upper part of the buttocks, and the outer side of the upper arm.[72] Injection locations need to be varied to prevent inflammation and lipodystrophy. Injections of at least two finger widths apart are recommended, and no injection site should be used more than once in a month. Absorption is most rapid when insulin is injected into the abdomen; it occurs more slowly when injected in the arms and even more slowly when injected in the thigh or buttocks. The exception is when a patient is exercising or receiving a massage.[103] Absorption under these circumstances will be greatly increased. In fact, exercise and massage are contraindicated in the area of injection for the length of the time that the drug is expected to be active. Injections in the abdomen are frequently used during the day, and the thigh and buttock locations are used in the evening so that insulin will persist longer in the circulation during the night.

Insulin is usually injected with a syringe specially calibrated for insulin and ultrafine needles (Figure 14-10).[72] Insulin pens combine an insulin container and a syringe in one device. The cartridges come prefilled, and the patient simply dials in the dose. Some are reusable and others are disposable. In a study in which patient preferences were compared, the prefilled, disposable pen was clearly preferred over the vial and syringe setup.[104] Jet injectors use a high-pressure jet of air to send a stream of insulin through the skin, eliminating the use of a needle.

Newer methods for insulin delivery include inhaled insulin (Exubera), a subcutaneous injection port, and continuous subcutaneous infusion. Inhalation of insulin is performed in a manner similar to the method used by patients with asthma.[105,106] The insulin comes in a dry powder form dispersed by aerosol as particles. The patient inhales the dry powder through the mouth into the lungs, and the drug then enters the bloodstream. The inhaler is about the size of a flashlight and dispenses regular insulin. Studies were performed with patients with type 2 diabetes who also take oral hypoglycemic agents, and they demonstrated improved glycemic control when inhaled insulin was given at premeal times. These studies were performed with individuals whose diabetes could not be controlled with the oral hypoglycemic agents alone. When inhaled insulin was added to the regimen of oral drugs, patients experienced significant reductions in glycosylated hemoglobin values, FPG levels, and postprandial glucose increases, compared with patients receiving only the oral drugs.[107] In addition, there was a marked reduction in fasting triglyceride levels. Adverse effects of inhaled insulin included weight gain, greater incidence of hypoglycemia, and a reduction in forced expiratory volume in one second (FEV_1). All of the hypoglycemic events, except one, were classified as mild to moderate. Only one event resulted in severe hypoglycemia, and third-party assistance was needed to provide a glucose source. Unfortunately, the marketing of this device manufactured by Pfizer was halted in 2007 due to low patient acceptance. A newer device, technosphere insulin (*Afresa*, Mannkind Corp) is currently under study.[108] So far, this drug has shown a rapid onset of action (10 minutes), compared with insulin lispro and the inhaled Exubera (30 minutes). Pulmonary function tests show no difference at the end of 2 years compared with values in individuals on the standard regimen. Time will tell if this method will be accepted by patients.

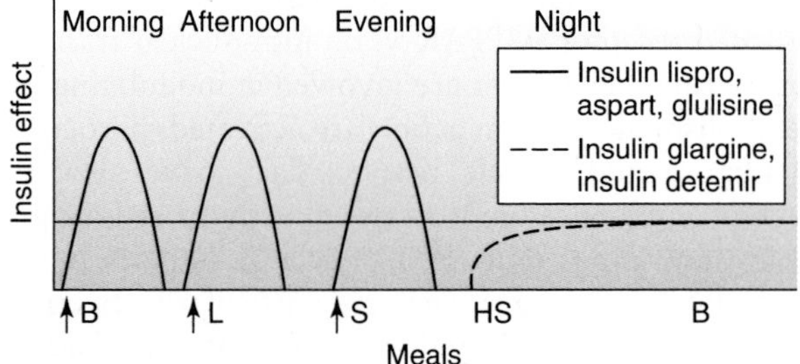

FIGURE 14-10 Premeal regular or ultra-short-acting insulin with bedtime long-acting, peakless insulin.

Continuous subcutaneous insulin infusion with external pumps is another alternative to multiple daily injections. These pumps provide continuous insulin infusion with supplemental regular insulin for mealtime. Doses can be adjusted fairly easily, allowing total flexibility with meals and snacks. A study in which multiple injections with the pen injector (NovoPen) were compared with subcutaneous continued infusion in patients with type 2 diabetes demonstrated similar glycemic control but significant improvement in satisfaction scores from the subjects who used the pump.[109] The safety profile was also similar between the groups in terms of hypoglycemic events, but a few users of the pump had to struggle with clogs and blockages. Similar results were seen in a study in which continuous insulin infusion was compared with multiple daily injections in children with type 1 diabetes.[109]

The use of a subcutaneous injection port is understudy to help improve glycemic control in children with type 1 diabetes.[110] A comparison between the Insuflon port and the use of a blood glucose meter with an alarm setup demonstrated that when children did not have to continuously inject themselves, they achieved a lower A_{1C} reading. This mode of administration took the fear of injections away and therefore resulted in more consistent and appropriate use of insulin that resulted in improve glycemic control in children.

Drugs Used in the Treatment of Type 2 Diabetes

Oral hypoglycemic agents and exenatide drugs are used by patients with type 2 diabetes who do not require insulin to prevent ketoacidosis, although insulin is often added as resistance increases. These drugs act to increase insulin secretion or to improve the sensitivity of tissues to insulin. They are classified according to whether they increase insulin secretion, improve insulin sensitivity, or block glucose uptake.

Biguanides (Metformin). Metformin is one of the most commonly used antidiabetic agents. It reduces gluconeogenesis in the liver and improves glucose utilization in skeletal muscle by increasing the number and activity of GLUT-4 transporters, thereby reducing insulin resistance.[111,112] It lowers A_{1C} by about 1 to 2%. Metformin does not stimulate insulin secretion, thus lowering the risk of hypoglycemia. It is often used as a first-line oral agent or in combination with a sulfonylurea (see discussion on sulfonylureas). In addition, this drug lowers cholesterol and triglyceride levels and may even help the patient lose weight.[113] Adverse effects include transient nausea and diarrhea. Lactic acidosis is a rare complication and might not be due to the drug but the underlying medical disorder. This drug is usually administered twice daily, with breakfast and then with dinner. Other formulations include the "XR" (extended release) and in combination with glyburide, glipizide, rosiglitazone, and pioglitazone.

Sulfonylureas. These agents block the ATP-sensitive K^+ channel in the beta cells of the pancreas.[114] This action depolarizes the cell and ultimately produces release of insulin, so they are considered insulin secretagogues. They reduce A_{1C} by approximately 1 to 2%. Examples include tolbutamide, glipizide, glimepiride, and glyburide.[115,116] They all have similar chemical structures and modes of action, so if a patient loses responsiveness to one sulfonylurea, he or she should be switched to a drug in another classification. Tolbutamide was the first sulfonylurea available and thus has been given the relative potency number of 1. Glipizide is considered a second-generation sulfonylurea and has a relative potency number of 100 relative to tolbutamide. The most common adverse effect is hypoglycemia, which is more likely to occur in malnourished older adults or those with liver abnormalities. Alcohol, skipped meals, and exercise might trigger hypoglycemia with these drugs.[117] In addition, they cause weight gain. However, there is a concern regarding cardiac protection with glyburide.[118,119] ATP-sensitive K^+ channels are also expressed in cardiac and vascular myocytes. Here, they are thought to be involved in the adjustment of vascular tone and myocardial contractility. Blocking this channel provides less protection of contractility during hypoxia. In addition, clinical studies have shown greater ischemia and more electrophysiologic abnormalities in patients taking glyburide compared with other sulfonylureas.

These drugs may be given once a day or in divided doses 15 to 30 minutes before a meal. Glipizide is now available as an extended release formulation called *Glucotrol XL*. Glyburide is also available in a fixed-dose combination with metformin. Used together, these drugs demonstrate better glycemic control than either drug alone.[120]

Repaglinide and Nateglinide (the glinides) are two other drugs that act in a similar manner to sulfonylureas but lack the sulfonylurea moiety.[116,121] They are rapidly absorbed and eliminated, so there is a lower risk of hypoglycemia than with standard sulfonylureas. In addition, they are relatively selective for the ATP-sensitive K^+ channel in the beta cells and do not affect these channels in cardiac tissue, thus reducing cardiac risk. They also produce less weight gain compared with sulfonylureas. They are given before a meal to reduce postprandial glucose rise.

Thiazolidinediones (Glitazones). The thiazolidinediones were developed as a result of the surprising finding that a clofibrate analog, ciglitazone, which was being developed for its lipid-lowering abilities, was found to lower blood glucose levels. Rosiglitazone and pioglitazone, two other drugs in this category, have since been developed for treatment of type 2 diabetes. These agents improve glycemic control by increasing insulin sensitivity in muscle, liver, and adipose tissue.[116] They produce a drop in A_{1C} by 1 to 2%.

One of the most interesting developments with the glitizones is that they appear to stabilize beta cell dysfunction, that is to slow the beta cell deterioration. In the Troglitazone in the Prevention of Diabetes TRIPOD study, it was found that troglitazone improved insulin sensitivity in Hispanic women who were previously diagnosed with gestational diabetes compared with women who received no preventive treatment.[122] The Pioglitazone Prevention of Type 2 Diabetes (PIPOD) trial, which was an extension of the TRIPOD trial, also demonstrated protection from diabetes in high-risk women. In addition, a delay in progression of type 2 diabetes was seen with rosiglitazone in the Diabetes Reduction Approaches with Ramipril and Rosiglitazone Medications (DREAM) trial.[123] This trial was quite significant, as it demonstrated that for every 1000 people treated with rosiglitazone for 3 years, 144 cases of diabetes were prevented. The PPAR-γ receptor has been found on the beta cells but the exact protective response has not been delineated yet. Since rosiglitazone also decreases blood pressure, a reduction in risk may have occurred through this mechanism. What is known, however, is that beta cell function begins to deteriorate approximately 12 years before diabetes is diagnosed and that at the time of diagnosis approximately 50% of beta cells would have been lost.[124] So the opportunity to preserve beta cells with these drugs offers a promising preventive treatment.

Thiazolidinediones bind to peroxisome proliferator–activated receptor-γ (PPAR-γ) on intranuclear transcription factors. Genes that are involved in modulating lipid metabolism and insulin action are activated, particularly in adipose and muscle tissues. They have also been shown to influence the beta cell directly by reducing the proinsulin/insulin ratio seen in type 2 diabetes but not produce hypoglycemia. They are particularly effective in patients who are obese with predominant central adiposity because of the association with insulin resistance.

Plasma triglyceride levels are reduced, HDL cholesterol levels are increased, and small LDL particles are transformed into larger particles that are less atherogenic.[125] These agents also have favorable effects on coagulation and blood pressure.

Adverse effects of the glitazones include weight gain, fluid retention, decreased bone mineral density, and possibly some cardiac involvement. A pooled analysis of some major trials has suggested that thiazolidinediones may be associated with increased hospital admissions for heart failure, although there was significant heterogeneity among these studies.[126,127] Due to fluid retention, these drugs are not recommended for patients with stage III or IV heart failure. Another concern is a possible increase in myocardial infarction (MI) with Avandia as determined by a meta-analysis of 42 studies performed by physicians at the Cleveland Clinic in Ohio in 2007.[128] This prompted an interim analysis of the Rosiglitazone Evaluated for Cardiac Outcomes and Regulation of Glycemia in Diabetes (RECORD) study, which was designed specifically to determine if there were any associated cardiac abnormalities with Avandia. The early analysis refuted any increase in MIs with this medication.[129] However, there is still no clear consensus as to the cardiac risk with these drugs. Unfortunately, in addition to creating a medical controversy, these studies have also added fuel to some political debates on the safety record of the FDA.[130] Apparently, the original meta-analysis was sent directly to the *New England Journal of Medicine* prior to any notification to the FDA. The journal then asked two physicians who were critical of the FDA to write editorials on the meta-analysis, both of whom supported its findings. All of this took place before the FDA was either informed or could release a safety statement. This prompted some congressional hearings on the safety of Avandia. It is important to note that these adverse effects have not been seen with Actos, the other commonly used glitazone. In addition to cardiac monitoring, patients should have their liver transaminases monitored because the first clinically available glitazone (troglitazone) produced some fatal liver toxicity. This drug has since been withdrawn.[131] Another adverse effect may be reduced bone density and thus increased fracture risk. It is thought that increased PPAR-γ activity may trigger the multipotent mesenchymal stem cell to form into adipocytes rather than osteoblasts.[132]

Because insulin resistance precedes the development of type 2 diabetes and also leads to the decline in beta cell function, it is reasonable to suggest that either the thiazolidinediones or the biguanides be started very early at the first sign of disease.[116] Metformin exerts its effect primarily by decreasing glucose production, whereas the glitazones improve insulin-mediated uptake of glucose; therefore, it would seem that the first choice in the treatment of insulin resistance should be the thiazolidinediones. However, metformin has a better safety profile and produces weight loss, so the first agent of choice really depends on individual patient factors.

α-Glucosidase Inhibitors. Acarbose and miglitol inhibit GI absorption of carbohydrates by inhibiting the α-glucosidase enzymes in the intestines.[116] They reduce A_{1C} by only 0.5 to 1%. The drugs are taken just before meals and therefore lower the peak glucose levels seen after a meal. These drugs may also be given in combination with metformin, a sulfonylurea, or a glitazone. Adverse drug reactions include flatulence, diarrhea, and abdominal discomfort. Hypoglycemia may be a problem when the drug is administered with other agents but does not occur when α-glucosidase inhibitors are administered as monotherapy.

GLP-1 Analogs. Glucagon-like peptide-1 (GLP-1) is a hormone released from the GI tract (L cells in the jejunum and terminal ileum) in response to nutrient ingestion. It stimulates insulin secretion, which is the reason for the greater insulin release in response to an oral challenge than when glucose is given intravenously. This difference in insulin secretion is noted as the "incretin effect" and is two to three times greater than insulin secretion secondary to glucose infusion.[133] In addition to enhancing glucose-dependent insulin secretion, it suppresses glucagon secretion and slows gastric emptying. Patients with impaired glucose tolerance and type 2 diabetes have lower plasma GLP-1 levels compared with healthy controls.

The incretin hormones, GLP-1 and a similar hormone glucose-dependent insulinotropic polypeptide (GIP), have extraglycemic effects. Both have receptors on the pancreatic β-cells and have been found to inhibit their death in both animal and in vitro studies. And in humans, when using tests for β-cell function (intravenous glucose tolerance test, the hyperglycemic clamp with arginine stimulation, and the meal tolerance test), GLP-1 improved β-cell function and restored the first phase insulin secretion.[134] When human β-cells were cultured with and without GLP-1, cell morphology was maintained and cell death was slowed to a much greater extent with the cells bathed in GLP-1.[135] In addition, intracellular insulin content was higher in the treatment group compared with the control cells. Clearly, having adequate amounts of GLP-1 delays deterioration of β-cell function under certain conditions.

Endogenous GLP-1 has a very short half-life (less than 2 minutes), so an oral or even an IV form would not last long enough to stimulate insulin secretion.[136] It is rapidly degraded by the enzyme dipeptidyl peptidase-IV (DPP-IV). Therefore, a GLP-1 analog called *exenatide* (Byetta) has been developed. It is given by injection, 5 mcg twice a day for the first month, followed by 10 mcg twice a day.[137] Injections must be given within 60 minutes of a meal. Exenatide is available in an easy-to-administer disposable pen that releases a fixed dose. Each pen contains a 30-day supply of the drug and requires refrigeration between doses. It is easy to use, requiring no blood glucose monitoring and no adjustment for meal size or activity level. Adverse effects include nausea and vomiting, especially at the beginning of therapy. Since the drug slows gastric emptying, precautions should be taken when other drugs are administered at the same time, especially if their actions depend on quick absorption. In addition, if taken with a sulfonylurea, hypoglycemia may occur.

Exenatide when added to established oral hypoglycemic agents such as metformin or a sulfonylurea shows similar effectiveness to when insulin glargine is added to the same therapies. It is an effective alternative to adding insulin when oral hypoglycemic agents are no longer able to achieve good glycemic control in type 2 diabetes. It is not an option for individuals with type 1 diabetes since they do not have adequate insulin secretion. The advantage of using exenatide over insulin glargine is that it does not need to be titrated to any fasting blood glucose level or A_{1C} measurement. So there is no cumbersome dose adjustment involved, and there is less weight gain than with insulin.[138]

Dipeptidyl Peptidase-4 Inhibitors. As mentioned above, the enzyme dipeptidyl peptidase-IV (DPP-IV) is responsible for the degradation of GLP-1. Sitagliptin (Januvia) and saxagliptin (Onglyza) are DPP-IV inhibitors that extend the half-life of GLP-1 by inhibiting the enzyme for 24 hours. This results in a two- to three-fold increase in the circulating levels of GLP-1. The drugs are approved as monotherapy for the treatment of type 2 diabetes or as add-on drugs to metformin or thiazolidinediones. Both have shown to significantly lower A_{1C} and FPG level compared with placebo.[139] When added to metformin, the glucose profile measured over a 24-hour period shows significantly less postprandial glucose measures compared with metformin alone. The few adverse effects that have been reported include a slight increase in GI distress compared with placebo. There appears to be no increase in weight, but the weight reduction noted with exenatide is not seen with DPP-IV inhibitors.

Pramlintide (Symlin). Pramlintide is an analog of the β-cell hormone amylin that is secreted from the β-cell along with insulin. The hormone is absent in type 1 diabetes and exists at low levels in type 2 diabetes. Amylin has been shown to slow gastric emptying, increase satiety, and inhibit postprandial plasma glucagon secretion as well as hepatic glucose output.[140] It shares many of the characteristics of GLP-1. Since amylin has poor solubility, an amylinomimetic agent called *pramlintide* was developed.

Pramlintide is indicated for patients with type 1 diabetes as well as for patients with type 2 diabetes if they are taking insulin. The drug is given via subcutaneous injection before any meal of at least 250 kcal or more than 30 g of carbohydrates. If given along with insulin, the insulin dose must be reduced. Adverse effects include nausea and vomiting, and hypoglycemia when taken with insulin.

Selection of Agents for Type 2 Diabetes. Diet and exercise are the first-line treatments for type 2 diabetes; however, they often do not control blood glucose levels, and many clinicians are forced to prescribe drugs (Box 14-6 and Table 14-6). Popular initial choices for medications tend to be metformin or a sulfonylurea prescribed as monotherapy. However, only a small proportion of patients can achieve adequate glycemic control with one drug alone. As mentioned previously, there appears to be a good rationale for starting with an insulin sensitizer rather than an insulin secretagogue. Because the hallmark of type 2 diabetes is insulin resistance, it makes sense to begin therapy with a glitazone or with metformin, which improves insulin sensitivity, does not cause hypoglycemia, and can normalize the Hb_{A1C} levels. Given that this disease is progressive and glycemic control worsens with time, patients who initially respond to monotherapy will likely require combination therapy later. Either a sulfonylurea or a thiazolidinedione is then added to metformin. However, the oral incretins are other good choices. If A_{1C} is still not at a goal of 7% and the two oral hypoglycemic agents have been used maximally, then a third oral drug may be added. Other options at this point include adding exenatide or starting a long-acting insulin at bedtime. Generally, most patients with long-standing diabetes will end up on insulin, since the secretory capacity of the pancreas fails eventually.

Several clinical studies have proved the efficacy of the following combination therapies: metformin and rosiglitazone; pioglitazone and a sulfonylurea; and triple therapy with troglitazone, glyburide, and metformin.[141-143] These studies have demonstrated that combination therapy significantly improves FPG and lipid levels over those achieved with monotherapy. However, combination therapy is also associated with a greater risk of hypoglycemia.

Management of Nonglycemic Adverse Effects of Type 2 Diabetes. Complications associated with type 2 diabetes can be reduced with other medications. Management of cardiovascular disease with antihypertensive and lipid-lowering drugs has been shown to contribute significant clinical efficacy.[144] A subgroup analysis of 202 diabetic patients participating in the Scandinavian Simvastatin Survival Study who were given simvastatin demonstrated reduced major coronary heart disease events equal to the reductions seen in nondiabetic patients over a 5.5-year period.[145] The benefit of lowering cholesterol is viewed as being even more significant for diabetic patients who have coronary artery disease than for nondiabetic patients with the same disease process because diabetes magnifies the risk of atherosclerotic events. The Cholesterol and Recurrent Events (CARE) trial evaluated the effect of pravastatin compared with placebo in the prevention of recurrent cardiovascular events in 586 patients with diabetes and average cholesterol readings.[146] The patients with diabetes who received active drug experienced a significant reduction in cardiovascular events

BOX 14-6 Drug Effects on Glycemic Control

Drug Class	Mechanism of Action
Sulfonylureas/meglitinides	Increase insulin release
Metformin	Decreases gluconeogenesis/increases insulin sensitivity
Thiazolidinediones (PPAR-γ agonists)	Are insulin sensitizers
Alpha-glucosidase inhibitors	Inhibit glucose absorption
Incretins	Affect β-cells and non–β-cells
Insulin	Replaces

TABLE 14-6 Drugs for Diabetes

Drug Class	Drug	Mode of Administration	Comments
Insulin	Ultra-short-acting Aspart (Novolog), glulisine (Apidra), lispro (Humalog)	Injection	Onset<15 min Peak: 0.5–1.5 hr Effective Duration: 3 hr
	Regular insulin (Regular Novolin R, Regular Humulin R)	Injection	Onset: 0.5–1 hr Peak: 2–3 hr Effective Duration: 3–6 hr
	Intermediate-acting insulin NPH (NPH Humulin N, NPH Novolin N)	Injection	Onset: 2–4 hr Peak: 7–8 hr Effective Duration: 10–12 hr
	Long-acting insulin Glargine (Lantus), detemir (Levemir)	Injection	Onset: 1–2 hr Peak: Flat Effective Duration: 24 hr
Biguanide	Metformin (Glucophage, Glucophage XR)	Oral	Maximum therapeutic effect on A_{1C} % drop: –2.0
Sulfonylureas	Glyburide (DiaBeta, Micronase)	Oral	
	Glipizide (Glucotrol)	Oral	Maximum therapeutic effect on A_{1C} % drop –2.0
	Glimepiride (Amaryl)	Oral	Maximum therapeutic effect on A_{1C} % drop –1.9
Meglitinide	Repaglinide (Prandin)	Oral	Maximum therapeutic effect on A_{1C} % drop –1.0
	Nateglinide (Starlix)	Oral	Maximum therapeutic effect on A_{1C} % drop –0.5
Thiazolidinediones (PPAR-γ agonists)	Pioglitazone (Actos)	Oral	Maximum therapeutic effect on A_{1C} % drop –1.5
	Rosiglitazone (Avandia)	Oral	Maximum therapeutic effect on A_{1C} % drop –1.4
Amylin analogs	Pramlintide (Symlin)	Injection	
Incretins	Exenatide (Byetta)	Injection	
	Sitagliptin (Januvia)	Oral	
	Saxagliptin (Onglyza)	Oral	
Alpha-glucosidase Inhibitors	Acarbose (Precose)	Oral	Maximum therapeutic effect on A_{1C} % drop –0.75
	Miglitol (Glyset)	Oral	
Combinations	Glipizide plus metformin (Metaglip)	Oral	
	Glyburide plus metformin (Glucovance)	Oral	
	Rosiglitazone plus metformin (Avandamet)	Oral	

compared with those who received placebo. These studies were so convincing regarding the use of the statins in diabetes that the American College of Physicians developed guidelines on the management of hypercholesterolemia in persons with type 2 disease.[147] The recommendations call for the use of statins for the primary prevention of macrovascular complications in all patients with cardiovascular risk factors and diabetes. The Clinical Efficacy Assessment Subcommittee of the American College of Physicians cites many studies as evidence for this recommendation, several of which have been previously reviewed in this book: the Air Force Coronary Atherosclerosis Prevention Study/Texas Coronary Atherosclerosis Prevention Study (AFCAPS/TexCAPS), the Antihypertensive and Lipid-Lowering to Prevent Heart Attack Trial–Lipid-Lowering Trial (ALLHAT-LLT), the Cholesterol and Recurrent Events (CARE) trial, the Anglo-Scandinavian Cardiac Outcome Trial—Lipid Lowering Arm (ASCOT-LLA), and the Scandinavian Simvastatin Survival Study.

In addition to lowering cholesterol, reducing hypertension in patients with diabetes is paramount. There is a significant amount of evidence that angiotensin-converting enzyme (ACE) inhibitors improve cardiovascular outcomes in these patients. The Heart Outcomes Prevention Evaluation (HOPE) trial examined the effect of ramipril on the number of cardiac events in 3577 patients with diabetes.[148] This study was stopped 6 months early (after 4 to 5 years) when the evidence was overwhelming in favor of this therapy for diabetes. Treatment with ramipril reduced the risk of cardiac death by 37%, the risk of stroke by 33%, and the risk of MI by 22%. There was also a significant reduction in nephropathy with this treatment. In another study, losartan, an ACE-receptor blocker, was credited with significantly reducing the development of end-stage renal disease in patients with diabetes.[149] This study was a double-blind, placebo-controlled trial that included 1513 patients with type 2 diabetes. All subjects received maintenance therapy consisting of conventional antihypertensive agents, with the experimental group additionally receiving losartan. It is now the assumption that ACE inhibitors and ACE-receptor blockers have the potential to interfere with the development of more extensive coronary atherosclerosis, with alterations in the fibrinolytic system that impair reperfusion after an MI, and with diabetic neuropathy with sympathetic/parasympathetic imbalance, either directly by altering the renin–angiotensin system or indirectly through their hemodynamic effect such that the beneficial effects are experienced by a greater degree in the diabetic population.[149]

EXERCISE AND DIABETES TREATMENT: THERAPEUTIC CONCERNS

Physical activity plays a crucial role in attaining health and preventing disease. However, some critical principles need to be followed before exercising in the case of patients with diabetes. During physical activity, to meet energy requirements, skeletal muscles utilize their stores of glycogen and triglycerides, as well as FFAs from adipose tissue and glucose released from the liver. Glucose levels in healthy persons remain adequate during most physical activities to meet these energy requirements and also to preserve central nervous system function. However, it is difficult for an individual with diabetes to maintain the necessary metabolic adjustments. On the one hand, when there is an insufficient amount of insulin, the excessive release of the counterinsulin hormones glucagon and catecholamines, which normally occurs with exercise, will increase the already high levels of glucose and ketone bodies and may precipitate diabetic ketoacidosis. On the other hand, when there is a high plasma insulin level because of exogenous insulin injections, mobilization of glucose and other substrates that are released with exercise will be attenuated and hypoglycemia will be induced.

Exercise acts similarly to insulin by stimulating GLUT- 4 transporters in muscle and improves the pathways for glycogen storage.[150] In addition, regular exercise is associated with overall improved insulin sensitivity. However, exercise can be dangerous in that it can induce hypoglycemia. It is especially important for the patient with type 1 diabetes to be able to adjust his or her nutrition and insulin regimen for safe participation in recreational activities or sports. In particular, self-monitored blood glucose levels and the patient's response to physical activity need to be recorded, preferably at the same time every day. Hypoglycemia may occur during, immediately after, or several hours after exercise.

Insulin is the prototypical example of a drug injected subcutaneously that is affected by "local" activity or exercise. As discussed earlier, insulin is typically injected into the subcutaneous tissues of the abdomen, upper outer arms, upper outer legs, and buttocks. The fastest absorption is from the abdomen. The slowest absorption results from the buttocks area or when the drug is injected into areas of lipohypertrophy.[151-153] Exercise increases the absorption of both subcutaneously and intramuscularly injected drugs when the site of administration is into the tissues actively engaged in an activity, while drug absorption from inactive tissues is reduced. One hour of intermittent moderate cycling has been shown to increase regular insulin absorption from the thigh but not when the insulin is injected into the arm.[154] If exercise increases absorption and can lead to hypoglycemia, then the pre-exercise insulin injection should be decreased in dose. The goal should be to end the exercise session with a plasma glucose level similar to that measured before the preceding meal. This recommendation came from a study that evaluated premeal insulin dose reductions for postprandial exercises of varying intensities to prevent exercise-induced hypoglycemia in type 1 diabetes.[155] For this study, eight male patients receiving Ultralente as the basal injection and lispro as the premeal insulin exercised at 25% maximum oxygen consumption (VO_{2max}), 50% VO_{2max}, and 75% VO_{2max} on a cycle ergometer. Each subject acted as his own control in a crossover design, and each received a premeal insulin dose based on the number of carbohydrates expected to be consumed at the meal before exercise. Subjects performed the exercises after receiving a full dose of insulin—100% lispro—after receiving 50% of the lispro dose and again 25% for either 30 or 60 minutes. Venous blood samples were retrieved at 10- to 15-minute intervals for determination of plasma glucose, insulin, and glucagon levels. Glucose monitoring continued for 18 hours after the experiment but at a reduced frequency. Subjects were also studied during a period of rest instead of exercise at each of the designated insulin doses. The results demonstrated that the full premeal insulin dose was associated with increased hypoglycemia at all the exercise intensities and even at rest in some subjects. Reductions in the premeal insulin dose resulted in far fewer episodes of hypoglycemia. A similar concern regarding the reduction of medication has also surfaced when exercise is combined with the sulfonylureas.[117] A reduction in the dose of the oral hypoglycemic agent may also be needed.

Patients can supplement their exercise sessions with glucose to prevent hypoglycemia. However, this leads to the question: How much glucose supplementation should be given to a patient on insulin to avoid this drop in glucose level during and also after exercise? A few studies have attempted to answer this question. Nine subjects with type I diabetes who were maintained on a regimen of Humulin N (intermediate-acting insulin) and Lispro (short-acting insulin) prior to breakfast, were given 0 g, 15 g, or 30 g of glucose supplementation 15 minutes before a 60-minute session of cycling performed at 50% VO_{2max}.[156] In addition, the subjects received a dextrose infusion during exercise when their blood glucose level fell below 5 mmol/L. The amount of dextrose infused was then compared with the amount of glucose supplementation received prior to the exercise. It was then determined that 40 g of a glucose supplement ingested 15 minutes prior to exercise would maintain a safe blood glucose level during the 60 minutes of exercise. It is also significant to note that the exercise was performed 180 minutes after breakfast when the insulin was at its peak effect and that the insulin was injected into the abdomen. The American Diabetes Association (ADA) has recommended ingesting 15 g of carbohydrates for each hour of exercise, which falls below what was recommended in this study. The ADA also recommended administration of 15 to 20 g of glucose to any conscious individual experiencing hypoglycemia.[151,157] In another study, eight subjects with type 1 diabetes performed exercises of various intensities (ranging from 25% VO_{2max} to 75% VO_{2max}) for 30 and 60 minutes after a premeal dose of lispro (an ultra-short-acting insulin) plus a 600-kcal, 75-g carbohydrate breakfast.[155] The premeal dose of lispro also was varied, and each subject served as his own control. Exercise at all the stated intensities and durations produced a drop in glucose level but more than two thirds of subjects receiving the full lispro dose experienced hypoglycemia, including three who required a dextrose infusion for recovery. It was also observed that even at the lowest exercise intensity of 25%VO_{2max}, there was a significant drop in glucose level. The authors concluded that a reduction in premeal insulin is necessary when planning postmeal exercise. However, the exact reduction can only be determined on an individual basis and depends on the kilocalories consumed and energy expended. As a guideline, Schiffrin and Parikh recommended a 30 to 50% reduction in premeal regular insulin prior to moderate exercise for 45 minutes.[158]

An additional variable to consider when a patient on insulin exercises is the *type of insulin* utilized. A study showed that when glargine (long-acting basal insulin) was injected into the thigh, there was no increased absorption during intense exercise (65% of VO_{2max} for 30 minutes) compared with rest.[159] However, exercise does increase absorption of both regular and ultra-short-acting insulin.[154,156] Another variable is the *type of exercise*.[160] It has been shown that the drop in blood glucose level is less when the patient is performing intermittent high-intensity exercise compared with moderate continuous exercise. In this study, moderate exercise was determined to be continuous exercise performed for 30 minutes at 40% VO_{2max}; intermittent intense exercise was the same, except for the addition of a 4-second maximal sprint every 2 minutes.

Since the high glycemic response that occurs after food intake is more important in terms of microvascular risk than premeal levels, exercise should be performed after a meal.[98] In a study in which the effects that walking before and after a meal had on blood glucose levels were compared in patients with type 1 diabetes receiving intensive insulin therapy (premeal regular insulin and NPH at bedtime), walking after a meal was found to have a better effect on glycemic control.[161] Walking before breakfast was found to produce some hyperglycemia, probably resulting from secretion of catecholamines and glucagon on top of an already high glucose level. Walking an hour after a meal did not produce hypoglycemia, either because walking is a light aerobic exercise producing smaller effects on blood sugar levels than running or because the peak effect of regular insulin had not been reached when the subjects started walking. The peak effect of regular insulin does not occur until 2 hours after injection. However, this timing of exercise should not be generalized to all types of short-acting insulins because insulin lispro peaks at 1 hour, not at 2 hours. In a study in which the glycemic response of regular insulin was compared with that of insulin lispro during exercise 1 hour after a meal, insulin concentrations were higher and peaked earlier with a significantly higher drop in glucose level with lispro.[162] Therefore when timing exercise with food intake and insulin dose, the therapist must also consider the type of short-acting insulin the patient received and should not exercise the patient vigorously during the peak insulin times.

Since there are so many variables associated with injection of insulin and exercise, it is best to have patients routinely check their plasma glucose level before, during, and after exercise, and to eat and exercise at the same time every day. A regular routine plus a consistent caloric intake will help patients avoid hypoglycemia associated with exercise and insulin.

Some general guidelines that may help improve glycemic response to exercise and avoid hypoglycemia are as follows:

1. Good glycemic control must be attained before exercise.[163] If glucose is below 100 mg/dL, the patient should eat a snack. Exercise is contraindicated if FPG levels are >300 mg/dL and should be done with caution if the levels are >250 mg/dL.
2. Plasma glucose must be monitored before and after exercise to determine when food must be consumed. Monitoring during exercise may be necessary for long periods of activity. In addition, it is important for the patient to learn how the glycemic response varies with different exercises and under different conditions.
3. Carbohydrates should be consumed as needed to avoid hypoglycemia, and these foods should be readily available after exercise as well. A snack may be required for every 30 minutes of activity.
4. Glucose levels should be continuously and frequently monitored for up to 6 to 12 hours after exercise because exercise-induced hypoglycemia may occur even hours after activity has ended.
5. The premeal insulin dose should be reduced for postprandial exercise. Because exercise acts as insulin does and can trigger hypoglycemia, patients should be counseled to lower their pre-exercise insulin dose.
6. Exercise after meals improves glycemic control.
7. Do not perform massage or exercise and do not apply a modality to a body part that has recently received an injection of insulin.[103,159] These activities will hasten absorption and may cause hypoglycemia. Wait until the duration of action for that insulin injection is over.

In general, the principles cited in the list above for handling exercise in adults with diabetes also apply to children. Children may be prone to greater variations in glycemic control not only with exercise but also with play activities.[163] In the case of adolescents, monthly hormonal changes, particularly in girls, also make control of blood glucose levels challenging.[164]

ACTIVITIES 14

1. Discuss pharmaceutical and therapy options for the following patients. Include questions you would ask regarding medical history that would help make good treatment choices.

Patient A is a 52-year-old woman who has just passed through menopause. Her bone mineral density (BMD) is currently within normal limits, but she is at high risk for developing osteoporosis.

Patient B is an 82-year-old woman who has just completed rehab after a total hip replacement following a fall. She lives in a nursing home.

Patient C is a 22-year-old competitive runner. She is 5'10" but weighs only 110 lb. She has not had a menstrual period in more than a year, and bone density testing shows that she has a T-score of –2.7 at the femoral neck.

2. Discuss the available imaging studies that can be performed to monitor BMD.

3. A teenage girl with type 1 diabetes has been having bouts of hypoglycemia during the last period of the school day. There have even been two episodes when she became unconscious but responded to glucagon. She takes regular insulin with intermediate insulin every morning and again before supper.

Questions

A. What are the possible causes of this patient's hypoglycemia?

B. The timing of the glucose testing is very important. What information regarding this patient's insulin regimen is obtained by testing at the following times?

1. Fasting plasma glucose (FPG) taken before breakfast
2. Plasma glucose samples taken before lunch
3. Plasma glucose samples taken between 8:00 and 9:00 P.M.
4. Plasma glucose samples taken during the night

C. If this patient needed physical therapy, when would you schedule it?

D. This patient had an elevated glucose level at around 11:00 A.M. Which insulin dose should be adjusted?

E. List the symptoms of hypoglycemia.

F. Discuss some guidelines for exercising for a patient with diabetes.

4. A 62-year-old woman has had type 2 diabetes for more than 5 years. She has been taking glyburide twice daily but does not have good glycemic control. Her Hb_{A1C} level is 8.8%.

She has lost approximately 15 lb during the last 5 years, but her Hb_{A1C} level continues to climb even after the glyburide has been increased to the maximum allowable daily dose. What options should be discussed with the patient?

5. Discuss some factors that lead to poor compliance with self-monitoring for plasma glucose levels. Come up with some possible solutions.
6. Many drugs, including those commonly abused, increase or decrease glucose level. Review the literature to determine the effect of alcohol, amphetamines, sympathomimetics, marijuana, and cigarettes on glucose level. In addition, list five prescription drugs that increase glucose level and five prescription drugs that may lead to hypoglycemia.
7. Interview a patient with diabetes to find out how many hypoglycemic episodes he or she experiences in a year and what precautions should be taken to avoid them.

REFERENCES

1. Bono CM, Einhorn TA: Overview of osteoporosis: Pathophysiology and determinants of bone strength. Eur Spine J 12 (suppl 2):S90-S96, 2003.
2. Raisz LG: Pathogenesis of osteoporosis: Concepts, conflicts, and prospects. J Clin Invest 115(12):3318-3325, 2005.
3. Manolagas SC: Birth and death of bone cells: Basic regulatory mechanisms and implications for the pathogenesis and treatment of osteoporosis. Endocr Rev 21(2):115-137, 2000.
4. Alliston T, Derynck R: Interfering with bone remodelling. Nature 416:686-687, 2002.
5. Takayanagi H, Kim S, Matsuo K, et al: RANKL maintains bone homeostasis through c-Fos-dependent induction of interferon-β. Nature 416:744-749, 2002.
6. Clarke BL, Khosla S: Disorders of calcium metabolism and bone mineralization. In Waldman SA, Terzic A, editors: Pharmacology and therapeutics: Principles to practice, Philadelphia, 2009, Saunders.
7. Bushinsky DA, Monk RD: Calcium. Lancet 352:305-311, 1998.
8. Taxel P, Kaneko H, Lee SK, Aguila HL, Raisz LG, Lorenzo JA: Estradiol rapidly inhibits osteoclastogenesis and RANKL expression in bone marrow cultures in postmenopausal women: A pilot study. Osteoporosis Int 19:193-199, 2008.
9. D'Ippolito G, Schiller PC, Ricordi C, Roos BA, Howard GA: Age-related osteogenic potential of mesenchymal stromal stem cells from human vertebral bone marrow. J Bone Miner Res 14(7):1115-1122, 1999.
10. Parhami F, Tintut Y, Beamer WG, Gharavi N, Goodman W, Demer LL: Atherogenic high-fat diet reduces bone mineralization in mice. J Bone Miner Res 16(1):182-188, 2001.
11. Weinstein RS, Chen JR, Powers CC, et al:, Promotion of osteoclast survival and antagonism of bisphosphonate-induced osteoclast apoptosis by glucocorticoids. J Clin Invest 109(8):1041-1048, 2002.
12. O'Brien CA, Jia D, Plotkin LI, et al: Glucocorticoids act directly on osteoblasts and osteocytes to induce their apoptosis and reduce bone formation and strength. Endocrinology 145(4):1835-1841, 2004.
13. Weinstein RS, Manolagas SC: Apoptosis and osteoporosis. Am J Med 108(2):153-164, 2000.
14. Gourlay ML, Brown SA: Clinical considerations in premenopausal osteoporosis. Arch Intern Med 164(6):603-614, 2004.
15. The International Society for Clinical Densitometry (website). http://www.iscd.org/Visitors/patient/patientinformation.cfm#bone. Accessed September 22, 2009.
16. Cummings SR, Bates DW, Black DM: Clinical use of bone densitometry. JAMA 288(15):1889-1897, 2002.
17. National Osteoporosis Foundation: What does the numbers mean? (website). http://www.nof.org/osteoporosis/bmdtest.htm. Accessed September 22, 2009.
18. Cummings SR, Black DM, Thompson DE, et al: Effect of alendronate on risk of fracture in women with low bone density but without vertebral fractures: Results from the Fracture Intervention Trial. JAMA 280(24):2077-2082, 1998.
19. WHO Fracture Risk Assessment Tool (website). http://www.shef.ac.uk/FRAX/tool.jsp?locationValue=9. Accessed September 22, 2009.
20. Lindsay R, Gallagher JC, Kleerekoper M, Pickar JH: Effect of lower doses of conjugated equine estrogens with and without medroxyprogesterone acetate on bone in early postmenopausal women. JAMA 287(20):2668-2676, 2002.
21. Villareal DT, Binder EF, Williams DB, Schechtman KB, Yarasheski KE, Kohrt WM Bone mineral density response to estrogen replacement in frail elderly women: A randomized controlled trial. JAMA 286(7):815-820, 2001.
22. Rossouw JE, Anderson GL, Prentice RL, et al: Risks and benefits of estrogen plus progestin in healthy postmenopausal women: Principal results from the Women's Health Initiative randomized controlled trial. JAMA 288(3):321-333, 2002.
23. Reid IR, Ames RW, Evans MC, Gamble GD, Sharpe SJ: Long-term effects of calcium supplementation on bone loss and fractures in postmenopausal women: A randomized controlled trial. Am J Med 98:331-335, 1995.
24. Dawson-Hughes B, Harris SS, Krall EA, Dallal GE: Effect of calcium and vitamin D supplementation on bone density in men and women 65 years of age or older. N Engl J Med 337(10):670-676, 1997.
25. Prince RL: Diet and the prevention of osteoporotic fractures. N Engl J Med 337(10):700-702, 1997.
26. Delmas PD: Treatment of postmenopausal osteoporosis. Lancet 359:2018-2026, 2002.
27. Solomon DH, Rekedal LA, Cadarette SM: Osteoporosis treatments and adverse events. Curr Opin Rheumatol 21(4):363-368, 2009.
28. Black DM, Thompson DE, Bauer DC, et al: Fracture risk reduction with alendronate in women with osteoporosis: The Fracture Intervention Trial. J Clin Endocrinol Metab 85(11):4118-4124, 2000.
29. Bone HG, Hosking D, Devogelaer JP, et al: Ten years' experience with alendronate for osteoporosis in postmenopausal women. N Engl J Med 350(12):1189-1199, 2004.
30. Black DM, Schwartz AV, Ensrud KE, et al: Effects of continuing or stopping alendronate after 5 years of treatment: The Fracture Intervention Trial Long-term Extension (FLEX): A randomized trial. JAMA 296(24):2927-2938, 2006.
31. Ste-Marie LG, Sod E, Johnson T, Chines A: Five years of treatment with risedronate and its effects on bone safety in women with postmenopausal osteoporosis. Calcif Tissue Int 75:469-476, 2004.
32. Abramowicz M: Once-a-week alendronate (Fosamax). In The Medical Letter, New Rochelle, NY, 2001, The Medical Letter, Inc.
33. Clemett D, Spencer CS: Raloxifene: A review of its use in postmenopausal osteoporosis. Drugs 60(2):380-411, 2000.
34. Delmas PD, Bjarnason NH, Mitlak BH, et al: Effects of raloxifene on bone and mineral density, serum cholesterol concentrations, and uterine endometrium in postmenopausal women. N Engl J Med 337(23):1641-1647, 1997.
35. Barrett-Connor E, Grady D, Sashegyi A, et al: Raloxifene and cardiovascular events in osteoporotic postmenopausal women. JAMA 287(7):847-857, 2002.
36. Cauley JA, Norton L, Lippman ME, et al: Continued breast cancer risk reduction in postmenopausal women treated with raloxifene: 4-year results from the MORE trial. Multiple

outcomes of raloxifene evaluation. Breast Cancer Res Treat 65(2):125-134, 2001.

37. Abramowicz M: Raloxifene for postmenopausal osteoporosis. In The Medical Letter, New Rochelle, NY, 1998, The Medical Letter, Inc.
38. Abramowicz M: Drugs for prevention and treatment of postmenopausal osteoporosis. In Treatment guidelines from the medical letter, New Rochelle, NY, 2002, The Medical Letter, Inc.
39. Cummings SR, Ettinger B, Delmas PD, et al: The effects of tibolone in older postmenopausal women. N Engl J Med 359(7):697-708, 2008.
40. Anedda FM, Velati A, Lello S, et al: Observational study on the efficacy of tibolone in counteracting early carotid atherosclerotic lesions in postmenopausal women. Horm Res 61(1):47-52, 2004.
41. Bots ML, Evans GW, Riley W, et al: The Osteoporosis Prevention and Arterial effects of tibolone (OPAL) study: Design and baseline characteristics. Control Clin Trials 24(6):752-775, 2003.
42. Mueck AO, Lippert C, Seeger H, Wallwiener D: Effects of tibolone on human breast cancer cells and human vascular coronary cells. Arch Gynecol Obstet 267(3):139-144, 2003.
43. Chesnut CH 3rd, Silverman S, Andriano K, et al: A randomized trial of nasal spray salmon calcitonin in postmenopausal women with established osteoporosis: The prevent recurrence of osteoporotic fractures study. Am J Med 109:267-276, 2000.
44. McClung MR, Lewiecki EM, Cohen SB, et al: Denosumab in postmenopausal women with low bone mineral density. N Engl J Med 354:821-831, 2006.
45. Rosen CJ, Bilezikian JP: Anabolic therapy for osteoporosis. J Clin Endocrinol Metab 86(3):957-964, 2001.
46. Holloway L, Butterfield G, Hintz RL, Gesundheit N, Marcus R: Effects of recombinant human growth hormone on metabolic indices, body composition, and bone turnover in healthy elderly women. J Clin Endocrinol Metab 79(2):470-479, 1994.
47. Whitehead HM, Boreham C, McIlrath EM, et al: Growth hormone treatment of adults with GH deficiency: Results of a 13 month placebo controlled cross-over study. Clin Endocrinol (Oxf) 36:45-52, 1992.
48. Biller BM, Sesmilo G, Baum HB, Hayden D, Schoenfeld D, Klibanski A: Withdrawal of long-term physiological growth hormone (GH) administration: Differential effects on bone density and body composition in men with adult-onset GH deficiency. J Clin Endocrinol Metab 85(3):970-976, 2000.
49. Morley P, Whitfield JF, Willilck GE: Parathyroid hormone: An anabolic treatment for osteoporosis. Curr Pharm Des 7:671-687, 2001.
50. Ghiron LJ, Thompson JL, Holloway L, et al: Effects of recombinant insulin-like growth factor-I and growth hormone on bone turnover in elderly women. J Bone Miner Res 10(12):1844-1852, 1995.
51. Baumann BD, Wronski TJ: Response of cortical bone to antiresorptive agents and PTH in aged ovariectomized rats. Bone 16(2):247-253, 1995.
52. Andreassen TT, Ejersted C, Oxlund H: Intermittent parathyroid hormone (1-34) treatment increases callus formation and mechanical strength of healing fractures. J Bone Miner Res 14(6):960-968, 1999.
53. Neer RM, Arnaud CD, Zanchetta JR, et al: Effect of parathyroid hormone (1-34) on fractures and bone mineral density in postmenopausal women with osteoporosis. N Engl J Med 344(19):1434-1441, 2001.
54. Cosman F, Nieves J, Zion M, Woelfert L, Luckey M, Lindsay R: Daily and cyclic parathryoid hormone in women receiving alendronate. N Engl J Med 353:566-575, 2005.
55. Chan KA, Andrade SE, Boles M, et al: Inhibitors of hydroxymethylglutaryl-coenzyme A reductase and risk of fracture among older women. Lancet355(9222):2185-2188, 2000.
56. Pasco JA, Kotowicz MA, Henry MJ, et al: Statin use, bone mineral density, and fracture risk. Arch Intern Med 162(5):537-540, 2002.
57. Ettinger B, Bilezikian JP: For osteoporosis, are two antiresorptive drugs better than one? J Clin Endocrinol Metab 87(3):983-984, 2002.
58. Johnell O, Scheele WH, Lu Y, Reginster JY, Need AG, Seeman E: Additive effects of raloxifene and alendronate on bone density and biochemical markers of bone remodeling in postmenopausal women with osteoporosis. J Clin Endocrinol Metab 87(3):985-992, 2002.
59. Bone HG, Greenspan SL, McKeever C, et al: Alendronate and estrogen effects in postmenopausal women with low bone density. J Clin Endocrinol Metab 85(2):720-726, 2000.
60. Black DM, Bilezikian JP, Ensrud KE, et al: One year of alendronate after one year of parathyroid hormone (1-84) for osteoporosis. N Engl J Med 353:555-565, 2005.
61. Zimmet P, Alberti KG, Shaw J: Global and societal implications of the diabetes epidemic. Nature 4141. 782-787, 2001.
62. National Center for Chronic Disease Prevention and Health Promotion: Behavioral Risk Factor Surveillance System: (website). http://apps.nccd.cdc.gov/brfss/display.asp?cat=DB&yr=2008&qkey=1363&state=US. Accessed September 24, 2009.
63. The Centers for Disease Control and Prevention Diabetes Data & Trends: (website). http://www.cdc.gov/diabetes/statistics/prev/national/figpersons.htm. Accessed September 24, 2009.
64. Zhang Y, Dall TM, Mann SE, et al: The economic costs of undiagnosed diabetes. Popul Health Manag 12(2):95-101, 2009.
65. American Diabetes Association: Diagnosis and classification of diabetes mellitus. Diabet Care 31 (suppl 1):S55-S60, 2008.
66. American Diabetes Association: Diagnosis and classification of diabetes mellitus. Diabetes Care 32(suppl 1):S62-S67, 2009.
67. Shah S, Kublaoui BM, Oden JD, White PC: Screening for type 2 diabetes in obese youth. Pediatrics 124(2):573-579, 2009.
68. Sreekumar R, Halvatsiotis P, Schimke JC, Nair KS: Gene expression profile in skeletal muscle of type 2 diabetes and the effect of insulin treatment. Diabetes 51(6):1913-1920, 2002.
69. Roglic G, Colhoun HM, Stevens LK, Lemkes HH, Manes C, Fuller JH: Parental history of hypertension and parental history of diabetes and microvascular complications in insulin-dependent diabetes mellitus: The EURODIAB IDDM Complications Study. Diabet Med 15(5):418-426, 1998.
70. Insulin resistance syndrome. Mayo Clin Women's Healthsource 6:11, 2002.
71. Sheehan JP, Diabetes Technology & therapeutics. Diabetes Technol Ther. Aug; 6(4):525-533, 2004.
72. Margolis S, Saudek CD: The Johns Hopkins White Papers on Diabetes, Baltimore, Maryland, 2002, Johns Hopkins Medical Institutions.
73. Levin SR, Coburn JW, Abraira C, et al: Effect of intensive glycemic control on microalbuminuria in type 2 diabetes. Veterans Affairs Cooperative Study on Glycemic Control and Complications in Type 2 Diabetes Feasibility Trial Investigators. Diabetes Care 23(10):1478-1485, 2000.
74. The Diabetes Control and Complications Trial (DCCT): Effect of intensive diabetes management on macrovascular events and risk factors in the diabetes control and complications trial. Am J Cardiol. 75:894-903, 1995.
75. Stratton IM, Adler AI, Neil HA, et al: Association of glycaemia with macrovascular and microvascular complications of type 2 diabetes (UKPDS 35): Prospective observational study. Br Med J 321(7258):405-412, 2000.

76. Way KJ, Katai N, King GL: Protein kinase C and the development of diabetic vascular complications. Diabet Med 18:945-959, 2001.
77. Standards of Medical Care in Diabetes. Diabetes Care 32(suppl 1):S13-S61, 2009.
78. The Expert Committee on the Diagnosis and Classification of Diabetes Mellitus: Report of the Expert Committee on the Diagnosis and Classification of Diabetes Mellitus. Diabetes Care 21(1S):5S-19S, 1998.
79. Hughes S: ADVANCE does not confirm ACCORD results: Heartwire 2008. (website). http://www.medscape.com/viewarticle/570243. Accessed 3/15/10.
80. Skyler JS, Bergenstal R, Bonow RO, et al: Intensive glycemic control and the prevention of cardiovascular events: Implications of the ACCORD, ADVANCE, and VA Diabetes trials: A position statement of the American Diabetes Association and a scientific statement of the American College of Cardiology Foundation and the American Heart Association. J Am Coll Cardiol 53(3):298-304, 2009.
81. Fineberg SE, Bergenstal RM, Bernstein RM, Laffel LM, Schwartz SL: Use of an automated device for alternative site blood glucose monitoring. Diabetes Care 24(7):1217-1220, 2001.
82. Newman SP, Cooke D, Casbard A, et al: A randomised controlled trial to compare minimally invasive glucose monitoring devices with conventional monitoring in the management of insulin-treated diabetes mellitus (MITRE), Health Technol Assess 13(28): iii-iv, ix-xi. 1-194, 2009.
83. Garg SK, Potts RO, Ackerman NR, Fermi SJ, Tamada JA, Chase HP: Correlation of fingerstick blood glucose measurements with GlucoWatch Biographer glucose results in young subjects with type 1 diabetes. Diabetes Care 22(10):1708-1714, 1999.
84. Guyton AC, Hall JE: Textbook of medical physiology (10th ed.), Philadelphia, 2000, W.B. Saunders Company.
85. Page AJ, et al: Drugs and the endocrine and metabolic systems. In Page C, Hoffman B, Curtis M, Walker M, editors: Integrated pharmacology, Philadelphia, 2006, Mosby.
86. Cooppan R, Weissman PN: Evolutions in insulin therapy: Current perspectives on treatment design, Medscape Medical News 2007. (website). http://www.medscape.com/viewprogram/7838. Accessed 3/15/10.
87. Owens DR, Zinman B, Bolli GB: Insulins today and beyond. Lancet 358:739-746, 2001.
88. Homko C, Deluzio A, Jimenez C, Kolaczynski JW, Boden G: Comparison of insulin aspart and lispro: Pharmacokinetic and metabolic effects. Diabetes Care 26(7):2027-2031, 2003.
89. Insulin aspart: A new rapid-acting insulin. Med Lett 43:1115, 2001.
90. Home PD, Barriocanal L, Lindholm A: Comparative pharmacokinetics and pharmacodynamics of the novel rapid-acting insulin analogue, insulin aspart, in healthy volunteers. Eur J Clin Pharmacol 55(3):199-203, 1999.
91. Allen J: Insulins. In Prescriber's letter, Stockton, CA, 2002, Therapeutic Research Center.
92. Rizza RA, Vella A: Diabetes mellitus. In Waldman SA, Terzic A, editors: Pharmacology and therapeutics: Principles to practice, Philadelphia, 2009, Saunders.
93. Wang F, Carabino JM, Vergara CM: Insulin glargine: A systematic review of a long-acting insulin analogue. Clin Ther 25(6):1539-1540, 2003.
94. Jones MC, Patel M: Insulin detemir: A long-acting insulin product. Am J Health Syst Pharm 63(24):2466-2472, 2006.
95. Rosenstock J, Park G, Zimmerman J: Basal insulin glargine (HOE 901) versus NPH insulin in patients with type 1 diabetes on multiple daily insulin regimens. U.S. Insulin Glargine (HOE 901) Type 1 Diabetes Investigator Group. Diabetes Care 23(8):1137-1142, 2000.
96. Insulin administration. Diabetes Care 27:S106-S107, 2001.
97. Rosenstock J: Insulin therapy: Optimizing control in type 1 and type 2 diabetes. Clin Cornerstone 4(2):50-64, 2001.
98. Home PD: Therapeutic targets in the management of type 1 diabetes. Diabetes Care 18(suppl 1):S7-S13, 2002.
99. Riddle MC: Timely initiation of basal insulin. Am J Med 116(3 suppl 1):3-9, 2004.
100. Frier BM: How hypoglycaemia can affect the life of a person with diabetes. Diabet Metab Res Rev 24:87-92, 2008.
101. McKenry LM, Salerno E: Drugs affecting the endocrine system. In Pharmacology in nursing, Philadelphia, 2003, Mosby.
102. National Diabetes Information Clearinghouse (NDIC) (website). http://diabetes.niddk.nih.gov/dm/pubs/hypoglycemia/. Accessed September 28, 2009.
103. Linde B: Dissociation of insulin absorption and blood flow during massage of a subcutaneous injection site. Diabetes Care 9(6):570-574, 1986.
104. Korytkowski M, Bell D, Jacobsen C, Suwannasari R; FlexPen Study Team: A multicenter, randomized, open-label, comparative, two-period crossover trial of preference, efficacy, and safety profiles of a prefilled, disposable pen and conventional vial/syringe for insulin injection in patients with type 1 or 2 diabetes mellitus. Clin Ther 25(11):2836-2848, 2003.
105. Cefalu WT, Skyler JS, Kourides IA, et al: Inhaled human insulin treatment in patients with type 2 diabetes mellitus. Ann Intern Med 134(3):203-207, 2001.
106. Rosenstock J, Zinman B, Murphy LJ, et al: Inhaled insulin improves glycemic control when substituted for or added to oral combination therapy in type 2 diabetes: a randomized, controlled trial. Ann Intern Med 143(18):549-558, 2005.
107. Weiss SR, Cheng SL, Kourides IA, Gelfand RA, Landschulz WH; Inhaled Insulin Phase II Study Group: Inhaled insulin provides improved glycemic control in patients with type 2 diabetes mellitus inadequately controlled with oral agents. Arch Intern Med 163(19):2277-2282, 2003.
108. Potocka E: ADA 2009. New inhaled insulin has rapid onset of action with no adverse effect on lung function, in American Diabetes Association 69th Scientific Sessions. New Orleans, Louisiana, 2009, ADA.
109. Raskin P, Bode BW, Marks JB, et al: Continuous subcutaneous insulin infusion and multiple daily injection therapy are equally effective in type 2 diabetes: A randomized, parallel-group, 24 week study. Diabetes Care 26(9):2598-2603, 2003.
110. Burdick P, Cooper S, Horner B, Cobry E, McFann K, Chase HP: Use of a subcutaneous injection port to improve glycemic control in children with type 1 diabetes. Pediatr Diabetes 10(2):116-119, 2009.
111. Bailey CJ: Biguanides and NIDDM. Diabetes Care 15(6):755-772, 1992.
112. Stumvoll M, Nurjhan N, Perriello G, Dailey G, Gerich JE: Metabolic effects of metformin in non-insulin-dependent diabetes mellitus. N Engl J Med 333(9):550-554, 1995.
113. DeFronzo RA, Goodman AM: Efficacy of metformin in patients with non-insulin-dependent diabetes mellitus. N Engl J Med 333(9):541-549, 1995.
114. Akiyoshi M, Kakei M, Nakazaki M, Tanaka H: A new hypoglycemic agent, A-4166 inhibits ATP-sensitive potassium channels in rat pancreatic beta-cells. Am J Physiol 268:E185-E193, 1995.
115. Hu S, Wang S, Fanelli B, et al: Pancreatic b-cell KATP channel activity and membrane-binding studies with nateglinide: A comparison with sulfonylureas and repaglinide. J Pharm Exp Ther 293(2):444-452, 2000.
116. Weissman PN: Reappraisal of the pharmacologic approach to treatment of type 2 diabetes mellitus. Am J Cardiol 90(5):42-50, 2002.

117. Larsen JJ, Dela F, Madsbad S, Vibe-Petersen J, Galbo H: Interaction of sulfonylureas and exercise on glucose homeostasis in type 2 diabetic patients. Diabetes Care 22(10):1647-1654, 1999.
118. Riddle MC, editorial: Sulfonylureas differ in effects on ischemic preconditioning—Is it time to retire glyburide? J Clin Endocrinol Metab 88(2):528-530, 2003.
119. Wascher TC, Boes U: Ischemia in type 2 diabetes: Tissue selectivity of sulfonylureas and clinical implications. Metabolism 52(8):3-5, 2003.
120. Glyburide/metformin (Glucovance) for type 2 diabetes. Med Lett 42:1092, 2000.
121. Repaglinide for type 2 diabetes mellitus. Med Lett 40:1027, 1998.
122. Buchanan TA, Xiang AH, Peters RK, et al: Preservation of pancreatic beta-cell function and prevention of type 2 diabetes by pharmacological treatment of insulin resistance in high risk Hispanic women. Diabetes 51:2796-2803, 2002.
123. Effect of rosiglitazone on the frequency of diabetes in patients with impaired glucose tolerance or impaired fasting glucose: A randomised controlled trial. Lancet 368(9541):1096-1105, 2006.
124. Butler AE: β-cell deficit and increased β-cell apoptosis in humans with type 2 diabetes. Diabetes 52:102-110, 2003.
125. Lebovitz HE: Rationale for and role of thiazolidinediones in type 2 diabetes mellitus. Am J Cardiol 90(5, suppl 1):34-41, 2002.
126. Eurich DT, McAlister FA, Blackburn DF, et al: Benefits and harms of antidiabetic agents in patients with diabetes and heart failure: systematic review. Br Med J 335(7618):497, 2007.
127. Lincoff AM, Wolski K, Nicholls SJ, Nissen SE: Pioglitazone and risk of cardiovascular events in patients with type 2 diabetes mellitus: a meta-analysis of randomized trials. JAMA 298(10):1180-1188, 2007.
128. Nissen SE, Wolski K: Effect of rosiglitazone on the risk of myocardial infarction and death from cardiovascular causes. N Engl J Med 356(24):2457-2471, 2007.
129. Home PD, Pocock SJ, Beck-Nielsen H, et al: Rosiglitazone evaluated for cardiovascular outcomes—an interim analysis. N Engl J Med 357(1):28-38, 2007.
130. Nainggolan L, Rosiglitzaone meta-analysis continues to drive controversy in second week. 2007. (website). www.theheart.org. Accessed May 31, 2007.
131. Gale EA: Lessons from the glitazones: A story of drug development. Lancet 357:1870-1875, 2001.
132. Monami M, Cresci B, Colombini A, et al: Bone fractures and hypoglycemic treatment in type 2 diabetic patients. Diabetes Care 31(2):199-203, 2008.
133. Gautier JF, Fetita S, Sobngwi E, Salaün-Martin C: Biological actions of the incretins GIP and GLP-1 and therapeutic perspectives in patients with type 2 diabetes. Diabetes Metab 31:233-242, 2005.
134. Mudaliar S, Henry RR: Incretin therapies: Effects beyond glycemic control, Eur J Intern Med 122:S25-S36, 2009.
135. Farilla L, Bulotta A, Hirshberg B, et al: Glucagon-like peptide 1 inhibits cell apoptosis and improves glucose responsiveness of freshly isolated human islets. Endocrinology 144(12):5149-5158, 2003.
136. Triplitt C, Chiquette E: Exenatide: From the Gila monster to the pharmacy. J Am Pharm Assoc 46(1):44-55, 2006.
137. Kruger D: Exenatide: A novel therapy for the treatment of type 2 diabetes. Medscape Diabetes Endocrinol 7(2), 2005.
138. Viswanathan P, Chaudhuri A, Bhatia R, Al-Atrash F, Mohanty P, Dandona P: Exenatide therapy in obese patients with type 2 diabetes mellitus treated with insulin. Endocr Pract 13(5):444-450, 2007.
139. FDA approves new drug treatment for type 2 diabetes. 2009. (website). http://www.fda.gov/NewsEvents/Newsroom/PressAnnouncements/ucm174780.htm. Accessed September 28, 2009.
140. Kruger D, Gloster MA: Pramlintide for the treatment of insulin-requiring diabetes mellitus. Drugs 64(13):1419-1432, 2004.
141. Fonseca V, Rosenstock J, Patwardhan R, Salzman A: Effect of metformin and rosiglitazone combination therapy in patients with type 2 diabetes mellitus: A randomized controlled trial. JAMA 283:1695-1702, 2000.
142. Kipnes MS, Krosnick A, Rendell MS, Egan JW, Mathisen AL, Schneider RL: Pioglitazone hydrochloride in combination with sulfonylurea therapy improves glycemic control in patients with type 2 diabetes mellitus: A randomized, placebo-controlled study. Am J Med 111(1):10-17, 2001.
143. Yale JF, Valiquett TR, Ghazzi MN, Owens-Grillo JK, Whitcomb RW, Foyt HL: The effect of a thiazolidinedione drug, troglitazone, on glycemia in patients with type 2 diabetes mellitus poorly controlled with sulfonylurea and metformin: A multicenter, randomized, double-blind, placebo-controlled trial. Ann Intern Med 134(9):737-745, 2001.
144. Estacio RO, Jeffers BW, Gifford N, Schrier RW: Effect of blood pressure control on diabetic microvascular complications in patients with hypertension and type 2 diabetes. Diabetes Care 23(suppl 2):B54-B64, 2000.
145. Pyörälä K, Pedersen TR, Kjekshus J, Faergeman O, Olsson AG, Thorgeirsson G: Cholesterol lowering with simvastatin improves prognosis of diabetic patients with coronary heart disease: A subgroup analysis of the Scandinavian Simvastatin Survival Study (4S). Diabetes Care 20(4):614-620, 1997.
146. Goldberg RB, Mellies MJ, Sacks FM, et al: Cardiovascular events and their reduction with pravastatin in diabetic and glucose-intolerant myocardial infarction survivors with average cholesterol levels: Subgroup analyses in the Cholesterol and Recurrent Events (CARE) trial. Circulation 98(23):2513-2519, 1998.
147. Snow V, Aronson MD, Hornbake ER, Mottur-Pilson C, Weiss KB; Clinical Efficacy Assessment Subcommittee of the American College of Physicians: Lipid control in the management of type 2 diabetes mellitus: A clinical practice guideline from the American College of Physicians. Ann Intern Med 140(8):644-649, 2004.
148. Heart Outcomes Prevention Evaluation (HOPE) Study Investigators Effects of ramipril on cardiovascular and microvascular outcomes in people with diabetes mellitus: Results of the HOPE study and MICRO-HOPE substudy. Lancet 355:253-259, 2000.
149. Brenner BM, Cooper ME, de Zeeuw D, et al: Effects of losartan on renal and cardiovascular outcomes in patients with type 2 diabetes and neuropathy. N Engl J Med 345(12):861-869, 2001.
150. Rice B, Janssen I, Hudson R, Ross R: Effects of aerobic or resistance exercise and/or diet on glucose tolerance and plasma insulin levels in obese men. Diabetes Care, 22(5):684-691, 1999.
151. Association AD: Insulin administration. Diabetes Care 27(suppl 1):S106-S107, 2004.
152. Neufer PD, Dohm GL: Exercise induces a transient increase in transcription of the GLUT-4 gene in skeletal muscle. Am J Physiol 265(6 Pt 1):C1597-C1603, 1993.
153. Hällsten K, Yki-Järvinen H, Peltoniemi P: Insulin- and exercise-stimulated skeletal muscle blood flow and glucose uptake in obese men. Obes Res 11(2):257-265, 2003.
154. Koivisto VA, Felig P: Effects of leg exercise on insulin absorption in diabetic patients. N Engl J Med 298(2):79-83, 1978.

155. Rabasa-Lhoret R, Bourque J, Ducros F, Chiasson JL: Guidelines for premeal insulin dose reduction for postprandial exercise of different intensities and durations in type 1 diabetic subjects treated intensively with a basal bolus insulin regimen (ultralente-lispro). Diabetes Care 24(4):625-630, 2001.
156. Dubé MC, Weisnagel SJ, Prud'homme D, Lavoie C: Is early and late post-meal exercise so different in type 1 diabetic lispro users? Diabetes Res Clin Pract 72(2):128-134, 2006.
157. American Diabetes Association updates: Guidelines for medical nutrition therapy. Diabetes Care 31(suppl 1):S61-S78, 2008.
158. Schiffrin A, Parikh S: Accommodating planned exercise in type I diabetic patients on intensive treatment, Diabetes Care. 8(4):337-342, 1985.
159. Peter R, Luzio SD, Dunseath G:, Effects of exercise on the absorption of insulin glargine in patients with type 1 diabetes. Diabetes Care 28(3):560-565, 2005.
160. Guelfi KJ, Jones TW, Folurnier PA: New insights into managing the risk of hypoglycaemia associated with intermittent high-intensity exercise in individuals with type 1 diabetes mellitus. Sports Med 37(11):937-946, 2007.
161. Yamanouchi K, Abe R, Takeda A, Atsumi Y, Shichiri M, Sato Y: The effect of walking before and after breakfast on blood glucose levels in patients with type 1 diabetes treated with intensive insulin therapy. Diabetes Res Clin Pract 58(1): 11-18, 2002.
162. Yamakita T, Ishii T, Yamagami K, et al: Glycemic response during exercise after administration of insulin lispro compared with that after administration of regular human insulin. Diabetes Res Clin Pract 57(1):17-22, 2002.
163. American Diabetes Association: Physical activity/exercise and diabetes. Diabetes Care 27(suppl 1):S58-S62, 2004.
164. DeWitt DE, Dugdale DC: Using new insulin strategies in the outpatient treatment of diabetes. JAMA 289(17):2265-2269, 2003.

SECTION V

Neurologic Pharmacology

15

Drugs for Epilepsy and Attention-Deficit/Hyperactivity Disorder

Barbara Gladson

OVERVIEW OF EPILEPSY

Epilepsy is a disorder characterized by seizures, which may appear in various forms, depending on the locations affected in the brain.[1] A seizure is the outward expression of a sudden excessive electrical discharge of neurons, with firing rates between 200 and 900 Hz, many times the activity of normal neurons. A seizure may appear as a brief lapse in attention or as a convulsive episode lasting for several minutes. Seizures involving the motor cortex produce convulsions, those involving the hypothalamus produce autonomic changes, and those involving the reticular formation in the brainstem produce a loss of consciousness.

Seizures may occur as a result of fever, alcohol withdrawal, head trauma, stroke, a brain tumor, central nervous system (CNS) infections, or epilepsy.[1] Epilepsy, however, is the only disorder characterized by recurrent spontaneous seizures. In more than 50% of cases of epilepsy, the cause is unknown, and this is called *primary* or *idiopathic epilepsy*. Epilepsy related to a particular event is called *secondary epilepsy*. The principal causes of secondary epilepsy in children are injury at birth and metabolic disease. Traumatic brain injury is the primary cause in adults.

Diagnosis of epilepsy requires careful clinical observation of the seizure in progress, an adequate patient history, and an electroencephalogram (EEG), which detects excessive electrical discharges in the brain (Figure 15-1).[1] A computed tomography (CT) or magnetic resonance imaging (MRI) scan may also assist in the diagnosis, particularly if a structural lesion is present.

Types of Epilepsy

Epileptic seizures are divided into two main classes: partial seizures and generalized seizures (Box 15-1).[2] They are further divided into simple seizures, if consciousness remains intact, or complex seizures, if consciousness is lost.

Partial seizures originate in a localized area of one cerebral hemisphere. The discharge begins locally and ends locally. The simple partial seizure has a primary sensory component (odor or taste), or some autonomic discharge, without loss of consciousness. However, there may be some focal motor symptoms, depending on the anatomic region affected. In the complex partial seizure, loss of consciousness may occur. If the anatomic insult is in the motor cortex, it is called *Jacksonian epilepsy*. This consists of repetitive jerking movements of a specific muscle group, which can, on occasion, spread to involve much of the body. The psychomotor seizure often has its foci in the temporal lobe and may show stereotypical purposive movements or automatisms (e.g., chewing movements, hand rubbing, patting movements, or hair combing). This type of seizure may last for a few minutes, and the patient has no memory of it when he or she recovers.

In *generalized seizures*, the neuronal discharge involves both cerebral hemispheres. Immediate loss of consciousness occurs as a result of involvement of the reticular formation. There are six types of generalized seizures:

1. The most common type is the *tonic–clonic seizure*. This seizure begins with a sudden rigid extensor spasm, causing the patient to fall to the ground, with rigidity lasting for 10 to 30 seconds. Respiration ceases; and defecation, micturition, or salivation may occur. This is followed by the clonic phase in which there is a rhythmic flexor spasm lasting 2 to 4 minutes. The spasm gradually lessens, but the patient may remain unconscious for a few more minutes. Alertness occurs slowly, with the patient feeling ill and confused at first.
2. *Tonic seizures* consist of tonic contractions of certain muscle groups and altered consciousness, but no progression to the clonic phase.
3. *Clonic seizures* are characterized by repetitive clonic jerks without a tonic component. Both types of seizures last only seconds.

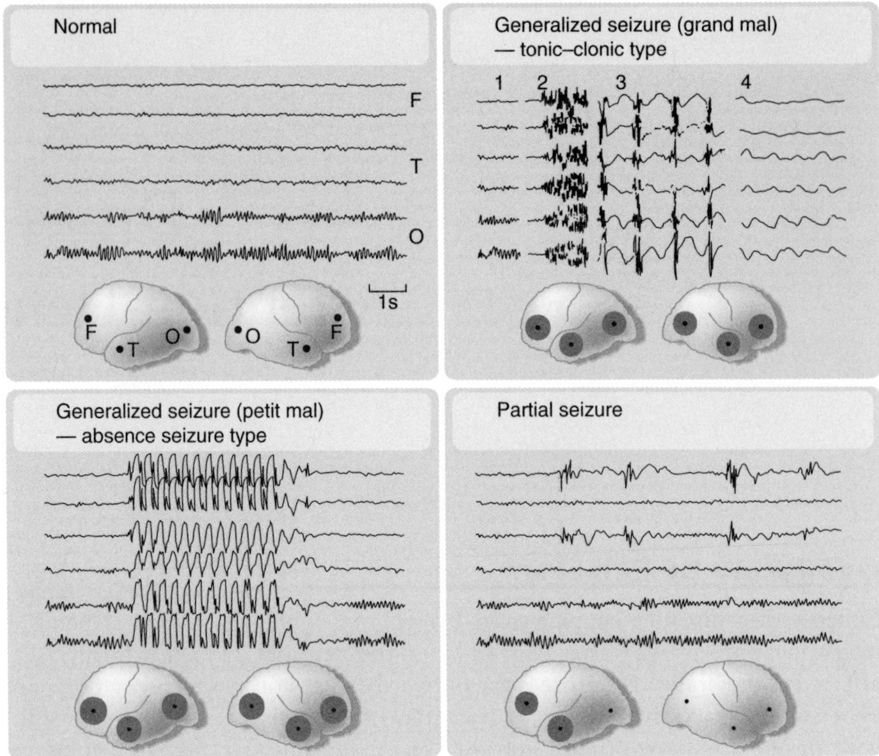

FIGURE 15-1 Electroencephalograph (EEG) records in epilepsy. **A**, Normal EEG recorded from frontal (F), temporal (T), and occipital (O) sites on both sides, as shown in the inset diagram. The α-rhythm (10/s) can be seen in the occipital region. **B**, Sections of EEG recorded during a generalized tonic–clonic (grand mal) seizure. 1, Normal record; 2, onset of tonic phase; 3, clonic phase; 4, postconvulsive coma. **C**, Generalized absence seizure (petit mal) showing sudden brief episode of 3/s "spike and wave" discharge. **D**, Partial seizure with synchronous abnormal discharges in left frontal and temporal regions. *(From Eliasson SG, Hardin WB, Prensky AL:* Neurological pathophysiology *(2nd ed.). New York, 1978, Oxford University Press; Rang HP, Dale DC, Ritter JM, Moore JL: Antiepileptic drugs. In Rang HP, Dale DC, Ritter JM, Moore JL, editors:* Pharmacology, *New York, 2003, Churchill Livingstone.)*

BOX 15-1 International Classification of Seizures

Partial Seizures

Description

Short alterations in consciousness, repetitive unusual movements (chewing or swallowing movements), psychological changes, and confusion.

Simple seizures

- No impaired consciousness
- Motor symptoms (most commonly face, arm, or leg)
- Hallucinations of sight, hearing, or taste, along with somatosensory changes (tingling)
- Autonomic nervous system responses
- Personality changes

Complex seizures

- Impaired consciousness
- Memory impairment
- Behavioral effects
- Purposeless behaviors
- Aura, chewing and swallowing movements, unreal feelings, bizarre behavior
- Tonic, clonic, or tonic–clonic seizures

Generalized Seizures

Description

Most often seen in children and commonly characterized by temporary lapses in consciousness lasting a few seconds. Staring off into space, daydreaming, and inattentive look are common symptoms. Patients may exhibit rhythmic movements of their eyes, head, or hands but do not convulse. May have several attacks per day.

- Both cerebral hemispheres involved
- Tonic, clonic, myotonic, atonic, or tonic–clonic seizures and infantile spasms possible
- Brief loss of consciousness for a few seconds with no confusion
- Head-drop or falling-down symptoms

From Lilley LL, Harrington D, Snyder JS: Antiepileptic agents. In *Pharmacology and the nursing process*, (4th ed.). St. Louis, 2005, Mosby.

4. *Absence seizures* occur most often in children. They are less dramatic in presentation but may occur more frequently than tonic–clonic seizures. An absence seizure consists of an abrupt, brief loss of consciousness with amnesia. The patient suddenly stops whatever he or she is doing, even ceasing to finish a sentence, and stares blankly for a few seconds. Some mild clonic movements, such as eye blinking and slight changes in postural tone, may occur. The patient recovers quickly with no ill feeling.
5. *Atonic seizures*, also known as *drop attacks*, are characterized by a sudden reduction in muscle tone of selective muscle groups, leading to head dropping or dropping of a limb. Duration is 10 to 30 seconds.
6. *Myoclonic seizures* are characterized by a single contraction or multiple sudden, brief, contractions confined to the face, trunk, or extremities, again lasting only seconds (Box 15-2).

Neural Mechanisms and Models of Epilepsy

The underlying neuronal mechanism of epilepsy is not well understood. It is thought that excitation of neurons will spread unless normally prevented from doing so by inhibitory devices. Thus a seizure can occur if excitation is increased or inhibition is reduced. Glutamate, an excitatory amino acid that activates N-methyl-D-aspartate receptors, is believed to be increased in areas where seizures originate.

Animal models are available, but none match the human form of epilepsy exactly.[1] There are mice that convulse briefly in response to certain sounds, baboons that show seizures in response to certain visual stimuli, and a group of beagles with an inherited disorder that resembles the human form of epilepsy. In addition, chemical and electrical means can be used to produce a seizure in an animal. Local application of penicillin crystals in the brain may result in a partial seizure, and the convulsant drug pentylenetetrazol can produce a generalized seizure. It has been found that drugs that inhibit these convulsions are effective against absence seizures and that drugs that inhibit electrically induced seizures are helpful for tonic–clonic seizures. There is also a kindling model that may evoke seizures that more closely resemble the human versions more than the drug or chemical model.[3] Low-intensity electrical stimulation is applied to the amygdala with implanted electrodes. Normally, this would not evoke a seizure, except that when the stimulation is repeated daily for several days, seizures may begin to occur spontaneously. The seizures are blocked by glutamate antagonists.

ANTIEPILEPTIC DRUGS

The main mechanisms of action of the current antiepileptic drugs (AEDs) are the augmentation of gamma (γ)-aminobutyric acid (GABA) activity and the blockade of sodium (Na^+) or calcium (Ca^{2+}) channels.[1] Similar to drugs for cardiac arrhythmias, the purpose of AEDs is to prevent abnormal and excessive discharge without inhibiting normal transmission.

Many of the AEDs have multiple effects on neuronal activity; however, some predominant effects for each drug can be delineated.[4] Many drugs control seizures by acting on voltage-gated sodium channels and are particularly effective for treating tonic–clonic seizures and complex partial seizures. Other drugs act on voltage-gated calcium channels in the thalamus and are effective for treating absence seizures. Additionally, the benzodiazepines and barbiturates act at the GABA-gated chloride channel to provide some inhibition of the spreading excitation. Some newer drugs target glutamate receptors directly.

AEDs may produce changes in the brain that provide neuroprotection from seizure damage in addition to action on specific ion channels and neurotransmitters.[5] It has been believed for years that seizure activity can facilitate additional seizures by producing abnormal structural and neurochemical processes. It is also known that status epilepticus can result in hippocampal and cerebral damage, although it is not certain that tonic–clonic and complex partial seizures cause brain damage. Animal models are currently being used to determine

BOX 15-2 Factors Associated with Seizure Activity

Preseizure (Possible Provoking Stimuli)	Activity During Seizure	Postseizure Events
Emotional stress	Aura	Confusion
Sleep deprivation	Rhythmic behavior of face or extremities	Fatigue in a partial seizure
Flashing lights	Tonic movements or posturing observed	Focal weakness or diminished sensation as stiffening
Recent illness	Clonic movements	Headache
Drugs	Incontinence	Physical injury
Alcohol withdrawal	Tongue biting	
Fever	Rhythmic flexion and extension of limbs	Hypoglycemia

Adapted from Brodie MJ, Kwan P: Staged approach to epilepsy management, *Neurology* 58(suppl 5):S2–S8, 2002.

whether the drugs are anti-epileptogenic, neuroprotective, or both.

Relatively few drugs are available for the treatment or control of seizures compared with drugs for treatment of conditions such as hypertension and angina. In fact, before 1990, only six major AEDs were available to treat all forms of epilepsy.[6] These older AEDs include carbamazepine, phenobarbital, phenytoin, primidone, valproic acid, and ethosuximide. Although they are helpful for some, many patients have seizures that are refractory to treatment or require combination therapies for effectiveness. The other problem with these drugs is that several are hepatic enzyme inducers, resulting in numerous drug–drug interactions, such as those with warfarin, oral contraceptives, calcium channel antagonists, and some chemotherapeutic agents; these drugs also affect how sex steroids and vitamin D are metabolized.[7]

The problems in pharmacokinetics and effectiveness with the older AEDs have led investigators to the discovery of at least seven new AEDs within the past 10 years. However, the majority of the new AEDs are approved only for adjunctive treatment.[8] This is because the studies evaluated by the U.S. Food and Drug Administration (FDA) were conducted with patients who had refractory seizures and continued to receive their original antiseizure medication but were given either placebo or the study drug as an adjunct. These studies, for the most part, are flawed because they were conducted with patients whose seizures were refractory to their original medicines and thus would be presumed to be more difficult to treat. Additionally, these patients do not represent patients with a new diagnosis of epilepsy seeking first-time help from a neurologist. Nevertheless, many clinical investigators are using the new AEDs off label as monotherapy.

Phenytoin

Phenytoin is one of the primary drugs for controlling all seizures except absence seizures. It alters conductance at potassium (K^+) and calcium (Ca^{2+}) channels, but its primary action is blocking of the Na^+ current. It is also used in the treatment of trigeminal neuralgia and related neuralgias.

Adverse effects from phenytoin include rashes, hirsutism, hepatitis, gingival hyperplasia, and a coarsening of facial features. The hirsutism and changes in facial features may be due to elevated androgen levels produced by the drug. The gingival hyperplasia occurs only in portions of the gum that have teeth. Good oral hygiene may help to minimize this effect and periodontal disease as well. Endocrine effects such as hyperglycemia and osteomalacia may also occur. The hyperglycemia is due to inhibition of insulin secretion, and the osteomalacia is due to inhibition of Ca^{2+} absorption through the intestines and accelerated hydroxylation of vitamin D to its inactive forms.[9] Arrhythmias and hypotension, which are adverse effects related to the drug's action on Na^+ channels in the heart, can also occur. Phenytoin also has an excitatory effect on the cerebellar–vestibular system, resulting in nystagmus, ataxia, and dizziness. These effects plus additional CNS effects—including blurred vision, hyperactivity, silliness, confusion, sedation, and coma—are dose related. Long-term use may produce megaloblastic anemia and hypoprothrombinemia and hemorrhage caused by vitamin K deficiency. Many of the drug–drug interactions are connected to phenytoin's metabolism. The enzymes that metabolize this drug become saturated at levels close to the usual effective dose. So any increase in dose will remain active in blood, leading to an excessively high level. On the other end of the spectrum, some drugs decrease phenytoin's effects by inducing hepatic microsomal enzymes, producing a decrease in antiseizure activity. Excessive or long-term consumption of alcohol can significantly reduce phenytoin's effectiveness. Phenytoin itself is an enzyme inducer. Other drugs increase phenytoin's effect by displacing the drug from its protein-binding sites. Because of all these potential problems, there is a move away from this drug, which has been the mainstay of treatment for seizure disorders for years.

Barbiturates (Phenobarbital, Primidone)

Barbiturates inhibit seizure activity by increasing the threshold for neuronal firing. They also enhance inhibition by activating the GABA receptors.[10] Primidone is a prodrug that is metabolized in the liver to phenobarbital and phenylethylmalonamide, both of which have antiseizure properties. These drugs provide effective treatment for tonic–clonic and partial seizures, but their long list of adverse effects prevents them from being chosen as first-line agents.

The majority of adverse effects are related to CNS depression. These drugs usually produce drowsiness, depression, inattention, confusion, and ataxia; but in some cases, they cause excitation. They may also cause skin rashes and hematologic effects such as megaloblastic anemia and osteomalacia, similar to the adverse effects of phenytoin. They should not be taken during pregnancy because they can produce congenital malformations and coagulation problems in the newborn. Also, lower intelligence scores have been noted in children whose mothers took phenobarbital during pregnancy. Phenobarbital is a P450 enzyme inducer, so not only does some tolerance for this drug develop, but it is also affected by other enzyme-inducing drugs. This drug is as effective as phenytoin for the treatment of generalized tonic–clonic seizures but less effective for partial seizures. It continues to be used as a third-line agent. The only advantage to using this drug is that it has the longest half-life of all the older AEDs, allowing for once-a-day dosing.

Carbamazepine

Carbamazepine has a structure similar to that of the tricyclic antidepressants, although pharmacologically it resembles phenytoin by blocking voltage-gated Na^+ channels.[1] But it does not induce the same cosmetic adverse effects produced by phenytoin. This drug is highly effective in the treatment of all partial seizures, including complex partial seizures and tonic–clonic seizures, and it is currently the second most commonly prescribed AED after phenytoin.

Drowsiness, fatigue, vertigo, ataxia, diplopia, hyperirritability, and respiratory depression are related to its depressive effects on the CNS. Gastrointestinal (GI) reactions include nausea, vomiting, and dry mouth. Dry mouth is related to the anticholinergic effects of carbamazepine. More severe reactions involve the skin, cardiovascular, and hematologic systems. Skin reactions include rashes, urticaria, photosensitivity, and altered skin pigmentation. Congestive heart failure, syncope, hypertension, and hypotension are some of the cardiovascular reactions, which may be related to the excessive secretion of antidiuretic hormone with concomitant hyponatremia. Hematologic reactions include aplastic anemia, agranulocytosis, and thrombocytopenia. Lastly, this drug is an enzyme inducer, so when it is taken with other drugs, it may make them less effective.

Valproic Acid (Sodium Valproate)

Valproate is one of the first "broad-spectrum antiseizure drugs being effective against tonic–clonic, absence, atonic, and myoclonic events." It is the drug of choice for absence seizures and is also used for migraine prophylaxis. Valproic acid stimulates glutamic acid decarboxylase, which is needed to synthesize GABA from glutamate, resulting in an increase in the concentration of GABA in the synapses.[11] In addition, it prevents reuptake of GABA and limits sodium entry into rapidly firing neurons. Valproate is the drug of choice for absence seizures.

The CNS depressive effects of valproic acid are less severe than those of the other antiseizure agents. However, adverse effects still include drowsiness, sedation, headache, dizziness, ataxia, confusion, and some visual disturbances. Valproic acid also produces thinning of the hair in about 10% of patients.[1] Hematologic reactions occur as a result of inhibition of platelet aggregation and lead to bleeding, and there are also some reports of liver damage. GI disturbances are common but may be minimized when the drug is taken with food.

Ethosuximide

Ethosuximide works by increasing the seizure threshold by blocking the T-type calcium currents in the thalamus. This type of current controls the depolarization threshold and may be intimately involved in the generation of absence seizures; however, more studies are needed.[12] Ethosuximide is well tolerated, having few adverse effects, with the exception of headache, fatigue, and some GI problems. Agranulocytosis has been reported.

Lamotrigine

The exact mechanism of action of lamotrigine is unknown, but it is believed to block Na^+ channels, reduce Ca^{2+} influx, and inhibit the release of excitatory amino acids, glutamate, and aspartate.[13] It is approved as adjunctive therapy, usually with carbamazepine or phenytoin, for the treatment of partial seizures. Although it has been approved for monotherapy in the United Kingdom because some studies have shown similar efficacy and better tolerability compared with carbamazepine, it is mostly used as an add-on drug for generalized seizures, with significant efficacy in the treatment of absence seizures. This drug is also being studied for use in the treatment of depression and bipolar disorder. Lamotrigine does not induce or inhibit the P450 enzymes, so it can be used safely with a variety of drugs. Adverse drug reactions include dizziness, diplopia, ataxia, headache, and rashes.

Gabapentin

Gabapentin acts on a unique receptor that has not yet been identified.[14] It is structurally related to GABA but has no affinity for the GABA, glutamate, N-methyl-D-aspartate, kainate, glycine, cholinergic, dopamine (D_1 or D_2), 5-hydroxytryptamine (5-HT), opiate, voltage-gated Ca^{2+}, or Na^+ channel receptors. For several years, researchers were not sure how this drug achieved its action. Just recently, it was discovered to bind to the $\alpha 2\delta$ subunit of the presynaptic voltage-dependent Ca^{2+} channel on neurons. This results in a reduction of neurotransmitters, including glutamate, acetylcholine, and noradrenaline. In addition, it produces a reduction in substance P release, which is probably why it is effective in the treatment of neuropathic pain.[15] Gabapentin is used as an adjunct in the treatment of partial and tonic–clonic seizures and is also used to reduce pain in neuropathic pain syndromes.[16]

Adverse effects of gabapentin are relatively minor and include sedation and ataxia. Patients also might experience dizziness and nystagmus. Because this drug does not undergo metabolism, it does not interfere with the breakdown of any other antiseizure medications.

Pregabalin is very similar to gabapentin but has improved bioavailability.[10] It requires twice-a-day dosing, which is an improvement on the three-times-per-day dosing for gabapentin.

Levetiracetam

Levetiracetam belongs to a new class of antiseizure medications recently approved by the FDA.[17] Originally it was found to be ineffective based on a standard animal screening model. However, it was later found to be effective in the treatment of focal seizures. It works by blocking N-type Ca^{2+} channels in the hippocampus.[10]

This drug is extremely well tolerated but has adverse effects resulting from CNS depression, similar to those of other antiseizure medications (i.e., dizziness, headache, and fatigue). Studies show a higher rate of rhinitis during treatment with this drug compared with placebo in clinical trials, but it is not known whether this adverse effect is related to the drug. Levetiracetam is not metabolized by cytochrome P450 enzymes, and therefore fewer drug–drug interactions may be expected.

Oxcarbazepine

Oxcarbazepine is a new drug on the U.S. market that became available in 1999.[17] It is structurally related to carbamazepine with similar action. Oxcarbazepine is a prodrug that is converted into the primary active metabolite monohydroxy derivative, which is not metabolized by the P450 enzymes as is carbamazepine, so there is less potential for drug interactions. It is approved for monotherapy and adjunctive use in the treatment of partial seizures in adults and for adjunctive therapy in children. This drug produces adverse effects similar to those of carbamazepine, but they are less frequent and milder. Hepatic and hematologic problems have not been reported, but dizziness and sedation are present.

Other Antiepileptic Drugs

Topiramate, tiagabine, and zonisamide were approved for use in the United States in the late 1990s and early 2000s.[1] Topiramate appears to be the "jack-of-all-trades" of antiseizure medications. It blocks Na^+ channels, enhances the action of GABA, and inhibits glutamate activity. Tiagabine is an analog of GABA that can advance through the blood–brain barrier. It also functions to inhibit the reuptake of GABA. Last, zonisamide is a new drug to the United States but has been approved in Japan since 1989. It binds to voltage-dependent Na^+ channels inducing inactivity and then delays the channel's return to the open state.[10] It also may block T-type Ca^{2+} channels.

GENERAL APPROACH TO THE MANAGEMENT OF EPILEPSY

Patients with epilepsy start with one drug and then increase the dose gradually until they are either free of seizures or the adverse effects become intolerable.[4] If the first drug fails to control the seizures or the patient cannot tolerate the adverse effects, either another drug is tried or the dose of the first is lowered and a second drug is added. The choice of drug depends on the seizure type, age of the patient, psychiatric history, other disease states, and concomitant use of other medication (Table 15-1). Most patients with a partial-onset seizure disorder are initially given drugs that block voltage-dependent Na^+ channels, such as phenytoin, carbamazepine, and oxcarbazepine.[18] Second-line choices and add-ons include gabapentin, lamotrigine, levetiracetam, valproic acid, and the other newer agents. However, ethosuximide is not effective in treating focal epilepsy. Drugs commonly used for generalized seizures include lamotrigine and valproic acid, with lamotrigine being favored because of its fewer adverse effects, and ethosuximide or valproate for absence seizures (Figures 15-2 and 15-3).

The appropriate drug may also be chosen on the basis of the "differences" matched to the patient.[10] If the patient has a comorbid condition such as a migraine, the choice may be topiramate. If the patient is obese, topiramate may be chosen, since it produces less weight gain. If rapid onset of action is necessary, then the choice might be zonisamide or valproate, and lastly, if cost is an issue, then the choice would be an older agent such as phenytoin, carbamazepine, or phenobarbital.

TABLE 15-1 Efficacy of Selected Antiepileptic Drugs for Different Seizures

Drug	Partial	Tonic–Clonic	Absence	Myoclonic	Atonic
Phenobarbital	+	+	0	?	?
Phenytoin	+	+	–	–	0
Carbamazepine	+	+	–	–	0
Valproate	+	+	+	+	+
Ethosuximide	0	0	+	0	0
Gabapentin	+	+	–	–	0
Lamotrigine	+	+	+	+	+
Topiramate	+	+	?	+	+

+, Efficacy; 0, ineffective; –, negative effect (enhances seizure activity); ?, unknown efficacy.
Adapted from Brodie MJ, Kwan P: Staged approach to epilepsy management, *Neurology* 58(suppl 5):S2–S8, 2002.

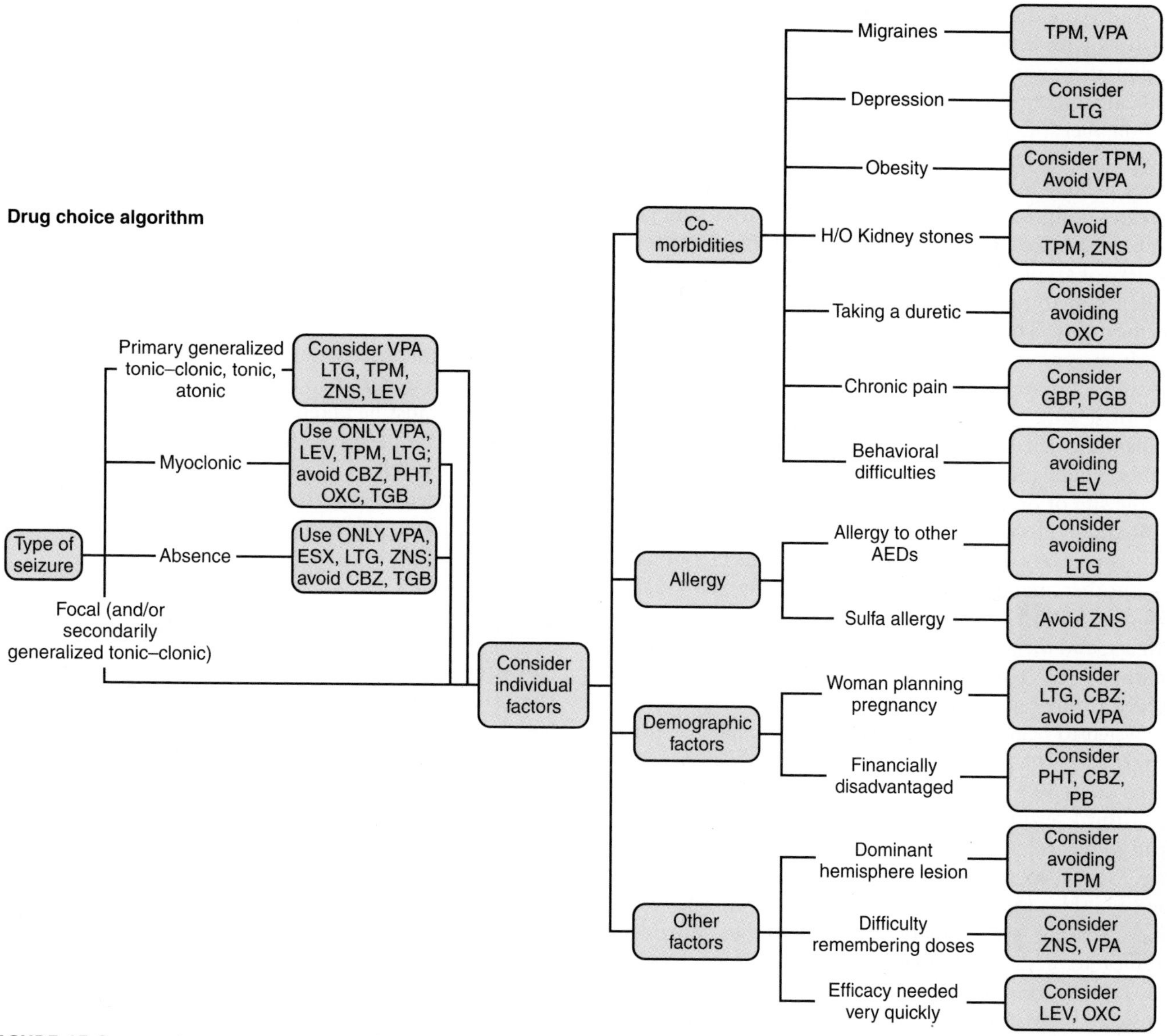

Drug choice algorithm
Type of seizure
Primary generalized tonic–clonic, tonic, atonic
Consider VPA LTG, TPM, ZNS, LEV
Myoclonic
Use ONLY VPA, LEV, TPM, LTG; avoid CBZ, PHT, OXC, TGB
Absence
Use ONLY VPA, ESX, LTG, ZNS; avoid CBZ, TGB
Focal (and/or secondarily generalized tonic–clonic)
Consider individual factors
Co-morbidities
Migraines
TPM, VPA
Depression
Consider LTG
Obesity
Consider TPM, Avoid VPA
H/O Kidney stones
Avoid TPM, ZNS
Taking a duretic
Consider avoiding OXC
Chronic pain
Consider GBP, PGB
Behavioral difficulties
Consider avoiding LEV
Allergy
Allergy to other AEDs
Consider avoiding LTG
Sulfa allergy
Avoid ZNS
Demographic factors
Woman planning pregnancy
Consider LTG, CBZ; avoid VPA
Financially disadvantaged
Consider PHT, CBZ, PB
Other factors
Dominant hemisphere lesion
Consider avoiding TPM
Difficulty remembering doses
Consider ZNS, VPA
Efficacy needed very quickly
Consider LEV, OXC

FIGURE 15-2 Drug choice algorithm. *LTG*, lamotrigine; *TPM*, topiramate; *ZNS*, zonisamide; *LEV*, levetiracetam; *VPA*, valproate; *OXC*, oxcarbazepine; *TGB*, tiagabine; *ESX*, ethosuximide; *CBZ*, carbamazepine; *GBP*, gabapentin; *PGB*, pregabalin. *(Redrawn from Mintzer S: Seizure disorders. In Waldman SA, Terzic A, editors:* Pharmacology and therapeutics: Principles to practice, *Philadelphia, 2009, Saunders.)*

Epilepsy treatment algorithm
Continue Rx for ≥ 2 yrs
Continued seizure freedom
Consider withdrawal of Rx (depending on many factors)
Seizure-free without side effects
Recurrent seizures
Seizure-free without side effects
Choose appropriate drug (see Fig. 45-3)
Titrate to low-moderate dose
Assess response to treatment
Continued seizures at low-moderate dose
Assess compliance (history, serum levels)
Compliant with Rx
Increase from low-moderate dose to moderate-high dose
Side effects at low-moderate dose
Continued seizures or side effects
Patient has failed 1 or 2 drugs
Alternative treatment needed
Patient has failed 2-3 drugs
Refer to epilepsy center to verify diagnosis, consider other treatment options

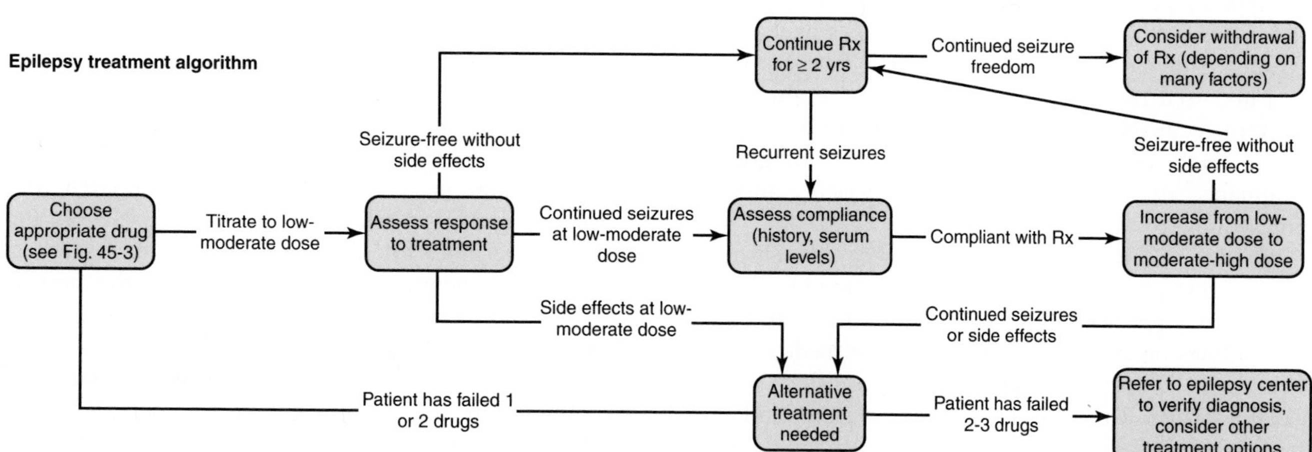

FIGURE 15-3 *(Redrawn from Mintzer S: Seizure disorders. In Waldman SA, Terzic A, editors:* Pharmacology and therapeutics: Principles to practice, *Philadelphia, 2009, Saunders.)*

Approximately 60 to 70% of patients become free of seizures with a first- or second-choice antiseizure medication as monotherapy.[4] The remainder of patients have difficult-to-control seizures but may respond to combination therapy, particularly when drugs with different mechanisms of action are used. Some effective combinations include valproate with ethosuximide for absence seizures, valproate with lamotrigine for partial and generalized seizures, and lamotrigine with topiramate for a variety of atypical seizures. However, some patients have epilepsy that remains refractory to their combination medications. These patients may be candidates for epilepsy surgery or a vagus nerve stimulator. In addition, because current technology can be used to identify the site of seizure onset in some patients and can detect an impending seizure, it may be possible in the future to deliver small amounts of antiseizure medications directly to the site of origin to avert an episode.

Regular blood level monitoring of the AEDs is not only necessary for minimizing toxic effects but also as another management tool. Monitoring the plasma concentration is necessary for maximizing therapeutic effects, and the plasma concentration is important information to have before a second or even a third drug is added to the regimen.

When to begin treatment with AEDs remains controversial.[19,20] The seizure recurrence rate has been reported to be 20 to 80%. After two tonic–clonic seizures, the risk of a third seizure may be as high as 85%. Factors that lead to recurrence are a family history of seizures, neurologic deficit, cognitive dysfunction, and abnormal findings on EEG. Head trauma accounts for 5% of epilepsy cases and 20% of symptomatic cases. This has provoked studies to determine whether the prophylactic use of AEDs after trauma can reduce the occurrence of epilepsy.[21] Using animals, investigators were able to determine that administering valproic acid 20 to 30 minutes after head trauma on a one-time basis reduced the incidence of post-traumatic epilepsy. Early administration of the drug was critical to its success.

Certain types of seizures are also more likely to recur. An unprovoked, single, prolonged seizure is likely to be repeated and require medication, but a febrile seizure does not need treatment. Partial seizures are also more likely to recur. Noncompliance with the drug program after a single seizure is high, but patients show greater compliance after the second seizure experience and are more willing to take medication.

When to withdraw medication is also a difficult decision.[22] Most physicians prefer a seizure-free interval of 2 to 5 years, absence of abnormalities on EEG, and normal findings on a neurologic exam before medication is withdrawn. Withdrawal must be accomplished slowly because sudden withdrawal may result in status epilepticus. Most recurrences, however, develop within the first 6 months after withdrawal and many are observed within the first year. Childhood-onset epilepsy has a better prognosis than adult-onset epilepsy. Reasons to withdraw medications include a desired pregnancy (because many of the drugs are teratogenic) or intolerable adverse effects such as sedation in school-age children or adolescents. Seizure control with medication is desired in cases where the patient cannot risk seizure activity, for example, a person who needs to drive to work or operate dangerous equipment. Drug withdrawal is performed slowly over a period of 3 to 6 months to avoid recurrence, but epilepsy of long duration (more than 6 years) before control may warrant continuation of therapy.

Poor compliance with the drug regimen is a problem that leads to recurrence of seizure activity.[23] Many of these drugs must be taken multiple times per day. This is disruptive to a person's lifestyle, particularly for a child who must be removed from the classroom for dosing. New extended-release formulations are available for carbamazepine, phenytoin, and valproic acid and are expected to improve compliance.

Treatment of Status Epilepticus

Status epilepticus is defined as a function of time. The clinical presentation is 30 minutes of continuous seizure activity or two or more seizures within this time frame without regaining of full consciousness.[24] Lorazepam and diazepam are the first-line treatments for status epilepticus and are given along with a loading dose of phenytoin.[6] Both are given intravenously. Fosphenytoin is a prodrug of phenytoin and is a good alternative. It is water soluble, making infusion easier and faster. If the seizure is refractory to these drugs, intravenous midazolam or propofol may be added. Supportive care is also given in the form of maintaining an airway, providing ventilation, and ensuring that the patient is safe.

Is There a Superior Antiepileptic Agent?

Neurologists and patients were pleased when the newer AED agents were released on the market. They were expected to be superior to the traditional drugs in efficacy and adverse effect profile, especially for patients who continued to experience breakthrough seizures. However, there has been a lack of clinical trials comparing new agents with older ones. Gabapentin, lamotrigine, and oxcarbazepine have each been compared with carbamazepine as monotherapy for partial seizures and found to be more tolerable but no more or less effective.[25,26] The newer agents do not affect the hepatic enzymes and therefore produce fewer drug–drug interactions and adverse effects than do the older agents. Of the newer agents, only felbamate, which is used infrequently for only the most refractory seizure disorders, is associated with serious organ toxicity. However, in terms of efficacy, there seems to be little difference between the newer and older drugs (Table 15-2).

TABLE 15-2 Antiseizure Drugs

Drug	Main Site of Action	Main Use	Predominant ADR
Phenytoin (Dilantin)	Na^+ channel	All types of seizures, except absence seizures	Gum hypertrophy, hirsutism, megaloblastic anemia, sedation, ataxia, vertigo
Carbamazepine (Tegretol)	Na^+ channel	All types of seizures, except absence seizures	Sedation, ataxia, liver failure, water retention
Valproate (Depakene)	Na^+ channel; Inhibits GABA reuptake	Absence seizures	Nausea, weight gain, hair loss, less sedating
Ethosuximde (Zarontin)	Ca^{2+} channel	Absence seizures	Nausea, less sedating
Phenobarbital (Luminal)	Na^+ channel	All types of seizures, except absence seizures	Sedation, ataxia, depression
Lamotrigine (Lamictal)	Na^+ channel	All seizure types	Dizziness, sedation, skin rashes
Gabapentin (Neurontin)	$\alpha 2\delta$ subunit of the presynaptic voltage-dependent Ca^{2+} channel	Partial seizures	Sedation
Tiagabine (Gabitril)	Inhibits GABA reuptake	Partial seizures	Sedation
Topiramate (Topamax)	Na^+ channel	All types of seizures, except absence seizures	Sedation
Levetiracetam (Keppra)	Blocks N-type Ca^{2+} channels in the hippocampus	Partial seizures	Less sedating
Zonisamide (Zonegran)	Na^+ channel	Partial seizures	Less sedating, weight loss

ADR, adverse drug reaction; Na^+, sodium; GABA, gamma aminobutyric acid; Ca^{2+}, calcium.

Therapeutic Concerns

The major adverse effects that will affect rehabilitative treatment and attainment of goals include sedation, dizziness, and ataxia. Some of these drugs also produce a moderate amount of cognitive slowing, particularly topiramate.[27] Patients may develop some tolerance for the sedating qualities, but if seizures are difficult to control and a patient is receiving a high dose of medication, this tolerance may not be recognized. Another adverse effect that needs to be recognized is the presence of skin rashes. In most cases, the drug will be withdrawn, but if the patient is allowed to continue using the medication, skin care is important. It has to be realized that physical therapy modalities and massage may exacerbate the condition. Because bone marrow depression and vitamin K deficiency, which lead to depression of clotting factors, may occur with some antiseizure agents, the presence of bruising or bleeding must be reported. Infection control measures and careful handling procedures must be instituted.

There are special concerns for women taking AEDs. Negative interactions between the drugs and the endocrine system may affect ovarian function, produce polycystic ovary disease (PCOD), increase weight, and reduce fertility.[28] If a woman taking these drugs becomes pregnant, there is a 4 to 6% greater risk of the infant having a neural tube defect.[29] In addition, the effect of these drugs on bone health is a real concern, particularly in postmenopausal women.

Therapists should also be able to recognize seizures and maintain a record of the number and quality of events witnessed during a therapy session.[19] In most therapy centers, an incident report may need to be completed, especially if a fall was involved.

ATTENTION-DEFICIT/HYPERACTIVITY DISORDER

Attention-deficit/hyperactivity disorder (ADHD) is present in 6 to 9% of children, with 60 to 80% continuing to have this disorder into adulthood.[30] ADHD commonly occurs with a variety of behavioral disorders, including conduct disorder, oppositional defiant disorder, depression, anxiety, and many developmental disorders. There are three subtypes of ADHD: (1) the inattentive type, (2) the hyperactive-impulsive type, and (3) the combined type. The American Academy of Pediatrics uses criteria from the *The Diagnostic and Statistical Manual of Mental Disorders,* Fourth Edition, Text Revision (DSM-IV-TR) diagnostic criteria for ADHD in childhood. For a positive diagnosis, symptoms must be present before the age of 7 and observed in many environments such as home and school. See Box 15-3 for the diagnostic criteria.

The etiology of ADHD is most likely a combination of environmental, genetic, and biologic factors.[31] Prenatal and perinatal exposure to cigarettes or alcohol increases the risk of ADHD two to three times. Having a parent with ADHD increases the risk eight times. In a study of dizygotic and monozygotic twins, genetics accounted for a 75% contribution.[32]

BOX 15-3 Diagnostic Criteria for ADHD

Criterion	Clinical Presentation
Inattention	Often makes careless mistakes in schoolwork or other activities
	Often cannot focus attention on tasks
	Often does not seem to listen when addressed directly
	Often has difficulty with organization
	Often avoids activities that take mental effort for a sustained period
	Often loses things
	Is easily distracted
	Is forgetful
Hyperactivity	Often fidgets with hands, cannot sit still
	Often leaves the seat in a classroom
	Often has difficulty playing or engaging in leisure activities quietly
	Often talks constantly
Impulsivity	Often blurts out answers before questions have been completed
	Often has difficulty awaiting turn
	Often interrupts

The presences of six symptoms causing functional impairment in at least two settings over 6 months confirms a diagnosis.
Adapted from Dopheide JA, Pliszka SR: Attention-deficit-hyperactivity disorder: An update, *Pharmacotherapy* 29(6):656–679, 2009.

There appears to be a plethora of information regarding the behavioral aspects of ADHD but little information on the neurochemical or anatomic anomalies associated with this disorder. Brain imaging and EEG studies have not shown clear differences between control subjects and children with ADHD, nor is there a particular defect solely associated with this disorder.[33] Structural MRI studies have shown that children with ADHD have a reduced brain volume, especially in the corpus callosum, caudate, and cerebellar areas.[34] Despite aggressive treatment, there is no reversal of this abnormality. However, there are some neurochemical explanations for this disorder. Dopamine dysfunction in the prefrontal cortex, particularly decreased activity of dihydroxyphenylalanine (DOPA) decarboxylase, has been seen in adults with ADHD.[35] However, researchers are not sure whether this dysfunction is responsible for the ADHD or represents a secondary change caused by the ADHD experienced in childhood. An extension of this dopamine dysfunction theory includes mention of a defect in glutamate-stimulated release of dopamine in the nucleus accumbens that results in dopamine hypofunction.[36] Other investigators are looking for a candidate gene, possibly one involved in the expression of the dopamine (D_4) receptor to describe the neurobiology of the subtype of ADHD that continues into adulthood.[37] Increased expression of dopamine transporters has been observed in adults with ADHD.[38] It has also been determined that dopamine, epinephrine, and norepinephrine all have activity at the D_4 receptor sites, which helps explain the usefulness of some drugs in treating this disorder. Specifically, it has been found that therapeutic doses of methylphenidate (a commonly used medication for ADHD) blocks more than half the dopamine transporters, thus increasing extracellular dopamine levels.[39] A further complication to our understanding of ADHD is related to the theory that the motor (hyperactivity) and cognitive (inattention) predominance of symptoms may represent two separate dysfunctions related to insults in different parts of the brain.[40] Specifically, the hyperactivity may result from dysfunction at the subcortical sites in which insufficient dopamine produces a "reverse parkinsonism" or excessive motor output through loss of inhibition. The lack of attention and diminished memory might relate to lesions in the prefrontal cortex. This is further supported clinically by the divergence of dose–response curves for motor and cognitive effects produced by the stimulant agents. The theories are complicated by the fact that little reference has been made to the role of presynaptic autoreceptors and how increased dopaminergic activity affects them. Clearly, understanding of this disorder is in its infant stage.

Drug Treatment for ADHD

Medications are the foundation of treatment for children and adults with ADHD, in addition to support groups, specialized educational planning, and focused therapies.[37] Stimulants, antidepressants, and antihypertensive medications are among the most commonly used agents for this disorder, and the stimulants in particular are considered to be first-line agents.

Stimulant Therapy (Methylphenidate, Amphetamine). CNS stimulants are used to reduce the hyperactivity, impulsivity, and inattentiveness that characterize ADHD behavior (Table 15-3). At first, the use of these agents for hyperactivity seems counterintuitive. These drugs are sympathomimetic, producing increased mental alertness and wakefulness and decreased fatigue. However, they also produce nervousness and heightened motor activity, symptoms that are already seen in the ADHD population. As mentioned previously, explanations are uncertain, but what is clear is that stimulants significantly improve behavior as judged by both parents and teachers.[40] In addition, they reduce restless behavior and improve memory, although to a greater extent in subjects who do not have comorbid symptoms such as anxiety.[41,42]

Both D-amphetamine and methylphenidate bind to the dopamine and norepinephrine transporters, blocking the reuptake of dopamine. In addition D-amphetamine facilitates the release of dopamine.[40] These drugs are used to treat ADHD in both children and adults.[43] However, outcomes are variable, and approximately 30% of patients do not respond to medication or cannot tolerate the adverse effects. Children with tic symptoms may experience a worsening of this condition.[44]

TABLE 15-3 Stimulant Medications for ADHD

Duration	Form of Administration	Methylphenidates	Amphetamine
Short-acting Administered twice daily or three times daily	Tablet	Ritalin Methylin Focalin	Adderall Dexedrine Dextrostat Desoxyn
	Chewable tablet	Methylin	None
	Liquid	Ritalin Methylin	Dextrostat
Intermediate acting Administered once every morning or twice daily	Tablet	Ritalin SR Methylin ER Metadate ER	None
Long-acting Administered once every morning	Tablet Capsule that may be crushed and sprinkled on food Skin patch	Concerta Metadate CD Ritalin LA Focalin XR Daytrana	Dexedrine Spansule Adderall XR Vyvanse None

Adapted from Rader R, McCauley L: Current strategies in the diagnosis and treatment of childhood attention-deficit/hyperactivity disorder, *Am Fam Physicians* 79(8):657–665, 2009.

There have been increasing concerns over possible long-term consequences of stimulant use. The first is that use of stimulant medication in early childhood will lead to the development of substance abuse later in life.[45] However, a meta-analysis of six studies that included 674 patients receiving medication and 360 control subjects indicated that the children who were treated for ADHD with stimulants had a reduction in substance abuse. Another concern is the possibility of growth retardation with stimulant therapy.[44] Unfortunately, the studies that address this issue have some intrinsic flaws, and the question remains unanswered. Some retrospective studies have shown a height reduction of 3 to 4 cm after 3 years of treatment when patients were matched with untreated siblings. However, a prospective study performed with female subjects demonstrated that methylphenidate had no effect on height. In none of these studies was final adult height examined.

Methylphenidate and D-amphetamine are both short-acting compounds with onset of action in about 30 to 60 minutes. Peak effect occurs in 1 to 2 hours and lasts for 2 to 5 hours. Newer intermediate and extended-release preparations of both drugs prolong the duration of action to between 8 and 12 hours.[46,47] Short-acting drugs may be used to help the child with certain specific activities but long-acting formulations eliminate the need for dosing during the school hours and cover late afternoon homework time. In addition, they improve compliance and eliminate some of the moodiness and headaches associated with peaks in plasma level reported by patients taking drugs with short durations of action. Treatment begins at a low dose and then is titrated up over 2 to 4 weeks until an adequate response is achieved.

Short-term adverse effects include reduced appetite, insomnia, nervousness, and GI dysfunction. In adults, hypertension is a problem, and D-amphetamine and methylphenidate should not be prescribed to an individual with borderline or above-normal blood pressure. The stimulants are associated with increased aggression and may precipitate tics or psychotic symptoms. Some cardiac fatalities have been documented, so patients with congenital cardiac conditions should be carefully monitored.[48]

The effects of the stimulant drugs used for ADHD resemble the actions of cocaine, and therefore these drugs present a risk of abuse when they are taken in an unauthorized manner.[49,50] They are listed as schedule II controlled substances. Because many children and adults take stimulant drugs for ADHD, these drugs are widely available and can be obtained easily, although illegally. Some reports in the literature have documented the abuse of methylphenidate. When methylphenidate is used for recreational purposes, the tablets are often crushed, and the powder is then sniffed. In other cases, the powder has been mixed with liquid and administered intravenously. Under these conditions, the drug creates euphoria and therefore a very high abuse potential.

Atomoxetine. Atomoxetine is a nonstimulant drug approved for use in children 6 years of age and older, as well as in adults. It is a very selective presynaptic norepinephrine reuptake inhibitor and thus has little influence over other neurotransmitters, which limits its adverse effects. It is the first nonstimulant drug to be approved by the FDA for ADHD. Several small trials have shown that atomoxetine is superior to placebo and equal to methylphenidate in efficacy.[51-53] Adverse effects of atomoxetine include insomnia and hypertension in adults and abdominal pain, decreased appetite, dizziness, and vomiting in children. Some growth disturbances may also be associated with this drug because mean height and weight have been seen to have declined in children treated with this drug for more than 18 months. Also, some suicidal ideation has occurred with this drug. As for most new drugs, further study is warranted.

Antidepressants for the Treatment of ADHD. Tricyclic antidepressants have been shown to be effective in treating ADHD but not superior to stimulants. Their mechanism of action in ADHD relates to their action of catecholamine reuptake. The advantages to the tricyclic antidepressants include reducing comorbid mood disorders, a longer half-life, and a low abuse potential. In addition, they do not exacerbate tic disorders. The disadvantages of tricyclic antidepressants are their anticholinergic and cardiac adverse effects. Other antidepressants under study for ADHD include venlafaxine and bupropion (see Chapter 18).[44,54] Both appear to be effective in patients with comorbid mood disorders. Bupropion which inhibits the reuptake of dopamine, serontonin, and norepinephrine has also been used off label in the treatment of ADHD (Box 15-4).

α_2-Noradrenergic Agonists (Clonidine, Guanfacine). α_2-Agonists have been used for years in the treatment of ADHD. Clonidine has been used as monotherapy or in conjunction with methylphenidate in children with both ADHD and tic disorder.[44] These drugs maybe useful when ADHD is combined with conduct disorder. In addition, α-agonists help lessen insomnia, since they have a sedative effect.

Therapeutic Concerns with Drugs for ADHD

When patients with ADHD are receiving rehabilitative therapy, it is particularly important for therapists to assess behavior and attention span. This assessment is important not only because the patient must be cooperative and follow instructions for therapy to be successful but also because therapists must determine whether the patient is taking the medication properly. Because methylphenidate is a CNS stimulant and has recently become an abused drug, some patients may decide to sell their drugs rather than take them. If this becomes a concern, the therapist can discuss this with the prescribing physician by framing the conversation in terms of the patient's inattentive or impulsive behavior.

BOX 15-4 Nonstimulant Treatment for ADHD

Second-line agents	Atomoxetine (Strattera)
Third-line agents	Bupropion (Wellbutrin)
	Imipramine (Tofranil)
	Desipramine (Norpramin)
	Clonidine (Catapres)
	Guanfacine (Tenex)

Other assessments that should be performed include measurement of resting and exercise blood pressures and heart rate. Vital signs may be elevated, especially in adults, as a result of stimulant therapy. In addition, questioning the patient about angina is important. Angina may occur if the patient combines the stimulants with caffeine or other sympathomimetic agents and exercise. Other adverse effects to look for are loss of appetite and insomnia. Therapists are uniquely qualified to offer suggestions for combating insomnia. Biofeedback and relaxation exercises as well as proper positioning for sleep can be helpful.

Therapists should consult with the patient's physician and teacher about providing the same structure during therapy sessions as that provided in the school setting. Therapy can complement the educational goals outlined for the classroom, and therapists can follow through with the same reward system to foster successful behavior.

ACTIVITIES 15

1. You are treating a 16-year-old boy for chondromalacia patella. He is performing a sitting knee extension exercise when he begins to have a tonic–clonic seizure. Describe what you are witnessing. Construct a seizure diary for the patient and family to assist them in recording seizure episodes.
2. Interview a pediatric therapist who has worked with children with epilepsy. Discuss what impact seizure medication has had on a particular patient he or she has treated.
3. You are treating a patient who is taking methylphenidate. In addition to your rehabilitation assessments, what other items should be evaluated?

REFERENCES

1. Lilley LL, Harrington D, Snyder JS: Antiepileptic agents. In Lilley LL, Harrington D, Snyder JS, editors: Pharmacology and the nursing process, St. Louis, 2007, Mosby.
2. Rang HP, et al: Antiepileptic Drugs, in Rang HP, Dale MM, Ritter JM, Flower R, editors: Pharmacology, New York, 2007, Churchill Livingstone.
3. Post RM: Neurobiology of seizures and behavioral abnormalities. Epilepsia 45(suppl 2):5-14, 2004.
4. Brodie MJ, Kwan P: Staged approach to epilepsy management. Neurology 58(suppl 5):S2-S8, 2002.
5. Duncan JS: The promise of new antiepileptic drugs. Br J Clin Pharmacol 53(2):123-131, 2002.
6. French JA, Kanner AM, Bautista J, et al: Efficacy and tolerability of the new antiepileptic drugs, I: Treatment of new-onset epilepsy: Report of the TTA and QSS subcommittees of the American Academy of Neurology and the American Epilepsy Society. Epilepsia 45(5):401-409, 2004.
7. Patsalos PN, Fröscher W, Pisani F, van Rijn CM: The importance of drug interactions in epilepsy therapy. Epilepsia 43(4):365-385, 2002.
8. LaRoche SM, Helmers SL: The new antiepileptic drugs. JAMA 291(5):605-614, 2004.

9. Ali II, Schuh L, Barkley GL, Gates JR: Antiepileptic drugs and reduced bone mineral density. Epilepsy Behav 5:296-300, 2004.
10. Mintzer S: Seizure disorders. In Waldman SA, Terzic A, editors: Pharmacology and therapeutics: Principles to practice, Philadelphia, 2009, Saunders.
11. Johannessen CU, Johannessen SI: Valproate: Past, present, and future. CNS Drug Rev 9(2):199-216, 2003.
12. Posner EB, Mohamed K, Marson AG: Ethosuximide, sodium valproate or lamotrigine for absence seizures in children and adolescents. Cochrane Database Syst Rev 3(CD003032), 2003.
13. Hurley SC: Lamotrigine update and its use in mood disorders. Ann Pharmacother 36(5):860-873, 2002.
14. McLean MJ, Gidal BE: Gabapentin dosing in the treatment of epilepsy. Clin Ther 25(5):1382-1406, 2003.
15. Taylor CP, Angelotti T, Fauman E: Pharmacology and mechanism of action of pregabalin: The calcium channel alpha$_2$-delta subunit as a target for antiepileptic drug discovery. Epilepsy Res 73:137-150, 2007.
16. Pappagallo M: Newer antiepileptic drugs: Possible uses in the treatment of neuropathic pain and migraine. Clin Ther 25(10):2506-2538, 2003.
17. McAuley JW, Biederman TS, Smith JC, Moore JL: Newer therapies in the drug treatment of epilepsy. Ann Pharmacother 36:119-129, 2002.
18. Beydoun A, Passaro EA: Appropriate use of medications for seizures. Postgrad Med 111(1):69-82, 2002.
19. Prego-Lopez M, Devinsky O: Evaluation of a first seizure. Postgrad Med 111(1):34-48, 2002.
20. Sirven JL: Antiepileptic drug therapy for adults: When to initiate and how to choose. Mayo Clin Proc 77(12):1367-1375, 2002.
21. Benardo LS: Prevention of epilepsy after head trauma: Do we need new drugs or a new approach? Epilepsia 44(suppl 10):27-33, 2003.
22. Specchio LM, Beghi E: Should antiepileptic drugs be withdrawn in seizure-free patients? CNS Drugs 18(4):201-212, 2004.
23. Pellock JM, Smith MC, Cloyd JC, Uthman B, Wilder BJ: Extended-release formulations: Simplifying strategies in the management of antiepileptic drug therapy. Epilepsy Behav 5:301-307, 2004.
24. Manno EM: New management strategies in the treatment of status epilepticus. Mayo Clin Proc 78(4):508-518, 2003.
25. Brodie MJ, Richen A, Yuen AWC: Double-blind comparison of lamotrigine and carbamazepine in newly diagnosed epilepsy. Lancet 345:476-479, 1995.
26. Dam M, Ekberg R, Løyning Y, Waltimo O, Jakobsen K: A double-blind study comparing oxcarbazepine and carbamazepine in patients with newly diagnosed, previously untreated epilepsy. Epilepsy Res 3(1):70-76, 1989.
27. Loring DW, Meador KJ: Cognitive side effects of antiepileptic drugs in children. Neurology 62:872-877, 2004.
28. Tatum WO 4th, Liporace J, Benbadis SR, Kaplan PW: Updates on the treatment of epilepsy in women. Arch Intern Med 164:137-145, 2004.
29. Yerby MS: Management issues for women with epilepsy: Neural tube defects and folic acid supplementation. Neurology 61(6 suppl 2):S23–S26, 2003.
30. Dopheide JA, Pliszka SR: Attention-deficit-hyperactivity disorder: An update. Pharmacotherapy 29(6):656-679, 2009.
31. Spencer TJ, Biederman J, Wilens TE, Faraone SV: Overview and neurobiology of attention-deficit/hyperactivity disorder. J Clin Psychiatry 63(suppl 12):3-9, 2002.
32. Farone SV, Perlis RH, Doyle AE: Molecular genetics of attention deficit/hyperactivity disorder. Biol Psychiatry 57:1313-1323, 2005.
33. American Academy of Pediatrics: Clinical Practice Guideline: Diagnosis and evaluation of the child with attention-deficit/hyperactivity disorder. Pediatrics 105:1158-1170, 2000.
34. Zametkin A, Liotta W: The neurobiology of attention-deficit/hyperactivity disorder. J Clin Psychiatry 59:17-23, 1998.
35. Ernst M, Zametkin AJ, Matochik JA, Jons PH, Cohen RM: DOPA decarboxylase activity in attention deficit hyperactivity disorder adults. A [fluorine-18] fluorodopa positron emission tomographic study. J Neurosci 18(15):5901-5907, 1998.
36. Russell VA: Dopamine hypofunction possibly results from a defect in glutamate-stimulated release of dopamine in the nucleus accumbens shell of a rat model for attention deficit hyperactivity disorder—the spontaneously hypertensive rat. Neurosci Biobehav Rev (27):671-682, 2003.
37. Wilens TE, Biederman J, Spencer TJ: Attention deficit/hyperactivity disorder across the lifespan. Ann Rev Med 53:113-131, 2002.
38. Madras BK, Miller GM, Fischman AJ: The dopamine transporter: Relevance to attention deficit hyperactivity disorder (ADHD). Behav Brain Res 130:57-63, 2002.
39. Sergeant JA, Geurts H, Huijbregts S, Scheres A, Oosterlaan J: The top and the bottom of ADHD: A neuropsychological perspective. Neurosci Biobehav Rev 27:583-592, 2003.
40. Solanto MV: Dopamine dysfunction in AD/HD: Integrating clinical and basic neuroscience research. Behav Brain Res 130:65-71, 2002.
41. Tannock R, Ickowicz A, Schachar R: Differential effects of methylphenidate on working memory in ADHD children with and without comorbid anxiety. J Am Acad Child Adolesc Psychiatry 34(7):886-896, 1995.
42. Waxmonsky J: Assessment and treatment of attention deficit hyperactivity disorder in children with comorbid psychiatric illness. Curr Opin Pediatr 15(5):476-482, 2003.
43. Lutton ME, Leach L, Triezenberg D: Does stimulant therapy help adult ADHD. J Fam Pract 52(11):888-889, 2003.
44. Daley KC: Update on attention-deficit/hyperactivity disorder. Curr Opin Pediatr 16(2):217-226, 2004.
45. Wilens TE, Faraone SV, Biederman J, Gunawardene S: Does stimulant therapy of attention-deficit/hyperactivity disorder beget later substance abuse? A meta-analytic review of the literature. Pediatrics 111(1):179-185, 2003.
46. McCracken JT, Biederman J, Greenhill LL, et al: Analog classroom assessment of a once-daily mixed amphetamine formulation, SLI381 (Adderall XR), in children with ADHD. J Am Acad Child Adolesc Psychiatry 42(6):673-683, 2003.
47. Dexmethylphenidate (Focalin) for ADHD. In Abramowicz M, editor: The Medical Letter, New Rochelle, NY, 2002, The Medical Letter, Inc.
48. Wilens TE, Prince JB, Spencer TJ, Biederman J: Stimulants and sudden death: What is a physician to do? Pediatrics 118:1215-1219, 2006.
49. Swanson JM, Volkow ND: Serum and brain concentrations of methylphenidate: Implications for use and abuse. Neurosci Biobehav Rev 27:615-621, 2003.
50. Volkow ND, Fowler JS, Wang GJ, Ding YS, Gatley SJ: Role of dopamine in the therapeutic and reinforcing effects of methylphenidate in humans: Results from imaging studies. Eur Neuropsychopharmacol 12:557-566, 2002.
51. Atomoxetine (Strattera) for ADHD. In Abramowicz M, editor: The Medical Letter, New Rochelle, NY, 2003, The Medical Letter, Inc.
52. Kratochvil CJ, Heiligenstein JH, Dittmann R, et al: Atomoxetine and methylphenidate treatment in children with ADHD: A prospective, randomized, open-label trial. J Am Acad Child Adolesc Psychiatry 41(7):776-784, 2002.
53. Eiland L, Guest AL: Atomoxetine treatment of attention-deficit/hyperactivity disorder. Ann Pharmacother 38:86-90, 2004.
54. Hornig-Rohan M, Amsterdam JD: Venlafaxine versus stimulant therapy in patients with dual diagnosis ADD and depression. Prog Neuropsychopharmacol Biol Psychiatry 26:585-589, 2002.

16

Antispasticity Medications and Skeletal Muscle Relaxants

Sue Ann Sisto

Several pharmacologic agents are available for patients with spasticity who have upper motor neuron syndrome and also for those who have muscle spasms. This chapter first reviews the neurophysiology of muscle tone and spasms; this is followed by a description of agents commonly used to treat spasticity. Because spasticity is present in any upper motor neuron disease, such as stroke, spinal cord injury (SCI), or cerebral palsy (CP), this section does not focus on one diagnostic group selectively.

PHYSIOLOGY OF SPASTICITY AND MUSCLE SPASMS

A widely accepted definition of spasticity is that it is a velocity-dependent increased resistance to passive stretch.[1] Although the pathophysiology of spasticity is poorly understood, the final common pathway is overactivity of the alpha motor neuron.[2] This is unlike dystonia, which is not dependent on sensory input but, rather, on supraspinal output or efferents not involved in the reflex arc.[3] In 2001, the National Institutes of Health (NIH) defined spasticity, through an interdisciplinary workshop, as hypertonia with resistance to externally imposed movement that increases with increasing speed and varies with the direction of joint movement and/or is above a threshold speed or joint angle. Spasticity results from a lesion along the path of the corticospinal tracts. These pyramidal tracts include the motor pathways of the cortex, basal ganglia, thalamus, cerebellum, brainstem, central white matter, and spinal cord.[4] The term *parapyramidal* can be used to describe upper motor neuron fibers that travel near the pyramidal fibers, modulating tone and movement.[5] The term *extrapyramidal* refers to fibers associated with the basal ganglia and clinical findings of Parkinson's disease.[4] Spasticity is a result of an imbalance between the afferent excitatory pathway and the descending inhibitory pathway after central nervous system (CNS) damage.[6]

FACTORS IN DETERMINING TREATMENTS OF SPASTICITY

In 2009, a group of rehabilitation experts published professional practices and recommendations for drug treatments of spasticity.[7] These recommendations suggest that before beginning pharmacologic treatment for increased tone, a detailed evaluation plan be followed to determine the true impact of spasticity. First, spasticity should be measured using the Ashworth scale or the Tardieu scale. Spasms can be measured by the Penn scale. A further analysis should follow considering such factors as the impact of hypertonia on range of motion (ROM), pain, difficulties with hygiene measures provided by caregiver or taken by self, and movement impairments. A separate analysis should also include the patient's personal goals identified by asking the patient how the spasticity is problematic, what other concomitant limitations exist, and whether the spasticity predominates in one muscle group or is more widespread. Note should be taken of common nociceptive triggers that increase spasticity, such as pain and pressure ulcers. Finally, while this chapter focuses on the pharmacology of the treatment of spasticity and muscle spasms, drug treatments should be considered as only one component of the therapeutic program, which may include physical therapy, orthotics or other technical aides, and orthopedic surgery or neurosurgery.

SPASTICITY

Medications to resolve excessive muscle tone are numerous, but few have been established to reduce disability. The adverse effects of a drug should be considered when the effect of the drug on a patient is evaluated. The mechanisms and anatomic sites of action are not yet well understood. The consensus is that they either alter the functions of neurotransmitters or neuromodulators in the CNS or have an action on the peripheral neuromuscular sites. CNS function could include suppression of excitation through glutamate or by enhancement of inhibition either through gamma (γ)-aminobutyric acid (GABA) or glycine.[8]

To avoid potential adverse effects, pharmacotherapy for spasticity is generally initiated at low doses and then gradually increased. Ideally, therapy is optimal at the lowest dose. Baclofen, diazepam, tizanidine, and dantrolene are currently approved for use in patients with spasticity. In addition, clonidine (usually in combination therapy), gabapentin, and botulinum toxin (BTX) have shown efficacy; however, more studies are needed to confirm their efficacy. Intrathecal baclofen (ITB), administered via a surgically implanted pump and reservoir, may provide relief to patients with severe refractory spasticity.[2]

Centrally Acting Agents for Spasticity

Examples of centrally acting agents include diazepam, baclofen, and tizanidine. Their mechanisms of action are dissimilar, and therefore they are described separately. However, all three are useful in reducing spasticity of spinal origin (spinal cord and multiple sclerosis [MS]), in which there is less sensitivity to their sedating effects.

Diazepam (Valium). Diazepam is indicated for the management of anxiety disorders or for short-term relief of symptoms of anxiety.[9] However, it is also a useful adjunct for the relief of skeletal muscle spasms caused by reflex spasms of a local pathologic condition (such as inflammation of muscles or joints or trauma injury); spasticity caused by upper motor neuron disorders (such as CP and paraplegia); athetosis; stiff person syndrome; and tetanus (Table 16-1). Stiff person syndrome is a rare neurologic disorder with autoimmune features. It is characterized by progressive, severe muscle rigidity or stiffness, most prominently affecting the spine and lower extremities.[10] In addition, injectable diazepam is a useful adjunct in the treatment of status epilepticus and severe recurrent convulsive seizures.[9] Contraindications include the use of diazepam in the treatment for MS and known hypersensitivity to benzoidiazapines; diazepam is not recommended for use in children under 6 months of age. The drug is rarely justified for use in pregnant women or in women with childbearing potential who may be pregnant.

The antispasticity effects of benzodiazepines are achieved by binding to the $GABA_A$-gated chloride channel.[9] Diazepam binds in the brainstem, reticular formations, and spinal pathways with a particular predilection for the higher pathways. It is considered to be an intermediate-to-long–acting benzodiazepine because of its half life of 20 to 80 hours. The duration of its half life is dependent on the metabolism of one active intermediate, desmethyldiazepam, and two minor active metabolites. In animals, diazepam appears to act on parts of the limbic system—the thalamus and the hypothalamus—and induces calming effects. It has no demonstrable peripheral autonomic blocking action, nor does it produce extrapyramidal adverse effects; however, at higher doses, transient ataxia can occur. Diazepam was found to have transient cardiovascular depressor effects in animals.[9]

Adverse effects most commonly reported are drowsiness, fatigue, and ataxia. Infrequently encountered adverse effects are confusion, constipation, depression, diplopia, dysarthria, headache, hypotension, incontinence, jaundice, changes in libido, nausea, changes in salivation, skin rash, slurred speech, tremor, urinary retention, vertigo, and blurred vision. Cutson et al[11] examined the

TABLE 16-1 Efficacy of Selected Antispasticity Medications and Adverse Effects

	MS	SCI	Stroke	TBI	CP	Adverse Effects
Dantrolene	+	+	++		+	Decreased walking speed, muscle weakness, hepatotoxicity
Oral baclofen	++	+	+/–			Decreased walking speed, muscle weakness, sedation, lowered threshold for seizures
Intrathecal baclofen	+	+	+	?	?	Decreased walking speed, muscle weakness, sedation, lowered threshold for seizures, pump malfunction
Diazepam	+	+	+/–		+	Decreased walking speed, marked sedation, cognitive slowing, hypotension
Tizanidine	++	+	+	?		Minor muscular weakness, sedation, dry mouth, dizziness, hypotension, liver dysfunction

+, Effective in a double-blind study; ++, demonstrated effectiveness in a double-blind comparative study; +/–, effectiveness was modulated by annoying side effects; ?, effectiveness established in open trials; *empty block*, indicates lack of information up to 1997; *MS*, multiple sclerosis; *SCI*, spinal cord injury; *TBI*, traumatic brain injury; *CP*, cerebral palsy.

Adapted from Gracies J, Nance P, McGuire J, Simpson DM: General pharmacological treatments for spasticity. Part II: General and regional treatments, *Muscle Nerve Suppl* 6:S61–S92, 1997.

effect of a single dose of diazepam on a spectrum of balance measures in healthy older adults and found that benzodiazepines affect neuromuscular processing related to balance control. They observed increased muscle latency in response to sudden perturbations, which are suggested to have an effect on the oligosynaptic spinal reflex distinct from the sedation.[11] This finding would suggest caution in the dosing of diazepam, when a patient with spasticity already has limitations in static or dynamic balance without pharmacologic intervention, as this may further limit functional tasks such as sitting, standing, and walking. In children, sedation is the most common adverse effect, but occasionally, increased drooling, ataxia, and cognitive dullness has been observed.[12]

Paradoxical reactions such as acute hyperexcited states, anxiety, hallucinations, increased muscle spasticity, insomnia, rage, and sleep disturbances have been reported; should these occur, the drug should be discontinued.[9] Because of isolated reports of neutropenia and jaundice, periodic blood counts and liver function tests are advisable during long-term therapy. Minor changes in electroencephalographic (EEG) patterns, usually low-voltage fast activity, have been observed in patients during and after diazepam therapy and are of no known significance.

Concomitant use of barbiturates, alcohol, or other CNS depressant increases CNS depression with increased risk of apnea and is thus a significant contraindication.[9] For example, if diazepam is to be combined with other psychotropic agents or anticonvulsant drugs, careful consideration should be given to the pharmacology of the agents to be used—particularly that of known compounds that may potentiate the action of diazepam, such as phenothiazines, narcotics, barbiturates, and antidepressants.

Benzodiazepines can have a hypotensive effect. Kitajima et al[13] found that after diazepam administration, systolic and mean blood pressure decreased significantly; they concluded that the hypotensive effect of diazepam is mainly due to the central mechanism rather than an alteration in autonomic cardiovascular control. The protein binding characteristic of the pharmacology of diazepam is clinically significant in SCI and stroke because a low serum albumin level is often associated with these conditions. Consequently, diazepam could be more toxic in these circumstances.[8] Diazepam is relatively devoid of autonomic effects and thus may be an effective medication for SCI spasticity.

As always, dosing depends on indication and severity and is adjusted to achieve the maximal benefit with the lowest dose (2–10 mg, 3–4 times/day). Lower doses with gradual increases should be given to older adults or those taking other sedatives (2 mg 1–2 times/day gradually increasing as tolerated).[9] Doses for children range from 1 to 10 mg given three to four times per day. Severe spasticity associated with local pathologic conditions, CP, athetosis, stiff person syndrome, or tetanus may be treated with 5 to 10 mg of diazepam, administered via the intravenous route initially; then 5 to 10 mg may be administered in 3 to 4 hours, at which time the intramuscular route could be used, if necessary.[9] If diazepam is administered to infants or young children for tetanus spasm, respiratory assistance should be available in case breathing becomes depressed.

Abrupt cessation of benzodiazepines can result in withdrawal symptoms similar in character to those noted with barbiturates and alcohol withdrawal (convulsions, tremor, abdominal and muscle cramps, vomiting, and sweating).[9] The more severe withdrawal symptoms have usually occurred only in those patients who had received excessive doses over an extended period. Generally, milder withdrawal symptoms (e.g., dysphoria and insomnia) have been reported after abrupt discontinuation of benzodiazepines taken continuously at therapeutic levels for several months. Consequently, after extended therapy, abrupt discontinuation should generally be avoided, and a gradual dose tapering schedule should be followed.

Beard et al[14] conducted a systematic review to identify drug treatments currently available for the management of spasticity and pain in MS and evaluated their clinical effectiveness and cost-effectiveness. Evidence of the effectiveness of oral diazepam in the treatment of spasticity is limited. Many of the interventions identified are not approved for the alleviation of pain or spasticity in MS, and the lack of evidence relating to their effectiveness may also limit their widespread use. Diazepam is widely prescribed to persons with SCI to treat muscular spasticity.[15] Because diazepam binds in both the reticular formation and spinal polysynaptic pathways, it appears to produce lesser response in patients with complete SCI.[16]

With regard to the use of diazepam in children, Cruikshrank and Eunson[17] reported three cases where intravenous diazepam was used successfully with planned ITB withdrawal. This finding was significant in these cases due to the potential life-threatening risk of baclofen withdrawal syndrome. The authors reported these cases to illustrate the potential benefit of diazepam with elective baclofen withdrawal. The quality standards subcommittee of the American Academy of Neurology and the practice committee of the Child Neurology Society published an evidenced-based review of the efficacy and safety of pharmacologic treatments of childhood spasticity.[18] This review identified diazepam as effective in treating generalized childhood spasticity in the short term, but little to no evidence was available on adverse motor effects; caution in the use of diazepam should therefore be exercised due to its toxicity.

Drugs Affecting Skeletal Muscle and Calcium Stores

Agents that act at the skeletal muscle level cause changes peripherally instead of at the neural level. Dantrolene is the only agent in this category that has been approved as a general pharmacologic treatment for spasticity. It is used when muscle overactivity is diffuse or when the number of muscles affected precludes local treatment.

Dantrolene Sodium (Dantrium). Dantrolene produces relaxation of the muscle by interfering with calcium flux at the sarcoplasmic reticulum, thereby interfering with the excitation–contraction coupling process. Dantrolene generally affects skeletal muscle fast-twitch fibers to a greater extent than the slow-twitch fibers, but it will affect both fiber types.[9] It does not appear to affect the neural input to the muscle, the neuromuscular junction, or the excitable muscle membranes themselves.[19] Indirect CNS effects sometimes cause drowsiness, dizziness, and generalized weakness. The duration of dantrolene depends on the dose. Its biologic half life is 8.7 hours after a 100-mg dose. The drug's metabolic patterns appear to be similar in adults and children.[9]

In chronic disability due to upper motor neuron disease or injury, dantrolene is used when spasticity limits rehabilitation goals. A reduction in spasticity can enhance function, nursing care, and usefulness of braces and can reduce painful clonus that may disturb sleep. Dantrolene is not indicated for treatment of skeletal muscle spasms in rheumatic disorders.

The dose of dantrolene should be maintained for at least 4 to 7 days to determine the patient's response. Some patients do not respond until higher doses are used. Dosing should begin with 25 to 50 mg once a day and increase to 25 mg three times a day (tid), 50 mg tid, and 100 mg tid. Doses higher than 100 mg four times daily (qid) should not be used. Pediatric doses are 5 mg once daily, increased to 0.5 mg tid, 1 mg tid, and 2 mg tid or 12 mg/kg/day. If no benefits are derived within 45 days, administration of dantrolene should be discontinued.[9]

Dantrolene is contraindicated when spasticity is required for upright posture, balance, or locomotion.[19] In such cases, reduction in spasticity would result in loss of function. Spasticity of spinal origin responds less favorably to dantrolene because of the resultant weakness. Few studies have evaluated this effect. One study of patients with spasticity of spinal origin demonstrated a decrease in severity of spasticity; however, the reduction in strength outweighed the benefit.[20]

The most frequently occurring adverse effects of dantrolene are drowsiness, dizziness, weakness, general malaise, fatigue, and diarrhea.[9] These are generally transient, occurring early in treatment, and can often be obviated by beginning with a low dose and increasing the dose gradually until an optimal regimen is established. Diarrhea may be severe and may necessitate temporary withdrawal of the drug. If diarrhea recurs on readministration of dantrolene, therapy should probably be discontinued permanently. Dantrolene has the advantage of having minimal cognitive adverse effects and modest drug interactions.[21]

Several precautions should be taken when patients are prescribed dantrolene. Patients should not use dantrolene when they have pulmonary dysfunction such as chronic obstructive pulmonary disease, severe cardiac dysfunction such as myocardial disease, or certain forms of liver disease. Because of the potential for hepatotoxicity, dantrolene should be used with caution, and liver function should be monitored.[21,22] The risk for hepatotoxicity appears greatest among women 35 years and older and patients taking more than 300 mg daily. The risk may increase when dantrolene is combined with some other medications.

Dantrolene is used in patients with stroke, CP, and MS and may be preferable for these indications because sensitivity in terms of sedation appears to be higher in spasticity of cerebral origin (stroke) (see Table 16-1). Steinberg et al. found a decrease in clonus in patients treated with dantrolene for hemiparetic spasticity. This was accompanied by improvements in gait and personal care abilities.[23] Less improvement was noted in resistance to passive stretch. A study in which oral agents for treatment of spasticity in CP were compared indicated that dantrolene compared favorably with diazepam and baclofen in reducing spasticity.[24] A brief withdrawal of dantrolene for a period of up to 2 days should result in exacerbation of symptoms and confirm the clinical impression or patient self-report of symptoms of spasticity. In one study, when patients with hemiparesis stopped taking dantrolene, a significant decrement in motor performance occurred, suggesting the benefit of dantrolene in treating spasticity of central origin.[25] Some studies indicate that dantrolene acts favorably in combination with other agents. Dantrolene was compared with diazepam in a double-blind study of children with spasticity. The combination of the two drugs was suggested to be most effective.[25]

Drugs Acting on the γ-Aminobutyric Acid$_B$ Receptors

The pharmacologic control of spasticity is believed to result from the reduction of inhibitory mechanisms, namely, GABA-mediated or glycine-mediated antagonism of excitatory mechanisms, or both. GABA receptor sites are widely present in the CNS and therefore are amenable to pharmacologic manipulation.[6]

Baclofen (Lioresal). Baclofen is a structural analog of GABA but does not bind to the $GABA_A$ receptor but rather to the more recently identified $GABA_B$ receptor, both presynaptically and postsynaptically. When the drug binds to the GABAergic interneuron, membrane hyperpolarization blocks the influx of calcium into the presynaptic terminal, thus reducing neurotransmitter release.[9] Postsynaptic binding of the drug on the Ia sensory afferent terminal also produces hyperpolarization and increases potassium influx so that inhibition is enhanced. $GABA_B$ receptors may inhibit gamma motor neuron activity and reduce muscle spindle sensitivity. The net effect is inhibition of monosynaptic and polysynaptic spinal reflexes.

Baclofen is useful for the alleviation of spasticity resulting from MS, particularly for the relief of flexor spasms and associated pain, clonus, and muscle rigidity.[8] Patients should have reversible spasticity so that baclofen treatment will aid in restoring residual function. Baclofen may also be of some value in patients with spinal cord injuries and spinal diseases, but it is not indicated in the treatment of skeletal muscle spasm resulting from rheumatic disorders.

Very few double-blind, placebo-controlled studies of baclofen have been performed.[26] However, the efficacy of oral baclofen has been established for MS and SCI, and the efficacy of ITB has been established for MS, SCI, and stroke (see Table 16-1). This is not to say that these medications are not effective in treating other conditions associated with spasticity but only that placebo-controlled studies of patients with other conditions have not been performed. However, a recent double-blind randomized trial examined the efficacy and tolerability of baclofen in spastic palsy compared with that of eperisone.[27] Eperisone (Myonal) is an antispastic agent that has an effect on skeletal muscles and vascular smooth muscles by blocking sodium channels and suppressing the activity of γ-motor neurons.[28] It is only available in Japan, India, and the Far East. In this study, both baclofen and eperisone significantly improved functionality of lower limbs versus baseline, but only eperisone improved this parameter in the upper limbs. Both drugs reduced muscular tone, but only eperisone improved ROM in joints. Both treatments reduced the 10-meter walking time, but this effect was evident at week 2 with eperisone only. For tolerability, no differences were observed between eperisone and baclofen in any parameters. The authors concluded that compared with baclofen, eperisone might be associated with some additional clinical benefits.

A recent review of the evidence on the use of oral baclofen in children also indicated the existence of only a few studies that had conflicting results. One such study reviewed was a double-blind crossover trial in 20 children 2 to 6 years old receiving a dose of 10 to 60 mg/day. This study found a reduction in spasticity measured by the Ashworth scale; after 28 days of treatment, 14 patients improved at least one level and 5 improved more than one level. Spasticity improvement was demonstrated by increased passive ROM (11 patients); however, of the patients who walked without assistance prior to treatment, 10 patients showed no significant functional improvement.[29] Another study with similar dose, age group, and design reported improvement on the Goal Attainment Scale, but not in spasticity measured by the Tardieu scale or functional benefits measured by the Pediatric Evaluation of Disability Inventory at 12 weeks, roughly twice as long as the Milla et al study.[29,30] More recently, Dai et al studied oral baclofen versus tizanidine in a pilot study on children with CP who had spastic equinus, all of whom received botulinum toxin (BTX) injections.[31] After 2- to 4-week follow-up evaluations over 12 weeks, the authors reported that the tizanidine group had significantly better results compared with the baclofen group. This study suggested that a combination of botulinum toxin type A with oral tizanidine is more effective with fewer adverse effects than a combination of botulinum toxin type A and oral baclofen for treating spastic CP. However, one study by van Doornik et al found that oral baclofen increased the voluntary neuromuscular activation of plantar flexors in children with spasticity caused by CP and suggested that antispasticity agents could even facilitate strength training.[32]

The optimal oral dose of baclofen requires titration. Therapy should be started at a low dose and increased gradually until the optimal effect is achieved (usually between 40 and 80 mg daily).[8] The following dosage schedule is suggested: 5 mg tid for 3 days and subsequently increasing by 5 mg every 3 days. Thereafter, additional increases may be necessary, but the total daily dose should not exceed 80 mg (20 mg qid). As always, the lowest dose compatible with the optimal response is recommended. If benefits are not evident after a reasonable trial period, the drug should be slowly withdrawn. Baclofen has general CNS depressant properties as evidenced by increased somnolence, ataxia, and cardiac and respiratory depression. Baclofen may also impair attention and memory and produce confusion, particularly in older adults and in patients with brain injuries.[33] Baclofen may also interfere with neural recovery because of its GABA central pathways, lower the seizure threshold, and cause withdrawal syndrome.[25,26,33,34] Patients should be cautioned about the additive effects of baclofen and alcohol and other CNS depressants. Like other antispasticity drugs, baclofen should not be used when spasticity is needed to maintain upright posture.[35] In general, patients who have had a stroke do not tolerate the drug well.[25]

Another CNS effect may be hallucination.[9] Baclofen also induces muscle weakness, which may be a more significant problem for the functional patient than for the patient with severe impairment.[8] Increased gait disturbances have been reported in patients with MS receiving baclofen, presumably as a result of induced weakness or underlying weakness that becomes apparent after spasticity is reduced or removed.[36,37] Sudden withdrawal of oral baclofen may result in seizure, hallucination, and rebound spasticity with fever. Milla et al also reported adverse effects in 25% of the children and adolescents studied, where participants demonstrated somnolence or sedation (20%) and hypotonia (15%) that resolved after drug discontinuation.[29]

Intrathecal Baclofen (ITB). To treat spasticity of spinal cord origin, long-term infusion of baclofen may be prescribed to patients with severe spasticity that is unresponsive to oral antispasticity medication or to those who experience intolerable CNS adverse effects at effective doses.[38] Patients with spasticity caused by traumatic brain injury should wait at least 1 year after the injury before long-term ITB therapy is considered.

Long-term intrathecal administration of baclofen entails subcutaneous implantation of a pump in the abdominal wall with the catheter tip placed in the subarachnoid space (Figure 16-1).[39] Usually, the tip is placed between T12 and L1, but if a patient has significant upper extremity spasticity, the tip may be placed in the midthoracic area. Because the drug is delivered directly into the spinal cord, in order to reduce overall systemic effects, higher concentrations are placed in the target area at lower doses than those used with the oral route. The intrathecal dose is only 1% of the oral dose. The pumps can be programmed to infuse the drug at a constant rate or can be titrated according to the patient's individual needs; for example, a patient may be given a greater concentration at night to relieve night spasms (Figure 16-2).

Before pump insertion, patients must demonstrate a positive clinical response to a baclofen screening injection of a bolus dose.[39] For this "ITB screening trial," patients are usually admitted to the hospital for 1 to 3 days. The trial begins with an initial Ashworth screening, often performed by the physical therapist, followed by a 50-mcg intrathecal injection for adults and a 25-mcg injection for children. The therapist returns after 1 hour to repeat the Ashworth screening and then every 2 hours for the next 8 hours. If the Ashworth scores do not drop, a higher dose (75 mcg) is administered the following day. If the scores remain the same, a 100-mcg dose may be given on the third day. A maximum dose of up to 150 mcg is allowed for adults, but it is capped at 100 mcg for children. The goal of each injection is a decrease of 1 point in the Ashworth score and maintenance of this score over two consecutive assessments. Hypotonia, even if greater than desired, is a positive result on the screening test.[39] If this goal is achieved without respiratory or other complications, then the pump is offered to the patient.

The onset of action of an intrathecal bolus dose of baclofen in adults is generally 30 minutes to 1 hour after injection.[9] The peak spasmolytic effect is seen at approximately 4 hours after dosing, and the effects may last 4 to 8 hours; however, this may vary, depending on drug dose and severity of symptoms. Similar responses are seen in pediatric patients.

The pharmacokinetics of cerebrospinal fluid (CSF) clearance of baclofen injection calculated from intrathecal bolus or continuous infusion studies approximates CSF turnover.[9] After a bolus lumbar injection of 50 or 100 mcg or intrathecal infusion of baclofen injection, the average CSF clearance is approximately 30mL/hr. Limited pharmacokinetic data suggest that a lumbar cisternal concentration gradient of about 4:1 is established along the neuraxis during baclofen infusion. Absorption may be dose dependent, being reduced with increasing doses. The mean absorption and half life of baclofen is 3.5 hours.[8]

After the pump is implanted, the patient will stay in the hospital for a few days.[39] Often, the patient is required to remain supine in bed for the first 2 to 3 days to prevent headaches and CSF leaks. With continuous infusion using the pump, baclofen injection's antispastic action is first seen at 6 to 8 hours after initiation of infusion. Maximum activity is observed in 24 to 48 hours. If swelling occurs at the site of either the pump incision or the back incision, an Ace bandage is fitted around the abdomen. For the first few weeks, an abdominal binder may be used when the patient sits up. At this point, the patient must be instructed that transfers and mobility will feel very different. Transfer training should be provided to family members of low-functioning patients, and training with assistive devices should be provided to

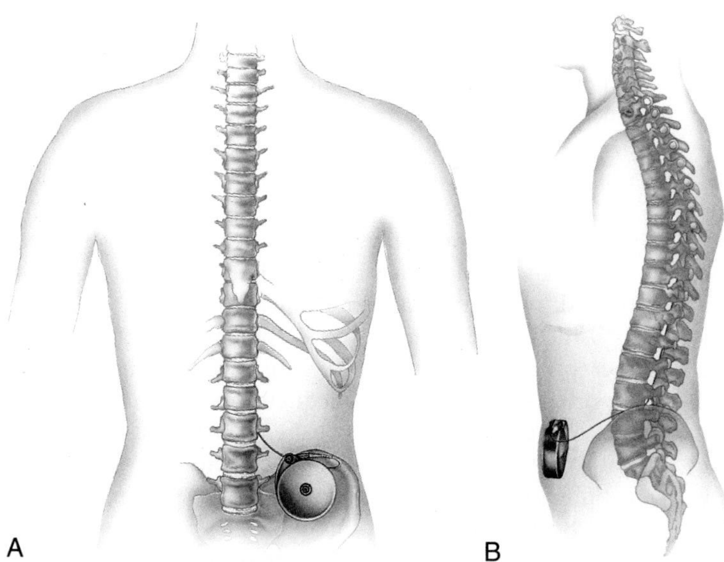

FIGURE 16-1 The pump is surgically implanted in the abdominal region (*front view*). The pump is connected to a catheter that is tunneled under the skin, around to the spine, and enters the intrathecal space (*side view*). (*Courtesy Medtronic, Inc.*)

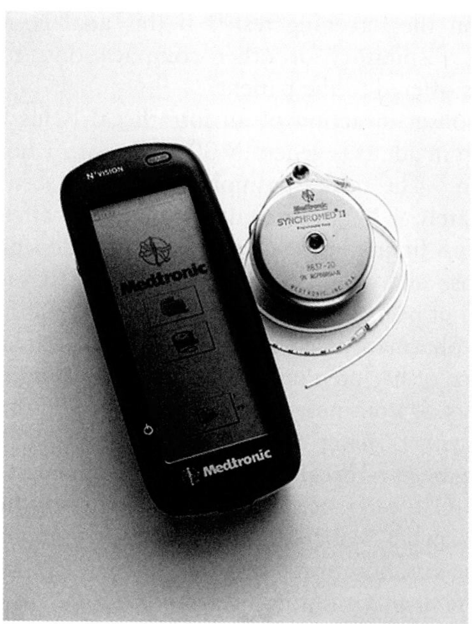

FIGURE 16-2 SynchroMed programmable infusion pump (*foreground*). (*Courtesy Medtronic, Inc.*)

ambulatory patients; however, actual rehabilitation will be on hold for a few weeks until healing occurs.

The intensity and frequency of therapy depend on underlying weakness, motor control, and, in the real world, insurance coverage. A thorough evaluation performed after pump implantation will likely show that the patient has very different impairments and functional limitations than he or she had before implantation.[39] Splints and seating systems will need to be reassessed, and new assistive devices may be considered. New goals will be established, and depending on the patient, may range from feeding and oral motor skills to wheelchair mobility or even driving and sport activities. However, for any patient, balance and safety issues are paramount as the patient learns to adjust to the new muscle tone. Modalities such as ultrasound and electrical stimulation may be used but not over or near the pump site.

The postimplantation titration period requires determination of the initial total daily dose. This dose should be double the screening dose that produced the positive clinical effect delivered over 24 hours.[8] Adult patients with SCI or stroke should have the daily dose increased by 10% to 30% (SCI) or 5% to 15% (stroke) after the first 24 hours until the desired clinical effect is achieved. Maintenance therapy requires periodic refills, and the daily dose for a patient with SCI may increase by 10% to 40%, then be reduced if the patient experiences any adverse effects. The allowable increase in daily dose for a patient with stroke or brain injury is less and should only be increased by 5% to 20%, then reduced if any adverse effects occur. Bowden and Stokic reported the advantages of using clinical and neurophysiologic testing of strength and spasticity when titrating both oral and ITB in incomplete SCI.[40] These authors demonstrated that the control of spasticity could be achieved without detrimental effects on strength in incomplete SCI and suggested the need for including strength testing in comprehensive clinical assessment of spasticity. They also reported the convergent validity between clinical and neurophysiologic assessments during ITB dose titration, thus providing objectivity and sensitivity and facilitating decision making during ITB titration.

For most patients, the dose must be gradually increased over time to maintain effectiveness.[7] A sudden requirement for an increase in dose usually means a kink in the catheter or a pump malfunction. Dose adjustment may be titrated to maintain some degree of spasms for circulation and to prevent deep vein thrombosis. Concomitant administration of oral baclofen should be decreased and eliminated to avoid an overdose.

The pump will need to be refilled approximately every 3 months, and refilling takes about 30 to 45 minutes.[38] A syringe is inserted through the subcutaneous tissue into the pump. The pump should emit a soft beep when the volume decreases to a certain level to warn the patient when the drug level is low. A beeping sound will also occur when the battery gets low, which usually occurs between 4 and 5 years.

Complications associated with the pump include infection, dislodgment, kinking or blocking of the catheter, and pump failure.[8,38,39] One study reviewed 174 cases of children with CP in their facility between 1996 and 2007 and found a 31% rate of complications requiring surgery within a 3-year follow-up period; however, both parents and children reported a high rate of satisfaction with ITB therapy. With the exception of infection, any of these complications may produce symptoms of an overdose or withdrawal.[41] All medical personnel and caregivers should be instructed in recognizing the signs and symptoms of an overdose, the procedures to follow if there are signs of an overdose, and ways to manage the pump and the injection site. Signs of an overdose include sedation, confusion, hypotonia, urinary hesitancy, respiratory depression, and even coma. Signs associated with withdrawal include increased spasticity and dystonia, hyperthermia, pruritus, agitation, hallucinations, multiple organ system failure, and death. Death is rare but has been seen with sudden withdrawal, caused by the pump running out of baclofen or a clogged catheter. Patients and caregivers should be diligent in keeping appointments for programming and monitoring of the infusion system and pump alarms and refilling the pump to avoid the risk of withdrawal syndrome.

With regard to evidence supporting or refuting ITB therapy for the treatment of spasticity, Delgato et al. reported that data are inadequate concerning the use of continuous ITB as an antispasticity treatment in children with CP.[18] CSF leaks, seromas, catheter-related complications, and wound infection occur frequently, and other, milder complications occur less frequently. One study in this review was a retrospective study of the safety of ITB in 200 children; this study found that 11% had CSF leakage, 7% had catheter-related problems, and 5.5% developed infections.[42] Still, this consensus group did not support or refute the use of ITB in children and adolescents. In adults, Kofler et al reported limitations of ITB for eight individuals with spastic hemiparesis following stroke.[43] They found that ITB reduced spasticity in a dose-dependent manner irrespective of its origin, and it may alleviate pain if it arises from increased muscle tone. Additionally, they reported that a functional benefit may result in ITB as it can uncover "subclinical" motor control that had been masked by spasticity. However, as with all antispasmodics, when a patient uses antigravity patterns for ambulation in the absence of more complex motor control, ITB could cause loss of residual walking ability. A Cochrane review of pharmacologic interventions for spasticity following spinal cord injury by Taricco included two studies that found ITB effective in reducing spasticity as measured by the Ashworth scale as well as on activities of daily living (ADL) scales, compared with placebo and without adverse events.[44]

With regard to the use of oral baclofen in the treatment of spasticity, the majority of studies have demonstrated efficacy in the reduction of hypertonicity in patients with SCI and MS; however, improvement in physical functions, such as ambulation or ADLs, has not been demonstrated.[26] In a Scandinavian study of patients with MS, no significant functional improvement was observed among those treated with baclofen.[37] This agent seems most effective in those with spasticity of spinal pathogenesis. There is no doubt that baclofen decreases spasticity and painful spasms in a variety of neurologic conditions; however, many studies have failed to demonstrate improvement in gait and ADLs. This lack of functional gain may be due to variations in study design and difficulty in making comparisons between studies because of the wide variety of outcome measures used. The outcome measures themselves may be the problem in that they do not always identify the specific daily activity that the patient deems most important in terms of individual improvement. Others have reported that limitation in functional gains could be due to muscle weakness that overrides the gains in reduction in stiffness from baclofen.[26]

A recent study of the effects of baclofen on motor units paralyzed by chronic spinal cord injury demonstrated that the median motor unit tetanic forces were significantly weaker in those individuals who were using baclofen versus those who did not or controls. In other words, compared with those with cervical injuries who were not taking baclofen and to healthy controls, the entire thenar muscle was weaker and more fatiguable because it took more electrical stimulation to generate the same force when on baclofen versus not on baclofen. The authors concluded that the short-term benefits of baclofen must be weighed against the long-term need for more rehabilitation to return to the preinjury state in chronic SCI.[45]

Drugs Acting on the α_2 Receptor

Centrally acting α_2 adrenoceptor agonists are primarily used to reduce blood pressure. However, because they interact with these receptors both spinally and supraspinally, they can also be used to reduce tone.

Tizanidine (Zanaflex). Tizanidine is a centrally acting α_2-adrenergic agonist that presumably decreases spasticity by increasing presynaptic inhibition of spinal motor neurons. It acts on group II sensory afferents, decreases the impact on excitatory transmission, and facilitates glycine.[46] The effect is greatest on polysynaptic pathways rather than on monosynaptic spinal reflexes, skeletal muscle, or the neuromuscular junction. Therefore presynaptic inhibition occurs. Clonidine is another drug in this category that is primarily used for lowering blood pressure.

Tizanidine tablets and capsules are bioequivalent to each other under fasting conditions, but not under fed conditions, as determined by changing the plasma concentrations.[9] Food also increases the extent of absorption for both the tablets and capsules. The amount absorbed with food is significantly greater for the tablet than for the capsule.

Those sensitive to the ingredients of tizanidine should not use it, and it should be used with caution if renal or hepatic disease is present. Monitoring of aminotransferase levels is recommended during the first 6 months of treatment (e.g., baseline, 1, 3, and 6 months) and periodically thereafter, based on clinical status. Because of the potential toxic hepatic effect of tizanidine, the drug should be used only with extreme caution in patients with impaired hepatic function.[9]

Tizanidine's peak plasma concentration occurs 1 to 2 hours after dosing, and its half life is 2.5 hours.[9] The starting dose for tizanidine is 2 to 4 mg at bedtime, increasing to a maximum of 36 mg/day. A slow titration program is often best tolerated.

Commonly reported adverse effects include somnolence, asthenia, dizziness, dry mouth, and hypotension.[9] Hypotension can be seen within 1 hour after dosing and peaks 2 to 3 hours after dosing; it can also be associated, at times, with bradycardia, orthostatic hypotension, light-headedness or dizziness, and, rarely, syncope. The hypotensive effect has been measured after administration of single doses of 2 mg; therefore advancement of doses should be based on hypotensive signs and symptoms. Tizanidine can also produce sedation that appears to be dose related; sedation may be noted approximately 30 minutes after dosing and peaks at 1.5 hours afterward. Tizanidine use has been associated with hallucinations. Formed, visual hallucinations or delusions have been reported. Additionally, tizanidine can have cardiovascular effects. Caution is advised when tizanidine is to be administered to patients receiving concurrent antihypertensive therapy and should not be used with other α_2-adrenergic agonists. Prolongation of the QT interval and bradycardia were noted in patients with chronic toxicosis. Still, studies comparing tizanidine with other agents suggest that it is better tolerated than baclofen and diazepam.[47] It is less likely to weaken the muscles but is still of concern because it may slow neural recovery in patients with brain injury.[25]

The therapeutic profile of antispastic drugs must be evaluated in comparison with existing drugs. Lataste et al. reviewed the efficacy and tolerability of tizanidine with those of baclofen and diazepam, the most widely used antispastic agents, for a variety of diagnoses and target symptoms associated with spasticity.[48] More than 20 double-blind, comparative studies between 1977 and 1987 included a total of 777 patients with spasticity from various causes. Tizanidine emerged as a valuable drug in the treatment of spasticity related to cerebral and spinal disorders. Groves et al. conducted a meta-analysis of the antispastic efficacy and tolerability of tizanidine compared with baclofen or diazepam.[49] As measured by Ashworth scores, tizanidine had spasticity-reducing effects similar to those of both baclofen and diazepam. Muscle strength was affected less by tizanidine than by baclofen and diazepam, and tizanidine was judged to have greater tolerability. More recently (2006), a Cochrane review was conducted to examine the effects of pharmacologic interventions on spasticity in spinal cord injury. [44] This review reported one study that compared tizanidine with placebo (118 patients with SCI) and showed significant effects on Ashworth scores but not on ADLs, and significant rates of adverse effects such as drowsiness were noted.

The efficacy of tizanidine in the treatment of MS has been shown. In a multicenter trial, a significant decrease in spasticity was seen as measured by the Ashworth scale and the knee swing pendulum test, compared with placebo.[50] A good reduction in tone was seen in stroke-related and traumatic brain injury–related spasticity without effects on the strength of muscle force, tendon reflexes, or clonus.[47] More recently, Kamen et al. conducted a review of studies of tizanidine in the treatment of spasticity in spinal cord injury, stroke, and MS.[51] In their review, the authors included clinical trials that demonstrated the efficacy of tizanidine comparable with that of baclofen or diazepam, with global tolerability data favoring the use of tizanidine. They further suggested its combination with baclofen as a logical avenue for improved spasticity control.

Therapeutic Concerns Regarding the Use of Oral Antispasticity Medications

Baclofen, dantrolene, diazepam, and tizanidine continue to be the most commonly used oral systemic agents in the treatment of spasticity.[8] All these medications are nonspecific and produce a variety of adverse effects. The most troublesome effects are related to sedation and weakness, both of which interfere with therapeutic intervention and attainment of functional goals. Fine-tuning the dose often takes time because drug benefit in terms of reducing muscle tone must be balanced against the sedating or weakening effects of the drug.

The other issue is the less than optimal spasticity rating scales that are used to determine drug efficacy.[26] Often, a reduction in tone is achieved but without improvement in results of standardized tests of gross motor or functional performance. The test may not address the specific individual's improvements, or perhaps, there are simply not enough functional gains achieved with the medication. More likely, it is a problem with the standardized tests because patient and caregiver reports often indicate improvements with medication.

The third issue to consider before a drug trial is proper patient selection.[39] Are there severe contractures that would require orthopedic surgery even after the institution of drug therapy, and is surgery available to the patient? Does the patient have adequate underlying strength, particularly trunk strength? Does the patient need tone for function? Patients who ambulate and can perform hip and knee flexion and ankle dorsiflexion may not benefit from drug intervention. In addition, intensive physical therapy is also needed along with drug therapy to help the patient develop new motor patterns and functional abilities. Thus many factors need to be considered, especially if the patient opts for intrathecal drug application.

Consideration should also be given to the combinations of oral and injectable medications. For example, Dai et al. studied oral baclofen versus tizanidine in a pilot study of children with CP who had spastic equinus, all of whom received BTX injections.[31] The authors reported after 2- to 4-week follow-up evaluations over 12 weeks that the tizanidine group had significantly better results compared with the baclofen group. This study suggested that the combination of botulinum toxin type A with oral tizanidine is more effective with fewer adverse effects than is the combination of botulinum toxin type A and oral baclofen for spastic cerebral palsy.

Finally, it is best to consider that GABAergic agents such as benzodiazepines (and baclofen) may have harmful effects on the body during the recovery phase, as has been observed in animal models. This should prompt great caution in their use in patients in the recovery phase (in acute-phase stroke or during an MS relapse). There is no evidence that a tizanidine–baclofen combination is of value.[7]

Drugs Affecting the Neuromuscular Junction and Nerve Fibers

Local treatments for spasticity include those agents that are administered directly to the region of interest.[52] Several agents can be administered for chemodenervation, a method of injection directly into the muscle or nerve for the intended treatment effect. Two local treatments for spasticity are discussed: botulinum toxins and alcohols, including ethanol and phenol.

Chemodenervation. Pharmacologic neuromuscular blockades, such as botulinum toxins and alcohol injections, are collectively defined as chemodenervation.[52] These interventions are used to produce focal effects rather than the systemic effects that oral medications may have.

Chemical Neurolysis. Reports of use of phenol to perform peripheral and intramuscular nerve blocks were published in the 1960s.[53] A nerve block is the application of a chemical to impair nerve function, either for the short term or permanently. A percutaneous block of a peripheral nerve trunk produces chemical neurolysis and damage to the nerve by demyelinating it, thereby weakening the muscle.[54] Ethanol can also be used for nerve blocks to produce neurolysis (Table 16-2).

Ethyl alcohol is a powerful drug, causing extraction of lipids from the neuron and precipitation of proteins.[54] The use of 100% alcohol can cause edema of Schwann cells and axons with separation of the myelin sheath. Eventually, wallerian degeneration begins without differential action on specific nerve roots.[53] Phenol injections or nerve blocks are often used for their clinical effect on larger proximal muscle groups because the nerve injected often supplies multiple muscles and therefore can have a greater effect for a given dose.[55]

Neurolysis to reduce spasticity is preferable to use of other agents when there is no hope of recovery of function in the injected muscle.[54] If a person with SCI is not expected to have a return of function, either because of the neurologic completeness or the chronicity of the injury, neurolysis may be chosen so that several muscles could benefit from a permanent reduction in activation. Alternatively, a combination of neurolysis and BTX may produce more desirable effects when there is significant spasticity in many muscles. BTX decreases spasticity by affecting the fusimotor system and muscle spindle, whereas phenol decreases spasticity by affecting the α-motor fibers within the fusimotor system.[55-59]

Injection of phenol and alcohol chemoneurolysis requires great skill and a cooperative patient. The injection techniques for neurolytic blocks involve use of small portable stimulators.[60] The anode is attached behind the limb, and the cathode is a hollow Teflon-coated needle that is attached to the stimulator. The bare needle tip serves to localize the stimulation site to which the neurolytic agent, such as phenol or alcohol, flows. The needle is directed toward the nerve trunk or at an electrically active site. The phenol is then injected in locations where the current can be reduced to approximately 0.5mA (milliampere) while still producing a palpable contraction.

Initially, after the injection, the limb may be erythematic and warm as a result of the sympathetic block in the nerve distribution. The sites of neurolytic blocks could include mixed sensorimotor nerves, such as the musculocutaneous nerve to decrease elbow flexion and the median nerve to decrease finger flexion. Other examples are injection at the obturator nerve to decrease hip adduction, injection at the sciatic nerve to address the hamstrings, and injection at the tibial nerve to decrease clonus and equinus at the ankle.[60] The clinical implications of these sites are improvement in hygiene or functional mobility.

Elovic et al. outlined the advantages and disadvantages of alcohol and phenol as chemical denervating agents.[61] The advantages of these agents are that (1) they are less expensive than BTX, (2) there is a rapid onset of action, (3) they can facilitate serial casting, (4) their strong potency allows for use of large muscle groups,

TABLE 16-2 Local Treatments for Spasticity

Drug	Mechanism	Site of Injection	Structure Blocked	Onset	Duration	Adverse Effects
Ethyl alcohol (>10%)	Tissue destruction	Intramuscular, perineural	Sensory and motor nerves; muscle; neuromuscular junction	<1 hr	2–36 mo	Pain at intramuscular injection site; pain and dysesthesia perineurally; microcirculatory damage; permanent nerve palsy; tissue necrosis
Phenol (>3%)	Tissue destruction	Intramuscular, perineural	Sensory and motor nerves; muscle; neuromuscular junction	<1 hr	2–36 mo	Pain at intramuscular injection site; pain and dysesthesia perineurally; microcirculatory damage; pain and dysesthesia perineurally; permanent nerve palsy; tissue necrosis
Botulinum toxin	Blocks acetylcholine release	Intramuscular	Neuromuscular junction	24–72 hr	3–6 mo	Rarely, distant paralysis; otherwise, no major risk

Adapted from Gracies J, Nance P, McGuire J, Simpson DM: Traditional pharmacological treatments for spasticity. Part I: Local treatments, *Muscle Nerve Suppl* 6:S61–S92, 1997.

(5) their effect on the sensory fibers can further decrease spasticity through the reflex pathway, (6) there are fewer injection sites (thus more spastic muscles can be treated at one time compared with BTX), (7) there are fewer challenges for storage, and (8) the patient can be reinjected or given a booster in less than 3 months.

Elovic at al indicated that the disadvantages of alcohol and phenol as chemical denervating agents include (1) risk of dysesthesias, (2) muscle fibrosis, (3) need for patient sedation, (4) scarring, (5) risk of granuloma, (6) reduction of contractility of muscle during voluntary movement, (7) postinjection discomfort, (8) more discomfort during the procedure, and (9) the procedure requiring more skill and time compared with BTX.[61]

Clinical experience indicates that caution should be exercised when injections are administered to patients who are receiving anticoagulation therapy because of the potential for bleeding at the injection site. Another factor to consider is that if patients already demonstrate significant weakness or flaccidity, the use of this modality may decrease function instead of improving it.[52] Careful assessment is needed because mild weakness may be overshadowed by spastic musculature. Chemodenervation could further weaken these muscles, potentially reducing function. Therefore other muscles must be capable of compensating for the functional control of the muscles weakened by injection. Elovic et al suggested the value of diagnostic blocks as predictors of responses.[61] This allows the clinician to determine the effects of longer-lasting interventions, diagnose contractures that will not respond to chemodenervation or neurolysis, and identify any undesirable effects such as excessive muscle weakness, and it allows the patient to experience the potential benefit of reduced muscle hyperactivity and pain.

Finally, if the muscle to be injected crosses an area where there are joint deformities or other restrictions, there will likely be few gains.[52] Reducing muscle spasticity cannot increase limb mobility if the restriction is primarily orthopedic in nature. Additionally, although not substantiated in the literature, in cases in which significant, chronic muscle shortening is present, the mobility gains from chemodenervation are likely to be more protracted compared with cases in which muscle shortening is limited or spasticity is acute.

If a nerve trunk is selected for neurolytic injection to produce a more complete blockade of muscle activity, there is a greater risk of partially involving the sensory nerves causing dysesthesias. Where there is complete sensory loss, such as in SCI with American Spinal Injury Association A classification, complete neurolysis may be less likely to produce dysesthesias.[62] Treatments for dysesthesias include oral glucocorticoids such as prednisone, tricyclic antidepressants, carbamazepine, and gabapentin; transcutaneous electrical nerve stimulation; and repeat blockades.[62,63]A repeat blockade may be helpful because the dysesthesia may be caused by an incomplete initial blockade of sensory fibers. However, chemical neurolysis with alcohol or phenol is often unsuccessful when the procedure is repeated more than a few times, theoretically because of fibrous tissue formation at the injection site.[64] There is also an increased risk of dysesthesias and phlebitis when more distal and deeper muscles are injected with phenol.[56]

In general, adverse effects associated with neurolytic blockades include painful injections, chronic dysesthesia, necrosis of muscle, and necrosis of the intimal lining of arteries. The disadvantage of both drugs is the risk of sensory involvement. A positive result from these injections is that stretch reflexes tend to be more affected than strength, unless muscle necrosis is present. Because studies on both alcohol and phenol injections are limited, many clinicians today prefer to treat local muscle overactivity with BTX.

Botulinum Toxin (BTX). There are seven neurotoxins produced by *Clostridium botulinum* designated by the letters A through G.[52,65] They are genetically distinct but have overlapping sequences of homology. Botulinum toxin type A (BoNT-A) has been used for years to reduce muscle overactivity, and more recently, Botulinum toxin type B (BTX-B) has been introduced. BoNT-A blocks peripheral nerve cholinergic synaptic transmission. Axonal conduction remains unaffected. The toxin blocks the release of acetylcholine by binding to the presynaptic nerve ending, which is followed by an internalization of the toxin by endocytosis, which, in turn, blocks exostosis or release of the neurotransmitter. The mechanism for neurotransmitter blockade is not completely understood, but BTX selectively cleaves a protein called SNAP-25, which is responsible for the fusion of neurotransmitter vesicles at the nerve terminal. The complexity of this mechanism may explain why there is a relatively slow onset of action of BoNT-A. The effect of BoNT-A on individual nerve terminals is irreversible; therefore recovery of neuromuscular control occurs only when nerve sprouting creates new terminal formation. If symptoms recur, re-injection is necessary.[55]

BoNT-A is packaged in glass vials containing 100 units.[52] A unit is not a measure of weight but of potency. One unit of BoNT-A is equivalent to the amount of toxin that can kill 50% of a group of 18- to 20-g female Swiss-Webster mice. Two types of BoNT-A are available: Botox manufactured by Allergan, Inc. in the United States; and Dysport, manufactured by Speywood Pharmaceuticals in England and available in Europe. Botox is the more potent preparation. Doses must be adjusted depending on the type of toxin injected. In addition, the dose of BTX is based on adjusted patient weight, muscle size, and desired effect. The onset of action is 24 to 72 hours, although the clinical effect is seen more often in 2 to 3 days.[53] The maximum recommended dose for humans is 300 to 400 units of Botox in any one session and no more than 400 units over a 3-month period (Table 16-3). The median lethal dose

TABLE 16-3 Botulinum Toxin A Dosing Recommendations: A Comparison Between Adult and Pediatric Doses

Abnormal Pattern	Muscles Involved	Botox Pediatric Dosing (units/kg)	No. of Injection Sites/Muscle (Pediatrics)	Botox Adult Dosing (units/visit)	No. of injection Sites/Muscle (Adult)
Adducted/internally rotated shoulder	Pectoralis major and minor	2	2–3	75–150	4
	Latissimus dorsi	2	2	50–150	4
	Teres major	2	1–2		
Flexed elbow	Brachioradialis	1	1	25–75	2
	Biceps	2	2–3	50–200	4
	Brachialis	2	1–2	25–75	2
Flexed wrist	Flexor carpi radialis	1–2	1	25–100	2
	Flexor carpi ulnaris	1–2	1	10–50	2
Fist	Flexor digitorum superficialis	1–2	1–2	25–75	4
	Flexor digitorum profundus	1–2	1–2	25–100	2
Flexed hip	Iliacus	1–2	1–2	50–150	2
	Rectus femoris	3–4	2	75–200	3
Flexed knee	Medial hamstrings	3–6	3–4	50–150	3
	Gastrocnemius	3–6	2–4	50–150	4
	Lateral hamstrings	2–3	1–2	100–200	3
Adducted thighs	Adductor brevis/longus/magnus	3–6	1–2	75–300	6/leg
Equinovarus foot	Medial and lateral	3–6	1–2	50–200	4
	Gastrocnemius	2–3	1–2	50–100	2
	Soleus	1–3	1	50–150	3
	Tibialis anterior	1–2	1	50–200	2
	Tibialis posterior	1–2	1	50–100	4
	Flexor digitorum longus/brevis				

Dosing Guidelines: 400 units = total maximum dose per visit for adults; 400 units or <12 units/kg = total maximum dose per visit for children; 50 units = maximum dose per injection site.

Adapted from Russman BS, Tilton A, Gormley ME: Cerebral palsy: A rational approach to a treatment protocol and the role of botulinum toxin in treatment, *Muscle Nerve Suppl* 6:S181–S206, 1997; and Brin MF, and the Spasticity Study Group: Dosing, administration, and a treatment algorithm for use of botulinum toxin A for adult-onset spasticity, *Muscle Nerve Suppl* 6:S208–S220, 1997.

(LD_{50}) in humans is not known but has been determined in monkeys and is approximately 40 units/kg with either intramuscular or intravenous administration. An antitoxin is available if complications occur.

BoNT-A should be diluted with preservative-free 0.9% saline solution and used within 4 hours.[57] Dilution, needle size, and injection site per muscle vary according to clinician preference. BoNT-A injections can be guided by muscle palpation, with electromyography, or by electrical stimulation with a Teflon-coated needle. Some have suggested that injecting near the motor end plate produces greater denervation, but these areas can be difficult to locate because of variability of location.[56,58] Electromyography can be used to determine injection sites, especially during complex activities such as gait to identify where muscles are overactive. Deeper muscles or muscles not under volitional control can demonstrate improved clinical benefit when identified with electrical stimulation.[59] Typically, when the needle is inserted to locate the muscle by using electrical stimulation, the same site is used for the insertion of the needle for BoNT-A injections. When BoNT-A is injected into the proximal muscles, a much larger dose is needed to have a clinical effect, based on muscle size, compared with that needed for smaller muscles. Because there is a limited safe dosage of the total BoNT-A allowable every 3 months, the clinician can use the entire dosage on one or two larger proximal muscles.

After numerous injections of BoNT-A, some patients may develop antibodies, thereby rendering the injections ineffective. However, if only the minimum dose of 400 units is used and injections are given at 3-month intervals, this can be minimized.[52] Swelling can occur at or around the injection site, especially in the lower leg, and should be treated with cold compresses and an elastic wrap to minimize it. Dysphagia has also been reported to be an adverse effect of BoNT-A in the treatment of cervical dystonia, presumed to be related to toxin diffusion from an injection into the sternocleidomastoid muscle.[66] Weakness, however, is the most common adverse effect with the use of BoNT-A. The toxin does spread to neighboring muscles and possibly into the CNS by retrograde transmission. This may be of concern when injections are given to large muscles that may be needed for functional tasks. Therefore when treatment with BoNT-A is considered, it is important to make sure that loss of muscle function will not limit functional capacity. For example, in the quadriceps group, injection to the rectus femoris may decrease knee extension during the swing phase of gait while still preserving knee extension during stance through the action of the other recti. Because of potential loss of hip flexion after injection to the rectus femoris, sufficient strength of the iliopsoas muscles must be available to compensate.

Long-term effects of BoNT-A injections have been reported, but they are isolated and distinct problems without an overall pattern.[52] Gallbladder emptying has been slowed by these injections. There have also been reports of brachial plexus problems after sternocleidomastoid injections and a report of urinary incontinence after injections for lower extremity spasticity. Changes in muscle fiber size have been reported but seem to have little clinical significance.

Hyman et al reported that the two most frequent adverse events in patients treated with BoNT-A were hypertonia (new or worsening spasticity after the drug wears off) of injected and/or noninjected muscles and weakness of noninjected muscles caused by spread of the drug.[67] The authors reported that this could have been attributed to normal variation in the disease state in the study sample (patients with MS).

BoNT-A is used for a variety of conditions that produce muscle overactivity.[52,67] The list is long and includes strabismus, blepharospasm, hemifacial spasm, cervical dystonia, writer's cramp, tremors, tics, and, of course, spasticity related to CNS injury or disease. The U.S. Food and Drug Administration (FDA) has recently approved Botox under the label "Botox Cosmetic" for the treatment of frown lines.

Intramuscular injections of BTX have been found to reduce the muscle tone of extremities in patients with stroke, brain injury, SCI, neurodegenerative diseases, and MS. Richardson et al conducted a randomized, placebo-controlled trial of BoNT-A injection to the upper and lower limbs of patients with stroke, head injury, incomplete SCI, tumors, and CP.[68] The authors identified improvements in the Ashworth scale of spasticity severity, passive ROM, motor scores, and subjective ratings of severity. This underscores the notion that BoNT-A can alleviate spasticity, regardless of cause.

In the cases in which functional recovery cannot be reasonably expected, BoNT-A has been demonstrated to be effective in increasing mobility to improve personal care and hygiene activities. Examples include reducing adductor spasticity for improved hygiene activities in the genital region and in positional flexor spasticity for improved hand hygiene activity and dressing.[67-72]

There are numerous reports of reduction in muscle tone after an injection of BoNT-A for a variety of diagnoses. In patients with SCI, Keren et al found that the injection of 200 to 300 units of BTX into the lower limbs was effective in reducing spasticity and improving gait.[73] Wilson et al performed a three-dimensional gait analysis on a single subject with traumatic brain injury who received BoNT-A in the ankle plantar flexors.[74] The subject demonstrated improved kinematic angles, such as knee extension and ankle dorsiflexion, throughout the gait cycle. Additionally, increased stride time and gait velocity were exhibited. Yablon et al studied the effect of BoNT-A on upper limb spasticity in 21 patients with traumatic brain injury, categorized as either acute or chronic.[70] Chemodenervation combined with physical therapy exercises such as passive ROM exercises and modalities significantly improved ROM and significantly reduced spasticity as measured by the Ashworth scale of spasticity severity.

Wissel et al evaluated two doses—a high dose and a low dose—of BoNT-A in a randomized double-blind study of children and teenagers with spastic gait caused by CP.[75] Both the high-dose group and the low-dose group demonstrated significant improvement in muscle spasticity and knee ROM, but a high dose was needed for significant improvement in ankle ROM, gait velocity, and stride length after injection. However, 200 units of BoNT-A distributed to four to five muscles per leg was better than 100 units without significant adverse effects. Koman et al conducted a randomized, double-blind, placebo-controlled clinical trial on BoNT-A for lower limb spasticity in CP.[76] Approximately 50% to 60% of the children with CP in the BoNT-A group demonstrated significantly higher physician rating scores (specifically the ankle component of gait), greater ROM (increased between 3 and 7 degrees), and a significant reduction in the M response. In the recent consensus statement by Delgado et al the authors reported that although there is sufficient evidence to recommend BoNT-A as an effective antispasticity treatment in children with CP, its beneficial effects on function, ease of caregiving, activity, and participation need to be established.[18] More data about safety and long-term effects are also needed.

BTX has also been shown to reduce spasticity in neurodegenerative diseases. Spasticity resulting from MS was evaluated by Hyman et al who studied adductor spasticity.[67] After 4 weeks, the authors found that 1500 units of Dysport resulted in statistically significant improvement in maximal distance between the knees, indicating reduced adductor muscle tone. Hyman et al recommended that the clinical dose of 500 to 1000 units, divided between both legs, was best because the group that received 1500 units sometimes demonstrated too much weakness.[67] Giladi and Honigman reported on a single case of BoNT-A injection into one leg of a patient with Parkinson's disease to alleviate freezing of gait.[77] The freezing of gait was determined to have been due to focal foot dystonia. After injections to the extensor hallicis longus and gastrocnemius, the patient reported almost complete reduction in gait hesitation.

Hesse et al studied 12 patients with stroke and chronic hemiparesis using electronic goniometry and electromyography and found that approximately 75% of these patients demonstrated a more normal temporal pattern of muscle activity with a prominent reduction in premature activity of the plantar flexors after BoNT-A injection.[78] Brashear et al performed a placebo-controlled clinical trial of 126 patients with stroke and upper-limb spasticity.[79] The injections produced a significant decrease in wrist and finger muscle tone as measured by the Ashworth scale of spasticity severity, especially during week 4 of a 12-week protocol.

Considerations for the Physical Therapist. The physical therapist should expect that the patient may show diminished function initially after a BTX injection as a result of uncovering of weakness in the antagonist muscles. The therapist should pay particular attention to safety issues while the patient adapts to the new reduced muscle tone. Use of physical therapy modalities over the injection site is contraindicated for at least 10 days.

MUSCLE RELAXANTS

Muscle relaxants are drugs typically used for relaxation of spasms caused by musculoskeletal injury. The two agents covered in this section are cyclobenzaprine, an oral agent, and the topical agent dichlorodifluoromethane. These drugs are typically used for the treatment of low back pain resulting from muscle spasms, certain types of pain resulting from tight muscles such as the hamstrings, headache related to muscle tension, and referred pain caused by trigger points.

Cyclobenzaprine Hydrochloride (Flexeril)

Cyclobenzaprine improves the signs and symptoms of skeletal muscle spasm. Additional improvements can be seen in the reduction of local pain and tenderness, increased ROM, and less restriction in ADLs. Improvements can be seen as early as the first day of therapy.

Cyclobenzaprine relieves skeletal muscle spasm locally without interfering with muscle function and therefore is ineffective in treating spasms of CNS origin. Animal studies show that cyclobenzaprine acts at the brainstem rather than at the spinal cord. The net effect of cyclobenzaprine is a reduction of tonic somatic motor activity, influencing both gamma (γ) and alpha (α) motor systems.[9] Orally administered cyclobenzaprine is well absorbed but has a lengthy elimination time. Its half life is between 1 and 3 days.

Cyclobenzaprine is used as an adjunct to physical therapy and rest for the treatment of muscle spasms, which are most often caused by an acute musculoskeletal injury. Its benefit is indicated by reduction of pain and tenderness, increased ROM, and improvement in ADLs. Cyclobenzaprine should only be used for a short period, about 2 to 3 weeks. There is inadequate evidence of long-term use because it is beneficial in treating acute injuries.

Cyclobenzaprine is contraindicated during the immediate recovery phase of myocardial infarction, arrhythmias, heart block or other conduction disturbances, and congestive heart failure. Additionally, the drug should not be used if hyperthyroidism is present because of the drug's atropine-like action. Similarly, cyclobenzaprine should be used with caution in patients with a history of urinary retention, in those with glaucoma or increased intraocular pressure, and in those taking anticholinergic medication.[9] Cyclobenzaprine can enhance the effects of alcohol and barbiturates and other CNS depressants.

The usual dosage of cyclobenzaprine is 10 mg three times a day, with a range of 20 to 40 mg a day in divided doses. Dose should not exceed 60 mg a day. Use of cyclobenzaprine for periods longer than 2 or 3 weeks is not recommended.[9] The most common adverse effects reported by patients who take cyclobenzaprine are drowsiness, dry mouth, and dizziness. Less frequent adverse effects are fatigue or tiredness, asthenia, nausea, constipation, dyspepsia, unpleasant taste, blurred vision, headache, nervousness, and confusion.

Cyclobenzaprine was compared with diazepam and placebo in double-blind trials for efficacy in treating spasms and pain in the neck and low back. Clinical improvement over 2 weeks was statistically significant in all treatment groups with a preference for cyclobenzaprine. The most striking improvements recorded were seen in electromyographic findings, which showed statistically significant changes for this group.[80] Borenstein and Korn conducted randomized controlled trials to assess the efficacy and tolerability of cyclobenzaprine 2.5, 5, and 10 mg tid, compared with placebo, in patients with acute musculoskeletal spasm.[81] Neither study included a nonsteroidal anti-inflammatory drug (NSAID) as an active control, which is frequently prescribed along with cyclobenzaprine. Cyclobenzaprine 2.5 mg tid was not significantly more effective than placebo, but the cyclobenzaprine 5- and 10-mg tid regimens were associated with significantly higher mean efficacy scores compared with placebo. Cyclobenzaprine 5 mg tid was as effective as 10 mg tid and was associated with a lower incidence of sedation. Katz and Dube reported that cyclobenzaprine was found to have a more rapid onset of action than diazepam and was associated with few serious adverse experiences.[82] The authors concluded that cyclobenzaprine represents a cost-effective approach to the management of acute muscle spasms, primarily because of the rapid symptomatic relief that it provides.

Dichlorodifluoromethane: (Fluori-Methane)

Dichlorodifluoromethane is a vapocoolant spray intended for topical use.[8] It is used for the management of pain and muscle spasms and myofascial pain and for the prevention of pain caused by muscular injections. In the case of muscle spasms, the spray sweeps should move from the muscle origin to the insertion. In the case of a trigger point, sweeping the target and referral zone is advisable. During the spraying procedure, the muscle is passively stretched, and the stretch is gradually increased with successive sweeps. As this is continued, a new resting length of the muscle is achieved. This new resting length should eliminate muscle spasms and trigger point pain. After the muscle has been rewarmed, the spraying procedure can be repeated until the pain is significantly reduced or eliminated. The technique can be followed with the application of a heat pack to enhance the warming. Postural and relaxation exercises or any other therapeutic technique to reduce the primary source of the muscle spasms and pain should be applied.[9]

Dichlorodifluoromethane spray can also be used for preinjection analgesia. The spray is applied to minimize cutaneous sensation before injection and has been demonstrated to be a useful technique in children to reduce the anxiety associated with injections.[83]

This product should not be used in individuals who are hypersensitive to dichlorodifluoromethane. It is especially contraindicated in individuals with vascular insufficiencies because the drop in surface temperature may result in further vessel constriction. Dichlorodifluoromethane should be used with caution to avoid inhalation of vapors, especially when applied around the face and neck, such as when it is used for facial neuralgia.[83] Contact with the eyes should be avoided, and use of the drug should never be prolonged as to take a region to the frost point. It must be remembered that the contents of the bottle are under pressure and therefore should be stored in a cool dry place (not over 120°F) away from high-frequency ultrasound equipment.

The application of dichlorodifluoromethane for myofascial pain involves three steps—evaluation, spraying, and stretching—which, if performed in the proper sequence, produce optimal results.[84] Evaluation is done to determine whether the pain is due to muscle spasms or a trigger point. The spraying phase involves positioning the patient in a comfortable position and covering the eyes and nose if spraying will be done near the face. The spraying technique involves inverting the bottle at least 12 inches (30 to 45 cm) away from the target area and pressing the valve to release a stream of vapocoolant spray. The stream should be applied at an oblique angle parallel to the muscle belly fibers in rows about 2 to 3 cm apart and at a rate of 10 cm/sec until the entire muscle is covered. Passive stretching is then performed.

Though extremely rare, cutaneous sensitization is possible. Also rare is skin discoloration or pigment change. Apart from these, there are relatively few adverse effects of the topical treatment, as long as the nose and eyes are protected when dichlorodifluoromethane is applied around the face.

EXERCISES

1. Review the literature on botulinum toxin (BTX), and discuss the advantages BTX has over alcohol and phenol injections. Discuss patient selection issues.
2. A 12-year-old boy with a diagnosis of CP (spastic quadriplegia) has been taking baclofen for the past 6 months. After careful titration, 20 mg qid (oral) was determined to be the optimal dosage. At this dosage, the patient needed only minimal assistance for dressing and was independent in both transfers and hygiene activities. In addition, the patient progressed to independent ambulation with a rolling walker. However, over the last several weeks, there has been an increase in rigidity and spasticity of the lower extremities. The patient now requires moderate assistance for all dressing and hygiene activities, and ambulation is now too slow to be functional. The patient's mother reports that he is very distressed over his loss of function. Today, however, his condition has worsened and appears to be different from what it was in previous weeks. She brings him to the emergency department because he is confused, weak, and very lethargic.

   Questions

   A. Why did this patient develop increased spasticity after 6 months of improved function?
   B. Are the patient's current symptoms due to the adverse effects of the drug, drug withdrawal, or drug overdose?
   C. How should this patient's spasticity be managed without causing drowsiness or muscular weakness?
   D. Describe the role of the physical therapist in an "intrathecal baclofen screening trial."
3. Identify the most probable pharmacologic management of spasticity in the following cases:
   A. Recent stroke (months) with the goal of increasing active finger extension
   B. Recent stroke (months) with severe spasticity of the arm and leg
   C. Nonrecent stroke (years) with upper extremity spasticity greater than the lower extremity
   D. MS with widespread spasticity of the lower extremities
4. What factors must the therapist consider before referring a patient for pharmacologic management of spasticity?

REFERENCES

1. Lance JW: Spasticity: Disordered motor control, Chicago, 1980, Yearbook Medical Publishers.
2. Kita M, Goodkin DE: Drugs used to treat spasticity. Drugs 59:487-495, 2000.
3. Denny-Brown D, Feldman RG: Historical aspects of the relation of spasticity to movement. In Feldman RG, Young RR, Koella WP, editors: Spasticity: Disordered motor control, Chicago, 1980, Yearbook Medical Publishers.
4. Ivanhoe CB, Reistetter TA: Spasticity: The misunderstood part of upper motor neuron syndrome. Am J Phys Med Rehabil 83:S3-S9, 2004.
5. Sehgal N, McGuire JR: Beyond Ashworth: Electrophysiologic quantification of spasticity. Phys Med Rehabil Clin N Am 9: 949-979, 1998.
6. Francisco GE, Kothari S, Huls C: GABA agonists and gabapentin for spastic hypertonia. Phys Med Rehabil Clin N Am 12:875-888, 2001.
7. Yelnik AP, Simon O, Bensmail D, et al: Professional practices and recommendations: Drug treatments for spasticity. Ann PhysRehabilitat Med 52:746-756, 2009.
8. Gracies JM, Nance P, Elovic E, McGuire J, Simpson DM: Traditional pharmacological treatments for spasticity. Part II: General and regional treatments. Muscle Nerve Suppl 6:S92-S120, 1997.
9. Mosby: Mosby's drug consult, St Louis, MO, 2005, Mosby.
10. Murinson BB: Stiff-person syndrome. Neurologist 10:131-137, 2004.
11. Cutson TM, Gray SL, Hughes MA, Carson SW, Hanlon JT: Effect of a single dose of diazepam on balance measures in older people. J Am Geriatr Soc 45:435-440, 1997.
12. Patel, DR, Soyode O: Pharmacologic interventions for reducing spasticity in cerebral palsy. Indian J Pediatr 72(10):869-872, 2005.
13. Kitajima T, Kanbayashi T, Saito Y, et al: Diazepam reduces both arterial blood pressure and muscle sympathetic nerve activity in humans. Neurosci Lett 355:77-80, 2004.
14. Beard S, Hunn A, Wight J: Treatments for spasticity and pain in multiple sclerosis: A systematic review. Health Technol Assess 7: iii, ix-x:1-111, 2003.
15. Broderick CP, Radnitz CL, Bauman WA: Diazepam usage in veterans with spinal cord injury. J Spinal Cord Med 20:406-409, 1997.
16. Davidoff RA: Antispasticity drugs: Mechanisms of action. Ann Neurol 17:107-116, 1985.
17. Cruikshrank M, Eunson P: Intravenous diazepam infusion in the management of planned intrathecal baclofen withdrawal. Dev Med Child Neurol 49(8):626-628, 2007.
18. Delgado MR, Hirtz D, Aisen M, et al: Practice parameter: Pharmacologic treatment of spasticity in children and adolescents with cerebral palsy (an evidence-based review): Report of the Quality Standards Subcommittee of the American Academy of Neurology and the Practice Committee of the Child Neurology Society. Neurology 74(4):336-343, 2010.
19. Elovic E: Principles of pharmaceutical management of spastic hypertonia. Phys Med Rehabil Clin N Am 12:793-816, 2001.
20. Glass A, Hannah A: A comparison of dantrolene sodium and diazepam in the treatment of spasticity. Paraplegia 12:170-176, 1974.
21. Zafonte R, Lombard L, Elovic E: Antispasticity medications: Uses and limitations of enteral therapy. Am J Phys Med Rehabil 83:S50-S58, 2004.
22. Chan CH: Dantrolene sodium and hepatic injury. Neurology 40:1427-1432, 1990.
23. Steinberg F, Ferguson K: Effect of dantrolene sodium on spasticity associated with hemiplegia. J Am Geriatr Soc 23:70-73, 1975.
24. Krach L: Pharmacotherapy of spasticity: Oral medications and intrathecal baclofen. J Child Neurol 16:31-36, 2001.
25. Ketel W, Kolb M: Long term treatment with dantrolene sodium of stroke patients with spasticity limiting return of function. Curr Med Res Opin 9:161-169, 1984.
26. Pierson SH: Outcome measures in spasticity management. Muscle Nerve Suppl 6:S36-S60, 1997.
27. Bresolin N, Zucca C, Pecori A: Efficacy and tolerability of eperisone and baclofen in spastic palsy: A double-blind randomized trial. Adv Ther 26(5):563-573, 2009. Epub 2009.
28. Sakai Y, Matsuyama Y, Nakamura H, et al: The effect of muscle relaxant on the paraspinal muscle blood flow. Spine 33(6):581-587, 2008.
29. Milla PJ, Jackson AD: A controlled trial of baclofen in children with cerebral palsy. J Int Med Res 5:398-404, 1977.
30. Scheinberg A, Hall K, Lam LT, O'Flaherty S: Oral baclofen in children with cerebral palsy: A double-blind cross-over pilot study. J Paediatr Child Health 42:715-720, 2006.
31. Dai AI, Wasay M, Awan S: Botulinum toxin type A with oral baclofen versus oral tizanidine: A nonrandomized pilot comparison in patients with cerebral palsy and spastic equinus foot deformity. J Child Neurol 23(12):1464-1466, 2008.
32. van Doornik J, Kukke S, McGill K, Rose J, Sherman-Levine S, Sanger TD: Oral baclofen increases maximal voluntary neuromuscular activation of ankle plantar flexors in children with spasticity due to cerebral palsy. J Child Neurol 23(6):635-639, 2008. Epub 2008.
33. Castellano C, Brioni JD, McGaugh JL: Post-training systemic and intra-amygdala administration of the GABA-B agonist baclofen impairs retention. Behav Neurol Biol 52(2):170-179, 1989.
34. Terrence CF, Fromm GH, Roussan MS: Baclofen: Its effect on seizure frequency. Arch Neurol 40:28-29, 1983.
35. Taricco M, Adone R, Pagliacci C: Pharmacological interventions for spasticity following spinal cord injury. Cochrane Database Syst Rev 2:CD001131, 2000.
36. Nielsen JF, Sinkjaer T: Peripheral and central effect of baclofen on ankle joint stiffness in multiple sclerosis. Muscle Nerve 23:98-105, 2000.
37. Orsnes G, Sorensen P, Larsen T: Effect of baclofen on gait in spastic MS patients. Acta Neurol Scand 101:244-248, 2000.
38. Meythaler JM, Guin-Renfroe S, Brunner RC, Hadley MN: Intrathecal baclofen for spastic hypertonia from stroke. Stroke 32(9):2099-2109, 2001.
39. Barry MJ, Shultz BL: Intrathecal baclofen therapy and the role of the physical therapist. Pediatr Phys Ther 12:77-86, 2000.
40. Bowden M, Stokic DS: Clinical and neurophysiologic assessment of strength and spasticity during intrathecal baclofen titration in incomplete spinal cord injury: Single-subject design. J Spinal Cord Med 32(2):183-190, 2009.
41. Borowski A, Littleton AG, Borkhuu B, et al: Complications of intrathecal baclofen pump therapy in pediatric patients. J Pediatr Orthop 30(1):76-81, 2010.
42. Motta F, Buonaguro V, Stignani C: The use of intrathecal baclofen pump implants in children and adolescents: Safety and complications in 200 consecutive cases. J Neurosurg 107:32-35, 2007.
43. Kofler M, Quirbach E, Schauer R, Singer M, Saltuari L: Limitations of intrathecal baclofen for spastic hemiparesis following stroke. Neurorehabil Neural Repair 23(1):26-31, 2009. Epub 2008.
44. Taricco M, Pagliacci MC, Telaro E, Adone R: Pharmacological interventions for spasticity following spinal cord injury: Results of a Cochrane systematic review. Eur Medicophys 42(1):5-15, 2006.
45. Thomas CK, Häger-Ross CK, Klein CS: Effects of baclofen on motor units paralysed by chronic cervical spinal cord injury. Brain 133(Pt 1):117-125, 2010.

46. Skoog B: A comparison of the effects of two antispastic drugs, tizanidine and baclofen, on synaptic transmission from muscle spindle afferents to spinal interneurons in cats. Acta Physiol Scand 156:81-90, 1996.
47. Wallace JD: Summary of combined clinical analysis of controlled clinical trials with tizanidine. Neurology 44:S60-S68; discussion S68-S69, 1994.
48. Lataste X, Emre M, Davis C, Groves L: Comparative profile of tizanidine in the management of spasticity. Neurology 44:S53-S59, 1994.
49. Groves L, Shellenberger MK, Davis CS: Tizanidine treatment of spasticity: A meta-analysis of controlled, double-blind, comparative studies with baclofen and diazepam. Adv Ther 15:241-251, 1998.
50. Nance PW, Sheremata WA, Lynch SG, et al: Relationship of the antispasticity effect of tizanidine to plasma concentration in patients with multiple sclerosis. Arch Neurol 54:731-736, 1997.
51. Kamen L, Henney HR III, Runyan JD: A practical overview of tizanidine use for spasticity secondary to multiple sclerosis, stroke, and spinal cord injury. Curr Med Res Opin 24(2):425-439, 2008.
52. Gracies JM, Elovic E, McGuire J, Simpson DM: Traditional pharmacological treatments for spasticity. Part I: Local treatments. Muscle Nerve Suppl 6:S61-S90, 1997.
53. Little JW, Micklesen P, Umlauf R, Britell C: Lower extremity manifestations of spasticity in chronic spinal cord injury. Am J Phys Med Rehabil 68:32-36, 1989.
54. Bell KR: The use of neurolytic blocks for the management of spasticity. Phys Med Rehabil Clin N Am 6:885-895, 1995.
55. On AY, Kirazli Y, Kismali B, Aksit R: Mechanisms of action of phenol block and botulinus toxin type A in relieving spasticity: Electrophysiologic investigation and follow-up. Am J Phys Med Rehabil 78:344-349, 1999.
56. McGuire JR: Effective use of chemodenervation and chemical neurolysis in the management of poststroke spasticity. Top Stroke Rehabil 8:47-55, 2001.
57. O'Brien CF: Injection techniques for botulinum toxin using electromyography and electrical stimulation. Muscle Nerve Suppl 6:S176-S180, 1997.
58. Shaari CM, Sanders I: Quantifying how location and dose of botulinum toxin injections affect muscle paralysis. Muscle Nerve 16:964-969, 1993.
59. Comella CL, Buchman AS, Tanner CM, Brown-Toms NC, Goetz CG: Botulinum toxin injection for spasmodic torticollis: Increased magnitude of benefit with electromyographic assistance. Neurology 42(4):878-882, 1992.
60. Bell KR: The use of neurolytic blocks for the management of spasticity. Phys Med Rehabil Clin N Am 6:885-895, 1995.
61. Elovic EP, Esquenazi A, Alter KE, Lin JL, Alfaro A, Kaelin DL: Chemodenervation and nerve blocks in the diagnosis and management of spasticity and muscle overactivity. Phys Med Rehabilitat 1(9):842-851, 2009.
62. Glenn MWJ: Practical management of spasticity in children and adults. In Glenn M, editor: Nerve blocks, Philadelphia, 1990, Lea & Febiger.
63. Kirshblum S: Treatment alternatives for spinal cord injury related spasticity. J Spinal Cord Med 22:199-217, 1999.
64. Bakheit A: Management of muscle spasticity. Crit Rev Phys Med Rehabil 8:235-252, 1996.
65. Brin MF: Botulinum toxin: Chemistry, pharmacology, toxicity, and immunology. Muscle Nerve Suppl 6:S146-S168, 1997.
66. Jankovic J, Schwartz K, Donovan DT: Botulinum toxin treatment of cranial-cervical dystonia, spasmodic dysphonia, other focal dystonias and hemifacial spasm. J Neurol Neurosurg Psychiatry 53:633-639, 1990.
67. Hyman N, Barnes M, Bhakta B, et al: Botulinum toxin (Dysport) treatment of hip adductor spasticity in multiple sclerosis: A prospective, randomised, double blind, placebo controlled, dose ranging study. J Neurol Neurosurg Psychiatry 68:707-712, 2000.
68. Richardson D, Sheean G, Werring D, et al: Evaluating the role of botulinum toxin in the management of focal hypertonia in adults. J Neurol Neurosurg Psychiatry 69:499-506, 2000.
69. Snow BJ, Tsui JK, Bhatt MH, Varelas M, Hashimoto SA, Calne DB: Treatment of spasticity with botulinum toxin: A double-blind study. Ann Neurol 28:512-515, 1990.
70. Yablon SA, Agana BT, Ivanhoe CB, Boake C: Botulinum toxin in severe upper extremity spasticity among patients with traumatic brain injury: An open-labeled trial. Neurology 47(4):939-944, 1996.
71. Bakheit AM, Pittock S, Moore AP, et al: A randomized, double-blind, placebo-controlled study of the efficacy and safety of botulinum toxin type A in upper limb spasticity in patients with stroke. Eur J Neurol 8:559-565, 2001.
72. Bhakta BB, Cozens JA, Chamberlain MA, Bamford JM: Impact of botulinum toxin type A on disability and caregiver burden due to arm spasticity after stroke: A randomised double blind placebo controlled trial. J Neurol Neurosurg Psychiatry 69:217-221, 2000.
73. Keren O, Shinberg F, Catz A, Giladi N: Botulin toxin for spasticity in spinal cord damage by treating the motor endplate [in Hebrew]. Harefuah 138:204-208, 270, 2000.
74. Wilson DJ, Childers MK, Cooke DL, Smith BK: Kinematic changes following botulinum toxin injection after traumatic brain injury. Brain Inj 11:157-167, 1997.
75. Wissel J, Heinen F, Schenkel A, et al: Botulinum toxin A in the management of spastic gait disorders in children and young adults with cerebral palsy: A randomized, double-blind study of "high-dose" versus "low-dose" treatment. Neuropediatrics 30:120-124, 1999.
76. Koman LA, Mooney JF III, Smith BP, Walker F, Leon JM: Botulinum toxin type A neuromuscular blockade in the treatment of lower extremity spasticity in cerebral palsy: A randomized, double-blind, placebo-controlled trial. BOTOX Study Group. J Pediatr Orthop 20:108-115, 2000.
77. Giladi N, Honigman S: Botulinum toxin injections to one leg alleviates freezing of gait in a patient with Parkinson's disease. Mov Disord 12:1085-1086, 1997.
78. Hesse S, Krajnik J, Luecke D, Jahnke MT, Gregoric M, Mauritz KH: Ankle muscle activity before and after botulinum toxin therapy for lower limb extensor spasticity in chronic hemiparetic patients. Stroke 27:455-460, 1996.
79. Brashear A, Gordon MF, Elovic E, et al: Intramuscular injection of botulinum toxin for the treatment of wrist and finger spasticity after a stroke. N Engl J Med 347:395-400, 2002.
80. Basmajian JV: Cyclobenzaprine hydrochloride effect on skeletal muscle spasm in the lumbar region and neck: Two double-blind controlled clinical and laboratory studies. Arch Phys Med Rehabil 59:58-63, 1978.
81. Borenstein DG, Korn S: Efficacy of a low-dose regimen of cyclobenzaprine hydrochloride in acute skeletal muscle spasm: Results of two placebo-controlled trials. Clin Ther 25:1056-1073, 2003.
82. Katz WA, Dube J: Cyclobenzaprine in the treatment of acute muscle spasm: review of a decade of clinical experience. Clin Ther 10:216-228, 1988.
83. Cohen Reis E, Holubkov R: Vapocoolant spray is equally effective as EMLA cream in reducing immunization pain in school-aged children. Pediatrics 100:E5, 1997.
84. Travell J: Identification of myofascial trigger point syndromes: A case of atypical facial neuralgia. Arch Phys Med Rehabil 62:100-106, 1981.

17

Pharmacologic Management of Degenerative Neurologic Disorders

Lee Dibble

INTRODUCTION

The focus of this chapter is on degenerative diseases of the nervous system. Although great time and detail could be spent on the wide spectrum of neurodegenerative disorders, the discussion in this chapter is limited to three specific pathologic conditions. The three conditions covered here—Parkinson's disease (PD), multiple sclerosis (MS), and Alzheimer's disease (AD)—all have unclear etiologies, although a genetic predisposition and environmental exposure appear to play a part in all three cases.

Because no distinct causative agent has been identified in any of these conditions, the current pharmacologic management focuses on addressing body system abnormalities imposed by the disease (neurotransmitter dysfunction in PD and AD and immune system dysfunction in MS). In addition, because these conditions are progressive, the needs for pharmacologic management may change over time. The sections on each of these disorders include discussions of basic epidemiology and pathology, followed by treatments targeted at the impaired system. Given the unclear etiologies of these disorders, in each section, a discussion of treatments targeted at slowing neuronal loss (neuroprotection) is provided for each of the three conditions.

PARKINSON'S DISEASE: EPIDEMIOLOGY AND PATHOLOGY

PD is common among older people, affecting more than 1 in every 100 people over the age of 75 years and 1 in every 1000 people over the age of 65 years.[1] Globally, it is estimated that 10 million older people have PD.[2] As a result of an increasing proportion of the population being older than 60 years, it has been estimated that by the year 2020, more than 40 million people in the world will have PD.

The primary movement deficits associated with PD are akinesia (delayed initiation of movement), bradykinesia (slowness of movement), postural instability, rigidity, and tremor.[2] The neurochemical origin of these movement disturbances is a neurotransmitter imbalance in the basal ganglia, a region of the brain thought to be critical in the production of voluntary movement (specifically the execution of well-learned automatic movements). The neurotransmitter imbalance develops in the motor circuit from the frontal lobe to the basal ganglia to the motor cortex as a result of progressive death of dopamine-producing neurons in the substantia nigra pars compacta of the basal ganglia. The cause of the selective neuronal death that occurs is not known, although current theories support the interaction of environmental exposure and a genetic predisposition to PD. Considerable evidence suggests that the interplay of genetics and the environment leads to mitochondrial dysfunction and oxidative damage, which contribute to neuronal death. The result of dopaminergic cell loss is a disruption of the fine balance of dopamine, acetylcholine, gamma (γ)-aminobutyric acid (GABA), and other neurotransmitters in the basal ganglia and in the projections of the basal ganglia throughout the central nervous system (CNS).[2]

Despite little knowledge regarding the cause of the neurotransmitter imbalance, medical management of PD does result in improved movement abilities and reductions in most of the primary movement deficits. Pharmacologic management of PD can be divided into several categories: (1) dopamine replacement, (2) increasing dopamine stimulation, and (3) modulation of nondopaminergic systems. Treatments targeted at these categories strive to restore a neurochemical balance in the basal ganglia and its functionally connected areas. The following sections describe the pharmacologic mechanisms of action and the positive and negative effects of these medications. This section on PD ends with a discussion of the effects of the medications on movement abilities and a discussion of pharmacologic treatments targeted toward neuroprotection so that the degradation of the neurons within the basal ganglia is slowed.

Dopamine Replacement

In 1960, studies of cadaveric brains of individuals who had extrapyramidal movement disorders suggested that the loss of dopamine in a portion of the basal ganglia was characteristic in persons with PD.[3,4] This neuroanatomic finding led to experimentation with dopamine replacement as a means of treating persons with PD. Although dopamine was determined to be the neurotransmitter that is deficient in the basal ganglia in patients with PD, dopamine did not cross the blood–brain barrier and therefore was ineffective in reducing the cardinal symptoms associated with PD (the motor impairments of bradykinesia, tremor, rigidity, and postural instability). However, the utility of the dopamine precursor levodopa (L-dopa) was studied and found to be effective.[5] As opposed to dopamine, L-dopa is able to cross the blood–brain barrier, and it then undergoes enzymatic conversion to dopamine.[6-8] At present, dopamine replacement with L-dopa is the most effective and widely used treatment for PD.[9-11] Levodopa is available as an oral medication that is coupled with a dopamine decarboxylase inhibitor (carbidopa or benserazide) to minimize metabolism outside of the CNS (Figure 17-1).

Positive Effects of Dopamine Replacement on Movement Tasks. The majority of studies describe the benefits of pharmacologic therapy in PD in terms of outcomes on the Unified Parkinson's Disease Rating Scale (UPDRS).[12,13] Although the UPDRS is the primary outcome measure used to judge symptomatic relief in studies of dopamine agonists and other medications, studies of L-dopa have included more sensitive measures of bradykinesia, tremor, rigidity, and postural instability.[13,14]

Dopamine replacement results in substantial increases in overall movement velocity compared with the off-medication state. This improved movement velocity appears to be due in part to the improved magnitude of agonist muscle action potentials as determined by electromyography (EMG). Although dopamine replacement improves the magnitude of the initial agonist EMG bursts, dopamine replacement appears to have little effect on the temporal aspects (burst duration, multiple agonist bursts, timing of antagonist bursts) of EMG control.[15-34] Therefore dopamine replacement may preferentially affect only one of the determinants of force generation and is limited in its ability to improve muscle activation in patients with PD.[33,35-41]

Studies of the effects of dopamine replacement on tremor have demonstrated a 50% reduction in tremor amplitude.[42-44] Although results of these studies support the effectiveness of dopamine replacement in reduction of tremor, other reports have indicated little or no response to dopamine replacement and better responses to other medications (e.g., anticholinergics). Such findings suggest that tremor associated with PD may have multiple causes with contributions from both dopaminergic and nondopaminergic pathways.[42]

Studies which examined PD rigidity consistently demonstrated reductions in tonic EMG activity as a result of dopamine replacement. Such findings suggest that the active muscle contribution to rigidity is diminished by dopamine replacement.[26,27,44,45]

Although force production and coordination of anticipatory postural tasks have been shown to improve in response to dopamine replacement, control of the center of mass during reactive postural control tasks is adversely affected.[46-49] Specifically, dopamine replacement appears to diminish distal lower extremity background postural tone and lower the magnitude of reactive EMG bursts in response to displacements of the surface on which subjects are standing. The functional consequences of this abnormality are that dopamine replacement may reduce the ability of a patient with PD to react appropriately and regain his or her balance if pushed.[47-56]

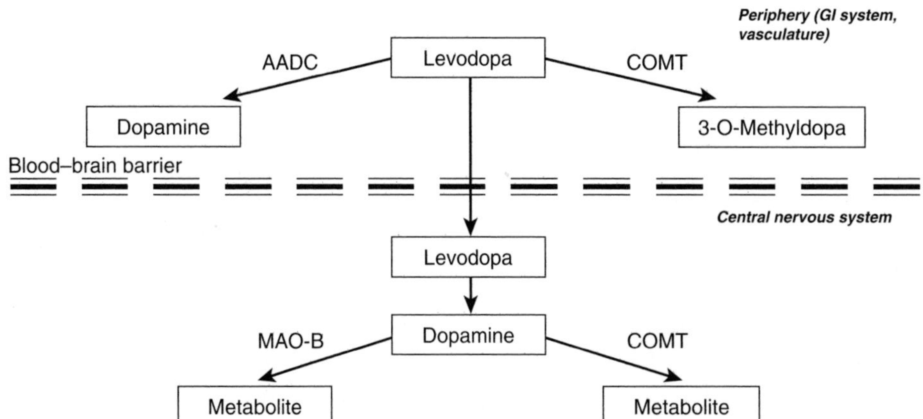

FIGURE 17-1 Orally ingested levodopa can be broken down in the periphery (gastrointestinal system or blood) by amino acid decarboxylase (AADC) or catechol-O-methyl transferase (COMT). Such breakdown will lead to adverse effects such as nausea, vomiting, diarrhea, and orthostatic hypotension and will decrease the effective dose reaching the brain. Coupling of levodopa with carbidopa (an AADC inhibitor) diminishes peripheral adverse effects and increases the effective dose reaching the brain. In addition, once levodopa enters the brain, inhibition of monoamine oxidase B (MAOB) and COMT will slow the synaptic breakdown of dopamine.

Negative Effects of Dopamine Replacement on Movement Tasks. Although the positive effects of dopamine replacement are well documented, it is not a benign treatment. Despite its widespread use and effectiveness, dopamine replacement can cause significant adverse effects.

Immediate Effects of Dopamine Replacement. Stimulation of dopamine receptors within the gastrointestinal (GI) system and the vasculature can immediately lead to nausea, vomiting, and anorexia and to hypotension, respectively. The oversupply of dopamine to nondeficient areas within the CNS contributes to the GI effects (through stimulation of the chemoreceptor trigger zone) and can also lead to adverse cognitive and psychiatric effects (anxiety, obsessive compulsive behaviors, insomnia, psychoses, nightmares, hallucinations, paranoia, and confusion).[57]

Long-Term Effects of Dopamine Replacement. Chronic exposure to exogenous sources of dopamine may contribute to the advent of movement-related complications. The most common types of movement-related complications are dyskinesias and motor fluctuations (wearing-off and on-off phenomena).[58,59] Dyskinesias are dynamic involuntary movements that are classically choreoathetotic in nature. The functional impact of dyskinesias can vary from negligible to completely disabling.[60,61] A thorough discussion of dyskinesias and other motor fluctuations is beyond the scope of this chapter. For additional information, readers are referred to recent journal supplements dealing specifically with dyskinesias (*Annals of Neurology*, 2008; *Movement Disorders*, 2008).[62,63]

Dyskinesias and motor fluctuations have been reported in as many as 84% of individuals with PD.[57,64] Although these problems are typically not observed on initiation of dopamine replacement, some authors have reported the onset after as few as 18 to 28 months of dopamine replacement therapy. Clinical observations indicate that the majority of patients with PD will experience dyskinesias and motor fluctuations after more than 5 years of dopamine replacement therapy.[65,66]

The pathophysiology of dyskinesias and motor fluctuations is thought to result from chronic exposure to the nonphysiologic stimulation of dopamine receptors.[58,59] Under normal neural functioning, dopamine release within the basal ganglia is a tonic process with intermittent changes in synaptic concentrations. With the advance of PD, dopaminergic transmission within the basal ganglia becomes a more phasic process, dependent on exogenous sources of dopamine via L-dopa, which results in neurophysiologic abnormalities in pathways through the basal ganglia.[11,67-69]

Recent research has suggested that persons with dyskinesias undergo a conversion in the way that the basal ganglia respond to dopamine replacement compared with persons without dyskinesias. As a result, dopamine receptors become supersensitized, creating an altered functional state of the basal ganglia that allows overactivity of connections from the basal ganglia to the frontal lobe.[70,71]

As the severity of PD progresses, the therapeutic effect of each L-dopa dose lasts a progressively shorter time (Figure 17-2).[72] Patients with PD must resort to taking L-dopa more often for the same level of relief from symptoms. The dose that previously gave them relief from their motor symptoms for several hours becomes effective for progressively shorter periods (what is referred to as the "wearing-off phenomenon"). Initially, these wearing-off periods may occur on a predictable schedule, such as end-of-dose deteriorations. With additional disease progression, the response to L-dopa becomes more unpredictable, and patients with PD may fluctuate between an effective medication state for management of motor symptoms (the "on-medication state") and complete ineffectiveness of the medication and

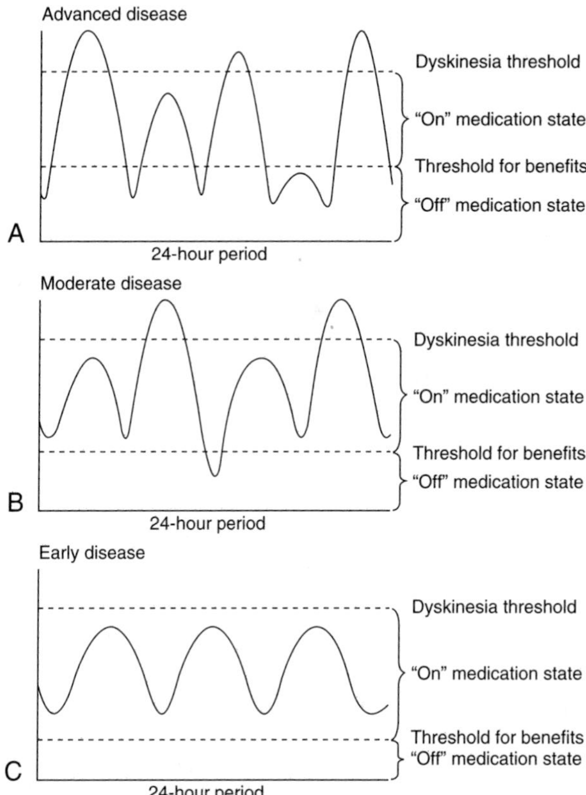

FIGURE 17-2 Schematic of the relationship between levodopa dosage and the clinical effects as Parkinson's disease (PD) progresses. **A**, In early PD, there is a prolonged therapeutic response to a given dose without exceeding the dyskinetic threshold, and no off-medication times are present. **B**, In moderate PD, the duration of therapeutic effect for a given dose may be narrowed. Thus more frequent dosing for the same clinical effect is necessary. Variability in medication responses may begin with intermittent but often predictable off-medication periods and dyskinesias. **C**, In severe PD, variability of response may be the rule rather than the exception. There may be periods of ineffective response, followed by dyskinetic responses at the same dose. The duration of effective therapeutic response may be greatly narrowed and often will be accompanied by dyskinesias.

immobility (the "off-medication state") in a matter of minutes. The motor manifestations of these off-medication periods are often freezing, falls, stiffness, and bradykinesia. Because these motor fluctuations are often related to overall L-dopa dose, pharmacologic management of these movement-related complications involves the manipulation of other antiparkinsonian medications (dopamine agonists, enzymatic inhibitors, anticholinergics). Through careful, individually determined combinations of medications, neurologists can maximize function while minimizing the L-dopa dosage.[65,66]

Despite consistent exposure to pulsatile dosing, not all persons with PD experience dyskinesias and motor fluctuations.[66,72] Factors identified in the literature as playing a role in the development of dyskinesias and motor fluctuations include the following: (1) The severity of PD when dopamine replacement is initiated (patients with more functional involvement, at Hoehn and Yahr stage III, are more likely to have dyskinesias and motor fluctuations); (2) the duration of dopamine replacement therapy (more than 5 years of therapy is associated with a greater likelihood of dyskinesias and motor fluctuations); (3) the age at diagnosis (age less than 60 years is associated with a greater likelihood of dyskinesias and motor fluctuations); (4) the cumulative L-dopa dose; and (5) a large initial dopamine replacement response.[57,59,63,65,66,72]

Although the presence of dyskinesias and motor fluctuations complicates the clinical treatment of the patient with PD, dyskinesias and motor fluctuations may have positive aspects. Generally, it appears that the development of dyskinesias is associated with a better long-term prognosis for functional independence because individuals with dyskinesia have a greater capacity to respond to pharmacologic treatment. [62,63,65,66,72]

The composite effects of disease progression and the long-term effects of dopamine replacement may eventually limit the clinical usefulness of L-dopa in many individuals. Despite these negative effects, in some cases, the reduction in cardinal movement impairments far exceeds the problems with the medication. For this reason, many patients with PD choose to endure any short- or long-term negative effects in exchange for the improved movement abilities and lessened disability.[10,11,73,74]

In an effort to diminish the adverse effects of pulsatile exposure to exogenous L-dopa, there are experimental efforts examining the delivery of dopamine replacement medication via intraduodenal infusion. Recent results from these studies suggest that these methods of delivery are successful in reducing motor fluctuations and dyskinesias.[75]

Increasing Dopamine Receptor Stimulation

Two classes of medications work to increase the stimulation of postsynaptic dopamine receptors (Table 17-1). The first (dopamine agonists) operate through the direct stimulation of dopamine receptors, whereas the second class of drugs (enzymatic inhibitors) exert their action through reduced breakdown of dopamine within the synapse.[74,75]

Dopamine Receptor Agonists. Dopamine agonists produce their symptomatic effects in PD by binding directly with postsynaptic dopamine receptors.[75] This class of drugs includes bromocriptine mesylate, pergolide mesylate, pramipexole, and ropinirole hydrochloride (Table 17-2). They are currently used in early PD as monotherapy and in late PD as a means of lowering L-dopa doses and therefore minimizing dyskinesias and motor fluctuations.[76-82] Recently, they have gained popularity because they have a much longer half-life than L-dopa, which creates more sustained stimulation of dopamine receptors and less phasic stimulation. Given the theorized role of pulsatile stimulation of dopamine receptors in the generation of dyskinesias, this may reduce the progression of motor complications.[76-82]

As an alternative to oral medications, two dopamine agonists are available with alternative routes of drug delivery. First, apomorphine has been approved for subcutaneous injection as a rapidly and powerfully acting dopamine agonist medication. It is currently indicated for use as a "rescue" medication for the treatment of unexpected off-medication periods. In addition, the dopamine agonist ropinirole is available as a transdermal patch that is currently approved for use in Europe.

Short-term studies have shown that dopamine agonists are effective in early as well as later stages of PD, both as monotherapy and as adjuncts to L-dopa.[11,76-82] Pramipexole and ropinirole have an advantage over older dopamine agonists in that they do not stimulate the serotonin receptors and thus do not cause some of the adverse effects of the other dopamine agonists. All dopamine agonists can cause symptoms similar to those of L-dopa, but these symptoms are usually transient.[83] This class of drugs must be used with caution in older patients, who may experience CNS effects such as confusion and cognitive impairment.

Enzymatic Inhibitors. Enzymatic inhibitors inhibit monoamine oxidase type B (MAOB) and catechol-O-methyl transferase (COMT), resulting in greater serum L-dopa levels. This increases the amount of time available for L-dopa to cross the blood–brain barrier. The bioavailability of L-dopa is approximately doubled in combination with these drugs.

Selegiline hydrochloride is an MAOB inhibitor that acts clinically by inhibiting dopamine metabolism in the brain.[75] Selegiline improves motor performance, activities of daily living (ADLs), and total scores on the UPDRS. In addition, it reduces the incidence of motor fluctuations, and some studies have shown that it delays the need for L-dopa therapy. Although selegiline does not stop the progression of PD, the delay in the need for L-dopa that it causes has been interpreted by some as a sign of a neuroprotective benefit. Selegiline may be used early in the illness because of its potential neuroprotective effects. As

TABLE 17-1 Common Drugs Used for Parkinson's Disease

Drug	Primary PD Deficits Addressed	Common Adverse Effects	Starting Dosage
Dopamine Replacement			
Levodopa-carbidopa (Sinemet)	Bradykinesia, tremor, rigidity	Dizziness, nausea, psychiatric problems, dyskinesias	25/100 mg three times daily
Increasing Dopamine Receptor Stimulation			
Bromocriptine (Parlodel)	Bradykinesia, tremor, rigidity	See Table 17-2	1.25 mg twice daily
Pergolide (Permax)	Bradykinesia, tremor, rigidity	See Table 17-2	0.05 mg at bedtime
Pramipexole (Mirapex)	Bradykinesia, tremor, rigidity	See Table 17-2	0.125 mg three times daily
Ropinirole (Requip)	Bradykinesia, tremor, rigidity	See Table 17-2	0.25 mg three times daily
Selegiline (Eldepryl)	Bradykinesia, tremor, rigidity	Insomnia, headaches, sweating, dyskinesias	0.5 mg twice daily
Rasagiline (Azilect)	Bradykinesia, tremor, rigidity	Insomnia, headaches sweating, dyskinesias	0.5 mg once daily
Tolcapone (Tasmar)	Bradykinesia, tremor, rigidity	Dizziness, orthostasis, diarrhea, dyskinesias	100 mg three times daily
Entacapone (Comtan)	Bradykinesia, tremor, rigidity	Dizziness, orthostasis, diarrhea, dyskinesias	200 mg
Apomorphine (Apokyn)	Bradykinesia, freezing, rigidity	Dizziness, orthostasis, diarrhea, dyskinesias	Subcutaneous injection 0.2 mL
Modulating Nondopaminergic Systems			
Amantadine (Symmetrel)	Bradykinesia, rigidity	Confusion, nausea, hallucination	100 mg twice daily
Trihexyphenidyl (Artane)	Tremor, rigidity	Confusion, dry mouth, nausea	0.5 to 1 mg twice daily
Biperiden (Akineton)	Tremor, rigidity	Confusion, dry mouth, nausea	
Procyclidine (Kemadrin)	Tremor, rigidity	Confusion, dry mouth, nausea	
Benztropine (Cogentin)	Tremor, rigidity	Confusion, dry mouth, nausea	1 to 2 mg twice daily

TABLE 17-2 Dopamine Agonists Used in Parkinson's Disease: Properties and Adverse Effects

	Bromocriptine (Parlodel)	Pergolide (Permax)	Pramipexole (Mirapex)	Ropinirole (Requip)
Initial dosage	1.25 mg bid	0.05 mg	0.125 mg tid	0.25 mg tid
Half-life	10–12 hours	16–24 hours	8 hours	6 hours
Potential Adverse Effects				
Somnolence	+	++	+++	++
Insomnia	+	++	++++	+
Dizziness or lightheadedness	+++	+++	+++	++
Hallucinations or confusion	+++	++	++	++
Headache	+++	+++	—	++
Orthostasis	+++	+++	++	+++
Nausea	++++	++++	++++	++
Constipation	—	++	++	—

bid, two times per day; *tid*, three times per day; +, incidence of 1 to 5%; ++, incidence of 6 to 15%; +++, incidence of 16 to 25%; ++++, incidence of greater than 25%.

patients with PD begin to take L-dopa, selegiline can be used as an adjunct, especially for those experiencing wearing-off effects. Its effectiveness, when combined with low doses of L-dopa, is comparable with that of a higher L-dopa dose and also to doses given at more frequent intervals.[75,80,84]

Selegiline is generally well tolerated, and there are few dietary restrictions compared with the nonselective monoamine oxidase inhibitors (MAOIs) (see discussion of MAOIs in Chapter 18). GI adverse effects and exacerbation of peptic ulcers may occur. When selegiline is administered with L-dopa, dopaminergic adverse effects are often increased (e.g., hallucinations, nausea, orthostatic hypotension). In addition, because of the role of MAOBs in the metabolism of serotonin, selegiline cannot be given in conjunction with tricyclic antidepressants and selective serotonin reuptake inhibitors (SSRIs). Because of its CNS effects, it must be used with caution in older patients.[80,84]

One of the concerns regarding the oral delivery of selegiline has been the production of amphetamine metabolites. For this reason, it may predispose patients to insomnia, so it is most commonly taken in the morning.[75,80,84] More recently, selegiline has become available in an orally dissolving tablet (ODT) formulation. This mode of delivery allows for the transmucosal absorption of the medication and has the advantages of increasing the drug's bioavailability and reducing the concentrations of amphetamine metabolites.

Rasagiline, a more recently available MAOB, is currently used in isolation as monotherapy in early PD and also as a means of helping to manage motor fluctuations in more advanced cases. Initial research with rasagiline suggested that newly diagnosed patients who took rasagiline monotherapy early in PD had reduced functional decline compared with a delayed-start group.[80] These results were interpreted as potential evidence for the neuroprotective effect of the drug and prompted a larger placebo-controlled trial to examine neuroprotective outcomes. This research is currently ongoing.

COMT inhibitors are one of the newest classes of drugs for PD and include entacapone and tolcapone.[75,84-88] In addition, the combination formulation Stalevo, which is a combination of L-dopa, carbidopa, and entacapone, reduces L-dopa breakdown to 3-O-methyldopa in the periphery, and thus increases the amount of L-dopa that crosses the blood-brain barrier. Thus when given in conjunction with L-dopa, COMT inhibitors may increase CNS delivery of dopamine and therefore reduce the L-dopa dose necessary for a given clinical effect. Pharmacokinetic studies have shown that they increase the area under the plasma L-dopa concentration-time curve but not peak levels of L-dopa. They also provide a more controlled concentration of L-dopa, thereby decreasing pulsativity. Such a mechanism is potentially ideal for patients with peak dose dyskinesias and motor fluctuations.[75,84-88] Currently, these drugs appear particularly useful for patients with "brittle" PD (i.e., those who fluctuate between off-medication and on-medication states frequently throughout the day). Research is ongoing to determine whether this will reduce progression of motor complications and to determine whether these drugs are indicated for both early and fluctuating PD.[75,84-88]

Because COMT inhibitors work by improving and prolonging dopamine stimulation, their adverse effects are similar to those seen with L-dopa. These drugs may trigger dyskinesias or produce cognitive impairments (e.g., hallucinations). Nausea and diarrhea are also common adverse effects. In addition, there have been a small number of reports of fatal liver damage with tolcapone, which led to a temporary withdrawal in Europe. In the United States, the U.S. Food and Drug Administration (FDA) and also drug manufacturers have mandated monitoring of liver function and the package labeling has been changed to state that the drug should be reserved for patients who have severe movement abnormalities and who are not appropriate candidates for other available pharmacologic therapy.[75,84-88]

Modulating Nondopaminergic Systems

In addition to drugs that primarily interact with the dopaminergic system, there are several medications that seek to normalize the unopposed actions of other neurotransmitter systems. These may be used as monotherapy or in conjunction with drugs that modulate the dopaminergic system.

Amantadine. In 1969, the anti-influenza drug amantadine was serendipitously discovered to have antiparkinsonian effects (see Table 17-1).[43,75,84] The exact mechanism of action has not been determined, but it probably acts as a glutamate antagonist. In addition, it may exert its effect through the enhanced release of stored dopamine, inhibition of presynaptic reuptake, or dopamine receptor agonism. It is commonly used as monotherapy in early, mild PD, and it appears to be most effective in patients whose bradykinesia, akinesia, or rigidity is more prominent than tremor. Because amantadine has an additive effect with L-dopa, it can be used in combination with L-dopa in patients with moderate PD who are experiencing "wearing-off" effects. The drug's adverse effects include nausea, insomnia, hallucinations, and autonomic symptoms.[43,75,84]

Anticholinergics. Before the discovery of L-dopa, anticholinergics were the only drugs available to treat PD.[43,75,89] This class of drugs includes trihexyphenidyl, benztropine mesylate, procyclidine, biperiden, and diphenhydramine. Anticholinergics reduce the relative cholinergic excess produced by dopamine deficiency, thereby counterbalancing the reduced dopaminergic influence on the output neurons of the basal ganglia. They are most effective in patients with mild PD whose tremor is more prominent than rigidity or akinesia.[43,75,89]

Anticholinergics appear to have little effect on bradykinesia. Although they can be beneficial in some patients, their adverse effects are significant. Mucosal secretions may be inhibited, causing dry mouth and skin. Because they antagonize cardiac cholinergic receptors, tachycardia is another adverse effect. Other anticholinergic adverse effects include dilation of pupils, increased intraocular pressure, and GI and genitourinary motility inhibition. Urine retention, especially in men with prostatic hypertrophy, is often a problem.[43,75,89]

Neuroprotection

Considerable evidence suggests that mitochondrial dysfunction and oxidative damage may play a role in the pathogenesis of PD.[80,90-91] One area of intense research interest is the search for compounds that can modulate cellular energy metabolism and exert antioxidative effects. The aim of neuroprotective therapy is to prevent further dopaminergic cell death, thereby slowing or halting disease progression. The objective of neuroprotection trials is to prove decreased loss of dopaminergic neurons from the basal ganglia in patients receiving the potentially neuroprotective agent. This type of proof is impossible to obtain in vivo, so researchers currently use outcome measures, such as clinical rating scales (e.g., the UPDRS), time to clinical endpoints (e.g., time until L-dopa therapy is required in previously untreated patients), radionuclide imaging (i.e., single photon emission computed tomography (CT) and positron emission tomography, PET), and mortality rates.[80,90-91]

Recently, The Committee to Identify Neuroprotective Agents in Parkinson's (a committee formed by the United States National Institute of Neurologic Disorders and Stroke) reviewed potential neuroprotective agents for PD.[75,80,90-91] The committee concluded that at least a dozen compounds should be candidates for further clinical trials. These included, but were not limited to, MAOB inhibitors (selegiline, rasagiline), dopamine agonists (ropinirole, pramipexole), and coenzyme Q-10. Two groups of prescription medications (MAOB inhibitors and dopamine agonists) and two supplements (vitamin E and coenzyme Q-10) are discussed in terms of their potential neuroprotective abilities.[80,90-91]

Monoamine Oxidase Type B Inhibitors. The MAOB inhibitor selegiline inhibits production of a free radical metabolite and has been found to be neuroprotective in an animal model.[9,10] To examine the potential neuroprotective abilities of selegiline and vitamin E, the Deprenyl and Tocopherol Antioxidative Therapy of Parkinsonism Trial included a comparison of selegiline with placebo in persons with untreated PD.[80,90-91] Although a 9-month delay in the need for L-dopa in selegiline-treated patients was observed, follow-up interpretation determined this benefit to be due to the drug's symptomatic effects. With long-term follow-up (10 years), no difference in mortality rate between the two treatment groups was seen. Subsequent studies have demonstrated equivocal or conflicting results. In fact, a recent meta-analysis of the results of all selegiline trials in early PD showed no statistically significant increase in the mortality rate among those treated with selegiline. Currently, selegiline is considered to have a limited neuroprotective benefit. The neuroprotective abilities of another MAOB inhibitor, rasagiline, are currently being examined.[80,90-91]

Dopamine Agonists. Recent evidence from in vitro and animal models of PD suggests that dopamine agonists have neuroprotective effects. As follow-up to these observations, two studies have examined the neuroprotective effects of two dopamine agonists (ropinirole and pramipexole) through the use of radionuclide imaging.[92,93] The findings of these studies showed reduced decline in radionucleotide markers of dopamine function in the dopamine agonist groups. These findings were initially interpreted to indicate neuroprotective effects. However, subsequent evaluation of the findings has called the methods into question, and at this time, none of the dopamine agonist drugs are indicated for slowing of disease progression.[75,80-82,90-91]

Vitamin E and Coenzyme Q-10. Epidemiologic researchers have examined the associations between dietary intake of vitamin E and the risk of PD.[80,90-91] In two large longitudinal studies conducted in the United States, there was no evidence that the use of vitamin E reduced the risk of PD. However, higher intake of dietary vitamin E was associated with a significantly lower risk of PD. Because of the inherent weaknesses of epidemiologic methods for determining cause and effect, the lower risk of PD should be interpreted cautiously and may be due to other unidentified dietary or lifestyle factors. As mentioned earlier, the Deprenyl and Tocopherol Antioxidative Therapy of Parkinsonism Trial examined the effects of selegiline and vitamin E on early PD over a 5-year period. The benefits of vitamin E could not be confirmed by this trial.[90,91]

In addition to vitamin E, coenzyme Q-10 has received recent attention as a potential neuroprotective agent. In a recent multicenter, placebo-controlled trial, participants taking 1200 mg of coenzyme Q-10 were found to have developed less disability than those receiving placebo (as measured by the UPDRS). Further studies are needed with larger samples, long-term follow-up, and a broader range of outcome measures to confirm these preliminary findings.[90,91]

Changes in Pharmacologic Management with Disease Progression

Generally, PD signs and symptoms appear to decrease as a result of use of medications such as dopamine agonists; however, the most potent effect on movement abilities is from dopamine replacement. Although dopamine replacement will result in reductions in the cardinal movement impairments associated with PD, it will not restore movement control to normal levels, and the response to dopamine replacement may vary among individuals. Specifically, bradykinesia, tremor, and rigidity are all reduced to variable degrees.[9-11,75,78,79,86]

After being treated with L-dopa for more than 5 years, the majority of individuals will demonstrate some form of movement-related complications, such as dyskinesias and wearing-off phenomena.[65-66,73] As a result of these complications, pharmacologic treatment of these individuals may be changed. Patients with PD who begin experiencing movement-related complications may be switched to controlled-release formulations of dopamine replacement medications in an effort to provide more prolonged stimulation to dopamine receptors. Other options are treatment with dopamine agonists, enzymatic inhibitors, or other medications as a means of lowering the overall L-dopa dose.[9-11,75,78,79,86]

Clinical Practice Considerations

Given the fact that medications for the treatment of PD produce a profound effect on the motor system, there are therapeutic concerns regarding the drugs and physical therapy practice. Obviously, the timing of physical therapy services is important to consider because intervention would be useless if it did not take place during peak effect of the drug. However, there are also some concerns that exercising the patient who is taking dopamine may negatively affect absorption.

Timing of Physical Therapy Treatment with Medications. Despite the lack of specific examinations of the effects of medications on responses to exercise, research demonstrating improvements in UPDRS items related to ADLs implies that exercise/rehabilitation training should take place while patients with PD are in an on-medication state.[94] Most individuals with mild to moderate PD demonstrate improved movement competencies within 1 to 1.5 hours of taking their dopamine replacement medication. If physical therapy is scheduled during optimal medication effects, the improved movement competencies seen during on-medication states should allow patients with PD to participate to a greater degree in rehabilitative efforts.[94]

Effect of Exercise on Dopamine Pharmacotherapeutics. An additional clinical concern is the relationship of exercise to L-dopa absorption, utilization, and subsequent motor effects. Physical therapists will likely treat patients with PD who experience a variety of effects of exercise on the physiologic effect of their dopamine replacement medications (in some, exercise improves medication effects; in others, exercise decreases medication effects).[95-98] Synthesis of the results of the few studies that have examined this issue suggests that as a result of aerobic exercise, L-dopa absorption improves. However, in the literature there is a lack of agreement regarding whether there is an increased demand for L-dopa during exercise. One study demonstrated a decrease in the duration and severity of dyskinesias during exercise.[95] Large intersubject variability and small sample sizes limit the conclusions that can be drawn from this research.[95-98] Additional research with larger samples, control for severity and subtype of PD (tremor predominate versus akinetic rigid predominate), and comparison of exercise types (aerobic training versus strength training) is needed to better understand this issue.

MULTIPLE SCLEROSIS: PATHOLOGY AND CLINICAL PRESENTATION

MS is an inflammatory, degenerative disease of the CNS, which is usually progressive and eventually results in permanent neurologic damage and disability.[99,100] The onset of MS is often very gradual, and the wide variety of symptoms that can occur overlap to some extent with those of other neurologic disorders. For this reason, establishing a definitive diagnosis of MS is not straightforward, and there is often a significant period of latency between the onset of clinical signs and symptoms and the point at which clinically definite MS is diagnosed.[101,102] Relative to many neurodegenerative diseases, the average age of onset for MS is early (20 to 40 years), and there is generally a 2:1 predominance in women over men.[103,104]

The clinical presentation of MS is generally characterized by periods of impaired neurologic function interspersed with periods of complete or partial recovery. Such disease behavior has led MS to be categorized according to the pattern and progression of neurologic function. In the majority of patients (up to 85%) with MS, the disease will initially follow a relapsing–remitting course (i.e., relapses separated by periods of remission). Of these patients, approximately 50 to 60% will have secondary progressive MS within 10 to 15 years.[99] A small percentage (15%) of patients with MS will experience a gradual worsening of neurologic function from the outset. This form of the disease is known as primary progressive MS.[105,106] Exacerbations typically develop slowly over hours to several days, persist for several days or weeks, and then gradually remit.

The development of MS lesions is thought to be a consequence of alterations in normal immune regulation, leading to the development and proliferation of T cells that react to myelin and/or oligodendrocytes. These activated T cells cross the blood–brain barrier and enter the CNS, where they encounter the antigen (i.e., myelin). An inflammatory process is initiated, and this process involves the release of inflammatory mediators, generation of acute edema, and neural tissue injury.[107]

Recent research is challenging the classic descriptions of the pathogenesis and progression of MS. MS is no longer considered to be simply an autoimmune demyelinating disease. Although autoimmune processes are critical to the development of the neuronal lesions, a genetic predisposition, coupled with environmental exposures (perhaps mediated by a viral or other infectious disease vector), contributes to the development of the disease.[107-110] In addition to the classically described demyelination, it is now clear that substantial axonal injury within active MS lesions is a central pathologic feature. Within the past decade, clinical and laboratory studies have demonstrated that axonal injury occurs very early in the disease process and appears to contribute significantly to the accumulation of disability associated with disease progression. It is now theorized that axonal transection is the pathologic correlate of the irreversible neurologic impairment seen in MS. The relationship between axonal damage and other components of the pathologic features, such as demyelination and remyelination, are the focus of current research.[111-114]

Examination of CNS tissue of individuals with MS reveals multiple sharply demarcated plaques.[100] The demyelinating lesions and axonal damage of MS can occur in the white matter throughout the CNS but most commonly in the optic nerves, white matter tracts of the periventricular regions, brainstem, cerebellar tracts, and spinal cord. The consequences of demyelination for neuronal conduction reflect the functional anatomy of impaired saltatory conduction at affected sites and account for many of the observed signs and symptoms. Common signs and symptoms may include blurred vision, upper motor neuron signs (spastic muscle weakness, hyperreflexia, positive Babinski response), nystagmus, dysarthria, ataxia, autonomic dysfunction, and sensory abnormalities (from internal capsule or spinal cord lesions).

Outcome Measures Used for Multiple Sclerosis Drug Studies

In human studies of MS medications, several different outcome measures are used. These include magnetic resonance imaging (MRI), relapse rate, and the Kurtzke Expanded Disability Severity Scale (EDSS)[115,116] (Box 17-1). There appears to be a relationship between these outcome measures in that MRI activity and relapse rate during the initial phase of the disease have been found to correlate to some extent with the degree of long-term disability.[117,118]

Magnetic Resonance Imaging. MRI is used to visualize MS lesions and to distinguish between old lesions (from

BOX 17-1 Kurtzke Expanded Disability Status Scale

Score	Description
0.0	Normal neurologic examination
1.0	No disability, minimal signs in one FS
1.5	No disability, minimal signs in more than one FS
2.0	Minimal disability in one FS
2.5	Mild disability in one FS or minimal disability in two FS
3.0	Moderate disability in one FS or mild disability in three or four FS; fully ambulatory
3.5	Fully ambulatory but with moderate disability in one FS and more than minimal disability in several others
4.0	Fully ambulatory without aid, self-sufficient, up and about some 12 hours a day despite relatively severe disability; able to walk without aid or rest some 500 meters
4.5	Fully ambulatory without aid, up and about much of the day, able to work a full day, may otherwise have some limitation of full activity or require minimal assistance; characterized by relatively severe disability; able to walk without aid or rest some 300 meters
5.0	Ambulatory without aid or rest for about 200 meters; disability severe enough to impair full daily activities (work a full day without special provisions)
5.5	Ambulatory without aid or rest for about 100 meters; disability severe enough to preclude full daily activities
6.0	Intermittent or unilateral constant assistance (cane, crutch, brace) required to walk about 100 meters with or without resting
6.5	Constant bilateral assistance (canes, crutches, braces) required to walk about 20 meters without resting
7.0	Unable to walk beyond approximately 5 meters even with aid, essentially restricted to wheelchair; wheels self in standard wheelchair and transfers alone; up and about in wheelchair some 12 hours a day
7.5	Unable to take more than a few steps; restricted to wheelchair; may need aid in transfer; wheels self but cannot carry on in standard wheelchair a full day; may require motorized wheelchair
8.0	Essentially restricted to bed or chair or perambulated in wheelchair but may be out of bed itself much of the day; retains many self-care functions; generally has effective use of arms
8.5	Essentially restricted to bed much of day; has some effective use of arms; retains some self-care functions
9.0	Confined to bed; can still communicate and eat
9.5	Totally helpless, bed-ridden; unable to communicate effectively or eat/swallow
10.0	Death due to MS

EDSS steps 1.0 to 4.5 refer to people with MS who are fully ambulatory.
EDSS steps 5.0 to 9.5 are defined by the impairment to ambulation.
FS, functional system; *MS*, multiple sclerosis.
From Kurtzke JF: Rating neurologic impairment in multiple sclerosis: An expanded disability status scale (EDSS), *Neurology* 33(11):1444–1452, 1983: www.nationalmssociety.org: Accessed June 17, 2005.

previous MS exacerbations) and new or active lesions (where inflammation and demyelination are ongoing).[119] Typically used with the contrast agent gadolinium, MRI has proved to be highly valuable in assessing the effects of potential disease-modifying drugs. The use of MRI in the monitoring of disease progression has led to the understanding that disease activity is likely present in the absence of corresponding clinical symptoms (in the order of 5 to 10 times more new or active lesions than the number of clinical relapses observed).[120,121]

Relapse Rate. The frequency of exacerbations/relapses is used to determine whether medications reduce the progression of disease activity. The initial studies of interferon β_{1a} (IF-β_{1a}) in MS involved the evaluation of change in the exacerbation rate.[118]

Expanded Disability Severity Scale. For most studies, significant progression of disability has been defined as an increase of one or more points on the Kurtzke EDSS, a standard measure of disability used in clinical studies of MS, sustained for at least 6 months.[115] The EDSS quantifies disability in eight functional systems and allows neurologists to assign a functional system score in each of these. The functional systems are pyramidal, cerebellar, brainstem, sensory, bowel and bladder, visual, cerebral, and other.

Disease-Modifying Drug Therapies

Pharmacologic therapies developed for the treatment of MS can be divided into two main categories: (1) drugs for the treatment of acute relapses (corticosteroids) and (2) drugs that affect the disease course (collectively termed *disease-modifying drugs*). The latter group can be subdivided into those with broad immunosuppressive effects (e.g., methotrexate and mitoxantrone) and those with immunomodulatory effects (IF-β and glatiramer acetate [GA]). At this time, the class of medications considered to be disease-modifying drugs includes three commonly used interferon medications (two types of IF-β_{1a}, one type of IF-β_{1b}), one medication that modifies the immune response to myelin basic protein (GA), and one chemotherapeutic agent (mitoxantrone).

Interferons. The belief that MS had a virus-mediated component contributed to the study of interferons in reducing the number of exacerbations in specific groups of patients with MS. First studied for efficacy in the late 1970s, IF-β has subsequently been shown to have antiviral, anti-inflammatory, and immunomodulatory properties.[122] Evidence in support of an immunomodulatory mechanism of action comes from both laboratory and clinical studies, which have shown that IF-β has dose-dependent actions on a variety of mediators that inhibit MS disease activity. These processes include the inhibition of proinflammatory cytokines and stimulation of the production of the anti-inflammatory cytokines.[123,124]

Phase III drug trials of all of the available interferon medications have shown these medications to be effective in reducing lesion accumulation, relapse frequency, and progression of disability. However, questions remain regarding the relative merits of different types of interferons, the most effective route of delivery, the frequency of dosing, and the dose–response relationship for individual interferon medications (Table 17-3).[125-129]

In recent years, it has become increasingly apparent that the demyelination and axonal damage that appear to lead to irreversible disability actually begin very early in the course of the disease. For this reason, it has been suggested that in order to prevent axonal damage, interferon therapy be initiated as soon as possible after the diagnosis of MS is made. Recent evidence appears to indicate that initiation of interferon treatment with signs of clinically silent MRI lesions (subclinical demyelination) may slow the progression to clinically definite MS.[130-133]

Glatiramer Acetate. GA is a synthetic protein mixture of random polymers containing glutamic acid, tyrosine, lysine, and alanine. It appears to simulate myelin basic protein, a component of the myelin that insulates nerve fibers in the brain and spinal cord. Through a mechanism that is not completely understood, this drug seems to block myelin-damaging T cells by acting as a myelin decoy. Potential mechanisms of action suggested for GA include the alteration of immune function and reduction of inflammation via a T-cell receptor pathway and/or a neuroregenerative/protective action.[134-137]

In controlled clinical trials with relapsing-remitting MS, GA appears to have positive effects on MRI measures (reduction of new lesions, prevention of re-enhancement of old lesions, and potentiation of reparative mechanisms), as well as effects on clinical measures (reduction of relapses and slowing disability) compared with placebo.[138-143] Similar to interferon treatment, recent evidence appears to indicate that initiation of GA treatment with signs of clinically silent MRI lesions (subclinical demyelination) may slow the progression to clinically definite MS.[130]

Although the mechanisms of action of GA and IF-β are not completely understood, multiple lines of research suggest that they work through different immunologic pathways. For this reason, if a patient with MS does not respond to IF-β, it is possible that he or she will respond to GA, and vice versa. When GA is compared with IF-β, the advantage of GA treatment is the absence of important adverse effects (flu-like symptoms), but the disadvantage is the need for daily administration.

Mitoxantrone. Mitoxantrone belongs to the general group of medicines called antineoplastics. Before its approval for use in MS, it was used only to treat certain forms of cancer. It acts in MS by suppressing the activity of T cells and other immune system cell types thought to be involved in the degradation of the myelin sheath and axonal damage.

The use of mitoxantrone for the treatment of MS was evaluated in a series of studies in Europe during the

TABLE 17-3 Drugs Approved for Treatment of Multiple Sclerosis

Drug Name (Trade Name)	Class of Medication	Common Adverse Effects	Type of MS Indicated	Dosage/Frequency/Route of Administration
Interferon-β_{1a} (Avonex)	Immunomodulator	Flu-like symptoms (fever, chills, sweating, muscle aches, and tiredness)	RRMS	30 mcg/once per week/ intramuscular injection
Interferon-β_{1a} (Rebif)	Immunomodulator	Flu-like symptoms (fever, chills, sweating, muscle aches, and tiredness)	RRMS	44 mcg/3 times per week/ subcutaneous injection
Interferon-β_{1a} (Betaseron)	Immunomodulator	Flu-like symptoms (fever, chills, sweating, muscle aches, and tiredness)	RRMS	250 mcg/every other day/ subcutaneous injection
Glatiramer acetate (Copaxone)	Immunomodulator	Skin reactions (itching, inflammation), nausea, upset stomach, muscle weakness or stiffness, flushing, chest/joint pain	RRMS	20 mg/every day/subcutaneous injection
Mitoxantrone (Novantrone)	Antineoplastic	Immunosuppression, heart muscle damage*	SPMS, PRMS, worsening RRMS	Four times a year by IV infusion in a medical facility. Lifetime limit of 8-12 doses (12 mg/m2 every 3 months)

MS, multiple sclerosis; *RRMS*, relapsing remitting multiple sclerosis; *SPMS*, secondary progressive MS; *PRMS*, progressive, relapsing MS.
*The total lifetime dose of mitoxantrone is limited in order to avoid possible heart damage. Patients taking mitoxantrone should have regular tests of their heart function. Mitoxantrone cannot be used by patients with pre-existing heart problems, liver disease, and certain blood disorders.

1990s. The results of these studies indicate that mitoxantrone delays the time to first treated relapse and time to disability progression and also reduces the number of treated relapses and number of new lesions detected by MRI.

On the basis of the findings from these studies, the FDA approved mitoxantrone in October 2000 for reducing neurologic disability and/or the frequency of clinical relapses (attacks). Because of its significant adverse effect profile, the indications are limited to specific subgroups of patients. These groups are as follows:[144-146]

1. Patients with secondary progressive MS (MS that has changed from relapsing–remitting MS to progressive MS at a variable rate)
2. Progressive-relapsing MS (disease characterized by a gradual increase in disability from onset with clear, acute relapses along the way)
3. Worsening relapsing–remitting MS (disease characterized by clinical attacks without complete remission, resulting in a stepwise worsening of disability)

As with other chemotherapeutic drugs, there are potential adverse effects of mitoxantrone on healthy tissues in the body. These include cardiotoxicity, liver dysfunction, and treatment-related acute leukemia.[147,148]

Because of these adverse effects, monitoring for potential cardiac, hematologic, and hepatic complications is necessary. The potential for cardiac complications dictates that mitoxantrone be prescribed only to patients with normal cardiac function, and evaluation of cardiac output is necessary before treatment is started. In addition, periodic cardiac monitoring is required throughout the treatment period. The lifetime cumulative dose is limited to 140 mg/m^2 (approximately 8 to 12 doses over 2 to 3 years). Because mitoxantrone can increase the risk of infection (by decreasing the number of protective white blood cells) and damage the liver, blood counts and liver enzyme levels are determined before each dose is given.

Emerging Medications

Monoclonal Antibodies. The monoclonal antibody natalizumab was recently approved by the FDA for reduction in the frequency of clinical relapses in relapsing forms of MS.[149] In the initial analyses of the ongoing trials, natalizumab reduced the relapse rate by up to 66% and reduced the development of new MRI-detected brain lesions. In addition, a greater proportion of patients receiving natalizumab remained relapse-free compared with those receiving the control drug. In more recent analyses of results, dramatic reductions in measures of disease activity were found in those taking natalizumab, compared with those taking placebo (37% of subjects demonstrated no disease activity in the treatment group compared with 7% in the placebo control group).[150]

Natalizumab is given every 4 weeks by infusion into a vein. It is designed to interfere with the movement of T cells across the blood–brain barrier and into the brain and spinal cord. The most common adverse effects include headache, fatigue, urinary tract infection, depression, lower respiratory tract infection, joint pain, and abdominal discomfort. Currently, no information on long-term safety is available. Additional research examining the effects of monoclonal antibodies (alemtuzumab, natalizumab) on MS is ongoing.

There have been a small number of specific adverse events associated with natalizumab treatment. Few individuals have developed a viral infection of the brain (progressive multifocal leukoencephalopathy [PML]) which has led to severe disability or death in those persons affected. The precise risk of developing PML has not been determined but appears to be less than 1 in 1000 based on the most recent data. Clinicians should monitor persons taking natalizumab for symptoms associated with PML and immediately report these to the referring provider should they occur. The typical symptoms associated with PML progress over the course of days to weeks and can include clumsiness and progressive weakness on one side of the body, disturbances of vision, and changes in thinking, memory, and orientation leading to confusion and personality changes.[151]

In addition to natalizumab, there are a number of other monoclonal antibody medications that are currently being examined in clinical trials. These medications, along with several others that are in late phase clinical trials demonstrate promise as new disease-modifying medications for persons with MS (Box 17-2).[151]

Symptomatic Treatment

Two of the most common complaints of patients with MS are the presence of abnormal fatigue (estimated to be present in nearly 90% of patients with MS) and motor signs such as spasticity (estimated to be present in more than 60% of patients with MS). Although treatments of spasticity are discussed elsewhere in this text, pharmacologic treatment of fatigue warrants further discussion.[152-154]

BOX 17-2 Experimental Drugs for the Treatment of MS

Drug Name	Proposed Mechanism of Action
Alemtuzumab	Selectively depletes T lymphocytes
Cladribine	Selectively depletes T and B lymphocytes
Daclizumab	Reduces T-lymphocyte immune response Increases presence of natural killer cells
Dimethylfumarate	Induces expression and production of anti-inflammatory cytokines
Fingolimod	Reduces circulating lymphocytes Induces upregulation of neurotropic factors
Laquinimod	Induces upregulation of neurotropic factors
Rituximab	Selectively depletes B lymphocytes

Fatigue is one of the most common symptoms of MS and is often rated by patients with MS as the most disabling symptom.[155] Fatigue is especially bothersome in MS because it can potentiate other symptoms: It may reduce cognition, increase depression, or further limit physical abilities. Several drugs have been examined to determine their effect on what is thought to be CNS-mediated fatigue in patients with MS. Although no medications have been approved by the FDA for the treatment of MS-related fatigue, in an expert opinion paper from the U.S. National Multiple Sclerosis Society, the off-label uses of four specific drugs (modafinil, amantadine, pemoline, and methylphenidate) are discussed.[155]

Modafinil is a CNS α-adrenergic receptor agonist with wakefulness-promoting properties. Its FDA-approved use is for the treatment of excessive daytime sleepiness in persons with narcolepsy. Studies in patients with MS-related fatigue demonstrate reductions in fatigue severity scale scores and improvements in self-rated feelings of fatigue, quality of life, and overall satisfaction with treatment.[156] The typical prescription of modafinil is 50 to 100 mg to be taken in the morning. The dose is then gradually increased to achieve optimal benefit with minimal adverse effects (which include appetite suppression, headache, insomnia, nervousness, and restlessness). The recommended daily dose is 400 mg.[157,158]

Amantadine is an antiviral agent whose primary use is as an antiparkinsonian drug. It has been used to treat MS-related fatigue for approximately 20 years.[154] More than 20% of mild to moderately disabled patients with MS experience significant reductions in fatigue while taking amantadine. The recommended dose of amantadine is 100 mg in the morning and 100 mg in the early afternoon.

Two specific CNS stimulants have been used to treat MS-related fatigue.[159-161] Pemoline is preferred to other stimulants because it appears to be less addictive; however, it is not recommended as a first-line therapy for MS-related fatigue because of its limited efficacy and the high risk of adverse effects (e.g., irritability, anxiety, hyperactivity, anorexia, and liver dysfunction). Although study results have been contradictory, pemoline may be an effective therapy for patients with MS who do not respond to amantadine or modafinil. Lastly, the stimulant methylphenidate has been used. Although methylphenidate's primary use is for the treatment of attention disorders in children, it appears to be effective and well tolerated with few adverse effects. The patient should be observed for the adverse effects of overstimulation, such as anxiety and tachycardia, which are possible with methylphenidate.

ALZHEIMER'S DISEASE: PATHOLOGY AND EPIDEMIOLOGY

AD is a progressive, neurodegenerative disease characterized by protein abnormalities in the brain. The damage associated with AD begins in the entorhinal cortex, which is near the hippocampus and has direct connections to it. It then proceeds to the hippocampus, a structure deep in the brain that helps to encode memories, and then to other areas of the cerebral cortex that are used in thinking and making decisions.

The characteristic symptoms of AD include memory loss, language deterioration, impaired ability to mentally manipulate visual information, poor judgment, confusion, restlessness, and mood swings. Eventually, AD destroys cognition, personality, and the ability to function. The early symptoms of AD, which include forgetfulness and loss of concentration, are often missed because they resemble natural signs of aging. AD is clinically characterized by a global decline of cognitive function that cannot be accounted for by acute delirium or depression. In comparison with other potential causes of decreased cognition, AD progresses slowly but consistently and leaves patients in the end stage of the disease bedridden, incontinent, and dependent on custodial care. Death occurs, on average, 9 years after diagnosis.

More than 12 million individuals worldwide have AD, and AD accounts for most cases of dementia that are diagnosed after the age of 60. AD is the most common cause of dementia among people 65 years and older, and it is estimated that up to four million people now have AD. For every 5-year age group beyond 65, the percentage of people with AD doubles. By 2050, 14 million older Americans are expected to have AD.[162-167]

An understanding of the neuronal pathophysiology associated with AD is critical to the understanding of current treatments, potential neuroprotective agents, and emerging lines of pharmacologic management. A broad view of the etiology and pathology of AD is that AD arises from a series of genetic and/or environmental cellular stressors that increase with age. These stressors can include, but may not be limited to, inherited genetic mutations, free radical oxidative stress, reduced energy metabolism, excitotoxicity, and mitochondrial dysfunction. Regardless of the original causes, a cascade of biochemical abnormalities leads to cellular dysfunction, failure of neurotransmission, cell death, and a common clinical outcome. The defining neuropathologic hallmarks of AD are extracellular plaques containing the β-amyloid peptide and intracellular neurofibrillary tangles containing abnormally phosphorylated tau (τ)-protein grouped into filaments.[168,169]

Amyloid Plaques and Neurofibrillary Tangles

In AD, amyloid plaques accumulate in the critical parietal, temporal cortex, and hippocampus areas associated with memory and learning functions. In a manner similar to atherosclerotic plaques in arteries, amyloid deposits can develop into β-amyloid plaques that damage the cell walls of neurons.[170] These plaques trigger an inflammatory cascade, which ultimately results in loss of synapses, pruning of dendrites, decreased neurotransmitter release (especially acetylcholine), and cell death.

Healthy neurons have an internal support structure made up in part of microtubules. These microtubules act to guide molecules from the neuronal cell body to the axon terminals and back. A specific protein, τ, makes these microtubules stable. In AD, τ is chemically altered and begins to pair with other τ-threads, and they become tangled up together. When this happens, the microtubules disintegrate, collapsing the neuron's transport system. This may result first in malfunctions in communication between neurons and later in the death of the cells.

Neuronal Cell Death and Neurotransmitter Depletion

Although it is not clear whether β-amyloid plaques and neurofibrillary tangles themselves cause AD or whether they are a byproduct of the AD process, they appear critical in the process, given that the load and distribution of these protein abnormalities correlate with the severity and manifestation of AD.[171,172] The intracellular and extracellular abnormalities caused by β-amyloid plaques and neurofibrillary tangles are associated with loss of synaptic density and neuronal death. Degeneration of neurons dramatically reduces the production of the neurotransmitter acetylcholine. A loss of 60 to 90% of acetylcholine activity results in memory impairment. Other neurotransmitters depleted in AD include serotonin, somatostatin, and norepinephrine. Receptors for these neurotransmitters are also reduced.

Symptomatic treatment of AD focuses on manipulation of neurotransmission. The greatest success has been obtained by blocking the enzyme acetylcholinesterase.[173] More recently, one medication that targets an N-methyl-D-aspartate (NMDA) pathway has become available.

Treatment of Mild to Moderate Alzheimer's Disease

Cholinergic neurotransmission within the cerebrum plays an important role in cognition. In AD, the central cholinergic system, particularly in the hippocampus and entorhinal cortex, has reduced functional capacity as well as loss of neurons. This has led to the hope that improving the remaining cholinergic neurotransmission would minimize symptoms of AD.[174] Acetylcholinesterase inhibitors (AChEIs) appear to do this through their inhibition of acetylcholinesterase, the major enzyme that degrades acetylcholine.

This class of drugs may help delay or prevent symptoms from becoming worse for a limited time and may help control some behavioral symptoms.[174] However, as AD progresses, the brain produces progressively less acetylcholine; therefore AChEIs may eventually lose their effect. AChEI medications currently approved for use in the United States are tacrine, donepezil, rivastigmine, and galanthamine (Table 17-4).

In virtually all randomized placebo-controlled trials of AChEIs versus placebos, untreated patients showed significant decline in cognition and function. In contrast, treated patients tended not to show this response. This preservation of function is an important therapeutic outcome. Although all AChEIs would be considered "beneficial" in the treatment of AD, at this time, studies in which different AChEIs were directly compared showed no evidence of superiority of one agent over another with cognitive, behavioral, or functional outcomes.[175,176] In addition, it should be noted that although AChEIs appear to delay admission to nursing homes, they are not neuroprotective and offer little clinical improvement when the Mini-Mental Status Examination score drops below 12.[177]

Treatment of Moderate to Severe Alzheimer's Disease

One NMDA antagonist, memantine, is approved for the treatment of moderate to severe AD. The apparent mechanism of action of memantine involves regulation of glutamate concentrations, thereby reducing excitotoxic neuronal injury. Memantine appears to delay the progression of cognitive and physical functioning deficits associated with moderate to severe AD. Because NMDA antagonists work very differently from cholinesterase inhibitors, the two types of drugs can be prescribed in combination. Combining memantine with other AD drugs may be more effective than any single therapy, and in fact, one controlled clinical trial has demonstrated that patients receiving donepezil plus memantine perform better on cognitive and physical functioning measures than do patients receiving donepezil alone. Recent studies of persons with moderate to severe AD have demonstrated functional improvement, slowing of the rate of cognitive decline, and a reduction in care dependence.[178-182]

Preventive Treatment

Neuroprotection has been suggested as a means of preventing or slowing the progression of AD. Two specific classes of prescription drugs have been suggested as a means of neuroprotection for patients with AD. These are statins and antiamyloid treatments. While there have been encouraging observations from epidemiologic studies and animal experiments, subsequent prospective trials are demonstrating limitations of these types of medications in the prevention of AD. [183,184] Regardless of the outcome of these prospective trials, additional insights have been gained regarding the roles of inflammation and cholesterol metabolism in the pathogenesis of AD. Such insights will likely lead to effective treatments in the future.

Statins. Despite conflicting results of prospective trials, the theoretical rationale for statin use remains compelling. The hypothesized mechanism of action of the statin medications is the alteration of amyloid regulation. People with high systolic blood pressure, elevated low-density lipoprotein (LDL) levels, or elevated apolipoprotein E levels in midlife have three times the risk of AD in later life.[185-188] Epidemiologic studies have demonstrated that statin medications used to control hyperlipidemia may be associated with a lower incidence of AD. Future prospective studies will provide greater insights into the potential efficacy of statins in the treatment of AD.

Antiamyloid Strategies. Animal studies of antiamyloid treatments initially generated excitement when it was observed that long-term immunization of a mouse model of AD resulted in much less β-amyloid being deposited in the brains of the mice. Similar transgenic

TABLE 17-4 Drugs Approved for Treatment of Alzheimer's Disease

Drug Name (Trade Name)	Class of Medication	Common Adverse Effects	Possible Drug Interactions	Recommended Dosage
Donepezil (Aricept)	Cholinesterase inhibitor	Headache, generalized pain, fatigue, dizziness, nausea, vomiting, diarrhea, insomnia, increased frequency of urination	Drugs with anticholinergic action†*	5–10 mg/day
Galantamine (Reminyl)	Cholinesterase inhibitor	Nausea, vomiting, diarrhea, weight loss	Drugs with anticholinergic action†*	8–24 mg/day
Rivastigmine (Exelon)	Cholinesterase inhibitor	Nausea, vomiting, weight loss, upset stomach, muscle weakness	Drugs with anticholinergic action*	1.5–6 mg/day
Memantine (Namenda)	NMDA antagonist	Dizziness, headache, constipation, confusion	Other NMDA antagonists such as amantadine, dextromethorphan	5–20 mg

NMDA, N-methyl-D-aspartate.
*These drugs include atropine, benztropine, trihexyphenidyl, paroxetine, amitriptyline, fluoxetine, and fluvoxamine.

mice that had been immunized also performed better on memory tests than did a group of these mice that had not been immunized.[189-191]

These results led to preliminary studies in humans to test the safety and effectiveness of the vaccine. However, initial studies of the immune response in β-amyloid vaccine had to be stopped because of a high incidence of encephalitis in treatment subjects.[192] Subsequent research has demonstrated that despite a reduction in amyloid load, clinical measures of dementia continued to decline. These findings call into question the role of amyloid accumulation in the progression of the neurodegeneration of AD.[192]

Symptomatic Management

Because AD affects memory and mental abilities, it begins to change a person's emotions and behaviors. More than 70% of patients with AD eventually have one or more behavioral symptoms that contribute substantially to patient morbidity and caregiver distress. The common behavioral symptoms include sleeplessness, wandering and pacing, aggression, agitation, anger, depression, hallucinations, psychosis, and delusions. Some of these symptoms may become worse in the evening, a phenomenon called *sundowning*, or during daily routines, especially bathing. A variety of medication classes are used to treat behavioral symptoms. Antipsychotic, antiseizure, and SSRIs are used to treat psychoses and other psychiatric or behavioral symptoms in AD, although treatment guidelines are not well defined. Anecdotally, medications in these classes have been shown to reduce psychoses and behavioral symptoms in patients with AD, although the evidence is inconclusive for many medications. Adverse effects vary substantially across these medication classes. A full discussion of the pharmacologic management of AD behavioral symptoms with noncholinergic medications is beyond the scope of this chapter, and readers should refer to recent reviews for more in-depth discussions of this topic.[193,194]

ACTIVITIES 17

1. There are several symptoms associated with MS that have devastating effects on patients' quality of life. These symptoms include fatigue, bowel and bladder dysfunction, sexual dysfunction, weakness, visual problems, psychiatric issues, pain, spasticity, and tremor. Review the literature regarding pharmacologic and nonpharmacologic methods for reducing these symptoms. Discuss the anticipated effects of these medications on your treatment as well as how the potential adverse effects may affect your treatment plan.
2. Mr. H. is a 40-year-old man you are treating for shoulder impingement. During history taking, he relates that he has just been diagnosed with MS. His neurologist prescribed a disease-modifying medication (IF-β_{1a}), but Mr. H. is not taking it because he does not like the way it makes him feel. During your treatments, he asks you about the benefits of taking medications when he currently does not have any neurologic symptoms. In addition, he wonders what other medication options are available to him. Discuss your responses to Mr. H.
3. Ms. C. is a 65-year-old woman who has been referred to therapy for evaluation and treatment of her right knee. She reports that she was rushing to cross the street and tripped at the curb and fell. She was transported to University Hospital by ambulance and subsequently seen in the emergency department for an evaluation. X-ray films showed no fracture but did reveal moderate joint narrowing. Ms. C. was sent home with an Ace wrap and instructed to ice and elevate the leg for the next 24 hours. She was also given aspirin to take every 4 to 6 hours for pain. One week later, she went to see her general practitioner for further evaluation. Her right knee continued to be swollen and painful and therefore she asked to see a physical therapist.

   Medical History: Hypertension × 5 years

   Social History: Married, two grown children, homemaker, no smoking or alcohol abuse

   Medications: Hydrochlorothiazide, aspirin

   Examination: The patient presents with swelling in the right knee with limited range of motion (ROM) (30–80/20–85). The left knee is slightly limited (10–100/10–110). She is ambulating with a cane in her right hand. It has been borrowed from a friend and is too long. In general, her gait is very slow, and she shows decreased movements in the lower limbs, hip, knee, and ankles bilaterally.

   As you proceed with your evaluation, you notice resting tremors of the hands. When you ask the patient about this, she reports that they developed about 1 year ago but have gotten much worse since the fall. You complete the evaluation and call the physician to discuss the tremors.

   The patient returns to the clinic 1 week later. She reports having had a full neurologic workup, which revealed early Parkinson's disease (PD). She has started to receive rasagiline and coenzyme Q-10. The patient continues with physical therapy for 2 more weeks on a program of electrical stimulation to her quadriceps, knee active and passive ROM exercises, and gait training. ROM of the right knee improves and is equal in range to the left.

   Questions

   A. What symptoms of PD are displayed by this patient?
   B. What are the goals of drug therapy in PD?
   C. Given the diagnosis of PD, what other interventions might be helpful?
   D. Is there any problem with the drug combination that she is currently receiving?

4. Two years later, Ms. C. returns to your clinic with the chief complaint that her PD has worsened. She is currently taking, levodopa, rasagiline and ropinirole, and Sinemet. She reports having some good days, but most are bad. She has difficulty performing her chores, continues to have resting tremors, and now shows rigidity of the right upper extremity and general difficulty in initiating movements. Further evaluation shows a shuffling gait with decreased trunk and arm movements.

Questions

A. Considering her current level of functioning with Sinemet, levodopa, rasagiline and ropinirole therapy, what drug therapy would you recommend at this time?

B. How will you schedule therapy, given the possibility of drug-related fluctuations in function?

C. What information should you regularly send to the neurologist that would help in determining what combination of medicines Ms. C. should be receiving as maintenance therapy?

5. Ms. C complains about how her medications work well on one day and do not work well on other days. Upon further questioning, you discover that she is taking dopamine replacement medications and intermittantly takes them with her protein shakes in the morning. Why may this affect the action of her medications? What advice will you provide to this patient regarding her dietary habits and her medications?

6. You periodically assess a patient who has dementia with Lewy bodies. What concerns do you have about the effect of his dementia medications (acetylcholinesterase inhibitors) on his PD symptoms?

REFERENCES

1. Shoenberg BS: Epidemiology of movement disorders. In Marsden CD, Fahn S, editors: Movement disorders (2nd ed.), London, 1987, Butterworth.
2. Marsden CD: Parkinson's disease. J Neurol Neurosurg Psychiatry 57:672-681, 1994.
3. Hornykiewicz O: Historical aspects and frontiers of Parkinson's disease research. Adv Exp Med Biol 90:1-20, 1977.
4. Hornykiewicz O: How L-dopa was discovered as a drug for Parkinson's disease 40 years ago. Wien Klin Wochenschr 113(22):855-862, 2001.
5. Cotzias GC, Papavasiliou PS, Gellene R: Experimental treatment of parkinsonism with L-dopa. Neurolog 18(3):276-277, 1968.
6. Cotzias GC: L-dopa for parkinsonism. N Engl J Med 278(11):630-631, 1968.
7. Cotzias GC, Papavasiliou PS, Gellene R: Modification of parkinsonism: Chronic treatment with L-dopa. N Engl J Med 280(7):337-345, 1969.
8. Cotzias GC, Papavasiliou PS, Gellene R: L-dopa in Parkinson's syndrome. N Engl J Med 281(5):272, 1969.
9. Lang AE, Lozano AM: Parkinson's disease. First of two parts. N Engl J Med 339(15):1044-1053, 1998.
10. Lang AE, Lozano AM: Parkinson's disease. Second of two parts. N Engl J Med 339(16):1130-1143, 1998.
11. Metman LV, Konitsiotis S, Chase TN: Pathophysiology of motor response complications in Parkinson's disease: Hypotheses on the why, where, and what. Mov Disord 15(1):3-8, 2000.
12. Ramaker C, Marinus J, Stiggelbout AM, Van Hilten BJ: Systematic evaluation of rating scales for impairment and disability in Parkinson's disease. Mov Disord 17(5):867-876, 2002.
13. Gordon AM, Reilmann R: Getting a grasp on research: Does treatment taint testing of parkinsonian patients? Brain 122 (Pt 8):1597-1598, 1999.
14. Berardelli A, Rothwell JC, Thompson PD, Hallett M: Pathophysiology of bradykinesia in Parkinson's disease. Brain 124(Pt 11):2131-2146, 2001.
15. Berardelli A, Dick JP, Rothwell JC, Day BL, Marsden CD: Scaling of the size of the first agonist EMG burst during rapid wrist movements in patients with Parkinson's disease. J Neurol Neurosurg Psychiatry 49(11):1273-1279, 1986.
16. Blin O, Ferrandez AM, Pailhous J, Serratrice G: Dopa-sensitive and dopa-resistant gait parameters in Parkinson's disease. J Neurol Sci 103(1):51-54, 1991.
17. Ferrandez AM, Blin O: A comparison between the effect of intentional modulations and the action of L-dopa on gait in Parkinson's disease. Behav Brain Res 45(2):177-183, 1991.
18. O'Sullivan JD, Said CM, Dillon LC, Hoffman M, Hughes AJ: Gait analysis in patients with Parkinson's disease and motor fluctuations: Influence of levodopa and comparison with other measures of motor function. Mov Disord 13(6):900-906, 1998.
19. Robertson LT, Hammerstad JP: Jaw movement dysfunction related to Parkinson's disease and partially modified by levodopa. J Neurol Neurosurg Psychiatry 60(1):41-50, 1996.
20. Shan DE, Lee SJ, Chao LY, Yeh SI: Gait analysis in advanced Parkinson's disease: Effect of levodopa and tolcapone. Can J Neurol Sci 28(1):70-75, 2001.
21. Baroni A, Benvenuti F, Fantini L, Pantaleo T, Urbani F: Human ballistic arm abduction movements: Effects of L-dopa treatment in Parkinson's disease. Neurology 34(7):868-876, 1984.
22. Burleigh-Jacobs A, Horak FB, Nutt JG, Obeso JA: Step initiation in Parkinson's disease: Influence of levodopa and external sensory triggers. Mov Disord 12(2):206-215, 1997.
23. Cioni M, Richards CL, Malouin F, Bedard PJ, Lemieux R: Characteristics of the electromyographic patterns of lower limb muscles during gait in patients with Parkinson's disease when OFF and ON L-Dopa treatment. Ital J Neurol Sci 18(4):195-208, 1997.
24. Corcos DM, Chen CM, Quinn NP, McAuley J, Rothwell JC: Strength in Parkinson's disease: Relationship to rate of force generation and clinical status. Ann Neurol 39(1):79-88, 1996.
25. Forssberg H, Johnels B, Steg G: Is parkinsonian gait caused by a regression to an immature walking pattern? Adv Neurol 40:375-379, 1984.
26. Johnson MT, Mendez A, Kipnis AN, Silverstein P, Zwiebel F, Ebner TJ: Acute effects of levodopa on wrist movement in Parkinson's disease. Kinematics, volitional EMG modulation and reflex amplitude modulation. Brain 117 (Pt 6):1409-1422, 1994.
27. Johnson MT, Kipnis AN, Coltz JD, et al: Effects of levodopa and viscosity on the velocity and accuracy of visually guided tracking in Parkinson's disease. Brain 119 (Pt 3):801-813, 1996.
28. Morris M, Iansek R, Matyas T, Summers J: The pathogenesis of gait hypokinesia in Parkinson's disease. Brain 117:1169-1181, 1994.
29. Morris M, Iansek R, Matyas T, Summers J: Stride length regulation in Parkinson's disease. Normalization strategies and underlying mechanisms. Brain 119:551-568, 1996.

30. Morris M, Iansek R. Characteristics of motor disturbance in Parkinson's disease and strategies for movement rehabilitation. J Human Mov Sci 15(5):649-669, 1996.
31. Morris ME, Matyas TA, Iansek R, Summers JJ: Temporal stability of gait in Parkinson's disease. Phys Ther 76(7): 763-777; discussion 778-780, 1996.
32. Murray M, Sepic S, Gardner G, Downs W: Walking patterns of men with parkinsonism. Am J Phys Med 57:278-294, 1978.
33. Robichaud JA, Pfann KD, Comella CL, Corcos DM: Effect of medication on EMG patterns in individuals with Parkinson's disease. Mov Disord 17(5):950-960, 2002.
34. Weinrich M, Koch K, Garcia F, Angel RW: Axial versus distal motor impairment in Parkinson's disease. Neurology 38(4): 540-545, 1988.
35. Pastor MA, Jahanshahi M, Artieda J, Obeso JA: Performance of repetitive wrist movements in Parkinson's disease. Brain 115 (Pt 3):875-891, 1992.
36. Glendinning DS, Enoka RM: Motor unit behavior in Parkinson's disease. Phys Ther 74(1):61-70, 1994.
37. Kakinuma S, Nogaki H, Pramanik B, Morimatsu M: Muscle weakness in Parkinson's disease: isokinetic study of the lower limbs. Eur Neurol 39(4):218-222, 1998.
38. Nogaki H, Fukusako T, Sasabe F, Negoro K, Morimatsu M: Muscle strength in early Parkinson's disease. Mov Disord 10(2):225-226, 1995.
39. Nogaki H, Kakinuma S, Morimatsu M: Muscle weakness in Parkinson's disease: A follow-up study. Parkinsonism Relat Disord 8(1):57-62, 2001.
40. McAuley JH, Corcos DM, Rothwell JC, Quinn NP, Marsden CD: Levodopa reversible loss of the Piper frequency oscillation component in Parkinson's disease. J Neurol Neurosurg Psychiatry 70(4):471-476, 2001.
41. Pedersen SW, Oberg B: Dynamic strength in Parkinson's disease. Quantitative measurements following withdrawal of medication. Eur Neurol 33(2):97-102, 1993.
42. Deuschl G, Raethjen J, Baron R, Lindemann M, Wilms H, Krack P: The pathophysiology of parkinsonian tremor: A review. J Neurol 247(suppl 5):V33-V48, 2000.
43. Koller WC: Pharmacologic treatment of parkinsonian tremor. Arch Neurol 43(2):126-127, 1986.
44. Burleigh A, Horak F, Nutt J, Frank J: Levodopa reduces muscle tone and lower extremity tremor in Parkinson's disease. Can J Neurol Sci 22(4):280-285, 1995.
45. Dietz V: Neurophysiology of gait disorders: Present and future applications. Electroencephalogr Clin Neurophysiol 103(3): 333-355, 1997.
46. Rogers MW: Motor control problems in Parkinson's disease. Contemporary Management of motor control problems: Proceedings of the II Step Conference, Alexandria, VA, 1991, American Physical Therapy Association.
47. Horak FB, Frank J, Nutt J: Effects of dopamine on postural control in parkinsonian subjects: Scaling, set, and tone. J Neurophysiol 75(6):2380-2396, 1996.
48. Frank JS, Horak FB, Nutt J: Centrally initiated postural adjustments in parkinsonian patients on and off levodopa. J Neurophysiol 84(5):2440-2448, 2000.
49. Johnson MT, Kipnis AN, Lee MC, Loewenson RB, Ebner TJ: Modulation of the stretch reflex during volitional sinusoidal tracking in Parkinson's disease. Brain 114 (Pt 1B):443-460, 1991.
50. Benecke R, Rothwell JC, Dick JP, Day BL, Marsden CD: Simple and complex movements off and on treatment in patients with Parkinson's disease. J Neurol Neurosurg Psychiatry 50(3):296-303, 1987.
51. Fattapposta F, Pierelli F, Traversa G, et al: Preprogramming and control activity of bimanual self-paced motor task in Parkinson's disease. Clin Neurophysiol 111(5):873-883, 2000.
52. Fattapposta F, Pierelli F, My F, et al: L-dopa effects on preprogramming and control activity in a skilled motor act in Parkinson's disease. Clin Neurophysiol 113(2):243-253, 2002.
53. Ingvarsson P, Johnels B, Lund S, Steg G: Coordination of manual, postural, and locomotor movements during simple goal-directed motor tasks in parkinsonian off and on states. Adv Neurol 45:375-382, 1987.
54. Ingvarsson PE, Johnels B, Steg G, Olsson T: Objective assessment in Parkinson's disease: Optoelectronic movement and force analysis in clinical routine and research. Adv Neurol 80:447-458, 1999.
55. Johnels B, Ingvarsson PE, Steg G, Olsson T: The Posturo-Locomotion-Manual Test. A simple method for the characterization of neurological movement disturbances. Adv Neurol 87:91-100, 2001.
56. Johnels B, Ingvarsson PE, Matousek M, Steg G, Heinonen EH: Optoelectronic movement analysis in Parkinson's disease: Effect of selegiline on the disability in de novo parkinsonian patients—a pilot study. Acta Neurol Scand Suppl 136:40-43, 1991.
57. Rajput AH, Fenton ME, Birdi S, et al: Clinical-pathological study of levodopa complications. Mov Disord 17(2):289-296, 2002.
58. Bedard PJ, Blanchet PJ, Levesque D, et al: Pathophysiology of L-dopa-induced dyskinesias. Mov Disord 14(suppl 1):4-8, 1999.
59. Kostic V, Przedborski S, Flaster E, Sternic N: Early development of levodopa-induced dyskinesias and response fluctuations in young-onset Parkinson's disease. Neurology 41(2 (Pt 1):202-205, 1991.
60. Linazasoro G: Physiopathology of parkinsonism and dyskinesias: Lessons from surgical observations [in Spanish]. Neurologia 16(1):17-29, 2001.
61. Nutt JG, Gancher ST: Parkinson's disease dyskinesias. Neurology 44(6):1187; author reply 1187-1188, 1994.
62. Fahn S: How do you treat motor complications in Parkinson's disease: Medicine, surgery, or both? Ann Neurol 64(suppl 2): S56-S64, 2008.
63. Fox SH, Lang AE: Levodopa-related motor complications—Phenomenology. Mov Disord 23 (suppl 3):S509-S514, 2008.
64. Chase TN, Mouradian MM, Engber TM: Motor response complications and the function of striatal efferent systems. Neurology 43(12 suppl 6):S23-S27, 1993.
65. Encarnacion EV, Hauser RA: Levodopa-induced dyskinesias in Parkinson's disease: Etiology, impact on quality of life, and treatments. Eur Neurol 60(2):57-66, 2008.
66. Thanvi B, Lo N, Robinson T: Levodopa-induced dyskinesia in Parkinson's disease: clinical features, pathogenesis, prevention and treatment. Postgrad Med J 83(980):384-388, 2007.
67. Wenzelburger R, Zhang BR, Poepping M, et al: Dyskinesias and grip control in Parkinson's disease are normalized by chronic stimulation of the subthalamic nucleus. Ann Neurol 52(2):240-243, 2002.
68. Wenzelburger R, Zhang BR, Pohle S, et al: Force overflow and levodopa-induced dyskinesias in Parkinson's disease. Brain 125(Pt 4):871-879, 2002.
69. Nutt JG, Gancher ST, Woodward WR: Does an inhibitory action of levodopa contribute to motor fluctuations? Neurology 38(10):1553-1557, 1988.
70. Blanchet PJ, Calon F, Morissette M, et al: Regulation of dopamine receptors and motor behavior following pulsatile and continuous dopaminergic replacement strategies in the MPTP primate model. Adv Neurol 86:337-344, 2001.
71. Rascol O, Sabatini U, Brefel C, et al: Cortical motor overactivation in parkinsonian patients with L-dopa-induced peak-dose dyskinesia. Brain 121 (Pt 3):527-533, 1998.
72. McColl CD, Reardon KA, Shiff M, Kempster PA: Motor response to levodopa and the evolution of motor fluctuations

in the first decade of treatment of Parkinson's disease. Mov Disord 17(6):1227-1234, 2002.
73. Levodopa: Management of Parkinson's disease. Mov Disord 17(suppl 4):S23-S37, 2002.
74. Tintner R, Jankovic J: Treatment options for Parkinson's disease. Curr Opin Neurol 15(4):467-476, 2002.
75. Samanta J, Hauser RA: Duodenal levodopa infusion for the treatment of Parkinson's disease. Expert Opin Pharmacother 8(5):657-664, 2007.
76. Clarke CE: Dopamine agonist monotherapy in early Parkinson's disease. Hosp Med 64(1):8-11, 2003.
77. Gerlach M, Double K, Reichmann H, Riederer P: Arguments for the use of dopamine receptor agonists in clinical and preclinical Parkinson's disease. J Neural Transm Suppl 65:167-183, 2003.
78. Grimes DA, Lang AE: Treatment of early Parkinson's disease. Can J Neurol Sci 26(suppl 2):S39-S44, 1999.
79. Mendis T, Suchowersky O, Lang A, Gauthier S: Management of Parkinson's disease: A review of current and new therapies. Can J Neurol Sci26(2):89-103, 1999.
80. Antonini A, Barone P: Dopamine agonist-based strategies in the treatment of Parkinson's disease. Neurol Sci 29 (suppl 5):S371-S374, 2008.
81. Schwarz J: Rationale for dopamine agonist use as monotherapy in Parkinson's disease. Curr Opin Neurol 16(suppl 1):S27-S33, 2003.
82. Tintner R, Jankovic J: Dopamine agonists in Parkinson's disease. Expert Opin Investig Drugs 12(11):1803-1820, 2003.
83. Stocchi F, Vacca L, Onofrj M: Are there clinically significant differences between dopamine agonists? Adv Neurol 91:259-266, 2003.
84. Romrell J, Fernandez HH, Okun MS: Rationale for current therapies in Parkinson's disease. Expert Opin Pharmacother 4(10):1747-1761, 2003.
85. Gordin A, Kaakkola S, Teravainen H: Position of COMT inhibition in the treatment of Parkinson's disease. Adv Neurol 91:237-250, 2003.
86. Melamed E, Zoldan J, Galili-Mosberg R, Ziv I, Djaldetti R: Current management of motor fluctuations in patients with advanced Parkinson's disease treated chronically with levodopa. J Neural Transm Suppl 56:173-183, 1999.
87. Rinne JO, Ulmanen I, Lee MS: Catechol-O-methyl transferase (COMT) inhibitors in patients with Parkinson's disease: Is COMT genotype a useful indicator of clinical efficacy? Am J Pharmacogenomics 3(1):11-15, 2003.
88. Tolosa E: Advances in the pharmacological management of Parkinson disease. J Neural Transm Suppl (64):65-78, 2003.
89. Wasielewski PG, Burns JM, Koller WC: Pharmacologic treatment of tremor. Mov Disord 13(suppl 3):90-100, 1998.
90. Mandel S, Grunblatt E, Riederer P, Gerlach M, Levites Y, Youdim MB: Neuroprotective strategies in Parkinson's disease: An update on progress. CNS Drugs 17(10):729-762, 2003.
91. Stocchi F, Olanow CW: Neuroprotection in Parkinson's disease: Clinical trials. Ann Neurol 53(suppl 3):S87-S97, 2003.
92. Whone AL, Watts RL, Stoessl AJ, et al: REAL-PET Study Group. Slower progression of Parkinson's disease with ropinirole versus levodopa: The REAL-PET study. Ann Neurol 54:93-101, 2003.
93. Parkinson Study Group: Dopamine transporter brain imaging to access the effects of promixpexole vs levodopa on Parkinson disease progression. JAMA 287:1653-1661, 2002.
94. Morris ME: Movement disorders in people with Parkinson disease: A model for physical therapy. Phys Ther 80(6):578-597, 2000.
95. Reuter I, Harder S, Engelhardt M, Baas H: The effect of exercise on pharmacokinetics and pharmacodynamics of levodopa. Mov Disord 15(5):862-868, 2000.
96. Goetz CG, Thelen JA, MacLeod CM, Carvey PM, Bartley EA, Stebbins GT: Blood levodopa levels and unified Parkinson's disease rating scale function: With and without exercise. Neurology 43(5):1040-1042, 1993.
97. Mouradian MM, Juncos JL, Serrati C, Fabbrini G, Palmeri S, Chase TN: Exercise and the anti-parkinsonian response to levodopa. Clin Neuropharmacol 10(4):351-355, 1987.
98. Carter JH, Nutt JG, Woodward WR: The effect of exercise on levodopa absorption. Neurology 42(10):2042-2045, 1992.
99. Weinshenker B: The natural history of multiple sclerosis. Neurol Clin 13:119-146, 1995.
100. Keegan B, Noseworthy J: Multiple sclerosis. Annu Rev Med 53:285-302, 2002.
101. McDonald W, Compston A, Edan G, et al: Recommended diagnostic criteria for multiple sclerosis: Guidelines from the International Panel on the Diagnosis of Multiple Sclerosis. Ann Neurol 50:121-127, 2001.
102. Poser C, Brinar V: Diagnostic criteria for multiple sclerosis. Clin Neurol Neurosurg 103:1-11, 2001.
103. Confavreux C, Aimard G, Devic M: Course and prognosis of multiple sclerosis assessed by the computerized data processing of 349 patients. Brain 103:281-300, 1980.
104. Weinshenker B, Bass B, Rice G, et al: The natural history of multiple sclerosis: A geographically based study. I. Clinical course and disability. Brain 112:133-146, 1989.
105. Sweeney V, Sadovnick A, Brandejs V: Prevalence of multiple sclerosis in British Columbia. Can J Neurol Sci 13:47-51, 1986.
106. Thompson A, Polman C, Miller D, et al: Primary progressive multiple sclerosis. Brain 120:1085-1096, 1997.
107. Compston A, Coles A: Multiple sclerosis. Lancet 359:1221-1231, 2002.
108. Skegg D: Multiple sclerosis: Nature or nurture? Br Med J 302:846-847, 1991.
109. Wingerchuk D, Weinshenker B: Multiple sclerosis: Epidemiology, genetics, classification, natural history, and clinical outcome measures. Neuroimaging Clin N Am 10:611-624, 2000.
110. Compston A, Sawcer S: Genetic analysis of multiple sclerosis. Curr Neurol Neurosci Rep 2:259-266, 2002.
111. Trapp BD, Peterson J, Ransohoff RM, Rudick R, Mork S, Bo L: Axonal transection in the lesions of multiple sclerosis. N Engl J Med 338:278-285, 1998.
112. Trapp B, Ransohoff R, Rudick R: Axonal pathology in multiple sclerosis: Relationship to neurologic disability. Curr Opin Neurol 12:295-302, 1999.
113. Trapp B, Ransohoff R, Fischer E, Rudick R: Neurodegeneration in multiple sclerosis: Relationship to neurological disability. Neuroscientist 5:48-57, 1999.
114. De Stefano N, Narayanan S, Francis G, et al: Evidence of axonal damage in the early stages of multiple sclerosis and its relevance to disability. Arch Neurol 58:65-70, 2001.
115. Kurtzke JF: Rating neurologic impairment in multiple sclerosis: An expanded disability status scale (EDSS). Neurology 33(11):1444-1452, 1982.
116. Hobart J, Freeman J, Thompson A: Kurtzke scales revisited. Brain 123(Pt 5):1027-1040, 2000.
117. O'Riordan J, Thompson A, Kingsley D, et al: The prognostic value of brain MRI in clinically isolated syndromes of the CNS. A 10-year follow-up. Brain 121:495-503, 1998.
118. Brex P, Ciccarelli O, O'Riordan J, Sailer M, Thompson A, Miller D: A longitudinal study of abnormalities on MRI and disability from multiple sclerosis. N Engl J Med 346: 158-164, 2002.

119. Rovaris M, Filippi M: Contrast enhancement and the acute lesion in multiple sclerosis. Neuroimaging Clin N Am 10:705-715, 2000.
120. McFarland H, Frank J, Albert P, et al: Using gadolinium-enhanced magnetic resonance imaging lesions to monitor disease activity in multiple sclerosis. Ann Neurol 32:758-766, 1992.
121. Miller D, Albert P, Barkhof F, et al: Guidelines for the use of magnetic resonance techniques in monitoring the treatment of multiple sclerosis. US National MS Society Task Force. Ann Neurol 39:6-16, 1996.
122. Cook S, Dowling P: Multiple sclerosis and viruses: An overview. Neurology 30:80-91, 1980.
123. Revel M, Chebath J, Mangelus M, Harroch S, Moviglia G: Antagonism of interferon beta on interferon gamma: Inhibition of signal transduction in vitro and reduction of serum levels in multiple sclerosis patients. Mult Scler 1(suppl 1): S5-S11, 1995.
124. Hohlfeld R: Biotechnological agents for the immunotherapy of multiple sclerosis. Principles, problems and perspectives. Brain 120:865-916, 1997.
125. Durelli L, Verdun E, Barbero P, et al: Independent Comparison of Interferon (INCOMIN) Trial Study Group. Every-other-day interferon beta-1b versus once-weekly interferon beta-1a for multiple sclerosis: Results of a 2-year prospective randomised multicentre study (INCOMIN). Lancet 359:1453-1460, 2002.
126. Durelli L, Verdun E, Barbero P, Bergui M, Versino E, Ghezzi A, Montanari E, Zaffaroni M: Independent Comparison of Interferon (INCOMIN) Trial Study Group. Every-other-day interferon beta-1b versus once-weekly interferon beta-1a for multiple sclerosis: Results of a 2-year prospective randomised multicentre study (INCOMIN). Lancet. 2002. Apr 27;359(9316):1453-1460.
127. Benatar M: Interferon beta-1a and beta-1b for treatment of multiple sclerosis. Lancet 360:1428; author reply 1428-1429, 2002.
128. Panitch H, Goodin DS, Francis G, et al: Randomized, comparative study of interferon beta-1a treatment regimens in MS: The EVIDENCE Trial. Neurology 59:1496-1506, 2002.
129. Clanet M, Radue EW, Kappos L, et al: A randomized, double-blind, dose-comparison study of weekly interferon beta-1a in relapsing MS. Neurology 59:1507-1517, 2002.
130. Clerico M, Faggiano F, Palace J, Rice G, Tintorè M, Durelli L: Recombinant interferon beta or glatiramer acetate for delaying conversion of the first demyelinating event to multiple sclerosis. Cochrane Database Syst Rev 16(2):CD005278, 2008.
131. Kappos L, Freedman MS, Polman CH, et al: Effect of early versus delayed interferon beta-1b treatment on disability after a first clinical event suggestive of multiple sclerosis: A 3-year follow-up analysis of the BENEFIT study. BENEFIT Study Group. Lancet 370(9585):389-397, 2007.
132. Polman C, Kappos L, Freedman MS, et al: Subgroups of the BENEFIT study: risk of developing MS and treatment effect of interferon beta-1b. BENEFIT investigators. J Neurol 255(4):480-487, 2008.
133. Coyle PK: Early treatment of multiple sclerosis to prevent neurologic damage. Neurology 71(24 suppl 3):S3-S7, 2008.
134. Duda PW, Schmied MC, Cook SL, Krieger JI, Hafler D: Glatiramer acetate (Copaxone) induces degenerate, Th2-polarized immune responses in patients with multiple sclerosis. J Clin Invest 105:967-976, 2000.
135. Chen M, Gran B, Costello K, Johnson K, Martin R, Dhib-Jalbut S: Glatiramer acetate induces a Th2-biased response and crossreactivity with myelin basic protein in patients with MS. Mult Scler 7:209-219, 2001.
136. Schori H, Kipnis J, Yoles E, et al: Vaccination for protection of retinal ganglion cells against death from glutamate cytotoxicity and ocular hypertension: Implications for glaucoma. Proc Natl Acad Sci 98:3398-3403, 2001.
137. Schwartz M: Physiological approaches to neuroprotection. Boosting of protective autoimmunity. Surv Ophthalmol 45(suppl 3):S256-S260; discussion, S273-S276, 2001.
138. Bornstein M, Miller A, Slagle S, et al: A pilot trial of Cop 1 in exacerbating-remitting multiple sclerosis. N Engl J Med 317(7):408-414, 1987.
139. Johnson KP, Brooks BR, Cohen JA, et al: Copolymer 1 reduces relapse rate and improves disability in relapsing-remitting multiple sclerosis: Results of a phase III multicenter, double-blind placebo-controlled trial. The Copolymer 1 Multiple Sclerosis Study Group. Neurology 45(7):1268-1276, 1995.
140. Johnson KP, Brooks BR, Cohen JA, et al: Extended use of glatiramer acetate (Copaxone) is well tolerated and maintains its clinical effect on multiple sclerosis relapse rate and degree of disability. Copolymer 1 Multiple Sclerosis Study Group. Neurology 50(3):701-708, 1998.
141. Johnson KP, Brooks BR, Cohen JA, et al: Sustained clinical benefits of glatiramer acetate in relapsing multiple sclerosis patients observed for 6 years. Copolymer 1 Multiple Sclerosis Study Group. Mult Scler 6(4):255-266, 2000.
142. Wolinsky JS, Narayana PA, Johnson KP: United States open-label glatiramer acetate extension trial for relapsing multiple sclerosis: MRI and clinical correlates. Multiple Sclerosis Study Group and the MRI Analysis Center. Mult Scler 7(1):33-41, 2001.
143. Comi G, Filippi M, Wolinsky JS: European/Canadian multicenter, double-blind, randomized, placebo-controlled study of the effects of glatiramer acetate on magnetic resonance imaging-measured disease activity and burden in patients with relapsing multiple sclerosis. European/Canadian Glatiramer Acetate Study Group. Ann Neurol 49(3):290-297, 2001.
144. Hartung HP, Gonsette R, Konig N, et al: Mitoxantrone in progressive multiple sclerosis: A placebo-controlled, double-blind, randomised, multicentre trial. Lancet 360:2018-2025, 2002.
145. Hartung HP, Gonsette R, Konig N, et al: Therapeutic effect of mitoxantrone combined with methylprednisolone in multiple sclerosis: A randomised multicentre study of active disease using MRI and clinical criteria. J Neurol Neurosurg Psychiatry 62:112-118, 1997.
146. Hartung HP, Gonsette R, Konig N, et al: Randomized placebo-controlled trial of mitoxantrone in relapsing-remitting multiple sclerosis: 24-month clinical and MRI outcome. J Neurol 244:153-159, 1997.
147. Ghalie RG, Mauch E, Edan G, et al: A study of therapy-related acute leukaemia after mitoxantrone therapy for multiple sclerosis. Mult Scler8:441-445, 2002.
148. Ghalie RG, Edan G, Laurent M, et al: Cardiac adverse effects associated with mitoxantrone (Novantrone) therapy in patients with MS. Neurology 59:909-913, 2002.
149. Youssef S, Stuve O, Patarroyo JC, et al: The HMG-CoA reductase inhibitor, atorvastatin, promotes a Th2 bias and reverses paralysis in central nervous system autoimmune disease. Nature 420(6911):78-84, 2002.
150. Vollmer T, Key L, Durkalski V, et al: Oral simvastatin treatment in relapsing-remitting multiple sclerosis. Lancet 363:1607-1608, 2004.
151. Havrdova E, Galetta S, Hutchinson M, et al: Effect of natalizumab on clinical and radiological disease activity in multiple sclerosis: A retrospective analysis of the Natalizumab Safety and Efficacy in Relapsing-Remitting Multiple

Sclerosis (AFFIRM) study. Lancet Neurol 8(3):254-260, 2009.

152. Gasperini C, Cefaro LA, Borriello G, Tosto G, Prosperini L, Pozzilli C: Emerging oral drugs for multiple sclerosis. Expert Opin Emerg Drugs 13(3):465-477, 2008.
153. Miller A, Bourdette D, Cohen JA, et al: Multiple sclerosis. Continuum 5:120-133, 1999.
154. Krupp LB, Rizvi SA: Symptomatic therapy for underrecognized manifestations of multiple sclerosis. Neurology 58 (suppl 4):S32-S39, 2002.
155. Krupp LB: Mechanisms, measurement, and management of fatigue in multiple sclerosis. In Thompson AJ, Polman C, Hohfeld R, editors: Multiple sclerosis: Clinical challenges and controversies, London, 1997, Martin Dunitz.
156. Medical Advisory Board of the National Multiple Sclerosis Society: Expert opinion paper: Treatment recommendations for physicians—Management of MS-related fatigue. New York, 2002, National Multiple Sclerosis Society. Available at http://www.nationalmssociety.org/pdf/forpros/Expert_fatigue.pdf: Accessed June 14, 2005.
157. Zifko UA, Rupp M, Schwarz S, Zipko HT, Maida EM: Modafinil in treatment of fatigue in multiple sclerosis. Results of an open-label study. J Neurol 249:983-987, 2002.
158. Rammohan KW, Rosenberg JH, Lynn DJ, et al: Efficacy and safety of modafinil (Provigil®) for the treatment of fatigue in multiple sclerosis: A two center phase 2 study. J Neurol Neurosurg Psychiatry 72:179-183, 2002.
159. Weinshenker BG, Penman M, Bass B, Ebers GC, Rice GPA: A double-blind, randomized, crossover trial of pemoline in fatigue associated with multiple sclerosis. Neurology 42:1468-1471, 1992.
160. Steinman L, Martin R, Bernard C, et al: Multiple sclerosis: deeper understanding of its pathogenesis reveals new targets for therapy. Annu Rev Neurosci 25:491-505, 2002.
161. Wiendl H, Kieseier BC: Disease modifying therapies in multiple sclerosis: An update on recent and ongoing trials and future strategies. Exp Opin Invest Drugs 12:689-712, 2003.
162. Bachman DL, Wolf PA, Linn RT, et al: Incidence of dementia and probable Alzheimer disease in a general population: the Framingham Study. Neurology 43:515-519, 1993.
163. Jorm AF, Jolley D: The incidence of dementia: A meta-analysis. Neurology 51:728-733, 1998.
164. Kawas C, Gray S, Brookmeyer R, et al: Age-specific incidence rates of Alzheimer disease: The Baltimore Longitudinal Study of Aging. Neurology 54:2072-2077, 2000.
165. Brookmeyer R, Gray S, Kawas C: Projections of Alzheimer disease in the United States and the public health impact of delaying disease onset. Am J Public Health 88:1337-1342, 1998.
166. Ernst RL, Hay JW: Economic research on Alzheimer disease: A review of the literature. Alzheimer Dis Assoc Disord 11(suppl 6):135-145, 1997.
167. McKhann G, Drachman D, Folstein M, et al: Clinical diagnosis of Alzheimer disease: Report of the NINCDS-ADRDA Work Group under the auspices of Department of Health and Human Services Task Force on Alzheimer Disease. Neurology 34:939-944, 1984.
168. Cotman CW, Anderson AJ: A potential role for apoptosis in neurodegeneration and Alzheimer's disease. Mol Neurobiol 10:19-45, 1995.
169. Mattson MP, Bruce AJ, Mark RJ: Amyloid cytotoxicity and Alzheimer's disease: Roles of membrane oxidation and perturbed ion homeostasis. In Brioni JD, editor: Pharmacological treatment of Alzheimer's disease: Molecular and neurobiological foundations, New York, 1997, Wiley-Liss.
170. Selkoe DJ: The genetics and molecular pathology of Alzheimer's disease: Roles of amyloid and the presenilins. Neurol Clin 18:903-922, 2000.
171. Arriagada PV, Growdon JH, Hedley-Whyte ET, et al: Neurofibrillary tangles but not senile plaques parallel duration and severity of Alzheimer's disease. Neurology 42:631-639, 1992.
172. Giannakopoulos P, Hof PR, Michel JP, et al: Cerebral cortex pathology in aging and Alzheimer's disease: A quantitative survey of large hospital-based geriatric and psychiatric cohorts. Brain Res Brain Res Rev 25:217-245, 1997.
173. Francis PT, Palmer AM, Snape M, Wilcock GK: The cholinergic hypothesis of Alzheimer's disease: A review of progress. J Neurol Neurosurg Psychiatry 66:137-147, 1999.
174. Mayeux R, Sano M: Treatment of Alzheimer's disease. N Engl J Med 341:1670-1679, 1999.
175. Mohs RC, Doody RS, Morris JC, et al: A 1-year, placebo-controlled preservation of function survival study of donepezil in AD patients. Neurology 57:481-488, 2001.
176. Winblad B, Engedal K, Soininen H, et al: A 1-year, randomized, placebo-controlled study of donepezil in patients with mild to moderate AD. Neurology 57:489-495, 2001.
177. O'Brien JT, Ballard CG: Drugs for Alzheimer's disease. Br Med J 323:123-124, 2001.
178. Winblad B, Poritis N: Memantine in severe dementia: Results of the M-BEST study (benefit and efficacy in severely demented patients during treatment with memantine). Int J Geriatr Psychiatry 14:135-146, 1999.
179. Reisberg B, Doody R, Stöffler A, et al: Memantine in moderate-to-severe Alzheimer's disease. N Engl J Med 348: 1333-1341, 2003.
180. Ferris SH, Schmitt FA, Doody RS, et al: Long-term treatment with the NMDA antagonist, memantine: Results of a 24-week, open-label extension study in moderate to severe Alzheimer's disease [abstract]. Neurology 60(suppl 1):A414, 2003.
181. Farlow MR, Tariot PN, Grossberg GT, et al: Memantine/donepezil dual-therapy is superior to placebo/donepezil therapy for treatment of moderate to severe Alzheimer's disease [abstract]. Neurology 60(suppl 1):A412, 2003.
182. Hartmann S, Möbius HJ: Tolerability of memantine in combination with cholinesterase inhibitors in dementia therapy. Int Clin Psychopharmacol 18:81-85, 2003.
183. Hirohata M, Ono K, Yamada M: Non-steroidal anti-inflammatory drugs as anti-amyloidogenic compounds. Curr Pharm Des 14(30):3280-3294, 2008.
184. Sano M, Grossman H, Van Dyk K: Preventing Alzheimer's disease: Separating fact from fiction. CNS Drugs 22(11):887-902, 2008.
185. Kivipelto M, Helkala EL, Laakso MP, et al: Midlife vascular risk factors and Alzheimer's disease in later life: Longitudinal, population based study. Br Med J 322:1447-1451, 2001.
186. Moroney JT, Tang MX, Berglund L, et al: Low-density lipoprotein cholesterol and the risk of dementia with stroke. JAMA 282:254-260, 1999.
187. Wolozin B, Kellman W, Ruosseau P, Celesia GG, Siegel G: Decreased prevalence of Alzheimer disease associated with 3-hydroxy-3-methyglutaryl coenzyme A reductase inhibitors. Arch Neurol 57:1439-1443, 2000.
188. Yaffe K, Barrett-Connor E, Lin F, Grady D: Serum lipoprotein levels, statin use, and cognitive function in older women. Arch Neurol 59:378-384, 2002.
189. McGuinness B, Craig D, Bullock R, Passmore P: Statins for the prevention of dementia. Cochrane Database Syst Rev (2):CD003160, 2009.

190. Schenk D, Barbour R, Dunn W, et al: Immunization with amyloid-beta attenuates Alzheimer-disease-like pathology in the PDAPP mouse. Nature 400:173-177, 1999.
191. Weiner HL, Lemere CA, Maron R, et al: Nasal administration of amyloid-beta peptide decreases cerebral amyloid burden in a mouse model of Alzheimer's disease. Ann Neurol 48:567-579, 2000.
192. Holmes C, Boche D, Wilkinson D, et al: Long-term effects of Abeta42 immunisation in Alzheimer's disease: Follow-up of a randomised, placebo-controlled phase I trial. Lancet 372(9634):216-223, 2008.
193. Hogan DB, Bailey P, Black S, et al: Diagnosis and treatment of dementia: Nonpharmacologic and pharmacologic therapy for mild to moderate dementia. Can Med Assoc J 179(10):1019, 1026, 2008.
194. Ballard CG, Gauthier S, Cummings JL, et al: Management of agitation and aggression associated with Alzheimer disease. Nat Rev Neurol (5):245-255, 2009.
195. Foster JK, Verdile G, Bates KA, Martins RN: Immunization in Alzheimer's disease: naïve hope or realistic clinical potential? Mol Psychiatry. 2009 Mar;14(3):239-251.

ADDITIONAL RESOURCES

The following are comprehensive resources with greater specificity than those provided in this chapter:

Fillit HM, O'Connell AW: Drug discovery and development for Alzheimer's disease, New York, 2000, Springer.
Fillit HM, O'Connell AW, Refolo LM: Strategies for drug discovery for cognitive aging and Alzheimer's disease., *J Mol Neurosci* 19(1-2):1-3, 2002.
Qizilbash N, Schneider LS: Practical recommendations and opinions on therapies for cognitive symptoms and prognosis modification. In Qizilbash N, Schneider LS, Chui H, et al, editors: *Evidence-based dementia practice*, London, 2002, Blackwell.
Schneider LS, Tariot PN: Cognitive enhancers and treatments for Alzheimer's disease. In Tasman A, Kay J, Lieberman JA, editors: *Psychiatry* (2nd ed.), London, 2003, John Wiley and Sons.
Zlokovic BV: Alzheimer's disease (AD) has been classified and treated as a neurodegenerative disorder, *Adv Drug Deliv Rev* 54:1533-1537, 2002.
Zlokovic BV: Vascular disorder in Alzheimer's disease: Role in pathogenesis of dementia and therapeutic targets, *Adv Drug Deliv Rev* 54:1553-1559, 2002.

18

Drug Treatment for Depression and Anxiety

Giovanni Carracci and Arnold Williams

DEPRESSION

Depression is an extremely common condition with a high prevalence worldwide and is associated with a fair amount of morbidity and mortality.[1] Community surveys on depression in Europe have shown 1-year prevalence rates from 1.4% in rural Germany to as high as 9.3% in Finland.[2] One survey from Japan indicated that 53.4% of first-year university students were depressed.[3] Chronic depression is frequently associated with dysfunction in interpersonal, marital, occupational, and family functioning, so many more individuals are affected by this disorder than just those who are classified as depressed.[4]

Depression is a disorder of mood, as opposed to a disorder of thought or reality. Symptoms range from mild and hardly noticeable to severe with hallucinations and delusions. The majority of depressions include some of the following symptoms: low mood, loss of interest in pleasurable activities, loss of motivation, loss of libido, pessimism, feelings of helplessness, hopelessness, fatigue, sleep disturbances, poor self-esteem, suicidal thoughts, and disturbances in food intake.[5] Two major categories of depression outlined in the fourth edition of the *Diagnostic and Statistical Manual of Mental Disorders (DSM-IV)* are dysthymic disorder and major depressive disorder, chronic type.[4] *Major depressive disorder* is defined by the above-mentioned symptoms for a period of 2 weeks or more and can be classified as mild, moderate, or severe. Severe depression can be present with or without psychotic features.[6] *Dysthymic disorder* is a mild chronic depression defined by the presence of more depressive moments than not for at least 2 years, the persistence of the depression for longer than 2 months, and an insidious onset. Patients with dysthymic disorder can display several of the symptoms of depression, but dysthymic disorder is usually characterized by more of the cognitive aspects of depression (low self-esteem, hopelessness), affective (low mood), and social dysfunction (loss of motivation and social withdrawal) than disturbances in sleep or appetite. In addition, the *DSM-IV* recognizes the diagnostic importance of symptoms that begin with an early onset, before the age of 21 years. For an actual diagnosis, the *DSM-IV* requires the presence of two of the following symptoms: fatigue or decreased energy, insomnia or hypersomnia, increased or decreased appetite, low self-esteem, poor concentration, and difficulty with decision making.[4]

Individuals with dysthymic disorder may also experience exacerbations in mood disturbance that meet the criteria for a major depressive episode. In fact, 75 to 90% of patients with dysthymic disorder report having had a major depressive episode previously.[4] Approximately 25% of patients given a diagnosis of a major depressive episode report having pervasive dysthymic disorder. For some patients, this may represent different phases of a single disease that waxes and wanes, depending on environmental stressors, rather than two distinct conditions. Those patients who are actually given a diagnosis of a major depressive episode may display the full gamut of symptoms described in the *DSM-IV*. However, one of the difficulties with classifying any of the depressions is that there is no "biologic feature" or laboratory value that separates one type from another. Psychological tests can help with the diagnosis, but few primary care doctors will take the time to administer them. Therefore, the classification system is based on subjective descriptions of symptoms.

Distinctions have been made between other types of depressive syndromes; for example, *unipolar affective disorder* involves mood being in the same direction (depression), as opposed to *bipolar affective disorder*, in which the primary mood may be either depression or mania but may include periods when the opposite affect is interspersed. Unipolar affective disorder is further divided into *reactive depression*, precipitated by a stressful life event, and *endogenous depression*, which is unrelated to external stress and has a familial component. There is a diagnosis called *adjustment disorder*, which can have symptoms of depression, anxiety, or both but does not meet the criteria for another formal *DSM-IV* diagnosis; the diagnosis is used to acknowledge the presence of these symptoms due to external stress, as described here, and can have features of depression, features of anxiety, or both.[100] In some cases, symptoms of depression can be pinpointed directly to a certain time of year, a condition referred to as *seasonal affective disorder (SAD)*.

At least three aspects of depression underline the urgency for a rapid diagnosis and initiation of treatment. Suicide is a consequence of depression and is the eighth leading cause of death in the United States and the third leading cause of death among children between the ages of 5 and 14 years.[1] Depression can lead to significant medical morbidity. There is evidence that depression affects cardiovascular health, resulting in a greater mortality rate among patients who have experienced a myocardial infarction (MI).[7] Depression has also been linked to osteoporosis, peptic ulcer disease, and diabetes.[8] Even subthreshold psychiatric symptoms are associated with significant medical impairment.[9] Although several of these physical developments might be linked to an elevated cortisol level, which is a trend seen in patients with depression, they nevertheless highlight the physical manifestations of this mental illness. The third aspect of depression that demands concern is the chronicity of the disease. Studies have shown that many patients who experience a major episode of depression eventually have chronic disease.[4] This is particularly true if the depression is not appropriately treated or if the patient is undertreated. In the majority of medical illnesses, good therapeutic agents are developed as an outcome of having a thorough understanding of the biology of the condition. Unfortunately, little is known about the underlying mechanisms of depression.

Pathophysiology of Depression

The original biologic hypothesis of depression has been referred to as the monoamine hypothesis.[5] It was popularized in the early 1960s as a result of the observation that patients taking reserpine to lower blood pressure became depressed. Depression was also observed when reserpine was used in high doses for the treatment of schizophrenia. Reserpine inhibits storage and subsequent release of the amine neurotransmitters serotonin and norepinephrine from the presynaptic nerve endings in the brain. Reserpine is rarely used today, but it is credited with having helped establish a neurochemical basis for depression. According to this theory, depression is related to a deficiency or imbalance of norepinephrine or serotonin or a deficiency in transmission of these amines. In addition, catecholamine depletion caused by low levels of tryptophan, a precursor to serotonin, has been associated with depression. In two studies, limiting dietary intake of tryptophan was found to produce a relapse in patients being treated for depression.[10,11]

Evidence for the monoamine theory has been presented and accepted by many researchers in the field of psychiatry, mainly because pharmacologic evidence exists; limiting reuptake of these neurotransmitters with antidepressants increases their concentration at the synaptic cleft and reduces symptoms. However, research of many years has uncovered several inconsistencies in this theory. First, the biochemical effects of antidepressant drugs occur quickly, but their effects may take weeks to materialize. This suggests that relief of depression is related to a secondary adaptive change in the brain rather than to the direct action of the drug. A change in receptor sensitivity concurrent with a downregulation of the receptor is another theory that has been difficult to prove.

Current theories focus on the neuroendocrine system, as well as on signal transduction pathways and growth factors, in order to narrow down the pathophysiology of depression. Persistent stress is known to activate the sympathetic nervous system and the hypothalamus–pituitary–adrenal axis. Elevated levels of corticotrophin-releasing hormone (CRH) are implicated in the pathophysiology of depression; this has been borne out by studies showing that cortisol fails to reduce CRH levels in depressed patients. Some researchers have even proposed that subtypes of depression could be related to different levels of CRH. Further support is provided by the observation that a significant number of patients with Cushing's syndrome have depression and are also known to have hippocampal volume depletion correlated with cortisol hypersecretion, similar to that seen in patients with depression.[12-14] This has been described as stress-induced neuronal atrophy or impairment in neuroplasticity. Additionally, it has been shown that stress and glucocorticoids reduce cellular resilience, a process by which neuronal cells become more susceptible to certain abuse such as ischemia, hypoglycemia, and excitatory amino acid toxicity.[15] Some of the current antidepressants increase hippocampal neurogenesis and improve neuroplasticity. Dysfunctions in growth hormone, thyroid hormone release, opioid receptors, and substance P are also being explored. The addition of thyroid hormone to antidepressant treatment in refractory depression has been successful, and blockade of substance P receptors has also shown promise.[16-18]

Mechanism of Action of Antidepressants

In the absence of a definitive theory for the pathogenesis of depression, it is useful to look at some of the commonalities that exist among antidepressants to help explain at least some of the pathophysiology. In general, these drugs act by blocking the reuptake of either serotonin or norepinephrine (Figure 18-1).[19] Normally, the major mechanism by which neurotransmission is terminated is by reuptake of the transmitter from the synaptic cleft back into the nerve terminal. From there, the neurotransmitter is either metabolized or stored in vesicles for future release. Reuptake is performed by a transmembrane transporter that carries sodium (Na^+) and chloride (Cl^-) ions along with the neurotransmitter into the cell cytoplasm. By blocking the reuptake transporter with drugs, the excess neurotransmitter is allowed to accumulate in the synaptic cleft. The excess amounts of

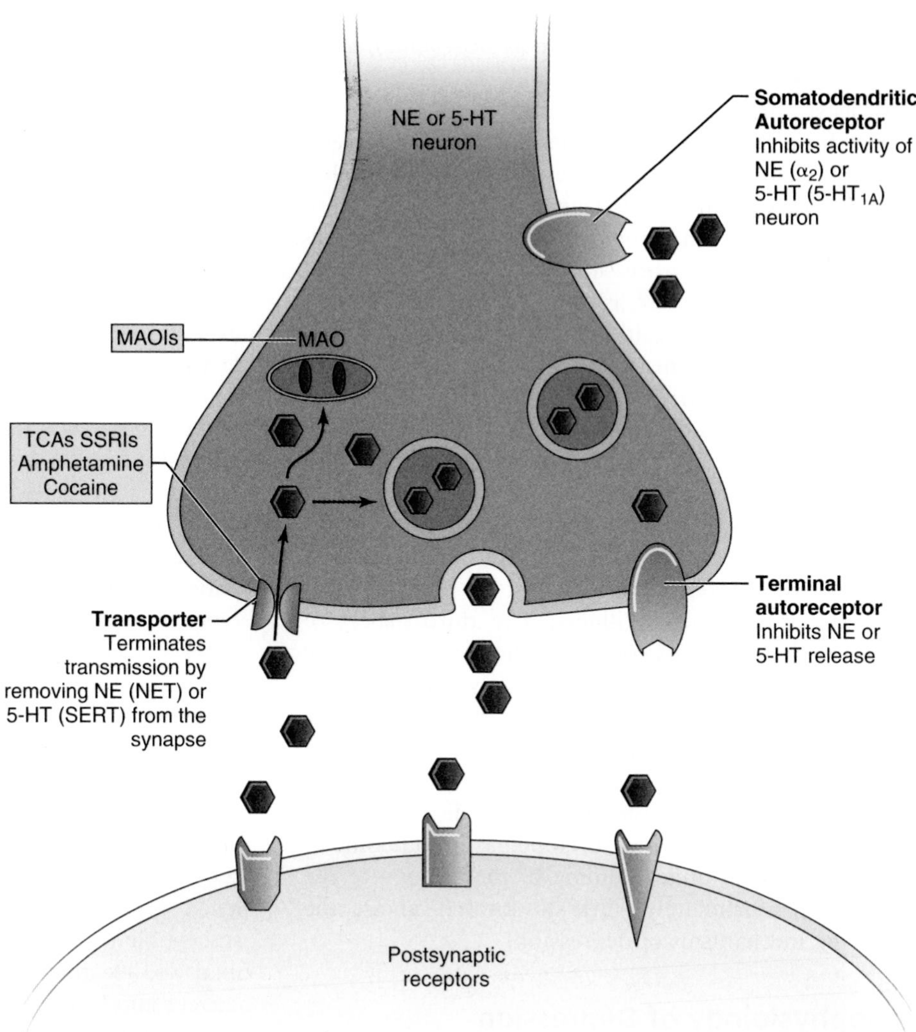

FIGURE 18-1 A noradrenergic or serotonergic synapse and sites at which some antidepressants may exert their actions. Tricyclic antidepressants, selective serotonin (5-HT) reuptake inhibitors, and some atypical antidepressants, as well as many other drugs such as amphetamine, act at the reuptake transporter (NET or SERT for norepinephrine [NE] or 5-HT, respectively). Monoamine oxidase (MAO), which is targeted by MAO inhibitors (MAOIs), is localized at the mitochondrial outer membrane. Somatodendritic and terminal autoreceptors regulate transmitter release through feedback inhibition of neuronal activity or inhibition of excitation–secretion coupling. The somatodendritic autoreceptors are innervated by recurrent collaterals from the same cell, by terminals from neighboring NE or 5-HT neurons, or by NE- or 5-HT–containing afferents from other brain regions. Dendritic release of transmitter may also activate somatodendritic autoreceptors. *(Adapted from Brody MJ, Larner J, Minneman KP, editors:* Human pharmacology: Molecular to clinical *(3rd ed.). St. Louis, 1998, Mosby.)*

serotonin or norepinephrine in the synaptic cleft lead to downregulation of their postsynaptic receptors. It is theorized that this downregulation of the receptors is ultimately responsible for the relief from depression.

Amphetamine and cocaine are similarly transported into the neuron by the transmembrane transporter.[19] However, this presents a problem because the transporters also allow reverse movement of serotonin and norepinephrine when the chemicals are displaced from the storage vesicles into the cytoplasm through the action of amphetamines. Therefore, it is extremely dangerous to combine antidepressants with an amphetamine. The result would be extremely high concentrations of the neurotransmitter in the synaptic cleft.

Another mechanism exerted by antidepressants is the desensitization of autoreceptors.[19] Somatodendritic and terminal autoreceptors regulate transmitter release through feedback inhibition. If excess neurotransmitter is released, the chemical makes its way to the autoreceptor and shuts down the nerve. These receptors are viewed as the neuron's shut-off switch in response to excessive firing. Drug desensitization of these autoreceptors would block this turn-off switch, allowing the neuron to continue firing and releasing the neurotransmitter. The result would be similar to blocking the reuptake of the neurotransmitter in that higher concentrations of the chemical in the synaptic cleft would produce a downregulation of the respective postsynaptic receptors.

Even though many of the older antidepressants focused on promoting higher neurotransmitter concentrations at the synaptic cleft, it has been determined that the availability of serotonin is critical to the relief of depression. A third mechanism by which antidepressants may achieve their goal is through the enhancement of norepinephrine release, which, in turn, enhances serotonergic cell firing. Norepinephrine acts on the α_1-receptor of the serotonin neuron to stimulate the firing and release of serotonin (Figure 18-2). The result is an elevated neurotransmitter concentration at the synaptic cleft and subsequent downregulation of the postsynaptic receptors.

Given the fact that antidepressants are effective in reducing the symptoms of depression in many patients, it is reasonable to speculate on the pathophysiology of this disorder on the basis of their mechanisms of action. The action of these drugs suggests that relief from depression may have to do more with the number of active receptors than with the absolute neurotransmitter concentration. This explanation fills in some of the gaps in the original monoamine hypothesis because downregulation of the receptors takes several weeks to occur; thus, even though elevated neurotransmitter release is observed fairly soon, the relief of depression occurs at a later date.

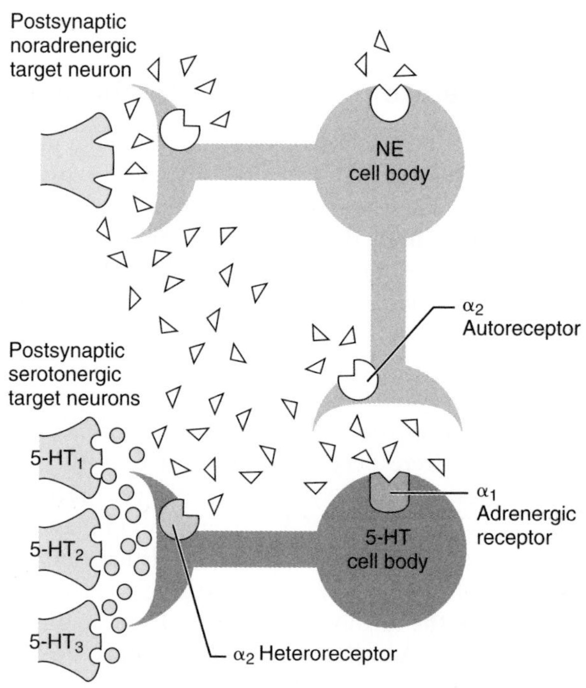

FIGURE 18-2 Mechanisms for noradrenergic control of serotonin (5-HT) release. The mechanism whereby modulation of norepinephrine (NE) release may alter 5-HT release is shown. α_2-Adrenergic autoreceptors regulate NE release by a negative feedback process. Activation of somatodendritic autoreceptors decreases noradrenergic neuronal activity, and activation of terminal autoreceptors decreases release of the neurotransmitter. Noradrenergic terminals innervate 5-HT cell bodies, where stimulation of postsynaptic α_1-adrenergic receptors activates 5-HT cell activity, increasing 5-HT release. α_2-Adrenergic receptors also exist as heteroreceptors on serotonergic terminals, where their activation inhibits 5-HT release. Thus a drug that blocks α_2-adrenergic receptors, but not α_1-adrenergic receptors, increases NE release, and thereby increases 5-HT release. *(Adapted from Brody MJ, Larner J, Minneman KP, editors:* Human pharmacology: Molecular to clinical *(3rd ed.). St. Louis, 1998, Mosby.)*

Tricyclic Antidepressants

Tricyclic antidepressants (TCAs) are a group of drugs that share a common three-ring chemical structure.[5] They are similar in structure to the phenothiazines (antipsychotic agents) except that they have an extra atom in the central ring (Figure 18-3). In fact, they were originally developed as antipsychotic drugs, but they were found to be useful only in reducing depression in schizophrenic individuals and not effective in reducing the psychosis.

Mechanism of Action of Tricyclic Antidepressants. As discussed previously, the main action of TCAs is to block the reuptake of serotonin and norepinephrine into the presynaptic terminal. Some are also effective at blocking dopamine uptake.[20] This is achieved by competitive inhibition of the binding site. However, the synthesis of neurotransmitters and their storage and release are not affected by these drugs.

Examples of TCAs include amitriptyline (also used to reduce pain in neurogenic pain syndromes), imipramine, nortriptyline, and clomipramine.[21] The choice of a TCA is based on the degree of sedation desired, or not desired, and the adverse effect profile (Table 18-1). For the most

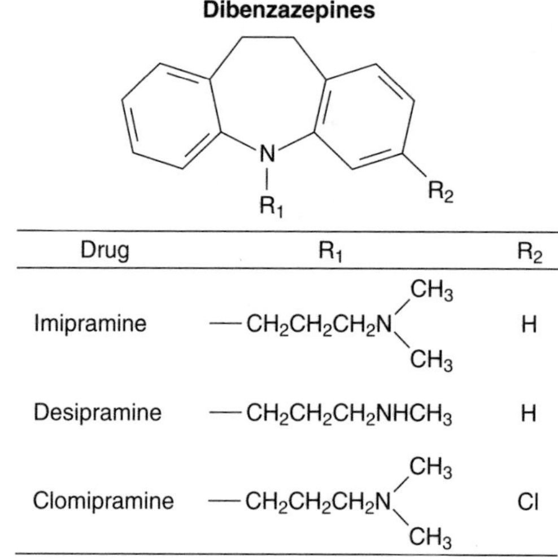

Drug	R_1	R_2
Imipramine	$-CH_2CH_2CH_2N(CH_3)_2$	H
Desipramine	$-CH_2CH_2CH_2NHCH_3$	H
Clomipramine	$-CH_2CH_2CH_2N(CH_3)_2$	Cl

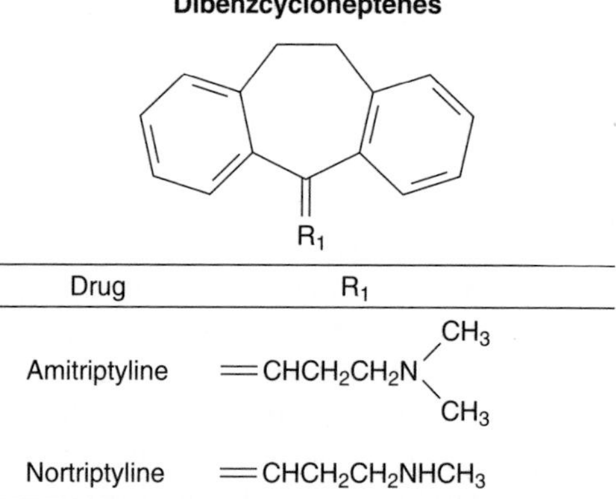

Drug	R_1
Amitriptyline	$=CHCH_2CH_2N(CH_3)_2$
Nortriptyline	$=CHCH_2CH_2NHCH_3$

FIGURE 18-3 Chemical structures of tricyclic antidepressants.

TABLE 18-1 Adverse Effect Profiles of Selected Antidepressant Drugs

Drug	Adverse Effects						
	Anticholinergic Effects	Drowsiness	Agitation	Orthostatic Hypotension	Arrhythmia	GI Effects	Weight Gain
Amitriptyline	4+	4+	0	4+	3+	0	4+
Desipramine	1+	1+	1+	2+	2+	0	1+
Imipramine	3+	3+	1+	4+	3+	1+	3+
Trazodone	0	4+	0	1+	1+	1+	1+
Bupropion	0	0	2+	0	0	3+	0
Fluoxetine	0	0	2+	0	0	3+	0
Paroxetine	0	0	2+	0	0	3+	0
Sertraline	0	0	2+	0	0	3+	0

Adapted from McKenry LM, Salerno E: *Mosby's pharmacology in nursing,* St Louis, 2003, Mosby .
Data were obtained from the following: Depression Guideline Panel: *Depression in primary care* (Vol 2.) Treatment of major depression. Clinical Practice Guideline #5. Rockville, MD, 2003, Department of Health and Human Services, Public Health Service, Agency for Health Care Policy and Research. DHCPR Pub. No. 93-0551.
0, Absent or seldom; 4+, very common; GI, gastrointestinal.

part, TCAs have equal effectiveness, with a success rate of approximately 60%, which is similar to that of other antidepressant agents.[1]

Adverse Drug Reactions Associated with Tricyclic Antidepressants. TCAs have varying affinities for histamine, muscarinic, and α_1-adrenoceptors.[5] In fact, the action at these neurochemical receptors is responsible for most of the adverse effects. TCAs act as antagonists at muscarinic receptors, producing dry mouth, constipation, urinary retention, blurred vision, and tachycardia. Blockade of histamine receptors produces sedation and weight gain, and the blockade at the adrenergic receptors produces orthostatic hypotension and dizziness. These adverse effects are especially problematic for the older patient because of the increased risk for falls. TCAs also produce sexual dysfunction, including decreased libido, abnormal ejaculation, and erectile dysfunction. Prolongation of the QT interval on an electrocardiogram (ECG) and its association with arrhythmia and sudden death pose another problem for the patient undergoing treatment with TCAs.[22,23] This may be associated with the inhibition of a cardiac potassium (K^+) channel in the ventricle known as the *human ether-a-go-go related gene* (HERG) channel. Because TCAs bind to plasma proteins, their effects tend to be enhanced by aspirin, which competes with them for binding to albumin. In addition, these drugs potentiate the effect of alcohol and other sedatives.

TCAs have a narrow safety index; overdose occurs at about five times the daily dose.[24] Toxic effects include shock, metabolic acidosis, arrhythmias and conduction defects, tremors, delirium, and bowel and bladder paralysis. In addition, because most of the drugs have a long half-life, if a person survives the initial overdose, he or she is still at risk for cardiac events 3 to 4 days later.

Selective Serotonin Reuptake Inhibitors

The discovery of the selective serotonin reuptake inhibitors (SSRIs) represented a major advance in psychopharmacology. These were among the first drugs in psychiatry to have been developed through a process of rational drug development. Many of the other psychopharmaceuticals were developed serendipitously. The choice to selectively block the serotonin uptake pump was based on the presumed relationship between serotonin and depression, anxiety disorders, and pain syndromes, as well as the pharmacodynamics of TCAs. In addition, they were developed to affect only the serotonin receptors (5-hydroxytryptamine [5-HT] receptors 5-HT_{1A}, 5-HT_{1D}, 5-HT_{2A}, 5-HT_{2C}, and 5-HT_3) and not other neuroreceptors. Unlike TCAs, SSRIs have no anticholinergic, histaminergic, or adrenergic properties. They also lack the cardiotoxic adverse effects commonly seen with TCAs. Another important advantage to these drugs is that they have a higher safety index than that of TCAs, but exactly how high an index has not been determined.[25]

Mechanism of Action of SSRIs. The leading hypothesis regarding the mechanism of action of these drugs is that they produce desensitization of the somatodendritic 5-HT_{1A} autoreceptors in the midbrain raphe nucleus. Desensitization of these receptors increases serotonin levels in critical areas of the brain. In addition, studies on paroxetine show that in young patients with depression (20 to 30 years old), there is a downregulation of the 5-HT_{2A}, but this downregulation is lessened in older subjects.[26,27]

Zimelidine, marketed by Astra, was the first SSRI to be developed.[25] It was approved for use in the early 1980s in Europe but was soon withdrawn because of reports of Guillain-Barré syndrome in some patients. Shortly after this withdrawal, fluoxetine and four other drugs in this category appeared on the market almost simultaneously: citalopram, sertraline, fluvoxamine, and paroxetine. The newest agent, escitalopram, has been released more recently. These are now among the most prescribed agents in medicine.

Although the SSRIs listed above have the same mechanism of action, there are some differences between them with regard to their inhibition of the cytochrome P450 enzymes.[25,28] Paroxetine and fluoxetine are modest inhibitors of these enzymes, whereas citalopram has little effect on them, indicating that it has fewer drug–drug interactions compared with the others. Paroxetine is viewed as having more adverse effects, particularly sexual dysfunction and weight gain.[29] Another difference among SSRIs is in their half-lives. Fluoxetine has a half-life of 1 to 4 days, longer than the other drugs. This is helpful for the patient demonstrating poor compliance because omission of one daily dose will have virtually no effect on concentration. There is also a prepared form of fluoxetine that is taken once per week, given its long half-life.[30] However, if it becomes necessary to switch to another drug (perhaps a TCA), the patient would have to endure a long washout period before the new drug could be administered.

Indications for Use of SSRIs. The number one indication for SSRIs is in the treatment of major depression. SSRIs are considered the first line of pharmacologic treatment for depression as well as for multiple anxiety disorders. Studies have shown the superiority of these agents compared with placebo, and several meta-analyses have indicated that TCAs and SSRIs have equal efficacy.[31,32] In addition, TCAs and SSRIs have similar time lines with regard to onset of action. However, the major difference between the two drug categories in these studies was that fewer patients discontinued their SSRIs because of adverse drug reactions (ADRs).[33]

SSRIs have also been the focus of other large studies examining their effectiveness in the treatment of obsessive compulsive disorder (OCD), social phobia, generalized anxiety disorder (GAD), panic disorder, post-traumatic stress disorder (PTSD), premenstrual syndrome, and eating disorders, as well as depression associated with medical illnesses. In fact, they have been shown to be superior to other drugs in the treatment of panic disorders, social phobia, and OCD; but for some of these disorders, a higher dose and longer duration of treatment may be necessary compared with the treatment for depression.[34-38] Treatment of these conditions also requires cognitive–behavioral therapy for improved efficacy. Expectations regarding SSRIs for the treatment of the eating disorders anorexia nervosa and bulimia nervosa have been lowered because clinical investigations with these drugs have resulted in mixed results. A lack of efficacy has been particularly observed in the treatment of patients with anorexia who are typically malnourished and underweight. It is theorized that the lack of adequate nutrients affects serotonin synthesis, which lowers treatment efficacy because once a normalization of weight is achieved, SSRIs reduce relapse rates.[39]

Adverse Effects of SSRIs. SSRIs have relatively few adverse effects compared with TCAs because they lack affinity for adrenergic, muscarinic, and histaminergic receptors. Minor ADRs include nausea, anorexia, and weight loss; but most patients develop tolerance to these effects with continued use. Gastrointestinal (GI) symptoms are exacerbated if these drugs are combined with a nonsteroidal anti-inflammatory drug.[40] Lasting adverse effects include sexual dysfunction, as well as bleeding due to inhibition of platelet aggregation.[29,41] Sexual dysfunction (erectile dysfunction and delayed ejaculation in men and anorgasmia in women) is a leading reason for switching to another type of antidepressant.[25,42] However, SSRIs, specifically fluoxetine, may be used in the treatment of premature ejaculation by exploiting its adverse effect on sexual function (Box 18-1).

Rarer ADRs include an association with the syndrome of inappropriate antidiuretic hormone (ADH) secretion and serotonin syndrome.[25,43] The syndrome of inappropriate ADH secretion results in hyponatremia, which may manifest as nervousness, agitation, and worsening of depression. Serotonin syndrome usually occurs from the interaction of two or more drugs that potentiate the central effects of serotonin.[44] It is characterized by changes in mental state, restlessness, hyperreflexia, diaphoresis, shivering, and tremors. It has occurred with the combination of SSRIs and monoamine oxidase inhibitors (MAOIs) (see discussion of monoamine oxidase inhibitors later in the chapter) and the combination of SSRIs and the diet drug fenfluramine. In addition, some other drugs with MAOI activity, for example, isoniazid, linezolid, dextromethorphan, tramadol, and St. John's Wort, can cause serotonin syndrome when they are taken with an SSRI. On very rare occasions, this syndrome has occurred with SSRIs alone. Treatment is immediate withdrawal of the SSRI and provision of supportive measures. Both inappropriate antidiuretic hormone (ADH) secretion syndrome and serotonin syndrome can result in death.

Other ADRs that seem just as troublesome to the patient include neurologic adverse effects. Several movement disorders, including akathisia, dystonia, dyskinesia, tardive dyskinesia, parkinsonism, and bruxism, have been reported.[45] Most of these ADRs were observed in patients who had some predisposition, a history of antipsychotic drug use, or existing neurologic diagnoses. Treatment strategies include lowering the dose, discontinuation of the drug, and addition of a benzodiazepine, anticholinergic, or β-blocker to reduce tremors. Other neurologic effects include the production or exacerbation of restlessness, agitation, anxiety, and headaches. Insomnia may also be a problem, but this can be treated by morning dosing.[46]

BOX 18-1 Adverse Effects of Antidepressants

Drug	Adverse Effects
Tricyclics	
Amitriptyline (Elavil) Desipramine (Norpramin) Doxepin (Sinequan) Imipramine (Tofranil)	Sedation, sleepiness, additive effects with other sedative drugs; tremor, insomnia; blurred vision, constipation, urinary hesitancy, confusion; orthostatic hypotension, conduction defects, arrhythmias; aggravation of psychosis, withdrawal syndrome; weight gain, sexual disturbances
Monoamine Oxidase Inhibitors	
Phenelzine (Nardil)—irreversible inhibitor Tranylcypromine (Parnate)—irreversible inhibitor Moclobemide—MAO-A selective; reversible inhibitor	Headache, drowsiness, dry mouth, weight gain, postural hypotension, sexual disturbances, interactions*
Serotonin Reuptake Inhibitors	
Citalopram (Celexa) Escitalopram (Lexapro) Fluoxetine (Prozac) Fluvoxamine (generic) Paroxetine (Paxil) Sertraline (Zoloft)	Anxiety, insomnia, gastrointestinal symptoms, decreased libido, sexual dysfunction, teratogenic potential with paroxetine
Second-Generation and Miscellaneous Drugs	
Mirtazapine (Remeron)	Somnolence, increased appetite, weight gain, dizziness
Trazodone (Nefazadone)	Drowsiness, dizziness, insomnia, nausea, agitation
Venlafaxine (Effexor)	Nausea, somnolence, sweating, dizziness, anxiety, sexual disturbances, hypertension
Duloxetine (Cymbalta)	Nausea, dry mouth, decreased appetite, insomnia, dizziness, sweating
Bupropion (Wellbutrin)	Dizziness, dry mouth, sweating, tremor, aggravation of psychosis, potential for seizures at high doses

*Interactions with tyramine-containing foods; interactions that cause serotonin syndrome.

Abrupt discontinuation of many drugs produces some unpleasant withdrawal symptoms, and SSRIs are not an exception to this.[47] The most common symptoms include GI problems, flu-like symptoms, disequilibrium, extrapyramidal symptoms, anxiety, crying spells, irritability, confusion, and sleep disturbances. Fluvoxamine and paroxetine have a greater risk of producing a withdrawal syndrome than the other drugs, possibly because paroxetine has some anticholinergic properties and sudden cessation of the drug could lead to a cholinergic rebound. Another explanation is that abrupt elimination of the drug would lead to a deficiency of serotonin or, at the very least, a neuronal dysregulation. In fact, sudden withdrawal of any of the antidepressants may create a stress response affecting many of the neuronal systems, which could cause further dysfunction and compromise the long-term outcome.[48] Patients with panic disorders are particularly susceptible to withdrawal syndrome.

SSRIs and Suicide: Are SSRIs Safe for Children? Whether SSRIs increase the risk of suicide and whether they are safe for children are two debates that have emerged as a result of some case reports in the literature in 1990, as well as a "Dear Colleague" letter from the United Kingdom's Committee on Safety of Medicine.[49] In this letter, the committee advises physicians not to use paroxetine to treat childhood or adolescent depression.[50] The data (which were unpublished) leading to these recommendations came from three clinical trials presented to the U.S. Food and Drug Administration (FDA) by GlaxoSmithKline in a quest to gain approval for the use of paroxetine to treat OCD in children. According to *The Medical Letter*, which viewed the reports, in 1134 children, the effectiveness of paroxetine was no different from that of placebo. However, the treatment group did show significant emotional instability in the form of crying, mood alterations, suicidal thoughts, and attempted suicide. At present, only fluoxetine has been approved by the FDA for the treatment of depression in children, and only fluvoxamine and sertraline have been approved for the treatment of OCD in children. The FDA has followed the example of its counterpart in the United Kingdom by recommending that paroxetine not be prescribed to children.

To address concerns over the suicide rates with SSRIs, particularly as reported in mass media, the FDA recently reviewed suicide data for subjects who had participated in clinical trials of nine antidepressants, including SSRIs and some newer atypical antidepressants (fluoxetine, sertraline, paroxetine, venlafaxine, nefazodone, mirtazapine, sustained-release bupropion, extended-release venlafaxine, and citalopram).[49,51] Rates of suicide were tabulated for each of the drugs investigated. A total of 48,277 patients with depression participated in the trials, and 77 of them ended up committing suicide. The results demonstrated no difference in suicide rates between antidepressant-treated and placebo-treated individuals. In addition, there was no difference between the SSRIs and other types of antidepressants. The FDA concluded that the use of drugs from any class of antidepressants had little effect on suicide rates in these clinical trials. However, this report has a few problems that indicate further studies on this subject are needed. First, with regard to children, the FDA study did not distinguish children from adults, so there are no data on how many children committed suicide. Second, only data on completed suicides were collected but not those on attempts of suicide. In addition, there was no information offered on the percentage of subjects who experienced an increase in suicidal ideation. Third, randomized controlled trials (RCTs) designed to prove clinical efficacy are typically brief compared with the length of time a patient would be expected to be taking an antidepressant. Some suicides might not have been included simply because they occurred after the study had been terminated.[52]

Despite the FDA's current support of SSRIs, the debate between both sides of the argument continues. Physicians who argue that there is no increased risk of suicide with SSRIs report that many studies show a marked reduction in suicidal ideation.[53] They also argue that although written prescriptions for these drugs are growing worldwide, this has coincided with a decrease in suicides.[54] Others argue that if there were, in fact, an increase in suicides in some of the studies reviewed, it may have been a function of patient selection rather than a result of drug therapy.[55] Because patients who have a history of self-harm have an increased risk of suicide, if the studies did not include proper screening for this history, the review would represent a case of bias. In this case, what should be discussed are new therapeutic options for individuals who have resistant depression as opposed to the risk of suicide with SSRIs. Another point to consider is that many patients are undertreated and do not receive an adequate maintenance dose for a sufficient length of time. Perhaps the only conclusion that can be made from this ongoing debate is that further study on the safety of SSRIs is needed. The significant take-away message for therapists is to be alert for any increase in suicidal thoughts or behavior among their patients.

Returning to the issue of prescribing SSRIs to children, several studies have shown these drugs to be effective in the treatment of depression on at least a short-term basis.[50,56] Adverse effects have been similar to those reported in adults—nausea, nervousness, insomnia, and fatigue. However, increases in motor activity appear to be more prevalent in children than in adults. Although these issues do not seem to be very significant, there are some concerns about use of SSRIs in children. The first is that in some children SSRI therapy appears to suppress growth hormone secretion to an extent that replacement therapy with somatropin is necessitated.[57] Another concern is that the long-term effects of these drugs on the brain and personality development and behavior are still unknown.

A New Look at SSRIs from a Neurologist's Perspective. It has been determined that drugs that increase brain amine concentrations increase the rate and level of motor recovery from brain lesions in animals. In addition, single doses of fluoxetine and paroxetine have been shown to improve motor performance through practice in healthy individuals.[58] As a result of these discoveries, and on the basis of the fact that depression in stroke is associated with a poor outcome, several researchers have examined the effects of fluoxetine on motor and functional performance in patients who sustained ischemic strokes.[59] In one study, subjects who were unable to walk after an ischemic stroke in the area of the middle cerebral artery received physical therapy with placebo, with the norepinephrine reuptake inhibitor maprotiline, or with fluoxetine. Activities of daily living (ADLs) were assessed using the Barthel Index; the degree of neurologic impairment was assessed using a neurologic scale for subjects with hemiplegia; and mood was assessed using a depression rating scale. After 3 months of treatment, the greatest improvement in motor performance was observed in the fluoxetine group, and the poorest performance was seen in the maprotiline group.[57] In another study, a single dose of fluoxetine was given to patients in the early phases of recovery (2 weeks) after lacunar stroke.[60] Data were collected during a finger-tapping activity and during a nine-hole peg test of finger dexterity. Improvements were noted in speed of execution with fluoxetine, which also increased grip strength in the involved extremity as compared with placebo. The simplified explanation is that SSRIs, through the serotonin system, stimulate pyramidal cells. Other explanations include improved attention span with fluoxetine as well as its association with increased growth factors and other proteins that are involved in brain plasticity. The coupling of motor activity with drug administration as therapy after a stroke is an exciting concept. Studies are ongoing with SSRIs as well as with selective norepinephrine reuptake inhibitors.[61]

Serotonin and Norepinephrine Reuptake Inhibitors

In recent years, another controversy over selective versus multitransmitter antidepressants has erupted. TCAs have broad influence over many neurotransmitter systems and thus also produce many adverse effects. SSRIs produce few adverse effects, but technically they just alter the serotonergic system. Now a drug that functions between the two extremes of selectivity is available—venlafaxine.[62] Venlafaxine is very similar to TCAs but lacks their cholinergic and histaminergic properties. It is a potent serotonin reuptake inhibitor at low doses, but at higher doses, it also acts to block norepinephrine reuptake. It is a weak inhibitor of dopamine uptake but has no affinity for the other neurotransmitter systems. Its potential for anticholinergic and orthostatic hypotensive effects is minimal.

Venlafaxine has shown efficacy in the treatment of GAD, depression, and, at high doses, treatment-resistant depression. Traditionally, treatment of GAD has consisted of benzodiazepines, but the high comorbidity of GAD and depression has led to the use of antidepressants for this condition. In addition, results of recent studies suggest that GAD's pathophysiology relates to much more than just abnormalities of the gamma (γ)-aminobutyric acid (GABA) system and gives credence to the use of drugs with a broader pharmacologic spectrum.[63] Remission rates with extended-release venlafaxine for GAD have been consistently higher than those with placebo.[64,65] With regard to depression, venlafaxine has demonstrated superiority over SSRIs and placebo; remission rates are higher, and remission is reached, on average, after 2 weeks of treatment as opposed to 4 weeks.[66,68] Most of the adverse effects associated with venlafaxine are similar to those of SSRIs except that venlafaxine can also cause increases in blood pressure. Desvenlafaxine, the metabolite of venlafaxine, has also been approved for the treatment of major depressive disorder, with a similar adverse effect profile to venlafaxine.[69]

Mirtazapine is another antidepressant with broader activity than that of SSRIs. It is, in fact, labeled as a noradrenergic and specific serotonergic antidepressant.[5] This drug blocks α_2-autoreceptors on noradrenergic nerves and increases serotonergic neuronal firing by acting on the noradrenergic α_2-heteroreceptors sitting on the serotonin cell body. It is also a blocker at 5-HT_{2A} and 5-HT_3 receptors. This drug produces less nausea and anxiety and fewer headaches than do SSRIs, but because it has some affinity for muscarinic and histamine receptors, it produces an increase in appetite, weight gain, and sedation. Currently, the use of this drug is aimed at treating resistant depression and the prevention of relapses.[70] Comparative studies are needed to determine its effectiveness.

Atypical Antidepressants

Bupropion is a drug that resembles amphetamine in structure but is not clinically related to it. It appears to block the reuptake of dopamine and norepinephrine. Because of its action on the dopaminergic system, it has been used to treat addictions (primarily smoking) and also to relieve depression. Bupropion has been commonly used in adults as a secondary treatment of attention deficit/hyperactivity disorder (ADHD).[71] Also, because of its influence on the dopaminergic neurons, this drug is being investigated to determine its effect on periodic limb movement disorder brought on by the more traditional antidepressants.[72] Bupropion's ADRs include weight loss, nausea, increased sweating, tremor, and an increased risk of seizures, especially in persons with a prior diagnosis of bulimia nervosa.

Trazodone is another drug in this category. It blocks serotonin reuptake and also blocks postsynaptic serotonin receptors. However, it does have α_1-antagonist and antihistaminergic properties.[73] It is considered an antidepressant but is currently used in the treatment of insomnia, as it has shown some benefit in individuals with or without depression.[74] Its adverse effects include orthostatic hypotension, dizziness, and GI disturbances. A significant ADR for trazodone has been documented cases of priapism.[75] Atrial and ventricular arrhythmias have also been reported with this drug.

Monoamine Oxidase Inhibitors

MAOIs directly increase the activity of noradrenergic synapses by inhibiting the enzymes MAOA and MAOB, which are involved in the degradation of norepinephrine, dopamine, and serotonin.[5] These drugs were used with greater frequency years ago, but because of their adverse effects, they have largely been replaced by SSRIs and other agents listed previously. Adverse effects include central nervous system (CNS) excitation, restlessness, irritability, sleep loss, tremor, confusion, dry mouth, and urinary retention—many of which result from central and peripheral anticholinergic actions. When taken alone, a common response to blood pressure is orthostatic hypotension, which can also be dangerous in overdose.[76] In addition, hypertensive reactions are likely if a patient consumes foods containing tyramine. Tyramine is normally degraded by MAOA in the GI tract. However, if the enzyme is blocked, tyramine entering the circulation stimulates the release of norepinephrine. Foods rich in tyramine include cheese, beer, red wine, raisins, and avocados and must be avoided by patients taking these drugs. The exception is a new MAOI called moclobemide, which reversibly inhibits MAOA, as opposed to the irreversible inhibition produced by other drugs in this category. A risk of hypertension still exists, but higher levels of tyramine must be consumed before this occurs. Because of the risk of hypertension and several drug–drug interactions (cimetidine, meperidine, SSRIs, TCAs, and many over-the-counter-products), MAOIs are used only for drug-resistant or atypical depression.

Guidelines for the Use of Antidepressants and Therapeutic Concerns

The choice of antidepressant for a particular patient is usually made according to the drug's adverse effect profile and the relative risk posed by its drug–drug interactions. If a patient experiences a great deal of anxiety and insomnia, then an agent with a sedating effect is used. For patients who experience fatigue along with their depression, SSRIs are chosen. However, young or middle-aged men may reject these drugs, as they diminish libido. In addition, if a drug has been used successfully in the past, it is usually tried again with subsequent bouts of depression. However, a risk of intermittent treatment is that the drug's effectiveness may diminish with each use. If one antidepressant is not effective after a reasonable trial period (6 to 8 weeks), then another agent with a

TABLE 18-2 Pharmacologic Profile of Selective Antidepressants[1]

Drug	Sedative Action	Antimuscarinic Action	Block of Amine Pump for:		
			Serotonin	Norepinephrine	Dopamine
Amitriptyline	+++	+++	+++	++	0
Amoxapine	++	++	+	++	+
Bupropion	0	0	0	+, 0	+
Citalopram, Escitalopram	0	0	+++	0	0
Clomipramine	+++	++	+++	+++	0
Desipramine	+	+	0, +	+++	0
Doxepin	+++	+++	++	+	0
Duloxetine	0	0	+++	++	0
Fluoxetine	+	+	+++	0, +	0, +
Fluvoxamine	0	0	+++	0	0
Imipramine	++	++	+++	++	0
Maprotiline	++	++	0	+++	0
Mirtazapine[2]	+++	0	0	0	0
Nefazodone	++	+++	+, 0	0	0
Nortriptyline	++	++	+++	++	0
Paroxetine	+	0	+++	0	0
Protriptyline	0	++	?	+++	?
Sertraline	+	0	+++	0	0
Trazodone	+++	0	0, +	0	0
Venlafaxine	0	0	+++	++	0, +

From Potter, W.Z. and L.E. Hollister: Antidepressant agents. In Katzung BG, editor: *Basic and clinical pharmacology*, New York, 2007, McGraw Hill.
[1] 0 = none; + = slight; ++ = moderate; +++ = high; ? = uncertain.
[2] Significant α_2-adrenoceptor antagonism.

different neurotransmitter action is administered. For severe depression with psychotic symptoms, an antipsychotic may be prescribed, and the patient is re-evaluated to determine further treatment.[77]

Loss of effectiveness with intermittent use is the reason that many psychiatrists advocate continuous dosing even when symptoms improve. For patients with recurrent episodes of depression, it is usually recommended that the patient have continuous/indefinite treatment to prevent a relapse.[77]

The therapist treating patients taking antidepressants should always be aware of worsening symptoms. Patients should be assessed for appearance, behavior, speech, and level of interest. Negative changes in these areas, as well as any hypomania or manic behavior, should be reported to the physician because use of antidepressants may reveal undiagnosed bipolar illness. Blood pressure should be monitored for hypotension, and pulse should be checked for arrhythmias. Some TCAs and SSRIs may cause tremors, so performing fine motor tasks may be difficult. Success at strengthening activities may also be blunted because of sedation and a diminished level of alertness.

ANXIETY DISORDERS AND SEDATIVE AND ANXIOLYTIC DRUGS

The concept of anxiety has evolved to include a functional and normal mental state as well as a pathologic state or a symptom of a broader psychiatric disorder. Normal anxiety is useful in that it controls an animal's or human's response to a threat and assists in survival. Therefore, anxiety is a normal response under appropriate conditions, but it becomes pathologic when it is out of proportion to the situation.

The classification of anxiety disorders is based on the symptoms displayed by a patient. The *DSM-IV* divides anxiety disorders into the following categories: panic disorder without agoraphobia, panic disorder with agoraphobia (fearful avoidance), agoraphobia, specific phobia, social phobia (or social anxiety disorder), GAD, OCD, acute stress disorder, and PTSD. Anxiety can also be categorized as a state (short-lived and dependent on stressors in the environment) or a trait that is a long-lasting feature of a person's personality. Although anxiety disorders present in a number of different forms, they probably all have some common neurologic pathways.

There are several common somatic and psychological symptoms of anxiety.[63] Symptoms usually include a combination of somatic and psychological complaints. Patients might report restlessness, inability to relax, muscle aching or tension, fatigue, and some GI symptoms such as constipation or diarrhea or difficulty swallowing ("lump in the throat"). GAD usually occurs before the age of 40 years; this disorder is chronic, although symptoms may vary. During a panic attack, patients may describe other physical complaints including chest pain, palpitations, sweating, hyperventilation, hot flashes, nausea, tremor, or dizziness. Psychological issues reported include excessive worry, irritability, sleep disturbances, poor concentration, and fear.

Evidence regarding the neuroanatomy and neurochemistry of anxiety comes from animal studies that included stimulation and ablation of neuroanatomical areas, from human studies with magnetic resonance imaging (MRI) and positron emission tomography (PET), and from information derived from pharmacologic interventions.[78,79] The brainstem areas mediate the physiologic manifestations of anxiety, fear, and panic. The periaqueductal gray matter (PAG) receives descending afferents from the paralimbic cortex and limbic systems and afferents from the deep sensory structures. Stimulation of the ventrolateral PAG produces hypotension, bradycardia, and analgesia, whereas stimulation of the lateral PAG produces tachycardia, increased blood flow, and other manifestations seen in anxiety and panic. Direct stimulation of the locus coeruleus (a noradrenergic nucleus located lateral to the PAG) also produces anxious behavior and panic. Anxiolytic drugs and antiadrenergic drugs block the locus coeruleus. The hypothalamus, which receives input from the limbic system and the locus coeruleus, is central to the neuroendocrine response to anxiety through the activation of the hypothalamus–pituitary–adrenal axis and secretion of hormones involved in stress reactions. Another neuroanatomic area associated with anxiety is the limbic system, which has a central role in producing emotions. Within the limbic system lies the amygdala, which has widespread connections to other areas involved in anxiety and also has control over motor, neuroendocrine, autonomic, and respiratory responses seen during a panic attack. The amygdala has recently been recognized for its role in producing fear and therefore represents a target for anxiolytic agents.[80] Lastly, it has been shown that chronic stress and high levels of cortisol lead to a reduction in hippocampal volume, and the hippocampus also lies within the limbic system.

Most of the research into the neurochemistry of anxiety has centered on monoamines: serotonin, norepinephrine, and the GABA–benzodiazepine receptor complex. The noradrenergic theory of anxiety states that increased noradrenergic release leads to arousal.[81] There is supporting evidence based on the actions of amphetamines and cocaine as well as those of β-agonists in producing the peripheral symptoms of anxiety. Further support for the role of the sympathetic system in producing anxiety comes from the activation of the presynaptic α_2-adrenoceptors in the locus coeruleus. Blocking these α_2-receptors with yohimbine leads to anxiety, whereas administration of clonidine (an α_2-agonist) reduces sympathetic outflow and decreases anxiety.

A relationship between anxiety and the serotonergic system has been known to exist for a long time, but in the last decade, research into this area has dramatically increased. The impetus for this has come from the success of SSRIs in reducing depression and the realization that depression and anxiety often exist together.[82,83] However, this relationship is a very complex one. Increases in serotonin at the PAG are thought to reduce panic, but increases at the amygdala are thought to be anxiogenic. This is further complicated by the fact that at least in depression, it is not the absolute concentration of the neurotransmitter that is important, but rather the activity at, and the sensitivity of, the receptors. Some research suggests that activation of the 5-HT_{2C} receptor in the PAG exerts antipanic effects.[84] Explaining this complex concept is clearly beyond the scope of this text.

The association of anxiety with the GABAergic system has been demonstrated clinically by the efficacy of benzodiazepines in reducing acute anxiety. Alcohol, barbiturates, and benzodiazepines acting on the GABA-gated Cl^-channel produce a rapid anxiolytic action by inhibiting the release of many neurotransmitters.[85] Specifically, these agents facilitate the opening of the channel, allowing Cl^- ions to flow into the postsynaptic neuron and creating a more negative (inhibitory) membrane potential.[86] The benzodiazepines bind to the GABAA receptor, which is a pentameric complex containing 18 or more protein subunits.[87] A mutation in one of the α-subunits of a single amino acid eliminates benzodiazepine sensitivity. This information has been transformed into a series of experiments on transgenic mice in which this mutation was induced in four different α-subunits. Each of these mutations was responsible for eliminating one or two different effects of benzodiazepines. For example, a mutation in the α_1-subunit (the most widely expressed variant in the wild) eliminated the sedative and amnesic actions but not the anxiolytic effects, and a mutation on the α_2-subunit eliminated the anxiolytic effects but did not alter the sedative effects. It is hoped that these experiments will lead to more information on the role of abnormal benzodiazepine receptors in psychiatric disorders and assist in the development of partial agonists at the benzodiazepine receptor site that can reduce anxiety without producing sedation.[88]

Because it is clear that anxiety states can be affected by either the serotoninergic or the GABAergic system, another area of study is the interconnections between the two systems. There is evidence that administration of a single dose of an SSRI (citalopram) to healthy volunteers increases GABA concentrations.[89] In addition, a clinical interaction has been demonstrated by a reduction in serotonin function with a benzodiazepine and the return of anxiety when the drug is withdrawn, coinciding with serotonin function.[83] In the future, efficacy may result from developing compounds that exert GABAergic control over serotonin neurons.[90]

Barbiturates

Barbiturates are CNS depressants capable of producing effects that range from mild sedation and a reduction in anxiety to unconsciousness and death by respiratory and cardiac failure in a dose-dependent manner (Box 18-2).[5] They act at the GABAA receptor to enhance the action of GABA but at a different site from that targeted by benzodiazepines. Because of the risk of overdose and dependence, only a few barbiturates, with very specific indications, are used today. The ultra-short-acting thiopental is used to induce anesthesia and the longer-acting phenobarbital is used to control seizures.

Barbiturates are, for the most part, rapidly absorbed and have a quick onset of action because of their high lipid solubility.[91] Initially, patients experience dizziness, followed by sedation. The adverse effects are extensions of the CNS depression and include confusion, ataxia, and impairment of mental and psychomotor functions. All of these effects are increased if the drug is combined with other CNS depressants. Because of their lipid solubility, barbiturates tend to collect in the adipose tissue, only to be released slowly back into the circulation to again pass into the brain, and this is the cause for the "hangover" effect the next day. Paradoxical reactions consisting of excitement, confusion, and hostility may also occur and are more common in older adults. Other adverse effects that are not neurologically related include joint and muscle pain, vomiting, sore throat, fever, and angioedema.

Barbiturates are inducers of the P450 enzyme system, that is, they increase the activity of the enzymes that metabolize them.[92] Tolerance to the sedative-anxiolytic effect develops within 7 to 14 days, and use of these drugs for a period of just 1 month can lead to physical dependence. The drugs with the shorter half-life tend to be the more troublesome drugs because sudden discontinuation will produce a rapid and severe withdrawal syndrome. Sudden withdrawal produces anxiety, irritability, agitation, tremor, insomnia, and weakness.[93] Some patients may have generalized seizures or experience acute psychosis. This can also lead to death.[94] Cessation of administration of the longer-duration agents will produce a withdrawal syndrome that is slower in onset and less severe but of longer duration. For the purpose of avoiding severe withdrawal symptoms, patients are switched to a drug with a longer half-life, and then the dose is reduced by one eighth every 2 weeks.

BOX 18-2 Other Sedative Agents

Barbiturates
Amobarbital (Amytal)
Mephobarbital (Mebaral)
Pentobarbital (Nembutal Sodium)
Phenobarbital (Luminal Sodium)
Secobarbital (Seconal)

Miscellaneous Drugs
Buspirone (BuSpar): For treatment of anxiety
Flumazenil (Romazicon): Benzodiazepine antagonist
Midazolam (Versed): Used for surgical sedation

Benzodiazepines

The first benzodiazepine, chlordiazepoxide, was synthesized by accident in 1961 by Hoffman la Roche Laboratories.[5] As soon as its pharmacologic action was noted, it quickly became one of the most popular drugs worldwide. Benzodiazepines continue to be commonly prescribed, but because of tolerance and dependence issues, interest has begun to wane.[95] Expert panels have recommended a reduction in the use of benzodiazepines for anxiety disorders, with the exception of short-term use for acute anxiety and panic, but these drugs continue to be preferred by primary care physicians as first-line agents for all anxiety disorders except OCD.[96]

Like barbiturates, benzodiazepines act by binding to the GABAA receptor and facilitating the opening of the chloride channel. Therefore, their adverse effects are also similar to those of barbiturates but are milder.[97,98] Sedation, vertigo, dizziness, dysarthria, and ataxia are common effects, as are alterations in judgment, memory, and concentration. Tasks requiring speed and accuracy can be markedly disrupted. Older adults, in particular, are sensitive to the psychomotor impairments associated with these drugs, leading to an increased risk of falls, and the memory loss may be mistaken for dementia. Driving or operating heavy machinery can be dangerous under the influence of these drugs. Epidemiologic data indicate that benzodiazepines play a role in car accidents. Even though effects are strongly dose related, some benzodiazepines, such as diazepam, are more sedating than others. In addition, the longer-acting agents are more likely to produce excessive sedation, which can last for much of the day. Paradoxical arousal responses can also occur and present a major management problem. The patient may become panicky or anxious and may even become hostile or cry uncontrollably. Reduction in dose or total drug withdrawal may be needed to reverse the reaction.

Benzodiazepines have a few advantages over barbiturates in that they have a lower potential for abuse and fewer drug interactions and are associated with fewer fatalities. Overdose rarely ends in death unless a benzodiazepine is combined with other CNS depressants such as alcohol, opioids, or barbiturates. Antegrade amnesia—the inability to remember events that occur after dosing—may be considered either an adverse effect or a beneficial effect, depending on the patient and the desire to remember a medical procedure in which he or she has been sedated. They are the first line of treatment for alcohol withdrawal, which can be fatal if left untreated.[99]

At least 13 benzodiazepines are available. See Table 18-3 They have basically identical mechanisms of action, but differences in their pharmacokinetics exist. In addition, a few show some selectivity of action; for example, clonazepam possesses good anticonvulsant activity with less sedation. The main differences between the drugs are related to duration of action. Diazepam, chlordiazepoxide, and flurazepam have longer duration of action lasting 1 to 3 days because they are broken down to active metabolites that have additional half-lives. Lorazepam is considered an intermediate-acting drug with a half-life of 10 to 20 hours. Triazolam is a short-acting benzodiazepine with a half-life of only 2 to 4 hours.

Patients may develop tolerance (the need for increasing doses of the medication to have the same effect) to both the therapeutic effects and ADRs associated with benzodiazepines.[97,100] However, this tolerance issue is not as dramatic as that seen with narcotics. Patients receiving high doses or those who have taken the drugs for long periods can have severe or even fatal withdrawal reactions if the medication is stopped abruptly. Withdrawal symptoms begin 5 to 10 days after a long-acting drug is stopped (diazepam) and as soon as 48 hours after withdrawal of an intermediate-acting drug. Alprazolam, in particular, has been shown in several cases to produce significant withdrawal symptoms in patients. Also, there is a higher likelihood for tolerance and more difficulty in switching to another agent.[101] Withdrawal symptoms are similar to those of barbiturate withdrawal but may also include perceptual dysfunction such as photophobia, hyperacusis, and the feeling of being in constant movement. For the purpose of avoiding withdrawal, patients who have taken the short-acting drugs should be switched to longer-acting ones, and then the dosage should be reduced slowly over time (6 to 8 weeks). Slow withdrawal will also minimize the rebound insomnia that may occur with these agents.

Clinical Considerations with Benzodiazepines. Many patients take benzodiazepines for long periods. However, benzodiazepines are designed to treat symptoms of anxiety for short periods (no more than 3 to 4 months) while the patient works on the causative factors of a disorder.[102] Many older adults take the long-acting agents over an extended period, which leads not only to dependence but also to daily fatigue, ataxia, increased risk of falls, and problems with judgment.[103] This presents a challenge for the treating therapist because these adverse effects are not compatible with many of the rehabilitation goals, particularly strengthening interventions.

Benzodiazepines interfere with the sleep cycle, even though they are often prescribed for sleep disturbances.[73] The normal sleep cycle consists of non–rapid eye movement (non-REM) sleep and REM sleep. The non-REM portion is further divided into four stages, with the depth of sleep increasing from stage 1 to stage 4. Stages 3 and 4 together are known as *deep sleep*. Cycling between the stages occurs throughout the night, with each cycle lasting approximately 90 to 100 minutes. Most benzodiazepines reduce REM sleep but increase the time spent in the intermediate stages. The patient may end up sleeping more but not feeling any more rested. In addition, some researchers believe that reducing REM sleep results in an REM rebound along with vivid dreams and nightmares after the medication is withdrawn. Another problem is

TABLE 18-3 Drugs for Anxiety

Drug	Peak Blood Level (hours)	Elimination Half-Life* (hours)	Comments
Alprazolam (Xanax)	1–2	12–15	Rapid oral absorption
Chlordiazepoxide (Libruim)	2–4	15–40	Active metabolites
Clorazepate (Tranxene)	1–2	50–100	Prodrug
Diazepam (Valium)	1–2	20–80	Active metabolites
Eszopiclone (Lunesta)	1	6	Induces sleep (hypnotic)
Flurazepam (generic)	1–2	40–100	Active metabolites with long half-lives
Lorazepam (Ativan)	1–6	10–20	—
Oxazepam (generic)	2–4	10–20	—
Temazepam (Restoril)	2–3	10–40	—
Triazolam (Halcion)	1	2–3	Rapid onset; short duration of action
Zaleplon (Sonata)	<1	1–2	Induces sleep (hypnotic)
Zolpidem (Ambien)	1–3	1.5–3.5	Induces sleep (hypnotic)

Adapted from Trevor AJ, Way WL: Sedative-hypnotic drugs. In Katzung BG, editor: *Basic and clinical pharmacology*, New York, 2007, McGraw Hill,.
*Includes half-lives of major metabolites.

that the use of these drugs for more than 1 to 2 weeks leads to tolerance to their effect on sleep. At least five benzodiazepines have been approved by the FDA for the treatment of insomnia. They seem to span all categories with regard to duration of action. Triazolam is the shortest-acting drug but has been associated with rebound insomnia and excessive anterograde amnesia, as well as with confusion and bizarre behavior. The others are longer-acting drugs that lead to considerable daytime sedation, which is unacceptable to most patients. Zolpidem is actually a nonbenzodiazepine hypnotic that induces sleep at lower doses than benzodiazepines and has fewer effects on stage 4 and REM sleep. Less tolerance and less rebound insomnia are associated with this drug. It binds to the GABAA receptor but at a different site than the other drugs, so it lacks some of the properties of benzodiazepines. Zolpidem is devoid of the anticonvulsant, muscle relaxant, and antianxiety properties associated with benzodiazepines. Zaleplon and eszopiclone have recently joined zolpidem as sleep agents. They have longer half-lives than zolpidem but do not produce "day-after somnolence" or significant amnesia.

Azapirones (Buspirone)

Buspirone is a drug for the treatment of anxiety.[5] It does not bind to the GABAA receptor but instead is a partial agonist at the 5-HT_{1A} receptor. 5-HT_{1A} receptors are inhibitory presynaptic receptors and, when stimulated, actually reduce the firing of serotonin neurons. Buspirone offers several advantages over benzodiazepines because it does not produce sedation, amnesia, dependence, or tolerance.[104] However, it may take as long as 3 weeks to become active, and its effectiveness is not universal. Also, buspirone is commonly most effective with dosing multiple times per day, which can interfere with compliance.[105] Patients who have previously been treated with benzodiazepines do not do as well when they take buspirone. In addition, buspirone is no better than placebo when used for the prevention of panic attacks and has only a modest impact on social phobia, although greater efficacy is seen when it is combined with an SSRI. Its adverse effects are mild and consist of dizziness, headache, and lightheadedness.

SSRIs for Anxiety

The SSRIs are beginning to assume the leading role in the treatment of all types of anxiety. SSRIs are considered first line treatment for many anxiety disorders, including GAD, PTSD, OCD,[106] particularly when depression and anxiety occur together. They are the drugs of choice for the treatment of OCD and are good alternatives for treating anxiety in patients who have a history of substance abuse, panic, and social phobia.[107-109] In addition, they may be combined with a benzodiazepine for the treatment of acute anxiety; patients may then continue to take the SSRI while the benzodiazepine is being withdrawn. They are particularly useful for treating anxiety in older adults and for long-term anxiety management because benzodiazepines should be avoided in such cases.[63]

Venlafaxine for Anxiety

Extended-release venlafaxine has received approval for the long-term treatment of GAD.[110] It demonstrated efficacy for the treatment of GAD compared with placebo in a 6-month randomized controlled trial.[64,65] Further studies in which venlafaxine is compared with both SSRIs and buspirone are needed.

ACTIVITIES 18

1. A 32-year-old female patient has been attending physical therapy for the treatment of a herniated disc diagnosed 6 months ago. She has been in a great deal of pain and is depressed. Her husband has brought her to your clinic today because she started displaying "odd behavior" this morning. He would like your opinion on what is going on and your advice on how to handle this situation. You are quite alarmed when you see the patient. She appears to be very agitated and unaware of where she is, and she may be having hallucinations. Her husband reports that she recently began taking an antidepressant (2 weeks ago), but he cannot remember which one or how much of the drug was prescribed. He also states that his wife has not responded to the medication. You take the patient's pulse and determine that there are cardiac irregularities.

   Questions

   A. What is your immediate course of action?
   B. What additional information should you obtain from the patient or her husband?
   C. What do you think is happening?

2. Given the adverse effects associated with sedative-hypnotic drugs, what nonpharmacologic treatments can you offer a patient having difficulty falling asleep?
3. Many of our therapy patients receive prescriptions for benzodiazepines to reduce anxiety or as sleep aids. What adverse effects or reactions should they be monitored for?
4. Identify the ADRs of TCAs according to their receptor targets.

REFERENCES

1. Wong ML, Licinio J: Research and treatment approaches to "depression. Nat Rev Neurosci 2:343-351, 2001.
2. Lindeman S, Hamalainen J, Isometsa E, et al: The 12-month prevalence and risk factors for major depressive episode in Finland: Representative sample of 5993 adults. Acta Psychiatr Scand 102(3):178-184, 2000.

3. Tomoda A, Mori K, Kimura M, Takahashi T, Kitamura T: One-year prevalence and incidence of depression among first-year university students in Japan: A preliminary study. Psychiatry Clin Neurosci 54:583-588, 2000.
4. Klein DN, Santiago NJ: Dysthymia and chronic depression: Introduction, classification, risk factors, and course. J Clin Psychol 59(8):807-816, 2003.
5. Rang HP, Dale MM, Ritter JM, Moore JL: Pharmacology (5th ed.), New York, 2003, Churchill Livingstone.
6. American Psychiatric Association: Diagnostic and statistical manual of mental disorders (4th ed.), Washington D.C., 1994, American Psychological Association.
7. Roose SP: Treatment of depression in patients with heart disease. J Clin Psychol 54(3):262-268, 2003.
8. Brown SE, Varghese FP, McEwen BS: Association of depression with medical illness: Does cortisol play a role? J Clin Psychol 55(1):1-9, 2004.
9. Olfson M, Broadhead WE, Weissman MM, et al: Subthreshold psychiatric symptoms in a primary care group practice. Arch Gen Psychiatry 53(10):880-886, 1996.
10. Bell C, Abrams J, Nutt D: Tryptophan depletion and its implications for psychiatry. Br J Psychiatry 178(5):399-405, 2001.
11. Miller HL, Delgado PL, Salomon RM, et al: Clinical and biochemical effects of catecholamine depletion on antidepressant-induced remission of depression. Arch Gen Psychiatry 53(2):117-128, 1996.
12. Manji H, Drevets WC, Charney DS: The cellular neurobiology of depression. Nat Med 7(5):541-547, 2001.
13. Doris A, Ebmeier K, Shajahan P: Depressive illness. Lancet 354:1369-1375, 1999.
14. Dinan TG: Psychoneuroendocrinology of mood disorders. Curr Opin Psychiatry 14:51-55, 2001.
15. Manji H, Quiroz JA, Sporn J, et al: Enhancing neuronal plasticity and cellular resilience to develop novel, improved therapeutics for difficult-to-treat depression. J Clin Psychol 53(8):707-742, 2003.
16. Kramer MS, Cutler N, Feighner J, et al: Distinct mechanism for antidepressant activity by blockade of central substance P receptors. Science 281(5383):1640-1645, 1998.
17. Wahlestedt C: Reward for persistence in substance P research. Science 281(5383):1624-1625, 1998.
18. Joffe RT: Refractory depression: Treatment strategies, with particular reference to the thyroid axis. J Psychiatry Neurosci 22(5):327-331, 1997.
19. Frazer A, Morilak DA: Drugs for the treatment of affective (mood) disorders. In Brody MJ, Larner J, Minneman KP, editors: Human pharmacology: Molecular to clinical (3rd ed.), Philadelphia, 1998, Mosby.
20. Rampello LI, Nicoletti F, Nicoletti F: Dopamine and depression: Therapeutic implications. CNS Drugs 13(1):35-45, 2000.
21. McCleane G: Pharmacological management of neuropathic pain. CNS Drugs 17(14):1031-1043, 2003.
22. Witchel HJ, Hancox JC, Nutt DJ: Psychotropic drugs, cardiac arrhythmia, and sudden death. J Clin Psychopharmacol 23(1):58-77, 2003.
23. Ray WA, Meredith S, Thapa PB, Hall K, Murray KT: Cyclic antidepressants and the risk of sudden cardiac death. Clin Pharmacol Ther 75(3):234-241, 2004.
24. Kerwin R, Travis MJ, Page C, et al: Drugs and the nervous system. In Page C, Curtis MJ, Sutter MC, Walker MJ, Hoffman BB, editors: Integrated pharmacology (2nd ed.), Philadelphia, 2002, Mosby.
25. Vaswani M, Linda FK, Ramesh S: Role of selective serotonin reuptake inhibitors in psychiatric disorders: A comprehensive review. Prog Neuropsychopharmacol J Clin Psychol 27: 85-102, 2003.
26. Meyer JH, Kapur S, Eisfeld B, et al: The effect of paroxetine on 5-HT(2A) receptors in depression: An [(18)F] setoperone PET imaging study. Am J Psychiatry 158(1):78-85, 2001.
27. Benmansour S, Owens WA, Cecchi M, Morilak DA, Frazer A: Serotonin clearance in vivo is altered to a greater extent by antidepressant-induced downregulation of the serotonin transporter than by acute blockade of this transporter. J Neurosci 22(15):6766-6772, 2002.
28. Baumann P: Pharmacokinetic-pharmacodynamic relationship of the selective serotonin reuptake inhibitors. Clin Pharmacokinet 31:444-469, 1996.
29. Hirschfeld RM: Long-term side effects of SSRIs: Sexual dysfunction and weight gain. J Clin Psychiatry 64(suppl 18):20-24, 2003.
30. Weekly Prozac Formula Wins FDA Approval. Psychiatr News 36:33, 2001.
31. Anderson IM: Selective serotonin reuptake inhibitors versus tricyclic antidepressants: A meta-analysis of efficacy and tolerability. J Affect Disord 58:19-36, 2000.
32. Geddes JR, Freemantile N, Mason J, Eccles MP, Boynton J: SSRIs versus other antidepressants for depressive disorder. Cochrane Database Syst Rev 2(CD001851), 2000.
33. Song F, Freemantle N, Sheldon TA, Watson P, Long A, Mason J: Selective serotonin reuptake inhibitors: Meta-analysis of efficacy and acceptability. Br Med J 306(6879):683-687, 1993.
34. Vythilingum B, Cartwright C, Hollander E: Pharmacotherapy of obsessive-compulsive disorder: Experience with the selective serotonin reuptake inhibitors. Int Clin Psychopharmacol 15(suppl 2):S7-S13, 2000.
35. Mancini C, Van Ameringen M, Oakman JM, Farvolden P: Serotonergic agents in the treatment of social phobia in children and adolescents: A case series. Depress Anxiety 10(1): 33-39, 1999.
36. Boyer W: Serotonin uptake inhibitors are superior to imipramine and alprazolam in alleviating panic attacks: A meta-analysis. Int Clin Psychopharmacol 10(1): 45-49, 1995.
37. Wilander I, Sundblad C, Andersch B: Citalopram in premenstrual dysphoria: Is intermittent treatment during luteal phase more effective than continuous medication throughout the menstrual cycle? J Clin Psychopharmacol 18:390-398, 1998.
38. Berlant J: New drug development for post-traumatic stress disorder. Curr Opin Invest Drugs 4(1):37-41, 2003.
39. Kaye W, Gendall K, Strober M: Serotonin neuronal function and selective serotonin reuptake inhibitor treatment in anorexia and bulimia nervosa. J Clin Psychol 44(9):825-838, 1998.
40. de Jong JC, van den Berg PB, Tobi H, de Jong-van den Berg LT: Combined use of SSRIs and NSAIDs increases the risk of gastrointestinal adverse effects. Br J Clin Pharmacol 55(6): 591-595, 2003.
41. Serebruany VL, Glassman AH, Malinin AI, et al: Selective serotonin reuptake inhibitors yield additional antiplatelet protection in patients with congestive heart failure treated with antecedent aspirin. Eur J Heart Fail 5(4):517-521, 2003.
42. Masand PS. Tolerability and adherence issues in antidepressant therapy. Clin Ther. 2003;25(8):2289-2304.
43. Arinzon ZH, Lehman YA, Fidelman ZG, Krasnyansky II: Delayed recurrent SIADH associated with SSRIs. Ann Pharmacother 36(7):1175-1177, 2002.
44. Which SSRI? Med Lett Drugs Ther 45(1170):93-95, 2003.
45. Gerber P, Lynd LD: Selective serotonin-reuptake inhibitor-induced movement disorders. Ann Pharmacother 32(6): 692-698, 1998.
46. Jindal RD, Friedman ES, Berman SR, Fasiczka AL, Howland RH, Thase ME: Effects of sertraline on sleep architecture in patients with depression. J Clin Psychopharmacol 23(6): 540-548, 2003.
47. Ditto KE: SSRI discontinuation syndrome. Postgrad Med 114(2):79-84, 2003.

48. Harvey BH, McEwen BS, Stein DJ: Neurobiology of antidepressant withdrawal: Implications for the longitudinal outcome of depression. J Clin Psychol 54(10):1105-1117, 2003.
49. Teicher MH, Glod C, Cole JO: Emergence of intense suicidal preoccupation during fluoxetine treatment. Am J Psychiatry 147:207-210, 1990.
50. Are SSRIs safe for children? Med Lett Drugs Ther 45(1160) 53-54, 2003.
51. Khan A, Khan S, Kolts R, Brown WM: Suicide rates in clinical trials of SSRIs, other antidepressants, and placebo: Analysis of FDA reports. Am J Psychiatry 160(4):790-792, 2003.
52. Healy D, Whitaker C: Antidepressants and suicide: Risk-benefit conundrums. J Psychiatry Neurosci 28(5):331-337, 2003.
53. Lapierre Y: Suicidality with selective serotonin reuptake inhibitors: Valid claim? J Psychiatry Neurosci 28(5):340-347, 2003.
54. Hall WD, Mant A, Mitchell PB, Rendle VA, Hickie IB, McManus P: Association between antidepressant prescribing and suicide in Australia, 1991-2000: Trend analysis. Br Med J 326:1008-1011, 2003.
55. Montgomery SA, Dunner DL, Dunbar GC: Reduction of suicidal thoughts with paroxetine in comparison with reference antidepressants and placebo. Eur Neuropsychopharmacol 5(1):5-13, 1995.
56. Wagner KD, Ambrosini P, Rynn M, et al : Efficacy of sertraline in the treatment of children and adolescents with major depressive disorder: Two randomized controlled trials. JAMA 290(8):1033-1041, 2003.
57. Weintrob N, Cohen D, Klipper-Auerbach Y, Zadik Z, Dickerman Z: Decreased growth during therapy with selective serotonin reuptake inhibitors. Arch Pediatr Adolesc Med 156(7):696-701, 2002.
58. Loubinoux I, Pariente J, Rascol O, Celsis P, Chollet F: Selective serotonin reuptake inhibitor paroxetine modulates motor behavior through practice. A double-blind, placebo-controlled, multi-dose study in healthy subjects. Neuropsychologia 40:1815-1821, 2002.
59. Dam M, Tonin P, De Boni A, et al : Effects of fluoxetine and maprotiline on functional recovery in poststroke hemiplegic patients undergoing rehabilitation therapy. Stroke 27(7):1211-1214, 1996.
60. Pariente J, Loubinoux I, Carel C, et al: Fluoxetine modulates motor performance and cerebral activation of patients recovering from stroke. Ann Neurol 50:718-729, 2001.
61. Foster DJ, Good DC, Fowlkes A, Sawaki L: Atomoxetine enhances a short-term model of plasticity in humans. Arch Phys Med Rehab 87(2):216-221, 2006.
62. Guitierrez MA, Stimmel GL, Aiso JY: Venlafaxine: A 2003. update. Clin Ther 25(8):2138-2154, 2003.
63. Lydiard RB: An overview of generalized anxiety disorder: Disease state-appropriate therapy. Clin Ther 22(suppl A): A3-A24, 2000.
64. Gelenberg AJ, Lydiard RB, Rudolph RL, Aguiar L, Haskins JT, Salinas E: Efficacy of venlafaxine extended-release capsules in nondepressed outpatients with generalized anxiety disorder: A 6 month randomized controlled trial. JAMA 283(23): 3082-3088, 2000.
65. Rickels K, Pollack MH, Sheehan DV, Haskins JT: Efficacy of extended-release venlafaxine in nondepressed outpatients with generalized anxiety disorder. J Clin Psychiatry 157(6): 968-974, 2000.
66. Thase ME, Howland RH, Friedman ES: Treating antidepressant nonresponders with augmentation strategies: An overview. J Clin Psychiatry 59(suppl 5):5-12, 1998.
67. Entsuah AR, Huang H, Thase ME. Response and remission rates in different subpopulations with major depressive disorder administered venlafaxine, selective serotonin reuptake inhibitors, or placebo. J Clin Psychiatry. 2001; 62:869-877.
68. Thase ME, Entsuah AR, Rudolph RL: Remission rates during treatment with venlafaxine or selective serotonin reuptake inhibitors. Br J Psychiatry 178:234-241, 2001.
69. DeMartinis NA, Yeung PP, Entsuah R, Manley AL: A double-blind, placebo-controlled study of the efficacy and safety of desvenlafaxine succinate in the treatment of major depressive disorder. J Clin Psychiatry 68(5):677-688, 2007.
70. Thase ME, Nierenberg AA, Keller MB, Panagides J: Efficacy of mirtazapine for prevention of depressive relapse: A placebo-controlled double-blind trial of recently remitted high-risk patients. J Clin Psychiatry 62(10):782-788, 2001.
71. Wilens TE, Haight BR, Horrigan JP, et al: Bupropion XL in adults with attention-deficit/hyperactivity disorder: A randomized, placebo-controlled study. Biol Psychiatry 57(7): 793-801, 2005.
72. Nofzinger EA, Fasiczka AL, Berman SR, Thase ME: Bupropion SR reduces periodic limb movements associated with arousals from sleep in depressed patients with periodic limb movement disorder. J Clin Psychiatry 61(11):858-862, 2000.
73. Lenhart SE, Buysse DJ: Treatment of insomnia in hospitalized patients. Ann Pharmacother 35:1449-1457, 2001.
74. Nierenberg AA, Adler LA, Peselow E, Zornberg GL, Rosenthal M: Trazodone for antidepressant-associated insomnia. Am J Psychiatry 151:1069-1072, 1994.
75. Thompson JW Jr. Ware MR, Blashfield RK: Psychotropic medication and priapism: A comprehensive review, J Clin Psychiatry 51:430-433, 1990.
76. Thase ME, Trivedi MH, Rush AJ: MAOIs in the contemporary treatment of depression. Neuropsychopharmacology 12:185, 1995.
77. Raymond W. Lam, Sidney H. Kennedy, Sophie Grigoriadis, Roger S. McIntyre, Roumen Milev, Rajamannar Ramasubbu, Sagar V. Parikh, Scott B. Patten, Arun V. Ravindran: Canadian Network for Mood and Anxiety Treatments (CANMAT) Clinical guidelines for the management of major depressive disorder in adults: III. Pharmacotherapy, Journal of Affective Disorders, 117(1):S26-S43, 2009.
78. Tanev K: Neuroimaging and neurocircuitry in post-traumatic stress disorder: What is currently known? Curr Psychiatry Rep 5(5):369-383, 2003.
79. Sandford JJ, Argyropoulos SV, Nutt DJ: The psychobiology of anxiolytic drugs. Part 1: Basic neurobiology. Pharmacol Ther 88:197-212, 2000.
80. Davidson RJ: Anxiety and affective style: Role of prefrontal cortex and amygdala. J Clin Psychol 51:68-80, 2002.
81. Brunello N, Blier P, Judd LL, et al: Noradrenaline in mood and anxiety disorders: Basic and clinical studies. Int Clin Psychopharmacol 18(4):191-202, 2003.
82. Lader M: Recent developments in the treatment of anxiety and depression. Br J Clin Pharmacol 41(5):356-358, 1996.
83. Bell CJ, Nutt DJ: Serotonin and panic. Br J Psychiatry 172(6):465-471, 1998.
84. Jenck R, Martin RJ, Moreau JL: Animal models of panic disorder—Emphasis on face and predictive validity. Eur Neuropsychopharmacol 6(suppl 4):S4-S47, 1996.
85. Millan MJ, The neurobiology and control of anxious states. Prog Neurobiol 70:83-244, 2003.
86. Argyropoulos SV, Nutt D: The use of benzodiazepines in anxiety and other disorders. Eur Neuropsychopharmacol 9(suppl 6):S407-S412, 1999.
87. Rudolph U, Crestani F, Benke D, et al: Benzodiazepine actions mediated by specific √-aminobutyric acid A receptor subtypes. Nature 401:796-800, 1999.
88. Atack JR: Anxioselective compound acting at the GABA(A) receptor benzodiazepine binding site. Curr Drug Target CNS Neurol Disord 2(4):213-232, 2003.

89. Bhagwagar Z, Wylezinska M, Taylor M, Jezzard P, Matthews PM, Cowen PJ: Increased brain GABA concentrations following acute administration of a selective serotonin reuptake inhibitor. Am J Psychiatry 161(2):368-370, 2004.
90. Mohler H: Biochemical pharmacology of anti-anxiety drugs. Br J Clin Pharmacol 41(5):355-356, 1996.
91. Trevor AJ, Miller RD: General anesthetics. In Katzung BG, editor: Basic and clinical pharmacology New York, 2001, McGraw Hill.
92. Trevor AJ, Way WL: Sedative-hypnotic drugs. In Katzung BG, editor: Basic and clinical pharmacology (8th ed.), New York, 2001, McGraw Hill.
93. Karan LD, Benowitz NL: Substance abuse: Dependence and treatment. In Carruthers SG, Hoffman AR, Melmon KL, Nierenberg AA, editors: Melmon and Morrelli's clinical pharmacology (4th ed.), New York, 2000, McGraw-Hill.
94. Smith MC, Riskin BJ: The clinical use of barbiturates in neurological disorders. Drugs 42:365-378, 1991.
95. Costa e Silva JA: Introduction: The implications for public health of controls on the benzodiazepines. Eur Neuropsychopharmacol 9(suppl 6):S391-S392, 1999.
96. Uhlenhuth EH, Balter MB, Ban TA, Yang BK: Trends in recommendations for the pharmacotherapy of anxiety disorders by an international expert panel, 1992-1997. Eur Neuropsychopharmacol 9(suppl 6):S393-S398, 1999.
97. Lader M: Limitations on the use of benzodiazepines in anxiety and insomnia: Are they justified? Eur Neuropsychopharmacol 9(suppl 6):S399-S405, 1999.
98. Mattila MJ, Vanakoski J, Kalska H, Seppala T: Effects of alcohol, zolpidem, and some other sedatives and hypnotics on human performance and memory. Pharmacol Biochem Behav 59(4):917-923, 1998.
99. Kosten TR, O'Connor PG: Management of drug and alcohol withdrawal. N Engl J Med 348(18):1786-1795, 2003.
100. Verster JC, Volkerts ER: Clinical pharmacology, clinical efficacy, and behavioral toxicity of alprazolam: A review of the literature. CNS Drug Rev 10(1):45-76, 2004.
101. Chouinard G: Issues in the clinical use of benzodiazepines: Potency, withdrawal, and rebound. J Clin Psychiatry 65 (suppl 5)7-12, 2004.
102. McKenry LM, Salerno E: Antianxiety, sedative, and hypnotic drugs. In Pharmacology in nursing, Philadelphia, 2003, Mosby.
103. Cumming RG, Le Couteur DG: Benzodiazepines and risk of hip fractures in older people: A review of the evidence. CNS Drugs 17(11):825-837, 2003.
104. Argyropoulos SV, Sandford JJ, Nutt D: The psychobiology of anxiolytic drugs. Part 2: Pharmacological treatments of anxiety. Pharmacol Ther 88:213-227, 2000.
105. Chiaie RD, Pancheri P, Casacchia M, Stratta P, Kotzalidis GD, Zibellini M: Assessment of the efficacy of buspirone in patients affected by generalized anxiety disorder, shifting to buspirone from prior treatment with lorazepam: A placebo-controlled, double-blind study. J Clin Psychopharmacol 15:12, 1995.
106. Stein DJ, Ipser JC, Seedat S: Pharmacotherapy for post traumatic stress disorder (PTSD). Cochrane Database Syst Rev CD002795, 2006.
107. Drugs for depression and anxiety. Med Lett Drugs Ther 41(1050):33-38.
108. Ninan PT: Obsessive-compulsive disorder: Implications of the efficacy of an SSRI, paroxetine. Psychopharmacol Bull 37(suppl 1):89-96, 2003.
109. Blanco C, Raza MS, Schneier FR, Liebowitz MR: The evidence-based pharmacological treatment of social anxiety disorder. Int J Neuropsychopharmacol 6(4):427-442, 2003.
110. Allgulander C, Bandelow B, Hollander E, et al: WCA recommendations for the long-term treatment of generalized anxiety disorder. CNS Spectr 8(suppl 1):53-61, 2003.

19

Drug Treatment for Schizophrenia and Bipolar Illness

Najeeb Hussain and Carlos Jordan

ANTIPSYCHOTIC DRUGS AND SCHIZOPHRENIA

Antipsychotic drugs are also known as neuroleptic drugs, antischizophrenic drugs, or major tranquilizers. They are the main treatment intervention for schizophrenia and other psychoses and are characterized primarily by their dopamine receptor–blocking action. Although they are helpful for some patients, these drugs have some major shortcomings in terms of their effectiveness and adverse effect profile. Gradual improvements in drug treatment are being achieved, but major advances may have to wait until a more thorough understanding of this disease is obtained.

Etiology and Pathogenesis of Schizophrenia

Schizophrenia is a psychotic illness characterized by periods of psychosis (delusions and hallucinations) along with relatively chronic dysfunctions in mood, cognition, and social behavior.[1] It usually develops in adolescence or young adulthood and follows a relapsing and remitting course. Even though there are equal numbers of males and females affected, males tend to develop the disease earlier (by 2 to 4 years), have more severe symptoms, and are less responsive to medication than females.[2] In many cases, schizophrenia becomes chronic, progressive, and extremely disabling.

Symptoms of schizophrenia are characterized as either positive or negative, with the positive signs either a part of or signifying impending psychosis.[3] These include disturbances of reality and perception, bizarre behavior, hallucinations, and delusions. Hallucinations may be visual, olfactory, tactile, or auditory but are almost always auditory. In addition, there may be abnormal motor symptoms, echopraxia (imitation of another person's motor actions), posturing (assuming inappropriate or bizarre postures), and waxy flexibility (when the patient's limbs are placed in a position by another person and the patient remains in that position for an extended period). Negative symptoms include diminished speech, flattened emotions, apathy, attention problems, impaired problem solving, difficulty with abstract reasoning, and social withdrawal. Anxiety and depression may also be experienced by the patient with schizophrenia.

Several large-factor analytic studies of symptoms in representative treated and stable schizophrenic populations have consistently reported three clusters of symptoms in the illness: (1) positive psychotic symptoms (for example, hallucinations, delusions, and paranoia, including thought disorder and bizarre behavior), (2) cognitive dysfunction (for example, reductions in attention and executive function), and (3) negative symptoms (for example, anhedonia, asociality, and alogia).[4,5] The relative balance between positive and negative symptoms varies greatly among individuals and may help determine which antipsychotic agent might be most effective. Although the etiology, pathophysiology, or illness definition for *schizophrenia* have not been clarified, empirically derived treatments provide considerable symptomatic benefit for psychosis.[6,7] The exact cause of schizophrenia has not been identified, but twin studies demonstrate some genetic predisposition, although prenatal and birth complications (hypoxia, infection, exposure to toxins) have also been implicated.[2] There is a 1% incidence of schizophrenia among the general population, but the incidence increases within families; the incidence is between 6% and 17% among first-degree relatives and as high as 50% among identical twins. Many investigators have classified this disease as a neurodevelopmental one, but others argue against this because its clinical onset does not occur until young adulthood. Closer scrutiny reveals a long premorbid course of subtle symptoms and behaviors, beginning with mild motor, social, and cognitive impairments in infancy and early childhood.[8] This period is followed by a prodromal phase, which begins around puberty and is characterized by mood disturbances, impairments in attention and concentration, and suspicious thinking. During the premorbid course, the patient's personality may be cold, introverted, and aloof. This culminates in the onset of psychosis, followed by neuroprogressive deterioration. It is hypothesized that genetic abnormalities coupled with environmental insults produce defective connectivity between a number of brain regions, specifically, the midbrain, nucleus accumbens, thalamus, and temporo-limbic and prefrontal cortices. These functional deficits become unmasked during periods of stress and as a result of hormonal influences on the central nervous system (CNS) that occur during puberty.

Imaging studies of the brains of patients with schizophrenia have shown some commonalities, but it has not always been easy to determine whether these structural abnormalities cause the disease or result from the disease. However, ventricular enlargement along with cortical gray matter volume reductions (greater in the mesial temporal, temporal neocortical, and prefrontal regions) are consistent findings in patients with a recent diagnosis of schizophrenia.[9,10] In addition, these patients, including those who have had the illness for some time, show a reduction in blood flow in the prefrontal regions and a higher flow in the thalamus and cerebellum compared with healthy subjects.[11]

Neurochemical studies have implicated the dopamine and serotonin systems along with gamma (γ)-aminobutyric acid (GABA) and glutamate. However, most of the current theory regarding the neurochemistry of schizophrenia resulted from analyzing effects of antipsychotic and propsychotic drugs rather than the neurochemistry itself. The dopamine hypothesis is based on pharmacologic evidence that dopamine agonists produce or exacerbate the positive symptoms of schizophrenia.[12] An example is amphetamine, which causes the release of dopamine in the brain, and in humans, produces a behavioral syndrome similar to an acute schizophrenic episode. In addition, dopamine D_2-receptor agonists, such as bromocriptine, can produce similar effects in animals and exacerbate symptoms in patients who already have this disease. Drugs that block dopamine neural storage, such as reserpine, or drugs that act as dopamine antagonists are effective in reducing the positive symptoms of schizophrenia.

Dopamine is synthesized as a precursor to the catecholamines. It is metabolized by two enzymes: intraneurally by monoamine oxidase B and extraneuronally by catechol-O-methyl transferase (COMT). The final and primary metabolite of dopamine is homovanillic acid.

At least five types of dopamine receptors (D_1 to D_5) have been identified in the human brain.[13] D_1 and D_5 stimulate the formation of cyclic adenosine monophosphate by activating a stimulatory G-protein, whereas the other dopamine receptors activate an inhibitory G-protein. The dopamine pathways include the nigrostriatal tract, the mesolimbic/mesocortical tract, and the tuberoinfundibular tract (Figure 19-1). The nigrostriatal tract runs from the substantia nigra in the midbrain to the corpus striatum and is involved in motor control. The mesolimbic/mesocortical tract has cell bodies adjacent to the substantia nigra and runs to the limbic system and neocortex. It also supplies input to the medial surface of the frontal lobes and to the parahippocampus. This tract plays a crucial role in the regulation of behavior, particularly in the area of behaviors that are driven by reward. The tuberoinfundibular tract has cell bodies that lie in the arcuate nucleus and hypothalamus, projecting to the anterior pituitary. It is here that dopamine inhibits the release of prolactin. An overactivity in dopamine neurotransmission in the mesolimbic/mesocortical tract has been specifically implicated in schizophrenia.[2] However, the conclusion that there is an overabundance of dopamine should be avoided because schizophrenia may be associated with "dopamine dysregulation," that is, subcortical dopamine overactivity along with frontal dopamine underactivity.[14] In addition, there is no shortage of prolactin in patients with schizophrenia, which would be expected with an elevation of dopamine.

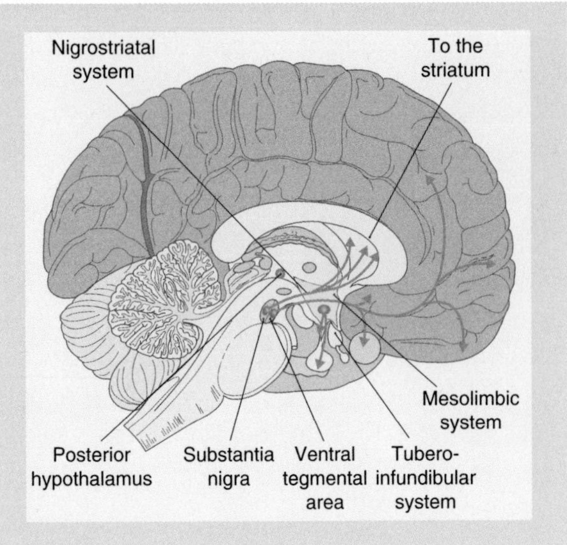

FIGURE 19-1 Dopamine pathways. These tracts include the nigrostriatal tract, the mesolimbic/mesocortical tract and the tuberoinfundibular tract. *(From Page C, Curtis MJ, Sutter MC, Walker MJ, Hoffman BB, editors:* Integrated pharmacology *(2nd ed.). Philadelphia, 2002, Mosby.)*

Patients with schizophrenia may have an increased density of D_2-receptors and show greater stimulation of these receptors after amphetamine challenge compared with healthy individuals.[14-16] Further studies with positron emission tomography (PET) and single-photon emission computed tomography (SPECT) demonstrate that these manifestations are present at the onset of the disease and in patients who have not been treated with antipsychotic medications. In addition, when antipsychotic drugs occupy 65 to 70% of the D_2-receptors, a short-term clinical response is often achieved.[17]

Glutamate has also been implicated in the pathogenesis of schizophrenia, largely by studies of the behavioral effects of N-methyl-D-aspartate (NMDA) receptor antagonists.[2,18] Administration of ketamine and phencyclidine produces psychotic symptoms in healthy subjects and exacerbates symptoms in patients with schizophrenia. NMDA receptor hypofunction can result in decreased inhibition of dopamine neurons, resulting in increased mesolimbic dopamine release.[19]

More recently, the serotonin system has become the focus of many studies on schizophrenia.[20] Quantitative differences in several 5-HT receptors have been found in schizophrenia by many investigators. There appears to be a reduction in the number of serotonin (5-hydroxytryptamine [5-HT_{2A}]) receptors in the prefrontal cortex of these patients and an increase in the number of 5-HT_{1A} receptors. There is evidence that the serotonin antagonist ritanserin is effective in reducing the negative symptoms of schizophrenia, as well as some of the adverse effects (extrapyramidal symptoms) of the typical antipsychotics. Further impetus to this theory comes from the fact that clozapine (an atypical antipsychotic agent) is an antagonist of the 5-HT_{2A} and 5-HT_{2C} receptors. Similar in some ways to the dopamine hypothesis, there may be a dysregulation in the serotoninergic system, resulting in areas of hypoinnervation and hyperinnervation, starting with early damage in the dorsal raphe.

Neuropeptides have also been added to the list of chemicals considered to be responsible for schizophrenia.[21] Neurotensin is a peptide neurotransmitter that coexists with norepinephrine and dopamine in neurons. Studies have shown a decreased neurotensin concentration in the cerebrospinal fluid in some patients with schizophrenia, which normalizes with treatment. Drugs that affect neurotensin levels are currently being explored.

Traditional (Typical) Antipsychotic Drugs

Several antipsychotic drugs are on the market today, but they basically fall into two categories (Table 19-1). The main categories are the "typical antipsychotics" (including chlorpromazine, haloperidol, fluphenazine, thioridazine) and the "atypical antipsychotics"; the atypical antipsychotics are further subdivided into those with a broad-profile receptor antagonist (clozapine, olanzapine, quetiapine), and the newer atypical antipsychotics "selective dopamine and serotonin receptor antagonists" (risperidone, ziprasidone, aripiprazole, paliperidone).[7] The term *atypical* has several meanings; it is used to describe the antipsychotic agents that have a receptor profile different from that of the typical drugs, those that produce fewer adverse effects, and those agents that have some impact on the negative symptoms of schizophrenia.

Mechanism of Action of Antipsychotic Agents. As is the case with many drugs, the original antipsychotic agent was discovered serendipitously by a French surgeon testing different compounds to alleviate stress in surgical patients. He tested promethazine, which appeared to have a calming but not a sedating effect. From promethazine (Phenergan) came chlorpromazine (Thorazine), the first antipsychotic agent.[1] Studies on chlorpromazine demonstrated that this drug blocked multiple receptor systems, including the histamine, catecholamine, acetylcholine, and serotonin systems. It is now clear that the drug's ability to block the D_2-receptor is largely responsible for the reduction in the positive symptoms of schizophrenia.[12]

The typical agents have relative affinities for the D_2-receptor and block this receptor in the midbrain, mesolimbic system, and basal ganglia.[12] The potency of these agents is correlated with their D_2-receptor–blocking ability in the mesolimbic/mesocortical pathways, but their adverse effects are often correlated with activity in the basal ganglia region. They reduce hallucinations and produce a calming effect without dulling intellectual function or impairing motor control. They are effective in reducing the positive symptoms of schizophrenia but less effective in relieving the negative symptoms. They may actually add to some of the negative symptoms by producing apathy and reducing initiative. The patient becomes slow to respond to external stimuli and may tend to fall asleep but is easily aroused. Because of their sedating effects, they are also used as tranquilizers to manage behavior in combative or agitated patients.

Other indications for the use of antipsychotic agents include nausea and vomiting, hiccups, Huntington's disease, and Tourette's syndrome.[22] Their antiemetic effect results from the blocking of the D_2-receptors in the chemoreceptor trigger zone in the medulla, and therefore they are often prescribed for nausea associated with anesthesia or chemotherapy. Chlorpromazine is also approved for the treatment of intractable hiccups and may be given orally, intramuscularly, or intravenously, depending on the severity of the condition. Pimozide is another conventional antipsychotic agent, which is approved by the U.S. Food and Drug Administration (FDA) for the treatment of Tourette's syndrome. Tourette's syndrome is believed to be caused by a hyperdopaminergic state and tends to respond to dopamine blockers. As with Tourette's syndrome, there is no cure for Huntington's disease, but the choreiform movements that characterize this illness are dampened by dopamine blockade. Lastly, these drugs may also be combined with narcotics to reduce chronic pain.

After diagnosis, patients are usually treated for a period of 4 to 6 weeks. If the response is positive, the patient may then be treated on a long-term basis with oral medications. Many patients become noncompliant as their condition improves, and depot preparations may then be necessary.[2] If treated appropriately early in the disease, many patients will experience a reduction in, and maybe even a remission of, psychotic behavior, although negative symptoms can persist. However, many

TABLE 19-1 Antipsychotic Agents

Drug	Class	Comments
Chlorpromazine (Thorazine)	First-generation antipsychotic	Highly sedating Skin problems
Fluphenazine (Prolixin)	First-generation antipsychotic	High probability of extrapyramidal effects Increased tardive dyskinesia Excessive weight gain Available as long-acting depot injection
Haloperidol (Haldol)	First-generation antipsychotic	High probability of extrapyramidal effects Available as long-acting depot injection
Thioridazine (Mellaril)	First-generation antipsychotic	Lowers seizure threshold
Thiothixene (Navane)	First-generation antipsychotic	Less risk of tardive dyskinesia than other first-generation drugs
Aripiprazole (Abilify)	Atypical antipsychotic	Minimal increase in prolactin
Clozapine (Clozaril)	Atypical antipsychotic	Excessive weight gain May cause agranulocytosis
Olanzapine (Zyprexa)	Atypical antipsychotic	Excessive weight gain Minimal increase in prolactin
Quetiapine (Seroquel)	Atypical antipsychotic	Minimal increase in prolactin
Risperidone (Risperdal)	Atypical antipsychotic	Available as long-acting depot injection
Ziprasidone (Geodon)	Atypical antipsychotic	Prolongs QTc

patients tend to discontinue drug therapy and subsequently experience a relapse. Improvements result when drug therapy resumes, but full recovery grows increasingly more difficult to achieve with each exacerbation. Another reason for the 4- to 6-week trial dosing period is that several weeks are needed for a drug's effect to surface, even though evidence of its receptor-blocking ability is immediate. This suggests that an increase in the number of D_2-receptors as a result of upregulation may be more important than the direct receptor-blocking ability.

Adverse Drug Reactions. Many adverse effects are associated with antipsychotic agents because the classic drugs act as antagonists in four major neurotransmitter receptor systems: the dopamine receptor family (D_2, D_3, and D_4), muscarinic cholinergic receptors (M1), α-adrenergic receptors (α_1 and α_2), and histamine receptors (H_1) (Box 19-1) (Table 19-2).[22] Lower-potency agents such as chlorpromazine require higher doses to achieve efficacy and therefore produce more adverse effects by interacting with other receptor systems. This results in more antihistaminergic, anticholinergic, and antiadrenergic effects, but chlorpromazine has fewer D_2-receptor–related adverse effects. Higher-potency agents such as haloperidol have more D_2-receptor–related movement effects but produce considerably fewer effects on other receptor systems. In general, the anticholinergic action of these drugs leads to dry mouth, blurred vision, constipation, urinary retention, tachycardia, a prolonged QRS interval, confusion, and exacerbation of glaucoma. Blockade of the α_1-receptors is associated with orthostatic hypotension, prolongation of the QT interval, reflex tachycardia, dizziness, incontinence, and sedation.

BOX 19-1 Antipsychotic Adverse Effects Related to Receptors and Systems

Receptor	Adverse Effects
α-Adrenergic blockade	Postural hypotension, dizziness, reflex tachycardia, problems with ejaculation
Dopamine blockade	Extrapyramidal symptoms, akathisia, tardive dyskinesia, dystonia
Antimuscarinic	Blurred vision, dry mouth, constipation, urinary retention, mydriasis
Endocrine	Prolactin secretion causing gynecomastia and galactorrhea, menstrual irregularities, increased appetite, decreased libido, sexual dysfunction, impaired temperature regulation
Histamine	Sedation, hypotension, weight gain
Hematologic	Agranulocytosis
Central nervous system	Sedation, neuroleptic malignant syndrome
Gastrointestinal	Constipation, paralytic ileus, hepatotoxicity, weight gain
Integumentary	Photosensitivity, hyperpigmentation, rash, pruritus

Histamine blockade leads to sedation and weight gain. Prescribing lower doses of these drugs, particularly if the D_2-receptor occupancies are in the therapeutic range, is recommended to minimize these effects, particularly for first-episode patients.[23]

Neuromuscular adverse effects are common and are due to the blockade of the D_2-receptors in the nigrostriatal dopaminergic pathway. These adverse drug reactions

TABLE 19-2 Characteristics of Antipsychotic Drugs

Drug	Receptor Affinity						Main Side Effects				Notes
	D_1	D_2	α adr	H_1	mACh	$5\text{-}HT_2$	EPS	Sed	Hypo	Other	
First Generation											
Chlorpromazine	++	+++	+++	++	++	++	++	++	++	Increased prolactin (gynecomastia) Hypothermia Anticholinergic effects Hypersensitivity reactions Obstructive jaundice	Phenothiazine class **Fluphenazine, trifluperazine** are similar but: • do not cause jaundice • cause less hypotension • cause more EPS Fluphenazine available as depot preparation
Thioridazine	+	++	+++	+	++	++	+	++	++	As chlorpromazine but does not cause jaundice	Phenothiazine class First drug with lower EPS tendency Withdrawn because of cardiac side effects
Haloperidol	+	+++	++	–	±	+	+++	–	++	As chlorpromazine but does not cause jaundice Fewer anticholinergic side effects	Butyrophenone class Widely used antipsychotic drug Strong EPS tendency
Flupenthixol	++	+++	++	++	–	+++	++	+	+	Increased prolactin (gynecomastia) Restlessness	**Clopenthixol** is similar Available as depot preparations
Second Generation (atypical)											
Sulpiride	–	+++	–	–	–	–	+	+	–	Increased prolactin (gynecomastia)	Benzamide class Selective D_2/D_3 antagonist Less EPS than haloperidol Poorly absorbed **Amisulpride** and **pimozide** (long acting) are similar
Clozapine	++	++	++	++	++	+++	–	++	+	Risk of agranulocytosis (~1%): regular blood counts required Seizures Sedation Salivation Anticholinergic side effects Weight gain	Dibenzodiazepine class Potent antagonist at D_4-receptors No EPS Shows efficacy in "treatment-resistant" patients Effective against negative and positive symptoms **Olanzapine** is similar, without risk of agranulocytosis, but questionable efficacy in treatment-resistant patients

D1 and *D2*, types of dopamine receptor; *EPS*, extrapyramidal side effects; *Sed*, sedation; *hypo*, hypotension; *adr*, adrenoreceptor; *mACH*, muscarine acetylcholine; *ECG*, electrocardiograph.
From Rang HP, Dale MM, Ritter JM, Moore JL. *Pharmacology*, 5th ed., New York: Churchill Livingstone; 2003.

(ADRs) are known as *extrapyramidal side effects* (EPSs) and include akathisia, parkinsonism, acute dystonias, and tardive dyskinesia.[24] Parkinsonism and the dystonias are associated with greater affinity for the D_2-receptor and are common among the typical antipsychotics, particularly haloperidol.[17] EPSs generally begin appearing when dopamine blockade at the D_2-receptor exceeds 75 to 80%.[25] The dystonias may appear as fixed muscle postures with involuntary spasms, clenched jaw, torticollis, protruding tongue, pharyngeal constriction, laryngospasm, or an oculogyric crisis (head back with mouth open and eyes staring upward).[24] Dystonia may begin early in treatment (within hours or days) and is more common in young male patients. The patient may also complain of tongue thickening, throat tightening, and difficulty speaking or swallowing. Such symptoms are treated immediately with an intravenous anticholinergic drug. Lowering the dose of the antipsychotic agent will then be necessary.

Pseudoparkinsonism may also appear early in the course of treatment.[1] It is more common in older patients, although it can occur at any age. Symptoms are identical to those of Parkinson's disease and can include muscle stiffness, shuffling gait, stooped posture, bradykinesia, resting tremor, and masked facies. These symptoms may be treated by dose reduction, addition of an anticholinergic drug, or switching to another drug that produces less motor involvement. Haloperidol and fluphenazine tend to produce more parkinsonian symptoms.

Akathisia is another early-onset adverse effect.[24] It refers to lower limb restlessness or the inability of a patient to stay still. It is also associated with repetitive, purposeless movements, such as finger tapping or pacing. It may be misdiagnosed as a worsening of psychosis and will become more pronounced if the antipsychotic dose is increased. Symptoms may be reduced by lowering the antipsychotic dose or adding an anticholinergic or a β-blocking drug. This is one of the most difficult EPSs to treat.

Tardive dyskinesia is considered a late-onset EPS.[22] It is characterized by involuntary choreoathetoid movements of the head, limbs, and trunk. Lateral jaw movements and "fly-catching" motions of the tongue tend to be the most common early signs of this disorder. This condition is thought to result from the upregulation of postsynaptic dopamine receptors in the basal ganglia. However, one additional explanation that is growing in popularity relates to the rate at which the drugs dissociate from the D_2-receptors.[25] With a rapidly dissociating compound, a surge of dopamine can overcome the block (act competitively), but a slowly dissociating compound will not respond to this surge. Because the atypical agents dissociate rapidly from the D_2-receptors, it is thought that brief surges of dopamine prevent the motor ADRs while having no affect on the antipsychotic actions of the drugs. Tardive dyskinesia has been reported with almost every antipsychotic agent, although the typical agents account for most of the cases, providing support to this dissociation theory. Tardive dyskinesia is also more common in older patients, with an incidence as high as 25%.[26] Unfortunately, this condition can be irreversible, lasting long after the offending drug has been discontinued.

EPSs, particularly tardive dyskinesia, have been refractory to treatment. However, some additional pharmaceutical agents may offer some benefit.[27] Several drugs used in the treatment of Parkinson's disease have the potential to reduce EPSs. These agents include anticholinergics (trihexyphenidyl), antihistaminics (diphenhydramine), and dopaminergic agents (amantadine). β-Blockers may also be effective in treating tremors, benzodiazepines for treating akathisia, and botulinum toxin for treating focal dystonias. Other options include reducing the dose of the antipsychotic agent, switching to a lower-potency neuroleptic, or administering clozapine, an atypical antipsychotic drug.

Neuroleptic malignant syndrome is another very serious adverse effect of antipsychotic drugs.[22] It is a life-threatening event characterized by fever (101°F to 107°F), muscle rigidity, autonomic instability (hypotension or hypertension, tachycardia, diaphoresis), and loss of consciousness. Renal failure caused by rhabdomyolysis also occurs. Bromocriptine (a D_2-receptor agonist) is used to reverse this syndrome, along with dantrolene to relax the skeletal muscles. The antipsychotic drug is also immediately withdrawn. This reaction may appear within a few days to weeks after treatment begins, but 80% of cases begin within the first 2 weeks. Risk factors include dehydration, poor nutrition, and the presence of mood disorders or organic brain syndromes. A 20% mortality rate is associated with neuroleptic malignant syndrome.

Additional adverse effects of the typical antipsychotic agents include dermatologic, hematologic, and endocrine dysfunction. Hypersensitivity rashes, most commonly maculopapular erythematous rashes on the trunk and face, and photosensitivity reactions that can lead to sunburn may be due to immune reactions.[22] Prolonged use of some of these drugs can lead to a blue-gray discoloration of the skin in areas exposed to sunlight. Hematologic adverse effects such as transient leukopenia and agranulocytosis may also occur, although these are rare. Because dopamine is inhibitory to prolactin release, D_2-receptor blockade leads to unopposed secretion of this hormone. Prolactin, in turn, is responsible for amenorrhea, galactorrhea, infertility, osteoporosis, and gynecomastia. Lastly, antipsychotic agents are known to reduce the seizure threshold and to provoke epileptic seizures.[28]

Therapeutic Concerns with Typical Antipsychotic Agents. Patients who are taking antipsychotic agents should be considered at risk for cardiac abnormalities as well as obesity, diabetes, and high cholesterol.[29,30] Many of these agents produce tachycardia, electrocardiographic (ECG) abnormalities, and cardiac arrhythmias. Prolongation of the QT interval and the associated torsades de pointes arrhythmia are particularly worrisome because they can lead to sudden death. These events are more common in patients taking moderate doses of antipsychotics, particularly thioridazine, as opposed to lower maintenance doses. Unfortunately, these issues have not been addressed clinically, but pharmacologists are called upon to evaluate potential antipsychotic agents for their effects on the ion channels involved in cardiac repolarization. For now, the clinical advice is to view these patients as having cardiac abnormalities, to monitor their vital signs, and to devise exercise protocols with this comorbidity in mind. In addition, because of the dermatologic adverse effects, physical therapists must exercise extreme caution when using heat or light modalities. Use of UV light is contraindicated.

Other concerns about these drugs include heat intolerance and impaired thermoregulation.[31] Antipsychotic agents and the condition of schizophrenia itself are related to several hyperthermic syndromes such as febrile catatonia, neuroleptic malignant syndrome, and heat stroke. These syndromes were recently studied when a group of patients were asked to ambulate on a treadmill at 3.2 mph at an ambient temperature of 40°C for 50 minutes. Rectal and skin temperatures were compared with those of healthy control subjects and were found to be statistically elevated. However, sweat production did not differ between the two groups, indicating that patients with schizophrenia may have an impaired ability to conduct heat from the core of the body to the periphery. Initial signs of heat injury include faintness, nausea, vomiting, headache, piloerection, chills, hyperventilation, muscle cramps, and an unsteady gait.[32] During rehabilitative therapy, patients should be encouraged to maintain adequate fluid intake, and if performing strenuous exercise, they should drink water more frequently than thirst dictates. Therapists should be aware that patients with mental disorders may not feel thirsty, even when they are dehydrated; however, the opposite condition of water intoxication is common in patients with schizophrenia. Some patients may even need to be temporarily restrained to keep them away from water fountains. However, if hydration is necessary, it should be achieved with water or a hypotonic glucose-electrolyte solution (e.g., Gatorade). Salt tablets are not recommended because fluid losses during exercise are much greater than electrolyte losses. Exercise sessions should only be conducted in a cool environment. If heat stroke occurs, cooling measures should begin immediately. The extent of neurologic damage is directly proportional to the duration and severity of the hyperthermia. Immersing the patient in ice and cold water or performing an ice massage can be quite helpful until emergency help arrives. Massage is necessary to counteract the vasoconstriction that occurs with cold application alone. Lastly, because the typical antipsychotic drugs have a high incidence of EPSs, the therapist must be particularly diligent in observing for any change in motor function. The presence of any tremors, akathisia, or dystonias—particularly of the oral–facial region—should be recorded and reported to the patient's physician.

Second-Generation Antipsychotics: Broad-Profile Receptor Antagonists (Atypical Antipsychotic Agents)

Atypical antipsychotic agents represent a new generation of antipsychotic drugs that have significantly fewer adverse effects, particularly a lower incidence of extrapyramidal effects and little hyperprolactinemia, block many monoamine and other G protein–coupled receptors in the brain and have a broad receptor affinity profile. Their spectrum of receptor antagonist activity is extensive, and their overall clinical action is neurochemically complex.[7] On the whole, they have a lower affinity for the D_2-receptor and a higher affinity for the D_4-receptor.[33] the lower incidence of parkinsonism appears to be related to less activity at the D_2-receptor. There is also less tardive dyskinesia. In addition, many of these drugs have antagonistic activity at the 5-HT_{2A} receptor, which is why the drugs may improve the negative symptoms of schizophrenia more than the original antipsychotic agents can.

Clozapine (Clozaril). The prototypical drug in this atypical or second-generation category is clozapine.[34] It was originally prescribed during the early 1970s; however, it was withdrawn soon after it appeared on the market as a result of several deaths caused by agranulocytosis. In the 1980s, it was reintroduced in North America, but with restrictions. Only patients unresponsive to other neuroleptics (failed response to at least three antipsychotic drugs) or those who have severe extrapyramidal symptoms are considered eligible for treatment with this drug and only with mandatory blood monitoring on a regular basis.

Studies performed in patients with drug-resistant schizophrenia have demonstrated the superiority of clozapine in reducing both positive and negative symptoms as compared with both chlorpromazine with benztropine and haloperidol.[35] Patients given clozapine were also less likely to withdraw from these studies and had fewer relapses.[36] In fact, the recognition that this drug produced minimal EPSs led to a re-evaluation of the models used for developing antipsychotic drugs. Until this time, it was assumed that a good antipsychotic drug had to block D_2-receptors at high occupancy and that EPSs would then be an expected outcome. However, clozapine challenged that belief when it was found to have a greater affinity for D_1- and D_4-receptors versus D_2-receptors. Clozapine appears to be effective in reducing psychosis when it occupies as few as 20% of the

D_2-receptors. This property explains the reduction in EPSs and also suggests that other receptors, not just the D_2-receptors, must be involved in reducing psychosis. A proposed role for the D_4-receptors in causing psychosis became an exciting concept, especially when it was determined that patients have a several-fold increase in the number of D_4-receptors.[37] However, experimental drugs with selective affinity for the D_4-receptor have not demonstrated any antipsychotic properties.[38]

One of the key studies on the efficacy of clozapine as compared with other atypical antipsychotics is the Clinical Antipsychotic Trials of Intervention Effectiveness (CATIE) study. In phase I of this study, roughly 1500 patients with schizophrenia were randomized to receive olanzapine, perphenazine, quetiapine, or risperidone, and then were followed up for effectiveness up to 18 months. Results showed that 74% of patients discontinued their study drug before the end of 18 months with the highest percentage in the quetiapine group and the lowest in the olanzapine group. Phase 2 then enrolled 99 patients who had discontinued treatment in phase I and randomly assigned them to either clozapine or one of the other atypical antipsychotic treatments. In this group of very ill patients, clozapine was remarkably effective and was substantially better than all the other atypical medications: 20 out of 45 patients (44%) who received clozapine were able to stay on clozapine for the rest of the study, whereas only 8 out of 45 patients (18%) who received another atypical antipsychotic medication were able to stay on that medication until study completion. The participants taking clozapine remained on it for an average of 10 months compared with an average of 3 months for those taking any of the three other medications (olanzapine, quetiapine, and risperidone). Those taking clozapine also had greater symptom reduction than those who took any of the other medications. Only one patient developed agranulocytosis (and was taken off clozapine).[39,40,41]

Some researchers believe that clozapine's high affinity for the 5-HT_{2A} receptor compared with the D_2-receptor could be a reason for the drug's success.[33] Some data indicate that the 5-HT_{2A} system can modulate the effects of the D_2-system, and this is a favored theory among many researchers. However, there are some gaps in this theory. Some of the typical antipsychotic agents also have high affinity for the 5-HT_{2A} receptors; pure 5-HT_2 receptor blockers have failed to reduce psychosis; and a new drug, amisulpride (available only in Europe), which is a pure D_2/D_3-antagonist without 5-HT_2 properties, has been shown to be quite effective. The profile of reduced dopamine receptor occupancy in striatum and increased serotonin receptor occupancy in cortex is characteristic of second-generation antipsychotics.[17]

Another theory proposed for the success of clozapine and the other atypical agents is related to how fast the drug can be dissociated from the D_2-receptors.[25] As described earlier, a lower affinity for the D_2-receptor and a fast dissociation allow the drug to enter into a competitive relationship with endogenous dopamine, thus avoiding EPSs and hyperprolactinemia.

Although clozapine appears to offer several advantages for patients with schizophrenia, it is plagued by many adverse effects. Agranulocytosis is defined as an absolute neutrophil count below 500 mm.[3] In 1975, 17 cases of this illness were reported in Finland, which resulted in the curtailment of clozapine use. When the drug was brought back to the market in 1990, a Clozaril National Registry was established to keep track of patients' medical status while they were taking the drug. Between 1990 and 1994, more than 99,000 patients were registered, but only 382 (0.38%) had agranulocytosis.[42] This is obviously a very small percentage of patients, and the good news is that once the drug is discontinued, leukopenia resolves within 14 to 24 days.

Some of the cardiac issues that are present with the typical antipsychotic agents are also part of the adverse effect profile for clozapine.[36] Tachycardia, orthostatic hypotension, and even some cases of sudden death from ventricular arrhythmias have been reported. In fact, cardiac issues may be more worrisome with this drug and with the other second-generation drugs than they were with the original agents. This is because weight gain, new-onset diabetes, and dyslipidemia are common events with these drugs. The weight gain, in particular, is troublesome, with an average gain of 6.9 ± 0.8 kg in 6 months.[43,44] Of the atypical agents, clozapine appears to produce the most weight gain, followed by olanzapine. In addition, the distribution of the weight is greater in the abdomen than in the hips and also greater in male patients than in female patients. The relative affinity for the H_1 receptor is to blame for this, although studies looking into the relationship between these drugs and the peptide hormone levels, ghrelin, leptin, and adiponectin are being conducted. Additional adverse effects include increased salivation and bedwetting.[45] The salivation is particularly problematic at night and necessitates frequent pillow-case changes.

Olanzapine (Zyprexa). Olanzapine is another second-generation antipsychotic agent.[46] Its chemical structure is very similar to that of clozapine, but it does not cause agranulocytosis. Specifically, this drug has affinity for D_2- and D_1-receptors, but the relative binding ratio is about 3:1, intermediate between haloperidol and clozapine. This reduced affinity for the D_2-receptor is responsible for fewer EPSs. Olanzapine also has affinity for the 5-HT_2 receptors, similar to that of clozapine, and it has affinity for muscarinic (M_1 to M_5) receptors, as well as for the α_1-adrenergic and H_1-histaminic receptors. Therefore, weight gain and subsequent diabetes occur frequently, with olanzapine rating second only to clozapine in terms of this adverse effect.[42] Postural hypotension, sedation, constipation, hyperlipidemia, dizziness, and akathisia also occur; but EPSs are rare at therapeutic doses.

Olanzapine has demonstrated efficacy similar to that of haloperidol in the treatment of first-episode psychosis and efficacy similar to that of clozapine in treatment-resistant schizophrenia; it is also associated with a slight adherence advantage over risperidone and the conventional antipsychotics.[47-49] The CATIE-I study found that olanzapine showed the greatest improvement in effectiveness, including a low rate of discontinuation, a greater initial reduction in psychopathology, a longer duration of successful treatment, and a lower rate of hospitalization for relapse among new-generation antipsychotics.

Quetiapine (Seroquel). Quetiapine also has a receptor binding profile similar to that of clozapine and hence displays many behavioral similarities, but with lower affinity for all of the receptors, especially the muscarinic receptors.[50] Quetiapine fails to potently upregulate D_2 dopamine receptors in striatum with chronic treatment, again suggesting its low affinity as a dopamine antagonist.[7] But it increases dopamine metabolites in the striatum as well as in the nucleus accumbens with acute administration; it shows an acute but short-lived action on increasing plasma prolactin in rats. Its efficacy is similar to that of the conventional antipsychotics, but the rates of EPSs are significantly lower. Its sleep-enhancing properties, probably derived from its potent 5-HT_{2A} activity, determine some portion of its prescription base. Major adverse effects include sedation and postural hypotension.

Preliminary imaging studies of quetiapine using PET show occupancy of 44% at 2 hours and of 27% at 12 hours at the dopamine receptor in the striatum. Quetiapine shows occupancy of 72% (2 hours), and 50% (24 hours) at the serotonin receptor in the cortex.[13] More recent imaging studies are consistent in demonstrating short-lived occupancy.

Quetiapine demonstrates antipsychotic action significantly greater than that of placebo in several controlled trials at doses of 150 to 750 mg/day and action equivalent to that of haloperidol.[39] Although this drug was initially recommended for use in schizophrenia at 300 mg/day, many clinicians suspect that a much higher dose is optimal, closer to or above 750 mg/day. Therapeutic action on positive and negative symptoms of psychosis has been demonstrated, with the magnitude of its antipsychotic effect significantly greater than placebo and equivalent to that of haloperidol.

The CATIE-1 study showed that quetiapine demonstrated effectiveness similar to the other atypical antipsychotics (except clozapine and olanzapine) but had the largest percentage of subjects who dropped out of the study. In CATIE-2, quetiapine was modestly but significantly less effective than olanzapine or risperidone. Studies show that quetiapine has actions on promoting sleep quality and efficacy in bipolar depression.[40]

Quetiapine appears to have a good safety profile compared with other drugs in its class. There are almost no motor adverse effects and no episodes of extrapyramidal adverse events beyond placebo. The most frequently observed adverse effects are sedation, somnolence, weight gain, and headache. However, the weight gain is lower than what is seen with either olanzapine or clozapine. No significant QTc prolongation has been seen with quetiapine.[7]

New Antipsychotics: Selective Dopamine and Serotonin Receptor Antagonists (Risperidone, Paliperidone, Ziprasidone, and Aripiprazole)

Selective dopamine and serotonin receptor blockers show effective antipsychotic action and preserve advantageous motor adverse-effect profiles. These second-generation drugs show greater serotonin than dopamine blockade, pharmacologically and in occupancy studies.[7]

Risperidone (Risperdal) and Paliperidone (Invega). Risperidone was the first atypical antipsychotic drug presented to and reviewed by the FDA in approximately 15 years. Risperidone has been widely prescribed for schizophrenia and is approved for treating bipolar disorder with psychosis as well.

Risperidone is a benzisoxazol derivative with high affinity for the 5-HT_{2A} and D_2-receptors. Its in vitro affinity for 5-HT_{2A} is 20 times higher than for D_2-receptors; its affinity for other serotonin receptor subtypes is lower. Risperidone has moderate affinity for α-l noradrenergic and H_1-histamine receptors.[46] It lacks significant affinity for cholinergic receptors, and for the D_1-receptor family. The major metabolite of risperidone, 9-hydroxyrisperidone, is active and has a receptor affinity profile similar to that of its parent compound. Given its extensive metabolism and the long half life of the metabolite, risperidone blocks serotonin and dopamine agonist–induced behaviors in animal studies, with greater serotonergic than dopaminergic potency. It has no anticholinergic activity in behavioral or neurochemical tests. Risperidone increases dopamine turnover in the frontal cortex and in the olfactory area but is less active in the striatum. It induces catalepsy in rats only at relatively high doses, but it induces dystonias in sensitized monkeys at clinically relevant concentrations.

Risperidone has been studied worldwide in patients who have active psychosis with schizophrenia. Its actions have been evaluated on positive and negative psychotic symptoms across a broad dose range (2–16 mg/day) in several large multicenter trials, with largely consistent findings. Risperidone treatment results in a significant reduction of positive and negative symptoms compared with placebo. In the CATIE-l study, risperidone showed modest but significantly lower effectiveness than olanzapine, whereas in the CATIE-2 study, they were similar in effectiveness but still less effective than clozapine.[39-41] The 9-0H metabolite of risperidone (developed as paliperidone; marketed as Invega) has pharmacologic effects that largely match those of risperidone.

Motor adverse effects with risperidone are the same as with placebo levels at doses below 6 mg/day. At doses above 10 mg/day, parkinsonism and akathisia are significant and probably similar to those with haloperidol. Anticholinergic drug use is also at placebo levels below 6 mg/day but progressively approaches the haloperidol use rate above 10 mg/day. Thus, below 6 mg/day of risperidone, parkinsonian motor adverse effects are minimal but rise thereafter. Agitation, anxiety, sedation, and insomnia have been reported with risperidone, but at rates similar to those of haloperidol. Hypotension was noted in normal volunteer studies but was not selectively noted in volunteers with schizophrenia. QTc is not affected by risperidone.[29] Hyperprolactinemia is common, and frank galactorrhea can occur with risperidone. Due to the mild weight gain that occurs, alterations in carbohydrate or lipid metabolism should be monitored.

Ziprasidone (Geodon). Ziprasidone was developed not only for its aminergic receptor–binding profile (5-HT_2, D_2) but also its unique reuptake blockade property with the serotonin and noradrenergic reuptake proteins. This has encouraged the speculation that ziprasidone will treat schizophrenia with depression and/or anxiety. Its affinity for the D_2 family of receptors is high, 10-fold higher than its affinity for the 5-HT_{2A} receptor. Ziprasidone is a partial agonist at the receptor and thereby increases extracellular dopamine in the medial frontal cortex. It also acts as an antagonist at its other receptors. It is unique among the new antipsychotics in showing moderate affinity for and inhibition of the 5-HT and norepinephrine receptor uptake proteins, comparable with the action of amitriptyline.[51] Moreover, it lacks significant affinity for the muscarinic M_1-receptor.

Ziprasidone has been associated with a low rate of motor adverse effects at all of the doses tested, indistinguishable from placebo. The drug produced significantly lower levels of parkinsonism and akathisia than did haloperidol. Moreover, anticholinergic drug prescriptions for motor adverse effects were at placebo levels (10–15%) across the range of ziprasidone doses and were lower than with haloperidol at any dose.[52] Moreover, in contrast to several other new antipsychotics, ziprasidone causes no significant weight gain, either in the short term or in extended (12-month) trials.[52] This advantage is substantial compared with other new antipsychotics in terms of cardiovascular health.[53,54] The advantage of ziprasidone on the metabolic adverse effects and weight gain was also documented in the CATIE trials.[39,40]

The most significant ziprasidone adverse effect is its mild but unequivocal effect on the QTc interval.[55] In a rigorously conducted study to evaluate the extent of this adverse effect, the average QTc prolongation time with ziprasidone at peak plasma levels, at its highest recommended dose, was 20.3 ms (95% Confidence Interval [CI]: 14.2–26.4), and this was not increased with a specific metabolic inhibitor (with ketoconazole: QTc 520.0 ms; 95% CI: 13.7–26.2). However, in its registration safety database of 7876 electrocardiograms from 3095 patients, only 2 individuals had a QTc interval of over 500 ms (a lower rate than with placebo). Of additional and critical relevance is the fact that ziprasidone has multiple routes of metabolic degradation, providing patients with protection against drug–drug interactions that increase ziprasidone plasma levels. Ziprasidone is currently marketed with the warning that it not be used in individuals with pre-existing heart disease.

Aripiprazole. Aripiprazole represents a novel antipsychotic agent with a unique receptor profile that differs from those of other agents. It exhibits partial agonist activity at the D_2-, D_3-, and 5-HT_{1A} receptors, but antagonist activity at the 5-HT_{2A} receptors.[56] A partial agonist minimizes excessive dopamine levels and increases low dopamine levels, which helps avoid overactivity and underactivity. Aripiprazole also has strong affinity for the presynaptic dopamine autoreceptor, which then acts to reduce neuron firing. Because of this unique profile, it is being called a dopamine–serotonin system stabilizer. Treatment with this drug is at least as effective as treatment with haloperidol but without the latter's EPSs, electrocardiographic changes, prolactin elevation, weight gain, or abnormalities in glucose or lipid metabolism.[57,58] However, aripiprazole can cause akathisia, insomnia, anxiety, headache, nausea, constipation, and lightheadedness.

Therapeutic Concerns with Atypical Antipsychotic Agents. Concerns with second-generation antipsychotic drugs rival or may even exceed those concerns with first-generation drugs.[59] Second-generation agents, with the exception of ziprasidone and aripiprazole, produce significant weight gain, hyperglycemia, and lipid abnormalities. Patients who regularly take these agents for schizophrenia should be considered to be at risk for cardiac abnormalities, so appropriate monitoring is necessary. These drugs may also produce heat intolerance similar to first-generation drugs, but this is less of a certainty.

Choice of Antipsychotics

For acute and first-episode psychosis, many psychiatrists still use a high-potency first-generation antipsychotic drug.[60] In cases of severe behavioral disturbances, a benzodiazepine can also be administered.

Current emphasis is on the early diagnosis and treatment of the first episode, as recent studies (but not all) have suggested that the longer the patient goes without treatment, the poorer the overall outcome will be. In addition, it is believed that the antipsychotic drugs not only treat the symptoms of psychosis but also contribute to neuroplasticity of the adult brain and help reduce future relapses.[61] Discontinuation after remission of the first episode of psychosis is also a controversial issue that is being debated.[62,63] Any decision regarding drug withdrawal needs to take into consideration the adverse effects of the drugs, as well as the high relapse rates—78% in the first year and 98% by the end of the second year without drug treatment. Another study demonstrated that the relapse rate among patients who discontinued drug therapy is five times greater than that among patients who continued to receive medication. If the decision to withdraw medication is made, discontinuation should be done very slowly, and the patient should be monitored carefully for an extended period. Because of the reduced incidence of EPSs with second-generation drugs, they are being favored for use in maintenance therapy.[36] The choice depends on the adverse effect profile because, with the exception of clozapine, they are all roughly equal in terms of efficacy. Clozapine is the drug of choice for treatment-resistant schizophrenia.

BIPOLAR DISORDER

Bipolar disorder is characterized by mood alterations that tend to fluctuate among recurrent episodes of mania, hypomania, and depression. Bipolar disorder is further divided into (1) bipolar I disorder, in which one or more manic episodes are accompanied by a history of one or more major depressive episodes, and (2) bipolar II disorder, in which major depressive episodes recur with one or more hypomanic or milder manic phases.[64] Specifically, a manic episode is defined as a period during which patients experience an abnormal, persistently elevated mood along with rapid speech, increased motor and speech activity, irritability, distractibility, decreased sleep, grandiose ideas, and possibly hallucinations and delusions. Hypomania is less well defined but consists of an elevated or irritable mood, lasting at least 4 days, and overactivity without psychotic thinking. A change in behavior must be noticeable by others and must not be due to substance abuse. This criterion is currently being challenged, as is the duration of the hypomania. Overactivity with other hypomanic symptoms present for only 1 day may soon be accepted.[65]

More recently, efforts have been directed toward defining a continuum of bipolar phenotypes, ranging from mild depression with brief hypomania to severe rapid cycling, to help link the type of disorder to its most effective pharmacologic agent. Additional terms involved in labeling of the variations include mixed episodes (characterized by a period of at least 1 week in which the patient displays symptoms of both mania and major depression), rapid cycling (in which four or more episodes of mania and depression occur in 1 year), and very rapid cycling (in which the fluctuations occur within days).[66]

Etiology and Pathophysiology

Bipolar disorder most commonly begins between the ages of 15 and 24 years, although there may be an extended period between the first episode and actual diagnosis and treatment.[66] Some patients are originally given a diagnosis of unipolar depression, only to have that diagnosis changed some time later after the induction of mania by a serotonin reuptake inhibitor.[67] Bipolar disorder affects men and women equally, with the exception of the very rapid cycling type, which is more prevalent in women. In addition, genetic factors are involved in this disorder, with a lifetime risk of 5 to 10% in first-degree relatives and a risk of 40 to 70% in monozygotic twins.

There are several theories on the pathophysiology of bipolar disorder, though none have been conclusively proven.[66] In the 1970s, the main theory was that this illness was caused by an imbalance between cholinergic and catecholaminergic activities. A lower concentration of choline (a precursor of acetylcholine) was found in the red blood cells of patients with bipolar disorder whose disease was primarily one of mania. Another theory was that levels of a serotonin metabolite were diminished, implicating the serotonergic system in this affective disorder. A third theory was that electrolyte fluxes caused by deficits in the sodium/potassium-adenosine triphosphatase (Na^+/K^+-ATPase) pump are responsible for bipolar disorder. Hormonal abnormalities, specifically abnormalities in the hypothalamic–pituitary–thyroid axis, are associated with major depression and bipolar disorder; and hypothyroidism is especially associated with the rapid cycling variant of bipolar illness.[68] The two major theories that are currently drawing the most attention are (2) increased signaling via second-messenger systems in the circuitry between the prefrontal-subcortical and limbic areas and (2) a decreased number of glial cells in the prefrontal cortex.[69]

Increased signal activity has been detected in both the cyclic adenosine monophosphate and phosphatidylinositol cascade along with elevations in G-proteins, particularly in the prefrontal cortex of patients with bipolar disorder.[69] Because G-proteins are involved in numerous neurotransmitter receptor families, multiple systems are affected, including dopamine receptors (D_1, D_2); adrenergic receptors (α_2, β_1, and β_2); a serotonin receptor (5-HT_1); a histamine receptor (H_2); GABA; and multiple peptide systems. It is unclear whether a reduction in glial cells causes the disorder or it is an outcome of the disorder. Glial cells maintain metabolic and ionic homeostases and also sequester glutamate; therefore, their loss could lead to excitatory damage.[70] It is too early to accurately identify the significance of these findings, but because lithium (the major pharmacologic agent used to treat bipolar disorder) appears to offer some neuroprotective function for glial cells and also reduces signal transduction intermediates, finding a connection between the two main themes with regard to the pathophysiology of bipolar disorder has become prominent.[71]

Drug Treatment of Bipolar Disorder

The treatment of bipolar illness has traditionally involved immediate treatment of the affective episode (manic, mixed, or depressive) and prophylactic treatment to prevent relapses.[66] For improvement in the mental health of patients with this illness, a combination of drugs is usually necessary; exactly which ones depend on the major affective component present at the time. The term *mood stabilizer* has been adopted by psychiatrists to classify some of these drugs; however, there has been no consensus on the exact definition.[72] Some suggest that a drug is a mood stabilizer if it is effective in decreasing the severity and duration of a particular incident without cycling to the other polarity. Others have proposed that this term means that a drug is effective in treating both manic and depressive symptoms. A third proposition states that for a drug to be classified as a mood stabilizer, it must have efficacy in four areas: (1) treatment of acute mania, (2) treatment of acute depression, (3) prevention of mania, and (4) prevention of depression. For the purposes of this book, the more liberal definition of the term will be used, that is, improving the current condition while not facilitating the opposite affective profile. Thus, lithium, some antiepileptic agents, and the atypical antipsychotics are considered to be mood stabilizers.

Lithium. Lithium has been the main drug for the treatment of bipolar disorder for more than 50 years. It is used to treat acute mania and mixed episodes and to prevent relapse to either a manic or a depressive state; it is also used with other agents to treat the resistive depressive state.[13] It has superior efficacy compared with placebo in the treatment of the acute manic state and has efficacy comparable with that of other agents listed previously.[73] In addition, lithium treatment reduces the risk of relapse by 40 to 61%.[74] However, lithium appears to be more effective in patients who have a more manic profile.

There are multiple theories regarding lithium's mechanism of action, but much research has been focused on its role as a noncompetitive inhibitor of inositol monophosphatase, depleting inositol in the frontal cortex.[75] Inositol is a major player in several signal transduction cascades, profoundly affecting many neurotransmitter systems in the brain. A reduction in inositol would subsequently reduce the synthesis of second messengers, such as diacylglycerol and inositol 1,4,5-triphosphate. It has been suggested that lithium only affects activated second-messenger systems so that the basal release of inositol is not altered; thus there is no effect on control subjects. Another role for lithium is related to its neuroprotective properties over glial cells. Specifically, this drug reduces neurotoxicity by facilitating increased glutamate uptake into glial cells.[69]

Many adverse effects are associated with lithium treatment.[75] Patients report polydipsia, polyuria, nausea, diarrhea, and fine tremor. Other effects include weight gain, edema, and acne. Long-term effects include polyneuropathy, hypothyroidism, hyperparathyroidism, and diabetes insipidus. Lithium inhibits vasopressin action in the kidneys, so renal function must be monitored. In fact, baseline renal lab tests (blood urea nitrogen [BUN], creatinine level) as well as thyroid function tests and an electrocardiogram (for patients older than 40 years) are recommended. Renal function should be assessed every 2 to 3 months, and thyroid function should be assessed twice during the first 6 months of treatment. After the first 6 months, testing is recommended twice per year.

Lithium has a narrow therapeutic index, so plasma levels must be monitored frequently.[75] Levels should be checked every 5 days after a change in dose and every 2 to 3 months during maintenance therapy. Symptoms of lithium toxicosis include nausea, vomiting, coarse tremor, ataxia, dysarthria, confusion, and sedation. In the later stages of toxicosis, when plasma levels increase further, adverse effects include impaired consciousness, nystagmus, muscle twitching, hyperreflexia, renal failure, and cardiac arrhythmias. If lithium toxicosis occurs, the drug should be stopped, and measures such as dialysis should be taken to help facilitate elimination of the drug. Lithium is also involved in several drug–drug interactions. All nonsteroidal anti-inflammatory drugs, except aspirin, increase plasma lithium levels by interfering with excretion. Diuretics act similarly. Cardiac drugs such as digoxin and angiotensin-converting enzyme (ACE) inhibitors increase the risk of neurotoxic effects because of their electrical membrane effects.

Valproate and Divalproex Sodium. Divalproex and similar formulations of valproic acid have superior efficacy compared with placebo in the treatment of bipolar disorder and similar overall efficacy when compared with lithium.[73] These are antiseizure agents used primarily in the treatment of epilepsy; however, they deserve mention because they may be used in the treatment of bipolar disorder as either first-line agents or adjuncts in nonresponsive cases. They are particularly effective in patients who have experienced more depressive symptoms.[76] Their exact mechanism of action is not fully understood, but it is thought that these agents stimulate glutamic acid decarboxylase, which is needed to synthesize GABA from glutamate, resulting in an increase in the concentration of GABA in the synapses.[77] In addition, they prevent the reuptake of GABA and limit sodium entry into rapidly firing neurons.

Valproate is generally well tolerated during acute manic or mixed episodes.[80] Unlike lithium, it has a high therapeutic index. Common adverse effects include GI effects, sedation, ataxia, dysarthria, tremor, and a general cognitive slowing. Tremors may respond to β-blockers. Rare effects include pancreatitis, thrombocytopenia, and hepatic toxicity.

Carbamazepine. The anticonvulsant drug carbamazepine has been used to reduce mania and is considered an alternative agent for patients intolerant of or nonresponsive to lithium or valproate.[78] Carbamazepine has a tricyclic structure similar to that of TCAs but has markedly different neurochemical and adverse effect profiles. In terms of mechanism of action, it actually has many similarities to lithium. Carbamazepine inhibits inositol transport, thus affecting second-messenger systems. It also inhibits calcium influx through the NMDA receptors, blocks voltage-gated sodium channels, and increases limbic GABAB receptors.[79]

In several controlled trials, carbamazepine was found to be superior to placebo in its immediate antimanic efficacy, and it may have an overall response rate similar to that of lithium.[80,81] However, it appears to have a weaker antidepressant effect than lithium and is not as effective in preventing relapses in the classic bipolar disorder (bipolar type I). Patients with atypical or rapidly cycling disease may respond well to this drug.[82]

Adverse effects of carbamazepine include rash, drowsiness, blurred vision, ataxia, and occasional impairments in cognitive functioning.[79] Long-term use may produce agranulocytosis; thus any fever or infection should be reported immediately to the physician. This drug also induces its own metabolism, and therefore the patient may develop tolerance.

Antipsychotics. The antipsychotic medications mentioned for the treatment of schizophrenia and psychotic disorders have also been shown to have utility in the treatment of mood disorder. Of the antipsychotic medications, the FDA has approved olanzapine, ziprazadone, quetiapine, aripiprazole, clorapromazine and risperidal for the treatment of acute mania; quetiapine and olanzapine plus fluoxetine (Symbyax) for bipolar depression; and olanzapine and aripiprazole for bipolar maintenance treatment.[83]

Antipsychotic drugs are effective whether or not psychosis is present. Due to substantial variations in individual responsiveness, these medications are often selected for patients based on their adverse effect profile.[84] For more detailed information on individual adverse effects, see earlier discussion on antipsychotic drugs and schizophrenia.

Lamotrigine. Lamotrigine is a novel antiepileptic drug with acts in blocking voltage-sensitive Na^+ channels. It has been shown to be effective in bipolar disorder and has been FDA approved for maintenance treatment of bipolar depression, with studies showing efficacy in bipolar depression.[85] Lamotrigine has not been shown to be useful in treatment of acute mania.[86] It is generally well tolerated but has a small potential for a serious life-threatening rash at a rate of 0.3% in adult patients.[87] Any patient on lamotrigine with a rash associated with eyes, mouth or bladder discomfort, lymphadenopathy, or fever should go to an emergency room. In order to lower the risk of rash, a slow titration to target dose of medication is needed. It also has a high rate of more benign rashes in 10% of patients.[87] More rare adverse effects include headache, dizziness, diarrhea, somnolence, and fatigue.

Treatment of Bipolar Disorder with Various Symptom Profiles

Manic and mixed episodes of bipolar illness are emergencies and require hospitalization. The primary goal during this phase is a rapid reduction in mania with lithium, divalproex, carbamazepine, or an atypical antipsychotic, all of which show efficacy as monotherapy for acute mania. A benzodiazepine may also be added to control hyperactivity. Most patients will show a response to this regimen, defined rather loosely as a >50% reduction in mania. However, only a few patients will reach complete remission within a 3- to 4-week period, and thus combination therapy is often recommended.[73] Popular initial combinations include an atypical antipsychotic along with lithium, divalproex, or carbamazepine.[66]

Treatment of an acute bipolar depressive episode is more challenging. There is a substantial risk of suicide in these patients and also the risk of switching to mania if the episode is treated solely with an antidepressant.[88] Until recently, recommendations were to administer lithium as monotherapy and to avoid antidepressants if possible. More recently, quetiapine and the combination of olanzepine and fluoxetine (Symbyax) have been approved by the FDA for treatment of bipolar depression.[89,90] Studies of antidepressant treatment of bipolar are mixed, without much demonstration of efficacy.[83] Because bipolar disorder is a recurrent and lifelong disease, maintenance therapy is recommended as soon as the first manic episode is under control.[73] In a meta-analysis of randomized, placebo-controlled trials that evaluated maintenance therapy, lithium was found to be more effective than placebo in preventing all types of relapses, with greater efficacy in preventing a manic relapse.[91] In the bipolar type II disorder, lithium and carbamazepine were equally effective, but the combination of lamotrigine and lithium might be superior.[92]

There is some concern about neural adaptation to long-term lithium treatment because of evidence that perfusion to the limbic area is altered during long-term lithium maintenance therapy.[93]A patient who has been receiving lithium maintenance therapy for a long period may begin to experience adverse effects, and this will necessitate a reduction in dose. The ADR profile will improve, but the patient will more likely have a relapse. Therefore, some patients may be switched to another regimen for maintenance after their illness stabilizes. For this reason, there is renewed interest in combination drug regimens.[94] The combination of divalproex and lithium offers some safety advantages because their pharmacokinetic profiles do not overlap and there is the potential for lower, better-tolerated doses of lithium.[95] However, no matter what drug the patient is currently taking, if a switch is desired, the first drug must be discontinued slowly.

Therapeutic Concerns with Drugs for Bipolar Disorder

Because the majority of patients who have bipolar illness take lithium, it is prudent for the therapist to become familiar with the adverse effects associated with this drug, as well as the indicators of lithium toxicosis. Easily discernable red flags include the presence of tremors, nystagmus, muscle weakness or twitching, and hyperreflexia. Because these manifestations are motor abnormalities, the therapist should be adept at identifying them early on. In addition, the therapist should be concerned about osteoporosis (resulting from hyperparathyroidism) in patients who have been taking lithium for an extended period. Osteoporosis secondary to elevations in prolactin levels due to antipsychotic agents also must be noted, as well as the metabolic issues cited earlier in the chapter. A final concern is the worsening of the psychiatric condition. Because these patients cycle through different moods, it is important to be cognizant of the symptoms of depression, hypomania, and mania so that the patients can be directed to their psychiatrists before their behaviors become more difficult to manage.

ACTIVITIES 19

1. A significant number of adverse effects associated with the typical antipsychotic medications and some additional adverse effects of the atypical agents that will affect rehabilitation may develop. List the adverse drug reactions (ADRs) for each type of drug, and explain how they will affect treatment and how you should monitor for them.
2. One in three patients with bipolar disorder do not adhere to their medication regimen and this nonadherence to treatment is a frequent cause of relapse necessitating hospitalization. Review the literature and identify factors that affect treatment adherence. What are some strategies that can be used to improve treatment adherence?
3. Weight gain and the development of diabetes are common in patients taking antipsychotic medications. Discuss possible causes, and suggest some strategies to either prevent or minimize weight gain with these drugs.
4. What are some common comorbid conditions experienced by patients taking antipsychotic medications?

REFERENCES

1. Rang HP, Dale MM, Ritter JM, Moore JL, editors: Pharmacology (5th ed.), New York, 2003, Churchill Livingstone.
2. Lewis DA, Lieberman JA: Catching up on schizophrenia: Natural history and neurobiology. Neuron 28:325-334, 2000.
3. Pearlson GD: Neurobiology of schizophrenia. Ann Neurol 48:556-566, 2000.
4. Carpenter WT, Buchanan RW. Schizophrenia. N Eng Med 330(10):681-690, 1994.
5. Freedman R. N Engl J Med 349(18):1738-1749, 2003.
6. Gilmore JH. Understanding what causes schizophrenia: A Developmental Perspective. Am J Psychiatry 167(1):8-11, 2010
7. Taminga CA: Principles of the pharmacotherapy of schizophrenia. In Neurobiology of mental illness (3rd ed.). 23:329-347, 2009.
8. Lieberman JA, Perkins D, Belger A, et al: The early stages of schizophrenia: Speculations on pathogenesis, pathophysiology, and therapeutic approaches. Biol Psychiatry 50:884-897, 2001.
9. McCarley RW, Wible CG, Frumin M, et al: MRI anatomy of schizophrenia. Biol Psychiatry 45:1099-1119, 1999.
10. Goldstein JM, Goodman JM, Seidman LJ, et al: Cortical abnormalities in schizophrenia identified by structural magnetic resonance imaging. Arch Gen Psychiatry 56(6):537-547, 1999.
11. Kim JJ, Mohamed S, Andreasen NC, et al: Regional neural dysfunctions in chronic schizophrenia studied with positron emission tomography. Am J Psychiatry 157(4):542-548, 2000.
12. Kapur S, Mamo D: Half a century of antipsychotics and still a central role for dopamine D_2 receptors. Prog Neuropsychopharmacol Biol Psychiatry 27:1081-1090, 2003.
13. Kerwin R, Travis MJ, Page C, et al: Drugs and the nervous system. In Page C, Curtis MJ, Sutter MC, Walker MJ, Hoffman BB, editors: Integrated pharmacology (2nd ed.), Philadelphia, 2002, Mosby.
14. Laruelle M, Abi-Dargham A, Gil R, Kegeles L, Innis R: Increased dopamine transmission in schizophrenia: Relationship to illness phases. Biol Psychiatry 46:56-72, 1999.
15. Abi-Dargham A, Rodenhiser J, Printz D, et al: Increased baseline occupancy of D_2 receptors by dopamine in schizophrenia. Proc Natl Acad Sci USA 97(14):8104-8109, 2000.
16. Breier A, Su TP, Saunders R, et al: Schizophrenia is associated with elevated amphetamine-induced synaptic dopamine concentrations: Evidence from a novel positron emission tomography method. Proc Natl Acad Sci USA 94:2569-2574, 1997.
17. Kapur S, Zipursky R, Jones C, Remington G, Houle S: Relationship between dopamine D_2 occupancy, clinical response, and side effects: A double-blind PET study of first-episode schizophrenia. Am J Psychiatry 157(4):514-520, 2000.
18. Tsai G, Coyle JT: Glutamatergic mechanisms in schizophrenia. Annu Rev Pharmacol Toxicol 42:165-179, 2003.
19. Kegeles L, Abi-Dargham A, Zea-Ponce Y, et al: Modulation of amphetamine-induced striatal dopamine release by ketamine in humans: Implications for schizophrenia. Biol Psychiatry 48(7):627-640, 2000.
20. Brunello N, Masotto C, Steardo L, Markstein R, Racagni G: New insights into the biology of schizophrenia through the mechanism of action of clozapine. Neuropsychopharmacology 13(3):177-213, 1995.
21. Binder EB, Kinkead B, Owens MJ, Nemeroff CB: The role of neurotensin in the pathophysiology of schizophrenia and the mechanism of action of antipsychotic drugs. Biol Psychiatry 50:856-872, 2001.
22. Wilkaitis J, Mulvihill T, Nasrallah HA: Classic antipsychotic medications. In Schatzberg AF, Nemeroff CB, editors: Textbook of psychopharmacology (3rd ed.), Washington, D.C., 2004, American Psychiatric Publishing, Inc.

23. Kapur S, Remington G, Jones C, et al: High levels of dopamine D_2 receptor occupancy with low-dose haloperidol treatment: A PET study. Am J Psychiatry 153(7):948-950, 1996.
24. Woo TU, Zimmet SV, Wojcik J, Canuso CM, Green AI: Treatment of schizophrenia. InSchatzberg AF, Nemeroff CB, editors: Textbook of psychopharmacology (3rd ed.), Washington, D.C., 2004, American Psychiatric Publishing, Inc.
25. Kapur S, Seeman P: Does fast dissociation from the dopamine d(2) receptor explain the action of atypical antipsychotics? A new hypothesis. Am J Psychiatry 158(3):360-369, 2001.
26. Jeste DV, Lacro JP, Palmer B, Rockwell E, Harris MJ, Caliguiri MP: Incidence of tardive dyskinesia in early stages of low-dose treatment with typical neuroleptics in older patients. Am J Psychiatry 156(2):309-311, 1999.
27. Stanilla JK, Simpson GM: Drugs to treat extrapyramidal side effects. In Schatzberg AF, Nemeroff CB, editors: Textbook of psychopharmacology (3rd ed.), Washington, D.C., 2004, American Psychiatric Publishing.
28. Pisani F, Oteri G, Costa C, Di Raimondo G, Di Perri R: Effect of psychotropic drugs on seizure threshold. Drug Saf 25(2): 91-110, 2002.
29. Witchel HJ, Hancox JC, Nutt DJ: Psychotropic drugs, cardiac arrhythmia, and sudden death. J Clin Psychopharmacol 23(1):58-77, 2003.
30. Cavazzoni P, Mukhopadhyay N, Carlson C, Breier A, Buse J: Retrospective analysis of risk factors in patients with treatment-emergent diabetes during clinical trials of antipsychotic medications. Br J Psychiatry 47(suppl):S94-S101, 2004.
31. Hermesh H, Shiloh R, Epstein Y, Manaim H, Weizman A, Munitz H: Heat intolerance in patients with chronic schizophrenia maintained with antipsychotic drugs. Am J Psychiatry 157(8):1327-1329, 2000.
32. Prevention and treatment of heat injury. Med Lett Drugs Ther 45(1161):58-60, 2003.
33. Remington G: Understanding antipsychotic "atypicality": A clinical and pharmacological moving target. J Psychiatry Neurosci 28(4):275-284, 2003.
34. Kapur S, Remington G: Atypical antipsychotics: New directions and new challenges in the treatment of schizophrenia. Annu Rev Med 52:503-517, 2001.
35. Geddes JR, Freemantle N, Harrison P, Bebbington P: Atypical antipsychotics in the treatment of schizophrenia: Systematic overview and meta-regression analysis. Br Med J 321:1371-1376, 2000.
36. Marder SR, Wirshing DA. Clozapine: In Schatzberg AF, Nemeroff CB, editors: Textbook of psychopharmacology (3rd ed.), Washington, D.C., 2004, American Psychiatric Publishing.
37. Wong AHC, Van Tol HHM: The dopamine D_4 receptors and mechanisms of antipsychotic atypicality. Prog Neuropsychopharmacol Biol Psychiatry 27:1091-1099, 2003.
38. Kramer MS, Last B, Getson A, Reines SA: The effects of a selective D_4 dopamine receptor antagonist (L-745,870) in acutely psychotic inpatients with schizophrenia. Arch Gen Psychiatry 54:567-572, 1997.
39. McEvoy JP, Lieberman JA, Stroup TS, et al: Effectiveness of clozapine versus olanzapine, quetiapine, and risperidone in patients with chronic schizophrenia who did not respond to prior atypical antipsychotic treatment. Am J Psychiatry 163:600-610, 2006.
40. Stroup TS, Lieberman JA, McEvoy JP, et al: Effectiveness of olanzapine, quetiapine, risperidone and ziprasidone in patients with chronic schizophrenia following discontinuation of a previous atypical antipsychotic. Am J Psychiatry 163:611-622, 2006.
41. Stroup T S, McEvoy JP, Swartz MS, et al: The National Institute of Mental Health Clinical Antipsychotic Trials of Intervention Effectiveness (CATIE) Project: Schizophrenia trial design and protocol development. Schizophrenia Bull (29)1:15-31, 2003.
42. Honigfeld G: Effects of the clozapine national registry system on incidence of deaths. Psychiatr Serv 47(1):52-56, 1996.
43. Wirshing DA, Wirshing WC, Kysar L, et al: Novel antipsychotics: comparison of weight gain liabilities. J Clin Psychiatry, 1999. 60(6):358-363.
44. Lindenmayer JP, Czobor P, Volavka J, et al: Changes in glucose and cholesterol levels in patients with schizophrenia treated with typical or atypical antipsychotics. Am J Psychiatry 160(2):290-296, 2003.
45. Choice of an antipsychotic. Med Lett Drugs Ther 45(1172):102-104, 2003.
46. Schulz SC, Olson S, Kotlyar M: Olanzapine. In Schatzberg AF, Nemeroff CB, editors: Textbook of psychopharmacology (3rd ed.), Washington, D.C., 2004, American Psychiatric Publishing.
47. Diaz E, Neuse E, Sullivan MC, Pearsall HR, Woods SW: Adherence to conventional and atypical antipsychotics after hospital discharge. J Clin Psychiatry 65(3):354-360, 2004.
48. Bitter I, Dossenbach MR, Brook S, et al: Olanzapine versus clozapine in treatment-resistant or treatment-intolerant schizophrenia. Prog Neuropsychopharmacol Biol Psychiatry 28(1):173-180, 2004.
49. Lieberman JA, Tollefson G, Tohen M, et al: Comparative efficacy and safety of atypical and conventional antipsychotic drugs in first-episode psychosis: A randomized, double-blind trial of olanzapine versus haloperidol. Am J Psychiatry 160(8):1396-1404, 2003.
50. Lieberman JA: Quetiapine. In Schatzberg AF, Nemeroff CB, editors: Textbook of psychopharmacology (3rd ed.), Washington, D.C., 2004, American Psychiatric Publishing.
51. Seeger TF, Seymour PA, Schmidt AW, et al: Ziprasidone (CP-88,059): A new antipsychotic with combined dopamine and serotonin receptor antagonist activity. J Pharmacol Exp Ther 275(1):101-113, 1995.
52. Daniel DG: Tolerability of ziprasidone: An expanding perspective. J Clin Psychiatry 64(suppl 19):40-49, 2003.
53. Allison DB, Mentore JL, Heo M, et al: Antipsychotic-induced weight gain: A comprehensive research synthesis. Am J Psychiatry 156(11):1686-1696, 1999.
54. Bettinger TL, Mendelson SC, Dorson PG, Crismon ML, Olanzapine-induced glucose dysregulation. Ann Pharmacother 34(8):865-867, 2000.
55. Glassman AH, Bigger JT: Antipsychotic drugs: Prolonged QTc interval, torsade de pointes, and sudden death. Am J Psychiatry 158(11):1774-1782, 2001.
56. Yokoi F, Grunder G, Biziere K, et al: Dopamine D_2 and D_3 receptor occupancy in normal humans treated with the antipsychotic drug aripiprazole (OPC 14597): A study using positron emission tomography and [11C]Raclopride. Neuropsychopharmacology 27(2):248-259, 2002.
57. Kasper S, Lerman MN, McQuade RD, et al: Efficacy and safety of aripiprazole vs. haloperidol for long-term maintenance treatment following acute relapse of schizophrenia. Int J Neuropsychopharmacol 6(4):325-337, 2003.
58. Pigott TA, Carson WH, Saha AR, Torbeyns AF, Stock EG, Ingenito GG: Aripiprazole for the prevention of relapse in stabilized patients with chronic schizophrenia: A placebo-controlled 26-week study. J Clin Psychiatry 64(9):1048-1056, 2003.
59. Drugs for psychiatric disorders. Med Lett Treat Guide. 1(11)69-76, 2003.
60. Wyatt RJ, Damiani LM, Henter ID: First episode schizophrenia: Early intervention and medication discontinuation in the context of course and treatment. Br J Psychiatry 172(suppl 33):77-83, 1998.
61. Konradi C, Heckers S: Antipsychotic drugs and neuroplasticity: Insights into the treatment and neurobiology of schizophrenia. Biol Psychiatry 50:729-742, 2001.

62. Gitlin M, Nuechterlein K, Subotnik KL, et al: Clinical outcome following neuroleptic discontinuation in patients with remitted recent-onset schizophrenia. Am J Psychiatry 158(11):1835-1842, 2001.
63. Robinson DG, Woerner MG, Alvir JM, et al: Predictors of treatment response from a first episode of schizophrenia or schizoaffective disorder. Am J Psychiatry 156(4):544-549, 1999.
64. Angst J, Gamma A, Benzazzi F, Ajdacic V, Eich D, Rossler W: Diagnostic issues in bipolar disorder. Eur Neuropsychopharmacol 13:S43-S50, 2003.
65. Tillman R, Geller B: Definitions of rapid, ultrarapid, and ultradian cycling and of episode duration in pediatric and adult bipolar disorders: A proposal to distinguish episodes from cycles. J Child Adolesc Psychopharmacol 13(3):267-271, 2003.
66. Muller-Oerlinghausen B, Berghofer A, Bauer M: Bipolar disorder. Lancet 359:241-247, 2002.
67. Howland RH: Induction of mania with serotonin reuptake inhibitors. J Clin Psychopharmacol 16(6):425-427, 1996.
68. Bauer M, London ED, Silverman DH, Rasgon N, Kirchheiner J, Whybrow PC: Thyroid, brain and mood modulation in affective disorder: Insights from molecular research and functional brain imaging. Pharmacopsychiatry 36(suppl 3):S215-S221, 2003.
69. Vawter MP, Freed WJ, Kleinman JE: Neuropathology of bipolar disorder. Biol Psychiatry 48(6):486-504, 2000.
70. Sheline YI: Neuroimaging studies of mood disorder effects on the brain. Biol Psychiatry 54:338-352, 2003.
71. Bauer M, Alda M, Priller J, Young LT, International Group for the Study of Lithium Treated Patients (IGSLI): Implications of the neuroprotective effects of lithium for the treatment of bipolar and neurodegenerative disorders. Pharmacopsychiatry 36(suppl 3):S250-S254, 2003.
72. Bauer MS, Mitchner L: What is a "mood stabilizer"? An evidence-based response. Am J Psychiatry 161(1):3-18, 2004.
73. Keck PE, McElroy SL: Treatment of bipolar disorder. In Schatzberg AF, Nemeroff CB, editors: Textbook of psychopharmacology (3rd ed.), Washington, D.C., 2004, American Psychiatric Publishing.
74. Geddes JR, Burgess S, Hawton KD, Jamison K, Goodwin GM: Long-term lithium therapy for bipolar disorder: Systematic review and meta-analysis of randomized controlled trials. Am J Psychiatry 161(2):217-222, 2004.
75. Freeman MP, Wiegand C, Gelenberg AJ: Lithium. In Schatzberg AF, Nemeroff CB, editors: Textbook of psychopharmacology (3rd ed.), Washington, D.C., 2004, American Psychiatric Publishing.
76. Freeman TW, Clothier JL, Pazzaglia P, Lesem MD, Swann AC: A double-blind comparison of valproate and lithium in the treatment of acute mania. Am J Psychiatry 149(1):108-111, 1992.
77. Bowden CL: Valproate. In Schatzberg AF, Nemeroff CB, editors: Textbook of psychopharmacology (3rd ed.), Washington, D.C., 2004, American Psychiatric Publishing.
78. Hartong EG, Moleman P, Hoogduin CA, Broekman TG, Nolen WA: Prophylactic efficacy of lithium versus carbamazepine in treatment-naive bipolar patients. J Clin Psychiatry 64(2):144-151, 2003.
79. Ketter TA, Wang PW, Post RM: Carbamazepine and oxcarbazepine. In Schatzberg AF, Nemeroff CB, editors: Textbook of psychopharmacology (3rd ed.), Washington, D.C., 2004, American Psychiatric Publishing.
80. Weisler RH, Kalali AH, Ketter TA: A multicenter, randomized, double-blind, placebo-controlled trial of extended-release carbamazepine capsules as monotherapy for bipolar disorder patients with manic or mixed episodes. J Clin Psychiatry 65(4):478-484, 2004.
81. Small JG, Klapper MH, Milstein V, et al: Carbamazepine compared with lithium in the treatment of mania. Arch Gen Psychiatry 48(10):915-921, 1991.
82. Greil W, Kleindienst N, Erazo N, Muller-Oerlinghausen B: Differential response to lithium and carbamazepine in the prophylaxis of bipolar disorder. J Clin Psychopharmacol 18(6):455-460, 1998.
83. Stephen M. Strakowski: Approaching the challenge of bipolar depression: Results from STEP-BD. Am J Psychiatry 164:1301-1303, 2007.
84. Kaplan HI, Sadock BJ, editors: Kaplan & Sadock's comprehensive textbook of psychiatry (8th ed.), Baltimore, 2005, Lippincott Williams & Wilkins.
85. LAMICTAL® (lamotrigine), full prescribing information. In Physicians desk reference (63rd ed.), Montvale, NJ, 2009, GlaxoSmithKline Biologicals.
86. Thase ME: Maintenance therapy for bipolar disorder. J Clin Psychiatry 6;69(11):e32, 2008.
87. Robert EH, Stuart CY, Glen OG: The american psychiatric textbook of psychiatry (5th ed.), Arlington, 2008, American Psychiatric Publishing, Inc.
88. Keck PE, Nelson EB, McElroy SL: Advances in the pharmacologic treatment of bipolar depression. Biol Psychiatry 53(8):671-679, 2003.
89. SYMBYAX ® (olanzapine and fluoxetine HCL tablets), full prescribing information. In Physicians desk reference (63rd ed.), Montvale, NJ, 2009. Eli Lilly and Company.
90. Shelton RC: The combination of olanzapine and fluoxetine in mood disorders. Expert Opin Pharmacother 4(7):1175–1183, 2003.
91. Goodwin GM, Geddes DM: Latest maintenance data on lithium in bipolar disorder. Eur Neuropsychopharmacol 13:S51–S55, 2003.
92. Calabrese JR, Bowden CL, Sachs GS, et al: A placebo-controlled 18. month trial of lamotrigine and lithium maintenance treatment in recently depressed patients with bipolar II disorder. J Clin Psychiatry 64(9):1013-1024, 2003.
93. Perlis RH, Sachs GS, Lafer B, et al: Effect of abrupt change from standard to low serum levels of lithium: a reanalysis of double-blind lithium maintenance data. Am J Psychiatry 159(7):1155-1159, 2002.
94. Grof P: Selecting effective long-term treatment for bipolar patients: monotherapy and combinations. J Clin Psychiatry 64(suppl 5):53-61, 2003.
95. Bowden CL: Clinical correlates of therapeutic response in bipolar disorder. J Affect Disord 67:257-265, 2001.

ADDITIONAL RESOURCES

Goldsmith DR, Wagstaff AJ, Ibbotson T,Perry CM: Lamotrigine: A review of its use in bipolar disorder, Drugs 63:2029-2050, 2003.

Lieberman JA, Stroup TS, McEvoy JP, et al: Effectiveness of antipsychotic drugs in patients with chronic schizophrenia, N Engl J Med (353):1209-1223, 2005.

SECTION VI

Anti-Infective and Anti-Cancer Agents

20

Antimicrobial Agents

Wolfgang Vogel

CHARACTERISTICS AND CLASSIFICATION OF BACTERIA

Bacteria cause more infectious diseases than any other parasite, and bacterial infections cause substantial morbidity and mortality.[1] Therefore antibacterial drugs are among the most important groups of medicines that we possess, having substantially reduced or changed the course of many illnesses. In actuality, antibacterial agents belong to a larger group of drugs called *chemotherapeutic drugs*, defined as agents that have selective toxicity to invading parasites. In more recent times, the term *chemotherapy* has been used to refer to the treatment of cancer rather than infectious diseases, and *antibacterial agents* and *antibiotics* are substances that destroy or inhibit the growth and multiplication of microorganisms.

Although a detailed description of microbes is beyond the scope of this book, a brief review of bacteria and their classification is warranted. Bacteria are unicellular microorganisms that usually possess a rigid cell wall (in contrast to human cells which only posses a cell membrane). They lack a true cell nucleus but do contain two forms of deoxyribonucleic acid (DNA); one occurs in large loops and the other in small loops. The latter is referred to as *plasmid*, and its DNA can actually be exchanged among different bacteria. Bacteria possess all the basic subcellular organelles to make proteins, but bacterial ribosomes are somewhat different from their human counterparts. They rely on their host for metabolic substrates such as amino acids and glucose. Bacteria can be beneficial to the host (like some bacteria in the gut) but can exert harmful effects through a variety of mechanisms. They may release toxic substances or compete with the host for essential nutrients. They may also invade organ systems and interfere with their normal function or cause a tissue-damaging inflammatory or immune response.

Classifying Bacteria

Bacteria are classified according to their shape and histological staining.[2,3] Gram stain assists in the classification of bacteria by differentiating the bacteria with thick cell walls (gram-positive) from those with very thin walls but alcohol-labile or acetone-labile outer membranes (gram-negative) based on their susceptibility to staining with a combination of dyes. Gram-positive organisms stain purple or black, and gram-negative organisms stain pink. See Box 20-1 for the classification of many bacterial organisms.

In general, most gram-positive organisms are cocci, and most gram-negative organisms are rods. See Box 20-2 for the most common microorganisms and the infections they produce.

Bacterial Cell Wall Structure

Not only does the bacterial cell wall assist in classifying the organism as gram-positive or gram-negative, it plays an integral role in determining which antimicrobial agents will be effective (i.e., those that can successfully penetrate it).[1] The bacterial cell wall is somewhat rigid owing to the presence of polysaccharide structures called *peptidoglycans* (Figure 20-1). Gram-positive organisms have many layers of peptidoglycan strands and are also polar, having a negative charge. This strongly polar and charged layer favors the penetration of positively charged compounds.

Each peptidoglycan layer consists of multiple amino sugars that are cross-linked by short peptide side chains to form a latticework.[1] The cross-links are different for each type of bacteria. Synthesis of the peptidoglycan layer presents a challenge to the bacterium because it must use cytoplasmic materials to build a large insoluble wall that sits on the outside of the cell membrane. The bacterium constructs pieces of the hydrophilic wall intracellularly and then transports them via a large lipid carrier across the membrane. The synthesis, including the cross-linking, can be blocked at several stages by antibiotics. Specifically, the β-lactam antibiotics (e.g., penicillin) work by preventing the cross-linking peptides from binding to the amino sugar (Figure 20-2).

Within and directly below the peptidoglycan layer are the penicillin-binding proteins that offer a binding site for these drugs. However, also within the peptidoglycan strands are β-lactamases (sometimes called *penicillinases*), which provide a barrier to drug entry into the bacterium. β-Lactamases are produced by the bacterium and are enzymes that inactivate certain antimicrobial agent.

BOX 20-1 Classifications of Bacterial Microorganisms

Type	Shape	Examples
Gram-positive cocci	Spherical	*Staphylococcus aureus, Streptococcus pneumoniae*
Gram-negative cocci	Spherical	*Neisseria gonorrhoeae, Neisseria meningitidis*
Gram-positive bacilli	Rod shaped	*Clostridium tetani, Listeria* spp., *Clostridium perfringens, Clostridium difficile*
Gram-negative bacilli	Rod shaped	*Escherichia coli, Klebsiella pneumoniae, Pseudomonas aeruginosa, Shigella* spp., *Salmonella* spp., *Legionellae* spp. (legionnaires' disease)
Acid-fast bacilli	Rod shaped; retain color of certain stains even when exposed to acid; appear pink or red	*Mycobacterium tuberculosis, Mycobacterium leprae* (Hanson's disease, or leprosy)
Spirochetes	Corkscrew-shaped organisms that are able to move without flagella	*Borrelia burgdorferi* (Lyme disease), *Treponema pallidum* (syphilis)
Mycoplasma	Spherical-shaped organisms that lack a rigid cell wall	*Mycoplasma pneumoniae*
Rickettsiae	Intracellular bacterial parasites that appear like small gram-negative bacilli	*Rickettsia rickettsii* (Rocky Mountain spotted fever)
Actinomycetes	Gram-positive collection of microfilament rods	*Actinomyces israelii, Nocardia* spp.
Chlamydia	Atypical bacteria that stains similarly to *Mycobacterium tuberculosis*	—

The gram-negative organisms have an outer membrane containing lipopolysaccharide structures and also an inner cytoplasmic membrane.[1] The space between the two membranes is the periplasmic space, and it also contains β-lactamases. The presence of these two membranes offers quite a bit of resistance to drug entry. In fact, many drugs can only enter the bacterium through specialized aqueous pores existing in the cell wall. Thus, in general, it is more difficult to kill a gram-negative organism than a gram-positive organism.[4]

PROPERTIES OF ANTIBIOTICS

Properties of antibiotics, such as whether a drug is bacteriocidal or bacteriostatic and its antimicrobial spectrum of activity, help guide the physician in choosing the appropriate drug to treat an infection.

Selective Toxicity

Antibiotics possess selective toxicity by exploiting differences in the morphology between the host and bacteria because they affect the function of bacteria but have little effect on the host. Scientists have exploited these biochemical differences between bacteria and human cells to design drugs to attack targets that exist solely within the bacteria. For example, some of the drugs inhibit production of the cell wall as mentioned previously. These drugs will have little effect on the host because human cells do not contain the same rigid walls. Some other drugs target the bacterial ribosome, but this organelle is sufficiently different from human ribosomes. This selective toxicity enables antibiotics to have a high therapeutic index.

Bactericidal or Bacteriostatic

Antibiotics can be classified as either bacteriostatic or bactericidal.[5] Bacteriostatic drugs inhibit bacterial growth but do not actually kill the organisms (Figure 20-3). They depend on the body's immune system for that action. Bactericidal drugs will attain a high enough concentration in the body to kill the organisms. Which type of drug is used depends on the bacteria and certain host factors.

A bacteriostatic drug may be adequate to eradicate a simple infection in a healthy host but fail in a patient with a compromised immune system.[6] Tetracyclines are bacteriostatic agents that inhibit the growth of pneumococci; the actual destruction of the bacteria requires action of macrophages and neutrophils, which is unachievable in a patient with a low neutrophil count. The site of infection also influences the choice of a bactericidal agent versus a bacteriostatic agent. Certain sites are considered relatively protected from the host's immune responses. Bacteriostatic agents are associated with a high failure rate when used to treat infections in the cerebrospinal fluid, endocarditic vegetations, or another site that is difficult for the drug or immune system to access.

Bactericidal drugs are less dependent on the body's natural defenses, but they are effective in either a concentration-dependent or time-dependent manner.[7] Time-dependent killing depends on the drug concentration being maintained above a certain level for the majority of the dosing interval, whereas concentration-dependent killing depends on achieving a specific high concentration. Concentration-dependent drugs also exhibit a postantibiotic effect. This refers to a period in which growth of the bacteria ceases even after the antibiotic is withdrawn. The duration of the postantibiotic

BOX 20-2 Common Microorganisms Causing Infections

Body Site	Microorganisms	Gram Stain
Eyes	*Neisseria gonorrhoeae*	−
	Chlamydia trachomatis	
	Staphylococcus aureus	+
	Haemophilus spp.	−
	Streptococcus pneumoniae	+
	Pseudomonas aeruginosa	−
	Fungi	
	Herpes	
	Adenoviruses	
Oral cavity	Herpes	
	Candida	
	Actinomyces	+
	Anaerobic cocci	+
	Fusobacterium spp.	−
Throat	*Streptococcus pyogenes*	+
	Corynebacterium diphtheriae	+
	Arcanobacterium haemolyticum	+
	Neisseria gonorrhoeae	−
	Pseudomonas spp.	−
	Staphylococcus aureus	+
Lung (abscesses)	Anaerobic bacteria	
	Staphylococcus aureus	+
	Mycobacterium tuberculosis	
	Fungi	
Heart	Viridans group streptococci	+
	Staphylococcus aureus	+
	Enterococci	+
	Streptococcus agalactiae	+
Meninges	*Escherichia coli*	−
	Streptococcus pneumoniae	+
	Haemophilus influenzae	−
	Neisseria meningitidis	−
	Listeria monocytogenes	+
Brain (abscesses)	Anaerobic bacteria	−/+
	Nocardia	+
	Staphylococcus aureus	+
	Streptococci	+
Sinuses	*Haemophilus influenzae*	−
	Moraxella catarrhalis	−
	Streptococcus pneumoniae	+
	Streptococcus pyogenes	+
	Anaerobic streptococci	+
	Rhinoviruses	
	Coronaviruses	

Body Site	Microorganisms	Gram Stain
Ears	*Haemophilus influenzae*	−
	Streptococcus pneumoniae	+
	Moraxella catarrhalis	−
	Streptococcus pyogenes	+
Larynx-trachea	Respiratory viruses	
	Streptococcus pneumoniae	+
	Moraxella catarrhalis	−
Lungs	*Streptococcus pneumoniae*	+
	Haemophilus influenzae	−
	Staphylococcus aureus	+
	Mycoplasma pneumoniae	
	Legionella spp	
	Chlamydia psittaci	
	Mycobacterium tuberculosis	
	Enterobacteriaceae*	−
Bone (osteomyelitis)	*Staphylococcus aureus*	+
	Salmonella spp.	−
	Haemophilus influenzae	−
	Pseudomonas aeruginosa	−
	Escherichia coli	−
Urinary tract	*Staphylococcus saprophyticus*	+
	Enterobacteriaceae	−
	Enterococci	+
	Pseudomonas aeruginosa	−
Peritoneum (peritonitis)	Enterobacteriaceae	−
	Bacteroides spp.	−
	Anaerobic streptococci	+
	Enterococci	+
	Clostridium spp.	+
Skin	*Staphylococcus aureus*	+
	Herpes simplex	
	Clostridium perfringens	+
	Pseudomonas spp.	−
	Bacteroides spp.	−
	Enterobacteriaceae*	−
	Fungi	
Bloodstream (septicemia)	*Staphylococcus aureus*	+
	Streptococcus pyogenes	+
	Enterobacteriaceae*	−
	Pseudomonas aeruginosa	−
	Staphylococcus epidermidis	+
	Candida albicans	
	Haemophilus influenzae	−
	Streptococcus pneumoniae	+
	Neisseria meningitidis	−

From Brody MJ, Larner J, Minneman KP, editors: *Human pharmacology: Molecular to clinical* (3rd ed.). Philadelphia, 1998, Mosby.
+, Positive; −, negative. **E. coli, Klebsiella, Enterobacter, Serratia* species

effect is directly proportional to the concentration of drug entering the bacteria. This phenomenon allows flexible dosing and longer dosing intervals than those used with most other drugs. It also allows pulse dosing, which is the administration of a large concentration (much greater than needed to kill bacteria) at dosing intervals longer than the drug's half-life. This is different from what is done with most other drugs, particularly antiseizure medications, which are often given every half-life. Antibiotics may be given every 12 half-lives with no reduction in efficacy. The main reasons for this are the host's ability to tolerate high levels of antibiotics without significant toxic effects (i.e., a high therapeutic index) and the concentration-dependent killing.

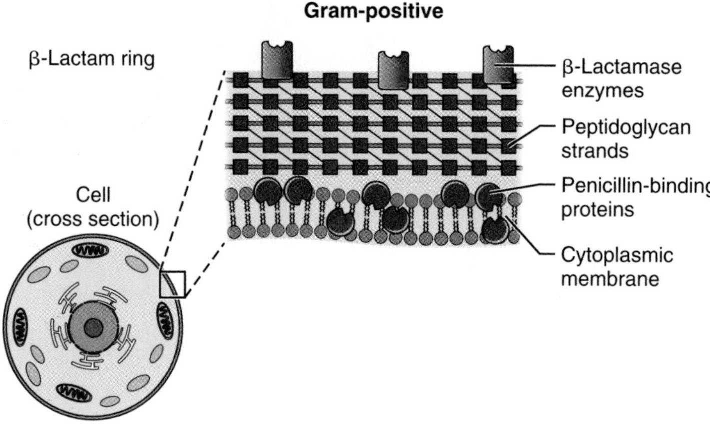

FIGURE 20-1 Outer coating of gram-positive (20 to 30 strands) and gram-negative bacteria showing a thinner (three to five strands) rigid peptidoglycan structure but an added outer membrane for gram-negative cells. β-Lactam drugs act by inhibiting the synthesis of the rigid peptidoglycan part of the cell wall.

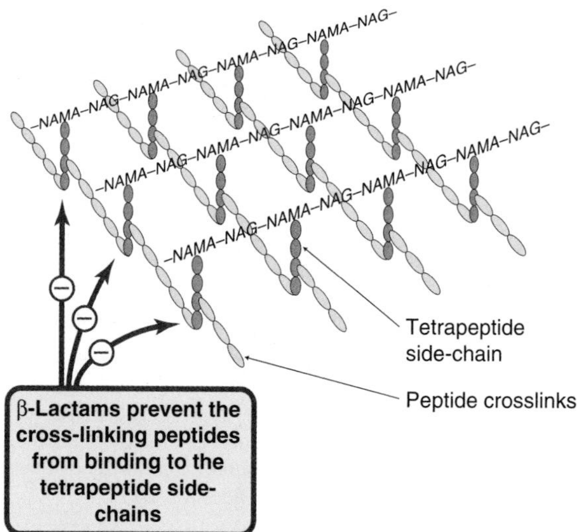

FIGURE 20-2 Schematic diagram of a single layer of peptidoglycan from a bacterial cell (e.g., *Staphylococcus aureus*) showing the site of action of the β-lactam antibiotics. In *S. aureus* the peptide cross-links consist of five glycine residues. Gram-positive bacteria have several layers of peptidoglycan. *NAMA*, N-acetylmuramic acid; *NAG*, N-acetylglucosamine. *(From Rang HP, Dale MM, Ritter JM, Moore JL, editors:* Pharmacology *(5th ed.) New York, 2003, Churchill Livingstone.)*

Antimicrobial Spectrum of Activity

Antibiotics that have activity against many different bacteria are called *broad-spectrum agents*. Those with activity against only a few organisms are called *narrow-spectrum agents*. In practice, broad-spectrum drugs are usually prescribed first, followed by a narrow-spectrum drug after the infecting organism has been identified. The initial drug choice is empiric and depends on the symptoms and location of infection. The exact identity, or a bacteria's susceptibility to a drug, is usually not known until 18 to 24 hours after an initial culture has been done.

One way to determine bacterial susceptibility to a drug is the disk diffusion method (Figure 20-4).[5] Paper discs impregnated with different antimicrobial agents are incubated in an Agar plate along with unknown bacteria obtained from a patient. The amount of drug placed on the disc is that which will provide a bacteria-free zone around the drug if the organism is susceptible. A bacteria-free zone of 14 mm or more implies that the organism is susceptible to the drug, whereas a zone of 11 mm or less implies some resistance.

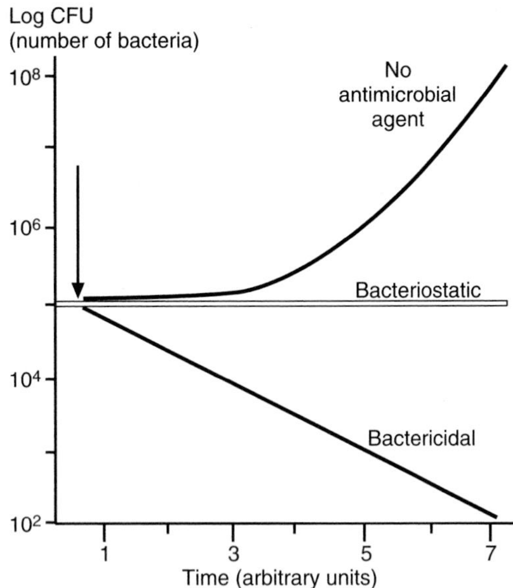

FIGURE 20-3 Bactericidal versus bacteriostatic antimicrobial agents. A typical culture is started at 105 colony-forming units (CFU) and incubated at 98.6°F (37°C) for various times (time in arbitrary units). In the absence of an antimicrobial agent, cell growth occurs. With a bacteriostatic agent added, no growth occurs, but the existing cells are not killed. If the added agent is bactericidal, 99.9% of the cells are killed during the standardized time. *(From Brody MJ, Larner J, Minneman KP, editors:* Human pharmacology: Molecular to clinical *(3rd ed.). Philadelphia, 1998, Mosby.)*

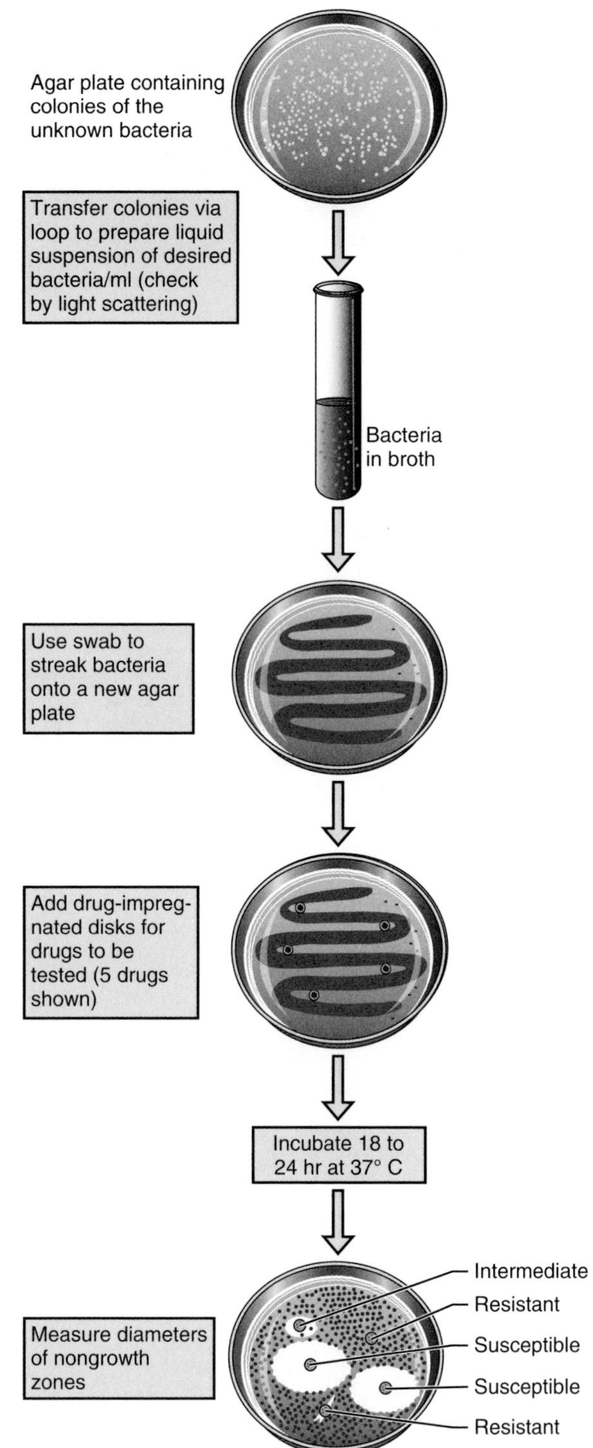

FIGURE 20-4 Disc diffusion method for testing bacteria for susceptibility to specific antimicrobial agents. *(Redrawn from Brody MJ, Larner J, Minneman KP, editors:* Human Pharmacology: Molecular to clinical *(3rd ed.). Philadelphia, 1998, Mosby.)*

DRUG-RESISTANT BACTERIA

Almost since the very beginning of antibiotic development, drug-resistant organisms have been emerging. To scientists who study evolution, this is no accident. Organisms frequently make biochemical or genetic changes to adapt to their environments.[1] Bacteria can multiply in as little as 20 minutes. Given this rapid rate of reproduction, it is conceivable that in a few hours there might be several generations of bacteria, and many may have undergone genetic mutations, making them more resistant to drugs. Repeated courses of antibiotics kill off the susceptible organisms but leave the more resistant strains unaffected.

Resistance to antibiotics can be either innate or acquired.[1] Some bacteria lack the transport mechanism that allows the antibiotic to enter the cell, making the drug useless in fighting this bacterial infection. This is an example of innate resistance. Acquired resistance occurs when gene mutations, either single or multiple, occur during multiple divisions and when one of them prevents the drug from entering the cell. This is called a *spontaneous mutation*. The probability of a spontaneous mutation is 1 per 106 to 108, which is low, but many more cells are present in an infection so that the probability of a mutation is actually higher.

Another form of acquired resistance involves extrachromosomal genetic material that exists in the cytoplasmic plasmids. Plasmids containing genes for resistance are referred to as *R plasmids*.[8] These R plasmids can exchange genetic information with DNA segments, and subsequently, these can be transferred to another bacterial cell.

The results of the previously mentioned genetic mutations produce several biochemical and physical alterations in bacteria that ultimately reduce the efficacy of antimicrobial agents. A significant example of resistance produced by genetic mutation is inactivation of the β-lactam antibiotics by the production of destructive enzymes.[9] These β-lactamases cleave the β-lactam ring of penicillins and cephalosporins which is responsible for the antibacterial activity. Staphylococci are the chief bacteria that produce β-lactamase through genes coding on plasmids. Synthesis of these enzymes is inducible, that is, it occurs only in the presence of a drug. Once produced, the enzymes can pass through the bacterial wall to inactivate antibiotic molecules in the surrounding medium. Scientists have developed some drugs to inactivate these β-lactamases, and, in part, some of the problem has been solved by the development of semisynthetic penicillins (methicillin) and new β-lactam antibiotics (monobactams and carbapenems) which are lactamase resistant.

Gram-negative organisms also produce β-lactamases via chromosomal genes or plasmid genes. The enzymes, however, are not free to enter the substrate; they remain fixed within the cell wall but still represent a formidable challenge to drugs by blocking access to the binding site. Another challenge is that production of these enzymes does not depend on the presence of the drug.

Another form of resistance occurs when the genetic mutation alters the drug-binding site. Obviously, if the drug cannot bind to its receptor, it will be unable to carry out its intended purpose. Other mutations prevent access of the drug to the binding site or actually produce a membrane transporter that actively pumps the antibiotic out of the cell.[4] This latter phenomenon has been seen in both gram-negative and gram-positive organisms.[10]

The main cause of antimicrobial resistance is overuse or inappropriate use of antibiotics[11] (Box 20-3). Bacteria face an onslaught of antibacterial agents so that the genetic mutations that have developed can be viewed as the organisms' acquired survival mechanism. The attacks from these drugs do not occur only in response to an illness or prophylactic treatment before surgery but are ubiquitous across the food chain and in the general environment. Antibiotics are commonly given to animals both as growth enhancers and as treatment for infection. Molecules are then passed down to offspring, appear in the feed, and end up on dinner tables. In addition, efforts to sterilize the environment by destroying bacteria indiscriminately with antibacterial soaps and cleaners are adding to the problem.

Control of antimicrobial resistance can be achieved but not without funding, research, and cooperation from those who care for the ill. The number one way to reduce resistance is to decrease antibiotic use. Accurate and rapid diagnostic equipment is needed to identify a bacterial organism so that treatment can begin with the appropriate drug.[12] As mentioned earlier, treatment is usually begun with a broad-spectrum agent until the offending bacterium is identified; this is followed by switching the patient to a narrow-spectrum agent. It would be more effective to start treatment with a narrow-spectrum but appropriate agent. Major efforts need to be directed toward surveillance of resistant bacteria, especially bacteria affecting the respiratory tract, because about 80% of antibiotic use in the community is related to respiratory tract infections.[13] Being able to differentiate a viral infection from a bacterial infection is also paramount, since most viral infections do not require therapy with an antibacterial drug. The second major way to reduce infection is through hygiene measures. This is particularly important for hospitals because bacteria can be transferred from one patient to another by health care workers. Each hospital needs an active infection control team to closely monitor hygiene practices and cleanup and sterilizing procedures, as well as the typical and atypical pathogens found in the facility.

BOX 20-3 Top Drugs of 2008

Rank	Drug
5	Amoxicillin
15	Azithromycin
26	Cephalexin
37	Levofloxacin
71	Amoxicillin/Clavulanate
141	Trimethoprim/Sulfmethoxazole
145	Penicillin VK
172	Ciprofloxacin
198	Doxycyline

Data from Lamb E: *Pharmacy Times*: pharmacytimes.com. Table shows the rank order of antibiotics among the 200 most widely prescribed drugs.

FACTORS TO CONSIDER IN THE CHOICE OF AN ANTIMICROBIAL AGENT

One of the major factors to consider in the choice of an antimicrobial agent is the identity of the bacterium that is causing the infection. Often, the offending agent is not known, but a knowledgeable physician may be able to make an educated guess. For example, a urinary tract infection in a sexually active woman is often due to *Escherichia coli.* Cellulitis is often caused by *Streptococcus pyogenes* or *Staphylococcus aureus.*

Several host factors also influence antibiotic choice (Box 20-4).[7] Allergies to certain drugs dictate that these medications be avoided. Hepatic and renal functions also need to be considered. Antibiotics are cleared by either the liver or the kidneys, and loss of function of either of these organs means that higher serum levels will be observed. Another factor is the age of the patient. Although most antibiotics are safe, some are contraindicated for infants and children and also for pregnant women. The site of infection represents another important host factor. Brain infections are difficult to treat because only a few antibiotics are able to penetrate the blood–brain barrier and enter the central nervous system in the required concentrations. Penicillins and

BOX 20-4 Bacterial, Host, and Drug Factors That Must Be Considered in Selection of Antibiotic Therapy

Bacterial Factors	Host Factors	Drug Factors
Identity of pathogens*	Site of infection	Activity against pathogen(s)*
Susceptibility of pathogens*	Allergies	Ability to get to site of infection
	Renal function	Potential for drug interactions
	Hepatic function	Available routes of administration
	Neutropenia	Dosing frequency (for outpatients)
	Digestive tract function	Taste (for liquid formulations)
	Other underlying diseases	Stability at different temperatures (for liquid formulations)
	Concomitant medication	Cost
	Pregnancy	
	Desired route of administration	

From Page C, Curtis MJ, Sutter MC, Walker MJ, Hoffman BB, editors: *Integrated pharmacology* (2nd ed.). Philadelphia, 2002, Mosby.
*Often not known at the start of therapy.

cephalosporins only cross into the brain when the meninges are inflamed. This problem also exists for the prostate gland, and infection in the prostate gland tends to require weeks to months of therapy. Kidney and urinary tract infections must be treated with antibiotics that remain in their active forms so that they are effective as they travel through the kidneys into the bladder and urethra.

SUPERINFECTION

Bacteria in the body compete with each other, and benign bacteria can suppress the development of pathogenic bacteria preventing their harmful effects. If other pathogenic bacteria invade a body and cause an infection, an antibiotic is used. This drug might now not only kill these invading bacteria but can also kill the benign bacteria. This allows the suppressed original pathogenic bacteria to grow and produce a secondary infection which usually occurs 1 to 2 weeks after start of the antibiotic therapy. This is called a *superinfection* or a *secondary infection* superimposed on the early one. One example is diarrhea caused by *Clostridium difficile* (described later on). This bacterium can be found in the intestines of about 5% of the population, but its growth is prevented by the rest of the intestinal flora and will not cause any problems. If a person suffers from an infection and is treated with an antibiotic, which also interferes with the normal intestinal flora and removes the growth-retarding factors of *C. difficile*, then these bacteria can multiply to large numbers and cause serious gastrointestinal (GI) problems.

MAJOR ANTIMICROBIAL AGENTS

Antibiotics may be classified in a variety of ways. Some are classified according to chemical structure, bacterial spectrum, or pharmacokinetic properties. However, most are classified according to the most common mechanisms of actions.

Bacterial Cell Wall Inhibitors

The class of drugs known as *bacterial cell wall inhibitors* is made up of the β-lactams (penicillins, cephalosporins, carbapenems, and monobactams) and glycopeptides. The β-lactam antibiotics have a four-member nitrogen-containing β-lactam ring carrying the antibacterial activity (Figure 20-5). They bind to the penicillin-binding proteins and inhibit the linking of the peptide chains to the bacterial cell wall. These drugs are bactericidal and kill in a time-dependent manner.

Penicillins. Penicillins consist of the β-lactam ring attached to a five-member thiazolidine ring.[14] Alterations of the side chains result in different antibacterial properties and thus different drugs. There are four types of penicillin drugs: (1) naturally occurring penicillin G and V, (2) antistaphylococcal penicillins, (3) aminopenicillins, and (4) antipseudomonal penicillins (Box 20-5).

Penicillin G is given parenterally, and penicillin V is given orally. Penicillin G will enter the cerebrospinal fluid when given in high doses to treat neurosyphilis and meningitis. However, these two drugs have a narrow spectrum and are active only against a few gram-positive and gram-negative cocci. They are useful for some streptococcal and meningococcal infections and syphilis, but resistance to these drugs is growing, particularly in the case of *Streptococcus pneumoniae*. In fact, shortly after the introduction of penicillin, many strains of staphylococci became resistant, primarily through the bacteria's production of β-lactamase. Resistance occurs also due to the modification of target penicillin-binding proteins.

Antistaphylococcal Penicillins. Antistaphylococcal penicillins are not inactivated by lactamase and specifically target β-lactamase–containing bacteria. Methicillin was the first antistaphylococcal drug developed; however, it is seldom used today because of a high incidence of allergic interstitial nephritis and the development of resistance. This particular resistance represents such a serious

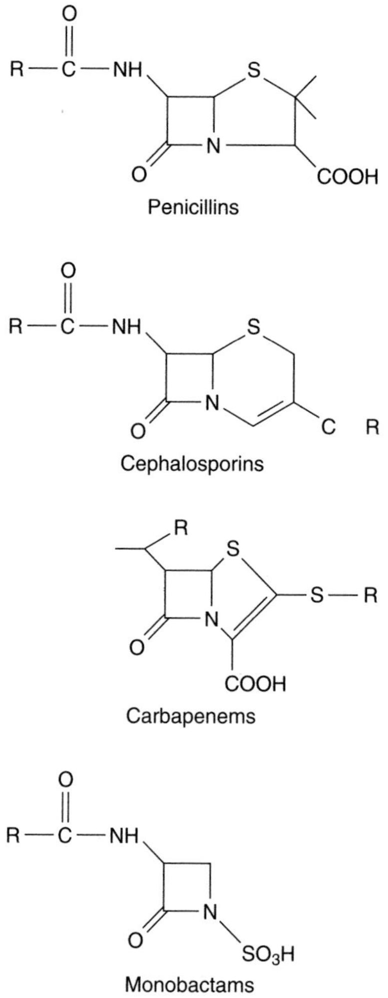

R—C(=O)—NH— [β-lactam–thiazolidine ring] —COOH
Penicillins

R—C(=O)—NH— [β-lactam–dihydrothiazine ring] —C R
Cephalosporins

R— [β-lactam–pyrroline ring] —S—R, COOH
Carbapenems

R—C(=O)—NH— [β-lactam ring] —N—SO_3H
Monobactams

FIGURE 20-5 Basic chemical structures of the four main classes of β-lactam antibiotics. R denotes sites where chemical substitutions are made to create individual drugs.

BOX 20-5 Classification of Penicillins

Classification	Examples
Standard penicillins	Penicillin G
	Penicillin V
Antistaphylococcal	Methicillin (Staphcillin)
	Nafcillin (Unipen)
	Oxacillin (Prostaphlin)
	Cloxacillin (Tegopen)
Aminopenicillins	Ampicillin (Principen)
	Amoxicillin (Amoxil, Trimox)
Antipseudomonal	Carbenicillin (Geocillin)
	Ticarcillin (Ticar)
	Piperacillin (Pipracil)
Other β-lactam antibiotics	Aztreonam (Azactam)
	Imipenem-cilastatin (Primaxin)
	Meropenem (Merrem)
	Ertapenem (Invanz)

problem for infectious disease specialists that this organism is known as methicillin-resistant *Staphylococcal aureus* (MRSA) (see discussion of MRSA later).

Aminopenicillins. Aminopenicillins are made by the addition of an amino group to the penicillin side chain. This enhances the activity of these drugs against gram-negative bacilli while still maintaining activity for cocci such as other penicillins. Specifically, aminopenicillins show activity against *E. coli*, *Proteus mirabilis*, and some strains of *Salmonella* and *Shigella*. The two most common aminopenicillins are ampicillin and amoxicillin. These drugs are also prescribed for respiratory tract infections because of their action against *Streptococcus pneumoniae* and *Haemophilus influenzae*.

Antipseudomonal Penicillins. Antipseudomonal penicillins have actions similar to those of the aminopenicillins but with extended activity against more gram-negative bacilli, including pseudomonads. A few have activity against anaerobic bacteria. However, none of the aminopenicillins or the antipseudomonal drugs has stable activity against staphylococcal β-lactamase.

β-Lactamase Inhibitors. Some drugs that lack antimicrobial activity but are strong inhibitors of β-lactamases have been developed.[15] These include clavulanate, sulbactam, and tazobactam. They are administered in combination with some antibiotic drugs; for example, clavulanate plus amoxicillin is called *augmentin*.[16,17] However, despite these advances, several strains of streptococci and staphylococci, including MRSA, remain resistant to penicillins.

Clinical Uses for Penicillins. Penicillins are the first-choice drugs for many infections. In general, they are active against many gram-positive and gram-negative cocci and some gram-negative bacilli. Penicillins are commonly used to treat bacterial meningitis caused by *Neisseria meningitidis* and *Streptococcus pneumoniae*; skin and soft tissue infections caused by *Streptococcus pyogenes* or *Staphylococcus aureus*; urinary tract infections caused by *E. coli*; and otitis media caused by *Streptococcus pyogenes* or *H. influenzae*; they are also used in the treatment of gonorrhea and syphilis. It is important to realize that this list is far from complete.

Adverse Drug Reactions Associated with Penicillins. The adverse effects of penicillins are relatively minor for most individuals compared with those of other drugs. They include GI discomfort and symptoms related to allergy, urticaria, joint swelling, and respiratory problems. However, if a patient is allergic to one of the penicillins, he or she will be allergic to all of them because they are all cross-sensitizing. Penicillins also have a high degree of cross-sensitivity with the cephalosporins for anaphylaxis. Oral penicillins tend to bind to food and are either degraded or have decreased absorption when taken with acidic juices and therefore should be either given 1 hour before a meal or 1 hour after a meal.

Cephalosporins. Cephalosporins are similar in structure to the penicillins except they have a six-member ring attached to the β-lactam ring (see Figure 20-5).[7] They are classified as first-, second-, and third-generation drugs according to their activity (see Box 20-6). First-generation drugs are active against gram-positive cocci and some gram-negative bacilli. Specifically, they fight streptococci, staphylococci, *E. coli*, *P. mirabilis*, and *Klebsiella pneumoniae*. They also perform well against skin and soft tissue infections caused by *S. pyogenes* and *S. aureus*. They are favored among surgeons for prophylaxis against infection after surgery. Examples include cefadroxil, cefazolin, and cephalexin.

Second-generation cephalosporins have activity against gram-positive cocci but are more effective than the first group against gram-negative bacteria. Some have action against *H. influenzae*, *Bacteroides fragilis*, and even some anaerobic organisms that are found in the GI tract. Examples include cefaclor, cefotetan, and cefoxitin.

Third-generation cephalosporins have the most activity against gram-negative bacilli, especially enterobacteriaceae, *Pseudomonas aeruginosa*, and *H. influenzae*. However, they have reduced activity against *S. aureus*. Some advantages of these drugs include being able to enter the central nervous system at concentrations high enough to treat bacterial meningeal infections and limited cross-reactivity (10%) with the penicillins, even though they are structurally related. Therefore these drugs are somewhat safer alternatives for patients allergic to penicillin. However, the cross-sensitivity for anaphylactic reactions is high. Examples in this category include ceftriaxone, ceftazidime, and a new oral third-generation drug called cefditoren.[18] Cefepime is a fourth-generation cephalosporin, and ceftobiprole, which shows some effectiveness against MRSA, is a fifth-generation cephalosporin.

Clinical uses of cephalosporins include septicemia, pneumonia, meningitis, biliary tract infection, skin infections, including diabetic foot infections, and sinusitis. Adverse events associated with these drugs include hypersensitivity reactions and GI disturbances, which are similar to those seen with penicillin. In addition, a few penicillin-sensitive individuals will experience some cross-reactions.

BOX 20-6 Cephalosporins

First Generation	Cefadroxil (Duricef)
	Cefazolin (Ancef)
	Cefmetazole (Zefazone)
	Cephalexin (Keflex)
	Cephradine (Velosef)
Second Generation	Cefaclor (Ceclor)
	Cefamandole (Mandol)
	Cefotetan (Cefotan)
	Cefuroxime (Zinacef)
Third Generation	Cefdinir (Omnicef)
	Cefixime (Suprax)
	Cefotaxime (Claforan)
	Ceftizoxime (Cefizox)
Fourth Generation	Cefepime (Maxipime)

Other β-Lactam Antibiotics. Carbapenems and monobactams are other β-lactam antibiotics that were specifically developed to treat β-lactamase–producing gram-negative organisms that are resistant to penicillins.[1] Monobactams consist of a single ring structure attached to a sulfonic acid group (see Figure 20-5). The only available monobactam is aztreonam, which only has activity against aerobic gram-negative bacilli, especially *P. aeruginosa*. This drug has no activity against gram-positive bacteria. An important property of this drug is that it is relatively nonallergenic and therefore can be used by patients who are allergic to penicillin or cephalosporin.[19]

Carbapenems have a very broad spectrum of activity against gram-positive, gram-negative, and some anaerobic organisms.[20] In addition, their activity is stable against many β-lactamases. Because of their broad effects, these drugs can be used to treat polymicrobial infections instead of two or more different antibiotics. Examples include imipenem, meropenem, and a new agent called ertapenem.

Glycopeptides. Vancomycin and teicoplanin are very potent bacterial cell wall inhibitors that lack a β-lactam ring.[1] These drugs act by binding to the terminal two alanine amino acids at one end of the peptidoglycan backbone, thus blocking elongation. Because they do not bind to the penicillin-binding proteins and do not have a β-lactam ring, they are not broken down by β-lactamase. The glycopeptides are active against gram-positive bacteria and are especially active against many resistant forms of streptococci and staphylococci. They are the drug of choice for methicillin-resistant staphylococci, penicillin-resistant pneumococci, and *C. difficile*.[21]

Vancomycin is given orally for the treatment of *C. difficile* because the drug cannot be absorbed from the GI tract, thus producing a high concentration at the target organ. Otherwise the drug is given intravenously.

Vancomycin is an extremely important arsenal in our war against bacteria. So far, only a few cases of resistance to vancomycin have been reported: *Enterococcus faecium* and a genetically based neonatal MRSA.[22,23] Because of its importance, indiscriminate use is discouraged. However, it is an excellent substitute treatment for patients with β-lactam allergy because there is no cross-reactivity between vancomycin and the β-lactam antibiotics.

The major adverse effect of vancomycin is an erythematous rash that is confined to the neck and upper trunk, called *red man syndrome*.[1] This reaction occurs when the drug is infused too quickly, creating a histamine reaction.

Bacitracin. Bacitracin inhibits cell wall production by blocking the recycling of the membrane lipid carrier which is needed to add on new cell wall subunits. For internal use, it is a prescription drug, but it can be obtained without a prescription for topical use. In this case, bacitracin is sold alone or in combination with polymyxin B (Polysporin) or with polymyxin B and neomycin (Neosporin). These ointments are used for the prevention and treatment of minor skin infections.

Inhibitors of Bacterial Cell Membrane Functioning

Polymyxin B and polymyxin E are drugs that injure the plasma membrane of gram-negative bacteria. They destroy its integrity and allow the escape of nutrients from the bacterial cell and allow the entry of toxic materials from the environment into the bacteria. Because they are quite toxic (neurotoxic and nephrotoxic), their use is limited to the treatment of skin infections, which allows topical application of the drugs.[7]

Antibiotics That Inhibit Bacterial Protein Synthesis

Bacterial protein synthesis takes place in the ribosomes.[1] Here, messenger RNA (mRNA), which provides the instructions for protein synthesis, and transfer RNA (tRNA), which physically brings the amino acids to the ribosome, synthesizes the various proteins (Figure 20-6). Because the bacterial ribosome is sufficiently different in structure from the mammalian ribosome, it represents a good target for drug action.

Aminoglycosides. Streptomycin, gentamicin, neomycin, and other aminoglycosides bind to bacterial ribosomes, causing misreadings of the mRNA genetic code.[1] These drugs enter the bacterial cells with the help of an oxygen-dependent transport system, which is not present in anaerobic bacteria or streptococci. They are active against many gram-negative bacilli, staphylococci, and mycobacteria. They are especially used for gram-negative enteric organisms in the treatment of sepsis. Resistance to these agents is becoming more problematic and develops by alterations in the bacterial cell wall or by the synthesis of aminoglycoside-modifying enzymes. These drugs are both nephrotoxic and ototoxic, depending on duration of use. The nephrotoxic effect is reversible, but the ototoxicity can be permanent. Because of these adverse effects, their use is limited to fighting *P. aeruginosa* and enterobacteriaceae.

Macrolides. Macrolides are primarily used to treat respiratory tract infections and are the drugs of choice for community-acquired pneumonia.[24] They work by binding to specific parts of the ribosome and inhibiting the formation of peptide bonds between amino acids and tRNA. They are active against streptococci, staphylococci, pneumococci, *Mycoplasma pneumoniae*, *Bordetella pertussis*, and legionellae. They are also the drugs of choice for treatment of chlamydial infections during pregnancy because tetracyclines are contraindicated. Erythromycin is the prototypical drug, but because it may cause excessive nausea and vomiting, it is poorly tolerated. Clarithromycin and azithromycin produce less severe GI effects.

Tetracyclines. Tetracyclines consist of four fused cyclic rings that bind to the ribosome in a manner that blocks binding of the tRNA to the mRNA-ribosome complex (Figure 20-7).[7] Thus the growing peptide chain is terminated. They offer broad activity against chlamydiae, mycoplasmas, spirochetes, rickettsiae, and legionellae. They have traditionally been used for the treatment of acne vulgaris. They bind strongly to developing bone, impairing growth, and also cause yellowing of teeth. They are contraindicated in pregnant and breast-feeding women and also in children younger than 8 years. Examples include tetracycline, doxycycline, and minocycline.

Streptogramins. Quinupristin and dalfopristin are members of a new family of antibiotics called streptogramins.[1] When administered individually, they show minimal antimicrobial action, but when given together intravenously, they are quite potent against gram-positive bacteria. Dalfopristin binds to the 50S subunit of the bacterial ribosome, changing its configuration and facilitating quinupristin binding. These drugs are new alternatives to the standard treatment for infections caused by multiresistant gram-positive bacteria, so they are quite important. When combined with other agents such as ampicillin or doxycycline, they mount an impressive attack against vancomycin-resistant *E. faecium*, another very resistant and dangerous organism.[25] Studies are ongoing to determine their effectiveness alone and in combination with other agents against MRSA. Adverse drug reactions include inflammation at the infusion site, GI effects, myalgias, and arthralgias.

Oxazolidinones. Linezolid is the first drug in a new category, the oxazolidinones, that inhibits bacterial protein synthesis at a step earlier than do other antimicrobials. Linezolid attaches to the 50S subunit at a position that interferes with tRNA binding.[26] It is active against penicillin-resistant pneumococci and *S. aureus*, resistant staphylococci including MRSA, and methicillin-resistant *S. epidermidis*.[27,28] So far, only rare resistance has been reported.

Glycilcyclines. Tigecycline is a new drug which is related structurally to the tetracyclines, is a wide spectrum drug showing activity against even some MRSA, and is given intravenously. It binds to the 30S ribosomal subunit and blocks the entry of tRNA into the ribosome, thus preventing amino acid incorporation into the protein chain (A). It is used against serious infections, including certain skin and abdominal infections, as well as community-acquired bacterial pneumonia. Adverse reactions include mild to moderate GI discomfort.

Antibiotics That Inhibit Bacterial DNA Synthesis or Break DNA Strands

Each strand of DNA consists of a series of sugars (deoxyribose) and phosphate molecules as the backbone, with either a purine (adenine [A] or guanine [G]) or a pyrimidine (cytosine [C] or thymine [T]) base attached.[1]

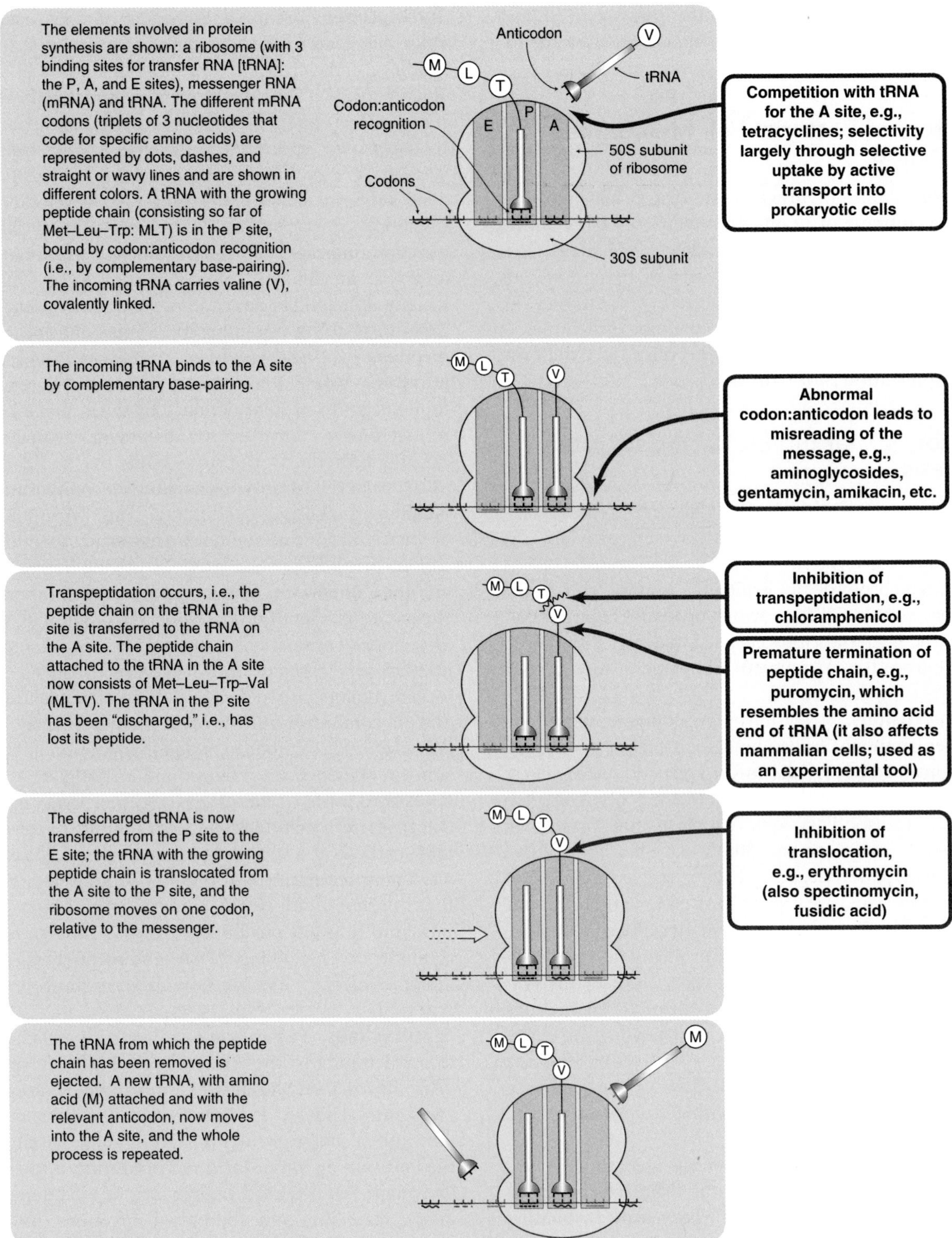

FIGURE 20-6 Schematic diagram of bacterial protein synthesis indicating the points at which antibiotics inhibit the process. *(From Rang HP, Dale MM, Ritter JM, Flower R, editors:* Pharmacology *(6th ed.). New York, 2007, Churchill Livingstone.)*

The base, sugar, and phosphate form the nucleotide. Two DNA strands are coiled together and held in place by hydrogen bonds linking purine and pyrimidine bases between G and C and between A and T on each strand (Figure 20-8). During DNA synthesis, each original DNA strand serves as a template for the formation of a new strand. The enzyme DNA polymerase copies the DNA strand by complementary base pairing.[29] Before this can occur, DNA gyrase, also known as *topoisomerase II*, produces a double-strand break in the DNA helix necessary for the separation of the two strands. The same enzyme is then responsible for resealing the

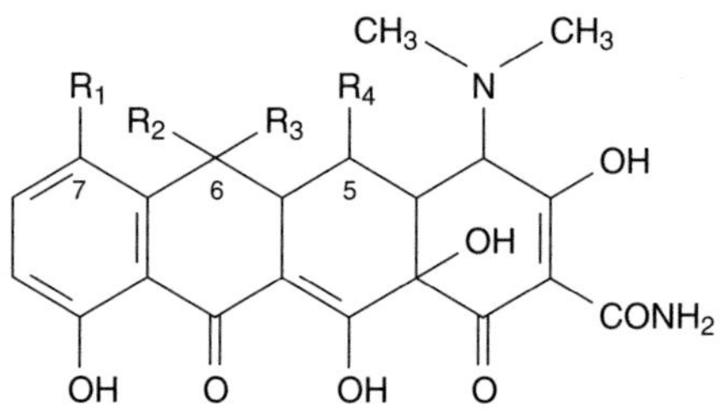

FIGURE 20-7 Chemical structure of tetracyclines. Substitutions at positions five, six, and seven result in different drugs, including the three common agents tetracycline, doxycycline, and minocycline.

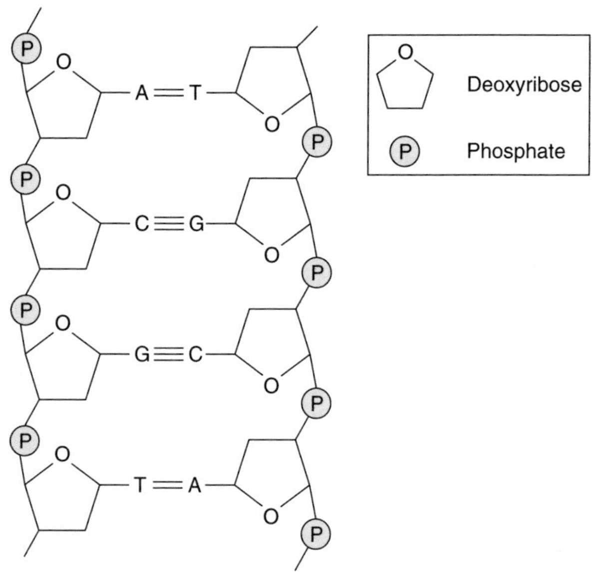

FIGURE 20-8 Structure of DNA. Each strand of DNA consists of a sugar-phosphate backbone with purine or pyrimidine bases attached. The purines are adenine (A) or guanine (G), and the pyrimidines are cytosine (C) or thymine (T). The sugar is deoxyribose. Complementarity between the two strands of DNA is maintained by hydrogen bonds (either two or three) between bases.

breaks and preventing tangling problems. If this enzyme is deactivated, the chromosomes remain intertwined during mitosis and are unable to separate. Inhibition of DNA gyrase is an important target for the fluoroquinolone antibiotics.

Fluoroquinolones. Fluoroquinolones inhibit DNA synthesis by blocking DNA gyrase.[1] They are active against aerobic gram-negative bacilli such as pseudomonads and gram-negative cocci. They can also penetrate difficult-to-reach areas such as the prostate gland. The most commonly used fluoroquinolone is ciprofloxacin. Cipro, as it is more commonly known, received attention in 2001 when it was used to treat anthrax infections.[30] It has a somewhat broader spectrum of activity than other fluoroquinolones and has excellent activity against enterobacteriaceae; gram-negative bacilli; and many organisms that are resistant to penicillins, cephalosporins, and aminoglycosides. Some clinical uses include complicated urinary tract infections, respiratory tract infections and otitis produced by pseudomonads, gonorrhea, bacterial prostatitis, cervicitis, and anthrax. The adverse effects of this drug include GI effects, dizziness, and headache, although arthralgias, myalgias, tendinitis, and tendon ruptures have been reported.[31] The most common site affected is the Achilles tendon; however, tendonitis has also been reported in the rotator cuff and patellar and quadriceps tendons. It is speculated that consistent overloading of the tendon during activities is to blame. Studies on the canine Achilles tendon have shown a decrease in fibroblast metabolism along with increased degrading activity when tendon specimens are incubated with ciprofloxacin.[32] The estimated incidence is 3.2 cases per 1000 patient years, and individuals aged 60 or over and those who are also taking corticosteroids or have undergone kidney, heart, or lung transplant surgery are predominantly affected.[32] It appears that patients are more susceptible to injury within the first 30 days following drug withdrawal. One case study of bilateral Achilles tendon pain associated with levofloxacin use has been reported in the physical therapy literature.[31] The author reported on a two-phase program that first aimed to reduce the loading stress on the tendon with crutches and an orthotic. Phase I continued for the first 6 weeks after medication withdrawal and was followed by Phase II consisting of progressive loading of the tendon over an additional 3-month period. Care was taken to protect the tendon from rupture while it was still susceptible to the degrading effects of the drug. Two other fluoroquinolones are gatifloxacin and moxifloxacin.[33]

Nitroimidazoles. Metronidazole acts by an uncertain mechanism but it is reduced in the mitochondria of bacteria, and the reduced intermediates seem to interact with bacterial DNA resulting in DNA strand breaks. It is active against anaerobic bacteria, especially *B. fragilis*, *C. difficile*, and certain protozoa (*Giardia lamblia*, *Entamoeba histolytica*, and *Trichomonas* species). It is the drug of choice for bacterial vaginosis and *C. difficile* and is also used in Crohn's disease. The adverse effects of these drugs include numbness in the hands and a disulfiram-like effect (vomiting with alcohol intake).

Antifolates. Antifolates interfere with the production of folate, which is necessary for the production of purine, and subsequently, DNA.[7] Humans can utilize folate obtained from dietary sources, but bacteria must synthesize folate from para-aminobenzoic acid (PABA), since folates do not penetrate the microorganisms. These antibiotics block enzymes involved in this folate pathway (Figure 20-9). Sulfonamides are used to treat bacterial conjunctivitis, urinary tract infections, and inflammatory bowel disease; and they are applied topically to prevent infection associated with burns. Because they are quite allergenic, producing a pruritic maculopapular rash, and have a high rate of bacterial resistance, they are rarely used. However, silver sulfadiazine and sulfamethoxazole are still used. In fact, sulfamethoxazole is combined with a drug called trimethoprim that blocks another step in

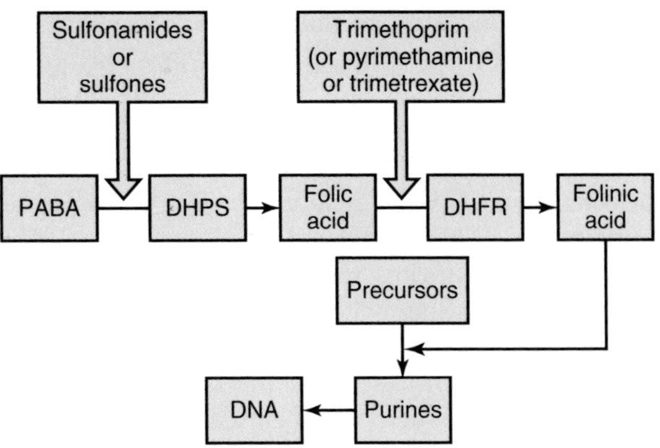

FIGURE 20-9 The folate biosynthetic pathway. Sulfonamides and sulfones compete with para-aminobenzoic acid (PABA) for dihydropteroate synthetase. Trimethoprim and the antiprotozoal drugs pyrimethamine and trimetrexate inhibit dihydrofolate reductase (DHFR).

this folate biosynthetic pathway. The combination is called *trimethoprim-sulfamethoxazole* (TMP-SMZ) and is also known as *co-trimoxazole*. This combination is effective against several gram-negative bacilli including *E. coli*, enterobacteriaceae, and *P. mirabilis*. TMP-SMZ is the drug of choice for urinary tract infections.

Silver sulfadiazine is a topical sulfonamide compound of silver nitrate and sodium sulfadiazine. It is useful against a wide range of gram-negative bacteria, especially *E. coli* and *P. aeruginosa*, and also against gram-positive bacteria such as *S. aureus* and *Candida* species. It is most useful as a topical agent for deep partial-thickness and full-thickness burns or large superficial partial-thickness injuries. In addition to its antimicrobial effect, it may accelerate wound healing.[34] It is applied with a gloved hand thickly enough that the wound cannot be seen. Dry gauze is then applied over the cream.

SOME SPECIFIC BACTERIAL INFECTIONS AND THEIR TREATMENT

Pathogenic microorganisms invade the body tissue by somehow evading normal host defenses. They multiply and create an infective process that usually consists of fever, chills, sweats, redness, pain, pus, and swelling. In addition, the white blood cell (WBC) count increases as the host begins to fight back. In most cases, the host's defense system and standard antibiotic treatment are enough to eradicate the infection. However, because of the ever-changing nature of bacteria, treatment of infection does not always follow a standard protocol.

Tuberculosis (TB)

Tuberculosis (TB) in its active form is estimated to affect eight million people, resulting in two million deaths every year.[35] In addition, it is estimated that more than two billion people have been infected with *Mycobacterium tuberculosis*, and many are not even aware of it because the bacteria can persist asymptomatically for long periods, finally causing an active infection years later (latent TB). Most individuals control the initial infection by mounting a cell-mediated immune response that prevents the disease but may leave some viable mycobacteria, resulting in clinical disease in 5 to 10% of cases. Primary disease can develop later in life, either by reactivation of the bacteria remaining from the initial infection or by the development of a subsequent infection.

The risk of developing TB is highly dependent on the host's immune status. Co-infection with human immunodeficiency virus (HIV) markedly increases the development of symptoms of both diseases.[36] In the year 2000, it was estimated that 11 million people were co-infected with HIV and *M. tuberculosis*, and in the same year, there were 500,000 new cases of active TB associated with HIV infection. The interaction between the two infections appears to be synergistic in that each increases the pathogenesis of the other. HIV infection promotes the progression to active TB in people with latent or recently acquired infection, and TB increases HIV viremia.

M. tuberculosis is transmitted by airborne particles in respiratory secretions when an infected person coughs, sneezes, or speaks. The bacteria are inhaled deep into the lungs and into the alveoli where they are engulfed by macrophages. However, the thick wall of the mycobacterium provides some resistance against the bacterial fighting mechanisms of the macrophages. The macrophages launch their own attack, with the result being *M. tuberculosis* uptake by the phagocytes into an immature phagosomal compartment, allowing the bacteria to replicate inside the macrophages.[37-39] At this point, the infection is controlled, and there are no clinical symptoms. However, the infection site can be identified by the presence of small granulomas characterized by a central area of mycobacteria-infected cells surrounded by other noninfected phagocytic cells and foamy giant cells (giant macrophages containing lipids). Lymphocytes are found around the periphery. The granuloma is sealed off from other tissue by a fibrotic capsule. The material is at first solid but becomes liquefied because of the continued multiplication of the bacilli. The liquefied granuloma may open up into a bronchus and infect the sputum. At this point, the patient is very infectious. Bacilli are ingested by macrophages and transported via the bloodstream and lymphatics to other areas. Eventually, fibrosis and calcification of the tissues render the disease inactive. However, there is a potential for reactivation years later.

Symptoms of TB include fever, night sweats, malaise, and weight loss. Productive cough and pleuritic pain are the pulmonary symptoms.[3] Up to 80% of patients without HIV infection show only pulmonary involvement, but the majority of patients with HIV infection show extrapulmonary symptoms involving the genitourinary tract, bones, joints, meninges, and peritoneum.

Treatment of active TB has two goals: (1) to cure the infection and (2) to prevent spread to others. Patients with active TB are kept in ventilated isolation rooms in which high-efficiency particulate air (HEPA) filtration and UV germicidal irradiation are provided.[40] Health care workers entering the room of an infected patient must wear personal respirators with HEPA-filtered masks that must be tested for proper fit annually to ensure close facial contact with the mask. Isolation may be discontinued when three consecutive sputum samples (taken on different days) are negative for the bacilli and the patient is improving clinically. This may take up to 3 weeks or longer if the patient is infected with a resistant strain.

The initial phase of treatment consists of at least three different medications, possibly four if the organism is suspected to be resistant, and includes isoniazid, rifampicin, pyrazinamide, and ethambutol.[1] This phase lasts a minimum of 2 months. The second, continuation phase lasts at least 4 months and consists of treatment with isoniazid and rifampin. If there is TB located in the bone or brain or if there is evidence of resistance, this phase is longer.

Antimycobacterial Drugs

Isoniazid. Isoniazid is the most critical drug for the treatment of TB. This drug inhibits the synthesis of mycolic acid, an important lipid constituent of the cell wall of the mycobacterium. It is absorbed well orally and even achieves concentrations in the cerebrospinal fluid to treat tuberculous meningitis. Common adverse effects include hepatitis and peripheral neuropathy, but hematologic changes, arthritic symptoms, and vasculitis have also been reported. In the treatment of active disease, this drug is always used in combination with rifampin plus at least one other antimycobacterial drug. Treatment is given two to three times per week for at least 6 months but may be as long as 12 months if the patient is also infected with HIV. Persons with a positive tuberculin skin test result but no evidence of TB on a chest X-ray film may be treated with isoniazid alone.[41] The protocol for this is isoniazid treatment two to three times a day for 6 to 9 months.

Rifampin. Rifampin is used along with isoniazid as a first-line agent against *M. tuberculosis*.[1] However, it is also used to treat other infections, such as *Mycobacterium leprae* (causes Hansen's disease), legionellae, *N. meningitidis*, *H. influenzae*, and staphylococci. Rifampin binds to the DNA-dependent RNA polymerase to inhibit RNA synthesis. Rifampin induces hepatic P450 enzymes, and therefore the metabolism of other drugs is increased. Other effects of these drugs include thrombocytopenia, nephritis, and orange discoloration of most secretions, including tears (which results in staining of contact lenses).

Pyrazinamide. Pyrazinamide is also a first-line agent against TB and is given along with rifampin and isoniazid.[1] It is a prodrug converted to pyrazinoic acid, which inhibits the enzyme fatty acid synthetase I, which is required by the bacterium to synthesize fatty acids. Its main adverse effect is hepatotoxicity.

Ethambutol. The fourth drug commonly included in this regimen is ethambutol. It is thought to inhibit the bacteria's production of RNA, but the exact mechanism is not known. It has some rather bizarre adverse effects, mainly on vision. It produces retrobulbar neuritis, which begins as red-green color blindness and progresses to a generalized loss of visual acuity.

Other Antimycobacterial Drugs. Other antimicrobial drugs are effective against TB, especially when given in combination.[42] Capreomycin is an aminoglycoside. Little is known about capreomycin's exact mechanism of action, but it is thought to inhibit protein synthesis by binding to the 70S ribosomal unit. Capreomycin also binds to components in the bacterial cell, which results in the production of abnormal proteins that are toxic to the microorganism. It can be injected in the event that a patient has difficulty with any of the standard drugs. Its adverse effects include renal failure and injury to the eighth cranial nerve, which causes deafness and ataxia. Cycloserine is a broad-spectrum agent that is bacteriostatic against the mycobacterium. Its primary mechanism of action is to inhibit cell wall synthesis. This drug primarily produces neurologic symptoms, including headache, depression, convulsions, and psychotic episodes.

Multidrug-Resistant Tuberculosis

Multidrug-resistant TB is a growing problem and a dangerous public health issue. It is defined as the presence of strains resistant to at least isoniazid and rifampin. Primary multidrug-resistant TB develops when a person acquires a strain of TB that is already resistant, whereas secondary multidrug-resistant TB develops in an individual who was noncompliant with treatment or who received inadequate treatment.[40] It is related both to noncompliance with treatment and HIV status. The noncompliance issue encompasses not only premature drug withdrawal but also treatment devoid of some of the key drugs used for TB.[40] In several parts of the world, the complete four-drug protocol is not available. Patients may receive only one of the four drugs, giving the mycobacterium an opportunity to develop resistance. Even in New York City, this has become a problem and is related to socioeconomic conditions. Poverty is a risk factor for TB, and from 1979 to 1993, the poverty rate in the city rose by almost 10%, corresponding to a 33% increase in the incidence of TB. In the United States, in the 1950s, drug resistance accounted for 1 to 2%, but by 1991, this had increased to 23%.

Several strategies have been developed to stem the growth of resistant TB.[43] An individual drug protocol is designed on the basis of the drugs "thought to be most sensitive." Medications are added one at a time until five effective drugs are found. More than five may be used if the sensitivity of the bacterium is unclear. Another strategy includes "directly observed therapy." This method refers to requiring patients to attend a local health clinic, where they can be directly observed taking their medication. If appointments are missed, the patient may then be incarcerated. In some cases, health care professionals visit the patient at home to ensure compliance with treatment. Other strategies include providing vouchers for transportation to the health clinic, food coupons, housing assistance, support groups, and educational activities.

Clostridium difficile

C. difficile is a gram-positive, spore-forming anaerobic bacillus that produces colitis, voluminous, infectious, and watery diarrhea; abdominal cramping; and sometimes fever.[44] Dehydration, electrolyte depletion, and other complications, including hemorrhage, reactive arthritis, sepsis, and death, may occur. *C. difficile* infection often occurs after administration of a broad-spectrum antibiotic but can also follow chemotherapy or immunosuppressive treatments. Antimicrobial agents are often to blame because they eradicate the normal GI flora needed to keep the *C. difficile* level to a minimum.[45] Older patients commonly have this illness after antibiotic treatment of a diabetic or vascular wound. Some individuals may be asymptomatic or only show mild symptoms but carry high levels of *C. difficile*. Patient-to-patient transmission occurs, and the organisms can be cultured from the hands, clothing, and stethoscopes of health care workers who have been in the rooms of infected patients. These bacteria can survive up to 5 months in the environment. Colonization occurs by the fecal–oral route. Ingested spores survive the acid environment of the stomach and grow in the colon. The drug of choice for *C. difficile* is intravenous metronidazole, with vancomycin coming in second.[46] Successful treatment of this infection has also been documented with intracolonic vancomycin.[21] This mode of administration eliminates the neurotoxicity and nephrotoxicity associated with this drug.

Methicillin-Resistant *Staphylococcus aureus*

Staphylococcus aureus is present on the skin of many people but generally does not cause a problem for those who are healthy. However, it is a significant threat to the sick and to the older adult population, particularly in the resistant form, methicillin-resistant *S. aureus* (MRSA). MRSA poses a significant health risk because it is immune to the effects of the standard first-line antibiotics used to treat *Staphylococcus* infections. MRSA spreads through direct contact, often from contamination of hands from hospital staff members to patients. It can also be spread through contact with contaminated surfaces in the environment. It can survive for long periods (up to 79 days) in dry environmental conditions, existing on paper, foil, cotton, Formica, and other surfaces.[47] In an effort to control these bacteria, patients with MRSA infections are usually isolated in single rooms. They remain in isolation until they are free from infection (three consecutive cultures taken on different days). Drug choices for the treatment of MRSA are becoming increasingly limited. For several years, vancomycin was one of the most effective remedies for this infection, but now there are several reports of vancomycin-resistant *S. aureus*. At the time of this writing, only two other drugs—linezolid and quinupristin/dalfopristin—have the approval of the U.S. Food and Drug Administration (FDA) for the treatment of MRSA. Of the two, linezolid is preferred because of its favorable pharmacokinetic properties. It is one of the few drugs with bioavailability nearing 100% for the oral form (making the transition from intravenous to oral administration easy), and it is metabolized without any P450 enzymes. In addition, the dosing interval is every 12 hours, and no dose adjustment is required for patients with renal problems. Fluoroquinolones, tetracyclines, and TMP-SMZ may occasionally be effective.[46] Linezolid, as well as other drugs used to treat resistant infections, must be used sparingly. Appropriate laboratory testing must be performed to ensure that the correct drugs are used to fight infection and to prevent indiscriminate use. Their use must be preserved for only difficult infections.

Pneumonia

Community-acquired bacterial pneumonia is often caused by *Streptococcus pneumoniae* (pneumococci).[48] In the United States, more than 15% of these bacteria are resistant to penicillin, and they are becoming increasingly resistant to cephalosporins, macrolides, and the fluoroquinolones. For treatment of *S. pneumoniae* infection, a fluoroquinolone (levofloxacin, gatifloxacin, or moxifloxacin) is the drug of choice. Doxycycline (a macrolide) is also recommended. Atypical pathogens, including *Mycoplasma pneumoniae*, *Chlamydia pneumoniae*, and *Legionellae pneumophila* cause up to 40% of cases of this community-acquired disease. To treat these atypical infections, a macrolide (e.g., erythromycin, azithromycin, or clarithromycin) is given.

Urinary Tract Infections

Uncomplicated cystitis is treated with a 3-day course of oral TMP-SMZ or a single dose of three double-strength tablets. In areas where there is TMP-SMZ–resistant

E. coli, a fluoroquinolone is substituted. When urinary tract infections have been acquired in a hospital or nursing home, the infectious agent is presumed to be resistant gram-negative bacilli, *S. aureus*, or enterococci. A fluoroquinolone, third-generation cephalosporin, or amoxicillin/clavulanic acid may be used.

ANTIMICROBIAL PROPHYLAXIS IN SURGERY

Antimicrobial prophylaxis can decrease the incidence of infection, particularly wound infection, after certain surgeries. However, this benefit must be weighed against risks such as adverse reactions, including allergic reactions, or the development of resistant bacteria. It is recommended for procedures associated with high infection rates such as those involving implantation of prosthetic material, those involving the GI tract, and those involving trauma in which the wound is already dirty.[49] Host factors, such as immunosuppression caused by diseases such as acquired immune deficiency syndrome (AIDS) or drugs such as steroids or immunosuppressant agents, and the presence of valvular and other cardiac diseases also warrant prophylaxis. Long preoperative hospitalizations are associated with increased risk of infection with a resistant organism, and therefore prophylaxis may be required. Antimicrobial prophylaxis to prevent bacterial endocarditis in patients with prosthetic heart valves, rheumatic heart disease, or other cardiac abnormalities is also recommended before dental procedures.

In most cases, a single intravenous or intramuscular dose of an antimicrobial administered between 30 and 60 minutes before the initial incision provides adequate tissue concentrations throughout the surgery. If the surgery is prolonged (more than 4 hours) or if major blood loss occurs, another dose is given. For "dirty surgery" such as that for a perforated abdominal cavity, a compound fracture, or a laceration caused by an animal or human bite, the use of antimicrobial drugs is considered to be therapy rather than prophylaxis and should be continued for several days. Cefazolin is recommended for many procedures because of its long half-life; however, in hospitals where MSRA is present, vancomycin may be used. For colorectal surgery and appendectomies, cefotetan is the drug of choice because it is more active against bowel anaerobes. Endocarditis prophylaxis commonly includes amoxicillin, cephalexin, azithromycin, or cefazolin. Many different protocols are used, depending on the type of surgery.

PROPER USE OF ANTIBIOTICS

It is important to take the antibiotic exactly as prescribed and to follow the label instructions as closely as possible. Certain drugs can be taken with meals or antacids (the latter are often used to counter stomach problems) while other drugs cannot, Thus, meals or antacids can weaken or even abolish their actions. The dosing schedule must be followed exactly. Too frequent dosing can enhance adverse reactions without providing extra benefits, while too infrequent dosing due to skipped doses allows tissue levels of the drug to fall below the effective threshold, thus allowing bacteria to recover and to multiply during these intervals. It is also important to follow the full course of drug therapy and not to stop early when clinical signs have improved or subsided. In this case, the remaining number of subclinical bacteria will be allowed to grow again and become clinically effective. The physician should be notified immediately if certain adverse reactions are noticed (e.g., skin rashes, diarrhea). Early cessation of the drug and use of another drug can then often reverse such adverse effects. Properly followed instructions can reduce or even prevent the occurrence of some adverse reactions and enhance the beneficial effects of these antibacterial drugs.

PREVENTING ANTIBIOTIC RESISTANCE AND SPREAD OF INFECTION

Antibiotic resistance was at one time confined to hospitals, but today it is quite prevalent in the community at large. One of the main reasons for this prevalence, as discussed previously, is related to the unnecessary use of antibiotics. See Box 20-7 for the most commonly prescribed antibiotics. In fact, it is thought that 20 to 50% of all antibiotic prescriptions are unnecessary.[13] To meet this challenge, several groups of physicians and scientists have come together to develop strategies for preventing the spread of infections and antibiotic resistance. One group, in particular, that has been very active in providing information to physicians, particularly those in the community, is the Alliance for the Prudent Use of Antibiotics.[50] One of the recommendations made by this group is "appropriate prescribing." This requires that physicians make use of diagnostic methods to identify the causative bacteria and then prescribe only the selected targeted-spectrum antibiotic. Care should be taken not to prescribe antimicrobials for viral infections, except in the case of people with weakened or suppressed immune systems. In addition, patients should receive appropriate medications such as decongestants, cough medicine, and antipyretics to reduce symptoms; and explanations should be provided regarding why an antibiotic might not be prescribed. The Centers for Disease Control and Prevention (CDC) has developed special prescription pads for patients with cold or flu explaining why antibiotics may not be prescribed.[13]

Strategies to prevent the spread of infection include detailed attention to hygiene before and after seeing a patient with an infection.[47] This includes disinfecting any equipment that comes in contact with the patient,

BOX 20-7 Other Antimicrobial Agents

Aminoglycosides
Amikacin (Amikin)
Gentamicin (Garamycin)
Kanamycin (Kantrrex)
Neomycin (Nebcin)
Streptomycin
Tobramycin (Nebcin)

Fluoroquinolones
Ciprofloxacin (Cipro)
Enoxacin (Penetrex)
Gatifloxacin (Tequin)
Levofloxacin (Levaquin)
Norfloxacin (Noroxin)

Macrolides
Azithromycin (Zithromax)
Clarithromycin (Biaxin)
Dirithromycin (Dynabac)
Erythromycin

Sulfonamides
Sulfadiazine
Sulfamethizole (Thiosulfil Forte)
Sulfamethoxazole (Gantanol)
Sulfisoxazole (Gantrism)

Tetracyclines
Demeclocycline (Declomycin)
Doxycycline (Vibramycin)
Minocycline (Minocin)
Oxytetracycline (Terramycin)
Tetracycline

Miscellaneous Antibiotics
Clindamycin (Cleocin)
Dapsone
Linezolid (Zyvox)
Metronidazole (Flagyl)
Quinupristin/dalfopristin (Synercid)
Spectinomycin (Trobicin)
Daptomycin (Cubicin)

especially if it will be used on another patient. Items left in the hospital room after a patient is discharged, such as the phone and bedside table also need attention. Other strategies are use of only disposable items and storing items away from other patients until the organisms have become nonviable. It is important to understand that nosocomial (hospital-acquired) pathogens can be transmitted not only from wet surfaces but also from dry ones.

One of the most effective ways to prevent infections is washing of hands, which should be done often with soap and for at least 30 seconds. Drying of the hands should be done with paper towels that must be discarded after use.

The widespread use of antibiotics in animals is another important reason for the creation of drug-resistant bacteria. Recently, the FDA is intensifying its efforts—in spite of protests from agricultural groups—to ban nontherapeutic use of antibiotics in healthy livestock for the sole purpose of promoting a more rapid growth. This unnecessary use is thought to contribute significantly to the emergence of drug-resistant bacteria.

ADVERSE EFFECTS OF ANTIBIOTICS AND THERAPEUTIC CONCERNS

The most common adverse effects of antimicrobial treatment are allergic reactions and GI problems such as nausea, vomiting, diarrhea, and abdominal discomfort. These symptoms are often minimized when the drug is taken with food, but some antibiotics will have reduced absorption if taken at mealtime. Other adverse effects include ototoxicity and nephrotoxicity if the drug is administered for long periods. In addition, tetracyclines, sulfonamides, and the fluoroquinolones all increase the patient's sensitivity to ultraviolet (UV) light. Nearly all the antibiotics can cause C. *difficile* enteritis.

Therapists must take extreme precautions when treating patients who are receiving metronidazole, vancomycin, linezolid, or quinupristin/dalfopristin. Administration of these drugs usually means that the patient has a resistant type of infection. Protection by means of mask, gown, and glove is often necessary, but this depends on the type of organism and whether the infection is spread by respiratory droplets or contact with infected bodily secretions.[23] Strict adherence to infection control measures, especially hand washing, is imperative, and any equipment that has been in contact with the infected patient, such as walkers and weights, must be disinfected. Therapists should also be aware of the psychological stress induced by isolation and refer the patient to the appropriate health care provider.[51]

ACTIVITIES 20

1. Briefly discuss one topical agent used for the treatment or prevention of wound infection commonly seen in a rehabilitative practice. Discuss the type of organism against which the drug is active, how the drug is administered, and any adverse effects that may occur. Also, if possible, report on any personal experience you have had with the drug and your thoughts on its effectiveness.
2. Discuss how therapists can help stop the spread of infection. What infection control strategies have been used in clinics with which you have been affiliated. Do you think physical therapists do enough to protect themselves and their patients against infections?
3. Search the literature for information regarding what clinical signs a patient should demonstrate before receiving a prescription for an antibiotic.
4. Visit the Web site of the Alliance for the Prudent Use of Antibiotics (http://www.apua.org). Review and discuss strategies for preventing infection after surgical procedures.

5. You are treating a patient who has been admitted in a nursing home following a recent thrombic stroke. The patient has a history of hypertension and painful osteoarthritis. The patient recently developed an upper respiratory tract infection and now is showing signs of pneumonia and was immediately placed on an extended-spectrum penicillin (piperacillin). What precautions should you take when treating this patient, and what lab values should be monitored?
6. Why is it important to follow exactly the instructions given by the physician or provided by the package insert when using antimicrobials?
7. What foods may help prevent superinfections such as vaginal yeast infections?

REFERENCES

1. Rang HP, Dale MM, Ritter JM, Moore JL, editors: Pharmacology (5th ed.), New York, 2003, Churchill Livingstone.
2. Livermore DM: The threat from the pink corner. Ann Med 35(4):226-234, 2003.
3. Infectious diseases. In Braunwald E, Fauci AS, Kasper DL, Hauser SL, Longo DL, Jameson JL, editors: Harrison's manual of medicine (15th ed.), New York, 2002, McGraw-Hill.
4. Poole K: Multidrug resistance in gram-negative bacteria. Curr Opin Microbiol 4:500-508, 2001.
5. Thielman NM, Neu HC: Principles of antimicrobial use. In Brody MJ, Larner J, Minneman KP, editors: Human pharmacology: Molecular to clinical, (3rd ed.), Philadelphia, 1998, Mosby.
6. Pankey GA, Sabath LD: Clinical relevance of bacteriostatic versus bactericidal mechanisms of action in the treatment of gram-positive bacterial infections. Clin Infect Dis 38(6): 864-870, 2004.
7. Shafran SD: Drugs and bacteria. In Page C, Curtis MJ, Sutter MC, Walker MJ, Hoffman BB, editors: Integrated pharmacology (2nd ed.), Philadelphia, 2002, Mosby.
8. Tan YT, Tillett DJ, McKay IA: Molecular strategies for overcoming antibiotic resistance in bacteria. Mol Med Today 6:309-314, 2000.
9. Amyes SG: Resistance to beta-lactams—the permutations. J Chemother 15(6):525-535, 2003.
10. Markham PN, Neyfakh AA: Efflux-mediated drug resistance in gram-positive bacteria. Curr Opin Microbiol 4:509-514, 2001.
11. Levy SB: Antimicrobial resistance: Bacteria on the defence. Br Med J 317:612-613, 1998.
12. Huovinen P, Cars O: Control of antimicrobial resistance: Time for action. Br Med J 317:613-614, 1998.
13. Hooton TM, Levy SB: Antimicrobial resistance: A plan of action for community practice. Am Fam Physician 63(6): 1087-1096, 2001.
14. Thielman NM, Neu HC: Bacterial cell wall inhibitors. In Brody MJ, Larner J, Minneman KP, editors: Human pharmacology: Molecular to clinical. Philadelphia, 1998, Mosby.
15. Klein JO: Amoxicillin/clavulanate for infections in infants and children: Past, present and future. Pediatr Infect Dis J 22 (suppl 8):S139-S148, 2003.
16. Augmentin XR. Med Lett Drugs Ther 45(1148):5-6, 2003.
17. White AR, Kaye C, Poupard J, Pypstra R, Woodnutt G, Wynne B: Augmentin (amoxicillin/clavulanate) in the treatment of community-acquired respiratory tract infection: A review of the continuing development of an innovative antimicrobial agent. J Antimicrob Chemother 53(suppl 1):13-20, 2004.
18. Cefditoren (Spectracef)—A new oral cephalosporin. Med Lett Drugs Ther 44(1122):5-6, 2002.
19. Leviton I: Separating fact from fiction: The data behind allergies and side effects caused by penicillins, cephalosporins, and carbapenem antibiotics. Curr Pharm Des 9(12):983-988, 2003.
20. Ertapenem (Invanz)—A new parenteral carbapenem. Med Lett Drugs Ther 44(1126):25-26, 2002.
21. Apisarnthanarak A, Razavi B, Mundy LM: Adjunctive intracolonic vancomycin for severe Clostridium difficile colitis: Case series and review of the literature. Clin Infect Dis 35:690-696, 2002.
22. Kikuchi K, Genetic basis of neonatal methicillin-resistant Staphylococcus aureus in Japan. Pediatr Int 45(2):223-229, 2003.
23. Slaughter S, Hayden MK, Nathan C, et al: A comparison of the effect of universal use of gloves and gowns with that of glove use alone on acquisition of vancomycin-resistant enterococci in a medical intensive care unit. Ann Intern Med 125(6):448-456, 1996.
24. Dunbar LM: Current issues in the management of bacterial respiratory tract disease: The challenge of antibacterial resistance. Am J Med Sci 326(6):360-368, 2003.
25. Brown J, Freeman BB: Combining quinupristin/dalfopristin with other agents for resistant infections. Ann Pharmacother 38(4):677-685, 2004.
26. Diekema DJ, Jones RN: Oxazolidinone antibiotics. Lancet 358:1975-1982, 2001.
27. Linezolid (Zyvox). Med Lett Drugs Ther 42(1079):45-46, 2000.
28. Ament PW, Jamshed N, Horne JP: Linezolid: Its role in the treatment of gram-positive, drug-resistant bacterial infections. Am Fam Physician 65(4):663-670, 2002.
29. Alberts B, Bray D, Lewis J, Raff M, Roberts K, Watson JD: Molecular biology of the cell, New York, 1989, Garland Publishing, Inc.
30. Post-exposure anthrax prophylaxis. Med Lett Drugs Ther 43(1116-1117):91-92, 2001.
31. Greene BL: Physical therapist management of fluoroquinolone-induced Achilles tendinopathy. Phys Ther 82(12):1224-1231, 2002.
32. van der Linden PD, Sturkenboom MC, Herings RM, Leufkens HG, Stricker BH: Fluoroquinolones and risk of Achilles tendon disorders: case-control study. Br Med J 324(7349): 1306-1307, 2002.
33. Gatifloxacin and moxifloxacin: Two new fluoroquinolones. Med Lett Drugs Ther 42(1072):15-17, 2000.
34. Edwards R, Harding KG: Bacteria and wound healing. Curr Opin Infect Dis 17(2):91-96, 2004.
35. Dye C, Scheele S, Dolin P, Patharia V, Raviglione MC: Consensus statement. Global burden of tuberculosis: Estimated incidence, prevalence, and mortality by country. JAMA 282:677-686, 1999.
36. de Jong BC, Israelski DM, Corbett EL, Small PM: Clinical management of tuberculosis in the context of HIV infection. Annu Rev Med 55:283-301, 2004.
37. Stewart GR, Robertson BD, Young DB: Tuberculosis: A problem with persistence. Nat Rev Microbiol 1:97-105, 2003.
38. Cosma CL, Sherman DR, Ramakrishnan L, The secret lives of the pathogenic mycobacteria. Annu Rev Microbiol 57: 641-676, 2003.
39. Chan J, Flynn J: The immunological aspects of latency in tuberculosis. Clin Immunol 110:2-12, 2004.
40. Paolo W, Nosanchuk JD: Tuberculosis in New York City: Recent lessons and a look ahead. Lancet 4:287-293, 2004.
41. Enarson DA: Use of the tuberculin skin test in children. Paediatr Respir Rev 5(suppl A):S135-S137, 2004.
42. Cohn DL: Treatment of latent tuberculosis infection. Semin Respir Infect 18(4):249-262, 2003.
43. Mukherjee JS, Rich ML, Socci AR, et al: Programmes and principles in treatment of multidrug-resistant tuberculosis. Lancet 363:474-481, 2004.

44. Mylonakis E, Ryan E, Calderwood SB: Clostridium difficile-associated diarrhea. Arch Intern Med 161:525-533, 2001.
45. Safdar N, Maki D: The commonality of risk factors for nosocomial colonization and infection with antimicrobial-resistant Staphylococcus aureus, Enterococcus, gram-negative bacilli, Clostridium difficile and Candida. Ann Intern Med 136: 834-844, 2002.
46. The choice of antibacterial drugs. Med Lett Drugs Ther 43(1111-1112):69-78, 2001.
47. Dietze B, Rath A, Wendt C, Martiny H: Survival of MRSA on sterile goods packaging. J Hosp Infect 49:255-261, 2001.
48. Thibodeau KP, Viera AJ: Atypical pathogens and challenges in community-acquired pneumonia. Am Fam Physician 69: 1699-1706, 2004.
49. Antimicrobial prophylaxis for surgery. Treat Guidel Med Lett 2(20):27-32, 2004.
50. Alliance for the Prudent Use of Antibiotics (website). http://www.apua.org. Accessed March 30, 2005.
51. Tarzi S, Kennedy P, Stone S, Evans M: Methicillin-resistant Staphylococcus aureus: Psychological impact of hospitalization and isolation in an older adult population. J Hosp Infect 49:250-254, 2001.

21

Antiviral Agents and Selected Drugs for Fungal Infections

Barbara Gladson and Wolfgang Vogel

TREATMENT OF VIRAL INFECTIONS

Viruses represent one of the smallest classes of microorganisms. Unlike bacteria, they can only replicate in the cells of their hosts. They can enter the body through the respiratory tract, gastrointestinal (GI) tract, or the skin or mucous membranes; and they can cross the placenta. Viruses may be transferred through the skin as a result of sharing of syringes, sexual contact, blood transfusions, or animal bites.

Virus Structure and Function

Viruses are extremely small parasites that consist of nucleic acids—ribonucleic acid (RNA) and deoxyribonucleic acid (DNA)—contained in a protein shell or capsid.[1] The protein shell plus the nucleic acid is called the *nucleocapsid*. In some viruses, the nucleocapsid is encased in a lipoprotein envelope. This entire structure is then called a *virion* (Figure 21-1). Some viruses also contain enzymes necessary to initiate replication in the host cell; however, for the most part, they use the host enzyme systems.

One of the most common viruses belongs to the Influenza family with Influenza A and B causing most of the human infections. Influenza A viruses are distinguished according to a set of proteins, hemagglutinin (H) and neuraminidase (N) proteins, of which there are 16H and 9N subtypes[2] (Figure 21-2). The genes for these proteins "mix and match," often creating new virus particles with tremendous antigenic variability. Specific mutations in the *H* gene can produce a new strain, and this is why a new flu vaccine must be engineered every year. Cross-species transmission of new H and N strains also occurs and was responsible for the H5N1 avian virus and the more recent "swine flu" virus. In the early 2000s, H3N1 appeared to be the most prevalent, but in 2009, the H1N1 (virus that causes swine flu) has clearly gained major attention. (See Treatment for the Flu, later in this chapter.)

Viral Entry and Uncoating

When a virion reaches a possible host cell, it attaches itself to the surface and prepares to deliver its capsid and enzymes in a form that favors replication.[3] The virion is extremely skilled at entering the host cell with minimal detection. The receptors on the host can be cytokines, neurotransmitters, hormones, ion channels, or membrane glycoproteins. Some host cell structures that are used as receptors include the CD4 glycoprotein on helper T lymphocytes for the human immunodeficiency virus (HIV), the acetylcholine receptor at the neuromuscular junction for the rabies virus, and major histocompatibility complexes for adenoviruses that produce a sore throat. The virion is aided by certain attachment factors and viral surface glycoproteins, which determine the cell types and tissues a virus can invade.

Many viruses depend on endocytosis to enter the host cell, including the adenovirus and the influenza virus.[3] One of the advantages to this method of entry is that the endocytic vesicles can cross the cytoskeleton and cytoplasm of the host cell. Another advantage is that the virus is exposed to an acidic environment in the endosome, which provides a trigger for the uncoating of the protein shell. Other viruses, especially those with a lipoprotein envelope, enter the cell by fusion and penetration.[3] Fusion proteins exist in the viral envelope and are triggered by receptor binding or low pH. Nonenveloped viruses penetrate the cell either by lysing part of the host membrane or by creating a channel or pore-like structure.

After the virus penetrates the host cell and has shed the coat, the nucleic acids must be transported to either the nucleus (for DNA viruses) or to specific cytosolic membranes.[3] At this point, endocytic vesicles can ferry the virus to the appropriate target, or the capsid itself can take advantage of certain motors within the cytoplasm, such as actin filaments. Actin has been found to pull virus-containing vesicles through the cytoplasm. Entering the nucleus represents the next challenge for the capsid, which must traverse through a nuclear pore to

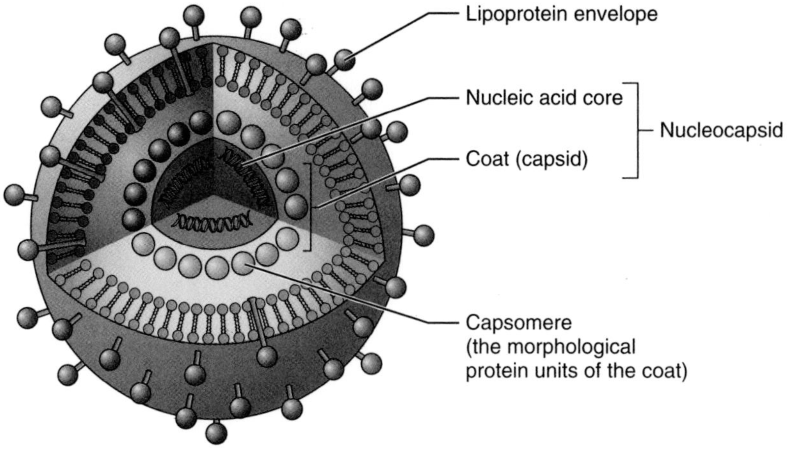

FIGURE 21-1 Schematic diagram of the components of a virus particle or virion. *(Adapted from Rang HP, Dale MM, Ritter JM, Moore JL, editors:* Pharmacology *(5th ed.). New York, 2003, Churchill Livingstone).*

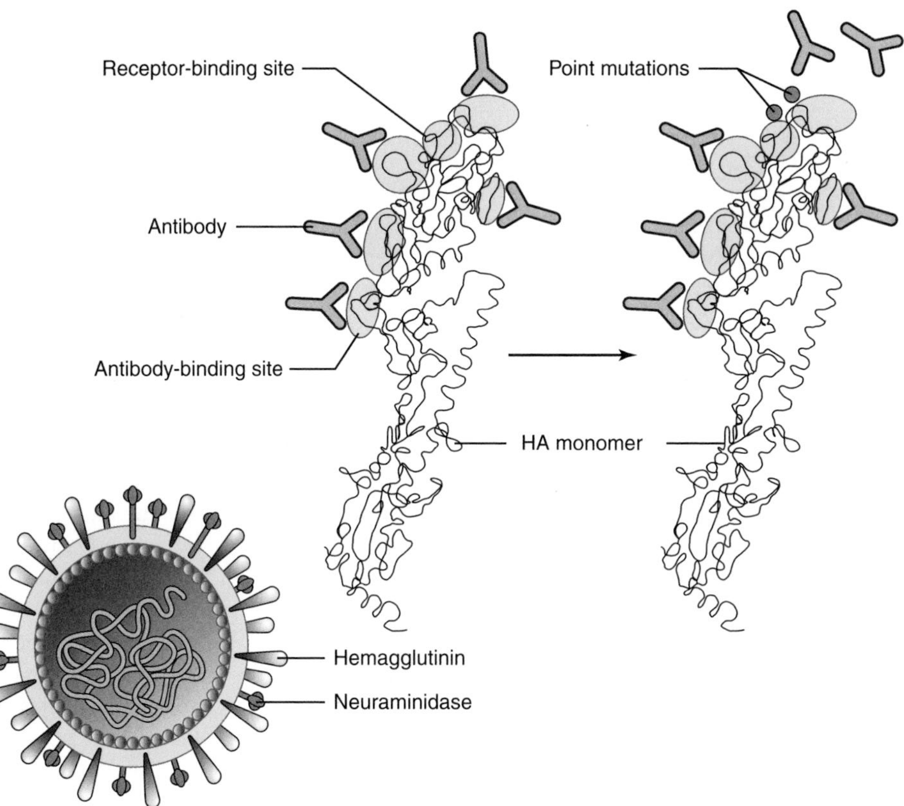

FIGURE 21-2 Viruses develop mutations in the genes that code for the formation of hemagglutinin (H) and neuraminidase (N) proteins. When these point mutations give rise to a new influenza strain it is called when the virus obtains a completely new H or N gene such as when the H3N2 virus mutated to the H1N1 virus. *Drawing in the text was adapted from N Engl J Med 2004; 350:218.*

reach the host's supply of DNA and RNA polymerases, as well as splice and modify the enzymes necessary for viral reproduction. Infection can also be transmitted directly from cell to cell with or without virus infection. Viruses, such as the measles virus, can often induce the fusion of infected cells with uninfected cells and pass the viral genes directly from cell to cell.

This simplified discussion highlights the mechanisms involved in viral entry into a cell. This is a complex multistep process involving many host and viral proteins that presumably can act as targets for antiviral agents. In the past, drug therapy was focused primarily on blocking viral replication. However, new drugs that target the entry and uncoating processes have been developed, specifically, an inhibitor against the influenza virus and an inhibitor against the fusion protein used by HIV-1.

Viral Replication. DNA viruses enter the host cell nucleus, and its DNA provides the directions for creation of a new virus. Transcription of the viral DNA into messenger RNA (mRNA) is carried out by the host cell RNA polymerase.[4] Translation of the mRNA into virus-specific proteins occurs next. Some of these proteins are then used to make the protein shell and envelope, and others are used to synthesize more viral DNA.

RNA viruses replicate in different ways. They must copy RNA molecules first by encoding their own RNA-dependent polymerase enzymes. The virus's RNA can then serve as its own mRNA, or the enzymes in the virion can synthesize its mRNA. Retroviruses are RNA viruses that were first known as *RNA tumor viruses* because infection leads to a permanent genetic change, making the cell cancerous.[4] They reverse the normal process in which DNA is transcribed into RNA. They contain a reverse-transcriptase enzyme (virus RNA–dependent DNA polymerase), which makes a DNA copy of the single-stranded viral RNA. This forms a DNA–RNA hybrid, which is then transcribed by the same enzyme into a double helix with two DNA strands. This DNA copy then integrates into a host cell chromosome. Large numbers of new viral RNA molecules are then constructed by the host cell RNA polymerase.

After synthesis of either viral DNA or viral RNA and the structural proteins, assembly of the coat proteins around the viral genome occurs, and the virion is ready to be released.[1] The mechanism of release may be budding or host cell lyses. The new viral particles are then free to infect other host cells. Examples of retroviruses include HIV and T-cell leukemia virus.

Host Warfare Against Viruses and Viral Defenses. The host cell launches a rather sophisticated campaign against an invading virus. There are a variety of innate and adaptive immune responses to viruses.[5] Innate immunity acts as the body's first line of defense and includes the skin and its mucosal barriers and a nonspecific inflammatory response. The nonspecific response involves the phagocytes (leukocytes), cytokines (interferons [IFNs] and tumor necrosis factor-α [TNF-α]), and natural killer (NK) cells. The IFNs are especially important, acting as messengers both within the immune system and between the immune system and other parts of the body, signaling invasion. In addition, IFNs have an important defense role against viruses. They are produced by virus-infected cells and act to interrupt the viral life cycle at many steps. They also coat the surrounding cells to make them more virus-resistant and upregulate major histocompatibility complex expression to target infected cells. The specific IFNs involved include interferon IFN-α and IFN-β, which become potent inducers of NK cell–mediated cytotoxicity.[6] NK cells, which are specialized lymphocytes, recognize virally infected cells and launch a direct attack, killing the organism by releasing lytic proteins on the infected cell, triggering the apoptotic pathway, and releasing cytokines.

In the adaptive immune response, the key cells are the lymphocytes: B cells, which produce antibodies; T cells, which are essential for the induction phase of the cell-mediated immune reaction; and cytotoxic T cells (derived from CD8 cells) (Figure 21-3). During the induction phase, the antigen is presented to the T lymphocytes on the surface of antigen presenting cells. At this point, the T cell becomes activated, meaning that it can now recognize the antigen. The T cell develops interleukin 2 (IL-2) receptors and also generates this IL. The T cells also give rise to two different subsets of helper cells, Th1 and Th2 cells. Each type of helper cell produces its own ILs. The Th2 cells produce cytokines, which stimulate B cells to proliferate and mature into plasma cells that produce antibodies. The effector phase is the antibody-mediated phase, in which the antibody recognizes the specific antigen and then activates several of the host's defense systems. Antiviral antibodies are observed late in most infections and are thought to be responsible for prevention of cell-to-cell spread. The additional host resources are reinforcement of the cell-mediated reactions and include CD8 cytotoxic T cells, which kill virus-infected cells; cytokine-releasing CD4 T cells, which stimulate macrophage killing; and memory cells, which are produced so that cells are ready to react more rapidly the next time the antigen invades.

Viruses use a variety of methods to overcome the host's immune reactions.[7] Viruses can limit the action of some cytokines by expressing a receptor on their cell surfaces to match the cytokine. These act as pseudoreceptors that bind cytokines, preventing them from reaching their real receptors. Another ploy is to express a major histocompatibility complex that NK cells are unable to recognize. Still another method is the production of viral proteins that interfere with apoptosis or programmed cell death.[8]

Antiviral Vaccines and Drugs

Viruses, for the most part, are difficult to eradicate for several reasons.[9] First, replication of the virus generally reaches its peak (host contains a large viral load) before any clinical symptoms appear. Second, the available antiviral drugs are virustatic as opposed to virucidal and depend on a normal host immune system for final viral destruction and a cure. A diseased host immune system will lead to impaired recovery and a prolonged and more severe illness. Third, drugs will usually never completely eradicate some of the viruses, since they can retreat into areas where they are protected from the immune system or can change in such a way to escape the detection of the immune system.[10] Here they can survive without clinical signs for long periods just to emerge again at later times. Shingles is a case in point, where the virus that produces chicken pox surfaces after many years of dormancy. Fourth, viruses using the host-cell metabolic processes present fewer specific viral target sites that can be selectively attacked by antiviral drugs. Thus, many of the drugs can also affect host cell metabolism and show more adverse reactions. Fifth, in vitro susceptibility testing for viruses is less predictive than testing sensitivity to antimicrobials. Finally, viruses like bacteria will develop drug resistance and render antiviral drugs slowly ineffective.

Vaccines. Vaccines are viral preparations that do not hurt the recipient but will stimulate the immune system so that it is prepared to more effectively fight infection of a particular virus later on. The term *vaccine* was derived from the latin term for cow (vacca) when it was discovered that administration of cow pox to humans could protect them later against smallpox. Today, viral vaccines basically contain either the killed or weakened

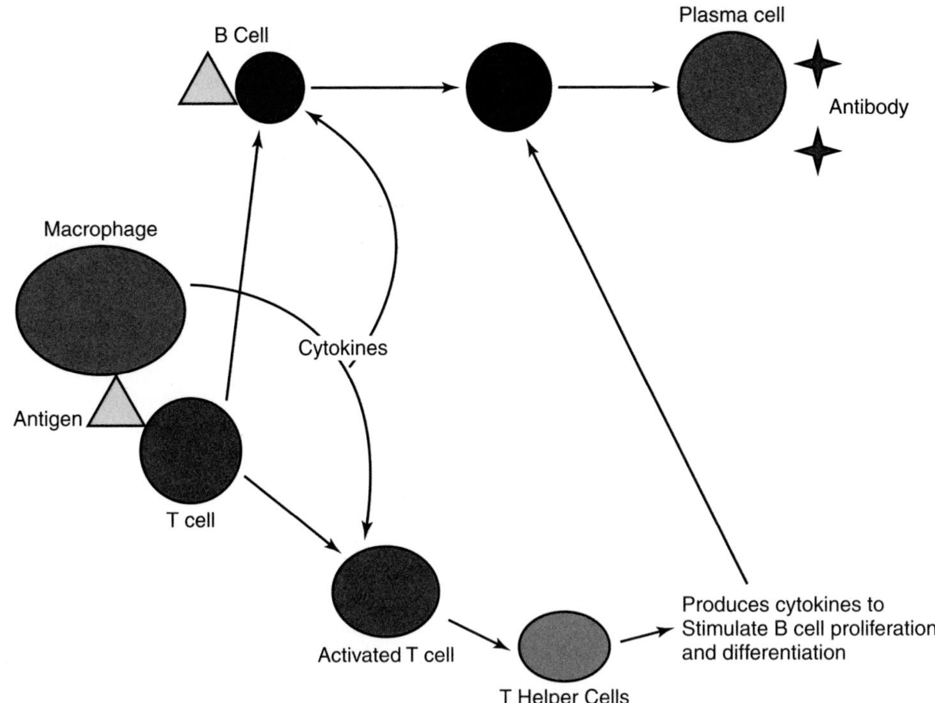

FIGURE 21-3 Simplified diagram of the induction and effector phases of lymphocyte activation, with the sites of action of immunosuppressants. Antigen-presenting cells (APC) ingest and process antigen (•) and present fragments of it (•) to naïve, uncommitted CD4 T cells in conjunction with major histocompatibility complex (MHC) class II molecules and to naïve CD8 T cells in conjunction with MHC class I molecules (-1), arming them. The armed CD4 T cells synthesize and express interleukin (IL)-2 receptors and release IL-2, which stimulates the cells by autocrine action, causing generation and proliferation of T helper zero (Th0) cells. Autocrine cytokines (e.g., IL-4) cause proliferation of some Th0 cells to produce Th2 cells, which are responsible for the development of antibody-mediated immune responses. These Th2 cells cooperate with and activate B cells to proliferate and eventually give rise to memory B cells (MB) and plasma cells (P), which secrete antibodies. Autocrine cytokines (e.g., IL-2) cause proliferation of some Th0 cells to produce Th1 cells, which secrete cytokines that activate macrophages (responsible for some cell-mediated immune reactions). The armed CD8 T cells also synthesize and express IL-2 receptors and release IL-2, which stimulates the cells by autocrine action to proliferate and give rise to cytotoxic T cells. These can kill virally infected cells. IL-2 secreted by CD4+ cells also plays a part in stimulating CD8+ cells to proliferate. Note that the "effector phase" depicted here relates to the "protective" deployment of the immune response. When the response is inappropriately deployed—as in chronic inflammatory conditions such as rheumatoid arthritis—the Th1 wing of the immune response is dominant, and the activated microphages (mα) release IL-1 and tumor necrosis factor-α (TNF- α), which, in turn, triggers the release of the various chemokines and inflammatory cytokines that have a major role in the pathogenesis of the disease. *(From Rang HP, Dale MM, Ritter JM, Moore JL, editors:* Pharmacology *(5th ed.). New York, 2003, Churchill Livingstone).*

(attenuated) viruses that still posses their specific antigenic sites and that can prime the immune system of the recipient without causing the disease. They are only effective prophylactically and are given alone or in combination. The problem is that a viral vaccine is relatively specific for one virus, while other viruses even of the same family causing the same disease will not be affected. The flu vaccine of 2009 contains only three of the most suspected viruses to cause the flu, while other flu viruses will not be affected and can still cause the disease. Vaccines have eradicated many dreadful viral diseases such as polio or have protected individuals from being infected with certain viruses such as the flu virus. They are relatively harmless with only very few individuals experiencing serious adverse reactions when proper precautions are taken, such as not giving the vaccines to individuals with egg sensitivities (because viruses are grown in an egg medium and vaccines can contain small amounts of their proteins). In spite of some opposition, medical professionals overwhelmingly feel that the benefits of vaccinations outweigh the risks by a large margin.

Antiviral drugs. Several sites that act as targets for drug action within the viral reproductive cycle are currently available (Figure 21-4).[9] Some drugs inhibit the uncoating of the virus, which is necessary to unleash the genome into the host cell. Other drugs block RNA and DNA replication as well as the production of viral proteins by inhibiting transcription and translation. Other drugs inhibit special proteases that cut newly synthesized proteins into such a length as needed for viral assembly. Some fairly new compounds on the market prevent the release and budding of new virions.

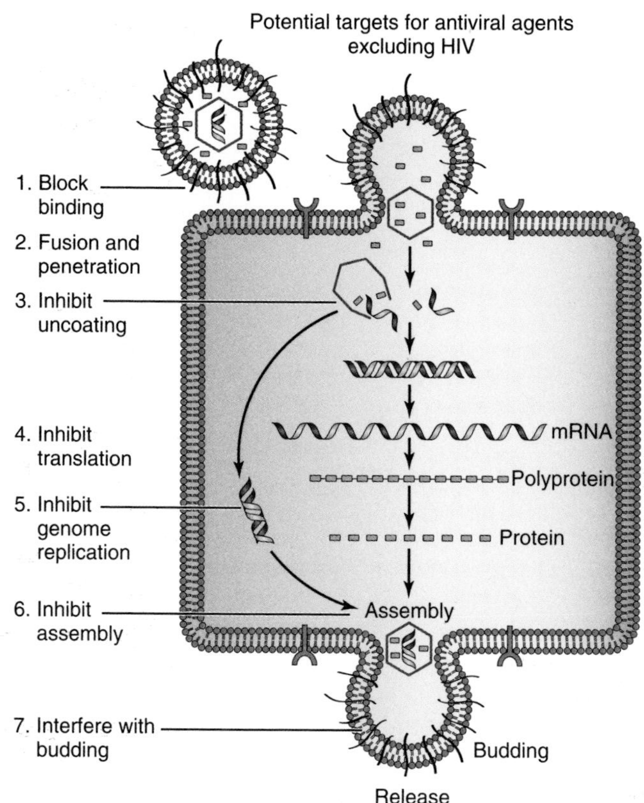

FIGURE 21-4 Targets for anti-viral drug action

Antiviral Agents That Inhibit Uncoating. Amantadine (Symadine), approved for the prevention of influenza A, and rimantadine (Flumadine) inhibit uncoating of the virus by blocking the hydrogen (H^+) channel, which would normally acidify the inside of the virion.[9] Acidification of the virion is necessary for uncoating. Both drugs are used to treat the influenza A virus but have no effect on influenza B and C viruses. Treatment must be initiated within 2 days of the start of illness to be 10 to 27% effective, but it may take at least 4 to 5 more days for the host to shed the virus. In the healthy individual, these drugs decrease flu duration by 1 day, and in the high-risk older patient, by 2.5 days.[11] Although a reduction in duration of 1 to 2.5 days does not seem very impressive, for the high-risk unvaccinated patient, these drugs could make a difference in overall morbidity and could significantly shorten hospital stay. The two drugs are equally effective in the treatment of flu and previously exhibited a 70% prophylactic efficacy in unvaccinated patients.[12] However, they are less effective in immunocompromised patients and may even produce resistant viral strains. Since the year 2000, the amount of adamantane-resistant viruses has grown to such an extent that during the 2004–2005 flu season, the majority of cases of H3N2 viruses from the United States and Canada were resistant.[13]

Adverse effects of amantadine and rimantadine are dose related.[14] Amantadine produces some mild reversible central nervous system (CNS) effects such as dizziness, insomnia, orthostatic hypotension, and slurred speech but can also produce livedo reticularis (a lace-like purplish discoloration of the lower extremities) caused by swelling of the small veins (venules) in the skin, which makes them more visible in older patients. This drug also enhances release of dopamine so it has a dopaminergic effect on the CNS and the cardiovascular system. Rimantadine is better tolerated, producing only some GI complaints.

Inhibitors of Viral Transcription. Interferons (IFNs) are the antiviral drugs that prevent transcription.[9] There are three classes of interferons—α, β, and γ—but only IFN-α and IFN-β are primary antiviral agents. Their mechanism of action is rather complex, but essentially they bind to cell surface receptors that activate Janus-activated kinases, further activating signal transducers and transcription to produce proteins that enhance cellular resistance to viruses. IFNs inhibit virus entry into cells, uncoating, and especially transcription of different viruses by inducing ribosomal enzymes that inhibit viral mRNA.

IFN-α_{2a} is useful against chronic hepatitis B virus (HBV), hepatitis C virus (HCV), Kaposi's sarcoma caused by human herpes virus,[9] and skin conditions associated with human papilloma virus (HPV).[14] IFN-α_{2b} (is also effective against HPV, HBV, and HCV. Commercial preparations of IFN-α are produced by recombinant DNA techniques. They are not orally bioavailable and must be administered either by intramuscular or subcutaneous injection or intravenously. For chronic HBV and HCV, subcutaneous injections three times a week for 48 weeks are recommended.

Adverse effects of IFNs include a flu-like syndrome, probably caused by the synthesis of IL-1.[9] Symptoms will lessen in severity after several weeks of treatment. Myelosuppression (neutropenia and thrombocytopenia), as well as some neurotoxic effects (headache, anxiety, and dizziness), may occur. However, fatigue is quite common and may be profound enough to interfere with rehabilitation. Autoimmune responses, primarily the development of autoantibodies against the thyroid gland and anti–double-stranded DNA, have also been reported with this therapy.[15] Clinical manifestations may include systemic lupus erythematosus (SLE) and thyroid disease. Depression is also a significant adverse effect of the IFNs.

Ribavirin is a guanosine analog that interferes with viral transcription by preventing elongation of mRNA.[16] Its mechanism of action is similar to that of acyclovir (see discussion of drugs that inhibit viral RNA or DNA replication) in that it acts as a chain terminator. It has been used as an aerosol to decrease morbidity in children with respiratory syncytial virus, bronchiolitis, and pneumonia. Oral ribavirin has been used as part of a combination treatment along with IFN-α (2a and 2b) for hepatitis C (hepatitis C virus). It directly inhibits HCV replication and reduces fatigue and hepatic inflammation. There is a high degree of synergistic action when ribavirin is given along with an interferon (Rebetron).

It is thought that ribavirin produces a mutation in the virus that makes it more susceptible to interferons.[2,17]

Intravenous (IV) ribavirin decreases mortality among patients with Lassa fever and hemorrhagic fever associated with hantavirus. In addition, it is also active against West Nile virus.[18] Because ribavirin accumulates in erythrocytes and produces hemolysis, one of the adverse effects is hemolytic anemia or disintegration of red blood cells. The drug is also carcinogenic and teratogenic in animals.

Drugs that Inhibit Viral RNA or DNA Replication (Chain Terminators). The prototypical drug that inhibits viral RNA or DNA replication is acyclovir (Zovirax). This drug undergoes intracellular phosphorylation to the active form, acyclovir triphosphate, by using first a virus-specific thymidine kinase and then subsequently host enzymes (Figure 21-5). Next, the active drug competes with deoxyguanosine triphosphate for the viral DNA polymerase. The drug becomes incorporated into the growing viral DNA chain, but because it is not a true nucleic acid (lacks a phosphodiester linkage for the next nucleic acid), chain termination occurs (Figure 21-6). Acyclovir and other drugs in this category, valacyclovir (Valtrex), penciclovir (Denavir), ganciclovir (Cytovene), and cidofovir(Vistide), are used to inhibit replication of herpes simplex virus (HSV-1 and HSV-2), varicella zoster virus (VZV), cytomegalovirus (CMV), and the Epstein-Barr virus (EBV).[14] They are somewhat effective against clinical infections but offer no immunity against latent infections. They all have slightly different sensitivities for different viruses; ganciclovir is more effective than acyclovir against CMV, and valacyclovir is more effective than acyclovir for the treatment of herpes. Valacyclovir is a prodrug of acyclovir with greater bioavailability, which allows a more convenient dosing schedule. For a genital herpes infection, this drug may be given two times a day for 5 days, instead of the more frequent dosing schedule required for acyclovir. It is also approved for once-a-day dosing to suppress frequently recurring herpes infections.

Adverse effects of acyclovir include neurotoxicity (lethargy, confusion, tremor, and seizures), but this drug is generally well tolerated. Discontinuation of the drug reverses the adverse effects.

Foscarnet is another drug in this category, but it inhibits viral DNA polymerase and HIV reverse transcriptase directly without undergoing any transformations.[9] It binds to and blocks the binding site for viral polymerase. It is a non-nucleoside herpes virus inhibitor because it does not resemble any of the purines or pyrimidines. Foscarnet is approved for the treatment of CMV retinitis in acquired immune deficiency syndrome (AIDS) and acyclovir-resistant HSV infections. Adverse effects include reversible serious organ toxicity, affecting the urinary tract, the CNS, and the hematologic system.

Drugs That Inhibit Viral Release. Zanamivir (Relenza) and oseltamivir (Tamiflu) inhibit influenza neuraminidase, which is necessary for cleaving the budding virion from its parent cell.[19] They prevent the spread of the virus and protect neighboring cells from being infected. They are equally effective against influenza A and B viruses, reducing the severity of illness by about 25 to 35% when treatment is initiated within 2 days of the onset of symptoms. They also reduce symptom duration by an average of 0.8 days in otherwise healthy adults and by 1 day in children.[20] In patients older than 65 years or in those who have chronic medical conditions, zanamivir reduced the duration of symptoms by 2 days, but

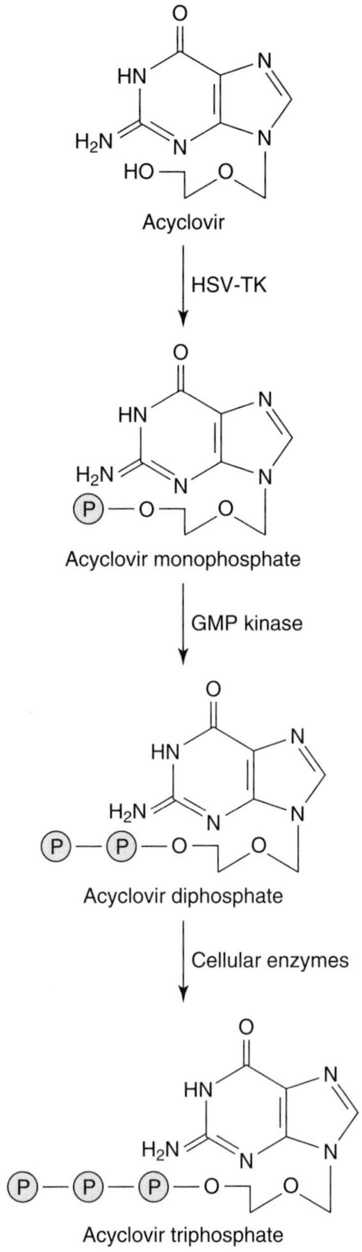

Acyclovir

HSV-TK

Acyclovir monophosphate

GMP kinase

Acyclovir diphosphate

Cellular enzymes

Acyclovir triphosphate

FIGURE 21-5 Enzymatic conversion of acyclovir to its monophosphate, diphosphate, and triphosphate forms. Herpes simplex virus thymidine kinase (HSV-TK) avidly catalyzes the formation of acyclovir monophosphate. Cellular kinases convert the monophosphate to the diphosphate and triphosphate forms. Acyclovir triphosphate is the active antiviral moiety.

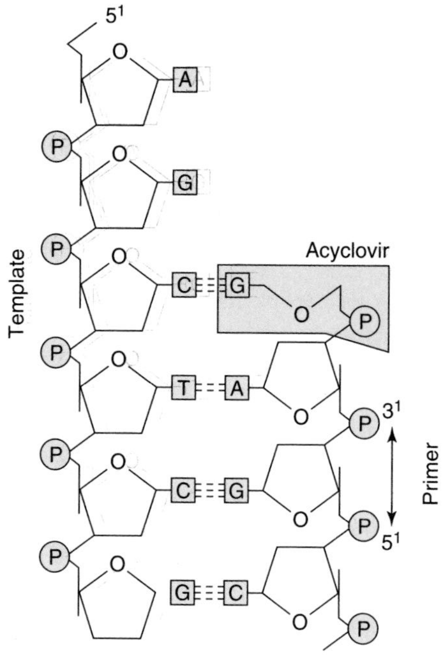

FIGURE 21-6 Representation of acyclovir triphosphate termination of DNA chain elongation. Absence of the 3′-C molecule on the acyclic ribose molecule precludes formation of the 3-5′-phosphodiester linkage needed to allow DNA chain elongation.

oseltamivir only reduced duration by 0.4 day. Postexposure prophylaxis for both drugs is 70 to 90%. Adverse effects include nausea and vomiting, but there have also been a few reports of bronchospasm.

Drug Treatment for the Flu

The seasonal flu is caused by viruses belonging to the large family of influenza viruses with types A, B, and C and their many subtypes. Presently, mostly A and B viruses seem to be responsible for the illness. The flu manifests itself basically as a usually high fever, muscle aches, sore throat, chills, tiredness, and headaches. The flu can be mild to severe, and older individuals with other diseases such as asthma, diabetes, and cardiac problems are at high risk of dying. The U.S. Center for Disease Control and Prevention (CDC) reported, as of November 7, 2009, 22,364 laboratory-confirmed influenza-associated hospitalizations and 877 laboratory-confirmed influenza-associated deaths for 2009.[20]

Often, lay people confuse the flu with the common cold, since many of the clinical signs are the same or similar. However, the two conditions are different; the common cold is caused by different viruses, such as the rhinoviruses or coronaviruses. There is no cure for the common cold and no antiviral drug therapy exists for a cure at this time.

Currently, treatment of the seasonal flu primarily is the use of zanamivir and oseltamivir, since prevalent viruses are now becoming resistant to amantadine and rimantadine.[21]

Swine flu is a special type of flu. The H1N1 virus that causes it is now the predominant flu strain worldwide, although it shows no signs of becoming more virulent and continues to produce mild-to-moderate symptoms in most people according to the CDC.[22] It is caused by a swine influenza virus (SIV) of the influenza family of viruses that is endemic in pigs but is mostly transferred from human to human. As of 2009, the known SIV strains include influenza C and the subtypes of influenza A known as H1N1, H1N2, H3N1, H3N2, and H2N3 (International Committee on Taxonomy of Viruses).[23] The symptoms of swine flu are similar to those of a typical flu except that nausea and vomiting might be more prevalent and only laboratory tests can definitively identify the presence of swine flu. Children, teenagers, and only older people with pre-existing illnesses such as chronic pulmonary problems, immunosuppression, or diabetes mellitus are at highest risk of contracting swine flu. Healthy older individuals show some resistance to the virus and so are much less at risk. These viruses respond to zanamivir and oseltamivir, and only in severe cases or emergencies is the use of a new drug called peramavir indicated. This drug interacts with influenza neuramidase and achieves higher and more effective tissue levels, since it is administered intravenously. These flu viruses are mostly resistant to amantadine and rimantidine.

The best way to prevent all types of flu is by getting vaccinated and washing hands frequently and thoroughly with soap.

Drug Treatment for Human Immunodeficiency Virus

HIV is a retrovirus that selectively targets the immune system, particularly the CD4+ T lymphocytes, severely compromising an individual's ability to prevent infection or certain types of cancer. There is currently no cure for this infection, but some drugs can reduce the viral load, giving the immune system a chance to recover function. Without treatment, most patients will die within 2 years after the onset of symptoms.[1] HIV infection is a global health problem, with at least 30 million people worldwide testing positive for HIV and with epidemic proportions, particularly in sub-Saharan Africa.[24] As of 2005, more than 40.3 million people have been found to be living with HIV, with over 3.1 million deaths reported in that year alone.[25] Although drugs are available, they do not reach everyone who needs them. Hence, the infection continues to spread.

Pathophysiology. Two distinct viruses, HIV-1 and HIV-2, actually produce AIDS. HIV-1 is responsible for most of the infections worldwide, but in West Africa, HIV-2 is predominant. The routes of transmission of the two viruses are the same: exchange of bodily fluids through sexual contact, sharing of syringes, exposure to infected blood, and vertical transmission from mother to fetus in utero and from mother to neonate during delivery and through breast milk.

Once infected, a patient may remain free of symptoms for a long time. Initially, the cytotoxic T lymphocytes are recruited to prevent the spread of HIV, mainly by killing HIV-infected cells. However, a depletion of noninfected T cells occurs as well.[26] Sources of T-cell production also fail, but the exact cause is not known. The virus continues to multiply, producing 1010 new particles each day, and many of these particles mutate to a slightly different form. The immune system tries to keep up with the viral load, but eventually the mutated virus escapes detection, the CD4 cell count decreases, and the immune system fails.

Disease Progression and Clinical Signs and Symptoms. There is much variation in the progression and clinical manifestations of AIDS. After exposure to the virus, an initial acute flu-like illness develops, resulting from the increase in HIV particles in the blood and the formation of antibodies.[27] This phase is known as *primary HIV infection* (Figure 21-7). Symptoms may include fever, diarrhea, arthralgias, headaches, maculopapular rash, and occasionally, neurologic symptoms such as meningitis, neuropathy, or encephalopathy. This syndrome is not specific and thus is rarely recognized as the beginning of AIDS. This is followed by the quiet stage as the cytotoxic cells reduce the viral load. However, virus replication continues, silently damaging the lymph nodes and depleting the CD4 lymphocytes and dendritic cells. This period of asymptomatic infection may last as long as 10 years, but eventually, the immune system fails and the signs of AIDS appear. As the disease progresses, the infected patient may demonstrate generalized lymphadenopathy, constitutional symptoms (fever, diarrhea, weight loss), hematologic abnormalities (anemia, thrombocytopenia, lymphopenia, and neutropenia), and dermatologic problems (dermatitis, candidiasis, and oral hairy leukoplakia).

AIDS is defined by the CD4 cell count and whether the patient has an AIDS-defining condition (opportunistic infection). Manifestations of AIDS are not common with CD4 cell counts above 500 cells/mm^3.[28] However, as this count drops, opportunistic infections develop. These infections include, but are not limited to, tuberculosis, toxoplasmosis, Kaposi's sarcoma, CMV infection, *Pneumocystis carinii* pneumonia, leishmaniasis, and cryptococcosis. They are more likely to develop when the CD4 cell count drops below 200 cells/mm^3.

Life Cycle of HIV. Several potential targets for anti-HIV drugs have been identified in the viral replication cycle of these viruses (Figure 21-8).[1] Step 1 in this cycle involves the binding of the virus to the host cell surface receptor. HIV recognizes the CD4 receptor on helper T lymphocytes and the CCR5 receptor on macrophages and dendritic cells. The surface glycoprotein, gp120, on the HIV envelope binds to these receptors and also to a chemokine co-receptor (CXCR4) on the T cell. After binding, the virion penetrates the cell and uncoats, exposing its RNA. At step 4, the viral RNA is converted to viral DNA by the reverse transcriptase enzyme. The virus draws from the infected cell's supply of deoxynucleosides (thymidine, guanosine, adenosine, and cytidine) to make a double-stranded DNA copy of the viral RNA. The viral DNA can then remain in the cytoplasm or be transported to the nucleus, where the viral DNA is integrated into the host DNA via the integrase enzyme. At step 6, transcription of the host cell's DNA and the viral DNA occurs and is followed by translation and production of viral proteins. However, these newly formed proteins are too long for viral assembly. Protease enzyme then hydrolyzes them into the proper smaller units and assembles them with the viral RNA to produce new virions. The last step is the budding and release of new HIV particles.

Antiretroviral Drugs. There are five types of anti-HIV drugs: (1) nucleoside reverse transcriptase inhibitors, (2) non-nucleoside reverse transcriptase inhibitors,

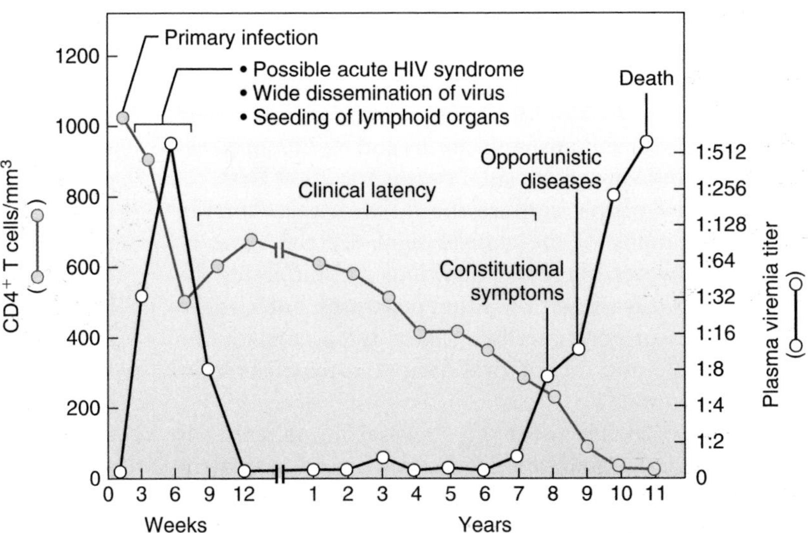

FIGURE 21-7 Schematic outline of the course of HIV infection. (CD4+ T cell titer is often given as cells/mm^3, which is equivalent to cells × 106 cells/L). *(Data from Pantaleo G, Graziosi C, Fauci AS. New concepts in the immunopathogenesis of human immunodeficiency virus infection,* N Engl J Med *328:327–335, 1993.)*

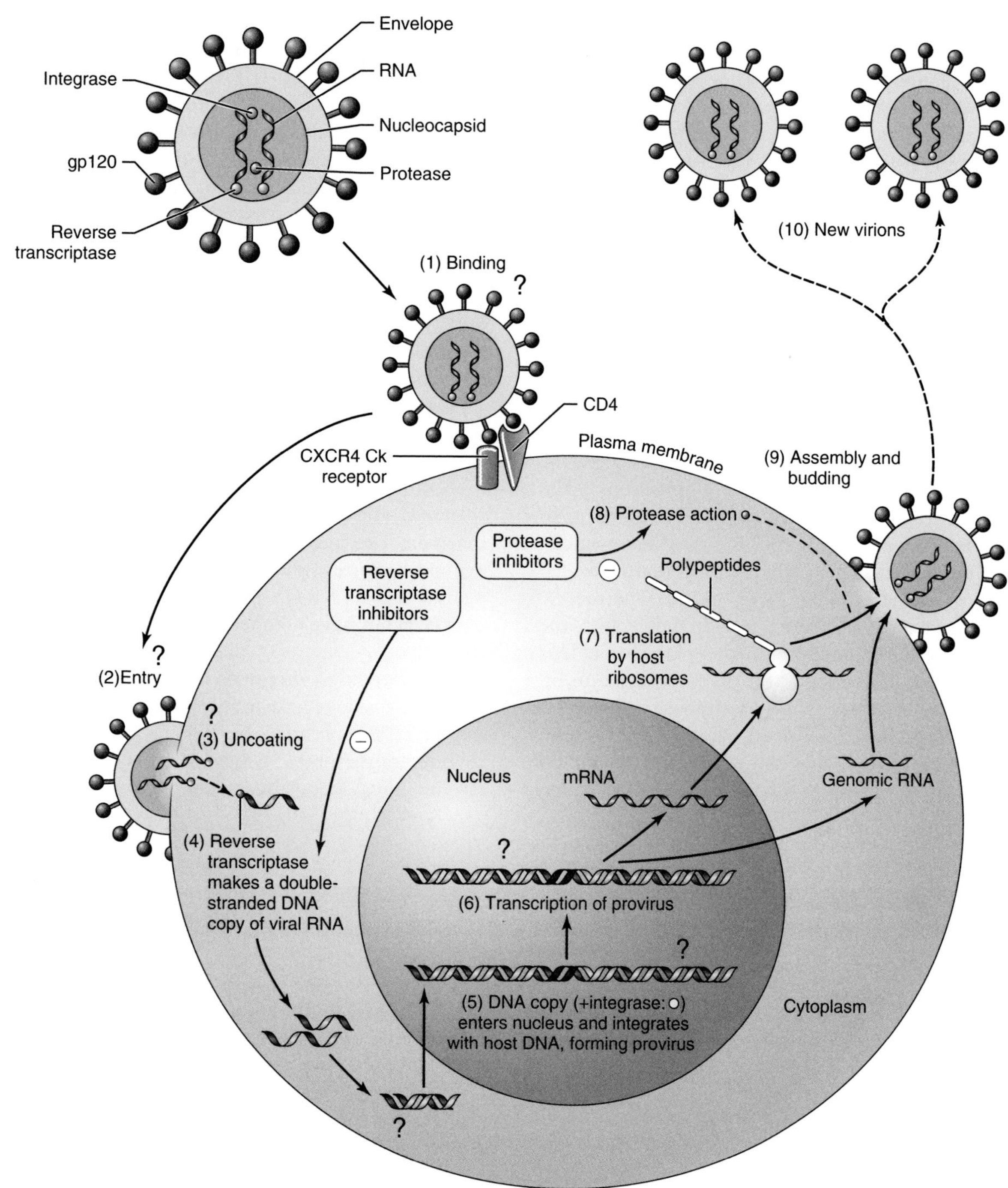

FIGURE 21-8 Schematic diagram of infection of CD4+ T cell by an HIV virion with the sites of action of the two main classes of drug and sites for possible new drugs. The 10 steps, from attachment to the cell to release of new virions, are shown. The virus uses the CD4 co-receptor and the chemokine (Ck) receptor CXCR4 as binding sites. Step 6, transcription, occurs when the T cell itself is activated; when this happens, transcription factor NF-κB initiates transcription of both host cell DNA and the provirus. Step 8, the action of the viral protease, involves the cleaving of the polypeptides into structural proteins and enzymes (integrase, reverse transcriptase, protease) for the new virion (the protease and thus the protease inhibitors actually act on the immature virions after budding). Sites of action of potential new drugs, each indicated by a question mark, include binding of the virion (by modification of the gp120-CD4 or gp120-CXCR4 interaction), entry of virion, uncoating of virion, translocation of viral complementary DNA into nucleus, integration of viral cDNA into host cell DNA, inhibition of the gene coding for the HIV core protein, and inhibition of budding.

(3) protease inhibitors (PIs), (4) fusion inhibitors, and (5) integrase inhibitors. Effective treatment requires the administration of a combination of these drugs, known as *highly active antiretroviral therapy* (HAART).[29] It is important for patients to understand that these medications do not cure HIV infection, and they should be reminded that while they are taking these drugs, they can still transmit the virus to others. In addition, patients

must continue to take these drugs to keep the viral load down and to raise CD4 cell counts. Viral rebound in the plasma and seminal fluids occurs after therapy interruption and results in a greater viral load compared with pretreatment viremia after early discontinuation of antiviral therapy (8 to 9 days after the initiation of therapy).[30,31] In one study, reintroduction of therapy resulted in a reduction in HIV-RNA, and in 1 to 2 months, approximately 50% of patients had undetectable HIV-RNA levels in plasma. An interruption to therapy may be acceptable under strict conditions: when the CD4 count is greater than 500 cells/mm^3 and if the patient has never suffered from a severe compromised immune system. However, most researchers feel that continuous HAART is needed to control the disease.[32]

Nucleotide Reverse Transcriptase Inhibitors. Nucleoside reverse transcriptase inhibitors (NRTIs) were the first group of drugs used to fight HIV infection.[29] The prototypical drug in this category is zidovudine (also known as *azidothymidine*, or AZT). It is a dideoxynucleoside analog that lacks a hydroxyl group that is needed to add bases to the growing DNA strand. The reverse transcriptase enzyme incorporates zidovudine into the growing chain, thus eliminating further elongation. This drug also has an inhibitory effect on the enzyme itself. Other drugs in this category include emtricitabine, lamivudine (Epivir), tenovir (Viread), didanosine (Videx), and stavudine (Zerit) with similar modes of action (Box 21-1).

Serious adverse effects are associated with most of the drugs in this category, with the exception of lamivudine, the best-tolerated anti-HIV drug. All of the drugs in this group have the potential to produce a fatal lactic acidosis and have been associated with fat redistribution and hyperlipidemia. Zidovudine causes anemia, neutropenia, myopathy, headaches, nausea, and vomiting. Myelosuppression is a major problem. Didanosine produces pancreatitis, diarrhea, and peripheral neuropathy. Stavudine is also associated with a high incidence of peripheral neuropathy. However, because HIV produces neuronal injury, including AIDS-related dementia, it is often difficult to determine whether this manifestation is disease related or an adverse effect of the drugs.[32,33]

Tenofovir disoproxil fumarate is a fairly new drug that has a slightly different structure than NRTIs; however, it has similar actions.[29] It is a nucleotide that is a phosphorylated nucleoside. This drug is generally well tolerated, although it produces nausea, vomiting, and diarrhea. The significance of this drug is that it is active against some resistant strains of HIV and is also active against HBV. NRTIs block the virus from attacking new cells but have no effect on cells that already contain the virus.

Non-nucleoside Reverse Transcriptase Inhibitors. Non-nucleoside reverse transcriptase inhibitors (NNRTIs) inhibit HIV replication by binding to a portion of the reverse transcriptase, which changes the shape of the enzyme, thus directly inactivating it.[29] The drugs that fall

BOX 21-1 Nucleoside/Nucleotide Reverse Transcriptase Inhibitors (NRTIs)

NRTI	Dose	Comments
Abacavir (ABC; Ziagen)	300 mg bid Coformulated products: Epzicom (ABC + 3TC) Trizivir (AZT + 3TC + ABC)	One of the most potent NRTIs and well tolerated; hypersensitivity reaction can occur
Didanosine (ddi; Videx)	400 mg qd (enteric-coated tablets) or 500 mg qd (powder)	Must be taken on empty stomach; irritates stomach; may lead to pancreatitis
Emtricitabine (ETC; Emtriva)	200 mg cap qd Coformulated product: Truvada (TDF + ETC) Atripla (TDF + FTC + EFV)	Active also against hepatitis B virus (HBV); well tolerated, qd dosing; risk of fulminant hepatitis; high resistance; hyperpigmentation
Lamivudine (3TC; Epivir)	150 mg bid Coformulated products: Epzicom (ABC + 3TC) Trizivir (AZT + 3TC + ABC) Combivir (AZT + 3TC)	
Stavudine (d4T; Zerit)	Either 30 or 40 mg bid, depending on weight	Well tolerated in short term; fatal lactic acidosis, peripheral neuropathy, lipoatrophy
Zidovudine (AZT; Retrovir)	300 mg bid	Prevents perinatal and occupational transmissions; high level of resistance; gastrointestinal intolerance; neutropenia, lipoatrophy, lactic acidosis, hepatic steatosis, fatigue, asthenia
Tenofovir (TDF; Viread)	300 mg qd Coformulated product: Truvada (TDF + FTC) Atripla (TDF + ETC + EFV)	Well tolerated; longer half-life; active against HBV; nephrotoxicity; may lead to osteoporosis

Adapted from Pham PA, Flexner CW: HIV infections and AIDS. In Waldman SA, Terzic A, editors: *Pharmacology and therapeutics: Principles to practice*, Philadelphia, Saunders, 2009.

within this category include etravirine, nevirapine, delavirdine, and efavirenz (Box 21-2). Combinations of NNRTIs with NRTIs or PIs at least have an additive effect in reducing HIV replication. HIV strains that are resistant to NRTIs may be sensitive to NNRTIs. Adverse effects include maculopapular rashes that require discontinuation of treatment in about 10 to 20% of patients. In addition, hepatitis and neuropsychiatric symptoms (vivid dreams, nightmares, and hallucinations) have been reported. CNS effects tend to occur between 1 and 3 hours after each dose but may subside within a few weeks. These drugs are metabolized by the cytochrome P450 enzyme system and therefore have many drug interactions, including a potential for interaction with PIs.

Protease Inhibitors. Protein inhibitors (PIs) bind to the protease enzyme of HIV-1 and HIV-2, preventing the breakdown of viral polyprotein into the components needed for viral assembly and budding.[29] The use of a PI in combination with other drugs has led to a marked improvement and prolonged survival, even in patients with advanced HIV infection. In addition, resistance to PIs requires more mutations for loss of effectiveness than does resistance to some other drugs. The drugs in this category include saquinavir (Invirase), tipranavir (Aptivus), ritonavir (Norvir), darunavir (Prezista), indinavir (Crixivan), nelfinavir (Viracept), and amprenavir (Agenarase) (Box 21-3). The principal adverse effects are GI symptoms and a syndrome of lipodystrophy.[34] This syndrome includes peripheral fat wasting, central obesity, high serum triglyceride and cholesterol levels, and insulin resistance. Because of these adverse effects, some physicians treating patients with AIDS discuss heart disease and myocardial infarctions (MIs) as new complications of HIV disease. Studies are ongoing to determine whether antidiabetes drugs could reduce lipodystrophy, but so far, they have not been useful.[35] However, some studies have demonstrated improvement in insulin levels when an NNRTI was substituted for a PI.[36]

BOX 21-2 Non-nucleoside Reverse Transcriptase Inhibitors (NNRTIs)

Drug	Dose	Comments
Delavirdine (DLV; Rescriptor)	400 mg tid	Low potency but some action against resistant forms
Efavirenz (EFV; Sustiva)	600 mg at bedtime but on an empty stomach during first 2 wk Coformulated product: Atripla (TDF + ETC + EFV)	High potency; well tolerated; central nervous system adverse effects common; hyperlipidemia
Nevirapine (NVP; Viramune)	200 mg qd × 14 days, then 200 mg bid	Efficacy similar to EFV; used to prevent perinatal transmission; severe hepatotoxicity; rash; resistance
Etravirine (ETR; Intelence)	200 mg bid with food	Active against most EFV- and NVP-resistant strains; many complex drug interactions

Adapted from Pham PA, Flexner CW: HIV infections and AIDS. In Waldman SA, Terzic A, editors: *Pharmacology and therapeutics: Principles to practice*, Philadelphia, Saunders, 2009.

BOX 21-3 Protease Inhibitors (PIs)

Drug	Dose	Comments
Atazanavir (ATV; Reyataz)	400 mg qd or ATV/r 300mg/100 mg qd	Good potency, no effects on lipids or gastrointestinal (GI) system; jaundice, drug interactions with PPIs, histamine-2 (H_2) blockers and antacids
Amprenavir (APV; Agenarase)	1400 mg bid liquid	Good activity against some resistive strains; rash
Fosamprenavir (FPV; Lexiva)	1400 mg bid or FPV/r 700/100 mg bid	Decreased pill burden; less effective in patients who have already taken PIs
Indinavir (IDV; Crixivan)	800 mg tid, with small meal or LDV/r 800/100 mg bid	Good potency; needs RTV boosting; nephrolithiasis; insulin resistance; retinoid effects
Lopinavir/ritonavir (LPV/r; Kaletra)	400/100 mg bid	Long-term efficacy is good; decreased pill burden; GI intolerance; high triglycerides and cholesterol
Nelfinavir (NFV; Viracept)	NFV 750 mg tid or NFV 1250 mg bid, with high fat meal	Less potent than NNRTIs and boosted PIs; depends on fatty foods for absorption, more diarrhea

Adapted from Pham PA, Flexner CW: HIV infections and AIDS. In Waldman SA, Terzic A, editors: *Pharmacology and therapeutics: Principles to practice*, Philadelphia, Saunders, 2009.

Fusion Inhibition. Enfuvirtide (Fuzeon) and maraviroc, also known as entry inhibitors, bind to the surface glycoprotein on the viral envelope and prevent the fusion of the virus to the host cell. These drugs, when given to patients already receiving a standard HIV protocol, resulted in a lowered viral load and higher CD4 cell counts compared with the protocol alone.[37] Maraviroc is given orally, and enfuvirtide is given by injection, which causes mild to moderate pain, erythema, induration, and cysts at the injection site. Other effects of enfuvirtide include eosinophilia and an increase in bacterial pneumonia. Because of the different mechanisms of action of NRTIs, NNRTIs, and PIs, these drugs are effective against viral particles that have become resistant to the older drugs and are usually reserved for patients who have experienced failures on the other regimens.

Integrase Inhibitors. Raltegravir is a new drug which interferes with the action of the enzyme integrase, which is necessary for the integration of viral genetic material into the human DNA.[38] Adverse reactions include diarrhea, fatigue, and headache. This drug is metabolized by glucuronidation and not by the P450 enzymes, making it less susceptible to drug–drug interactions.

Use of Antiretrovirals in Pregnancy. In the European nations and in the United States, the use of HAART in pregnant women has lowered the rate of mother-to-child transmission of HIV-1 from 25% to 1 to 2%.[39] However, in poorer countries where HAART is not available and breast-feeding and vaginal deliveries are standard practice (both of which facilitate transmission), mother-to-child transmission is a major component of the AIDS epidemic.[40]

Zidovudine is typically used during pregnancy to reduce transmission of HIV to the infant. When started at 14 to 32 weeks' gestation and continued for 6 weeks after delivery, transmission is reduced in the neonate from 26% to 8% globally.[29] This 8% is higher than what was reported in the previous paragraph because of the breast-feeding practices and lack of medications in developing nations, which lead to an overall risk of transmission as high as 15 to 25% at 18 to 24 months. For added protection, many clinicians are now offering zidovudine plus another NRTI and a PI. Single-dose nevirapine or single-dose lamivudine along with a short course of zidovudine (from weeks 32 to 36 of pregnancy) have shown the highest efficacy among women with CD4 cell counts of 200/mm^3 or less and viral loads of at least 2500 HIV-1 RNA copies/mL.[41] If infection is not detected until delivery, nevirapine can be administered to the mother during labor, and then zidovudine and nevirapine can be subsequently given to the infant for effective reduction in transmission.[43]

Combination Therapy for HIV. Potent combination drug regimens have proved to be the most efficacious approach to the treatment of HIV. Standard therapy for HIV infection requires at least a three-drug regimen. The goal of using multiple drugs is to stop the replication of the virus at a number of different steps in its reproductive cycle. It has also been found that administering just one or two drugs increases the chance of developing drug resistance. In fact, most resistance to treatment is due to partial suppression of the virus rather than acquisition of a resistant form.[43] In the United States, 50% of patients are resistant to at least one drug.[44] Combination therapy has also been found to be much more effective in reducing the viral load than sequential administration of the same drugs.

The most common regimens are as follows:

1. Two NRTIs + one NNRTI
2. Two NRTIs + ritonavir + another PI (ritonavir has been added to this protocol because it has been found to act as a PI enhancer.)[45]

Of these protocols, the one that appears to be most effective at this time is two NRTIs with one NNRTI, specifically zidovudine, lamivudine, and efavirenz.[46] The addition of a fourth drug has the potential to increase the potency of the regimen but may also be associated with increased toxic effects and increase the likelihood of drug-drug interactions (Box 21-4). The addition of a fourth drug may reduce adherence to the drug routine as well, and this may limit future treatment options if resistance develops, as many of the drugs are cross-resistant within the same category. A four-drug regimen, compared with the three-drug regimen of zidovudine, lamivudine, and efavirenz, was not significantly different in terms of the *length of time to failure*, defined as an increase in the viral load or viral rebound.[47] However, it is clear that much more work is necessary to determine the optimal protocol for controlling the viral load, particularly in light of developing drug resistance.

The optimal time to begin therapy has finally been determined. At one time, some clinicians were waiting until the CD4 cell count dropped below 200 cells/mm^3, and others began therapy when the count was at 500 cells/mm^3. Fear of development of resistance was the main factor that contributed to waiting until the CD4 cell count was at a critical level (200 cells/mm^3). It was believed that if a patient developed resistance to drugs early in the disease, there would be no medications left to try when the illness became critical. Treatment is now begun earlier, when the CD4 cell count drops to 350 cells/mm^3 or when opportunistic infections develop. Studies have shown that deferring treatment until the CD4 counts drop further is associated with "increased progression rates," although other factors such as the willingness of the patient to start and adhere to therapy, drug toxicity, pill burden, dosing schedule, sensitivity of the particular strain of HIV to treatment, and drug–drug interactions also help determine the optimal time for drug treatment to be initiated.[48,49]

Once the patient begins the treatment regimen, the viral load and CD4 cell counts should be tested. It is recommended that viral load testing be performed 2 to 8 weeks

BOX 21-4 **Drug-Drug Interactions with Anti-HIV Drugs**

Drug Affected	Interacting Drug	Effect
Midazolam, triazolam	All PIs, DLV and EFV	Significant increase in serum levels of affected drugs
Fentanyl	All PIs and DLV	Significant increase in serum levels of affected drugs
Antiarrhythmics	All PIs and DLV	Significant increase in serum levels of affected drugs
Calcium channel blockers	All PIs and DLV	Increase PR interval
Rifampin	All PIs	Serum level of PI is reduced
Simvastatin, lovastatin	All PIs and DLV	Marked increase in serum levels of affected drugs
Methadone	NVP, EFV	Decreased serum levels of methadone

Adapted from Pham PA, Flexner CW: HIV infections and AIDS. In Waldman SA, Terzic A, editors: *Pharmacology and therapeutics: Principles to practice*, Philadelphia, Saunders, 2009.
PI, protease inhibitor; *DLV,* delavirdine; *EFV,* efavirenz; *NVP,* nevirapine.

after therapy is started and then every 4 to 6 months throughout treatment.[50] CD4 cell counts should be done every 3 to 6 months throughout therapy. This count should increase, or at least not decrease, while the patient is taking medication. If the level decreases, it may mean that the drugs are not working and there is "regimen failure."

There are three types of regimen failure: (1) *virologic failure*, in which the virus is still detected in the blood 48 weeks after the start of treatment, or virus that was originally undetected becomes apparent; (2) *immunologic failure*, which reflects decreases in CD4 cell count; and (3) *clinical failure*, which indicates that physical health is deteriorating or the patient has acquired an HIV-related infection.[50] Virologic failure is the most common, and patients who maintain their present drug regimen despite this development usually experience immunologic failure within 3 years.

Adherence Issues. Therapy protocols for HIV were very difficult to follow in the past. Some of the drugs had to be administered with food, some had to be taken either 1 hour before meals or 2 hours after, and some had to be taken with large amounts of water.[29] In addition, some of the protocols required taking a large number of pills at the same time. The pill burden may have been as high as 18 pills per day. Many of the capsules were large and difficult to swallow, particularly if the patient had mucosal ulcers or oral candidiasis. Keeping track of when and how these drugs must be administered was a full-time job. When you add this to the adverse effects—particularly the severe nausea, vomiting, and diarrhea—it is not surprising that early in the history of HIV, patients had trouble being compliant with the program. In clinical studies, these drugs were effective in reducing the viral load and raising CD4 cell counts. However, when patients continued to take the drugs without the benefit of close supervision afforded by a clinical trial, many patients become noncompliant, and viral loads begin to climb. In one study, only about half the patients took all their antiretroviral medications as directed in terms of timing and dietary instructions during a preceding week.[51] However, the pill burden has been radically reduced in recent years due to the development of several once-daily fixed-dose combinations, for example, NRTI combinations of tenofovir or abacavir formulated with emtricitabine and lamivudine.[52] This has had profound ramifications on longevity—life expectancy between 2003 and 2005 increased to two thirds of that of the average healthy individual. A patient diagnosed with the disease at age 20 can now expect to live to approximately 49 years of age.[53]

Lipodystrophy. HIV-related lipodystrophy is the development of truncal obesity (central fat accumulation) also known as *lipohypertrophy*, with areas of localized lipoatrophy.[54] Additionally, patients may demonstrate an enlarged dorsocervical fat pad, increased circumference of the neck, and gynecomastia. Lipoatrophy may be exhibited in the face, arms, legs, and gluteal area. Patients may also have hyperlipidemia, hyperglycemia, and insulin resistance. Patients can exhibit predominantly one type, even though it is a less common occurrence.

Numerous drugs have been implicated in producing this condition, specifically the protease inhibitors ritonavir, saquinavir, and nelfinavir and the NRTIs stavudine and zidovudine. Not much is known about this condition, and the causes are speculative; however, some cases have been reported in patients who are drug naïve. In general, women are more susceptible than men, whites more than blacks, and older individuals more than their younger counterparts.

Treatment for lipodystrophy includes reducing drug dose or switching to another drug regimen altogether and adding medications for diabetes and cholesterol-lowering drugs. Additionally, patients may undergo liposuction, facial fat grafting, lipotransfer, and implantation of dermal fillers such as calcium hydroxylapatite (Radiesse), poly-L-lactic acid (Sculptra) and other soft tissue substances that have typically been designed to reduce the effects of aging skin.[55] One also cannot ignore the positive effects of exercise on this condition. Exercise has been shown to improve insulin sensitivity and to reduce truncal obesity in this condition.[56] Additionally, patients with HIV-associated lipodystrophy who performed aerobic exercise (three times/wk) at 70 to 85% HRmax and were on a special diet for a total of 12 weeks demonstrated a significant increase in peak oxygen uptake (VO_{2peak}) compared with the diet-only group.[57] Body mass index (BMI) and waist-to-hip ratio also showed significant changes compared with the control group. However, despite these functional improvements, no significant changes in triglycerides occurred. This is in contrast to some other studies that showed a reduction in cholesterol and triglycerides with exercise either for the same duration or 1 month longer.[58-61] All but one of these studies used a combination of aerobic and resistive exercises. None of the studies demonstrated consistent significant changes in CD4 cells, which indicated that moderate exercise did not change the patients' HIV status positively or negatively.

Other Therapeutic Concerns about HAART. The rehabilitation therapist may see patients with HIV because of some virus-related events or drug-related events, especially drug-related peripheral neuropathies and neurogenic pain, and the functional limitations they impose. Additionally, the drugs may cause fatigue and lactic acidosis that would interfere with exercise capacity. Therapists must approach therapy for patients with HIV as if they were "cardiac patients" and continue to follow appropriate principles of exercise physiology, including frequent monitoring of vital signs.

Hepatitis A

HAV is a common cause of acute viral hepatitis. It is transmitted via the oral-fecal route, which explains the high incidence in developing countries with poor sanitary conditions.[62] Clinical manifestations of this infection vary from mild myalgias, fevers, fatigue, and right upper quadrant pain, to hepatomegaly, jaundice, and peripheral edema and ascites. Fulminant hepatic failure may also occur within weeks of diagnosis in contrast to a much longer prodromal period with hepatitis B and C. However, it is often self-limiting and mild in nature. The virus replicates in the liver and then is excreted along with bile into the intestines. Fecal shedding then occurs within 1 to 4 weeks following infection. The period of greatest infectivity occurs just prior to hepatic injury.

Drug Treatment for Hepatitis A. Management of exposure and/or treatment can both occur through two routes. Passive immunoprophylaxis involves administering human immunoglobulin, which offers protection against viral transmission. It can provide protection for approximately 3 months after administration by injection. Immunoglobulins given within 2 weeks of suspected exposure can also confer protection.[62]

The HAV vaccine is a form of active immunoprophylaxis. There are currently two vaccines available in the United States: Havrix and VAQTA. Both are prepared from an inactivated virus and are highly effective. In addition, a combined HAV/HBV vaccine (Twinrix) is also available. This vaccine is recommended to individuals traveling to endemic areas, men who have sex with men, intravenous (IV) drug users, and those who work with nonhuman primates.

Hepatitis B

Hepatitis B is a major viral infection that can present across a clinical spectrum from an asymptomatic subclinical infection through a self-limiting illness to fulminant liver failure. HBV has infected two billion people worldwide and there are more than 350 million chronic carriers of HBV worldwide. HBV causes approximately 600,000 deaths annually.[63] If untreated or unresponsive to therapy, approximately 15% of patients with chronic HBV infections will develop cirrhosis of the liver, and 2 to 6% per year will develop hepatocellular carcinoma.[63] A prophylactic HBV vaccine has been developed but is unavailable to many.

Hepatitis B Virus. HBV is transmitted through blood and other bodily secretions and is 100 times more infectious than HIV.[64] HBV can remain alive outside the body in dried blood for more than 1 week. In the United States, transmission of the virus primarily occurs though sexual contact or IV drug use; but in Southeast Asia, China, and sub-Saharan Africa, hepatitis is primarily transmitted vertically from mother to child in the perinatal period. Progression to chronic HBV occurs in 25 to 30% of children and in 3 to 5% of adults.

HBV consists of double-stranded circular DNA enclosed in a nucleocapsid (core antigen), which is surrounded by an envelope (surface antigen).[64] The entire virus is also known as the *Dane particle*. HBV infects hepatocytes, and when it enters the nucleus, the genome encodes a DNA polymerase that also acts as a reverse transcriptase enzyme. The DNA provides a template for mRNA, which then undergoes transcription to produce other viral proteins, including a "pre-genomic" RNA. The HBV genome also produces a circulating protein called the *e antigen* that correlates with high viral replication and provides a useful laboratory marker for active disease. HBV replication is in excess of 1011 virions per day and has a high mutation rate. There are several HBV genotypes denoted with letters A through H.

Signs and Symptoms. Infection with HBV produces nausea, fatigue, low-grade fever, elevated liver transaminase levels, and right upper quadrant pain or epigastric pain.[65] Jaundice may also be present. Extrahepatic signs include myalgias, arthralgias, and urticaria. Symptoms do not occur immediately after exposure but have an incubation period of 1 to 4 months. In most cases, the host immune system can overcome the infection, and the illness subsequently resolves. However, some patients continue to have chronic HBV infection. In addition, about 1% of acute infections develop quickly into fulminant hepatic failure.

Chronic disease is defined as seropositivity for HBV surface antigen (HBsAg) for more than 6 months, HBV DNA levels >100,000 copies/mL, persistent elevation in liver enzyme levels, and detection of necrosis on a liver biopsy specimen.[65] Asymptomatic carriers are seropositive for HBV surface antigen (HBsAg) and seronegative for hepatitis B e antigen (HBeAg) and have lower levels of HBV DNA (<100,000 copies/mL). Patients who demonstrate resolution of the infection are seropositive for HBV core (Anti-HBc) and surface antibody (Anti-HBs) and seronegative for HBsAg. However, this chronic disease is fluid and patients can pass from one phase to another and back again. See Table 21-1.

Drug Treatment for Chronic Hepatitis B. Drugs for HBV fall mainly into two categories: (1) immune modulators (IFN-α_{2a} and IFN-α_{2b}) and (2) those that inhibit HBV replication (lamivudine and adefovir dipivoxil). The goals of therapy include lowering the viral load and preventing end-stage liver disease. The specific responses to therapy can be characterized as the "initial response" measured at 6 months or 12 months into treatment, "maintained response," in which the response was still present at the patient's last visit, and a "sustained response," which persists 6 months after the completion of therapy. A resolved infection is indicated by a sustained elimination of HBsAg.[66]

IFN-α_{2b} was approved as therapy for chronic HBV in 1992.[66,67] It appears to have the most success in patients who have low HBV DNA levels, elevated liver enzyme levels without fibrosis of the liver, and no HIV co-infection. Overall, approximately 46% of subjects who are treated with IFN-α_{2b} seroconvert from HBeAg to the antibody within the first year after treatment. However, even though they may lose their HBeAg seronegativity, a certain percentage of these patients will continue to be positive for HBsAg and experience further liver damage. To complicate treatment further, those that initially eliminate HBsAg, may have it return at a later date.[62] Elimination of HBsAg may only occur in approximately 3 to 8% of patients receiving IFN or the newer peginterferon. Long-term follow-up of IFN-treated patients demonstrated a 5-year survival rate of 95% in those who seroconverted but less than 50% in those patients who were still seropositive for HBeAg.[66] So, even though IFNs are quite helpful for a certain subset of patients with hepatitis B, many individuals do not benefit in the long term from this treatment. Some patients must stop taking the drug because of its adverse effects: flu-like symptoms, mood alterations, thyroid abnormalities, bone marrow suppression, and excessive fatigue. In addition, the rigorous dosing schedule—5 million units injected subcutaneously daily or 10 million units injected three times per week for 16 weeks—is difficult to tolerate. In some cases, dosing lasts a full year. Regular follow-up is still needed after seroconversion to monitor liver enzyme levels and the viral load.

In 2005, pegylated IFN, which allows for once-per-week dosing and improved compliance, was introduced. Pegylation is the process of attaching polyethyleneglycol (PEG) to the drug. This process increases half-life (approximately seven-fold) by reducing renal clearance and proteolytic decomposition.[62] In addition, so far, there have been few reports of antiviral resistance to this drug. There are currently two versions of this pegylated compound, peginterferon-α_{2a} (Pegasys) and peginterferon-α_{2b} (PEG-Intron).

Lamivudine is another first-line treatment for chronic hepatitis B. It was briefly discussed earlier in this chapter as a drug for HIV; this drug was also approved for treatment of hepatitis B in 1999. The drug inhibits the reverse transcriptase action of the DNA polymerase. Advantages over IFNs include a more rapid response, oral administration, and a good tolerability profile with fewer adverse effects. The disadvantages of this drug include uncertainty about the durability of HBeAg seroconversion and a high rate of antiviral resistance. The 3-year relapse rate has varied from 38 to 77%.[67,68]

Adefovir dipivoxil is the second nucleoside drug approved for the treatment of chronic HBV.[69] It has action similar to that of lamivudine in that it inhibits the DNA reverse transcriptase action. It was approved for use in 2002, so few long-term data on its efficacy or safety are available. It may be less effective than lamivudine but has a low rate of antiviral resistance. Adverse reactions have been described as being no different from those that occur with placebo.[69] The drug is administered orally for 48 weeks and demonstrates improved liver histologic findings in approximately 28% of patients who are HBeAg-seropositive compared with placebo. Other drugs include entecavir, telbivudine, and tenofovir, which are all available as oral preparations.[70] Of these, tenofovir may be the most potent and the most suitable for patients with lamivudine resistance and those who have had a poor response to the other nucleoside agents.

Studies using combination therapy are ongoing with preliminary reports showing little advantage to using more than one nucleoside agent. Unlike the drugs in combination therapy for HIV disease, all these agents act on the same target.

Even though drug therapy for patients with chronic hepatitis is available, the percentage of patients for whom drug therapy has long-term efficacy is not ideal. In most cases, these drugs do not achieve a complete cure or complete elimination of the virus from the body, but they substantially decrease the damage to the liver caused by the replication of the virus.

TABLE 21-1 Phases and Serology HBV Infection

	Acute HBV	Resolved HBV	Chronic HBV (HBeAg-positive)	Inactive HBsAg Carrier	Chronic HBV (HBeAg-negative)	Immune Tolerant	Immunized
HBeAg	+	—	+	—	—	+	—
HBsAg	+	—	+	+	+	+	—
HBV DNA	High HBV DNA	None detected in serum	High HBV DNA	Low	Moderate levels of HBV DNA	High HBV DNA	—
ALT	Elevated	Normal	Elevated	Normal Occasional flare	Elevated but fluctuates	Normal or minimal	Normal
Hepatic inflammation	Hepatic inflammation	Some evidence of fibrosis	Hepatic inflammation and fibrosis	Minimal fibrosis	Hepatic inflammation and fibrosis	Minimal inflammation	Normal
Comments	Immunoglobulin M (IgM) antibody to HBcAg	Loss of HBsAg and seroconversion to anti-HBs is indicative of complete response and recovery	—	Reactivation of viremia with immune suppression but without HBeAg	—	—	Positive for Anti-HBs

Adapted from Hoofnagle JH, Doo ET, Fleischer R, Lok ASF: Management of hepatitis B: Summary of a clinical research workshop. *Hepatology* 45:1056–1075, 2007.
ALT, alanine aminotransferase; *HBV*, hepatitis B virus; *HBeAg*, hepatitis B e antigen; *HBsAg*, hepatitis B surface antigen.

Hepatitis C

Hepatitis C is a leading cause of hepatic failure and mortality.[71] There are more than 170 million chronic carriers of hepatitis C worldwide. High prevalence rates are seen in Africa and Asia, with Egypt, Pakistan, and China having the highest rates. Because this virus is extremely robust, causing more than 85% of those infected to develop chronic infection, it has become a major health concern. Transmission occurs mostly through the bloodborne route (blood transfusions, organ transplantations, and IV drug use). As in the case of HBV, chronic infection with HCV is also associated with liver cirrhosis and hepatocellular carcinoma. HCV is associated with some autoimmune diseases, including arthritis and glomerulonephritis, as well, and it has been linked to diabetes mellitus, neuropathy, lymphoma, Sjögren's syndrome, and mixed cryoglobulinemia.

Hepatitis C Virus. HCV is an RNA virus that targets hepatocytes and possibly B lymphocytes.[71] Like HBV, it is a rapidly replicating virus producing 1010 to 1012 copies per day. Replication also occurs by an RNA-dependent RNA polymerase that lacks the ability to detect and repair mutations, so at any one time, an individual may have several forms of HCV. More than 90 genotypes have been identified and categorized into six main types, numbered from 1 to 6.[72,73] Subtypes are further identified by lowercase letters, with a, b, c, and so on. In fact, variability within a region of gene that codes for nonstructural proteins has significance, particularly in Japan where many individuals have an isolate called *subtype 1b*.[73] Unfortunately, this subtype confers resistance to IFN-α_{2b}. Types 1, 2, and 3 are most prevalent in Western Europe, North America, Australia, and Asia.

HCV encodes a single chain of 3011 amino acids, which then becomes 10 structural and regulatory proteins.[73] The structural components include the core and two envelope proteins. The envelope has a specialized region for binding to the CD81 marker expressed on hepatocytes and B lymphocytes. HCV also encodes a virus-specific helicase, a protease, and a polymerase for replication. All of these structures represent potential targets for drug therapy, but success in treatment has been difficult to achieve.

Signs and Symptoms. As in the case of HBV, diagnosis of HCV in the acute phase of infection is not common.[74] Symptoms usually occur within 7 to 8 weeks after infection, but many patients have either no symptoms or only mild complaints. Symptoms that do manifest are usually nausea, jaundice, right upper quadrant pain, and general malaise. Acute infection will lead to chronic disease in 74 to 86% of patients. Chronic infection leads to hepatic fibrosis and some nonspecific symptoms such as fatigue. Once the infection becomes chronic, a reduction in the viral load is unlikely. It may take 20 to 30 years to develop fulminant liver disease, but at least one third of patients become seriously ill in less than 20 years after infection. Progression of the disease depends on alcohol consumption, co-infection with HIV, male sex, and older age at the time of infection. Chronic HCV is also a major cause of hepatocellular carcinoma.[75]

Drug Treatment for HCV. Even though drug treatment has yielded disappointing results, the National Institutes of Health (NIH) recommends that all patients with chronic HCV be considered candidates for drug treatment. Factors that need to be taken into consideration are comorbid illnesses that would make drug treatment more dangerous, patient motivation, and HCV genotype. Treatment of HCV genotype 1 has a success rate of only 40 to 55%, but patients with HCV type 2 or 3 have a 70 to 80% treatment success rate, that is, they are asymptomatic and have minimal hepatic damage.[71]

In 1989, the first cases of HCV successfully treated with IFN-α were reported with great enthusiasm.[76] However, it quickly became apparent that there was a high rate of relapse. Later, it was shown that a combination of IFN-α_{2b} with ribavirin for 24 or 48 weeks resulted in normalization of liver enzyme levels and elimination of HCV RNA in 30 to 50% of previously untreated patients.[74] In addition, at the time, this combination yielded a sustained response two to three times over monotherapy with IFN.[77] The success rate of drug therapy for HCV has been further improved by the use of peginterferon plus ribavirin, demonstrating a sustained response rate to approximately 55% for genotype I.[79-81,] Comparison studies are ongoing to determine which IFN (2a or 2b) is more effective when paired with ribavarin.[82] Adverse effects of combination therapy are similar to those of IFN-α and include a flu-like syndrome, depression, alopecia, bone marrow depression, erythema at injection sites, cough, and ribavirin-induced anemia.

A combination of factors leads to the failure of IFN–ribavirin treatment to eradicate HCV and includes the genotype of the virus, the presence of marked liver disease, alcohol consumption, co-infection, and the remarkable ability of the virus to resist rigorous drug treatment.[82] In addition, it is now recognized that a genetic polymorphism that is prevalent in African Americans affects peginterferon efficacy.[83-85] It is likely that the problem in finding successful treatment for hepatitis has to do with our own lack of understanding about how this virus infects host cells and what strategies it uses to resist drug treatment. More research is therefore needed in this area.

Therapeutic Concerns about Antiviral Agents

Most individuals taking antiviral medications may be coping with a serious chronic illnesses. Constitutional symptoms, particularly of fatigue and general malaise, will affect a patient's performance in therapy. These symptoms may be exacerbated by drug therapy, particularly with the IFNs, which produce flu-like symptoms. However, these symptoms do respond to acetaminophen and symptom-modified activity and disappear with continued drug treatment.

Myelosuppression causing anemia may be caused by antiviral agents or by the illnesses themselves. In either case, it affects exercise performance. Hemoglobin levels tend to be reduced in patients with HIV, which, in turn, reduces maximal oxygen uptake and induces an earlier lactic acidosis threshold.[86] This higher lactate level is observed at lower exercise intensities, leading to hyperventilation and the sensation of dyspnea. Similar expectations are present in chronic hepatitis as well.

In terms of the effect of exercise on the viral load, there is evidence that prolonged intense training may impair some immune functions, such as neutrophil function, immunoglobulin levels, and NK cell cytotoxic activity.[86] Therefore, the viral load would be expected to increase during periods of intense workouts. These parameters have not been seen to increase with moderate exercise. However, patients with chronic infections need regular monitoring of their viral load and immune function. It is also recommended that persons with chronic hepatitis keep a record of their liver transaminase levels along with their activity levels and be prepared to reduce exercise intensity if the liver transaminase levels become elevated.[87,88] Participation in either contact sports or semicontact sports will also need to be limited if the patient has any palpable hepatomegaly or splenomegaly, and those patients who have extremely severe cirrhotic disease with ascites, jaundice, edema, bleeding varices, hypersplenism, or coagulopathy will only be able to participate in very-low-level activities.

Because many of the viral infections are transmitted through blood and secretions, therapists need to take appropriate measures to prevent transmission of pathogens during physical therapy intervention. Caring properly for exposed skin lesions and making sure all equipment is disinfected after use is important. Following guidelines for "standard precautions" is mandatory.

DRUGS AND FUNGAL INFECTIONS

Most of the large number of different fungi affect plants and do not cause serious human infection in healthy individuals. Minor infections, particularly in the cool and temperate climatic zones, include athlete's foot and oral or vaginal yeast infection.[1] These are somewhat bothersome infections but hardly life-threatening. However, in the last 20 years, there has been an upsurge of some serious systemic fungal infections, so a discussion of antifungal agents is necessary. The spread of fungal diseases has increased largely because of the pervasive use of broad-spectrum antimicrobials, which eliminate bacteria (nonpathogenic) that compete with fungi and suppress their growth. Another reason for the increase in fungal infections is the impaired immunity caused by HIV/AIDS or by immunosuppressive and chemotherapeutic agents. Fungal infections are also more common in older persons, patients with diabetes, pregnant women, and those with burn injuries.[89,90]

Fungal infections are referred to as *mycoses* and can be divided into *superficial infections* affecting the skin, nails, or mucous membranes and *systemic infections* affecting major organ systems.[1] Superficial fungal infections include dermatomycoses and candidiasis. Dermatomycoses are most commonly caused by *Trichophyton*, *Microsporum*, and *Epidermophyton* and produce various types of ringworm (tinea) (Table 21-2). Tinea cruris affects the groin, tinea pedis affects the feet, and tinea capitis affects the scalp. Superficial candidiasis is caused by a yeast-like organism that infects the mucous membranes, leading to oral thrush (mouth), vaginal candidiasis, or skin infection (diaper rash).

Serious systemic fungal diseases include cryptococcal meningitis, endocarditis, pulmonary aspergillosis, blastomycosis, histoplasmosis, and coccidiomycosis. The last three are considered primary infections, that is, they are not a result of immunosuppression.

Characteristics of Fungi

Fungi are considered to be plantlike parasitic microorganisms but lack chlorophyll and therefore cannot make their own food. Fungi reproduce by means of spores, but their reproductive process is still not completely understood.

Fungi consist of a cell wall, a cell membrane, and a nuclear division containing its DNA. The cell walls of most fungi consist of glycoproteins embedded within a polysaccharide scaffolding that includes a special compound 1,3 β-glucan.[90] The cell membrane also contains a special compound called *ergosterol* (the human membrane contains *cholesterol*). The DNA is, of course, fungi specific and has its own way of replication. The actions of most drugs are based on these differences.

Antifungal Agents

To be systemically effective, drugs usually need to achieve high concentrations that are not tolerated or only poorly tolerated by the patient. The three main classes of antifungal drugs are (1) polyene macrolides, (2) antifungal azoles, and (3) allylamines. A few other miscellaneous agents are also used to treat fungal infections.

Polyene Macrolide Antibiotics. Amphotericin B (Fungizone) is one of the original antifungal agents, developed in the 1950s. It binds to ergosterol and then produces a channel in the fungal cell membrane (Figure 21-9). This opening allows potassium and magnesium ions to flow out of the cell, leading to cell death.

Amphotericin B is considered a broad-spectrum agent and the drug of choice for the treatment of severe

TABLE 21-2 Mycotic Infections

Mycosis	Fungus	Endemic Location	Primary Tissue Reservoir	Transmission	Affected
Systemic Infection					
Aspergillosis	*Aspergillus* spp.	Universal	Soil	Inhalation	Lungs
Blastomycosis	*Blastomyces dermatitidis*	North America	Soil, animal droppings	Inhalation	Lungs
Coccidioidomycosis	*Coccidioides immitis*	Southwestern United States	Soil, dust	Inhalation	Lungs
Cryptococcosis	*Cryptococcus neoformans*	Universal	Soil, pigeon droppings	Inhalation	Lungs/meninges of brain
Histoplasmosis	*Histoplasma capsulatum*	Universal	Soil, bird and chicken droppings	Inhalation	Lungs
Cutaneous Infection					
Candidiasis	*Candida albicans*	Universal	Humans	Direct contact, non-susceptible antibiotic overgrowth	Mucous membrane/skin disseminated (may be systemic)
Dermatophytes, tinea	*Epidermophyton* spp., *Microsporum* spp., *Trichophyton* spp.	Universal	Humans	Direct and indirect contact with infected persons	Scalp, skin
Superficial Infection					
Tinea versicolor	*Malassezia furfur*	Universal	Humans	Unknown*	Skin

(From Lilley LL, Harrington S, Snyder JS, editors: *Pharmacology and the nursing process* (4th ed.). St Louis, 2005, Mosby)
**Malassezia* spp. are a usual part of the normal human flora and appear to cause infection in only select individuals.

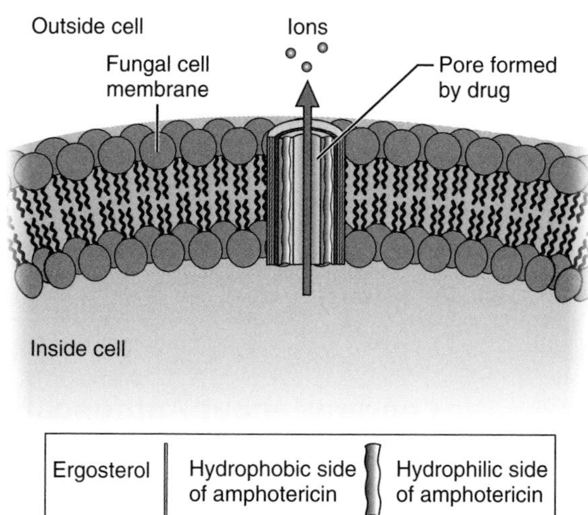

FIGURE 21-9 Mechanism of action of polyene antifungal agents. Binding to ergosterol damages the membrane with leakage of ions and irreversible fungal cell damage.

systemic fungal infections.[91] It is available in parenteral, topical, and oral forms. Topical forms are used for oral or cutaneous candidiasis. Oral formulations tend to be used for infections in the GI tract because this form of the drug is poorly absorbed and thus mostly stays in the GI tract near the site of infection. IV amphotericin is used for systemic fungal infections such as candidiasis, cryptococcosis, aspergillosis, and blastomycosis. The IV formulation is complexed with sodium deoxycholate, which causes significant adverse effects. There is an ongoing search for an improved formulation or a different delivery system.[92]

The adverse effects of amphotericin B include renal toxicity; impaired hepatic function; thrombocytopenia; and infusion-related effects such as tachycardia, chills, fever, tinnitus, and headache.[93] In addition, about one in five patients experiences vomiting. For some infections, daily IV treatment is needed, sometimes lasting for a period of 6 to 12 weeks. The drug is also highly irritating to the endothelium of the veins, sometimes resulting in thrombophlebitis after injection. Pretreatment with acetaminophen, antihistamines, and antiemetics may be provided to decrease these infusion-related adverse effects and thus make the duration of treatment more tolerable. Newer formulations of this drug—lipid-complexed agents—produce fewer complications. Amphotericin B has some annoying adverse effects, of which renal toxicity is the most common and also the most significant. Nearly 80% of patients treated with this drug experience renal impairment. Even after the drug is discontinued, impairment of glomerular filtration may remain.

Nystatin (Bio-Statin) is another polyene macrolide antibiotic, similar in structure to amphotericin, and it has the same mechanism of action.[92] Because it is poorly absorbed, its use is limited to *Candida* infections of the skin and GI tract. Oral administration may cause nausea, vomiting, diarrhea, and cramps, and topical application can lead to rash and urticaria. It is available as a lozenge for the treatment of oral candidiasis.[94]

Antifungal Azoles. Azoles inhibit ergosterol synthesis and interfere with the action of membrane-associated enzymes. They are a group of synthetic fungistatic agents with broad-spectrum activity.[92] Ketoconazole (Nizoraal), fluconazole (Diflucan), itraconazole (Sporanox), and miconazole (Micatin, Monistat-Derm) are mainly administered orally, although fluconazole and voriconazole are also available in IV forms. Miconazole, econazole (Spectazole), oxiconazole (Oxistat), sulconazole (Exelderm), and clotrimazole (Gyne-Lotrimin) are available in topical forms for use in the treatment of fungal skin infections and vaginal yeast infections.

Ketoconazole is a prototypical agent in this category, and it is used for treating serious, chronic, resistant mucocutaneous candidiasis, dermatophyte infections, and systemic infections, with the exception of fungal meningitis. Adverse effects include nausea, vomiting, photophobia, cardiac arrhythmias, rashes, hepatotoxicity, gynecomastia, and menstrual irregularities. Azoles also inhibit P450 enzymes and, in particular, decrease the metabolism and increase plasma concentrations of phenytoin, oral hypoglycemics, anticoagulants, and cyclosporine, leading to a number of drug-specific overdose reactions.

Allylamines. Terbinafine (Lamisil) also inhibits ergosterol synthesis by a different mechanism from that of azoles.[95,96] It is available as a topical cream, a gel, and a spray for the treatment of tinea pedis, tinea cruris, and tinea corporis. An oral formulation is available and is a popular mode for treating onychomycosis of the fingernails or toenails. It is quite lipophilic and therefore becomes concentrated in the dermis, epidermis, hair follicles, and adipose tissue within a few hours after oral administration. It enters the nail beds and distal nails, but this takes a few weeks. Treatment is required for 6 weeks for fingernail infections, and 12 weeks' treatment is needed for toenail infections.[97] After the drug is withdrawn, antifungicidal concentrations remain for several more weeks, reducing the chances of relapse. In a large clinical trial on onychomycosis and in a meta-analysis of randomized clinical trials, terbinafine demonstrated superior effectiveness compared with some other antifungal agents, including itraconazole.[94,95] Terbinafine also shows high efficacy in patients with high-risk conditions such as diabetes and those awaiting organ transplantations. In the treatment of tinea capitis, terbinafine was as effective in 4 weeks as griseofulvin (see following discussion on Other Antifungal Agents) was in 8 weeks.[98] The drug also works well when given in pulsed doses (administration of the drug for 1 week, followed by 3 weeks of no administration) for this condition. The cycle is repeated until the infection clears.[99] Adverse effects of terbinafine are mild but may include nausea, abdominal pain, and, less commonly, elevated liver enzyme levels. This drug is well tolerated, which is especially important, given the very long duration of treatment. Drugs with similar actions and profiles are butenafine (Mentax) and naftifine (Naftin).

Glucan Synthesis Inhibitors. Caspofungin (Cansidas), and micafungin (Mycarnine) are new drugs in a new category of antifungal agents called *echinocandins* or *glucan synthesis inhibitors*.[100] They act by inhibiting the synthesis of 1,3 β-glucan, a glucose polymer that is an important constituent in the fungal cell wall. This weakens the structure of the wall. These drugs are administered intravenously and are effective against candidiasis and some resistant forms of aspergillosis. Adverse effects are generally mild and reversible and include fatigue, vomiting, flushing, hypokalemia, eosinophilia, and proteinuria.

Other Antifungal Agents. Griseofulvin (Grisovin) is an oral, narrow-spectrum agent that acts by interfering with mitosis. It has been used to treat dermatophyte infections of the skin and nails and is the preferred agent for tinea capitis in children.[101,102] However, this drug is far from ideal. Tinea capitis requires treatment for 6 to 12 weeks, and some nail infections (tinea unguium, a dermatophyte infection of the nail) may require treatment for 12 to 24 months. In addition, relapse rates are high because the drug clears rapidly from the skin once it is discontinued.

Flucytosine (Ancobon) is another antifungal agent that is effective mostly against yeast infections.[93] Resistance is common with monotherapy, so it is often combined with amphotericin, particularly for treating cryptococcal meningitis. In fungal cells, flucytosine is converted to fluorouracil, which inhibits DNA synthesis. It is available in oral and IV forms. Infrequent adverse effects include GI disturbances, bone marrow depression, and alopecia.

Tolnaftate (Tinactin) is used topically and is available over the counter for treating a variety of minor skin problems. Its mechanism is unclear, but it seems to interfere with ergosterol synthesis.[102]

Therapeutic Concerns about Antifungal Agents

The main therapeutic concerns about antifungal agents are liver problems with elevated serum transaminase levels and renal damage. These concerns are especially important if patients are taking amphotericin B. An easy way to monitor for renal impairment is to have patients weigh themselves weekly and document any gain of more than 2 lb. Rapid weight gain may indicate retention of fluid caused by renal impairment.

Another general concern is the length of time required for treatment. Many patients have to take antifungal agents for 6 months to a year or longer, depending on the type of infection they have and their immune status. Continued motivation and diligence are often necessary for patients to complete the therapeutic protocol. Individuals who require IV medications spend a considerable amount of time with an infusion pump. The therapist must be sensitive to the psychosocial issues that may develop as a result of prolonged treatment and the impact they have on lifestyle.

ACTIVITIES 21

1. You are treating a patient with HIV for complaints of lower extremity weakness secondary to muscle wasting. The patient has a CD4 count of 250 and is currently taking Atripla (TDF + ETC + EFV).

Questions

A. Identify the individual drugs as well as their classification.
B. What are the adverse effects of these drugs?
C. Outline the patient's drug schedule.
D. What red flags should the therapist look for that warrant a call to the physician?
E. Are there any rehabilitative interventions that should be avoided when treating this patient?

2. The following are case vignettes of patients with HCV infection. Discuss the therapeutic options for treatment.

A. Mr. E. is a 40-year-old male who contracted HCV infection over 20 years ago, probably during a period of intravenous drug use. He received treatment for his addictions and has been clean and sober for the last 15 years. He reports experiencing fatigue but has no other specific complaints. Biopsy of his liver demonstrates moderate inflammation and fibrosis (3 out of a 4-point scale, with 0 being no fibrosis and 4 being cirrhosis).
B. Mr. J. is a 45-year-old construction worker who just found out that he is infected with HCV. He consumes large quantities of alcohol daily and has been in an alcohol detoxification unit at least two times in the past year. He refuses to go to AA (Alcoholics Anonymous) meetings. He also admits that during his drinking binges he had multiple sex partners, many of whom were prostitutes. Liver biopsy shows moderate inflammation, with level 3 fibrosis.
C. Ms. S. is a 45-year-old single mother with two young children. She contracted HCV (genotype 2) infection years ago in her teens from a blood transfusion. She has been asymptomatic for years but now complains of extreme fatigue and nausea. Her medical history is significant for chronic depression, and she is currently being treated with a selective serotonin reuptake inhibitor (SSRI). Her liver biopsy shows only minimal inflammation. She also works in the housekeeping department of a local hospital and has no family living close by.

3. What is meant by "boosted protease inhibitors"?

REFERENCES

1. Rang HP, Dale MM, Ritter JM, Moore JL, editors: Pharmacology (5th ed.), New York, 2003, Churchill Livingstone.
2. Lynch JP: Influenza and viral respiratory infections. In Waldman S, Terzic A, editors: Pharmacology and therapeutics: Principles to practice, Philadelphia, 2009, Saunders.
3. Smith AE, Helenius A: How viruses enter animal cells. Science 304(5668):237-242, 2004.
4. Alberts B, Bray D, Lewis J, Raff M, Roberts K, Watson JD: Molecular biology of the cell, New York, 1989, Garland Publishing, Inc.
5. Guidotti LG, Chisari FV: Noncytolytic control of viral infections by the innate and adaptive immune response. Annu Rev Immunol 19:65-91, 2001.
6. Biron CA, Nguyen KB, Pien GC, Cousens LP, Salazar-Mather TP: Natural killer cells in antiviral defense: Function and regulation by innate cytokines. Annu Rev Immunol 17: 189-220, 1999.
7. Tortorella D, Gewurz BE, Furman MH, Schust DJ, Ploegh HL: Viral subversion of the immune system. Annu Rev Immunol 18:861-926, 2000.
8. Polster BM, Pevsner J, Hardwick JM: Viral Bcl-2 homologs and their role in virus replication and associated diseases. Biochim Biophys Acta 1644(2-3):211-227, 2004.
9. Aoki FY, Rosser S: Drugs and viruses. In Page C, Curtis MJ, Sutter MC, Walker MJ, Hoffman BB, editors: Integrated pharmacology (2nd ed.), Philadelphia, 2002, Mosby.
10. Zelinskyy G, Dietze KK, Hüsecken YP, et al: The regulatory T-cell response during acute retroviral infection is locally defined and controls the magnitude and duration of the virus-specific cytotoxic T-cell response. Blood 114(15): 3199-3207, 2009.
11. Rothberg MB, Bellantonia S, Rose DN: Management of influenza in adults older than 65 years of age: Cost-effectiveness of rapid testing and antiviral therapy. Ann Intern Med 139(5): 321-329, 2003.
12. Couch RB: Prevention and treatment of influenza. N Engl J Med 343(24):1778-1787, 2000.
13. Deyde V, Garten R, Sheu T, et al: Genomic events underlying the changes in adamantane resistance among influenza A (H3N2). Influenza Other Respir Viruses 3(6):297-314, 2009.
14. Balfour HH: Antiviral drugs. N Engl J Med 340(16):1255-1268, 1999.
15. Krause I, Valesini G, Scrivo R, Shoenfeld Y: Autoimmune aspects of cytokine and anticytokine therapies. Am J Med 115(5):390-397, 2003.
16. Drugs for non-HIV viral infections. Med Letter Drugs Ther 44(1126):28, 2002.
17. McHutchison JG, Lawitz EJ, Shiffman ML, et al: Peginterferon alfa-2b or alfa-2a with ribavirin for treatment of hepatitis C infection. N Engl J Med 361:580-593, 2009.
18. Jordan I, Briese T, Fischer N, Johnson YL, Lipkin WI: Ribavirin inhibits West Nile virus replication and cytopathic effect in neural cells. J Infect Dis 182:1214-1218, 2000.
19. Garman E, Laver G: Controlling influenza by inhibiting the virus's neuraminidase. Curr Drug Targets 5(2):119-136, 2004.
20. 2009-10 Influenza ('Flu) Season (website). http://198.246.98.21/flu/about/season/current-season.htm. Accessed March 16, 2010.
21. Cooper NJ, Sutton AJ, Abrams KR, Wailoo A, Turner D, Nicholson KG: Effectiveness of neuraminidase inhibitors in treatment and prevention of influenza A and B: Systematic review and meta-analyses of randomised controlled trials. Br Med J 326(7401):1235, 2003.
22. Frieden TR: Swine flu virus (website). http://www.cdc.gov/media/transcripts/2009/t091030.htm. March 16, 2010.
23. International Committee on Taxonomy of viruses (website). http://www.ncbi.nlm.nih.gov/ICTVdb/Images/index.htm. Accessed March 16, 2010.

24. Grant AD, De Cock K: HIV infection and AIDS in the developing world. Br Med J 322:1475-1478, 2001.
25. Pham PA, Flexner CW: HIV infections and AIDS. In Waldman S, Terzic A, editors: Pharmacology and therapeutics: Principles to practice, Philadelphia, 2009, Saunders.
26. McCune JM: The dynamics of CD4+ T-cell depletion in HIV disease. Nature 410:974-979, 2001.
27. Mindel A, Tenant-Flowers M: Natural history and management of early HIV infection. Br Med J 322:1290-1293, 2001.
28. Weller IVD, Williams IG: Antiretroviral drugs. Br Med J 322:1410-1412, 2001.
29. Drugs for HIV infection. Treat Guidel Med Lett 2(17):1-8, 2004.
30. de Jong MD, de Boer RJ, de Wolf F, et al: Overshoot of HIV-1 viraemia after early discontinuation of antiretroviral treatment. AIDS11(11):F79-F84, 1997.
31. Liuzzi G, D'Offizi G, Topino S, et al: Dynamics of viral load rebound in plasma and semen after stopping effective antiretroviral therapy. AIDS 17(7):1089-1092, 2003.
32. SMART Study Group, El-Sadr WM, Grund B, Neuhaus J, et al: Risk for opportunistic disease and death after reinitiating continuous antiretroviral therapy in patients with HIV previously receiving episodic therapy: A randomized trial. Ann Intern Med 149(5):289-299, 2008.
33. Lipton SA: Neuronal injury associated with HIV-1: Approaches to treatment. Annu Rev Pharmacol Toxicol 38:159-177, 1998.
34. Kaul M, Garden GA, Lipton SA: Pathways to neuronal injury and apoptosis in HIV-associated dementia. Nature 410: 988-994, 2001.
35. Carr A, Emery S, Law M, et al: An objective case definition of lipodystrophy in HIV-infected adults: A case-control study. Lancet 361:726-735, 2003.
36. Carr A, Workman C, Careyk D, et al: No effect of rosiglitazone for treatment of HIV-1 lipoatrophy: Randomised, double-blind, placebo-controlled trial. Lancet 363:429-438, 2004.
37. Koutkia P, Grinspoon S: HIV-associated lipodystrophy: Pathogenesis, prognosis, treatment, and controversies. Annu Rev Med 55:303-317, 2004.
38. Havlir, DV. HIV Integrase inhibitors—Out of the pipeline and into the clinic. N Engl J Med. 359(4):416-418. 2008
39. Lalezari JP, Henry K, O'Hearn M, et al: Enfuvirtide, an HIV-1 fusion inhibitor, for drug-resistant HIV infection in North and South America. N Engl J Med 348(22):2175-2185, 2003.
40. Coovadia H: Antiretroviral agents: How best to protect infants from HIV and save their mothers from AIDS. N Engl J Med 351(3):289-292, 2004.
41. World Health Organization: Anti-retroviral regimens for the prevention of mother-to-child HIV-1 transmission: The programmatic implications. World Health Organization; 2000. (website). http://www.who.int/reproductive-health/rtis/MTCT/. Accessed March 31, 2005.
42. Lallemant M, Jourdain G, Le Coeur S, et al: Single-dose perinatal nevirapine plus standard zidovudine to prevent mother-to-child transmission of HIV-1 in Thailand. N Engl J Med 351(3):217-228, 2004.
43. Taha TE, Kumwenda NI, Hoover DR, et al: Nevirapine and zidovudine at birth to reduce perinatal transmission of HIV in an African setting. JAMA 292(2):202-209, 2004.
44. Deeks SG: Treatment of antiretroviral-drug-resistant HIV-1 infection. Lancet 362:2002-2011, 2002.
45. Clavel F, Hance AJ: HIV drug resistance. N Engl J Med 350(10):1023-1035, 2004.
46. Walmsley S, Bernstein B, King M, et al: Lopinavir-ritonavir versus nelfinavir for the initial treatment of HIV infection. N Engl J Med 346(26):2039-2046, 2002.
47. Robbins GK, De Gruttola V, Shafer RW, et al: Comparison of sequential three-drug regimens as initial therapy for HIV-1 infection. N Engl J Med 349(24):2293-2303, 2003.
48. Shafer RW, Smeaton LM, Robbins GK, et al: Comparison of four-drug regimens and pairs of sequential three-drug regimens as initial therapy for HIV-1 infection. N Engl J Med 349(24):2304-2315, 2003.
49. Skolnik PR: HIV therapy—What do we know, and when do we know it? N Engl J Med 349(24):2351-2352, 2003.
50. When To Start Consortium, Sterne JA, May M, Costagliola D, de Wolf F, et al: Timing of initiation of antiretroviral therapy in AIDS-free HIV-1-infected patients: A collaborative analysis of 18 HIV cohort studies. Lancet 373(9672):1314-1316, 2009.
51. AIDSinfo: A Service of the U.S. Department of Health and Human Services (website). http://www.aidsinfo.nih.gov/guidelines/. Accessed June 28, 2004.
52. Nieuwkerk PT, Sprangers M, Burger DM, et al: Limited patient adherence to highly active antiretroviral therapy for HIV-1 infection in an observational cohort study. Arch Intern Med 161:1962-1968, 2001.
53. Willig JH, Abroms S, Westfall AOC, et al: Increased regimen durability in the era of once-daily fixed-dose combination antiretroviral therapy. AIDS 22(15):1951-1960, 2008.
54. Hogg R: Early combination antiretroviral treatment of HIV infection adds decades of life. Lancet 372:266-267,293–299, 2008.
55. Oh J, Hegele RA: HIV-associated dyslipidaemia: Pathogenesis and treatment. Lancet Infect Dis 7(12):787-796, 2007.
56. Davison SP, Timpone J Jr, Hannan CM: Surgical algorithm for management of HIV lipodystrophy. Plast Reconstr Surg 120(7):1843-1858, 2007.
57. Roubenoff R, Weiss L, McDermott A, et al: A pilot study of exercise training to reduce trunk fat in adults with HIV-associated fat redistribution. AIDS 13(11):1373-1375, 1999.
58. Lucrecia T, Eduardo S, Ricardo S, Nicia BM, Jarbas O, Jorge P: Exercise training in HIV-1-infected individuals with dyslipidemia and lipodystrophy. Ribeiro Med Sci Sports Exerc 38(3):411-417, 2006.
59. Yarasheski KE, Tebas P, Stanerson B, et al: Resistance exercise training reduces hypertriglyceridemia in HIV-infected men treated with antiviral therapy. J Appl Physiol 90:133-138, 2001.
60. Jones SP, Doran DA, Leatt PB, Maher B, Pirmohamed M: Short-term exercise training improves body composition and hyperlipidaemia in HIV-positive individuals with lypodystrophy. AIDS 15:2049-2051, 2001.
61. Thoni GJ, Fedou C, Brun JF, et al: Reduction of fat accumulation and lipid disorders by individualized light aerobic training in human immunodeficiency virus infected patients with lipodystrophy and/or dyslipidemia. Diabetes Metab 28: 397-404, 2002.
62. Herrine SK, Rossi S, Navarro VJ: Infectious hepatitis. In Waldman SA, Terzic A, editors: Pharmacology and therapeutics: Principles to practice, Philadelphia, 2009, Saunders.
63. World Health Organization: Hepatitis B. Fact Sheets (website). http://www.who.int/mediacentre/factsheets/fs204/en/index.html. Accessed November 18, 2009.
64. Rotman Y, Brown TA, Hoofnagle JH: Evaluation of the patient with hepatitis B. Hepatology 49:S22-S27, 2009.
65. Lin KW, Kirchner JT: Hepatitis B. Am Fam Physician 69: 75-82, 2004.
66. Hoofnagle JH, Doo ET, Fleischer R, Lok ASF: Management of hepatitis B: Summary of a clinical research workshop. Hepatology 45:1056-1075, 2007.
67. Niederau C, Heintges T, Lange S, et al: Long-term follow-up of HBeAg-positive patients treated with interferon alfa for chronic hepatitis B. N Engl J Med 334(22):1422-1427, 1996.

68. Lok ASF, McMahon BJ: Chronic hepatitis B: Update of recommendations. Hepatology 39(3):857-861, 2004.
69. Qaqish RB, Mattes KA, Ritchie DJ: Adefovir dipivoxil: A new antiviral agent for the treatment of hepatitis B virus infection. Clin Ther 25(12):3084-3099, 2003.
70. Rivkin A: Adefovir dipivoxil in the treatment of chronic hepatitis B. Ann Pharmacother 38:625-633, 2004.
71. Hepatitis Foundation International Online Learning Center (website). http://www.hepfi.org/learning/library/seeff/seeff_natural_history.htm. Accessed March 17, 2010
72. Eisen-Vandervelde A, Yao ZQ, Hahn YS: The molecular basis of HCV-mediated immune dysregulation. Clin Immunol 111:16-21, 2004.
73. Penin F, Dubuisson J, Rey FA, Moradpour D, Pawlotsky JM: Structural biology of hepatitis C virus. Hepatology 39(1): 5-19, 2004.
74. Lauer GM, Walker BD: Hepatitis C virus infection. N Engl J Med 345(1):41-52, 2001.
75. Omata M, Yoshida H: Prevention and treatment of hepatocellular carcinoma. Liver Transpl 10(S2):S111-S114, 2004.
76. McHutchison JG, Gordon SC, Schiff ER, et al: Interferon alfa-2b alone or in combination with ribavirin as initial treatment for chronic hepatitis C. Hepatitis Interventional Therapy Group. N Engl J Med 338(21):1485-1492, 1998.
77. Davis GL, Esteban-Mur R, Rustgi VK, et al: Interferon alfa-2b alone or in combination with ribavirin for the treatment of relapse of chronic hepatitis C. N Engl J Med 339(21): 1493-1499, 1998.
78. Hoofnagle JH: A step forward in therapy for hepatitis C. N Engl J Med 360(18):1899-1901, 2009.
79. Ward RP, Kugelmas M, Libsch KD: Management of hepatitis C: Evaluating suitability for drug therapy. Am Fam Physician 69(6):1429-1436, 2004.
80. Hadziyannis SJ, Sette H, Morgan TR, et al: Peginterferon-alpha-2a and ribavirin combination therapy in chronic hepatitis C: A randomized study of treatment duration and ribavirin dose. Ann Intern Med 140(5):346-355, 2004.
81. Camma C, Di Bona D, Schepis F, et al: Effect of peginterferon alfa-2a on liver histology in chronic hepatitis C: A meta-analysis of individual patient data. Hepatology 39(2): 333-342, 2004.
82. McHutchison JG, Lawitz EJ, Shiffman ML, et al: Peginterferon Alfa-2b or alfa-2a with ribavirin for treatment of hepatitis C infection. N Engl J Med 361(6): 580-593, 2009.
83. Pawlotsky JM: The nature of interferon-[alpha] resistance in hepatitis C virus infection. Curr Opin Infect Dis 16(6): 587-592, 2003.
84. Howell CD, Dowling TC, Paul M, et al: Peginterferon pharmacokinetics in African American and Caucasian American patients with hepatitis C virus genotype 1 infection. Clin Gastroenterol Hepatol 6:575-583, 2008.
85. Ge D, Fellay J, Thompson AJ, et al: Genetic variation in IL28B predicts hepatitis C treatment-induced viral clearance. Nature 461(17):399-401, 2009.
86. Stringer WW: Mechanisms of exercise limitation in HIV+ individuals. Med Sci Sports Exerc 32(7):S412-S214, 2000.
87. Mackinnon LT: Chronic exercise training effects on immune function. Med Sci Sports Exerc 32(7):S369-S376, 2000.
88. Harrington D: Viral hepatitis and exercise. Med Sci Sports Exerc 32(7):S422-S430, 2000.
89. Kauffman CA: Fungal infections in older adults. Clin Infect Dis 33:550-555, 2001.
90. Lionakis MS, Kontoyiannis DP: Glucocorticoids and invasive fungal infections. Lancet 362:1828-1838, 2003.
91. Masuoka J: Surface glycans of Candida albicans and other pathogenic fungi: Physiological roles, clinical uses, and experimental challenges. Clin Microbiol Rev 17(2):281-310, 2004.
92. Lilley LL, Harrington S, Snyder JS, editors: Antifungal agents. In Pharmacology and the nursing process (4th ed.), St Louis, 2005, Mosby.
93. Linden PK: Amphotericin B lipid complex for the treatment of invasive fungal infections. Exp Opin Pharmacother 4(11):2099-2110, 2003.
94. Eggimann P, Garbino J, Pittet D: Management of Candida species infections in critically ill patients. Lancet Infect Dis 3:772-785, 2003.
95. Sigurgeirsson B, Billstein S, Rantanen T, et al: L.I.O.N. Study: Efficacy and tolerability of continuous terbinafine (Lamisil) compared to intermittent itraconazole in the treatment of toenail onychomycosis. Lamisil vs. itraconazole in onychomycosis. Br J Dermatol 141(suppl 56):5-14, 1999.
96. Evans EG, Sigurgeirsson B: Double blind, randomised study of continuous terbinafine compared with intermittent itraconazole in treatment of toenail onychomycosis. The LION Study Group. Br Med J 318(7190):1031-1035, 1999.
97. Haugh M, Helou S, Boissel JP, Cribier BJ: Terbinafine in fungal infections of the nails: A meta-analysis of randomized clinical trials. Br J Dermatol 147:118-121, 2002.
98. Chan YC, Friedlander SF: New treatments for tinea capitis. Curr Opin Infect Dis 17(2):97-103, 2004.
99. Gupta AK, Adam P: Terbinafine pulse therapy is effective in tinea capitis. Pediatr Dermatol 15:56-58, 1998.
100. Wong-Beringer A, Kriengkauykiat J: Systemic antifungal therapy: New options, new challenges. Pharmacotherapy 23(11):1441-1462, 2003.
101. Klastersky J: Empirical antifungal therapy. Int J Antimicrob Agents 23:105-112, 2004.
102. Hainer BL: Dermatophyte infections. Am Fam Physician 67:101-108, 2003.
103. Ryder NS, Frank I, Dupont MC: Ergosterol biosynthesis inhibition by the thiocarbamate antifungal agents tolnaftate and tolciclate. Antimicrob Agents Chemother 29(5):858-860, 1986.

22

Cytotoxic Agents and Immune Modulation

Lillian Pliner and Tracie Saunders

ETIOLOGY AND PATHOPHYSIOLOGY OF CANCER

Cancer encompasses more than 300 diseases that are characterized by cellular transformation and uncontrolled cellular growth, with the potential to invade surrounding tissue and metastasize to sites distant from the site of origin.[1] Some other terms (*neoplasm, malignancy*, and *tumor*) have been used interchangeably with the term *cancer*, but technically, they have different meanings.[2] *Neoplasms* and *tumors* both refer to masses of new cells that show unrestrained growth. A neoplasm can be either benign or malignant. Benign tumors tend to be solid or encapsulated and slow growing, and they show no tendency to metastasize but may still cause death by growing into or pressing against vital tissue. A malignant tumor, however, is different in that it invades surrounding tissues, has an unpredictable rate of growth, and spreads by either direct extension into surrounding tissues or through the lymphatic system or circulating blood. The process by which normal cells are transformed into cancer cells is called *carcinogenesis* or *tumorigenesis* and is considered to be a complex multistep process arising from a single normal cell that undergoes a transformation (Figure 22-1).

Tissue categories for tumors include carcinomas, sarcomas, leukemias, and tissue of neural origin (Box 22-1).[2] Identifying the tissue of origin is extremely important because it often determines the type of chemotherapy that will be effective. Carcinomas originate from epithelial tissue, which is the tissue that lines body surfaces. Examples include the skin, the mucosal lining of the gastrointestinal (GI) tract, and the bronchial lining in the lungs. Sarcomas arise from connective tissue, which is composed of bone, cartilage, muscle, and vascular structures. Nerve tumors consist of constituents of the nerve tissue and exist in the cells of the central nervous system (CNS) or peripheral nervous systems. Lymphomas come from lymphocytes of the immune system located in lymphatic tissue; and leukemias arise from the blood-forming cells of the marrow (hematopoietic progenitor cells). Collectively, these two types of neoplasms are also known as *hematologic malignancies* because they are diffuse and usually do not form a distinct solid tumor.

In addition to the signs and symptoms produced by the loss of a particular tissue from the invasion of cancerous cells, neoplastic tissue may cause symptoms far from the tumor or its site of metastasis.[2] These clinical manifestations are referred to as *paraneoplastic syndromes* and may include hypercalcemia and syndrome of inappropriate antidiuretic diuretic hormone secretion in lung cancer; disseminated intravascular coagulation in leukemia; Cushing's syndrome in small cell lung cancer, neural tumors, and pancreatic cancer; or paraneoplastic cerebellar degeneration in lung, ovarian, and breast cancers. These syndromes may be caused by biologically active substances, for example, hormones, secreted by the primary tumor. Patients who experience these symptoms usually experience relief when the cancer treatment has been successful.

Principles of Cancer Cell Growth

Neoplastic growths are initiated by a variety of factors. Extrinsic factors such as exposure to chemical carcinogens play a significant role in many cancers, as do intrinsic factors such as genetic predisposition. Oncogenes—DNA sequences that code for proteins involved in tumorigenesis—are also at play.[3] Oncogenes may be overexpressed and promote proliferation of a neoplasm once cell growth has been initiated. In addition, proliferation can proceed without difficulty as a result of mutations or loss of tumor suppressor genes such as the *p53* gene, mutated DNA repair genes, or overexposure of antiapoptotic proteins such as Bcl-2.[4,5] The *p53* gene is responsible for halting DNA replication and initiates apoptosis. Loss of this gene allows the damaged DNA to replicate. High levels of Bcl-2 immortalize cancer cells because there is re-expression of certain enzymes that are usually lost in normal cells with each growth cycle. A great deal of research on gene therapy is being conducted to find methods to enhance the suppressor genes and inhibit Bcl-2.[6]

Cell Growth Cycle. Cancer cells spread by directly invading surrounding tissue or by traveling through the lymphatic or vascular circulation. Cancer cells express collagenases and other activators that help the cells

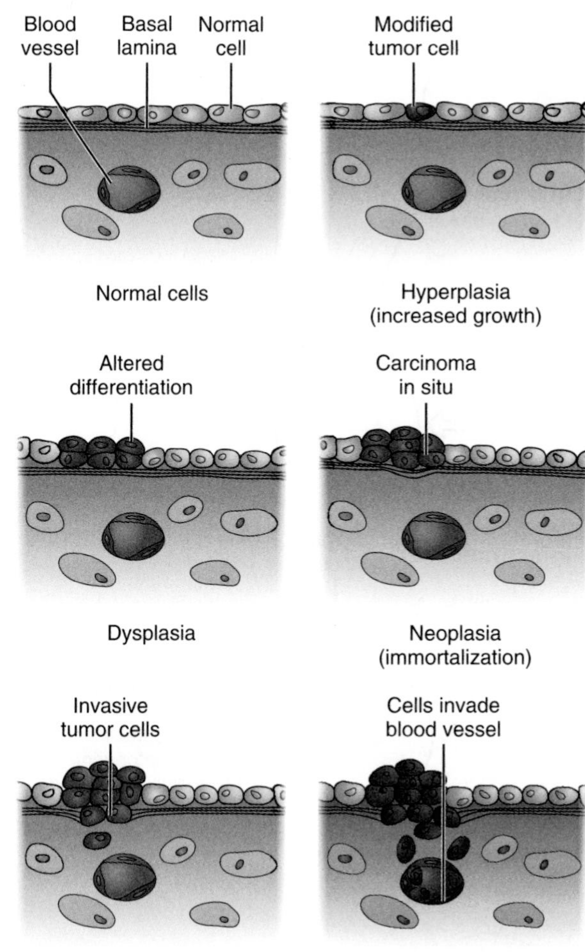

FIGURE 22-1 Hypothetical progression from normal to malignant cells.

BOX 22-1 Tumor Classification Based on Specific Tissue of Origin

Tissue of Origin	Malignant Tissue
Epithelial Carcinomas	
Glands or ducts	Adenocarcinomas
Respiratory tract	Small- and large-cell carcinomas
Kidney	Renal cell carcinomas
Skin	Squamous cell, epidermoid, and basal cell carcinoma; melanoma
Connective Tissue Sarcomas	
Fibrous	Fibrosarcoma
Cartilage	Chondrosarcoma
Bone	Osteogenic sarcoma (Ewing's tumor)
Blood vessels	Kaposi's sarcoma
Synovia	Synoviosarcoma
Mesothelium	Mesothelioma
Lymphatic Lymphomas	
Lymph tissue	Lymphomas (Hodgkin's disease and multiple myeloma)
Nerve	
Glial	Glioma
Adrenal medulla nerves	Pheochromocytoma
Blood	
White blood cells	Leukemia

From Lilley LL, Harrington D, Snyder JS, editors: *Pharmacology and the nursing process* (4th ed.), St Louis, 2005, Mosby.

move through tissues. Angiogenesis, the production of blood vessels supplying a tumor, is stimulated by factors such as vascular endothelial growth factor (VEG-F) and fibroblast growth factor, which helps create a scaffold that aids in the attachment of cells at metastatic sites. In addition, at any one time, neoplastic cells are actively dividing (progressing through a cell cycle period), differentiating, or at rest.

The process of cellular growth and reproduction has five distinct phases (Figure 22-2).[2] It occurs in both normal and malignant cells.

1. G0 is the resting stage, in which there is a temporary or permanent halt to cell proliferation. Since cells are not dividing in this phase, they are considered resistant to exposure from many chemotherapeutic agents.
2. G1 phase is the pre-DNA period, in which the proteins and RNA necessary for DNA production are synthesized.
3. S phase is when DNA synthesis occurs. During this time, the enzymes involved in DNA synthesis—DNA polymerase, RNA polymerase II, and topoisomerases I and II—become active. In addition, the enzymes involved in the folate pathway for purine and pyrimidine synthesis, such as dihydrofolate reductase, also become quite active.
4. G2 or the premitosis phase is when synthesis of the cellular and structural components needed for mitosis occurs. By the end of this phase, the usual numbers of chromosomes have doubled, and the cell is now prepared to actively divide.
5. The M phase (mitosis) is when cell division begins. This is the shortest phase of the cell life cycle and involves prophase, metaphase, anaphase, and telophase. At the conclusion of this phase, two daughter cells have been formed.

Each type of neoplastic cell runs through the cell cycle at a variable but rapid pace. Each phase takes only hours to complete (12 to 18 hours for some cells but as little as 1 to 2 hours for other cells). The entire cycle may take 48 to 72 hours. However, tumor growth is not linear. It has been described as "Gompertzian kinetics," which means that smaller tumors grow faster (exponentially) and larger tumors grow more slowly.[7]

CYTOTOXIC STRATEGY IN CANCER THERAPY

Knowledge of the cell cycle aids in identifying potential therapeutic agents that act on the cells during certain cycles of mitosis. Chemotherapy agents tend to be most

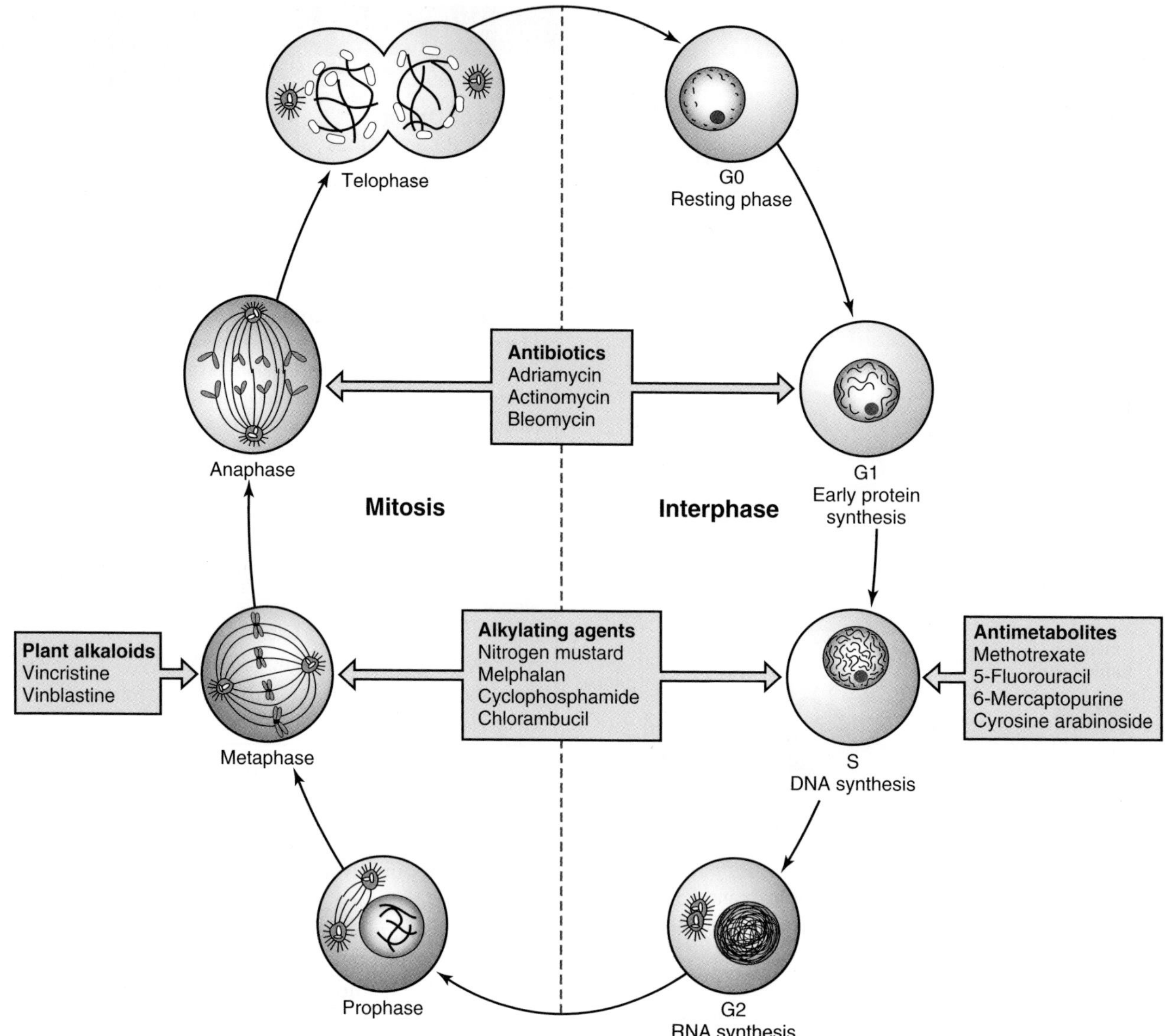

FIGURE 22-2 Phases of a cell cycle. Drugs are identified by where they exert their effects.

successful against cells that are cycling as opposed to those in the G0 stage at rest. Cell-cycle–specific (CCS) agents act on one particular phase of the cell cycle and have the greatest effect when given in divided but frequent doses or as a continuous infusion with a short cycle time.[8] These agents work more effectively on tumors with rapidly dividing cells. Cell-cycle–nonspecific (CCNS) agents act through the entire cycle, including the G0 resting phase.[8] These agents work more effectively on large slow-growing tumors and are given intermittently, allowing the patient to recover from dose-limiting toxicities.[8]

Chemotherapy agents kill a constant fraction of tumor cells with each treatment cycle.[1] This means that there will always be some cells that survive therapy. However, in theory, the idea is that each drug cycle will lower the tumor burden further so that eventually the patient's immune system can control the cancer. If the immune system cannot keep the cancer at bay, then the cells will continue to grow, although undetectably at first. This corresponds to the remission phase of cancer. By the time clinical symptoms recur or the tumor is detected, the tumor may have as many as 10^9 cells (about the size of a pea). Even if chemotherapy is resumed and is effective in killing 99.9% of cells, unfortunately there will still be plenty of cells left to multiply again. Hence, complete eradication of cancer cells is difficult.

CANCER THERAPY TREATMENT GOALS AND EVALUATION OF RESPONSE

The goals of cancer therapy include cure, control, and palliation. Cure refers to the "prolonged absence of detectable disease."[8] The combination of chemotherapy, biotherapy, radiation, and/or surgery is used when cure is the goal. Adjuvant therapy is offered to treat minimal disease or micrometastases in patients at high risk for recurrence. It is generally offered after a primary treatment modality such as surgery or radiation has been offered. Neoadjuvant therapy is offered prior to surgery or other treatment modalities to shrink the primary tumor and thus improve surgical resection and/or to decrease the likelihood of micrometastases.

Control or palliation therapy is offered when the possibility of a cure is not present. Control allows an extension of life when cure becomes an unrealistic goal. Therapy is geared toward the prevention of the growth of new cancer cells, even though complete elimination of the disease is not possible. Palliation refers to providing comfort to the patient when neither cure nor control is possible. Palliation therapies decrease tumor burden, improve quality of life, and relieve pain.

Therapy Response

There are several factors which affect an individual's response to therapy. The amount of tumor burden and the rate of tumor growth are important features which affect response. An inverse relationship exists between the number of tumor cells and the response to therapy, which implies that the smaller the tumor, the higher is the rate of response. Chemotherapeutic agents are more effective on rapidly growing tumors. Combinations of several chemotherapeutic agents with different mechanisms of action are superior to single-agent therapy because there is an increase in the number of cells killed at any given time. Combination chemotherapy may also use the principle of drug synergy to maximize the effects of another drug.[8] For example, leucovorin potentiates the cytotoxicity of 5-fluorouracil (5-FU). Delays in treatment or dose reductions may also have a negative impact on patient survival.

Tumor response is evaluated by objectively measuring the presence, reduction, or progression of the disease. This can be achieved by physical examination, surgery, radiologic examinations, and endoscopic or laparoscopic visualization. Serum or urine tumor markers may also be used to assist in this process. Common criteria used to evaluate radiologic response include Response Evaluation Criteria in Solid Tumors (RECIST). RECIST provides a consistent way to measure response to therapy. A complete response (CR) is the disappearance of all target lesions and no evidence of disease. A partial response (PR) is a 30% decrease in the sum of the longest diameter of the targeted lesions as compared with baseline. Progressive disease (PD) is at least a 20% increase in the longest diameter of the targeted lesion since the initiation of therapy or the appearance of one or more new lesions. Tumor markers that had been elevated prior to therapy should decrease significantly as the tumor responds positively to therapy.

CONSEQUENCES OF CANCER THERAPY

Chemotherapy targets cells that undergo extremely rapid cell division. However, the drugs are not selectively toxic because cancer cells are not the only actively proliferating cells in the human body. They affect the bone marrow, GI tract and buccal mucosa, reproductive organs, and hair follicles.[7] Hence, the adverse effects of most agents used for treating cancer include myelosuppression, more commonly known as bone marrow suppression (resulting in anemia, leukopenia, and thrombocytopenia); nausea and vomiting; diarrhea; stomatitis; amenorrhea with possible ovarian failure; lowered sperm count; and hair loss. These toxicities occur early in treatment and are generally reversible when treatment is discontinued and may be dose limiting. The gonadal dysfunction may or may not be reversible but tends to be less severe in prepubertal children. However, male patients at puberty are more susceptible than any other patient group. Chemotherapy agents may also produce secondary cancers later on. Specifically, a group of drugs called *alkylating agents* may produce hematopoietic malignancies. This is because these drugs cause permanent genetic mutations.

Contraindications for all cancer drugs include a very low white blood cell count, active infection, and poor nutritional or hydration status. The time at which white blood cells reach their lowest levels is called the *nadir* and may occur from 10 to 28 days after chemotherapy. Anticancer agents are withheld at this time, and the patient may be given prophylactic antibiotics and also special growth factors (see discussion of hematopoietic agents and stem cell replacement).

RESISTANCE TO CANCER THERAPY

Preventing drug resistance is one of the primary justifications for combination chemotherapy.[8] Resistance to chemotherapy may occur for several reasons. Cancer cells may inherently be resistant to chemotherapeutic agents or develop resistance over time when exposed to these agents. Cancer cells may produce abnormal transport mechanisms, resulting in decreased uptake of the drug.[9] Another transport problem that may occur is the development of an efflux pump.[10] This is a transport mechanism that pumps the drug out of the cell and is responsible for much of the multidrug-resistant cancers. If the drug makes it into a cell, enzymes may metabolize it to inactive forms. Enhanced DNA repair inside the cancer cell is another means by which carcinoma may develop resistance to chemotherapy.

In addition, some cancers are innately difficult to treat because of their locations. Brain cancers are more difficult to treat with chemotherapy because the drug must penetrate the blood–brain barrier. The testes represent another difficult area to treat because this tissue tends to be acidic, causing the drugs to become ionized, which decreases diffusion across the membranes. These areas are sometimes called *pharmacologic sanctuaries*.

CHEMOTHERAPY (ANTINEOPLASTIC) DRUG CLASSES

Drugs are classified according to their pharmacologic actions or their effects on cell reproduction. The major chemotherapy drug classes include alkylating agents, antimetabolites, antitumor antibiotics, hormonal therapies, mitotic spindle inhibitors, and various miscellaneous agents.

Alkylating Agents

The first class of drugs used to treat cancer comprises alkylating agents. These drugs are antineoplastics that are effective at various stages in the cell growth cycle, although they are most effective against rapidly growing cancer as well as rapidly growing normal body cells. Since they do not rely on the cell cycle to be effective, they are considered *cell cycle nonspecific*.

These agents work by one of three different mechanisms, all of which ultimately result in the disruption of DNA function and cell death. These agents covalently bind to DNA by nucleophilic substitution with an alkyl group (saturated carbon atom, for example, see Chapter 3) (Figure 22-3). Normally, the two DNA strands are linked together by the nucleic bases (adenine [A], guanine [G], thymine [T], or cytosine [C]) through covalent hydrogen bonds forming the molecular bridge between strands. The presence of an alkyl group, however, creates an abnormal chemical bond between adjacent DNA strands. These DNA cross-links are considered to be another classic characteristic of this drug class. Since alkylating agents chemically alter DNA, they are mutagenic. Therefore this class of agents can induce cancers that may not show up until years after exposure. The three categories of alkylating agents are classic alkylators (nitrogen mustards), nitrosoureas, and a group of probable alkylators (Table 22-1).

Class Alkylators. The most common subgroup of alkylating agents comprises nitrogen mustards. Mechlorethamine is a derivative of nitrogen mustard, which was originally discovered during World War I when mustard gas was used for chemical warfare. It is part of the MOPP (mechlorethamine, oncovorin, prednisone, and procarbazine) regimen for the treatment of Hodgkin's disease. Cyclophosphamide is among the most commonly used alkylating agents because it can be given orally as well as intravenously. Ifosfamide is a similar drug that has a longer half-life but is only available for parenteral administration.[11] A toxic metabolite of this drug is eliminated in the urine but not before it has caused damage to the bladder. Adequate hydration and intravenous injection of MESNA (sodium 2-mercaptoethane sulfonate) help inactivate the compound. MESNA binds to the irritant metabolites in the bladder to prevent cystitis.

Nitrosoureas. Carmustine and lomustine are nitrosoureas that act similar to classic alkylators by cross-linking strands of DNA to inhibit DNA and RNA replication. The cytotoxicity of these agents is greatest during cell division. These drugs are able to penetrate the CNS and attack brain tumors because of their lipid solubility properties.

Probable Alkylators. Cisplatin and carboplatin are heavy metals or platinum compounds that do not have an actual alkylating portion to their active molecule. These drugs are categorized as alkylating agents because both bind to purine bases in DNA and form intrastrand links.[12] The result is an unwinding of the DNA helix and ultimate cell inactivation. Carboplatin is better tolerated than cisplatin because it is associated with less vomiting.

The most common adverse effects of alkylating agents are related to the hematopoietic system causing myelosuppression (neutropenia, thrombocytopenia, and anemia). Myelosuppression is often dose dependent and cumulative. Nadir counts vary among agents; agents administered intravenously may reach the nadir within 1 to 2 weeks, whereas with oral alkylating agents, the nadir does not occur until 3 to 6 weeks. GI toxicities

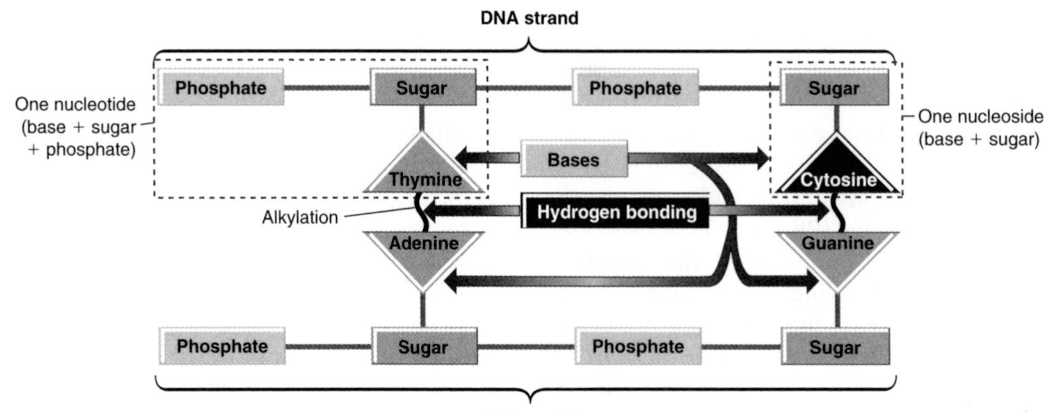

FIGURE 22-3 Organization of DNA and site of action of alkylating agents. *(From Lilley LL, Harrington D, Snyder JS, editors:* Pharmacology and the nursing process *(5th ed.), St Louis, 2007, Mosby.)*

such as nausea, vomiting, diarrhea, and mucositis are also drug and dose dependent. Other common adverse effects include alopecia, nephrotoxicity, ototoxicity, and peripheral neuropathy.

Antimetabolites

Antimetabolites are drugs that interfere with the formation of key biomolecules within the cell, including nucleotides, which are the building blocks of DNA. These drugs ultimately interfere with DNA replication and therefore cell division. Chemotherapeutic antimetabolites are cell-cycle–specific agents that imitate the actions of substances necessary for the synthesis of DNA, RNA, and protein. These agents are most effective against tumors that have a high growth rate and have several different cellular targets. The three classes are folate antagonists, purine antagonists, and pyrimidine antagonists (see Table 22-1).

Folate antagonists inhibit dihydrofolate reductase (DHFR), an enzyme involved in the formation of nucleotides. When this enzyme is blocked, nucleotides are not formed, which disrupts DNA replication and cell division. Methotrexate is the primary folate antagonist used as a chemotherapeutic agent. It may be used alone or in combination with other anticancer drugs. Leucovorin calcium (a lesser form of folic acid) is administered to protect normal cells from the antagonistic action of the drug, thus reducing toxicities to the patient. Purine antagonists function by inhibiting the production of the purine-containing nucleotides adenine and guanine. If a cell does not have sufficient amounts of purines, DNA synthesis is halted, and the cell cannot divide. In addition, it may be incorporated into the DNA molecule during DNA synthesis, which further interferes with cell division. Pyrimidine antagonists are thymidylate synthase inhibitors, which block DNA synthesis. Some of the pyrimidine has demonstrated activity in all of the phases of cell cycle activity. Toxicities vary, depending on the drug and the dose; however, myelosuppression is a common adverse effect of all of the antimetabolites, as are mucositis, diarrhea, nausea, vomiting, neurotoxicity, and nephrotoxicity.

Antitumor Antibiotics

Cytotoxic antibiotics are cell-cycle–nonspecific agents, although one phase may be favored over another, depending on the drug.[2] Most of these drugs act by intercalation, involving the insertion of the drug between the two strands of DNA. Specifically, a cytotoxic antibiotic binds to the base pairs, causing the DNA helix to assume an unstable structure. Many of these agents are topoisomerase II inhibitors. Topoisomerases are a group of enzymes that regulate the topologic (twisting and winding) state of a DNA double-strand molecule around itself. Topoisomerase enzymes are vital to DNA and RNA transcription and replication.[13] Doxorubicin and daunorubicin are examples of two antitumor antibiotics (see Table 22-1).

This class of drugs has vesicant properties and should be administered with extreme caution. Extravasation and tissue necrosis may occur if these agents leak from a vein into the subcutaneous tissue. Toxicities may be life threatening; cardiac tissue is extremely vulnerable to the iron-binding effect of these agents. The recommendation for total lifetime cumulative dose of doxorubicin is 400 mg/m2.[8] Doxorubicin is now available in a liposomal drug delivery system, which reduces systemic effects and increases the duration of action. Myelosuppression is to be expected and is often a dose-limiting factor when administering these agents. Other common adverse effects include nausea, vomiting, mucositis, alopecia, and what is known as "radiation recall phenomenon." In addition, these drugs may produce darkening of the palms and soles of the feet and a red discoloration of urine.

Hormone Therapy

Many tumors arise in organs or tissues that are hormone sensitive, that is, they may regress when a hormone is administered or when a hormone's action is blocked. Such cancers include those of the breast, ovary, endometrium, and prostate. The strategy in the treatment of these cancers is to reduce or block the source of the hormone or the receptor site where the hormone is active. An example is estrogen-sensitive breast cancer. To maintain the growth of the breast cancer, a supply of estrogen is needed. When a drug is given to block estrogen receptors, the tumor shrinks. In general, these drugs are more selective and less toxic than other chemotherapeutic agents.

Antiestrogen Therapy (Tamoxifen, Raloxifene). Tamoxifen is a mixed estrogen antagonist and agonist.[14] Tamoxifen binds to estrogen receptors and blocks estrogen activation in the breast. The result is a decrease in growth factors involved in the proliferation of breast tissue and an increase in certain antiproliferative proteins. Tamoxifen offers palliation and tumor regression in advanced metastatic disease and may produce a cure when given along with other agents in the early stages of the disease. In addition, tamoxifen has been shown to significantly reduce the incidence of breast cancer in women who are at high risk for the disease.[15] An advantage to the use of this drug is that it also produces estrogen-like effects in bone, so osteoporosis is not a problem with long-term treatment. Common adverse effects include nausea, irregular menstruation, vaginal bleeding, and menopausal symptoms such as hot flashes. In addition, there is a small increase in the risk of endometrial cancer because tamoxifen is an estrogen agonist in the uterus. Tamoxifen is also associated with a greater risk of venous thrombosis (see Chapters 13 and 14), so it is not given with to patients with cerebrovascular disease or

Text continues on page 392

TABLE 22-1 Chemotherapeutic Agents

Medication	Mechanism of Action	Cell Cycle Phase	Administration Route	Indications	Side Effects	Rehab Implications
Alkylating Agents – Classic Alkylators						
Mechlorethamine (nitrogen mustard, Mustargen®)	Blocks DNA replication and RNA transcription through alkylation; produces breaks in DNA as well as cross-linking of twin strands	Non-specific	Intravenous	Palliative treatment for Hodgkin's/Non-Hodgkin's lymphoma, chronic lymphocytic leukemia (CLL), chronic myeloid leukemia (CML), mycosis fungoides, bronchogenic carcinomas, polycythemia vera	Severe nausea, vomiting, anorexia, altered taste, bone marrow depression, pain at IV site, neurotoxicity, weakness, alopecia, hyperuricemia, ototoxicity, and gonadal atrophy	Acute nausea occurs within 30 minutes to 3 hours of infusion; the drug is a vesicant; health care providers must be protected from inadvertent contact; severe blistering occurs with contact to skin; bone marrow suppression places patients at risk for infection, bleeding, bruising; wash hands meticulously before caring for patients with low white blood cell (WBC) counts; limit activities for patients with platelets <50,000; assess numbness, tingling, decreased sensation of fingers and toes
Cyclophosphamide (Cytoxan®) Noncytotoxic form of nitrogen mustard	Similar activity to nitrogen mustard; transformed via liver enzymes to an active alkylating agent; prevents cell division by cross-linking DNA strands blocking replication		Oral, intravenous	Hodgkin/Non-Hodgkin's lymphoma, acute myeloid leukemia (AML), acute lymphocytic leukemia (ALL), CML, CLL, multiple myeloma, breast cancer, ovarian cancer, myeloma, neuroblastoma, retinoblastoma, mycosis fungoides, Ewing's sarcoma	Bone marrow depression, nausea, vomiting, alopecia, facial flushing and nasal stuffiness during infusion, hyperurecemia, hemorrhagic cystitis	Since the drug is not active when administered, it is not a vesicant; causes bladder irritation, so patients should be asked to void frequently to prevent hemorrhagic cystitis; bone marrow suppression places patients at risk for infection, bleeding, bruising; wash hands meticulously before caring for patients with low WBC counts; limit activities for patients with platelets <50,000
Ifosfamide (Ifex®) Nitrogen mustard derivative	Structurally similar to cyclophosphamide but has a longer half-life		Intravenous	3rd-line treatment for germ cell testicular cancer, Non-Hodgkin's lymphoma, sarcomas, leukemias	Bone marrow depression, nausea, vomiting, neurotoxicity, aloepecia, hemorrhagic cystitis; rare CNS toxicity	Toxic metabolite of the drug is eliminated in urine (acrolein); to prevent hemorrhagic cystitis, adequate hydration and IV MESNA are given to help inactivate the compound; bone marrow suppression places patients at risk for infection, bleeding, bruising; wash hands meticulously before caring for patients with low WBC counts; limit activities for patients with platelets <50,000; assess for changes in mentation which may be early sign of CNS toxicity; supervise ambulation, and ensure side rails of bed are up

Mephalan (Alkeran®) Derivative of mechlorethamine	Interferes with DNA replication and RNA transcription	Non-specific	Oral, intravenous	Hodgkin disease, CML, palliative care for multiple myeloma	Hypersensitivity, bone marrow depression, mild nausea, vomiting, bleeding, alopecia, hyperpigmentation of skin, mouth sores, gonadal atrophy, hyperuricemia	Bone marrow suppression places patients at risk for infection, bleeding, bruising; wash hands meticulously before caring for patients with low WBC counts; limit activities for patients with platelets <50,000
Chlorambucil (Leukeran®) Derivative of mechlorethamine	Bifunctional alkylating agent, closely related to mephalan in structure; displays a somewhat selective lympholytic action		Oral	CLL, Hodgkin's/non-Hodgkin's lymphoma	Bone marrow depression, nausea, vomiting, hyperuricemia, pulmonary fibrosis, seizures	Least toxic of alkylating agents; contraindicated in patients with history of seizure disorders; bone marrow suppression places patients at risk for infection, bleeding, bruising; wash hands meticulously before caring for patients with low WBC counts; limit activities for patients with platelets <50,000
Alkylating Agents – Nitrosoureas						
Carmustine (BCNU®) Lomustine (CCNU®)	Cross-link strands of DNA to inhibit DNA and RNA replication; highly lipid soluble so cross blood–brain barrier	Non-specific	Intravenous, Wafer, oral	Brain tumors, Hodgkin's/non-Hodgkin's lymphoma, CNS and multiple myeloma	Bone marrow depression, nausea, vomiting, pain at injection site, hepatic toxicity, pulmonary fibrosis, neurotoxicity	Bone marrow suppression places patients at risk for infection, bleeding, bruising; wash hands meticulously before caring for patients with low WBC counts; limit activities for patients with platelets <50,000; hyperpigmentation occurs if drug directly touches the skin; asses for shortness of breath (SOB), tachypnea, and nonproductive cough, which are early signs of pulmonary toxicity
Probable Alkylators						
Cisplatin	Platinum-containing inorganic compounds, which act as alkylating agents; primary mechanism is to cross-link DNA	Non-specific	Intravenous	Head and neck, testicular, ovarian, cervical cancers. Off-label uses include treatments for endometrial cancer, non–small cell lung cancer, and small cell lung cancer.	Bone marrow depression, nausea, vomiting, bleeding, alopecia, hyperpigmentation of skin, mouth sores, gonadal atrophy, hyperuricemia	Bone marrow suppression places patients at risk for infection, bleeding, bruising; wash hands meticulously before caring for patients with low WBC counts; limit activities for patients with platelets <50,000; assess for numbness, tingling, and decreased sensation of fingers and toes; assess for tinnitus and loss of balance
Carboplatin (Paraplatin®)	Platinum-containing inorganic compounds, which act as alkylating agents; primary mechanism is to cross-link DNA	Non-specific	Intravenous	Advanced ovarian cancer; off-label use includes treatments for endometrial cancer, non–small cell lung cancer, head and neck cancer, small cell lung cancer, and refractory acute leukemia	Bone marrow depression, nausea, vomiting, hyperuricemia, pulmonary fibrosis, seizures, mild peripheral neuropathies	Least toxic of alkylating agents; contraindicated in patients with history of seizure disorders; bone marrow suppression places patients at risk for infection, bleeding, bruising; wash hands meticulously before caring for patients with low WBC counts; limit activities for patients with platelets <50,000

Continued

TABLE 22-1 Chemotherapeutic Agents—cont'd

Medication	Mechanism of Action	Cell Cycle Phase	Administration Route	Indications	Side Effects	Rehab Implications
Antimetabolites – Folate Antagonists						
Methotrexate (Mexate®, Folex®, Rheumatrex®)	Inhibits enzyme dihydrofolate reductase (DHFR), which results in inhibition of DNA, RNA, and protein synthesis	Specific	Oral, intravenous, intramuscular, intrathecal	ALL, meningeal leukemia, lung, breast, and head and neck cancers, mycosis fungoides, non-Hodgkin's lymphoma, choriocarcinoma, osteogenic sarcoma; off-label use in bladder cancer	Bone marrow depression, nausea, vomiting, oral or gastrointestinal (GI) ulcerations, renal toxicity, neurotoxicity, liver toxicity, photosensitivity, rash, joint pains	Bone marrow suppression places patients at risk for infection, bleeding, bruising; wash hands meticulously before caring for patients with low WBC counts; limit activities for patients with platelets <50,000; patients require aggressive hydration to prevent renal toxicity; patients must stay out of the sun while receiving this medication; monitor for CNS changes
Pemetrexed (Alimta®)	Inhibits folate-dependent metabolic processes involved in the formation of thymidine and purine nucleotides which are essential for cell replication		Intravenous	Locally advanced or metastatic non–small cell lung cancer; in combination with cisplatin for malignant pleural mesothelioma	Bone marrow depression, fatigue, nausea, vomiting, chest pain, SOB, anorexia, stomatitis, diarrhea	Patients must be on vitamin supplementation with folic acid and vitamin B_{12} to reduce treatment related toxicities; bone marrow suppression places patients at risk for infection, bleeding, bruising; wash hands meticulously before caring for patients with low WBC counts; limit activities for patients with platelets <50,000
Antimetabolites – Purine Antagonists						
Fludarabine (Fludara®)	Inhibits DNA synthesis inhibiting DNA polymerase and ribonucleotide reductase	Specific	Intravenous	CLL; off-label use includes treatments for mycosis fungoides, non-Hodgkin's lymphoma, multiple myeloma, melanoma	Bone marrow depression, nausea, vomiting, bleeding, neurotoxicity, interstitial pneumonitis, diarrhea, tumor lysis syndrome	Bone marrow suppression places patients at risk for infection, bleeding, bruising; wash hands meticulously before caring for patients with low WBC counts; limit activities for patients with platelets <50,000; assess for SOB and nonproductive cough; monitor for numbness and tingling of fingers and toes; monitor for CNS changes
Cladribine (Leustatin®)	Phosphorylated to a 5'triphosphate derivative, which incorporates into susceptible cells; results in strand breaks and shutdown of DNA synthesis			Hairy cell leukemia; off-label use includes treatment for non-Hodgkin's lymphoma, CLL, Waldenstrom macroglobulinemia	Bone marrow depression, nausea, vomiting, hypersensitivity, neurotoxicity	Bone marrow suppression places patients at risk for infection, bleeding, bruising; wash hands meticulously before caring for patients with low WBC counts; limit activities for patients with platelets <50,000; may suffer from fatigue; exercise routines should be designed to provide frequent rest and conserve energy

Clofarabine (Clolar®)	Inhibits DNA synthesis by reducing cellular deoxynucleotide triphosphate collection through the inhibition of ribonucleotide reductase; inhibits DNA repair			Treatment of pediatric patients 1to 21 years old with relapse or refractory ALL after at least two prior regimens	Bone marrow suppression, nausea, vomiting, alopecia, cardiac toxicity, hepatobiliary toxicity, nephrotoxicity, capillary leak syndrome	
Antimetabolites – Pyrimidine Antagonists						
Cytrabine (cytosine arabinoside, ARA-C, Cytosar-U®)	Targets and kills cells undergoing DNA synthesis (S phase); inhibits DNA polymerase		Intravenous, intramuscular, intrathecal, subcutaneous	ALL, CML, meningeal leukemia; off-label use includes treatments for non-Hodgkin's lymphoma, MDS, and carcinomatous meningitis	Bone marrow depression, nausea, vomiting, mucositis, diarrhea, pruritus, CNS toxicity may be fatal.	Bone marrow suppression places patients at risk for infection, bleeding, bruising; wash hands meticulously before caring for patients with low WBC counts; limit activities for patients with platelets <50,000; assess for SOB and nonproductive cough; monitor for CNS changes; patients may have vision changes; patients may experience hypersensitivity reactions
Cytrabine liposomal (DepoCyt®) Formulation of cytrabine with sustained release properties	Converted to cytrabine-5'-triphosphate; interferes with cell division during S phase	Specific	Intrathecal	Lymphomatous meningitis	Nausea, vomiting, fever, back pain, confusion, headache	Patients must be on vitamin supplementation with folic acid and vitamin B_{12} to reduce treatment related toxicities; follow treatment implications for cytrabine–ARA-C as well
Fluorouracil (5-fluorouracil, 5-FU, Adrucil®)	Inhibition of DNA synthesis and RNA formation as a result of a decrease in thymine, resulting in cell death	Specific	Intravenous, topical	Cancers of colon, rectum, breast, stomach, pancreas, and head and neck; off-label use includes treatment for esophageal cancer	Bone marrow depression, nausea, vomiting, anorexia, diarrhea, mucositis, alopecia, photosensitivity, darkening of veins, nail changes	Bone marrow suppression places patients at risk for infection, bleeding, bruising; wash hands meticulously before caring for patients with low WBC counts; limit activities for patients with platelets <50,000; may suffer from fatigue; exercise routines should be designed to provide frequent rest and conserve energy; monitor for CNS changes; skin pigmentation may darken along vein or nails may darken; patients must stay out of sun while receiving medication

Continued

TABLE 22-1 Chemotherapeutic Agents—cont'd

Medication	Mechanism of Action	Cell Cycle Phase	Administration Route	Indications	Side Effects	Rehab Implications
Capecitabine (Xeloda®)	Prodrug of 5′-deoxy-5-fluorouridine, which is converted to 5-FU in vivo; inhibits DNA synthesis and RNA formation resulting in a decrease in thymine which is essential for DNA synthesis		Oral	Metastatic breast cancer, metastatic colon cancer	Diarrhea, hand-foot syndrome, nausea, vomiting, anemia, mucositis, increases in bilirubin	Severe diarrhea may result causing electrolyte imbalances; palmar–plantar erythrodysesthesia (hand-foot syndrome) may occur, causing painful erythema, blistering, and desquamation of the hands and feet; follow treatment implication for 5-FU as well
Floxuridine phosphate (FUDR®)	Inhibits DNA polymerase and ribonucleotide reductase resulting in inhibition of DNA synthesis		Intravenous	CLL; off-label use includes treatments for mycosis fungoides, multiple myeloma, melanoma, pancreatic care, hairy cell leukemia, non-Hodgkin's lymphoma	Bone marrow depression, nausea, vomiting, anorexia, darkening of the veins, hand-foot syndrome, abdominal pain, gastritis, hepatotoxicity	Bone marrow suppression places patients at risk for infection, bleeding, bruising; wash hands meticulously before caring for patients with low WBC counts; limit activities for patients with platelets <50,000; patient may suffer from fatigue; exercise routines should be designed to provide frequent rest and conserve energy
Gemcitabine (Gemzar®)	Converts to two metabolites intracellularly (gemcitabine diphosphate and gemcitabine triphosphate) both of which inhibit DNA synthesis; cell-cycle specific for S phase and G1/S phase boundary	Specific	Intravenous	1st line for locally advanced/metastatic pancreatic cancer, non–small cell lung cancer, metastatic breast cancer, advanced ovarian cancer	Bone marrow suppression, nausea, vomiting, rash, elevated liver function tests, cardiovascular events, rarely hemolytic uremia	Bone marrow suppression places patients at risk for infection, bleeding, bruising; wash hands meticulously before caring for patients with low WBC counts; limit activities for patients with platelets <50,000; patient may suffer from fatigue; exercise routines should be designed to provide frequent rest and conserve energy; may cause edema of the lower extremities; assess for shortness of breath, tachypnea, and hypertension

Antitumor Antibiotics						
Mitomycin (Mutamycin®)	Antibiotic produced from *Streptomyces caespitosus;* inhibits DNA synthesis	Non-specific	Intravenous	Pancreatic, gastric carcinoma; off-label use includes treatments for breast, bladder, colorectal, lung, head and neck, and cervical cancers, and CML	Bone marrow suppression, nausea, vomiting, anorexia, alopecia, mucositis, nephrotoxicity, pulmonary toxicity, fatigue, permanent sterility, peripheral neuropathy	Vesicant; health care providers must be protected from inadvertent contact, as severe blistering occurs with contact to skin; monitor for CNS changes; causes acute nausea and vomiting 1–2 hours after administration; assess for numbness and tingling of the fingers and toes; bone marrow suppression places patients at risk for infection, bleeding, bruising; wash hands meticulously before caring for patients with low WBC counts; limit activities for patients with platelets <50,000; patient may suffer from fatigue; exercise routines should be designed to provide frequent rest and conserve energy
Bleomycin (Blenoxane®)	Exact mechanism unknown; thought to bind to DNA thereby inhibiting DNA and RNA synthesis		Intravenous, subcutaneous, intramuscular, intracavitary	Testicular cancer, squamous cell cancer of head and neck, Hodgkin's and non-Hodgkin's lymphoma, cervical and vulvar cancers; off-label use includes treatments for Kaposi's sarcoma, soft-tissue sarcomas, endometrial, ovarian, bladder, and skin cancers	Pulmonary toxicity, hypersensitivity reactions, alopecia, photosensitivity, renal toxicity, pulmonary fibrosis, fever, chills	Assess for SOB, tachypnea, and nonproductive cough, which are early signs of pulmonary toxicity; may cause hypersensitivity reaction, so test dose is given before administration of scheduled dose
Dactinomycin (Actinomycin D®, Cosmegen®)	A product of *Streptomyces parvulus*; binds with DNA resulting in inhibition of DNA and RNA synthesis	Non-specific	Intravenous	Ewing's sarcoma, Wilm's tumor, testicular cancer, rhabdomyosarcoma, trophoblastic tumors, Kaposi's sarcoma, osteosarcomas	Bone marrow suppression, nausea, vomiting, alopecia, diarrhea, ovarian or sperm suppression, radiation recall, hypersensitivity reactions, alopecia, rashes	Vesicant; healthcare providers must be protected from inadvertent contact; severe blistering occurs with contact to skin; may cause severe nausea and vomiting within 2–5 hours of administration; monitor for CNS changes

Continued

TABLE 22-1 Chemotherapeutic Agents—cont'd

Medication	Mechanism of Action	Cell Cycle Phase	Administration Route	Indications	Side Effects	Rehab Implications
Antitumor Antibiotics – Anthracyclines						
Doxorubicin HCL (Adriamycin®, Rubex®)	Inhibition of DNA and RNA synthesis; inhibits the enzyme topoisomerase II; also intercalculation between base pairs in the DNA double helix	Non-specific	Intravenous	Breast, ovarian, prostate, stomach, small cell lung, and liver cancers, multiple myeloma, Hodgkin disease, non-Hodgkin's lymphoma, ALL, AML, Wilm's tumor	Bone marrow suppression, nausea, vomiting, alopecia, mucositis, dose-limiting cardiotoxicity, hand-foot syndrome, drug may cause the urine to turn red, ovarian or sperm suppression	Vesicant; health care providers must be protected from inadvertent contact; severe blistering occurs with contact to skin; bone marrow suppression places patients at risk for infection, bleeding, bruising; wash hands meticulously before caring for patients with low WBC counts; limit activities for patients with platelets <50,000; patient may suffer from fatigue; exercise routines should be designed to provide frequent rest and conserve energy; may see hand-foot syndrome in patients receiving Doxil®; assess for signs and symptoms of congestive heart failure; weight gain, lower extremity edema, SOB; urine may turn red 1–2 days after administration of the medication
Doxorubicin liposomal (Doxil®) Incorporates a polyethylene glycol derivative around a liposomal-coated core of doxorubcin	Inhibition of DNA and RNA synthesis; inhibits the enzyme topoisomerase II			AIDS-related Kaposi's sarcoma; off-label use includes treatments for metastatic breast and ovarian cancers		
Epirubicin (Ellence®)	Binds with DNA, thereby inhibiting DNA and RNA replication and transcription			Breast cancer		
Daunorubicin (Cerubidine®, Daunomycin®)	Interferes with DNA synthesis by binding to nucleic acids			ALL in adults, ALL in children		

Daunorubicin citrate liposomal (DaunoXome®) Aqueous solution of the citrate salt of daunorubicin encapsulated with liposomes	Interferes with DNA synthesis; liposomal formulation assists with protecting the encapsulated daunorubicin from chemical and enzymatic degradation			AIDS-related Kaposi's sarcoma		
Anti-tumor Antibiotics – Anthracyclines						
Idarubicin (Idamycin®)	Inhibition of DNA and RNA synthesis; interacts with the enzyme topoisomerase II	Non-specific	Intravenous	Acute non-lymphocytic leukemia, ALL in children	Bone marrow suppression, nausea, vomiting, alopecia, mucositis, dose-limiting cardiotoxicity, hand-foot syndrome, drug may cause the urine to turn red, ovarian or sperm suppression	Follow treatment implications for other antitumor antibiotics
Mitotic Spindle Inhibitors – Vinca Alkaloids						
Vinblastine (Velban®)	Acts late in G2 phase by binding to tubulin inhibits microtubule assembly blocking DNA production, and in M phase preventing cell division	Specific	Intravenous	Testicular cancer, Hodgkin's disease, non-Hodgkin's lymphoma, Kaposi's sarcoma, breast cancer	Bone marrow suppression, anorexia, peripheral neuropathy, constipation, paralytic ileus, anorexia	Irritant; may cause local irritation at injection site; use warm compresses to relieve pain; bone marrow suppression places patients at risk for infection, bleeding, bruising; wash hands meticulously before caring for patients with low WBC counts; limit activities for patients with platelets <50,000; may suffer from fatigue; exercise routines should be designed to provide frequent rest and conserve energy; assess for numbness and tingling of fingers and toes; may see changes in gait
Vincristine (Oncovin®)				Hodgkin's disease, non-Hodgkin's lymphoma, CML, ALL, sarcoma, breast cancer, small cell lung cancer, neuroblastoma, Wilm's tumor	Peripheral neuropathy, alopecia, constipation, paralytic ileus	

Continued

TABLE 22-1 Chemotherapeutic Agents—cont'd

Medication	Mechanism of Action	Cell Cycle Phase	Administration Route	Indications	Side Effects	Rehab Implications
Vinorelbine (Navelbine®)				Non–small cell lung cancer and breast cancer	Bone marrow suppression, alopecia, bronchospasms, fatigue, peripheral neuropathy, fatigue, shortness of breath	Follow treatment implications for other vinca alkaloids. Vesicant – Healthcare providers must be protected from inadvertent contact. Severe blistering occurs with contact to skin. May see changes in gait.
Mitotic Spindle Inhibitors – Taxanes						
Paclitaxel (Taxol®)	Stabilizes microtubules, inhibiting cell division; effective in G2 phase and M phase	Specific	Intravenous	Metastatic breast cancer, ovarian, non–small lung cancer and head and neck cancers; AIDS-related Kaposi's sarcoma	Bone marrow suppression, alopecia, peripheral neuropathy, hypersensitivity reaction, facial flushing, myalgia, fatigue, cardiac arrhythmias, fatigue, mucositis, diarrhea	Monitor for CNS changes; assess for numbness and tingling of fingers and toes; patient may experience acute hypersensitivity reactions
Paclitaxel protein-bound particles; albumin bound (Abraxane™)	Stabilizes microtubules, inhibiting cell division; effective in G2 phase and M phase	Specific	Intravenous	Metastatic breast cancer after failure of combination chemotherapy or relapse within 6 months of adjuvant therapy	Bone marrow suppression, neuropathy, myalgia, arthralgia, nausea, vomiting, aloepecia, mucositis	Bone marrow suppression places patients at risk for infection, bleeding, bruising; wash hands meticulously before caring for patients with low WBC counts; limit activities for patients with platelets <50,000; patient may suffer from fatigue; exercise routines should be designed to provide frequent rest and conserve energy
Docetaxel (Taxotere®)	Promotes the assembly and blocks the disassembly of microtubules, which prevents cancer cell division, causing cell death			Breast cancer, gastric cancer, prostate cancer, non–small cell lung cancer, head and neck cancer, and metastatic ovarian cancer	Alopecia, fluid retention, hypersensitivity reaction, nausea, vomiting, paresthesia, skin and nail changes	Follow treatment implications for paclitaxel; monitor for signs and symptoms of fluid retention i.e., swelling of lower extremities, hands and fingers; monitor for SOB during ambulation

Mitotic Spindle Inhibitors – Epipodophyllotoxin Derivatives						
Etoposide (VP16, VePesid®, Etopophos)	Induces irreversible blockage of cells in premitotic phases of cell cycle (late G2 and S phases); interferes with topoisomerase II enzyme reaction	Specific	Intravenous, oral	ALL, breast and testicular cancer, small-cell lung cancer, Hodgkin's disease, non-Hodgkin's lymphoma, multiple myeloma, Bone Marrow Transplant (BMT)	Bone marrow suppression, nausea, vomiting, alopecia, anorexia, orthostatic hypotension, hyperuricemia, hypersensitivity reaction, anaphylaxis, mucositis, diarrhea	Bone marrow suppression places patients at risk for infection, bleeding, bruising; wash hands meticulously before caring for patients with low WBC counts; limit activities for patients with platelets <50,000; patient may suffer from fatigue; exercise routines should be designed to provide frequent rest and conserve energy; monitor for signs and symptoms of pulmonary toxicity.
Teniposide (VM-26, Vumon®)	Causes single and double strand breaks in DNA preventing DNA synthesis; interferes with topoisomerase II enzyme reaction		Intravenous	Childhood ALL	Bone marrow suppression, hypotension, pulmonary toxicity, anaphylaxis, nausea, vomiting	
Mitotic Spindle Inhibitors – Topoisomerase-1 Inhibitors (Camtothecins)						
Irinotecan (Camptosar®)	Acts in S phase; inhibits topoisomerase I; causes double-strand DNA changes	Specific	Intravenous	Metastatic colorectal cancer	Diarrhea, bone marrow suppression, alopecia	Bone marrow suppression places patients at risk for infection, bleeding, bruising; wash hands meticulously before caring for patients with low WBC counts; limit activities for patients with platelets <50,000; patient may suffer from fatigue; exercise routines should be designed to provide frequent rest and conserve energy
Topotecan (Hycamtin®)				Metastatic ovarian cancer, small cell lung cancer	Bone marrow suppression, diarrhea, alopecia, nausea, vomiting, headache	

hypertension. Tamoxifen is not routinely given to premenopausal women because natural estrogen competes with tamoxifen for receptors, which will limit the drug's effectiveness.

Raloxifene is a compound similar to tamoxifen except that it is also an estrogen antagonist in endometrial tissue.[16] It is currently used to prevent postmenopausal osteoporosis but is also under study for the treatment of breast cancer. Initial studies show a reduction in new breast cancers by 50%, but further studies are needed to compare it with tamoxifen.

Aromatase Inhibitors (Exemestane, Letrozole). Postmenopausal women continue to have circulating estrogen levels even after the ovaries have shut down.[2] Estrogen is derived from the conversion of adrenal androstenedione and testosterone to estrone in the adrenal glands and fatty tissue by the aromatase enzyme. In many patients with breast cancer, aromatase activity is increased, which, in turn, is responsible for higher estrogen levels.

Aromatase inhibitors are generally nonsteroidal competitive inhibitors of the aromatase enzyme.[17] Reduction in this enzyme leads to reduced estrogen levels. Ongoing studies show that these drugs may be equivalent to tamoxifen as first-line therapy.[18,19] Adverse effects are fairly mild and include hot flashes, skin rashes, nausea, fatigue, headache, and dizziness.

Luteinizing Hormone–Releasing Hormone Agonists and Gonadotropin-Releasing Hormone Agonists. Leuprolide and goserelin are analogs of luteinizing hormone–releasing hormone (LHRH) and gonadotropin-releasing hormone (GRH), respectively.[2] These hormones control the secretion of luteinizing hormone (LH) and follicle-stimulating hormone (FSH) to stimulate sex hormone production in the testes and ovaries. FSH and LH are initially released, but continued dosing produces a drop in their levels. The result is regression of hormone-dependent tumors of the prostate, breast, endometrium, and ovaries. Adverse drug reactions are equivalent to those of menopause or castration. Both sexes experience hot flashes, weight gain, GI disturbances, osteoporosis, and loss of libido and muscle mass. Men experience erectile dysfunction and women breast atrophy and vaginitis. A flare-up of prostate cancer symptoms may occur initially and cause urinary retention.

Antiandrogens (Flutamide). Flutamide competitively inhibits binding of testosterone to androgen receptors in the testes and prostate gland. It is used in conjunction with leuprolide or goserelin in the treatment of prostate cancer. Adverse drug reactions include gynecomastia and GI discomfort.

Prednisone. Steroids (glucocorticoids, not anabolic steroids) can induce remission in acute lymphocytic leukemia and Hodgkin's and non-Hodgkin's lymphomas.[2] In particular, prednisone slows lymphocytic growth, produces lymphocytopenia, and reduces lymphoid tissue. Other steroids, such as dexamethasone, are used in cancer treatment to prevent extravasation injury during IV infusion of chemotherapeutic agents, to prevent hypersensitivity reactions to these drugs, and to retard emesis. Prednisone is also useful in reducing cerebral edema from a growing brain tumor or from edema induced by radiation.

Mitotic Spindle Poisons (Tubulin-Binding Agents)

Drugs in this category originate largely from plants: vinca alkaloids (vinblastine, vincristine, and vinorelbine) come from the periwinkle plant; epipodophyllotoxin derivatives (etoposide and teniposide) are semisynthetic derivatives from extracts of the mandrake plant; and taxanes (paclitaxel and docetaxel) are derived from the bark of the Western (Pacific) yew tree. In general, they are cell-cycle–specific agents working before and during mitosis to inhibit cell division. Vinca alkaloids are vesicants (see Table 22-1).

Vinca Alkaloids. Vinca alkaloids bind to the protein tubulin during the metaphase of mitosis.[20] Tubulin is a major protein that helps form the intracellular skeleton of the mitotic spindle. Binding to this protein prevents formation and assembly of the microtubules, and without mitotic spindles, cell division cannot proceed. Spindle disassembly is also promoted.

These agents can cause phlebitis or cellulitis if extravasation occurs during injection. Nausea, vomiting, diarrhea, and alopecia occur with both drugs; however, surprisingly, vincristine is not too myelosuppressive. All are extremely neurotoxic, producing paresthesias, painful peripheral neuropathy, loss of reflexes, foot drop, wrist drop, and ataxia. Specifically, these agents induce a nociceptor hyperresponsiveness to both heat and mechanical stimulation.[21] They may also induce the syndrome of inappropriate antidiuretic hormone secretion.

Epipodophyllotoxin Derivatives. Epipodophyllotoxin derivatives include etoposide and teniposide. These drugs are believed to kill cancer cells in the late S phase and the G2 phase of the cell cycle. Adverse effects include the usual GI and myelosuppressive symptoms, as well as liver and kidney toxicities.

Taxanes. Taxanes are a group of chemotherapy agents, including paclitaxel and docetaxel. Paclitaxel was originally isolated from the Western yew tree in 1958. However, because of purification and formulation problems, it did not reach the pharmacy until 25 years later; it is now made synthetically. This agent blocks cell growth by stopping mitosis. It binds to microtubules, but instead of promoting disassembly of the mitotic spindle like the vinca alkaloids, it promotes stability.[20,22] However, the result is the same in that the mitotic spindle becomes nonfunctional.

Common adverse effects are similar to other chemotherapeutic agents. However, these drugs may also produce neuropathic pain and peripheral neuropathy, which are common with cumulative doses and usually resolve after discontinuation of the medication. Paclitaxel is insoluble in water, so it must be emulsified in a substance called *Cremophor*. Anaphylactic reactions may result from the use of Cremophor in some individuals (dyspnea, chest pain, bronchospasm, urticaria, and hypotension); pretreatment with glucocorticosteroids and antihistamines can prevent this reaction.

Topoisomerase-1 Inhibitors (Camptothecins)

Topoisomerase-1 inhibitors are a newer class of chemotherapy agents consisting of two agents, topotecan and irinotecan.[23] Both are semisynthetic analogs of camptothecin, which was originally isolated from a shrub native to China. These drugs are cell-cycle–specific agents and bind to the DNA–topoisomerase-1 complex during the S phase. Normally, this complex creates temporary strand cleavage and then reattachment, which is necessary for the unwinding of DNA. Both drugs are used primarily to treat ovarian or colorectal cancers. Common adverse effects are similar to those of other chemotherapeutic agents and include GI disturbance and bone marrow depression. Irinotecan, in particular, is associated with severe diarrhea, which may occur acutely during drug infusion or may be delayed, beginning 2 to 10 days after infusion. The diarrhea can be quite severe and even life threatening. Aggressive treatment with atropine (acute) or loperamide (delayed) is necessary.

Miscellaneous Chemotherapeutic Agents

A variety of chemotherapeutic agents do not fall within the structural or mechanistic categories outlined previously but, nevertheless, are strong contenders in the fight against cancer.

Imatinib. Imatinib is a fairly new drug, approved for use as a chemotherapeutic agent by the U.S. Food and Drug Administration (FDA) in 2001.[24] It is primarily indicated for the treatment of chronic myelogenous leukemia (CML). CML results from a mutation in a pluripotent stem cell expressing a chromosome identified as the Philadelphia chromosome (a translocation of chromosomes 9 and 22, resulting in a shortened chromosome 22). This mutation produces progressive granulocytosis, marrow hypercellularity, and splenomegaly. CML is usually diagnosed in the chronic or stable phase, but within 4 to 6 years, an accelerated phase that leads to a fatal acute leukemia may occur. An accumulation of molecular abnormalities leads to the loss of terminal differentiation into a mature myeloid cell, and, instead, immature or blast cells are released from the bone marrow. Until now, treatment has consisted of stem cell transplantation and administration of hydroxyurea (a chemotherapeutic agent that closely resembles antimetabolite antineoplastics) or interferon (IFN); however, the cure rate with this treatment has been still less than 20%.[25]

The translocation of chromosomes produces a tyrosine kinase fusion gene called *BCR-ABL*, which phosphorylates proteins that drive cellular proliferation.[24] Imatinib inhibits *BCR-ABL*–mediated transfer of phosphate to its substrates. This drug is one of the first in a series of agents developed to target specific proteins expressed by human cancers. Imatinib inhibits or kills proliferating myeloid cell lines containing the *BCR-ABL* gene but with little harm to normal cells. In a group of 532 patients with CML in the chronic phase with whom IFN treatment had previously failed, 88% experienced a complete clinical response, and 30% experienced a complete genetic response.[26-28] Sixty-three percent of patients given imatinib during the accelerated phase of CML also demonstrated response to the drug, with 28% achieving a complete hematologic response and 14% achieving a complete genetic response. Patients in blast crisis did not fare as well, although 19% reverted to the chronic phase. Median duration of response in the chronic phase was 1 month; 6 months of treatment was necessary for patients in the accelerated phase. Adverse effects included nausea (55 to 68%), vomiting (28 to 54%), and diarrhea (33 to 49%). Edema—in the form of pleural effusion, ascites, or pulmonary edema—has also been reported, as well as neutropenia and thrombocytopenia, but these adverse effects were much less frequent than GI disturbances.

Combination Therapy

Most chemotherapy often consists of combinations of two or more drugs that are used together. Combinations of drugs have been proved to be better than single agents for treating most cancers, and a survival advantage has been shown when combinations are administered simultaneously rather than sequentially. When designing combination chemotherapy regimens, the drugs used in the combination protocols must show individual activity against the cancer in question and preferably not have overlapping toxic effects. A common protocol used for lymphoma is CHOP: *c*yclophosphamide, *h*ydroxydaunomycin (doxorubicin), *o*ncovin (vincristine), and *p*rednisone. Cyclophosphamide is an alkylating agent whose major toxic effects are myelosuppression and bladder irritation. Hydroxydaunomycin (doxorubicin) is an antibiotic whose major toxic effects are myelosuppression and cardiac toxicity. Oncovin (vincristine) is a vinca alkaloid with peripheral nerve toxicity but little myelosuppression (tubulin-binding drug). Prednisone shrinks lymphoid tissue; it has no myelosuppression but affects glucose metabolism and bone matrix formation. Other non–marrow-suppressive drugs, such as methotrexate with leucovorin rescue, may also be used with the CHOP protocol when blood cell counts are low. The reader should be aware that more than 200 drug combinations have been developed by oncologists.

Examples of other common drug combinations include the following:

MOPP (mechlorethamine/oncovin/procarbazine/prednisone)
CMF (cyclophosphamide/methotrexate/fluorouracil)
CAF (cyclophosphamide/doxorubicin/fluorouracil)

TUMOR IMMUNOTHERAPY

As knowledge of the immune system has grown, efforts have been directed at using the patient's own immune system for the destruction of cancer. Active immunotherapy refers to the administration of agents that mimic or enhance a patient's immune response (by giving IFNs and interleukins [ILs]) to recognize tumor-specific antigens. Passive immunotherapy involves giving active immunologic agents that can directly produce tumor regression. These agents include tumor vaccines, monoclonal antibodies (MABs), adoptive transfer of cytotoxic cells, and genetic manipulation. At this time, the majority of these interventions are either at their earliest stage of development or are experimental; nevertheless, they represent a new class of anticancer drugs called *biologic response modifiers*.[2] The current subclasses of biologic response modifiers include hematopoietic agents, IFNs, MABs, and ILs.

Normal Immune System

Although the immune system has been covered in various chapters in this text, a review at this point will be helpful and assist the reader in understanding biologic response modifiers. The immune system is vitally important in helping the body distinguish between self and an invading virus or bacterium.[2] However, even though tumors are not really foreign invaders, they may have undergone significant differentiation and may no longer resemble the cells from which they originated. Tumor cells also express markers on their surfaces that signal impending danger to the immune system. These chemical markers are called *tumor antigens*, and they label the cancer as non-self.

The major components of the immune system originate from the pluripotent stem cell and consist of humoral immunity, which is mediated by B cells producing antibodies, and cell-mediated immunity, which is mediated by T cells (Figure 22-4). Cytokines (IFNs and ILs) produced by T cells represent the specialized chemical communication system between the two components that fosters synchronization and coordination.

The humoral immune system has as its main component B lymphocytes, also known as *B cells*, which originate from bone marrow. When an antigen is detected, B cells mature into plasma cells, which then produce antibodies that bind to the antigen, inactivating it (Figure 22-5). B cells also produce memory cells that "study" the exact nature of the foreign invader, so the next time exposure to the antigen occurs, the system can launch a faster and stronger immune response.

The cell-mediated immune system consists of T lymphocytes, also known as *T cells* because they mature in the thymus. There are three main types of T cells: (1) cytotoxic T cells, which kill their targets by causing cell lysis; (2) T suppressor cells, which work in opposition to the cytotoxic cells to limit the actions of the immune system; and (3) T helper cells, the masters or directors of the entire system. T helper cells initiate the actions of other components of the immune system, such as lymphokines and cytotoxic T cells. Lymphokines are a subset of the cytokines produced by T lymphocytes. Through lymphokines, T cells help B cells to produce immunoglobulin G (IgG), activate monocytes, directly kill target cells, and mobilize the inflammatory response (Figure 22-6). The healthy individual has about two times as many T helper cells as T suppressor cells. There is speculation that an abundance of T suppressor cells permits tumor growth.

Additional cells of the immune system that function as active cancer killers include macrophages, neutrophils (polymorphonuclear leukocytes), lymphokine-activated killer cells, and natural killer (NK) cells.[29] NK cells contain perforin (a pore-forming protein), serine proteases, and other enzymes capable of lysing tumor cells. Lymphokine-activated killer cells are capable of lysing some tumors resistant to NK cells. Macrophages possess

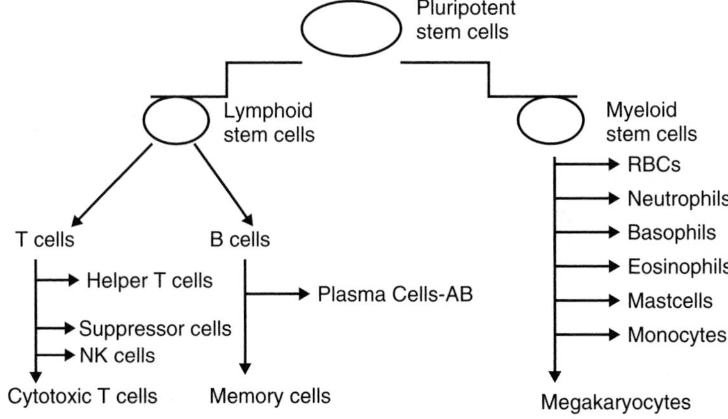

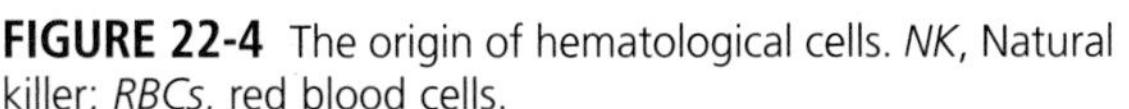
FIGURE 22-4 The origin of hematological cells. *NK*, Natural killer; *RBCs*, red blood cells.

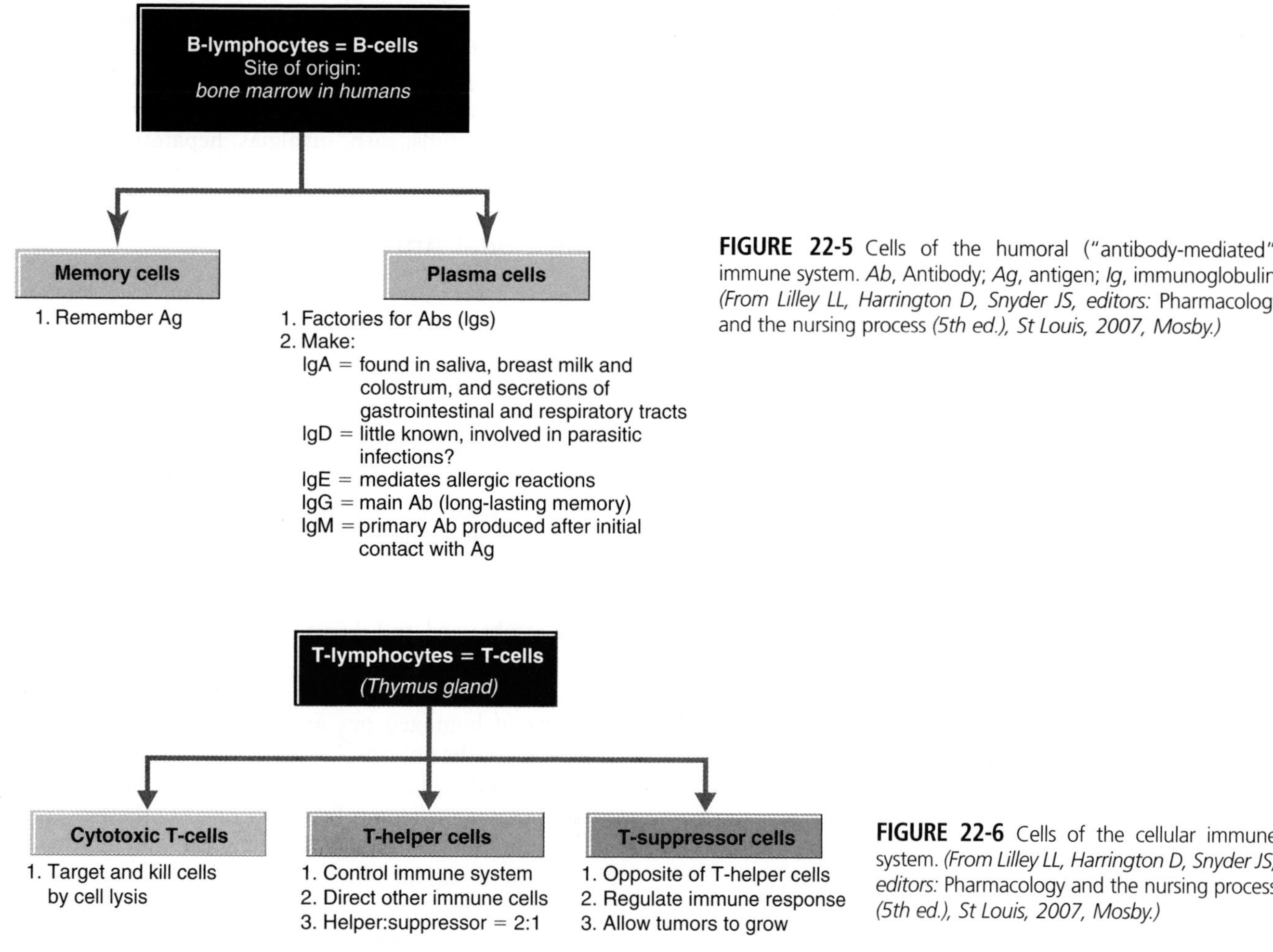

FIGURE 22-5 Cells of the humoral ("antibody-mediated") immune system. *Ab*, Antibody; *Ag*, antigen; *Ig*, immunoglobulin. *(From Lilley LL, Harrington D, Snyder JS, editors:* Pharmacology and the nursing process *(5th ed.), St Louis, 2007, Mosby.)*

FIGURE 22-6 Cells of the cellular immune system. *(From Lilley LL, Harrington D, Snyder JS, editors:* Pharmacology and the nursing process *(5th ed.), St Louis, 2007, Mosby.)*

some toxic properties, are capable of producing cytokines, and are also the cells that "present antigen to lymphocytes." Activation of many of these cells comes from the cytokines—ILs and IFNs.

Interferons

IFNs are proteins that have antiviral, antitumor, and immunomodulating properties (Box 22-2).[2] There are three types of IFNs: alpha (α), beta (β), and gamma (γ). The alpha subtype, from leukocytes, is used in the treatment of viral infections; the beta subtype is used in the treatment of multiple sclerosis; and the gamma subtype, produced by the cells of the immune system, is proinflammatory. In terms of designating IFNs, the word *alfa* is synonymous with the Greek letter *alpha* and seems to be used more frequently in clinical contexts.

The exact mechanism of action of IFNs in cancer is not known. Possibilities include oncogene modulation and activation of immune host defenses, resulting in an increase in cytotoxic T cells, helper T cells, NK cells, and antigen-presenting cells. IFN-α also has antiangiogenic effects on tumor endothelial cells by inhibiting fibroblast growth factors.

IFNs can be produced from genetically modified *Escherichia coli* bacteria by using recombinant DNA technology. There are currently six IFN-alfas, two IFN-betas, and one IFN-gamma. Specifically, IFNs involved in cancer treatment are the IFN-alfas: IFN-α_{2a}, pegIFN-α_{2a}, IFN-α_{2b}, pegIFN-α_{2b}, IFN-α_{n3}, and IFN-$\alpha_{con\text{-}1}$. As described in Chapter 20, "peg" refers to the IFN's attachment to hydrocarbon polyethylene glycol (PEG). This attachment reduces its antigenicity and prolongs its therapeutic effect.

In terms of chemotherapy, IFN-α_{2a} and IFN-α_{2b} have been used to treat hairy-cell leukemia and AIDS-related Kaposi's sarcoma. IFN-α_{2a} has also been used to treat chronic myelogenous leukemia, and IFN-α_{2b} has been

BOX 22-2 Interferon: Current FDA-Approved Indications

Antiviral Uses (Type of Interferon)
Condylomata acuminata (genital warts: HPV)
Hepatitis (alfa-2a*, alfa-2b*, alfacon-1)

Antineoplastic Uses (Type of Interferon)
Chronic myelogenous leukemia (α_{2a})
Follicular lymphoma (α_{2b})
Hairy-cell leukemia (α_{2a}, α_{2b})
Kaposi's sarcoma (α_{2a}, α_{2b})
Malignant melanoma (α_{2b})

Other Immunomodulatory Uses (Type of Interferon)
Chronic granulomatous disease (γ_{1b})
Multiple sclerosis (β_{1a}, β_{1b})
Osteopetrosis (γ_{1b})

From Lilley LL, Harrington D, Snyder JS, editors: *Pharmacology and the nursing process* (4th ed.), St Louis, 2005, Mosby.
FDA, U.S. Food and Drug Administration; *HPV*, human papilloma virus.
*Including pegylated dosage forms (pegIFNs).

used in the treatment of malignant melanoma and certain lymphomas. Adverse effects of these drugs include fever, chills, myalgias, headache, fatigue, neutropenia, GI disturbances, and elevated liver enzyme levels. Other adverse effects include cardiovascular (tachycardia, orthostatic hypotension, electrocardiographic [ECG] changes) and CNS disturbances (confusion, poor concentration, seizures, paranoid psychoses).

Interleukins

ILs are soluble proteins released from activated lymphocytes, especially NK cells. There are many different ILs (IL-2 through IL-8, IL-10, and IL-12), and more are being recognized as knowledge of the immune system grows. There are currently four ILs commercially available—three that are IL-2, which are used in cancer treatment, and a fourth, anakinra, which is, in fact, an IL-1 receptor blocker that is used in the treatment of rheumatoid arthritis.

The most widely used IL is aldesleukin. This is an IL-2 analog that binds to T-cell receptors to induce a differentiation into lymphokine-activated killer cells in the blood- and tumor-infiltrating lymphocytes in specific tumors. It may be used in the treatment of metastatic renal cell carcinoma in high or low doses. It is currently under investigation for use in the treatment of breast, ovarian, colon, brain, head and neck, and lung cancers.

Aldesleukin is associated with a syndrome known as *capillary leak syndrome*. This is a condition in which capillaries allow colloids, albumin, and other proteins to leak out of the vasculature. The result of this movement creates fluid overload in the surrounding tissues. Massive fluid retention can lead to respiratory distress, heart failure, and myocardial infarction (MI). These effects are reversible if the drug is promptly discontinued. Close patient monitoring is necessary, and visible edema or rapid weight gain needs to be immediately reported to the physician. Milder adverse effects include GI disturbances, fever, chills, rash, myalgias, hepatotoxicity, and eosinophilia.

Monoclonal Antibodies

MABs are genetically engineered murine (mouse), human, or chimeric (mouse–human) antibodies that are directed against certain specific antigens expressed on cancer cells—usually a specific protein that is overexpressed by the cancer cell and/or that is needed for the cancer cell to survive. Because specificity is high, destruction of other cells is limited; thus many adverse effects produced by traditional chemotherapeutic agents are avoided. MABs were originally made by immunizing a mouse with antigen and then removing the spleen several weeks later.[30] From the spleen, a mixture of lymphocytes and plasma cells was obtained and then fused in vitro with myeloma cells (cancerous B cells that produce large numbers of antibodies). This resulted in the production of significant amounts of homogeneous antibodies tailor-made to act against a specific antigen. Nowadays, these antibodies are manufactured using recombinant DNA techniques.

An MAB is made up of two regions: (1) the Fab fragment containing the antigen-binding site and (2) the Fc region containing the binding site for monocytes, macrophages, NK cells, and other similar effector cells. Using these regions, the antibody blocks tumor growth by several different mechanisms.[31] The traditional mechanism involves binding of the antibody to the antigen and activation of the complement components, opsonization by phagocytic cells, and then direct lysis. The second mechanism occurs when the MAB binds to the Fc receptors on macrophages or NK cells, resulting in the release of cytokines. A sort of cross-linkage forms among the effector cells, the MAB, and the tumor. Another method used by the MAB is to bind directly to the growth factor receptors on cancer cells. The drugs rituximab for B-cell lymphomas and trastuzumab for breast cancer both work in this manner.

Rituximab (Rituxan) was the first MAB to be approved for use in humans (Box 22-3). It binds to the CD20 antigen on the surface of normal and cancerous B lymphocytes.[32] It is primarily used against B-cell non-Hodgkin's lymphoma, but its use has expanded to include treatments for other lymphomas and chronic lymphocyte leukemia (CLL) as well. The CD20 antigen is a transmembrane protein that exists on almost all B cells—from the stage at which they become committed to becoming B cells up to the stage in which they become plasma cells. This marker does not exist on multiple myeloma cells, which arise from more mature B cells. The drawback to use of rituximab is that it also kills normal B cells.

BOX 22-3 Approved Monoclonal Antibodies and Their Indications

Monoclonal Antibody	Indication
Alemtuzumab (Campath)	Chronic lymphocytic leukemia
Bevacizumab (Avastin)	Colorectal cancer
Cetuximab (Erbitux)	Colorectal cancer; head and neck cancer
Gemtuzumab ozogamicin (Mylotarg)	Acute myeloid leukemia
Ibritumomab tiuxetan (Zevalin)	Non-Hodgkin's lymphoma
Rituximab (Rituxan)	Non-Hodgkin's lymphoma
Tositumomab (Bexxar)	Non-Hodgkin's lymphoma
Trastuzumab (Herceptin)	Breast cancer

Once rituximab binds to the CD20 marker, it is not exactly clear how cell death occurs. Complement activation occurs, but NK cells and cytokine secretion are also involved.[32] Unfortunately, resistance mechanisms are hard at work because not all the patients reach remission and because relapses are common. The response rate is 48%, with duration of response lasting about a year.[33] Response was significantly improved when the MAB was added to chemotherapy, resulting in complete response in 58% of patients and partial responses in 42%. In addition to flu-like symptoms during infusion, this drug can produce severe bronchospasm, angioedema, and hypotension.

Trastuzumab (Herceptin) is another MAB with a different mechanism of action. It has been approved for use in the United States since 1998 as a treatment for metastatic breast cancer. It is a genetically engineered anti–human epidermal growth factor receptor 2 (HER2) MAB that binds to the HER2 expressed on human breast cancer cells. Approximately 25 to 30% of patients with breast cancer have amplification of the *HER2* gene, resulting in overexpression of the HER2 protein. Abundance of this growth factor leads to rapid growth of the tumor and a particularly virulent and resistant form of the disease. Therefore blocking this receptor on the cancer cell appears to be a reasonable approach to treatment.

The initial studies on trastuzumab, when used as monotherapy in the first-line treatment of metastatic disease, demonstrated that the drug was not only effective but also produced improvements in quality-of-life measures.[34] This outcome measure has been chosen by many chemotherapeutic studies because in the majority of metastatic diseases, there is a prolongation of survival but no overall decrease in mortality rate. Any increase in survival should be matched by an improvement in function, or the drug would not be considered very effective. When trastuzumab was added to a regimen of chemotherapy, the overall response rate was 45%, compared with 29% for chemotherapy alone.[33,35] Specifically, the chemotherapeutic agents doxorubicin, paclitaxel, and vinorelbine all potentiate the effectiveness of trastuzumab.[36] Time to progression of disease was also significantly increased with combination therapy. However, when the drug is withdrawn, tumor growth resumes.

Adverse effects of trastuzumab are mild to moderate in severity and are usually infusion related.[37] Symptoms include fever, chills, nausea, and headache; but these usually dissipate during the infusion. In addition, symptoms are worse with the initial dose. However, cardiac dysfunction has been reported when trastuzumab is used in combination with chemotherapy, particularly anthracycline or doxorubicin.

Gemtuzumab ozogamicin (Mylotarg) is another MAB with a unique makeup.[2] The antibody is attached to the antineoplastic antibiotic ozogamicin. This complex binds to leukemic blast cells in the treatment of acute myelocytic leukemia. Attachment of the antibody portion of the drug leads to internalization of the compound. Once in the cell, the ozogamicin component is released into the lysosomes, which results in DNA damage.

Ibritumomab tiuxetan, like gemtuzumab ozogamicin, is also an interesting compound.[2] It is administered along with a radioactive isotope. The MAB binds to the CD20 antigen on the surfaces of normal as well as cancerous B lymphocytes. Once this binding occurs, the tiuxetan binds the radioisotope, which, in turn, damages the cell containing the drug. It is used to treat non-Hodgkin's lymphoma. Other MABs include cetuximab for the treatment of metastatic colorectal cancer and alemtuzumab for B-cell CLL.[38,39]

Hematopoietic Agents and Stem Cell Replacement

The hematopoietic agents are not directly involved in the killing of cancer cells but rather enhance the effects of chemotherapeutic agents by allowing higher and more frequent chemotherapy dosing with quicker recovery between antineoplastic cycles. They are also known as *colony-stimulating factors*, promoting the growth and differentiation of progenitor cells.

Colony-stimulating factors are produced by recombinant DNA technology and therefore are identical to natural, endogenously produced chemicals. They bind to receptors in bone marrow to increase the production of specific cell lines. Epoetin alfa is the synthetic version of erythropoietin that stimulates red blood cell production.[40] Darbepoetin alfa is a newer agent that has a longer duration of action.[41] Filgrastim and lenograstim stimulate the production of granulocytes and are also called *granulocyte colony-stimulating factors*.[42] Sargramostim stimulates the production of both granulocytes and macrophages and hence is known as *granulocyte-macrophage colony-stimulating factor*. Oprelvekin works slightly differently from the other colony-stimulating factors in that it is an IL-11 analog that stimulates megakaryocytes to produce platelets.

The benefits of these colony-stimulating factors include reduction in chemotherapy-induced neutropenia, thrombocytopenia, and anemia. Clinically, this results in reduced occurrence of fever, mouth sores, infections, antibiotic use, and hospital stay among patients with cancer receiving chemotherapy.[43] However, studies have not shown tremendous benefit unless the patient has a grade 4 neutropenia (defined as an absolute neutrophil count of <500 cells/mm^3) or a fever.[44] The administration of docetaxel in the treatment of metastatic disease illustrates how these drugs may be used.[45] The recommended dose and cycling of this drug is 100 mg/m^2 every 21 days. Neutropenia limits greater concentrations and a shorter dosing interval. However, in one small study, the addition of lenograstim reduced the dosing interval to once every 2 weeks. In general, filgrastim is given until the absolute neutrophil count is about 10,000/mm^3 after the neutrophil nadir.[2] Hematologic recovery (neutropenic status) may take as little as 7 days, whereas the return of hematologic status after straight chemotherapy may take 3 weeks or more.[46] This shortened time cuts down on mortality from infection and bleeding and also allows the next cycle of chemotherapy to begin earlier, if indicated.

In general, these stimulating factors are well tolerated, but there are a few things to watch out for. For example, erythropoietin may force the hematocrit and hemoglobin values to rise too high and too quickly, which will produce hypertension and seizures. There is also some concern that platelet-inducing agents might cause deep vein thrombosis (DVT) and pulmonary embolism (PE).[47]

The benefits of treatment with colony-stimulating factors may be more evident in patients undergoing hematopoietic stem cell mobilization or transplantation. Hematopoietic stem cell mobilization refers to the expansion of circulating stem cells in preparation for autologous and allogeneic peripheral blood stem cell replacements.[46] Administration of granulocyte colony-stimulating factor and granulocyte-macrophage colony-stimulating factor is used to cause the progenitor cells to leak into the circulation so that they can be collected. Chemotherapy agents may also be combined with growth factors because it has been observed that when the two therapies are combined, a synergistic effect occurs, resulting in substantially larger numbers of peripheral blood progenitor cells. In the early 1970s, it was observed that the use of chemotherapy agents with myelosuppressive, as opposed to myeloablative, characteristics produced a mobilization of hematopoietic stem cells from bone marrow about 2 weeks after recovery from the nadir. Cyclophosphamide and paclitaxel have been commonly used for this purpose.

In autologous transplantations, growth factors are administered first, followed by collection of the progenitor cells with leukapheresis. The wide gamut of stem cells include megakaryocytic, erythroid, and myeloid types as well as mature neutrophils. The patient then undergoes high-dose chemotherapy to eradicate malignant cells and to make space in bone marrow for new cells. This is followed by reinfusion of the patient's own progenitor cells, approximately 48 to 72 hours after the last chemotherapy dose. The neutropenia that occurs with stem cell transplantation may last from 9 to 21 days.[48] Persisting neutropenia usually indicates that the graft has failed. Mature T lymphocytes and lymphocyte subtypes may take a minimum of 6 months or as long as 2 years to recover, and B lymphocytes may also take up to 2 years to recover. Advantages of using growth factors include the avoidance of marrow harvesting from the iliac crest, enhanced engraftment, and the avoidance of graft-versus-host disease (GVHD).

CANCER THERAPY ADVERSE EFFECTS, RECOMMENDATIONS FOR TREATMENT, AND REHAB THERAPY IMPLICATIONS

Patients with cancer experience multiple symptoms, some related to the drugs and others related to the cancer, which may adversely affect their ability to continue taking the drugs. Uncontrolled symptoms are known to affect outcomes and quality of life. The focus of this section will be on individual symptoms; however, the therapist must understand that a single symptom may be related, directly or indirectly, to other symptoms. Focus should be on strategies for symptom management that both patients and their families can implement.

Anorexia

Patients with any type of cancer may experience anorexia. However, in patients with advanced disease, it is estimated to occur 60 to 70% of the time. *Anorexia* refers to a loss of appetite with subsequent reduction in food intake.[8] It is frequently one of the earliest manifestations of cancer and is known to improve with successful cancer therapy. Risk factors for the development of anorexia include advanced age and comorbid conditions such as diabetes and renal disease, uncontrolled pain, and the type of cancer therapy used. For example, patients receiving multimodality therapy (chemotherapy with radiation) are more at risk for developing nutritional complications due to the severity of the adverse effects from the treatment.

Several physiologic and psychological factors are also thought to play a part in the development of anorexia, which may be a consequence of the adverse effects of chemotherapy such as nausea and vomiting, taste changes, food aversions, appetite loss, or ulcerations of mucous membranes. Cancer-related anorexia may be related to the secretion of cytokines that circulate throughout the body and affect various regulatory systems involved in the control of hunger, satiety, and metabolism.[49] In addition, cancer processes are thought to cause abnormal neuronal or hormonal signals from the GI tract that directly influence the hypothalamic appetite centers. Psychological changes such as fatigue, anxiety, depression, anger or fear may also contribute to anorexia.

Signs and symptoms include unintentional weight loss of 10% within the last 6 months (5% if within the last month), dry flaky skin, muscle wasting, increasing debility, alterations in resting energy expenditure, pale skin or sclera, and unhealed wounds. Clinical consequences of anorexia result in compromise of other body functions, leading to weakness and fatigue, lower resistance to infection, and progression to cachexia. Cachexia is characterized by wasting of both adipose tissue and skeletal mass. Early detection of cachexia is important because it is associated with reduced quality of life, lower survival, and diminished response to chemotherapy.

Interventions to address anorexia depend on the contributing factors and the goal of cancer therapy for the patient. Treatments are generally decided in collaboration with a dietician who provides assistance with diet planning. The goal of treatment is to improve the patient's overall nutritional intake while changing the metabolic environment that contributes to the muscle and fat wasting. The use of aggressive nutritional supplementation may be necessary before drug therapy begins. This may include nasogastric feeding or central venous hyperalimentation (total parenteral nutrition); however, this is strongly discouraged in patients with advanced cancer. Pharmacologic therapy includes megestrol acetate (progestational agent), which has been shown to increase appetite, caloric intake, and weight, and glucocorticoids, which may be used to decrease nausea and improve appetite when used for a limited time.

Patient and family education should be provided to address any identified nutritional issues. Generally, patients are encouraged to eat small, frequent meals and incorporate high-protein foods into their diets. Foods should be marinated to disguise or enhance food flavors; hard candies and fresh fruit are useful to eliminate bad tastes in the mouth. The therapist should provide or assist patients with planning daily energy-conserving food-preparation activities. Patients should be provided with mild exercise routines and encouraged to perform them for about 20 minutes a day to stimulate muscles and increase strength.

Nausea and Vomiting (Emesis)

Approximately, 70 to 80% of all chemotherapy regimens are associated with chemotherapy-induced nausea and vomiting (CINV).[50] This remains a problematic symptom associated with the administration of cancer therapy. Uncontrolled nausea is known to negatively affect a patient's quality of life, so the key to treatment is aggressive and proactive anti-emetic therapy. The process of emesis occurs, sequentially or separately, in three phases: (1) nausea, (2) retching, and (3) vomiting.

Nausea is an unpleasant subjective feeling that is controlled by the autonomic nervous system. Symptoms often associated with nausea include dizziness, perspiration, pallor, tachycardia, and weakness. Retching follows nausea and is a rhythmic and spasmodic respiratory movement against a closed glottis with contractions of the abdominal muscles, chest wall, and diaphragm without any expulsion of gastric contents. This is controlled by the respiratory center, which is near the vomiting center, in the brain stem. Retching can occur without vomiting, but normally it generates the pressure gradient that leads to vomiting. Vomiting is the expulsion of contents from the stomach through the mouth and results from the stimulation of a complex process that involves the activation of various pathways and neurotransmitter receptors in an area of the brain referred to as the *vomiting center*. This reflex is not under voluntary control.

There are several risk factors that contribute to the development of CINV. The most significant one is related to the emetic potential of the chemotherapy regimen prescribed for the patient. Box 22-4 lists commonly used chemotherapeutic drugs according to their emetic potential. In regimens with multiple drugs, the combined emetic potential of all the drugs is higher than that of any drug alone. In addition, higher doses of the drugs listed have higher emetic potential. Other contributing risk factors which increase the risk of developing nausea and vomiting include age younger than 50 years, high level of anxiety prior to treatment, a history of motion sickness, severe nausea and vomiting with a previous course of treatment, and a feeling of generalized weakness after chemotherapy. Gender is another factor, and women are more likely than men to suffer from nausea and vomiting.

There are a number of antiemetic pharmacologic interventions that can help reduce vomiting.[51] Granisetron and ondansetron are selective antagonists at the 5-hydroxytryptamine 3 (5-HT3) receptor both in the CNS and at the peripheral sites in the GI tract. 5-HT3 receptors are present in abundance on vagal afferent neurons in the vomiting center and in the GI tract. These drugs can be given 30 minutes before chemotherapy and then at 2 and 4 hours after therapy. Aprepitant is another potent drug for the prevention of CINV. It is an NK1 receptor antagonist. This receptor, located at the

BOX 22-4 Emetic Potential of Some Chemotherapeutic Agents

Strong	Moderate	Low
Cisplatin	Daunorubicin	Vincristine
Cyclophosphamide	Cytarabine	Tamoxifen
Doxorubicin	Methotrexate	Bleomycin
Lomustine		Fluorouracil
Mechlorethamine		

brain stem nuclei of the dorsal vagal complex, binds the neuropeptide, substance P, a crucial regulator of vomiting. Dexamethasone is also used, but its exact mechanism for reducing emesis is unknown. The antipsychotic drug prochlorperazine reduces nausea and vomiting but is now used less frequently because of extrapyramidal reactions it causes and the availability of more effective drugs. Marijuana and tetrahydrocannabinol have also been used to control CINV.

Several nonpharmacologic interventions are also available and should be used in conjunction with antiemetic therapy. Behavioral interventions include progressive muscle relaxation, guided imagery, and biofeedback. Dietary interventions include encouraging the patient to eat small, frequent meals and avoiding spicy or highly fatty foods. Patients should avoid their favorite foods on the day of treatment and eat cold or room-temperature foods because they give off fewer odors than do hot foods. The therapist should work with the patient to choose a moderate form of daily aerobic exercise because this has been demonstrated to provide relief of nausea.[8]

Diarrhea and Mucositis

The epithelial lining of the GI tract is extremely sensitive to chemotherapy agents.[2] *Diarrhea* is defined as loose or watery stools and is a frequent adverse effect of some chemotherapeutic and biotherapeutic agents. Risk factors for the development of diarrhea are related to the type of agents administered; it occurs most frequently with the administration of topoisomerase inhibitors (irinotecan and topotecan) and 5-FU. The severity of the diarrhea is related to the specific agent, dose, schedule, and combination with other anticancer therapies. For example, up to 90% of patients undergoing chemotherapy and radiation therapy may experience diarrhea. If diarrhea cannot be controlled, the course of action may be to modify the dosing regimen or withhold the chemotherapeutic agent, which could compromise the benefit of the regimen. Management of diarrhea includes administration of antidiarrheal medications, such as loperamide or diphenoxylate HCL, with atropine sulfate. Patients are instructed to remain hydrated (8 to 10 glasses of clear fluid daily) and to eat foods containing pectin, such as bananas, avocados, and asparagus tips, which are all high in potassium. Other dietary interventions include eating a low-residue, low-fiber, low-fat diet and to avoid alcohol, caffeine-containing products, and tobacco.

Mucositis is a general term used to refer to the inflammation and ulceration of mucous membranes. *Stomatitis* or *oral mucositis* refers to inflammation of the mucous membranes of the oral cavity, including the lining of the mouth, pharynx, and esophagus. Oral inflammation causes pain with eating, speaking, and swallowing; thus many functional activities are affected. Stomatitis symptoms vary with each agent but generally develop within a few days of chemotherapy administration and persist for 2 to 3 weeks after treatment. Patients may complain of pain in the oral cavity before any other clinical manifestations, which progress from redness, cracking, and inflammation to bleeding and ulceration. It is estimated that approximately 40% of patients undergoing standard-dose chemotherapy develop mucositis.[8] The following classes of chemotherapy agents are known to contribute to the development of mucositis: antimetabolites, antitumor antibiotics, alkylating agents, and plant alkaloids. Several patient risk factors—age, gender, history of alcohol and tobacco use, baseline nutritional status, oral hygiene, and salivary gland function, just to name a few—may influence the development and severity of mucositis.

Currently, no standard exists for the prevention and treatment of oral mucositis. Most interventions are aimed at symptom relief. Treatment with topical anesthetics and antifungal drugs may be helpful in relieving pain and preventing infection. Most of the effort is focused on educating the patient on oral care protocols, which are essential in promoting good oral hygiene. Patients should be encouraged to use oral agents that promote cleansing and to frequently moisturize the oral cavity. In addition, patients should brush with a soft toothbrush, rinse the mouth frequently after eating, avoid irritating agents such as commercial mouthwashes that contain alcohol, hot and spicy foods, and beverages that contain alcohol.

Constipation

Constipation is a common problem in up to 35% of patients receiving chemotherapy and is most frequently related to the decreased motility of the large intestine. Several factors may contribute to the development of constipation. It may be a presenting clinical manifestation of cancer, an adverse effect of chemotherapeutic agents administered, or the result of tumor progression. It may also be unrelated to the cancer or to therapy. The most common cause of constipation in the patient with cancer is related to inadequate fluid intake and use of narcotic analgesics.

Pharmacologic agents that contribute to the development of constipation include vinca alkaloids and opioids. Vincristine and vinblastine may cause neurotoxicity that affects the smooth muscles of the intestines, which leads to decreased peristalsis and, in some patients, paralytic ileus. Opioids are known to cause decreased peristalisis and are the most common cause of medication-induced constipation. Chemotherapeutic agents which cause nausea and vomiting may also play a role because patients reduce their food intake, which decreases stool production and increases transit time causing stool to become hard and difficult to eliminate.

Management of constipation includes prescription and administration of laxatives. Patients receiving agents known to cause constipation, such as vinca alkaloids or opioids, are given a combination of a laxative and a stool softener prophylactically. Patients are encouraged to increase intake of fluids and fiber. The therapist should ensure that there is an increase in physical activities or passive exercise as appropriate. Encouraging the patient to regularly exercise stimulates intestinal motility and promotes the urge to defecate by helping to move the feces into the rectum.

Bone Marrow Suppression

Myelosuppression is the suppression of bone marrow activity. As a result, there can be a decrease in the number of circulating platelets (thrombocytopenia), white blood cells (neutropenia), and red blood cells (anemia) in the blood. Bone marrow suppression is the most common dose-limiting and certainly the most life threatening toxicity of chemotherapy. The frequency of occurrence varies depending on the chemotherapeutic agent administered. Box 22-5 outlines the myelosuppressive potential of chemotherapeutic agents.

Thrombocytopenia

Thrombocytopenia is an abnormally low number of circulating platelets in the blood. A normal platelet count is 150,000 to 400,000 cells/mm^3, and acute or delayed effects of chemotherapy decrease platelet production. Generally, chemotherapy administration is withheld when platelet levels are $<$90,000/mm^3 in solid tumors, which results in a delay of treatment and possible dose modification. Several chemotherapeutic classes—platinums (carboplatin and cisplatin) and taxanes (paclitaxel and docetaxel)—are known to cause thrombocytopenia as a dose-limiting toxicity. Other risk factors include combined modality therapy (chemotherapy plus radiation), disease that has infiltrated the bone marrow, elevated temperature leading to destruction of platelets, and comorbid conditions such as cirrhosis or infection.

Low levels of platelets, less than 20,000/mm^3, are associated with spontaneous and life-threatening bleeding in the GI tract and brain. Early clinical manifestations include the development of petechiae (tiny purplish dots) and ecchymoses (purplish bruises), indicating capillary microvascular bleeding, and overt bleeding causing nosebleeds, hematuria, or the presence of blood in the stool (GI bleeding). Patients may also experience bleeding from the mouth and gums after brushing the teeth. Platelet transfusions are usually given if active bleeding exists or the platelet count falls below 20,000/mm^3.

The rehabilitative therapist must maintain and reinforce bleeding precautions when the platelet count is $\leq$50,000/mm^3. Every effort should be made to ensure that the area where therapy is provided is safe and free from the potential for injury (e.g., falls and bumping into objects). Activity levels must be modified to ensure that patients do not injure themselves during exercise (Box 22-6). Activities that pose a high risk of injury, such as bicycle riding or contact sports, should be discouraged. Patients should be instructed to avoid wearing clothing that is restrictive. In addition, agents that impair platelet function, such as aspirin and nonsteroidal anti-inflammatory drugs (NSAIDs), should be avoided; and if the platelet count falls too low, oprelvekin can be added to the drug routine (see the discussion of hematopoietic agents and stem cell replacement).

BOX 22-5 Myelosuppressive Potential of Chemotherapeutic Drugs

Strong	Moderate	Mild
Vinblastine	Methotrexate	Bleomycin
Nitrosoureas	Fluorouracil	Vincristine
Cyclophosphamide	Etoposide	Tamoxifen
Doxorubicin		Hormone treatments
Mercaptopurine		
Ifosfamide		

Neutropenia

Neutropenia involves an abnormally low number of circulating neutrophils (white blood cells) in the blood. The normal neutrophil count is between 2500 and 7000/mm^3, and when the count falls below 1000/mm^3, the risk of developing an infection is increased. Profound neutropenia is an absolute neutrophil count (ANC) of $<$500/mm^3; this can lead to significant consequences for patients with cancer, including life-threatening infections, prolonged hospitalization stays, dose modifications, and dose delays.

The National Cancer Institute has defined four levels of neutropenia: (1) Grade 1 $<$lower limit of NML – 1500/mm^3; (2) Grade 2 $<$1500 to 1000/mm^3; (3) Grade 3 $<$1000 to 500/mm^3; and (4) Grade 4$<$500/mm^3 and/or life-threatening sequelae (septic shock, hypotension, acidosis, necrosis). *Febrile neutropenia* is defined as a

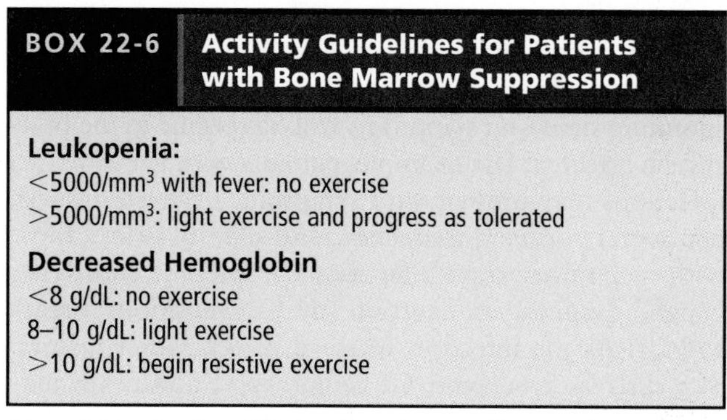

BOX 22-6 Activity Guidelines for Patients with Bone Marrow Suppression

Leukopenia:
<5000/mm^3 with fever: no exercise
>5000/mm^3: light exercise and progress as tolerated

Decreased Hemoglobin
<8 g/dL: no exercise
8–10 g/dL: light exercise
>10 g/dL: begin resistive exercise

Adapted from Goodman CC, Boissonnault WG, Fuller KS: Laboratory tests and values. In Goodman CC, Boissonnault WG, editors: *Pathology: Implications for the physical therapist,* New York, 1998, Saunders.

single temperature of 100.9°F (38.3°C) or a temperature higher than 100.4°F (38°C) that lasts over 1 hour and a total neutrophil count of less than 500/mm^3 or less than 1000/mm^3, with the cell count anticipated to drop to less than 500/mm^3 in the next 48 hours. Risk factors for developing febrile neutropenia include patient-related factors, including older age, female gender, poor nutritional status, decreased immune function, open wounds, and comorbidities such as diabetes. Treatment-related factors include a previous history of severe neutropenia with similar chemotherapy, type of chemotherapy (anthracyclines and platinum-based regimens, planned relative dose intensity greater than 80%, pre-existing neutropenia or lymphocytopenia, extensive prior chemotherapy, and concurrent or prior radiation. Cancer-related factors leading to febrile neutropenia include bone marrow involvement with tumor, advanced cancer, and elevated lactate dehydrogenase.

The incidence and severity of neutropenia varies according to agent, dose, and administration schedule.[8] For example, cell-cycle–specific agents generate rapid nadirs in 7 to 14 days; cell-cycle–nonspecific agents generate nadirs in 10 to 14 days. Concurrent chemotherapy and radiation therapy to areas with large bone marrow, highly myelosuppressive chemotherapy regimens, poor hepatic or renal function, poor nutrition, and tumor involvement of bone marrow may also contribute to the likelihood of neutropenia. In general, the lowest absolute neutrophil count occurs at approximately 10 to 14 days after treatment, which makes this the time when the patient is most susceptible to infectious agents. Recovery takes about 3 to 4 weeks. Chemotherapy will not be administered if the neutrophil count falls below 500/mm^3, the platelet count is below 100,000/mm^3, and/or the white blood cell count is below 4000/mm^3.[2]

If a chemotherapy regimen has a 20% or greater chance of causing neutropenia, granulocyte colony-stimulating factor will be administered 24 hours after the administration to prophylactically build up the granulocyte count to prevent infection. A granulocyte-macrophage colony-stimulating factor is also available (see discussion of hematopoietic agents and stem cell replacement). Both agents stimulate differentiation and proliferation of myeloid progenitor cells into granulocytes.

Often, the only sign of infection in the neutropenic patient is a fever of ≥100.4°F (≥38°C). Other corresponding signs and symptoms will be specific to the body system affected. For example, patients with urinary tract infections may present with symptoms of fever, dysuria, hematuria, urinary frequency, and cloudy urine; those with respiratory tract infections will present with fever, cough, dyspnea on exertion, and adventitious breath sounds. As the infection worsens, shock, adult respiratory distress syndrome, GI hemorrhage, and death may occur. The standard practice for patients presenting with neutropenic fever is to obtain a culture of the urine, blood, and all other potential sources of infection, perform a physical examination to try to pinpoint the source of infection, obtain a chest X-ray, and begin administration of empiric antibiotics that should include coverage for gram-positive and gram-negative organisms until the causative organism is identified.[52]

The Multinational Association of Supportive Care in Cancer (MASCC) has developed a risk model to predict an uncomplicated recovery or the development of serious complication following febrile neutropenia (Uys, 2004). This assessment is based on seven independent factors that contribute to increased morbidity (burden of illness, hypotension, chronic obstructive pulmonary disease, tumor type, dehydration, patient location, and age). Each of these items has a weighted score. When added together, a score of 21 or more indicates that the patient has a lower risk of complications.

The therapist should be alert for fever, sore throat, or chills in patients with cancer because these may be the first signs of infection.[2] When caring for the patient with neutropenia, it is important to ensure that protective measures for the patient have been implemented. From a therapy point of view, activity will need to be limited and skin integrity protected. Therapists who have recently had a contagious illness (e.g., cold) should avoid treating patients with neutropenia.

Anemia

Anemia is an abnormally low number of circulating red blood cells in the blood. The normal hemoglobin for an adult, depending on sex, ranges from 12 to 18 g/dL. The degree of anemia depends on the type of drug, dose, and frequency of treatment regimen; severe anemia (Hgb <8g/dL) is rarely seen when standard-dose chemotherapy is administered alone. Risk factors for anemia include prior or concomitant treatment with radiation therapy, acute bleeding or hemorrhage, renal dysfunction, poor nutrition, type of chemotherapy administered, and the concomitant use of other medications (i.e., alcohol, aspirin, NSAIDS, antibiotics, and anticonvulsants).

Patients presenting with mild anemia may be asymptomatic. The most common clinical manifestations include fatigue, irritability, headaches, pallor, and dyspnea with exertion. Once the underlying cause has been identified, treatment may include blood transfusions, iron supplementation for those with iron deficiencies, and the administration of epoetin alfa.

Erythropoietin is a hormone produced in the kidneys in response to tissue hypoxia. Sensors in the tubular cells of the kidneys are responsive to tissue oxygen content, and when hypoxia is present, they release erythropoietin. In bone marrow, erythropoietin binds to erythroid progenitor cells and activates tyrosine protein kinase signal pathways to stimulate cell proliferation into red blood cells. Recombinant erythropoietin (epoietin alfa) is now available (see discussion of hematopoietic agents and stem cell replacement) and is used to treat anemia caused by chronic renal failure, anemia associated with human immunodeficiency virus (HIV) infection, and chemotherapy-induced anemia in patients with cancer. For patients with cancer and anemia, the usual regimen is subcutaneous injections, once a week for 4 weeks.

The therapist should encourage the patient with anemia to rest periodically during therapy to conserve energy if he or she suffers from hypoxia. Patients should be encouraged to set short-term goals for activities of daily living (ADLs), and the therapist should develop exercise routines that support the identified goals. In addition, patients should be instructed on how to change positions slowly to prevent dizziness secondary to postural hypotension.

Fatigue

Cancer-related fatigue is defined as "a persistent, subjective sense of tiredness related to cancer or cancer treatment that interferes with usual functioning."[8] The exact cause is unknown, but it is speculated to result from muscle wasting caused by inflammatory cytokines or tumor necrosis factor (TNF). It tends to be more severe midway through the treatment cycle. Unfortunately, it is one of the most common complaints that patients make, and it seriously impacts ADLs and quality of life.

Fatigue is also inversely proportional to activity level, and it has been found to be reduced on days when patients exercise. The therapist should evaluate the ability of the patient to perform his/her ADLs and encourage the patient to balance exercise, rest, and energy. Efforts should be focused on assisting the patient to develop an individualized care plan that identifies strategies to address fatigue. For example, activities, including work, should be reorganized to decrease or eliminate low-priority activities. Recommendations for treatment include aerobic exercise programs at low intensity. Initially, patients may only be able to exert themselves for a few minutes, but if activity is continued, patients will experience lower levels of fatigue. Patients are encouraged to keep a diary, documenting the exercise mode, duration, intensity, heart rate, time of day, and any symptoms.

Pain

Pain is another symptom that may result from cancer or from chemotherapy. Most patients with cancer require some analgesic therapy while awaiting a response to chemotherapy. Regular administration of NSAIDs is the usual starting point for mild pain associated with cancer. However, the beneficial response of pain control needs to be balanced against the risks (GI problems, bleeding tendencies, kidney toxicity, and the masking of fever that indicates infection). When these drugs are no longer effective, a weak opioid may be added to or substituted for the NSAID. Codeine and hydrocodone, combined with aspirin or acetaminophen, are recommended. When combinations of codeine-like drugs and NSAIDs are not sufficient and pain is severe, strong opioids are recommended. Morphine, hydromorphone, oxycodone, and transdermal fentanyl are appropriate. These drugs can be administered in a variety of ways. Immediate-release preparations, which have a short latency and short duration, and controlled-release preparations such as MS Contin, which may be administered every 8 to 12 hours, are available. Transdermal fentanyl provides a stable level of pain control for up to 72 hours. NSAIDs may also be given along with these drugs.

Most patients require a basal, long-acting analgesic administered at regular intervals and a short-acting analgesic given on an as-needed basis for breakthrough pain. Patient compliance and the quality of analgesia are enhanced by regular administration. Oral transmucosal fentanyl (in the form of a lollipop) can provide relief from breakthrough pain within 5 minutes. This strategy promotes consistent therapeutic plasma levels that will keep pain at a minimum. Opioids may also be administered by several routes: orally, rectally, sublingually, subcutaneously, and epidurally.

Bone is one of the most common sites of metastases from breast, prostate, and lung cancers. Pain from bone lesions produces significant morbidity, and complete responses of bone lesions to chemotherapy are fairly rare. However, a partial response and disease stabilization can be achieved, particularly if surgery for stabilization of weight-bearing bones is possible. Bone pain has been described as "a unique pain state," involving neurochemical changes in afferent neurons. Mechanical allodynia often develops and becomes so severe that coughing, turning in bed, or even gentle limb movements can produce pain.[53] Bone pain is correlated with the extent of osteolysis. From a chemical standpoint, bone disease is related to the expression of dynorphin, a prohyperalgesic peptide. Treatment includes external beam radiation and bisphosphonates. Bisphosphonates inhibit bone reabsorption and have been shown to reduce morbidity in terms of pain, fracture, and hypercalcemia.[54,55]

Alopecia

Alopecia, or hair loss, occurs to some degree following administration of most chemotherapy drugs. The cells responsible for hair growth have high mitotic and metabolic rates. Approximately 90% of hair follicles on the scalp are in the growth phase of the hair cycle, which makes them extremely susceptible to injury from chemotherapeutic agents. Risk factors for alopecia are related to the type of cancer therapy administered and occur most frequently with the administration of cyclophosphamide, etoposide, ifosfamide, paclitaxel, vincristine, daunorubicin, doxorubicin, and bleomycin.[2] The extent of hair loss depends on the drug dose, infusion technique (bolus versus continuous infusion), mechanism of action of the drug, and the use of combination chemotherapy. Hair damage occurs at either the shaft or the root, and areas of sensitivity ranges from scalp (most sensitive) to pubic hair (least sensitive). Hair falls out spontaneously or during washing and combing. Many patients report waking up in the morning and finding a clump of hair on the pillow. Alopecia begins 7 to 10 days after treatment is initiated, with the peak effect seen at 2 months. Hair regrowth may take 3 to 5 months after completion of cancer therapy. Unfortunately, there is no known preventive treatment strategy. Patients are encouraged to take a before-treatment photograph so that a wig that closely matches their pretreatment hair type and color can be made. Instructions should be provided on strategies to manage hair loss such as avoiding vigorous brushing or avoiding perms and hair coloring. Patients should protect their scalp from the cold and the sun and should be reassured that even with continuing maintenance therapy, their hair will usually grow back, although color and texture may change.

Extravasation Injury

Extravasation is a rare but serious consequence of chemotherapy. If a vesicant chemotherapeutic agent leaks into tissue surrounding the vein, it may lead to severe tissue damage and sloughing.[2] In some cases, skin grafting will be necessary, and it may lead to a decline in limb functioning. The physical therapist may need to treat a patient for an upper extremity or hand injury. Only certified nurses can administer chemotherapeutic agents, and the patient's infusion site must be monitored very carefully during the administration. If extravasation occurs, administration of the drug must be stopped immediately and an antidote given. If a chemotherapy spill occurs while the therapist is providing treatment, a towel should be placed over the spill and the nurse contacted immediately. At no time should the care provider attempt to wipe off the chemotherapeutic agent without wearing proper personal protective equipment.

Organ Toxicity

Specific organ toxicity is another problem associated with chemotherapy and usually involves the kidneys, liver, heart, lungs, CNS, gonads, and even the brain.[2] Renal tubular necrosis can result from the use of cisplatin. Hydration and diuretics are necessary to ensure sufficient flow of urine to prevent this toxicity. Creatinine clearance from the kidneys, as well as serum creatinine values, must be monitored regularly. Liver toxicity may result from prolonged treatment with methotrexate or mercaptopurine. Cardiotoxicity is associated with anticancer antibiotics, especially doxorubicin and daunorubicin. It may be sudden in onset, irreversible, and fatal; or there may be transient ECG changes with delayed cardiomyopathy with congestive heart failure. Patients with pre-existing cardiac disease must be monitored very carefully. Frequent monitoring of left ventricular ejection fraction is warranted. Newer additions to the cancer pharmacopia, such as trastuzumab and the tyrosine kinase inhibitors, have also been found to cause cardiotoxicity, necessitating frequent monitoring of cardiac function.

Peripheral neuropathy, which is characterized by loss of deep tendon reflexes, paresthesias, motor weakness, and neuropathic pain, is commonly associated with vincristine and other mitotic spindle inhibitors.[21,56] It is a dose-limiting toxicity of three commonly used chemotherapeutic classes: platinols, vinca alkaloids, and taxanes. Improvement is slow and may take more than a year after drug withdrawal, and in some cases, the neuropathy is permanent. Evaluation of hand sensibility for light touch, moving touch, two-point discrimination, and vibration is helpful in the assessment of chemotherapy-induced neuropathy and is also useful for tracking sensory return.[57,58]

In general, red flags that may indicate organ toxicity include signs and symptoms of infection, yellowing of the skin, abdominal pain, decreased urine production, rapid respiration, poor skin turgor, skin lesions, and rashes. In addition, there is some evidence that chemotherapeutic agents can produce cognitive changes and even delirium.[59,60]

Secondary Malignancies

Secondary malignancies resulting from genetic damage caused by chemotherapy have become a concern among cancer survivors as they live longer because of improved treatments. The incidence of these cancers (usually leukemias) is greater when chemotherapy was originally combined with radiation therapy. The peak incidence of secondary leukemia is between 2 and 10 years after completion of treatment for the primary cancer and is greater among patients who were older than 40 years at the time of the initial cancer.

Hypersensitivity Reactions

Hypersensitivity reactions are not uncommon, but when they occur with chemotherapeutic drugs, they can present a significant challenge. Some mild reactions can be treated with diphenhydramine, acetaminophen, and steroids. Life-threatening reactions are treated with epinephrine, bronchodilators, and saline solution. If the reaction proves to be non–life threatening, infusion of the chemotherapeutic agent may be restarted after symptoms subside.

Performance Scale

Not every patient can tolerate the adverse effects of chemotherapy either physically or emotionally. Some attempts have been made to develop a simple performance scale to predict whether a patient will respond to chemotherapy and be able to tolerate the adverse effects. The Eastern Cooperative Oncology Group, a multicenter cooperative group for cancer studies, uses a simple ADL scale (Box 22-7).[61] If a patient has a performance status below 3, chemotherapy is not recommended, unless a response is highly likely and the patient is motivated enough to tolerate treatment. Level 3 corresponds to being in bed more than 50% of the time. Motivation is key because of the tremendous discomfort and pain associated with chemotherapeutic drugs. Patients often become noncompliant with treatment schedules because they are unable to tolerate the adverse effects of drug therapy. At this point, the patient must choose between therapeutic treatment and palliative treatment (symptom-controlling treatment).

Exercise and Chemotherapy

There is a strong rationale for exercising during chemotherapy, since exercising influences immune system parameters that are important in cancer defense and in protection from infection.[50] For example, neoplastic cells may be eliminated by cancer-cell–specific CD8+ cytotoxic cells or the natural killer (NK) cells of the immune system;[50] neutrophils (granulocytes) are important because of their activity in resisting infection, thus preventing an unnecessary and perhaps deleterious delay in chemotherapy. There is evidence that both these cell types and others are positively affected by exercise.

Natural killer cell counts and cytolytic activity vary with acute exercise as well as with training. A meta-analysis of 94 studies with more than 900 healthy volunteers showed that acute exercise produced elevations in NK cell count directly after exercise, followed by a slow drop and then a return to normal resting values within 24 hours.[62] With prolonged or very intensive exercise, these counts started to drop sooner, while the exercise period was still ongoing. This study also supported the theory that moderately intense exercise (as opposed to very intensive exercise) improves immune function, as demonstrated by an increase in resting NK cell count following the training period. Therefore it appears that acute and intensive bouts of exercise as well as chronic intensive workouts decrease immunity but that moderate exercise may enhance immunity.[63,64]

BOX 22-7 Eastern Cooperative Oncology Group (ECOG) Performance Status Scale

- 0: Normal Activity
- 1: Symptoms but ambulatory
- 2: Bed rest <50% of the time
- 3: Bed rest >50% of the time
- 4: Total bed rest

Adapted from Bakermeier RF, Qazi R: Basic concepts of cancer chemotherapy and principles of medical oncology. In Rubin P, editor: *Clinical oncology* (8th ed.), New York, 2001, Saunders.

In cancer survivors, regular exercise has been shown to increase natural killer cell cytotoxic activity, and acute exercise in this population has been related to leukocytosis and lymphocytosis.[65-70] Dimeo (1999) studied exercise training following peripheral stem cell transplantation demonstrating that exercise is associated with increased NK cell cytotoxic activity, increased neutrophil count, and greater phagocytotic capacity.[71] Exercise was also shown to be beneficial during chemotherapy; a study demonstrated that the traditional Chinese medicine, Qi-Gong therapy (a form of exercise in which the patient maintains a standing position with arms positioned as if they were hugging a tree trunk), significantly increased neutrophil count, compared with that in the control group, during the second and third weeks of a first cycle of chemotherapy in patients with breast cancer.[72] In another study, 8 weeks of exercise during chemotherapy was shown to produce a training effect, demonstrated by an elevation in VO_{2max}.[73] This training effect proves that exercise administered during chemotherapy can minimize deconditioning and debilitating adverse effects.

Supervised exercise during breast cancer treatment has also been shown to improve functional capacity, body composition, mood states, and symptoms of nausea and fatigue, and, in general, improve Quality of Life (QoL) measures.[74-78] Additionally, as mentioned above, some studies have demonstrated decreases in infection rate, elevated levels of some beneficial immune markers such as natural killer (NK) cells, and a decrease in the duration of neutropenia during treatment.

Although these studies demonstrated the numerous positive effects of exercise, it is difficult to make comparisons and interpret results, since there was a great deal of variability in study design, type of exercise, and frequency. The exercise studies that have been reviewed required a training frequency of three times per week for variable durations, for example, 6, 8, 10, and 16 weeks.[66,71,79,80] The modes of exercise in these studies varied as well; strength training was used in a study on prostate cancer, whereas other studies on breast cancer utilized either a combination of strength and aerobic training or just aerobic exercises.[69,71,81] Perhaps the biggest problem with reviewing the literature is that very few studies actually evaluated immune parameters, blood counts, and quality-of-life issues while the patient was receiving chemotherapy.[74,77,80] Most exercise studies have been performed on patients with breast cancer following chemotherapy.[50,69,70,82,83] The above literature review suggests that in patients undergoing chemotherapy and in cancer survivors exercise can be beneficial. However, the discussion also highlights the difficulty in determining the correct exercise prescription. Selecting the specific exercise prescription is also difficult, since cancer is not one disease with one type of treatment but rather comprises more than 100 different entities with a variety of treatment options. There are many variables, locations of cancer, chemotherapy protocols or surgical procedures, and individual patient factors such as level of fatigue, nausea, pain, muscle wasting and cachexia, and precancer physical capacity. Specific precautions need to be considered when prescribing exercise for patients with cancer undergoing chemotherapy. Besides abnormalities in complete blood counts, therapists must take into consideration any ataxia that might develop as a result of neuropathy from some of the drugs (taxanes and mitotic spindle inhibitors) that would contraindicate exercising on a treadmill. Bone metastases dictate avoidance of high-impact activities with increased fracture risk; activities such as swimming should be avoided by patients with neutropenia because of the increased risk of bacterial infection. Patients with joint pain, especially at the hip, that increases with activity should be referred back to their physicians. The presence of muscle wasting and sarcopenia may limit resistive training with all but very light weights. Cardiac monitoring, with a pulse oximeter, a blood pressure cuff, and a heart rate monitor, may also be a necessity with patients who have received anticancer antibiotics, especially doxorubicin and daunorubicin, as these drugs can cause congestive heart failure. Guidelines regarding when it is safe to exercise have been provided in the literature. These include a hemoglobin count of at least 10 g/mL, a platelet count of 50,000/mL, and an absolute neutrophil count (ANC) of $<500/mm^3$.

Prior to beginning an exercise program, therapists should obtain a detailed medical history and a history of present illness; the Revised Physical Activity Readiness Questionnaire (PAR-Q) should also be administered to assess readiness for exercise.[84] This assessment consists of seven questions about symptoms of cardiac disease, whether the patient feels dizziness, or if the patient has a bone or joint problem, all of which could be made worse by exercise. It also asks the patient to report use of any cardiovascular medications. If the patient answers yes to one or more questions, the physician's clearance is needed before participation in an exercise program. Other useful assessments are the Piper Fatigue Scale (PFS) and the Hospital Anxiety and Depression Scale (HADS). The PFS consists of 22 items that measure aspects of fatigue: severity, cognitive changes, mood, and so on. Each item is graded on a 0–10 scale, and then the results are summed and divided by the total number of items. The scores end up falling between 0 and 10, with greater fatigue corresponding to a higher earned score.[85-87] Other scales include the Fatigue Barriers Scale and the Fatigue Knowledge Scale. Similar to fatigue, depression and anxiety are common symptoms experienced by patients with cancer, both during and after treatment. The HADS can be used to rule out clinical depression.[88]

Once the patient's readiness to exercise is determined, a submaximal exercise test can be performed. This test will estimate the VO_{2max} or cardiorespiratory endurance from heart rate (HR) measurements. The target heart rate for training can be determined, usually between 40% and 60%.[89] Moderate intensity is recommended but depends on the current physical capacity and the adverse effects of treatment. Some guidelines include 50 to 75% VO_{2max} or $HR_{reserve}$, 60 to 80% HR_{max} or an RPE (rating of perceived exertion) of 11. Walking tends to be the preferred exercise, since it is functional; however, cycle ergonometry may be safer, depending on the presence of ataxia or the likelihood of dizziness. Elliptical training is another option. The recommended frequency of exercise is three to five sessions per week with a duration of 30 to 60 minutes per session. However, 30 minutes of exercise can be achieved in three 10-minute sessions if the patient cannot sustain the recommended dose. Some patients may only be able to sustain activity for a minute or two. On the basis of the patient's tolerance to exercise, fatigue level, and reaction to chemotherapy, exercise duration will need to be adjusted. To be safe, the target heart rate (THR) is 20 to 30 beats above resting, but signs and symptoms must be monitored closely. The guidelines for resistive training are less precise. It is generally recommended that the patient exercise using a specific level of resistance that will cause an overload, but, again, this is based on the patient's level of tolerance. The best rule of thumb is to use a gravitationally challenged position and an exercise overload that the patient can tolerate.

Red flags indicating that exercise must be halted include an abnormal HR or blood pressure (BP) response to exercise, pallor, dizziness, nausea, fatigue, and excessive sweating. The major warning symptoms prior to exercise include a resting HR above 100, shortness of breath (SOB), and a drop in diastolic BP from the normal resting rate. These are signs of anemia, and the physician needs to be called immediately. Throughout the training sessions, the patient should be monitored for a negative change in exercise performance and new or increasing bone pain. If these occur, a return to the physician is recommended.

The success of any exercise program depends largely on the motivation and perseverance of the patient. Unfortunately, sticking to an exercise regimen is difficult even for healthy individuals, and patients with cancer face greater barriers and challenges. Exercise studies in breast cancer survivors have reported adherence rates ranging from 52 to 89%. In a study of exercise during chemotherapy, 33% of the exercise group did not exercise at the prescribed levels.[90] Therapists must be both creative and pragmatic when designing a program for patients with cancer and have solutions that address the physiologic and psychological barriers as they develop in these patients. One suggestion is to prepare two exercise protocols for each patient—one that helps the patient progress to his or her target exercise level and another designed to match the patient's level of function on days when the effects of the chemotherapy are particularly troublesome. Psychologically, the patient will then not experience the added burden of worrying about an exercise session that may be too difficult and too uncomfortable. While helping patients inch ahead slowly, it is also extremely important to meet them at their levels of functioning.

IMMUNOSUPPRESSION

Drugs that are used to prevent organ or tissue rejection are known as *immunosuppressant agents*. Commonly used agents include cyclosporine, muromonab-CD3, tacrolimus, sirolimus, and basiliximab.[2,92] Steroids are often combined with these drugs for added immunosuppression. Each agent differs in its exact mechanism of action, but the result is always inhibition of T-cell activation. See Figure 22-7 for the sites of action of these agents. Patients who take these drugs become immunocompromised, similar to patients with acquired immune deficiency syndrome (AIDS) or patients with bone marrow depression resulting from high-dose chemotherapy. Thus, many of the concerns discussed earlier are also relevant in the case of the patient who has undergone transplantation surgery.

Immunosuppressant Agents

Cyclosporine is the primary agent used to prevent the rejection of a transplanted kidney, heart, liver, or bone marrow. It is also beneficial in the treatment of some autoimmune disorders. This is a potent drug that has a narrow therapeutic index. Acute nephrotoxicity is a common adverse effect that generally occurs within the first month of use. Reduction of the dose may reverse the toxicity. Some other effects include hepatotoxicity; hypertension (50% of patients); neurotoxicity, including tremors (20% of patients); hyperkalemia; hirsutism; glucose intolerance; and gingival hyperplasia.

Tacrolimus is similar to cyclosporine but more potent. It is used primarily to prevent liver rejection. It produces a lower incidence of rejection, and lower doses of glucocorticoids are needed, which reduces the incidence of infections. Because this agent is more potent, it also produces a greater incidence of nephrotoxicity and neurotoxicity compared with cyclosporine. Other toxic effects are similar to those caused by cyclosporine, except hirsutism and gingival hyperplasia. Sirolimus is very similar to tacrolimus in chemical structure and in mechanism of action. It is used to prevent organ rejection but also has been used as a coating on stents during angioplasty to prevent restenosis.

Basiliximab and daclizumab are both IL-2 receptor antagonists. They are MABs that bind to the IL receptor present on the cell surface of activated lymphocytes. Both drugs are used to prevent kidney rejection in a regimen that includes cyclosporine and a steroid. They are better tolerated than cyclosporine.

Muromonab-CD3 is another MAB directed against the CD3 antigen of the human T cell. It is unique for a variety of reasons. It is very similar to the antibodies naturally produced by the human body, but it is derived from mice. In addition, it is the only immunosuppressant agent indicated for the treatment of organ rejection once

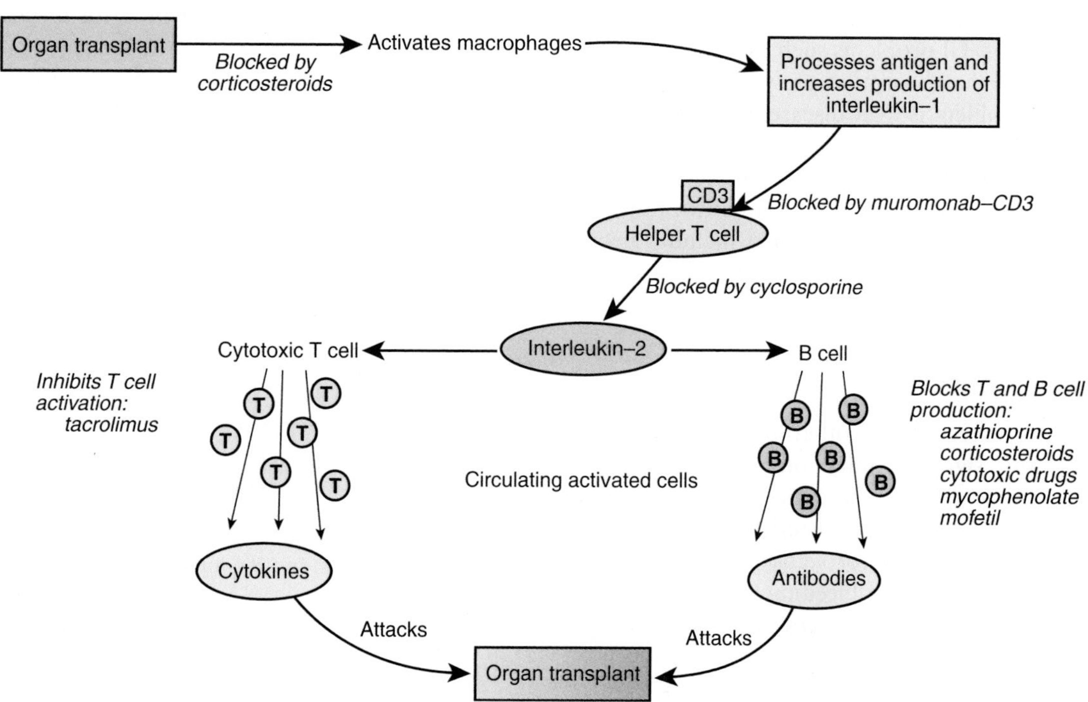

FIGURE 22-7 Sites of action for immunosuppressive agents. *(From McKenry LM, Salerno E.:* Mosby's pharmacology in nursing *(21st ed.), St Louis, 2003, Mosby.)*

it has started. However, because initial use is associated with cytokine release, it is necessary to premedicate the patient with methylprednisolone, diphenhydramine, and acetaminophen. This cytokine release syndrome leads to flu-like illness. A high fever as well as seizures, encephalopathy, and cerebral edema may occur.

Implications for the therapist are similar to those outlined for some of the chemotherapeutic agents. Therapists must watch for signs of infection and bone marrow depression. Therapists must also watch for signs of graft-versus-host disease (GVHD), which can be devastating.

Graft-versus-Host Disease

Acute GVHD occurs very quickly after transplantation or bone marrow infusion. It is caused by alloantigen-activated donor T cells that travel into target organs and cause tissue destruction.[92] It is the primary cause of morbidity and mortality among transplant recipients. In terms of hematopoietic cell transplantation, it causes death in 15 to 40% of patients. Symptoms include hepatitis, dermatitis, and GI problems. The rashes are maculopapular and often begin on the palms and soles. This syndrome results from inflammatory cytokines and has been called *cytokine storm* because of the continued release of cytokines.

Chronic GVHD develops in 15 to 50% of patients who survive 3 months after transplantation.[92] It involves multiple organ toxicity. The skin becomes fragile, and rashes also occur. Nails become fragile and cracked with vertical ridging, and hair becomes thin and delicate. Ocular symptoms include dryness, photophobia, and burning of eyes. The mouth becomes dry, a sensitivity to spicy food develops. GI problems such as reflux, dysphagia, diarrhea, and malabsorption as well as cholestasis occur. Another problem is liver disease. Chronic GVHD displays some musculoskeletal signs, including muscle cramps and fascitis (diminished slide of the skin over muscles).[93] Therapy may be required to monitor range of motion. Respiratory system involvement includes bronchiolitis; lastly, the immune system displays severe immunodeficiency.

Therapeutic Concerns

As with patients receiving chemotherapy, therapists must be alert for any signs of infection in patients with GVHD. The physician must be contacted immediately if fever, rash, sore throat, or unusual fatigue develops. Patients must be monitored for signs of bone marrow depression, such as increased bleeding or bruising. Frequent laboratory monitoring is necessary, and the drugs may be withheld if the leukocyte count drops below $30{,}000/mm^3$.

Patients who have undergone transplantation surgery must continue to receive immunosuppressants on a long-term basis. Adverse effects are unpleasant and often lead to noncompliance with treatment.[94] In addition to the hypertension or hypercholesterolemia, transplant recipients also experience changes in physical appearance and emotional baseline. Weight gain, sleep deprivation, tremors, hirsutism, sexual dysfunction, and psychiatric symptoms (depression and anxiety) may develop and affect the patient's quality of life. Therapeutic exercise can help deal with some of these adverse effects; gentle stretching modalities, conditioning programs, and biofeedback can help cope with drug-induced myalgias, weight gain, and some of the musculoskeletal symptoms of chronic GVHD. Patients should be scheduled for therapy at times when the facility is least crowded, and they should be kept away from those with a cold, infection, or other contagious illnesses.

ACTIVITIES 22

1. Multiple organ toxicity is a sign of graft-versus-host disease (GVHD). What are some of the early signs that indicate multiple organs are involved, and what dysfunction do they represent?
2. How would you monitor for the complications of multiple toxicity?
3. Provide some strategies that the therapist can implement to help protect the immunocompromised patient in the rehab clinic.
4. Chemotherapy agents are potentially hazardous not just to the patient but also to the caregiver who administers the drug. Therefore all drugs, vials, needles, syringes, and other equipment must be disposed of with extreme caution. Discuss some of the methods for drug disposal, as well as for disposal of body fluids that may contain chemotherapy agents.
5. Chemotherapy medications often cause neutropenia in the patient with cancer. What activities and/or foods should be avoided, and what is the neutropenic diet?
6. During the course of treatment with a mitotic spindle inhibitor, a patient complains of numbness and tingling in the hands and feet. What is the significance of this, and what is the treatment?

REFERENCES

1. McKenry LM, Salerno E: Principles of antineoplastic chemotherapy. In Mosby's pharmacology in nursing (21st ed.), St Louis, 2003, Mosby.
2. Lilley LL, Harrington D, Snyder JS. Antineoplastic agents. In Pharmacology and the nursing process (4th ed.), St Louis, 2005, Mosby.
3. Norman KL, Farassati F, Lee PWK: Oncolytic viruses and cancer therapy. Cytokine Growth Factor Rev 12:271-282, 2001.
4. Lane DP, Lain S: Therapeutic exploitation of the p53 pathway. Trends Mol Med 8(suppl 4):S38-S42, 2002.
5. Reed JC: Apoptosis-based therapies. Nat Rev Drug Discov 1: 111-121, 2002.

6. Sikic BI: New approaches in cancer treatment. Ann Oncol 10(suppl 6):149-153, 1999.
7. Eder JP: Drugs and neoplasms. In Page C, Curtis MJ, Sutter MC, Walker MJ, Hoffman BB, editors: Integrated pharmacology (2nd ed.), Philadelphia, 2002, Mosby.
8. Polovich M, White J, Kelleher, L: Chemotherapy and biotherapy guidelines and recommendations for practice (2nd ed.), Pittsburgh, 2005, Mafrica.
9. Damaraju VL, Damaraju S, Young JD, et al: Nucleoside anticancer drugs: The role of nucleoside transporters in resistance to cancer chemotherapy. Oncogene 22:7524-7536, 2003.
10. Kruh GD, Belinsky MG: The MRP family of drug efflux pumps. Oncogene 22:7537-7552, 2003.
11. Furlanut M, Franceschi L: Pharmacology of ifosfamide. Oncology 65(suppl 2):2-6, 2003.
12. Siddik ZH: Cisplatin: Mode of cytotoxic action and molecular basis of resistance. Oncogene 22:7265-7279, 2003.
13. Degrassi, F, Fiore M, Palitti F: Chromosomal aberrations and genomic instability induced by topoisomerase targeted antitumor drugs. Curr Med Chem Anti-Cancer Agents 4:317-325, 2004.
14. Osborne K: Drug therapy: Tamoxifen in the treatment of breast cancer. N Engl J Med 339(22):1609-1618, 1998.
15. Tamoxifen for prevention of breast cancer. Med Lett Drugs Ther 41(1043):1-2, 1999.
16. Cummings SR, Eckert S, Krueger KA, et al: The effect of raloxifene on risk of breast cancer in postmenopausal women. JAMA 281(23):2189-2197, 1999.
17. Piccart-Gebhart MJ: New stars in the sky of treatment for early breast cancer. N Engl J Med 350(11):1140-1142, 2004.
18. Toremifene and letrozole for advanced breast cancer. Med Lett Drugs Ther 40(1024):43-45, 1998.
19. Coombes RC, Hall E, Gibson LJ, et al: A randomized trial of exemestane after two to three years of tamoxifen therapy in postmenopausal women with primary breast cancer. N Engl J Med 350(11):1081-1092, 2004.
20. Dumontet C, Sikic BI: Mechanisms of action of and resistance to antitubulin agents: Microtubule dynamics, drug transport, and cell death. J Clin Oncol 17(3):1061-1070, 1999.
21. Tanner KD, Reichling DB, Levine JD: Nociceptor hyper-responsiveness during vincristine-induced painful peripheral neuropathy in the rat. J Neurosci 18(16):6480-6491, 1998.
22. Orr GA, Verdier-Pinard P, McDaid H, Horwitz SB: Mechanisms of taxol resistance related to microtubules. Oncogene 22:7280-7295, 2003.
23. Rasheed ZA, Rubin EH: Mechanisms of resistance to topoisomerase I-targeting drugs. Oncogene 22(47):7296-7304, 2003.
24. Savage DG, Antman KH: Imatinib mesylate: A new oral targeted therapy. N Engl J Med 346(9):683-693, 2002.
25. Druker BJ: ST1571 (Gleevec) as a paradigm for cancer therapy. Trends Mol Med 8(4):S14-S18, 2002.
26. Druker BJ, Talpaz M, Resta DJ, et al: Efficacy and safety of a specific inhibitor of the BCR-ABL tyrosine kinase in chronic myeloid leukemia. N Engl J Med 344(14):1031-1037, 2001.
27. Druker BJ, Sawyers CL, Kantarjian H, et al: Activity of a specific inhibitor of the BCR-ABL tyrosine kinase in the blast crisis of chronic myeloid leukemia and acute lymphoblastic leukemia with the Philadelphia chromosome. N Engl J Med 344(14):1038-1042, 2001.
28. Gleevec (STI-571) for chronic myeloid leukemia. Med Lett Drugs Ther 43(1106):49-50, 2001.
29. Papamichail M, Perez SA, Gritzapis AD, Baxevanis CN: Natural killer lymphocytes: Biology, development, and function. Cancer Immunol Immunother 53(3):176-186, 2003.
30. Kawabata TT: Immunopharmacology. In Brody MJ, Larner J, Minneman KP, editors: Human pharmacology: Molecular to clinical (3rd ed.), St Louis, 1998, Mosby.
31. Houghton AN, Scheinberg DA: Monoclonal antibody therapies: A "constant" threat to cancer. Nat Med 6(4):373-374, 2000.
32. Smith MR: Rituximab (monoclonal anti-CD20 antibody): Mechanisms of action and resistance. Oncogene 22:7359-7368, 2003.
33. White CA, Weaver RL, Grillo-Lopez AJ: Antibody-targeted immunotherapy for treatment of malignancy. Annu Rev Med 52:125-145, 2001.
34. Vogel CL, Cobleign MA, Tripathy D, et al: Efficacy and safety of trastuzumab as a single agent in first-line treatment of HER2-overexpressing metastatic breast cancer. J Clin Oncol 20(3):719-726, 2002.
35. Osoba D, Slamon DJ, Burchmore M, Murphy MB: Effects on quality of life of combined trastuzumab and chemotherapy in women with metastatic breast cancer. J Clin Oncol 20(14):3106-3113, 2002.
36. Mitchell MS: Combinations of anticancer drugs and immunotherapy. Cancer Immunol Immunother 52:686-692, 2003.
37. Bell R: Duration of therapy in metastatic breast cancer: Management using Herceptin. Anticancer Drugs 12:561-568, 2001.
38. Reynolds NA, Wagstaff AJ: Cetuximab: In the treatment of metastatic colorectal cancer. Drugs 64(1):109-118, 2004.
39. Harris M: Monoclonal antibodies as therapeutic agents for cancer. Lancet Oncol 5:292-302, 2004.
40. Erythropoietin (Procrit; Epogen) revisited. Med Lett Drugs Ther 43(1104):40-41, 2001.
41. Darbepoetin (Aranesp): A long-acting erythropoietin. Med Lett Drugs Ther 43(1120):109-110, 2001.
42. Martin-Christin F: Granulocyte colony stimulating factors: How different are they? How to make a decision? Anticancer Drugs 12:185-191, 2001.
43. Dale DC: Where now for colony-stimulating factors? Lancet 346:135-136, 1995.
44. Hoelzer D: Hematopoietic growth factors: Not whether, but when and where. N Engl J Med 336(25):1822-1824, 1997.
45. Culine S, Romieu G, Fabbro M, et al: Reducing the time interval between cycles using standard doses of docetaxel and lenogastrim support. Cancer 101:178-182, 2004.
46. Fu S, Liesveld J: Mobilization of hematopoietic stem cells. Blood Rev 14:205-218, 2000.
47. Fanucchi M, Glaspy J, Crawford J, et al: Effects of polyethylene glycol-conjugated recombinant human megakaryocyte growth and development factor on platelet counts after chemotherapy for lung cancer. N Engl J Med 336(6):404-409, 1997.
48. Trigg ME: Hematopoietic stem cells. Pediatrics 114(4): 1051-1057, 2004.
49. Inui A: Cancer anorexia-cachexia syndrome: Current issues in research and management, CA. Cancer J Clinicians 52:72-91, 2002.
50. Courneya KS: Exercise in cancer survivors: An overview of research. Med Sci Sports Exerc 35(11):1846-1852, 2003.
51. Grunberg SM, Hesketh PJ: Drug therapy: Control of chemotherapy-induced emesis. N Engl J Med 329(24):1790-1796, 1993.
52. Rolston K: Management of infections in the neutropenic patient. Annu Rev Med 55:519-526, 2004.
53. Clohisy DR, Mantyh PW: Bone cancer pain. Cancer 97 (suppl 3):866-873, 2003.
54. Fine PG: Analgesia issues in palliative care: Bone pain, controlled release opioids, managing opioid-induced constipation and nifedipine as an analgesic. J Pain Palliat Care Pharmacother 16(1):93-97, 2002.
55. Rogers MJ, Watts DJ, Graham R, Russell G: Overview of bisphosphonates. Cancer 80(8):1652-1660, 1997.
56. Tanner K, Levine J, Topp K: Microtubule disorientation and axonal swelling in unmyelinated sensory axons during vincristine-induced and painful neuropathy in rat. J Comp Neurol 395(4):481-492, 1998.

57. Ruppert M, Croarkin E: A review of four vibration sensation assessments used to examine chemotherapy induced neuropathy. Rehabil Oncol 21(3):11-18, 2003.
58. Perkins BA, Olaleye D, Zinman B, Bril V: Simple screening tests for peripheral neuropathy in the diabetes clinic. Diabetes Care 24(2):250-256, 2001.
59. Minisini A, Atalay G, Bottomley A, Puglisi F, Piccart M, Biganzoli L: What is the effect of systemic anticancer treatment on cognitive function? Lancet Oncol 5:273-282, 2004.
60. Fann JR, Sullivan AK: Delirium in the course of cancer treatment. Semin Clin Neuropsychiatry 8(4):217-228, 2003.
61. Bakemeier RF, Quazi R: Basic concepts of cancer chemotherapy and principles of medical oncology. In Rubin P, editor: Clinical oncology (8th ed.), New York, 2001, Saunders.
62. Moldoveanu AI, Shephard RJ, Shek PN: The cytokine response to physical activity and training. Sports Med 31(2): 116-144, 2001.
63. Wolach B, Gavrieli R, Ben-Dror SG, Zigel L, Eliakim A, Falk B: Transient decrease in neutrophil chemotaxis following aerobic exercise. Med Sci Sports Exerc 37(6):949-954, 2005.
64. Mackinnon LT: Chronic exercise training effects on immune function. Med Sci Sports Exerc 32(7):S369-S376, 2000.
65. Dimeo F, Fetscher S, Lange W, Mertelsmann R, Keul J: Effects of aerobic exercise on the physical performance and incidence of treatment-related complications after high-dose chemotherapy. Blood 90(9):3390-3394, 1997.
66. Dimeo F, Rumberger BG, Keul J: Aerobic exercise as therapy for cancer fatigue. Med Sci Sports Exerc 30(4):475-478, 1998.
67. Shore S, Shepard RJ: Immune responses to exercise in children treated for cancer. J Sports Med Physical Fitness 39:240-243, 1999.
68. Na YM, Kim MY, Kim YK, Ha YR, Yoon DS: Exercise therapy effect on natural killer cell cytotoxic activity in stomach cancer patients after curative surgery. Arch Phys Med Rehabilitat 81:777-779, 2000.
69. Fairey AS, Courneya KS, Field CJ, Bell GJ, Jones LW, Mackey JR: Randomized controlled trial of exercise and blood immune function in postmenopausal breast cancer survivors. J Appl Physiol 8:1534-1540, 2005.
70. Fairey AS, Courneya KS, Field CJ, Mackey JR: Physical exercise and immune system function in cancer survivors. Cancer 94:539-551, 2002.
71. Peters S, Lotzerich H, Niemeir B, Schule K, Uhlenbruck G: Exercise, cancer and the immune response of monocytes. Anticancer Res 15:175-180, 1995.
72. Yeh ML, Lee TI, Chen HH, Chao TY: The influences of Chan-Chuang Qi-gong Therapy on complete blood cell counts in Breast Cancer Patients treated with chemotherapy. Cancer Nurs 29(2):149-156, 2006.
73. Kim CJ, Kang DH, Smith BA, Landers KA: Cardiopulmonary responses and adherence to exercise in women newly diagnosed with breast cancer undergoing adjuvant therapy. Cancer Nurs 29(2):156-165, 2006.
74. Schwartz AL, Mori M, Gao R, Nail LM, King ME: Exercise reduces daily fatigue in women with breast cancer receiving chemotherapy. Med Sci Sports Exerc 33(5):718-723, 2001.
75. Segal R, Evans W, Johnson D, et al: Structured exercise improves physical functioning in women with stages I and II breast cancer: Results of a randomized controlled trial. J Clin Oncol 19(3):657-665, 2001.
76. Schwartz AL: Fatigue mediates the effects of exercise on quality of life. Quality Life Res 8:529-538, 1999.
77. Dimeo F, Stieglitz RD, Novelli-Fischer U, Fetscher S, Keul J: Effects of physical activity on the fatigue and psychologic status of cancer patients during chemotherapy. Cancer 85:2273-2277, 1999.
78. Winningham ML, MacVicar MG: The effect of aerobic exercise on patient reports of nausea. Oncol Nurs Forum 15(4):447-450, 1988.
79. Kolden GG, Strauman TJ, Ward A, et al: A pilot study of group exercise training (GET) for women with primary breast cancer: Feasibility and health benefits. Psycho-Oncology 11:447-456, 2002.
80. MacVicar MG, Winningham ML, Nickel JL: Effects of aerobic interval training on cancer patients' functional capacity. Nurs Res 38(6):348-351, 1989.
81. Segal R, Reid R, Courneya KS, et al: Resistance exercise in men receiving androgen deprivation therapy for prostate cancer. J Clin Oncol 21(9):1653-1659, 2003.
82. Burnham TR, Wilcox A: Effects of exercise on physiological and psychological variables in cancer survivors. Med Sci Sports Exerc 34(12):1863-1867, 2002.
83. Courneya KS, Mackey JR, McKenzie DC. Exercise for breast cancer survivors. The Physician and Sportsmedicine 30(8): 33-43, 2002.
84. http://www.shapeup.org/fitness/assess/parq1.php: Accessed November 9, 2009.
85. Borneman T, Piper B.F. Chih-Yi Sun V, Kodzywas M, Uman G, Ferrell B: Implementing the fatigue guidelines at one NCCN member institution: Process and outcomes. J Natl compr canc Netw·5(10):1092-1101, 2007.
86. Godin G, Lambert L, Owen N, Nolin B, Prud'homme D: Stages of motivational readiness for physical activity: A comparison of different algorithms of classification. Br J Health Psychol 9:253-267, 2004.
87. Godin G, Shephard RJ: A simple method to assess exercise behavior in the community. Can J Appl Sport Sci 10:141-146, 1985.
88. Vodermaier A, Linden W, Siu C: Screening for emotional distress in cancer patients: A systematic review of assessment instruments. J Natl Cancer Inst [Epub ahead of print] PubMed PMID: 19826136, 2009.
89. Whaley MH, Brubaker PH, Otto RM: ACSM's guidelines for exercise testing and prescription (7th ed.), New York, 2000, Lippincott Williams & Wilkins.
90. Pickett M, Mock V, Ropka ME, Cameron L, Coleman M, Podewils L: Adherence to moderate-intensity exercise during breast cancer therapy. Cancer Pract 10(6):284-292, 2002.
91. First MR, Fitzsimmons WE: New drugs to improve transplant outcomes. Transplantation 77(9):S88-S92, 2004.
92. Anasetti C: Advances in the prevention of graft-versus-host disease after hematopoietic cell transplantation. Transplantation 77(9):S79-S83, 2004.
93. Arai S, Vogelsang GB: Management of graft-versus-host disease. Blood Rev 14:190-204, 2000.
94. Galbraith CA, Hathaway D: Long-term effects of transplantation on quality of life. Transplantation 77(9):S84-S87, 2004.

SECTION VII

Special Topics in Pharmacology

23

Drugs for Gastrointestinal Disorders

Barbara Gladson

PHYSIOLOGIC CONTROL OF DIGESTION

Control of digestion represents a multisystem effort involving neuronal and hormonal regulation. Input from all of the involved systems coordinates the three phases of digestion.

Neuronal Control

The gastrointestinal (GI) tract can be viewed as a long, hollow tube surrounded by strong smooth muscle that propels food from one end to the other. Most of its length consists of five layers: (1) an inner mucosal layer, (2) a submucosal layer, (3) circular smooth muscle, (4) longitudinal smooth muscle, and (5) an outer serosal layer (peritoneum) continuous with the mesentery.[1,2] Two interconnected neural plexuses, which together are known as the *enteric nervous system*, that are contained within the wall of the GI tract provide neural input for smooth muscle contraction. The myenteric plexus is located between the circular muscle layer and the longitudinal muscle layer, and the submucosal plexus is located between the mucosal layer and the circular muscle layer.[3,4] Both plexuses receive preganglionic input from the parasympathetic fibers of the vagus nerve, where most of the fibers are cholinergic and excitatory, although some are inhibitory. Parasympathetic innervation to the colon also occurs from the sacral segments of the spinal cord via the pelvic nerve. Neurons within the plexus secrete acetylcholine (Ach) and norepinephrine as well as serotonin, purines, nitric oxide, and several peptides. Neural plexuses are concerned mainly with GI motility, but they also communicate with mechanoreceptors, which monitor wall stretch, and chemoreceptors, which check the osmolality, pH, and chemical composition of the contents.

The sympathetic system innervates the GI tract through thoracic ganglia as well as celiac, superior mesenteric, and inferior mesenteric ganglia. Control is exerted mainly by influencing the neural activity of the plexuses. The sympathetic system controls mucus secretion, decreases motility, and increases sphincter function. This system also increases the vascular smooth muscle tone of the vessels that supply the GI tract.

Hormonal Control

The GI tract is considered an endocrine organ because it produces hormones that pass through the portal circulation into the general circulation, only to return to exert influence on their organ of origin. One of the most important hormones produced by the GI tract is gastrin. Gastrin is produced by the mucosal G cells of the gastric antrum and duodenum.[5] Its primary function is to stimulate gastric acid secretion from the parietal cells, which aid in the digestion of food, particularly in the breakdown of protein. Gastrin also increases pepsinogen (which becomes pepsin when exposed to acid, another proteolytic enzyme) secretion, increases gastric blood flow, and increases gastric smooth muscle contraction. Growth of the mucosa of the stomach and of the small and large intestines is facilitated by gastrin, probably as a protective mechanism against acidity. The stimulus for gastrin production is vagal stimulation, which results from the intake of amino acids, alcohol, and calcium; whereas inhibition occurs in response to excessive acidity (pH below 2.5).

G cells and parietal cells are located within the deep pits and glands (oxyntic glands) of the stomach (Figure 23-1).[5] Parietal cells, which secrete intrinsic factor in addition to hydrocholoric acid, are located within the oxyntic gland in the deep neck region. The chief cells that secrete pepsinogen are located at the base of the gland, and mucous cells sit in the neck of the gland and also line the gastric surface. When stimulated, the acid from parietal cells that is mixed with pepsinogen makes its way up the glandular surface and then through the mucosal layer of the stomach.

Secretin is another GI hormone that is secreted by S cells in the mucosa of the duodenum and jejunum.[6] This hormone is released and activated when chyme enters the intestine with a pH less than 3. Secretin stimulates the pancreas to secrete a bicarbonate-containing solution. This is responsible for increasing the pH as food enters the intestine.

Cholecystokinin (CCK) is secreted from the duodenum and jejunum, particularly when the products of protein digestion and fatty acids arrive in the area.[6] This

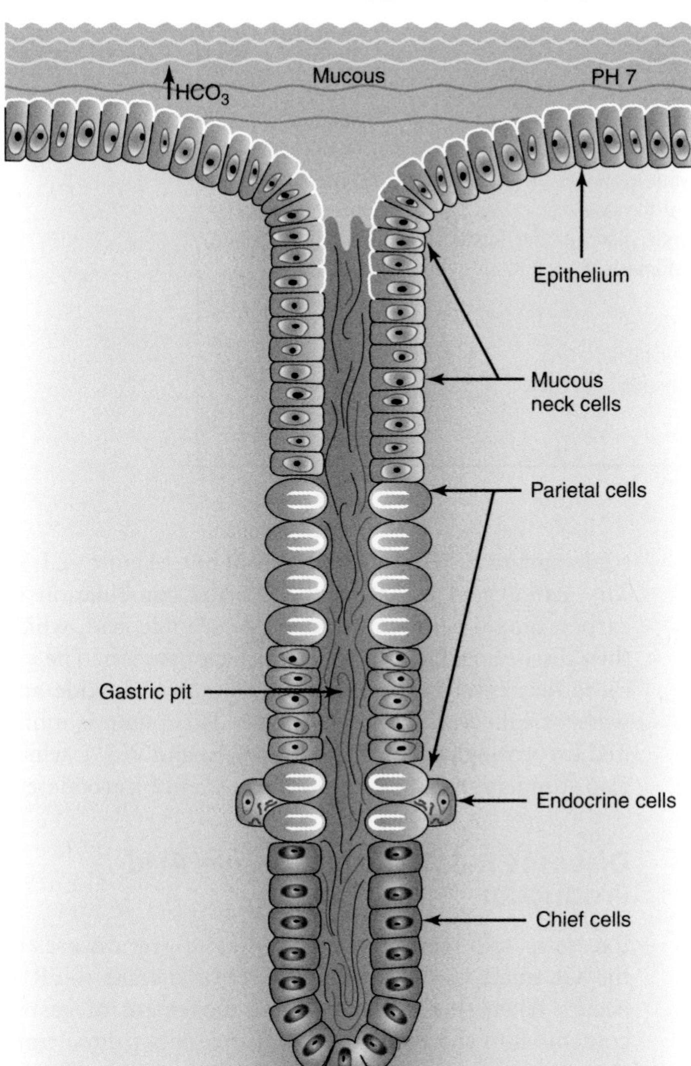

FIGURE 23-1 *(From Mejia A, Kraft WK:* Acid reflux and ulcer disease. *In Waldman SA, Terzic A, editors:* Pharmacology and therapeutics: Principles to practice, *Philadelphia, 2009, Saunders.)*

hormone stimulates contraction of the gallbladder to release its bicarbonate contents into the small intestine and also stimulates the secretion of pancreatic enzymes, which include trypsin, chymotrypsin, carboxypeptidase, and elastase. Pancreatic lipase is involved in the breakdown of triglycerides, forming micelles for easier absorption, and pancreatic amylase is the enzyme that breaks down carbohydrate.

A few other mediators of GI activity include somatostatin, gastric inhibitory peptide, motilin, ghrelin, and leptin. Somatostatin is released from D cells located in the gastric fundic and anthral mucosa.[5] It inhibits acid secretion from parietal cells and also histamine and gastrin release. Gastric inhibitory peptide is released from the intestinal mucosa in response to glucose and fats. It turns off gastric acid secretion in the stomach as the chyme passes into the intestine. Motilin stimulates intestinal motility. Leptin and ghrelin are hormones involved in satiety.[7-10] Leptin is secreted by adipocytes and is released in the presence of gastrin, CCK, secretin, and food, as well as in response to vagal nerve activity. Because of its role in creating fullness, it is being studied in relationship to obesity. Ghrelin may, in fact, have an opposite effect from that of leptin in that it is secreted in a fasting state, stimulates gastric acid secretion, and enhances food intake. Refer to Box 23-1 for a list of gastric mucosal cells, their locations, and their secretion.

Phases of Digestion

There are three main phases of digestion, the first of which begins even before food enters the mouth.[6,11] This is the *cephalic* or *psychic neural phase*. The smell, sight, or anticipation of food initiates the release of acid in the stomach. Parietal cells secrete acid to keep the pH between 1 and 4 for the denaturing of protein, the chief

BOX 23-1 Gastric Mucosal Cells and Their Secretions

Cell	Location	Secretion
Mucous cells	Isthmus of oxyntic gland in the cardiac and fundal (proximal) region and pyloric or antrum (distal) regions of the stomach	Mucous gel layer Mucin Prostaglandins
Parietal (Oxyntic) cells	Neck of oxyntic gland in the fundus and body of the stomach	Gastric acid Intrinsic factor
Chief cells	Base of oxyntic gland in the fundic region of stomach	Pepsinogen Renin Prostaglandin Leptin
Endocrine cells	Base of oxyntic glands	
G cells	Gastric antrum and duodenum	Gastrin
D cells		Somatostatin
Enterochromaffin-like cells		Histamine

cells secrete pepsinogen, and the mucoid cells secrete mucus that serves to protect the surface cells of the stomach from the digestive properties of the acid and enzymes.

The second phase is called the *gastric phase*. It begins when food comes into contact with the antrum. Gastrin is released as a result of stretching. Gastrin conveys information to the upper parts of the stomach to increase the secretion of gastric acid.

The third phase begins when the chyme enters the duodenum and is referred to as the *intestinal phase*. During this phase, the proteolytic enzyme activity in the stomach decreases, and acid secretion lessens. As the food moves into the intestine, a bicarbonate solution and pancreatic enzymes are released to further aid in digestion and absorption.

ACID-RELATED DISEASE AND ITS TREATMENT

Because the parietal cell secretes acid, it has become the target of many drugs for the treatment of acid-related disorders. The wall of the parietal cell contains three receptors, one for each of the following chemicals: ACh, histamine, and gastrin (Figure 23-2).[12] When histamine occupies the receptor, a cascade of events is initiated and results in the conversion of adenosine triphosphate (ATP) into cyclic adenosine monophosphate (cAMP), providing the energy for the proton (acid) pump. When either ACh or gastrin occupies the receptor, the signal to initiate the production of acid is the calcium ion. The proton pump is located in the parietal cell and can be blocked by histamine blockers, anticholinergic agents, and drugs called *proton pump inhibitors* (*PPIs*).

The pump itself transports chloride (Cl^-) into the stomach lumen along with potassium (K^+). K^+ is then exchanged for hydrogen (H^+) from within the cell by the energy derived from the potassium/hydrogen/adenosine triphosphatase (K^+/H^+-ATPase) pump (Figure 23-3). The actual acid is obtained from the combination of carbon dioxide and water to yield carbonic acid, which then dissociates into H^+ and a bicarbonate ion. The enzyme that catalyzes the binding of carbon dioxide and water is called *carbonic anhydrase*. This pump is inhibited by prostaglandins E_2 and I_2 (PGE_2 and PGI_2), which also stimulate the secretion of mucus and bicarbonate.

Diseases Related to Excessive Acid Production

Excessive acid secretion is related to several diseases of the GI tract. Gastroesophageal reflux disease (GERD) occurs when there is an upward movement of gastric contents into the esophagus.[13] This results from a transient relaxation of the lower esophageal sphincter. It may result from gastric distension after a large meal or delayed gastric emptying and may increase in frequency when alcohol or fatty food is consumed. The refluxed material is usually returned to the stomach by means of peristaltic waves. Regular reflux produces mucosal injury to the esophagus, resulting in hyperemia, inflammation, and heartburn. Other symptoms include belching and pain in the retrosternal or epigastric area, which may radiate to the throat, shoulder, or back. Pain usually occurs soon after eating and is exacerbated by bending at the waist, lying down, or anything that increases intra-abdominal pressure, for example, a tight belt or waistband.

Persistent GERD can lead to Barrett's esophagus,[14] a disease in which the esophagus displays strictures, scar tissue, spasms, and edema caused by repeated injury to the mucosa. Barrett's esophagus is associated with an increased risk of esophageal cancer.

The term *peptic ulcer disease* (*PUD*) refers to a group of ulcerative disorders that occur in the upper GI tract (stomach and duodenum). An ulcer can affect one or all

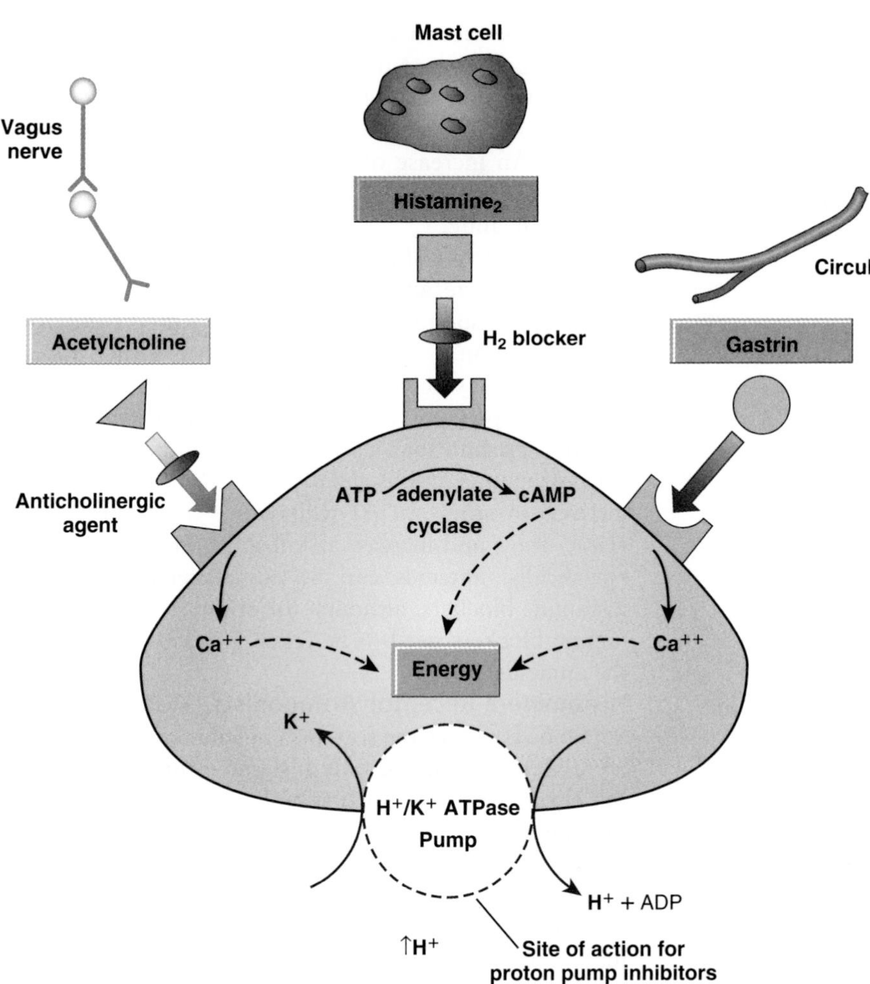

FIGURE 23-2 Parietal cell stimulation and secretion. *ADP,* Adenosine diphosphate; *ATP,* adenosine triphosphate; *cAMP,* cyclic adenosine monophosphate; H^+, hydrogen; H_2, histamine 2; K^+, potassium. *(From Lilley LL, Harrington S, Snyder JS, editors:* Pharmacology and the nursing process *(4th ed.). St. Louis, 2005, Mosby.)*

the layers of the stomach and duodenum. It may penetrate only the mucosal surface, or it can extend into the smooth muscle layers. Healing can occur, initially with scar tissue and later with the formation of a new muscle layer that is prone to further ulceration. Many cases of PUD result from *Helicobacter pylori* infection, although not everyone who is colonized by this bacterium develops PUD.[15] This is a gram-negative bacillus that lives within or beneath the mucosal layer and causes chronic gastritis. Gastritis and ulceration result from host immune responses to eradicate the organism, which induces proinflammatory cytokine expression and inflammation and also produces a reduction in somatostatin levels. Somatostatin inversely regulates gastrin production. Thus this bacterium indirectly increases gastrin and subsequent acid release.[16]

Aspirin and nonsteroidal anti-inflammatory drugs (NSAIDs) also account for many gastric and duodenal ulcers. It is estimated that approximately 25% of patients who are regular users of NSAIDs experience gastric distress, with some individuals developing ulceration and GI bleeding. A study showed that among patients who consume low to medium doses, the relative risk (RR) of developing a GI complication was 2.4 (95% confidence interval [CI] = 1.9–3.1); among those who consumed a high dose, the RR was 4.9 (95% CI = 4.1–5.8).[17] Although incidences of GI bleeding and mortality have been reduced over the last 10 years with the use of acid-controlling drugs and mucosal protectorants, complications secondary to NSAID use remain significant.[18] The pathogenesis of NSAID-induced PUD results from the inhibition of cyclooxygenase 1 (COX-1) in the GI mucosa.[19] Blockade of this enzyme limits the production of protective prostaglandins.

Pharmacologic Management (Acid-Suppressive Drugs)

Antacids, histamine blockers, and PPIs are the primary drugs used to suppress gastric hyperacidity. They represent three distinct mechanisms of action and therefore may be used in combination for more effective treatment (Box 23-2).

Antacids. The use of antacids dates back to the first century A.D. when they were used by ancient Greeks.[20] They would crush coral, which is calcium carbonate (the active ingredient in Tums) and use it to treat heartburn. Even though some excellent medications for acid-related

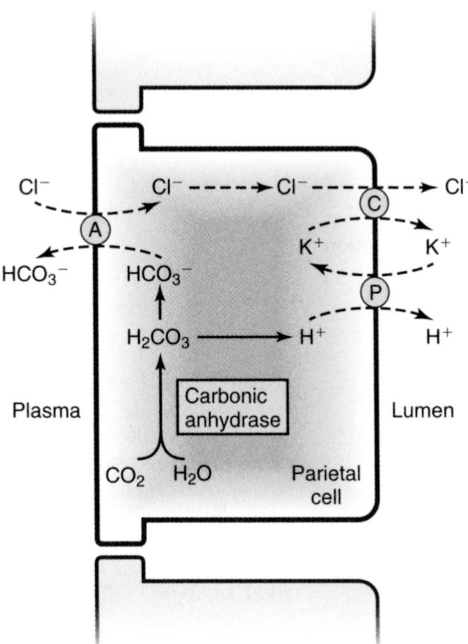

FIGURE 23-3 A schematic illustration of the secretion of hydrochloric acid by the gastric parietal cell. Secretion involves a proton pump (*P*), which is an H^+/K^+-ATPase pump, a symport carrier (*C*) for potassium (*K^+*) and chlorine (*Cl^-*), and an antiport (*A*), which exchanges Cl^- and HCO^{3-}. An Na^+/H^+ antiport at the interface with the plasma may also have a role (*not shown*).

BOX 23-2 Acid-Controlling Drugs

Drug	Pharmacologic Class
Cimetidine (Tagamet)	H_2 antagonist
Famotidine (Pepcid)	H_2 antagonist
Nizatidine (Axid)	H_2 antagonist
Ranitidine (Zantac)	H_2 antagonist
Aluminum hydroxide and magnesium hydroxide (Maalox, Mylanta)	Combination antacid
Calcium carbonate (Tums)	Antacid
Magnesium hydroxide (Milk of Magnesia)	Antacid
Omeprazole (Prilosec)	Proton pump inhibitor
Pantoprazole (Protonix)	Proton pump inhibitor
Rabeprazole (AcipHex)	Proton pump inhibitor
Esomeprazole (Nexium)	Proton pump inhibitor
Lansoprazole (Prevacid)	Proton pump inhibitor

diseases are available today, many people continue to take over-the-counter (OTC) antacid formulations.

Several basic preparations include aluminum-based, magnesium-based, and calcium-based preparations. A sodium bicarbonate–based solution is also available. The mechanism of action is to neutralize the gastric acidity.[21] However, it is also believed that antacids enhance the defensive properties of gastric mucosa by stimulating the secretion of mucus, prostaglandins, and bicarbonate. These actions result in reduction of pain and improved resistance to irritation.

Antacids are only modestly effective in healing of PUD, since frequent dosing is necessary, which reduces compliance. Therefore these drugs are typically not prescribed for PUD but, instead, are used for treating acid reflux.[22] An increase of pH from 1.3 to 3.5 with these agents produces symptomatic relief and allows for modest ulcer healing.[5]

Adverse effects of the antacids are minimal.[5] However, effervescent-type antacids (e.g., Alka-Seltzer) contain a great deal of sodium and should not be used regularly if a patient is on a sodium-restricted diet. Other adverse effects include some GI complaints. Magnesium preparations may produce diarrhea, and both aluminum and calcium preparations can produce constipation. Some drug–drug interactions can also occur with antacids. The increase in stomach pH will reduce the absorption of acidic drugs and increase the absorption of basic drugs. Specifically, antacids can be administered along with histamine blockers, although for optimal results, the histamine blockers need to be taken at least 1 hour before the antacids.

Histamine-2 Receptor Antagonists. Histamine-2 (H_2) antagonists reduce the secretion of stimulated acid.[5] They are able to inhibit not only histamine-stimulated release but also gastrin- and ACh-stimulated acid release, reducing the release of basal and some meal-related acids. These drugs promote the healing of ulcers, but unfortunately ulcers often reappear after therapy is stopped. Even with regular dosing, upregulation of the receptor may occur and limit the effectiveness of these drugs.[23]

The prototypical drugs in this category include cimetidine, ranitidine, famotidine, and nizatidine. These drugs are available in low doses over the counter. Generally, they are taken once daily in the evening. They are generally well tolerated but can produce diarrhea, dizziness, muscle pain, and rashes. Hypergastrinemia has also been reported. Cimetidine can cause gynecomastia because of its affinity for androgen receptors, and this drug also inhibits P450 enzymes and thus can slow down the metabolism of several drugs, including anticoagulants and some tricyclic antidepressants. A temporary rebound in acid secretion above pretreatment levels has been reported when these drugs are abruptly withdrawn. A surprising new finding has shown that famotidine can improve cardiac symptoms and ventricular remodeling in congestive heart failure.[24] The most probable explanation for this finding is the presence of H_2 receptors on cardiomyocytes. Further study is needed to determine if H_2 blockers will be included as part of standard care for heart failure.

Proton Pump Inhibitors. Omeprazole (now available OTC) was the first PPI on the market.[25] It irreversibly inhibits the H^+/K^+-ATPase pump on the parietal cell membrane, blocking the final step in acid secretion. Other drugs in this category include lansoprazole, pantoprazole, and rabeprazole. PPIs completely block both basal and stimulated acid secretion from the stomach, although they have little influence on H^+ secretion in other areas. These drugs are weak bases that need an acidic environment in order to become active, although rabeprazole is active in a wide range of pH readings. They become more effective with continued administration; acid secretion returns to baseline 3 days after withdrawal of the drug. PPIs have been approved for long-term use, but there is some concern that this treatment could facilitate more GI infections because it undermines the acidic environment, which offers some protection against invaders.

In numerous studies, omeprazole has been shown to be more effective than placebo in healing duodenal ulcers; it is also superior to H_2 receptor antagonists.[26] Its superiority extends to maintenance therapy as well. PPIs are superior in preventing bleeding with stress ulceration and reduce the need for further endoscopic therapy to treat upper GI bleeding. There appears to be little difference in effectiveness among the various PPIs. Adverse effects are minimal and similar to those of placebo or H_2 receptor blockers, but there have been some reports of *Campylobacter jejuni* enteritis and fungal infections.[27,28] There have also been some reports of cardiovascular abnormalities (angina, tachycardia, palpitations), musculoskeletal pain, fractures, and respiratory effects, mostly with lansoprazole and pantoprazole.[29,30]

Mucosal Protectors

The drugs that are currently available either enhance the protective mechanisms of the mucosa or provide a physical boundary over the surface of an ulcer.

Bismuth Chelate. Bismuth chelate offers numerous protective properties against an *H. pylori*–induced ulcer.[31,32] It is believed to coat the base of the ulcer, enhance prostaglandin synthesis, and increase gastric mucous epithelial cell growth. It also has a direct toxic effect on the bacillus. Blackening of the tongue and feces, as well as nausea and vomiting, are some adverse effects.

Sucralfate. Sucralfate is an aluminum salt of sucrose that is nonabsorbable. It is used to protect the mucosal lining in active stress ulcerations and chronic PUD. The term *stress ulcer* refers to a GI ulceration that develops during periods of major physiologic stress.[33] Patients who are at high risk for this ulcer include those with large surface area burns, trauma, liver failure, and acute respiratory distress syndrome (ARDS) and those undergoing major surgery. These ulcers appear in approximately 5 to 10% of patients receiving intensive care and result in perforation and bleeding.

Sucralfate acts locally by binding directly to the surface of the ulcer.[5] When it is exposed to an acid environment, the drug dissociates into aluminum hydroxide (an antacid) and sulfated sucrose. The sulfated molecules attach to the ulcer, forming a protective coating over the area. The drug is also thought to stimulate prostaglandin synthesis and release of mucus and bicarbonate.

One advantage of this drug is that it stays local and therefore does not interact with other drugs in the circulation; however, it can decrease the absorption of other medications. This interaction can be avoided by administering sucralfate separately, at least 2 hours after the administration of any other agent. Adverse effects are minor and include constipation and nausea.

Misoprostol. Misoprostol is a synthetic prostaglandin analog (PGE_2).[5] It is believed to inhibit acid secretion, enhance the production of mucus and bicarbonate, and maintain blood flow to the mucosa. It is used to prevent NSAID-induced ulcers. Diarrhea is a common adverse effect, but this drug also induces uterine contractions, so it is contraindicated in women who may become pregnant.

Management of *H. pylori* Infection

The presence of *H. pylori* infection leads to chronic gastritis, PUD, GERD, and gastric cancer.[34] Combination therapy is the standard regimen for the eradication of *H. pylori* and for the treatment of the associated ulcer. Because eradication of the bacterium decreases ulcer recurrence and enhances healing, antibiotics must be combined with acid-controlling drugs.[35] If *H. pylori* is not eliminated, ulcers recur in 50 to 90% of patients after antiulcer drugs are withdrawn. One of the first regimens for eliminating *H. pylori* included bismuth triple therapy consisting of colloidal bismuth, tetracycline, and metronidazole. This regimen demonstrated eradication rates above 80%. More recently, a PPI and two antibiotics (choice of clarithromycin, amoxicillin, and metronidazole) have been used, producing an eradication rate of 90%.[36] In fact, with good compliance, the bacterium may be eliminated in as little as 1 week. Efficacy depends on twice-a-day dosing of the PPI, not on which PPI is chosen. The classic quadruple regimen of bismuth triple therapy plus a PPI can also be used.

Management of Nonsteroidal Anti-inflammatory Drug–Induced Ulcers

The increasing trend toward administering NSAIDs and aspirin has led to a greater number of cases of PUD than has the presence of *H. pylori* infection.[37] Long-term NSAID use leads to gastritis and ulcerations, probably through blockade of prostaglandin production (see Chapter 11).[38] In some cases, *H. pylori* infection is present concomitantly with an NSAID-induced ulcer. In these cases, bacterial eradication alone is not adequate to prevent further bleeding.

Treatment regimens for *H. pylori* infection with NSAIDs initially include the eradication of the bacterium, followed by acid suppression therapy. NSAIDs should, however, be discontinued if possible. If they must be continued, it is imperative to have the patient continue acid suppression therapy, particularly with a

PPI. Misoprostol, available as a single agent or in combination with diclofenac, has been approved for the prevention of NSAID-induced ulcers, but the resulting diarrhea and abdominal cramping limit its use.[19] PPIs are now being recommended along with a gastroprotective drug when NSAIDs are needed. An alternative is to switch to the newer COX-2 inhibitors that are more GI friendly, even though they may pose additional cardiac risks.

NAUSEA AND VOMITING

Vomiting is the forceful expulsion of stomach contents through the mouth. It is usually preceded by nausea and repeated contractions of the abdominal muscles (retching). Vomiting can be a protective response to the ingestion of toxic chemicals or to an overdose of drugs but may also be an annoying or disabling adverse effect of medication. Vomiting accompanies many serious disease processes as well.

Although antiemetic drugs are quite helpful, it is important to acknowledge that even with treatment, nausea and vomiting from chemotherapy continue to occur in more than 50% of patients receiving strong emetogenic drugs such as cisplatin, and in more than 40% of patients receiving mild to moderately emetogenic drugs such as doxorubicin and cyclophosphamide. Because emesis can necessitate the withdrawal of chemotherapeutic agents, it is important that antiemetic drugs be used in conjunction with anticancer medications.

Neural Mechanisms Involved in Vomiting

Two separate areas in the medulla regulate vomiting.[39] The chemoreceptor trigger zone (CTZ) is located on the floor of the fourth ventricle of the cerebrum. Here the CTZ is exposed to both blood and cerebrospinal fluid and can respond to the presence of drugs and toxins.[40] The vomiting center, located in the dorsal reticular formation of the medulla, is responsible for the integration of signals from the GI tract, pharynx, vestibular system, and the CTZ (Figure 23-4). This area contains dopamine-2 (D_2) receptors, serotonin 5-HT_3 receptors, neurokinin-1 (NK_1) receptors, and opioid receptors. Hypoxia of this area produces vomiting, which accounts for events that occur during myocardial infarction or brain ischemia caused by increased intracranial pressure. Information from abdominal organs, the liver, the gallbladder, and other areas is communicated to the vomiting center through visceral afferent neurons. Mechanoreceptors located in the muscular wall of the stomach and chemoreceptors located in the mucosa of the upper GI tract also send information regarding the stretch and chemical makeup of the stomach to the vomiting center. The vestibular system, involved in motion sickness, contains muscarinic and histamine-1 (H_1) receptors. Irritation of the pharynx stimulates the gag-and-retch reflex via the vagus nerve and also can cause vomiting. The neurotransmitters involved in vomiting include dopamine, serotonin, and opioid receptors in the GI tract and the CTZ, norepinephrine, and ACh receptors in the vestibular center.

Antiemetic Drugs

Antiemetic drugs are mainly used to combat nausea and vomiting produced by many chemotherapy agents and illnesses related to vestibular motion. They include anticholinergic agents, antihistamines, neuroleptic agents, prokinetic drugs, serotonin inhibitors, and tetrahydrocannabinol (Box 23-3).[41] Steroids, with or without anxiolytics, may also be used.

Anticholinergics. Scopolamine is the primary anticholinergic drug used to prevent vomiting related to motion. It binds to ACh receptors on the vestibular nuclei located in the inner ear (labyrinths) and blocks the communication between this area and the vomiting center.[41]

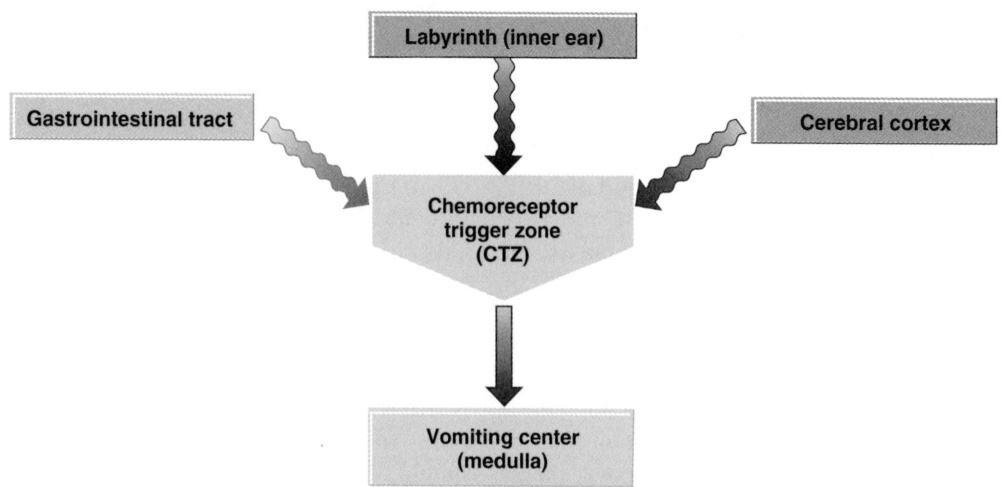

FIGURE 23-4 The various pathways and areas in the body that send signals to the vomiting center. *(From Lilley LL, Harrington S, Snyder JS, editors:* Pharmacology and the nursing process *(4th ed.). St. Louis, 2005, Mosby.)*

BOX 23-3 **Antiemetic Agents**

Drug	Mechanism of Action	Indication	Adverse Effects
Scopolamine (Transderm Scop)	Anticholinergic: blocks acetylcholine (ACh) receptors in the vestibular nuclei and reticular formation	Motion sickness	Dry mouth Blurred vision Drowsiness
Prochlorperazine (Compazine) Chlorpromazine (Thorazine) Metoclopramide (Reglan)	Neuroleptics: block dopamine in the chemoreceptor trigger zone (CTZ) center Metoclopramide also has peripheral effects; increases motility of esophagus, stomach, and intestine	Chemotherapy-induced vomiting, postoperative vomiting	Fatigue Motor restlessness Spasmodic torticollis Occulogyric crises
Meclizine (Antivert) Promethazine (Phenergan)	Antihistamines: block histamine-1 (H_1) receptors in the vestibular nuclei	Motion sickness	Sedation Dizziness
Ondansetron (Zofran) Granisetron (Kytril) Dolasetron (Anzemet)	Serotonin 5-HT_3 receptor antagonist: block serotonin receptors in the gastrointestinal tract, CTZ, and vestibular center	Chemotherapy-induced vomiting, postoperative vomiting	Headache Drowsiness
Dronabinol (Marinol) Nabilone (Cesamet)	Tetrahydrocannabinoids	Chemotherapy-induced vomiting	Drowsiness Dizziness Mood changes Postural hypotension Occasional hallucinations
Aprepitant (Emend)	Neurokinin-1 (NK_1) receptor antagonist: used in combination with 5-HT_3 receptor antagonists and steroids	Chemotherapy-induced vomiting, gastroparesis	Fatigue Dizziness Diarrhea Metabolized by Cytochrome P450 3A4 (CYP3a4) and may inhibit metabolism of other drugs metabolized by that enzyme, particularly some chemotherapeutic agents Increased international normalized ratio (INR)
Dexamethasone (Decadron)	Steroid	Chemotherapy-induced vomiting	Hyperglycemia Catabolic effects on connective tissue, muscle, peripheral fat, and skin Hypertension Immunosuppression Mood alterations

The most common form of scopolamine is a transdermal patch with a duration of action of up to 72 hours. The patch is applied to the hair-free skin behind the ear at least 4 hours before travel. Adverse effects include dizziness, drowsiness, blurred vision, dilated pupils, dry mouth, and difficulty with urination.

Neuroleptic Drugs. Neuroleptic drugs are antipsychotic agents that block dopamine receptors in the CTZ. Many of these drugs also have anticholinergic actions. Prochlorperazine and promethazine are commonly used for preventing nausea and vomiting during or immediately after surgery.[42] Adverse effects include orthostatic hypotension, tachycardia, blurred vision, dry eyes, and urinary retention. Long-term use produces extrapyramidal symptoms, akathisia, and tardive dyskinesia (see Chapter 19). Haloperidol and droperidol are commonly used for treating chemotherapy-induced vomiting.

Antihistamines. Cyclizine, dimenhydrinate, and diphenhydramine are H_1-blocking agents that act by inhibiting vestibular input to the CTZ.[43] Specifically, they block ACh binding to H_1 receptors in the vestibular nuclei and are used to treat motion sickness. Dizziness and sedation are the main adverse effects; therefore these drugs are not recommended for patients who will be driving.

Prokinetic Drugs. Prokinetic drugs block dopamine in the CTZ, but their primary action is to stimulate peristalsis, facilitating emptying of the stomach. Metoclopramide is used for treating delayed gastric emptying, GERD, and chemotherapy-related vomiting.[44] These drugs produce both central and peripheral antiemetic effects. Adverse effects include sedation, diarrhea, weakness, and prolactin release; with prolonged use, they cause extrapyramidal signs and motor restlessness. Patients taking prokinetic drugs may also experience hypotension, hypertension, and tachycardia. Other drugs in this category include trimethobenzamide and domperidone.

Serotonin Blockers. Serotonin antagonists that are used to prevent emesis specifically block the serotonin receptors in the GI tract, CTZ, and vomiting center.[45] They represent one of the newest classes of drugs for the prevention of nausea and vomiting caused by cancer chemotherapy. They include dolasetron, granisetron, ondansetron, and palonosetron.[46] They are equal in efficacy to a high dose of metoclopramide and can be administered in intravenous or oral formulations. Adverse effects include headache, dizziness, and diarrhea but no extrapyramidal effects. These drugs are usually administered 30 minutes before chemotherapy and often in conjunction with a steroid (dexamethasone).

Cannabinoids. Dronabinol, a schedule II controlled substance, is a synthetic derivative of THC (delta-9-tetrahydrocannabinol) used in the treatment of chemotherapy-related emesis.[47] It is also used as an appetite stimulant in patients with acquired immune deficiency syndrome (AIDS). Its antiemetic effects were originally observed in patients who were using marijuana during chemotherapy. This drug's mechanism of action in this role is unclear, but it may possess some antiadrenergic activity and block prostaglandin synthesis. It is considered a second-line agent in the treatment of emesis because of its adverse effects, which include ataxia, lightheadedness, blurred vision, dry mouth, weakness, tachycardia or bradycardia, and central nervous system (CNS) effects such as confusion, mood changes, and anxiety.

Corticosteroids. Corticosteroids, when used alone, are useful for decreasing emesis when mildly emetic chemotherapy drugs are administered but not with highly emetogenic agents.[41] The mechanism of action for this effect is poorly understood, but when steroids are combined with a serotonin blocker, this regimen is more effective than treatment with each drug alone. This combination is now standard practice for reducing chemotherapy-induced emesis.

Neurokinin-1 Receptor Antagonists. The category of NK_1 receptor antagonists contains several compounds that are currently under study for the treatment of emesis related to chemotherapy.[48] The focus of these drugs is to antagonize substance P. Substance P binds to the tachykinin NK_1 receptor and is capable of producing emesis through this mechanism. Aprepitant is approved by the U.S. Food and Drug Administration (FDA) for use with corticosteroids and selective serotonin receptor antagonists for the treatment of acute emesis and delayed emesis (more than 24 hours after infusion) associated with chemotherapy. When taken as monotherapy, aprepitant is no more effective than serotonin antagonists, but its usefulness is apparent in combination therapy. Adverse effects are mild but annoying. In comparison studies, hiccups occurred in 11% of patients receiving aprepitant compared with 6% of patients receiving the standard regimen.

Antinausea Drugs. Phosphorated carbohydrate solution, commonly sold under the name *Emetrol*, helps reduce nausea by working directly on the walls of the GI tract.[41] It appears to work by relaxing the smooth muscle. It is used for mild cases of nausea caused by intestinal flu or food-related causes.

DIARRHEA

Diarrhea refers to frequent passage of loose stools. The definition implies increased frequency, fluidity, and stool water excretion.[49] *Acute diarrhea* appears suddenly in a previously healthy person and lasts between 3 and 14 days.[50] Frequency of defecation is three or more times per day or 200 g of stool per day, and abdominal cramping is present. *Chronic diarrhea* refers to diarrhea lasting more than 3 to 4 weeks in conjunction with loss of appetite, fever, nausea, weight reduction, and fatigue.

Most cases of diarrhea are due to water and electrolyte imbalances in the intestinal tract.[51] Increased secretion of electrolytes and water into the lumen, loss of protein from the GI mucosa, and increased osmotic pressure in the intestine are all culprits. Underlying pathologic conditions associated with chronic diarrhea include irritable bowel syndrome (IBS), Crohn's disease, ulcerative colitis, bowel impaction with overflow, bacterial overgrowth, bile acid malabsorption, celiac disease, short bowel syndrome, laxative abuse, and diarrhea associated with diabetes. Other causes of fecal incontinence have to do with structural abnormalities, for example, weakness of the external anal sphincter and anorectal sensory loss, as well as use of some medications that reduce sphincter tone (anticholinergics such as tolterodine tartarate and oxybutynin and antispasticity drugs such as baclofen).[52]

Antidiarrheal Agents

Drugs that fall into the category of antidiarrheal agents include adsorbents, anticholinergics, intestinal flora modifiers, and opiates.

Adsorbents. Adsorbents coat the wall of the GI tract, bind to the diarrhea-causing bacteria, and then carry them out with the feces.[49] Examples of these agents include activated charcoal, bismuth subsalicylate, and attapulgite. The last two are commonly known as Pepto-Bismol and Kaopectate, respectively. Because bismuth subsalicylate is a salicylate similar to aspirin, it should be used with caution in children recovering from the flu or chickenpox because of the higher risk for Reye's syndrome. In addition, because it is an aspirin product, it has some of the same adverse effects, including increased bleeding time, GI bleeding, confusion associated with high doses, and hearing loss or tinnitus. Adsorbents decrease the effectiveness of many drugs, particularly digoxin, hypoglycemic drugs, and oral anticoagulants.

Anticholinergics. Anticholinergics reduce diarrhea by reducing peristalsis of the GI tract. Anticholinergic agents used for this purpose include atropine, hyoscyamine, and hyoscine.[49] They can be used in conjunction with adsorbents and opiates, but because of their adverse effects (see Chapter 5), they are rarely the first choice of treatment.

Intestinal Flora Modifiers. Intestinal flora modifiers are bacterial products obtained from *Lactobacillus* organisms.[49] They are normal occupants of the intestine that create an unfavorable atmosphere for the growth of certain kinds of diarrhea-causing bacteria. However, antibiotics destroy this normal flora and tip the balance in favor of the harmful organisms. *Lactobacillus acidophilus* returns the balance of the normal flora and suppresses the growth of harmful organisms, and it is available as an OTC remedy.

Opiates. Several opiates act as antidiarrheal drugs: codeine, loperamide (Imodium), and diphenoxylate (Lomotil).[53] Their mechanism of action in this venue is to decrease GI motility and propulsion. Slowing transit time increases the absorption of electrolytes and water. In addition, they can reduce the pain occurring with diarrhea. Loperamide can be obtained as an OTC medication, but others in this group require a prescription because they cross the blood–brain barrier. Opiates can be addictive and produce respiratory depression. Diphenoxylate is combined with a small quantity of atropine to prevent recreational opioid uses. In high quantities, the anticholinergic adverse effects will discourage abuse. Adverse effects of opiates include sedation, dizziness, constipation, nausea and vomiting, respiratory depression, bradycardia, hypotension, and urinary retention (see Chapter 11).

CONSTIPATION

Constipation is a movement disorder of the colon and rectum, which results in infrequent or painful defecation, hard stools, or a sense of incomplete evacuation. Chronic constipation consists of no more that two to three bowel movements per week with straining during more than 25% of the time.[54] It can be a symptom of a bowel impaction, or it can be due to some endocrine or neurogenic disorders. A sedentary lifestyle, a diet low in roughage or fluids, and certain medications can also be blamed. Constipation is usually managed by an improved diet, exercise, and use of laxatives. Surgical management is reserved for bowel impaction, organic or structural disorders of the bowel, or cancer.

Laxatives

Nonsurgical treatment of constipation can be divided into three categories: (1) improved fiber and fluid supplementation, (2) increased physical activity, and (3) pharmacologic treatment.[49] The pharmacologic approach involves the use of laxatives that may act by softening the feces or by increasing fecal movement through the colon and rectum. There are five basic types of laxatives and many are available as OTC medications (Figure 23-5 and Box 23-4).

Bulk-Forming Laxatives. Psyllium (Metamucil) and methylcellulose (Citrucel) act by increasing water absorption,

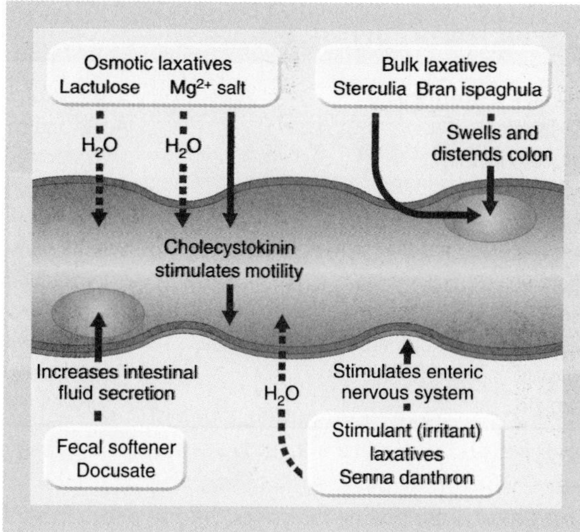

FIGURE 23-5 Mechanism of action of laxatives. Bulk laxatives absorb water and, on swelling, slowly distend the colon and increase peristaltic motility; osmotic laxatives enhance peristalsis by osmotically increasing the bowel fluid volume; stimulant (irritant) laxatives stimulate the enteric nervous system; fecal softeners increase intestinal fluid secretion. *(From Page C, Curtis AB, Sutter MC, Walker MJ, Hoffman BB, editors:* Integrated pharmacology *(2nd ed.). Philadelphia, 2002, Mosby.)*

which results in softening and increasing the bulk of the intestinal contents.[55] As the fiber swells, it distends the colon. This, in turn, results in increased peristalsis. These are relatively safe drugs that can be used on a prolonged basis and do not cause dependency. They are contraindicated in patients with abdominal pain and/or nausea and vomiting and must be consumed with a full glass of water to prevent esophageal obstruction and fecal impaction.

Emollient Laxatives. Emollient laxatives are also known as *fecal softeners* and *lubricant laxatives*.[54] Stool softeners such as docusate sodium (Colace) facilitate water and fat absorption into the stool, and lubricant laxatives such as mineral oil lubricate the fecal material and the wall of the intestine. Reabsorption of water back into the body is blocked. Adverse effects are minimal but can include skin rashes, decreased absorption of vitamins, and electrolyte imbalances. Staining of clothing can also occur when mineral oil is used.

Hyperosmotic Laxatives. Hyperosmotic laxatives work primarily in the large intestine by drawing fluid into the colon. Examples include glycerin, lactulose, and polyethylene glycol. Lactulose is a synthetic sugar that is not digested in the stomach or absorbed in the small intestine. However, it is metabolized in the large intestine into a hyperosmotic solution that draws fluid into the colon. Polyethylene glycol is a laxative used before diagnostic or surgical bowel procedures, but it is also prescribed for treating pediatric constipation.[56] It is a very potent laxative, producing almost complete gastric emptying. Adverse events associated with these agents include abdominal bloating, rectal irritation, and electrolyte abnormalities.

BOX 23-4 Laxatives

Laxative Category	Indication	Adverse Reactions
Bulk-forming (Citrucel, Fiberall)	Acute and chronic constipation, irritable bowel syndrome (IBS), diverticulosis	Flatulence, fluid disturbances
Emollient (Colace)	Acute and chronic constipation, fecal impaction	Decreased absorption of vitamins, electrolyte imbalance
Hyperosmotic (Fleet Babylax, polyethylene glycol, MiraLax)	Chronic constipation, bowel preparation for procedures	Abdominal bloating, rectal irritation, electrolyte imbalances
Saline (Epsom Salts, Milk of Magnesia, Fleet enema)	Chronic constipation, bowel preparation for procedures	Bloating, flatulence, electrolyte disturbances caused by salts
Stimulant (Senokot)	Acute constipation, bowel preparation for procedures	Abdominal discomfort and cramps

Saline Laxatives. Saline laxatives, like hyperosmotic laxatives, increase osmotic pressure by increasing water and electrolyte secretions into the small bowel.[57] What results is a very watery stool, which, in turn, stimulates peristalsis. Magnesium sulfate, magnesium citrate, and sodium phosphate (Fleet Enema) are drugs in this category. These drugs must be used with caution in patients with diminished cardiac or renal function caused by salts.

Stimulant Laxatives. Stimulant laxatives include natural extracts of plant products and also synthetic chemical agents that stimulate intestinal peristalsis. Senna is a commonly used stimulant available over the counter. It facilitates propulsive motility of the colon by stimulating the enteric nervous system. Other examples include casanthranol and bisacodyl. Long-term use of these products should be avoided due to the risk of dependence, as well as a "cathartic colon," which involves damage to the intestinal cells and progressive loss of colon function. Ultimately, the colon has reduced motility and dilation, and the underlying intestinal disease is exacerbated. However, this has been disputed by some.[55]

IRRITABLE BOWEL SYNDROME

IBS is characterized by a constellation of symptoms, including intermittent bouts of abdominal pain, bloating, diarrhea, and constipation.[58] In addition, several other complaints have been documented with this disorder, including sleep disturbances, depression, fibromyalgia, rheumatologic findings, and genitourinary dysfunction. Two subcategories exist: diarrhea-predominant IBS and constipation-predominant IBS, but these are rather poorly delineated.

The etiology and pathophysiology of IBS are unclear. There is no specific biologic marker, and the structural or physiologic abnormalities are not uniform among patients with IBS. Although there may be increased enterochromaffin cell numbers, decreased synthesis of 5-HT, and decreased expression of a serotonin reuptake protein inhibitor.[59] The current diagnostic criterion is recurrent abdominal pain of at least 6 months duration.[58] In addition, symptoms must have occurred for at least 3 days in a month and been associated with two or more of the following: improvement following defecation, change in stool frequency, and change in the appearance of the stool. There seems to be a genetic predisposition in some families, but in 30% of cases, patients had a preceding gastroenteric infection. Patients who develop IBS after gastroenteritis may show chronic mucosal lymphocytosis and enterochromaffin cell hyperplasia.[60,61] Some studies showed that after treatment for bacterial overgrowth, more than half the patients no longer met the diagnostic criterion of the disorder.[62] Patients do share a dysregulation of intestinal motor and sensory functions, with hypersensitivity of the GI tract to normal events, alterations in fluid and electrolyte balance in the bowel, and neuroendocrine disorders that contribute to impaired intestinal motility.[63] However, it is unclear whether IBS is primarily a CNS disorder with changes directed toward the intestines or an intestinal disorder in which abnormal afferent information is sent to the brain. About 70% of patients have mild disease, 25% have moderate disease, and 5% have severe disease. Psychosocial difficulties and lifestyle impairments are the factors that motivate patients to seek medical assistance.

Treatment for Irritable Bowel Syndrome with Constipation

Several agents are available to treat constipation-predominant IBS.

Bulking Agents. Fiber supplementation (psyllium or methylcellulose) can provide the needed bulk in some patients with constipation-predominant IBS.[64] The fiber decreases transit time through the gut, thus reducing bile salt concentrations in the colon. Because bile salts increase colonic contractions, this indirectly reduces pain. However, some patients with IBS may respond negatively to the fiber, and increased pain and bloating may occur. For these patients, fiber should be added slowly to the diet and a switch should be made to soluble fiber—found in fruits, vegetables, and legumes. Patients should consume 20 to 30 g/day of fiber.[65] In general, bulking agents improve bowel habits, but there are no significant differences compared with placebo with regard to the other complaints. If fiber therapy does not appear to be useful, other pharmacotherapy can be recommended; however, no single drug has been proved to be effective in the majority of cases of IBS.

Lubiprostone (Amitiza). This drug is a chloride channel receptor agonist and thus opens the chloride channel in the intestine.[54] It works by increasing liquid secretion into the intestine and also reduces transit time. It is one of the few drugs that improve the global symptoms of constipation-predominant IBS. The chief adverse effects are nausea and loose stools, but since it has just been released on the market, not enough time has passed to determine if other adverse effects are likely.

Serotonergic Agonists. Serotonin receptors located on enterochromaffin cells have a role in the initiation of peristalsis. Tegaserod (Zelnorm) is a partial serotonin agonist (5-HT_4) that increases intestinal motility, facilitating transit time through the bowel.[54] It is currently recommended for short-term use in women whose primary symptom is severe constipation. It is recommended for women because there were more women enrolled in the clinical studies and because tegaserod has questionable efficacy in men. This drug reduces bloating and abdominal pain and improves bowel habits compared with placebo. Diarrhea is the most common adverse effect. The drug may be temporarily withheld when diarrhea occurs. Overall, clinical trials of tegaserod demonstrate high quality in terms of methodology and show that this drug provides significant relief of global IBS symptoms compared with placebo. However, tegaserod was withdrawn from the market in 2007 because of increased risk of myocardial infarction and stroke. It now is available on a limited basis for treating severe cases of IBS and only in women younger than 55 years old who do not have risk factors for cardiovascular disease. The drug is thought to affect 5-HT_{1B} receptors causing vasoconstriction of the vascular wall. Currently, there are a few other serotonergic agonists under study that are thought to be extremely selective of the 5-HT_4 receptor, thus improving their safety profile.

Opioid Antagonists. Some opioid antagonists are being investigated for constipation related to pain medications and postoperative ileus.[54] Methylnaltrexone bromide is a μ-opioid blocker recently recommended for opiate-related constipation in terminally ill patients.

Treatment for Irritable Bowel Syndrome with Diarrhea

Opioid Agonists. Some studies on IBS have indicated that the opiate analogues diphenoxylate and loperamide have efficacy in the treatment of diarrhea-predominant IBS. However, in a systematic review on the management of IBS, loperamide was found to be effective but not more effective than placebo in the treatment of pain and overall symptoms.[66] The drug improves all symptoms of IBS as well as quality of life scores.

Last in this category is cholestyramine, a bile acid–binding agent that is normally used to lower cholesterol levels.[65] When some bile acids are eliminated, colonic contractions are reduced.

Antispasmodics. Antispasmodics used to treat IBS include drugs that act directly on the intestinal smooth muscle, anticholinergics, and calcium channel blockers. Mebeverine, which directly relaxes intestinal smooth muscle by blocking calcium channels, is currently not available in the United States. Dicyclomine (Bentyl) and hyoscyamine (Levsin) are anticholinergic agents. These drugs tend to be used on an as-needed basis before meals to avoid distention and postprandial cramping. The calcium channel blockers verapamil and nifedipine have also been useful in some patients to reduce pain and fecal urgency. Overall, antispasmodics decrease pain, but according to recent meta-analyses, they may not alter the symptoms of diarrhea or constipation.

Serotonin 5-HT_3 Receptor Antagonists. The serotonin receptor is of interest in the treatment of diarrhea-predominant IBS. Alosetron (Lotronex) is a serotonin receptor antagonist that slows transit time through the GI tract. This drug significantly reduces symptoms compared with placebo; however, in November 2000, the drug was withdrawn from the market. This resulted from reports of ischemic colitis and severe constipation leading to several hospital admissions and seven deaths. The drug was later reintroduced in June 2002 with restricted marketing for women with diarrhea-predominant IBS who fail to respond to other conventional therapies. In addition, the recommended starting dose was lowered.[58,67,68]

Other Therapies. Because stress and depression may exacerbate the symptoms of IBS, anxiolytic agents and tricyclic antidepressants (see Chapter 18) may be included in treatment.[69] Low-dose tricyclic antidepressants have been shown to be effective in reducing pain and may be useful in diarrhea-predominant IBS. This effect is probably related to the anticholinergic effects of these drugs.

Cognitive therapy and various behavioral therapies, in which patients learn how to identify and manage stressful events, are currently under study.[59] In a few facilities, biofeedback therapy has been offered to patients with IBS. Specifically, this modality is used to help patients sense changes in rectal distention and to help them regulate bowel habits (see the following section).

Probiotics, for example, *Lactobacillus B animalis* are considered live organisms that provide some health benefits when consumed. Original interest in these organisms came from observations of nineteenth century Eastern Europeans linking the health of Balkan peasants to a type of fermented milk drink frequently consumed by them.[70] Today, many individuals consume foods such as yogurt, miso, and tempeh, which are considered probiotic-rich foods. Although further study is needed, these live bacteria have been shown to limit the growth of harmful bacteria in the gut.[71] These agents also appear to exert a general anti-inflammatory effect by reducing cytokine influence, thereby modifying the lymphoid tissue in the intestine. A recent meta-analysis of 23 studies showed that probiotics exerted some improvement over global IBS symptoms.[70,72] However, this analysis was limited by different study designs and the use of different strains of bacteria, *Bifidobacterium infantis* 35624, *Lactobacillus acidophilus*, and *Lactobacillus helveticus*. Nevertheless, patients are encouraged to consume commercial products containing these bacteria.

THERAPEUTIC CONCERNS ABOUT GASTROINTESTINAL AGENTS

Some therapeutic concerns about drugs used to treat GI disorders influence therapy. However, the choice of therapeutic intervention is influenced by the specific disorder or symptoms experienced by the patient. For example, exercises performed in the supine position and those that increase intra-abdominal pressure should be provided with caution in patients with GERD.[73] These choices can exacerbate acid reflux, particularly if the therapy session is scheduled soon after a meal. In addition, bending over at the waist can increase reflux.

The other major concern about providing physical therapy to patients with GI problems is the presence of dehydration.[50] Significant vomiting and/or diarrhea cause fluid loss and electrolyte imbalances. Signs and symptoms of dehydration include absence of perspiration, tearing, and salivation; elevated body temperature; postural hypotension; dry skin and mucous membranes; headache; lethargy; sunken eyes; poor capillary refill; and skin turgor. Pulse may be rapid, and blood pressure may be low. Oral rehydration with a glucose-based electrolyte solution is recommended, except when the patient is severely dehydrated or comatose. In such cases, intravenous fluids should be administered. Otherwise, the patient should be encouraged to drink fluids and consume some salt, by eating soup or saltine crackers. Orange juice or bananas can be consumed to replace potassium.

On the other end of the spectrum, patients with constipation can be helped by therapy. Healthy eating and regular exercise promote good bowel habits. Moderate exercise can benefit patients with IBS and also those with colitis or Crohn's disease.[74] Exercise improves gastric emptying, but intense exercise can inhibit gastric emptying and disrupt GI absorption. In some cases, GI bleeding may occur with exercise.

Therapists may also find themselves involved in the treatment of constipation caused by pelvic floor dyssynergia. Approximately 50% of patients who complain of constipation have asynergic defecation. A paradoxical increase in anal pressure during straining occurs. This condition is diagnosed by the patient's inability to expel a rectal balloon and by pelvic floor magnetic resonance imaging (MRI) and evacuation scintigraphy. Biofeedback techniques, including sensory retraining and electromyography (EMG), are being investigated to help synchronize evacuation.[75,76] For sensory re-education, a water-filled balloon is inserted into the rectum and then slowly removed while the patient concentrates on its sensation and simultaneously tries to relax the anal sphincter and ease its evacuation. The EMG training is performed with either intraluminal electrodes or surface electrodes taped to the perianal skin. The patient watches the recording while first learning to relax the pelvic floor musculature. The patient also practices proper straining while keeping the pelvic floor muscles relaxed.

ACTIVITIES 23

1. Ms. R. is a 39-year-old woman with a history of epigastric pain. She feels relief after eating a meal and taking OTC antacid tablets. She has had this pain in the past but has never sought medical advice for it. She is a one-pack/day smoker and works as a busy executive in New York City. She runs six miles daily for physical and emotional benefits. The results of her physical examination are normal, except for epigastric tenderness and bilateral chondromalacia patella, which she has been self-treating with daily aspirin.

Questions

A. List questions you would ask the patient regarding her medical history and current symptoms.
B. What is the cause of the pain?
C. What is the treatment for this condition?
D. What are the physical therapy implications?
E. What should this patient know about smoking and H_2 blockers?

2. You are treating a 72-year-old woman for low back pain of unknown etiology. She also complains about suffering from constipation in the last 3 months and reports taking laxatives up to three times a day. She appears otherwise healthy, watches her weight, and exercises three times a week.

Questions

A. List the questions you would ask this patient about her medical history and current symptoms.
B. Why is long-term laxative use a problem?

3. Define *diabetic gastroparesis*, and discuss some agents that might be helpful in reducing symptoms.

4. Many common antacids are combinations of salts containing aluminum and magnesium. In which population of patients are such antacids contraindicated?

REFERENCES

1. Porth CM: Structure and function of the gastrointestinal system. In Essentials of pathophysiology, Philadelphia, 2004, Lippincott Williams & Wilkins.
2. Soybel DI: Anatomy and physiology of the stomach. Surg Clin N Am 85:875-894, 2005.
3. Goyal RK, Hirano I: Mechanisms of disease: The enteric nervous system. N Engl J Med 334(17):1106-1115, 1996.
4. Grundy D, Schemann M: Enteric nervous system. Curr Opin Gastroenterol 22:102-110, 2006.
5. Mejia A, Kraft WK: Acid reflux and ulcer disease. In Waldman SA, Terzic A, editors: Pharmacology and therapeutics: Principles to practice, Philadelphia, 2009, Saunders.
6. Guyton AC, Hall JE: Textbook of medical physiology (10th ed.), Philadelphia, 2000, W.B. Saunders Company.
7. Druce MR, Wren AM, Park AJ, et al: Ghrelin increases food intake in obese as well as lean subjects. Int J Obes Relat Metab Disord 29(9):1130-1136, 2005.
8. Druce MR, Neary NM, Small CJ, et al: Subcutaneous administration of ghrelin stimulates energy intake in healthy lean human volunteers. Int J Obes Relat Metab Disord 30(2):293-296, 2005.
9. Neary NM, Small CJ, Druce MR, et al: Peptide YY3-36 and glucagon-like peptide-17-36 inhibit food intake additively. Endocrinology 146(12):5120-5127, 2005.
10. Druce MR, Small C, Bloom SR: Mini-review: Gut peptides regulating satiety. Endocrinology 145:2660-2665, 2004.
11. Pandol SJ: Integrated response to a meal. J Parenter Enteral Nutr, 32(5):564-566.
12. Eswaran S, Roy MA: Medical management of acid-peptic disorders of the stomach. Surg Clin N Am 85:895-906, 2005.
13. Richter JE: Gastrooesophageal reflux disease. Best Pract Res Clin Gastroenterol 21:609-631, 2007.
14. Spechler SJ: Clinical manifestations and esophageal complications of GERD. Am J Med Sci 326(5):279-284, 2003.
15. Blaser MJ, Atherton JC: Helicobacter pylori persistence: Biology and disease. J Clin Invest 113(3):321-333, 2004.
16. Makola D, Peura DA, Crowe SE: Helicobacter pylori infection and related gastrointestinal diseases. J Clin Gastroenterol 41:548-558, 2007.
17. Garcia-Rodríguez LA, Hernandez-Diaz S: Relative risk of upper gastrointestinal complications among users of acetaminophen and nonsteroidal anti-inflammatory drugs. Epidemiology 12: 570-576, 2001.
18. Lanas A, García-Rodríguez LA, Polo-Tomás M, et al: Time trends and impact of upper and lower gastrointestinal bleeding and perforation in clinical practice. Am J Gastroenterol 104(7):1633-1641, 2009.
19. Hawkey CJ, Langman MJS: Non-steroidal anti-inflammatory drugs: Overall risks and management. Complementary roles for COX-2 inhibitors and proton pump inhibitors. Gut 52(4):600-608, 2003.
20. Lilley LL, Harrington S, Snyder JS: Acid-controlling agents. In Lilley LL, Harrington S, Snyder JS, editors: Pharmacology and the nursing process, St. Louis, 2007, Mosby.
21. Maton PN, Burton ME: Antacids revisited: A review of their clinical pharmacology and recommended therapeutic use. Drugs 57:855-870, 1999.
22. Tran T, Lowry AM: Meta-analysis: The efficacy of over-the-counter gastro-oesphageal reflux disease therapies. Aliment Pharmacol Ther 25:143-153, 2007.
23. Takeuchi K, Kajimura M, Kodaira M, Lin S, Hanai H, Kaneko E: Up-regulation of H2 receptor and adenylate cyclase in rabbit parietal cells during prolonged treatment with H2-receptor antagonists. Dig Dis Sci 44(8):1703-1709, 1999.
24. Kim J, Ogai A, Nakatani S, et al: Impact of blockade of histamine H2 receptors on chronic heart failure revealed by retrospective and prospective randomized studies. J Am Coll Cardiol 48(7):1378-1384, 2006.
25. Richardson P, Hawkey CJ, Stack WA: Proton pump inhibitors. Drugs 56(3):307-335, 1998.
26. Huang JQ, Hunt RH: Pharmacological and pharmacodynamic essentials of H2-receptor antagonists and proton pump inhibitors for the practising physician. Best Pract Res Clin Gastroenterol 15(3):355-370, 2001.
27. Neal KR, Scott HM, Slack RC, Logan RF: Omeprazole as a risk factor for campylobacter gastroenteritis: Case-control study. BMJ 312:414-415, 1996.
28. Leonard J, Marshall JK, Moayyedi P: Systematic review of the risk of enteric infection in patients taking acid suppression. Am J gastroenterol 102(9):2047-2056, 2007.
29. Der G: An overview of proton pump inhibitors. Gastroenterol Nurs 26(5):182-190, 2003.
30. Laine L: Proton pump inhibitors and bone fractures[quest]. Am J Gastroenterol 104(suppl 2):S21-S26, 2009.
31. Soll AH: Medical treatment of peptic ulcer disease: Practice guidelines. JAMA 275(8):622-629, 1996.
32. Gilster J, Bacon K, Marlink K, Sheppard B, Deveney C, Rutten M: Bismuth subsalicylate increases intracellular Ca2+, MAP-kinase activity, and cell proliferation in normal human gastric mucous epithelial cells. Dig Dis Sci 49(3):370-378, 2004.
33. Spirt MJ: Stress-related mucosal disease: Risk factors and prophylactic therapy. Clin Ther 26(2):197-213, 2004.
34. Kuipers EJ, Janssen MJR, de Boer WA: Good bugs and bad bugs: Indications and therapies for Helicobacter pylori eradication. Curr Opin Pharmacol 3:480-485, 2003.
35. Gisbert JP, Khorrami S, Carballo F, Calvet X, Gené E, Dominguez-Muñoz JE: H. pylori eradication therapy vs. antisecretory non-eradication therapy (with or without long-term maintenance antisecretory theray) for the prevention of recurrent bleeding from peptic ulcer. Cochrane Database Syst Rev (2):CD004062, 2004.
36. Chey WD, Wong BC: American College of Gastroenterology guideline on the managment of Helicobacter pylori infection. Am J Gastroenterol 102:1808-1825, 2007.
37. Sung JJ: Management of nonsteroidal anti-inflammatory drug-related peptic ulcer bleeding. Am J Med 110(1A):S29-S32, 2001.
38. Price AB: Pathology of drug-associated gastrointestinal disease. Br J Clin Pharmacol 56(5):477-482, 2003.
39. Hornby PJ: Central neurocircuitry associated with emesis. Am J Med 111(8 [suppl 1]):106-112, 2001.
40. Veyrat-Follet C, Farinotti R, Palmer JL: Physiology of chemotherapy-induced emesis and antiemetic therapy. Drugs 53(2):206-234, 1997.
41. Lilley LL, Harrington S, Snyder JS:, Antiemetic and antinausea agents. In Lilley LL, Harrington S, Snyder JS, editors: Pharmacology and the nursing process, St. Louis, 2007, Mosby.
42. Rang HP, Dale MM, Flower RJ: Antipsychotic drugs. In Rang HP, Dale MM, Flower RJ, editors: Rang and Dale's `pharmacology, New York, 2007, Churchill Livingstone.
43. Glare PA, Dunwoodie D, Clark K, et al: Treatment of nausea and vomiting in terminally ill cancer patients. Drugs 68(18):2575-2590, 2008.
44. Gumaste V, Baum J: Treatment of gastroparesis: An update. Digestion 78(4):173-179, 2008.
45. Aapro M: 5-HT3 receptor antagonists in the management of nausea and vomiting in cancer and cancer treatment. Oncology 69:97-102, 2005.
46. Navari RM: Pharmacological management of chemotherapy-induced nausea and vomiting: Focus on recent developments. Drugs 69(5):515-533, 2009.
47. Pisanti S, Malfitano AM, Grimaldi C, et al: Use of cannabinoid receptor agonists in cancer therapy as palliative and curative

agents. Best Pract Res Clinical Endocrinol Metab 23(1): 117-131, 2009.
48. Herrstedt J: Antiemetics: An update and the MASCC guidelines applied in clinical practice. Nature Clin Pract Oncol 5(1):31-43, 2007.
49. Lilley LL, Harrington S, Snyder JS: Antidiarrheals and laxatives. In Lilley LL, Harrington S, Snyder JS, editors: Pharmacology and the nursing process, St. Louis, 2007, Mosby.
50. Thielman NM, Guerrant RL: Acute infectious diarrhea. N Engl J Med 350:38-47, 2004.
51. Rao SSC: Pathophysiology of adult fecal incontinence. Gastroenterologoy 126:S14-S22, 2004.
52. Scarlett, Y: Medical management of fecal incontinence. Gastroenterology 126:S55-S63, 2004.
53. Baker DE: Loperamide: A pharmacological review. Rev Gastroenterol Disord 7(suppl 3):S11-S18, 2007.
54. Tack J, Müller-Lissner S: Treatment of chronic constipation: Current pharmacologic approaches and future directions. Clin Gastroenterol Hepatol 7(5):502-508, 2009.
55. Wald A: Appropriate use of laxatives in the management of constipation. Curr Gastroenterol Rep 9:410-414, 2007.
56. Bell EA, Wall GC: Pediatric constipation therapy using guidelines and polyethylene glycol 2250. Ann Pharmacother 38: 686-693, 2004.
57. Lembo A, Camilleri M: Current concepts in chronic constipation. N Engl J Med 349(14):1360-1368, 2003.
58. Longstreth GF, Thompson WG, Chey WD, Houghton LA, Mearin F, Spiller RC: Functional bowel disorders. Gastroenterology 130:1480-1491, 2006.
59. Moynihan NT: How do you spell relief for irritable bowel syndrome? J Family Pract 57(2):100-108, 2008.
60. Parry S, Forgacs I: Intestinal infection and irritable bowsel syndrome. Eur J Gastroenterold Heapatol 17:5-9, 2005.
61. Spiller RC, Jenkins D, Thornley JP, et al: Increased rectal mucosal enteroendocrine cells, T lymphocytes, and increased gut permeability following acute Campylobacter enteritis and in post-dysenteric irritable bowel syndrome. Gut 47:804-811, 2000.
62. Pimentel M, Chow EJ, Lin HC: Eradication of small intestinal bacterial overgrowth reduces symptoms of irritable bowel syndrome. Am J Gastroenterol 95:3503-3506, 2000.
63. Gershon MD: Nerves, reflexes, and the enteric nervous system: Pathogenesis of the irritable bowel syndrome. J Clin Gastroenterol 39(suppl):184-193, 2005.
64. Quartero AO, Meineche-Schmidt V, Muris J, Rubin G, de Wit N: Bulking agents, antispasmodic and antidepressant medication for the treatment of irritable bowel syndrome. Cochrane Database Syst Rev 2:CD003460, 2005.
65. Birrer RB: Irritable bowel syndrome. Dis Mon 48(2):101-144, 2002.
66. Brandt LJ, Bjorkman D, Fennerty MB, et al: Systematic review on the management of irritable bowel syndrome in North America. Am J Gastroenterol 97(11):S7-S26, 2002.
67. Cremonini F, Delgado A, Camilleri M: Efficacy of alosetron in irritable bowel syndrome: A meta-analysis of randomized controlled trials. Neurogastroenterol Motil 15:79-86, 2003.
68. Mayer EA, Bradesi S: Alosetron and irritable bowel syndrome. Expert Opin Pharmacother 4(11):2089-2098, 2003.
69. Mertz HR: Irritable bowel syndrome. N Engl J Med 349:2136-2146, 2003.
70. Shen YH, Nahas R: Complementary and alternative medicine for treatment of irritable bowel syndrome. Can Fam Physician 55:143-148, 2009.
71. Camilleri M: Probiotics and irritable bowel syndrome: Rationale, mechanisms, and efficacy. J Clin Gastroenterol 42:S123-S125, 2008.
72. Brenner DM, Moeller MJ, Chey WD, Schoenfeld PS: The utility of probiotics in the treatment of irritable bowel syndrome: A systematic review. Am J Gastroenterol 104(4):1033-1049, 2009.
73. Goodman CC: The gastrointestinal system. In Goodman CC, Boissonnault WG, Fuller JH, editors: Pathology implications for the physical therapist, Philadelphia, 2003, Saunders.
74. Bi L, Triadafilopoulos G: Exercise and gastrointestinal function and disease: An evidence-based review of risks and benefits. Clin Gastroenterol Hepatol 1(5):345-355, 2003.
75. Stessman M: Biofeedback: Its role in the treatment of chronic constipation. Gastroenterol Nurs 26(6):251-260, 2003.
76. Bassotti G, Chistolini F, Sietchiping-Nzepa F, de Roberto G, Morelli A, Chiarioni G: Biofeedback for pelvic floor dysfunction in constipation. BMJ 328:393-396, 2004.

24

Vitamins and Minerals

Jane Ziegler

BIOCHEMICAL FUNCTIONS OF VITAMINS AND MINERALS

Both vitamins and minerals play a central role in the many physiologic functions fundamental to life, including the metabolism of nutrients and the maintenance of cellular functions. Catabolism of vitamins does not provide energy, nor do vitamins serve as structural components of the body. Vitamin function is highly specific to each vitamin, and, as a result, the requirement of any vitamin from the diet is small. Although most vitamins share general characteristics, their chemical or functional components are very different. Some vitamins function as enzyme cofactors, some vitamins may also function as biologic antioxidants, and some function as cofactors in oxidation-reduction reactions. In addition, vitamins A and D function as hormones, and vitamin A is involved as a photoreceptive cofactor in the vision process.[1]

Macrominerals, or the major minerals, are distinguished from microminerals on the basis of their occurrence in the body. Several classification definitions have been established for macrominerals, including the requirement that a mineral constitute at least 0.01% of total body weight or about 5 g in a person who weighs 60 kg. A commonly used definition is the classification of the daily intake requirement of >100 mg per day. Macrominerals include calcium, phosphorus, magnesium, sodium, potassium, and chloride. Microminerals include iron, zinc, copper, selenium, chromium, iodine, manganese, molybdenum, and fluoride. The additional 19 ultratrace elements include arsenic, boron, nickel, silicon, vanadium, and cobalt, with estimated, established, or suspected requirements of <1 mg per day.[1]

Functionally, vitamins and minerals have several biochemical roles. Trace minerals are often involved in modulating enzyme activity or are components of enzyme prosthetic groups. As examples, zinc serves as a cofactor for over 100 enzymes; selenium is necessary in the form of selenocysteine within the enzyme glutathione peroxidase.[2] Vitamins or their metabolites may serve as coenzymes of metabolism in reactions critical for provision of energy and for protein and nucleic acid synthesis. Folic acid is part of the methyl group transfer, and riboflavin and niacin are involved in the reactions of the electron transport chain. In addition, some nutrients, such as zinc, provide genetic control. Zinc "fingers" bind to deoxyribonucleic acid (DNA) and assist in the regulation of receptor transcription for steroid hormones. Vitamin E, the carotenoids, and the minerals zinc, copper, and selenium also function as antioxidants or within antioxidant enzyme systems to dispose of products of oxidation.[2]

There has been a growing interest in the role vitamins and minerals may play in the prevention of chronic illnesses and in the optimization or enhancement of health.[2] People have become more knowledgeable about nutrition and the roles of these nutrients; however, information obtained from lay documents is not always well founded.[2] It is important for health professionals to understand the evidence of the essentiality of these nutrients to the metabolic processes and explore the need for supplementation in clinical situations where increased or monitored intake may be lead to improved clinical outcomes.

DEFINITION OF MULTIVITAMINS/ MULTIMINERALS

The term *multivitamin* includes hundreds of different products that contain various doses of vitamins and minerals.[3,4] This variety among multivitamins (MVMs) sold in the market place causes difficulty determining the use of these products.[5] Lack of standardization of vitamin and mineral dosages of over-the-counter MVMs also creates confusion for consumers.[5] Currently, there are no regulatory criteria for the content of MVMs, which further confuses the public and professionals alike. The 1994 Dietary Supplement Health and Education Act (DSHEA)[6] has not provided assistance with standardization, nomenclature, and safety considerations of MVMs. Adding to the confusion, various terms are used to describe the commercially available MVM products: *multivitamins, multiminerals, multies, multiple nutrients*, and *multivitamins/minerals; one-a-days*. A variety of products for specialized purposes (MVMs for women, men, older adults (male and female), menopause, or special health conditions, and so on) are also on the market. The types, dosages, and numbers of vitamins and minerals vary widely. Other ingredients such as herbals, botanicals, and fibers may also be added to the list of products on the market. Products may be available in a variety of forms—liquid, capsule, pill, or tablet—and add even more confusion to the choice of the consumer.[3]

USE OF MULTIVITAMINS/ MULTIMINERALS

Data on the use of MVM supplements have been collected on a nationally representative sample of the American population by the National Health and Nutrition Examination Survey (NHANES).[7] In the NHANES 1999–2000 survey, 52% of adults reported taking a dietary supplement within the past month, and 35% reported routine consumption of an MVM supplement.[8] Compared with earlier NHANES survey data, an increasing trend in supplement use has been seen.[8,9] The use of supplements has been found to contribute a significant percentage to the total vitamin and mineral intake among the American population.[9,10] Users of MVMs tend to use supplements on a daily basis, and approximately half the people who take supplements have done so for ≥2 years.[8] This use of supplements tends to be associated with several demographic subgroups and lifestyle characteristics.[11-14] Women, non-Hispanic whites, and individuals with a higher education level, those with a lower body mass index (BMI), and people who are physically active have a greater tendency to use MVM supplements.[8] In addition, individuals with a frequency of wine consumption of ≥5 times/month were associated with a greater use of supplements. Non-smokers were associated with a higher use of supplements compared with smokers. In general, use of MVMs is associated with the demographic characteristics of female gender, older age, higher level of education, regular physical activity, and being non-Hispanic white. Individuals with a higher BMI and smokers are less likely to use supplements.[10-13,15,16]

REFERENCE INTAKES OF VITAMINS AND MINERALS IN THE HEALTHY POPULATION

The United States and Canada have developed recommendations for the intake of vitamins and minerals for the healthy population.[17,18] These reference intakes have been based on observed nutrient intakes and on a small quantity of nutrient balance studies, laboratory tests of blood, and tissue status associated with certain levels of intake.[2] *Dietary Reference Intakes (DRI)*, published by the Institute of Medicine,[17,18] provides values which have been set for micronutrients at levels below which clinical deficiency states are progressively more likely to occur or at levels above which toxicities may develop. The values are set for populations, not for specific individuals, but are estimated to meet the requirements of almost all (97–98%) people within a specific age/gender group. DRIs were based on the nutritional intakes of healthy populations; therefore the diet typical of this population is expected to meet the necessary intake levels.[17,18] On this understanding, consuming a minimum of five servings of fruits and vegetables each day, in addition to a mixed diet providing adequate energy and protein, will provide adequate intake of nutrients over a period for most individuals.[2]

VITAMIN AND MINERAL BIOAVAILABILITY

The definitions of *bioavailability* and *bioequivalence* of MVMs are not standardized or scientific and regulatory definitions.[3] The term *bioavailability* is most commonly used to describe the process of absorption of a nutrient;[19] it is also used to describe the process of utilization of a nutrient.[20-22] This creates some problems, as this description may fail to include some of the beneficial effects or functions of a nutrient.[19] The functionality of a nutrient at the site(s) of action may also be a useful definition to consider.[23] The concept of bioequivalence is related to the concept of bioavailability,[23,24] as some nutrients may be absorbed equally but may not have the same biologic effect because of the differing chemical structures of the same nutrient.[19] For some nutrients, the DRIs are adjusted to account for differences in the activities of the different chemical sources of the vitamin.[17,18,25] One example is vitamin A, in which the different chemical sources of the vitamin are converted to vitamin equivalents when setting the *recommended dietary allowances (RDAs)*.[17] For some vitamins, the RDA, or *adequate intake (AI)*, is adjusted on the basis of the differences of bioavailability and bioequivalencies in mixed diets. Host factors within an individual can affect the bioavailability of MVMs.[3] For a particular nutrient, the nutritional status of the host may impact the regulation of the absorption or excretion of the nutrient (e.g., an iron-deficient individual will absorb more iron).[3] Host factors vary by the age, gender, and physiologic state of an individual.[21,22,26] Homeostatic mechanisms regulate the circulating concentrations of some nutrients within a very tight range and are insensitive to the ingested amount of the nutrient.[19] In addition, dosage may affect bioavailability, as with calcium, and the amount absorbed is inversely related to the amount of the dose.[19] The chemical form of the nutrient will also affect bioavailability and bioequivalence.[24] Nutrient–nutrient interactions may affect the bioavailability of the nutrient as well. For example, the presence of vitamin C enhances the bioavailability of inorganic iron, allowing iron to be absorbed more readily.[27] Magnesium and calcium both affect the bioavailability of iron, since the presence of either inhibits absorption.[27] Other factors such as excipients, fillers, coatings, and surfactants may impact how the nutrient is released into the system and the degree of release.[19]

RISKS OF INADEQUATE INTAKE OF VITAMINS AND MINERALS

Different groups of individuals are at a high risk for inadequate intake of vitamins and minerals, particularly those of lower socioeconomic status, as intakes of fresh fruits and vegetables are less in this population. Populations at risk include those with a known poor or limited food intake, for example, adolescents, who typically have a limited intake of dairy foods, and older adults, who may have inadequate vitamin D intake due to limited sun exposure.[2] In addition to the limited diet of older adults, intake or absorption may be affected by anorexia or chewing and swallowing difficulties, which may lead to clinical deficiencies of zinc, iron, vitamin C, and riboflavin.[28]

Certain population groups may have increased vitamin and mineral requirements, such as pregnant women, who require higher intakes of folate both before the pregnancy and during the first trimester.[18] Smokers need additional vitamin C, and people recovering from an injury, trauma, surgery, or illness will have multiple increases in nutrient requirements.[2]

MICRONUTRIENT STATUS CHANGES AS A RESULT OF DISEASE

People with acute as well as chronic diseases have an increased demand for nutrients, since during such times there is most likely a decreased intake. People with chronic inflammation, infections, or cancer as well as institutionalized older adults may have anorexia or a decreased appetite. Chronic alcohol abuse leads to malnutrition and multiple micronutrient deficiencies due to inadequate intake and decreased absorption of nutrients. However, aggressive nutritional support with carbohydrates can put the person with alcoholism at risk of acute thiamin deficiency and generalized refeeding syndrome deficiencies as well as hypokalemia, hypophosphatemia, and fluid overload.[29]

Acute infection, surgery, or trauma leads to increased energy expenditure and protein catabolism. Requirements of water-soluble vitamins and trace minerals are increased, as they function as coenzymes for the metabolic pathways involved in energy and protein metabolism.[2] An increased need for all nutrients is seen during recovery from illness or trauma; trace element deficiencies are more likely to occur during recovery after prolonged catabolism.[30] Loss of body fluids also leads to a loss of some micronutrients; the most common deficiency is of iron due to loss of blood during menstruation or other causes. Loss of zinc due to diarrhea, loss of fluids due to fistulas, and depletion of water-soluble vitamins and trace minerals due to burn exudates or dialysis can all occur.[30]

CONSEQUENCES OF NUTRITIONAL DEFICIENCIES OF VITAMINS OR MINERALS

Classic nutritional deficiencies have been well described in the literature. Individual micronutrient deficiencies result in specific physical or clinical signs and symptoms. Most clinical deficiency states, except specific single nutrient deficiencies, are relatively uncommon in the developed countries. The most common nutrient deficiencies are those of iron, vitamin D, folate, and vitamin B_{12}. These single nutrient deficiencies are relatively easy to recognize, diagnose, and confirm with laboratory tests and are treated with the appropriate supplementation and dosage.

Subclinical deficiencies, which are milder forms of deficiencies, are more common, and often multiple nutrients are deficient at one time. Subclinical deficiencies are thus difficult to recognize. The time frame over which a subclinical deficiency occurs will vary by the nutrient and depend on the body stores of the nutrient and the need for the nutrient in an individual. Metabolic pathways will begin to be affected as the intracellular concentration of the micronutrient begins to decline. For example, methyltetrahydrofolate (a form of folate) is required for the conversion of homocysteine to methionine, and vitamin B_{12} and vitamin B_6 are additionally required in the metabolism of homocysteine. The clinical benefits of the reduction of homocysteine through vitamin therapy has been investigated in relation to heart disease,[31,32] but the results of these studies have been conflicting.[33-35] The relationship between homocysteine metabolism and the treatment of high homocysteine levels with vitamin therapy remains a complex one, and reduction of atherosclerosis through decreased homocysteine levels has not been clearly demonstrated.[36]

Many of the micronutrients have antioxidant activities, and if these activities are suboptimal, oxidative damage to cells and tissues will result.[2] Oxidized low-density lipoprotein (LDL) is related to coronary artery disease incidence, and high intake of antioxidants has been related to a lower incidence of coronary artery disease. This led to the expectation that supplementation or an increased intake of antioxidants would result in decreased incidence and complications of coronary heart disease.[2] However, studies have failed to show any benefit from supplementation of antioxidant micronutrients.[37-39]

In a comprehensive review of studies on cardiovascular disease reduction, Kris-Everton et al concluded that disease risk reduction could be achieved through a well-balanced diet that is rich in whole grains, fruits, and vegetables, along with regular physical exercise.[40] No additional benefit was seen from supplementation with micronutrients above what was achieved from diet alone.[40]

The role of antioxidant supplements in cancer treatment is not clear. It seems likely that an increased intake of antioxidants would be helpful through the reduction of oxidation-induced mutations in the DNA of patients with cancer. However, studies have not supported this assumption but have suggested that a diet rich in antioxidants may minimize the risk of certain cancers. The use of specific antioxidant supplements requires additional research before they can be definitively recommended.[2] To date, research regarding the role of

MVMs in preventing morbidity or mortality from cardiovascular disease or cancer is not convincing.[41]

Reduction of age-related macular degeneration, but not age-related development or progression of cataracts, has been associated with antioxidant supplementation.[42,43] An approximately 25% reduction of age-related macular degeneration was seen with intake of a combination of antioxidants along with zinc.[42,43]

Infections are major causes of illness and death throughout the world. Since micronutrients are involved in a variety of functions within the immune system, supplementation of micronutrients in the immune-compromised population has been of interest to health care professionals. In a systematic review of MVM supplementation for infection by Stephen and Avenell, no significant difference was seen in the number of infectious occurrences in the older adult population between those who were supplemented and those not supplemented with MVMs.[44] It was concluded that larger clinical trials over a longer period of >6 months are needed. In particular, determining whether malnourished older adults will benefit from MVM supplementation over a longer duration of time is of particular concern.[44]

Because the widespread use of MVMs in the population may be possibly motivated by the hope of preventing chronic disease, full-scale trials of well-selected MVM supplements in specific population groups are needed.

ROLE OF MVM SUPPLEMENTS ON NUTRIENT ADEQUACY

The use of MVMs is common and may significantly contribute to the overall intake of nutrients.[45] Murphy et al found that the adequacy of 17 nutrients was similar when intake of food alone was compared with food intake plus MVM supplements.[45] The average prevalence of adequacy (defined as meeting the DRI) across all 17 nutrients was 74 ±25% in men who were nonusers of MVMs and 76±23% in users of MVMs. In women, nonusers and users of MVMs had an average prevalence of adequacy across the 17 nutrients of 72±27% and 75±25%, respectively. Even though the mean difference between users and nonusers of MVMs was only 2 to 3 percentage points, it was significant ($p<0.0001$).[45] Per single nutrient, the adequacy of vitamin A, vitamin E, and zinc were improved in those who were users of MVMs. Murphy suggested that information on the distribution of intakes of MVM products across all age groups is needed to determine if intake is excessive based on total intake from foods and MVMs.[45]

PREVALENCE OF INTAKES AT RISK OF BEING EXCESSIVE

Murphy et al also investigated the prevalence of intakes of nutrients that exceeded the *upper level intake (UL)*.[17,18,45] Data on intake of nutrients from both foods and MVM supplements were collected. Of those participants who did not take an MVM supplement, <5% reported intakes from food that exceeded the ULI and only for iron and zinc. When nutrients from MVMs were included in addition to those from food intake >10% of the participants had intakes that exceeded the ULI for the nutrients niacin, vitamin A, iron, and zinc.[45]

In optimizing the intake of vitamins and minerals, several factors need to be considered. If a person is able to consume an oral diet, then intake of vitamins and minerals is best achieved through a well-balanced diet that includes a variety of foods. If this "ideal" diet is not available or cannot be consumed, and there is concern that the diet is inadequate in vitamins and minerals, then an MVM supplement of all vitamins and minerals designed to meet 50 to 100% of the DRIs is recommended.[46]

In clinical deficiency states, any single nutrient that is deficient needs to be provided in the adequate dose and form. In chronic and acute illnesses, sufficient intake of all vitamins and minerals is necessary to prevent subclinical deficiency states. The patient's medical and diet histories should be reviewed when considering supplementation. To avoid subclinical deficiency states, an intake of vitamins and minerals that meets clinical needs, as supported by controlled clinical studies, should be provided. For evaluation of the micronutrient status, laboratory findings need to be interpreted along with an assessment of the disease state. Special attention and consideration should be given to micronutrients that are provided intravenously to ensure adequacy.[2]

The U.S. Food and Drug Administration (FDA) is notified of <1% of all adverse events associated with dietary supplements, including MVMs.[47] Adverse events related to intake of vitamins and minerals may be underreported because the majority of consumers presume MVMs to be safe and use them without the advice and supervision of health care professionals. In addition, most individuals are unaware of the FDA regulation with regard to adverse events.[47]

FOOD/NUTRIENT–DRUG INTERACTIONS

Provision of medical nutrition therapy includes the prevention and management of food/nutrient–drug interactions. Failure to recognize and control potential interactions can result in drug response failure, drug toxicity, and potential adverse events that can be life threatening. Numerous interactions between foods/nutrients (foods, nutrients and vitamin/mineral supplements) and drugs (both prescription and over-the-counter medications) occur. Some of these food/nutrient–drug interactions may not be clinically relevant or significant; however, some others may contribute to morbidity and may even result in a fatal reaction.[48,49] Awareness and understanding of potential interactions allow health care professionals to communicate potential consequences and interactions to patients in order to optimize the therapeutic effects of drugs, prevent therapeutic failures, and minimize adverse drug events.[48] Food/nutrient–drug interactions can occur in individuals of any age or health status. Vulnerable populations include older adults and children as well as those individuals who are immune compromised, critically ill, or with compensated physiologic reserves.[50] In addition, obesity being a major public health problem, adjustments of dosages for the obese population is of importance and concern, especially with regard to drugs with a narrow therapeutic index.[51]

A food/nutrient–drug interaction can be the result of physical, chemical, physiologic, or pathophysiologic relationship between a nutrient, multiple nutrients, or food in general and the drug.[52] Food/nutrient–drug interactions can be related to changes in the pharmacokinetic and pharmacodynamic profiles of various drugs, which can result in clinical complications or implications that may then impact the health of an individual.[53] Pharmacokinetic interactions include those effects preceding entry into the gastrointestinal (GI) tract (adding the drug to enteral feedings or crushing the medication and adding it to food for ease of swallowing), during absorption, during the distribution phase, during metabolism, and during elimination of the drug. These pharmacokinetic interactions make up the most common food/nutrient–drug interactions. Pharmacodynamic interactions are seen less frequently, but the absorption and metabolism phases of the drug are most vulnerable to the effect of food/nutrients.[53,54]

Most (~85%) marketed drugs are administered orally; therefore the food/nutrient–drug interactions that occur with the oral administration of a drug are of particular concern.[55] The physical and chemical characteristics of the drug itself need to be considered in relation to its potential interaction with food or nutrients.[54] Drugs within the same drug classification or different formulations of the same drug can result in different chemical characteristics and therefore result in different interactions.[54] Understanding and knowledge of the physiochemical properties of a drug tend not to be useful in predicting potential interactions of drugs with foods.[54] Practitioners and the pharmaceutical industry are responsible for communicating how drugs are administered and used and the importance of the relationship of food intake, use of MVMs, and lifestyle behaviors to the administration of drugs in order to ensure safety.[49]

Effects of Food/Nutrients on Drug Absorption

Food/nutrients may have considerable impact on the absorption of a drug.[48,56] The rate or degree of absorption of a drug can be affected in a variety of ways by foods or nutrients, resulting in decreased availability and delayed absorption rate and time to reach peak plasma drug concentration; however, overall bioavailability may, in some cases, remain unchanged.[53]

Delayed Absorption. Delayed absorption or a delayed rate of absorption can occur because of delayed gastric emptying and/or change in pH (increase) directly related to the secretion of hydrochloric acid occurring during ingestion of food.[53] A delay in gastric emptying will delay the onset of drug absorption occurring in the proximal small intestine.[47,53] This delay in drug absorption may also result in a delay in the onset of the therapeutic action of the drug. This may or may not be clinically significant and will vary by drug.[53]

Decreased Absorption. Drugs whose absorption is affected by food intake include drugs that are unstable in acidic or gastric fluids and those that interact or bind with dietary factors.[53] This results in a decreased systemic availability caused by either decreased GI absorption, increased hepatic first-pass metabolism, or increased clearance of the drug.[53,59] Some disease conditions are associated with a decrease in the bioavailability of drugs and need to be considered in drug management. Neuropathies, as those seen in diabetes mellitus, can cause delayed gastric emptying and may result in the decreased bioavailability of drugs. Decreased absorption of drugs is seen in a variety of inflammatory bowel diseases.[60] Viscosity or thickness—that of a drug suspension or resulting from the intake of soluble fiber used to regulate bowel movements or to impact glucose absorption—can result in reduced drug absorption.[61,62] The resulting chyme forms a physical barrier, reducing drug access to the absorptive surface of the GI tract.[61,62] The effects of viscosity on drug absorption varies widely, depending on the drug and the type of viscosity-inducing agent administered in combination with the drug.[61] The combination of bile acids and the drug may cause a physiochemical reaction in lipid-soluble or lipophilic drugs, resulting in reduced absorption.[53,63-65] Bile acid sequestrants, which are used to lower cholesterol, may also bind with the fat-soluble vitamins A, D, E, and K, which are then excreted adding to the intended effect of excretion of bile acids. Vitamin K is not stored in any significant amounts in the body; therefore, the use of bile acid sequestrants may lead to a deficiency of clotting factors, which results in excessive bleeding. These bile acid sequestrants also interfere with the absorption of folic acid, vitamin B_{12}, calcium, and iron.[53]

Increased or Accelerated Absorption. Drugs with poor solubility in gastric fluids exhibit a decrease in dissolution rate when consumed without food as there is less availability of hydrochloric acid to provide an acid environment for dissolution. When given with food, these drugs demonstrate an increase in absorption as the gastric contents become more acidic.[57] This increased absorption results from delayed gastric emptying (longer gastric residence time due to food intake and increased secretion of bile salts related to food intake), which may enhance the dissolution of the drug.[57] Also, the resulting increase in the volume of gastric fluid after food intake may enhance the solubility and dissolution of the drug.[66]

Absorption of a drug may be increased through the lowering of the first-pass metabolism by food.[67,68] Food may influence or change the blood flow to the splanchnic capillary bed, which results in increased absorption and a decrease in first-pass metabolism.[53,69,70] Food may affect the release of drug from some formulation types such as extended release and enteric-coated medications, which may be partially released if taken with food.[53,71]

Unchanged Absorption in the Presence of Food. If a drug is relatively insensitive to the changes in the GI tract that occur after eating, then absorption may be relatively unchanged. As overall absorption may not be affected, these drugs may be taken with or without food, allowing more flexibility and viability and a more practical option for individuals who may have difficulty swallowing, for example, by crushing a tablet or opening a capsule and mixing the drug with food.[53,72,73] This, however, is not an option for slow release agents.

Drug Bioavailability

Food–drug interactions can affect therapeutic effectiveness through a reduction in a drug's bioavailability.[74] Factors affecting bioavailability include the physicochemical properties of the drug, enantiomorphic composition of the drug, formulation type, timing of the meal in relation to drug dosing, composition of the meal, meal size, dose of drug, adsorbents, and concurrent intake of beverages.[53]

Physicochemical Properties. Physical and chemical interactions impact drug absorption when drugs are administered with meals or foods through alterations of GI physiologic conditions. The differences in the GI tract physiology may increase the potential for drug–nutrient interactions, which will affect the absorption process of the drug.[75] Within the different parts of the GI tract, pH and residence time vary and influence the amount of the dissolved drug available at the intestinal membrane for absorption. Within the GI lumen, alterations in gastric pH and emptying rate, changes in intestinal transit time, and changes in secretions from the intestine, pancreas, and liver (bile) will all impact the absorption of the drug.[75] GI residence times can influence the amount of drug released into solution and affect the duration of exposure to the absorptive surface.[53] Gastric emptying is affected by a variety of factors, including the volume of contents within the stomach, pH, calories consumed with the meal, osmolarity, viscosity, and temperature of the food or beverage.[75] Solid contents tend to empty more slowly than liquid contents, and the liquid calorie load of stomach contents will influence emptying time. Undissolved drug particles which are less than 1 to 2 mm in diameter empty with the liquid component; therefore, the extent of disintegration of the oral dosage form within the stomach may influence transit time.[75]

Composition of the Drug. Drugs may exist as a racemic mixture of R and S enantiomers (mirror images of each other), with different enantiomers having differing absorptive attributes and pharmacologic actions.[53] The desired pharmacologic activity usually resides in one enantiomer, while another may be responsible for either a different response or activity or an adverse effect. Examining the effects of food on both the racemate and the individual enantiomers of the drug is necessary to fully understand the drug's effect.[53]

Formulation Type and Meal Timing. Drug formulation type, whether conventional or a modified release formulation, impacts the bioavailability of drugs in fasting and fed states. The time a drug is administered in relation to a meal can influence the rate and the extent of drug availability. Drug administration before, during, or immediately after a meal may decrease the rate of drug availability most commonly due to delayed gastric emptying. Dietary patterns may have temporary effects on drug absorption, depending on the level and type of the interaction. Drugs causing gastric irritation may be buffered if taken just before or immediately after a meal.[76] When a drug is administered in relation to a meal, the stability of the drug may be impacted, as some drugs need to be taken before a meal when gastric secretion and gut motility are reduced.[77] Some drugs are best taken 1 hour before or 2 hours after a meal to allow for the least acidic environment and the shortest gastric emptying time. Meals may also decrease the protein binding of some drugs, which leads to an increase in the distribution of the drug.[78] Understanding the relationship of the timing of meals to the delivery of the drug assists in determining when to take a drug in relation to meals and snacks.

Meal Composition. The fat content of the meal can significantly increase the bioavailability of a drug. This increase in bioavailability is thought to be the result of increased secretion of bile salts, pancreatic secretions, digestive enzymes, and gastric hormones after a meal high in fat.[67,79,80] The reverse is true for other drugs that may have reduced bioavailability when consumed with a high fat meal.[81] The effect of dietary fat strongly depends on whether the drug is absorbed via the portal route or the lymphatic route.[82] With the lymphatic route of absorption, dietary fat appears to enhance the absorption of the dissolved drug,[82] whereas in the portal vein route of absorption, dietary fat results in an enhancement of lipophilic drugs through improved dissolution.[82] A drug formulation with an excellent food dissolution profile is therefore less likely to be affected by a high-fat meal.[82] A drug may bind with dietary protein, which results in enhanced absorption due to increased luminal amino acid concentrations, which, in turn, results in an increased upregulation or increased activity of the L-amino acid transporter.[83] Dietary fiber, especially soluble fiber, can decrease the absorption of some drugs. In contrast, the intake of insoluble fiber may result in the binding of some drugs, leading to poor absorption.[53,84,85]

Meal Size and Dose Size. The size of a meal and its effect on drug absorption has not been well researched;

TABLE 24-1 Vitamin/Mineral–Drug Interactions

	Vitamin or Mineral Affected	Drug	Type of Interaction or Mechanism of Action
Changes in absorption of the vitamin or mineral	Thiamin, riboflavin, B_6, B_{12}, vitamin K, biotin, and potassium	Antibiotics in general	Bacterial flora changes, which may result in bacterial overgrowth (reduced synthesis) and malabsorption
	Calcium	Tetracyclines	Chelation of drug and calcium through the formation of an insoluble, nonabsorbable complex, resulting in poor absorption of calcium
	Sodium, potassium, calcium, vitamin B_{12}, vitamin K	Neomycin	Mucosal injury, resulting in decreased absorption of nutrients
	Vitamins A, D, E, K, B_{12}, beta-carotene, folic acid, niacin, calcium, iron, and zinc	Bile acid sequestrants	Adsorption to anion exchange resin, resulting in decreased absorption of nutrients
	Vitamin B_{12}	Colchicine	Gastrointestinal (GI) mucosal changes or injury, resulting in decreased absorption through inhibition of intestinal enzymes or transport mechanisms
	Vitamin C, iron	Anti-inflammatory drugs	GI mucosal changes or injury, resulting in decreased absorption of nutrients
	Most vitamin and minerals	Most antineoplastics	GI mucosal changes or injury, resulting in decreased absorption of nutrients
	Vitamin B_{12}, folic acid, iron, and zinc	H_2-receptor antagonists	Decreased gastric acid secretion, resulting in decreased absorption of nutrients
	Vitamin B_{12}, folic acid, and zinc	Proton pump inhibitors	Decreased secretion of gastric acid, resulting in decreased absorption of nutrients
	Phosphate, vitamin B_{12}, folic acid, iron, and zinc	Aluminum and magnesium hydroxides	Precipitation, decreased secretion of gastric acid, resulting in decreased absorption of nutrients
	Vitamin B_{12}, folic acid, iron, and zinc	Sodium bicarbonate	Decreased gastric acid secretion, resulting in decreased absorption of nutrients
	Folic acid	Pancreatin	Decreased absorption
Changes in metabolic activities	Vitamin K	Anticoagulants, antibiotics (cephalosporins)	Reduced reductase/carboxylation activities; increased risk of thrombosis
	Vitamin B_6, calcium	Antituberculosis	Decreased pyridoxal kinase; decreased hepatic/renal vitamin D hydoxylation
	Folic acid	Antibiotics (trimethorprim)	Folate antagonist
	Folic acid Vitamin D Calcium	Anticonvulsants, phenobarbital/phenytoin	Increased hepatic microsomal enzymes, which change vitamin D metabolites
	Vitamin B_6	Antihypertensives (hydralazine HCL)	Decreased pyridoxal kinase
	Folic acid	Antihypertensives, diuretics (triamterene/hydrocholorothiazide)	Decreased dihydrofolate reductase, resulting in decreased utilization of folate
	Folic acid	Anti-inflammatory (prednisone/prednisolone)	Decreased hepatic/renal reductase
	Folic acid	Antiarthritic, anti-inflammatory (sulfasalazine), antiarthritic, NSAID (sulindac)	Inhibition of dihydrofolate reductase in the GI tract
	Folic acid	Antiarthritic, antineoplastic (methotrexate)	Folate antagonist
	Niacin	Statins	Increased risk of myopathy or rhabdomyosis
	Vitamin D, calcium	Antisecretory H_2-antagonist (famotidine)	Decreased hepatic/renal vitamin D hydroxylation
	Vitamin D, calcium	Antisecretory, antiulcer (lansoprazole)	Decreased hepatic/renal vitamin D hydroxylation
	Vitamin B_{12}	Tricyclic antidepressants	Decreased flavin adenine dinucleotide
	Vitamin B_{12}	Antipsychotics	Decreased flavin adenine dinucleotide
Changes in excretion	Sodium, potassium, chloride, calcium, chromium, magnesium, zinc, thiamin, B_6	Loop diuretics	Increased renal excretion due to decreased renal reabsorption
	Sodium, potassium, magnesium, zinc	Thiazide diuretics	Increased renal excretion due to decreased renal reabsorption
	Sodium, calcium	Triamterene/hydrochlorothiazide	Increased renal excretion due to decreased renal reabsorption
	Folic acid	Acetylsalicylic acid	Competition for binding sites

Adapted from Chernoff: Drug-induced alterations in nutrient kinetics. In *Geriatric nutrition*, Sudbury, MA, 2006, Aspen Publishers, Table 16-8; Yetley EA: Reported interactions of vitamins and minerals with drugs, *Am J Clin Nutr* 85(suppl):269S–276S, 2007, Table 2.

however, the size of a meal may impact drug bioavailability, as gastric emptying may be affected. In addition to the sizes of meals, the components of meals play a role in the resulting drug availability. The pharmacokinetics of a drug, not necessarily its bioavailability, will also be affected by the size of the drug dose.[53]

Beverages/Fluids. Beverages such as alcohol (beer, wine, liquors), caffeine-containing drinks, milk, milk-based beverages, fruit and vegetable juices, mineral waters, and soda, all make up fluid intake. Insoluble chelates are formed between specific drugs and the calcium present in milk. Even small volumes of milk can severely impact the absorption of some drugs such as tetracycline. Caffeine is hydrophilic and impacts gastric emptying. The absorption rate of caffeine increases as dose increases. Mixing drugs with juices and other beverages (sodas) may also affect the absorption of drugs due to the resultant decreased gastric pH. Grapefruit juice has been shown to be a potent inhibitor of the metabolism of many drugs through the selective down regulation of the intestinal cytochrome P450 (CYP) 3A4 isoenzyme, which leads to an increase in serum concentrations of these medications.[48] If drug absorption is affected by fluid intake, the rate of drug absorption may be decreased when large volumes of fluids are taken. The gastric emptying rate can be slowed by phosphoric acid and sugar, cold temperature of beverages may result in reduced rate of blood flow within the intestine, and gas in the beverage can increase the mixing and motility actions of the GI tract. However, liquids may cause a faster dissolution of drug or result in an osmotic effect or change in the surface area of the intestinal mucosa, thus altering drug absorption.[48]

Drug–Nutrient Interactions

Drug–nutrient interactions can be described as a change in the kinetics or dynamics of a drug or a vitamin, mineral, or nutrient constituent, or a change or compromise in the nutritional status of an individual as a result of a drug.[50] Multiple factors can create a drug–nutrient interaction and make a drug less effective, increase the potency or action of a drug, or cause unanticipated adverse effects.[3] Certain medications may also decrease the effectiveness of vitamins or minerals. Unfortunately, little research exists on drug–vitamin or drug–mineral interactions and the level and grade of evidence varies widely among studies. Supplement manufacturers are not required to evaluate potential drug–supplement interactions, and the only mechanism in place to report adverse events is voluntary reporting to the FDA MedWatch Program.[86] If an interaction is determined, it is more likely that the information on the interaction is included on the drug label rather than on the label of the supplement.[3] This is of concern due to the large number of MVMs commonly consumed.

Vitamin metabolism may be affected by medication use. Antibiotics destroy beneficial bacteria in the GI tract that synthesize vitamin K. Prophylactic vitamin K therapy may be provided to patients undergoing long-term antibiotic therapy in order to maintain vitamin K status. Anticoagulants inhibit the synthesis of vitamin K–dependent clotting factors II, VII, IX, and X; therefore, large volumes of foods high in K during anticoagulant therapy may decrease or negate the effect of the anticoagulant. A diet "consistent" in vitamin K is therefore recommended. As vitamin K is involved in bone function, those on long-term therapy with anticoagulants may have lowered bone density.[1]

Long-term anticonvulsant therapy places patients at risk for vitamin D deficiency and may result in rickets or osteomalacia. Phenytoin interferes with the metabolism of vitamin D in the liver; other drugs may also interfere with vitamin D metabolism.[87]

Methotrexate is an antagonist of folic acid and acts to destroy cancer cells, which also require folic acid for DNA replication. Isoniazid and levo-dopa (L-dopa) form complexes with vitamin B_6, which are then excreted by the kidney. A B_6 supplement is sometimes added to the drug regimen to correct B_6 deficiency, but this will decrease drug effectiveness. In addition, vitamin B_6 deficiency results in an inability to convert tryptophan to nicotinic acid, which can result in niacin deficiency. Isoniazid is similar in structure to niacin; therefore, the body reduces the production of this vitamin, and thus the vitamin deficiency disease of pellagra can be an adverse effect of isoniazid therapy.[88]

Concurrent administration of MVMs and medications may lead to interactions that alter the absorption, metabolism, or excretion of drugs or nutrients. Some interactions will have more severe effects than others, with some being fatal reactions. Health care providers must be familiar with drug–food/nutrient interactions and counsel their patients according to the medication and diet normally consumed (Table 24-1).

ACTIVITIES 24

1. You have been asked to see a 73-year-old man, who presents with a 15-year history of hypertension; status post myocardial infarction; status post coronary artery bypass graft (CABG, three-vessel), and type 2 diabetes mellitus. In addition, there is a history of smoking (1 pack/day) and a history of alcohol abuse.

   Lab values: Fasting blood glucose (FBG) 200 mg/dL, hemoglobin A_{1C} (HgA_{1C}) 11%, blood urea nitrogen (BUN) 20, creatinine 1.4

   Medications: atenolol, clopidogrel, aspirin, captopril, glimepiride

   A. List potential drug–drug, drug–nutrient interactions.

   B. What are the concerns with regard to alcohol use?

REFERENCES

1. Gropper SS, Smith JL, Groff JL: Advanced nutrition and human metabolism (5th ed.), Belmont, CA, 2009, Wadsworth.
2. Shenkin A: Micronutrients in health and disease. Postgrad Med J 82:559-567, 2006.
3. Yetley EA. Multivitamin and multimineral dietary supplements: Definitions, characterization, bioavailability, and drug interactions. Am J Clin Nutr 85(suppl):269S-276S, 2007.
4. Rock CL: Multivitamin-multimineral supplements: Who uses them? Am J Clin Nutr 85(suppl):277S-279S, 2007.
5. Rosenberg IH: Challenges and opportunities in the translation of the science of vitamins. Am J Clin Nutr 85(suppl):325S-327S, 2007.
6. Dietary Supplement Health and Education Act of 1994. Public Law 103-417. 103rd Congress (website). http://www.fda.gov/opacom/laws/dshea.html#sec3: Accessed February 3, 2009.
7. National Health and Examination Survey. NHANES (website). http://www.cdc.gov/nchs/nhanes.htm: Accessed March 30, 2009.
8. Radimer K, Bindewald B, Hughes J, Ervin B, Swanson C, Picciano MF: Dietary supplement use by US adults: Data from the National Health and Nutrition Examination Survey, 1999–2000. Am J Epidemiol 160:339-349, 2004.
9. Ervin RB, Wright JD, Kennedy-Stephenson J: Use of dietary supplements in the United States. 1988–1994, Hyattsville, MD, 1999, National Center for Health Statistics.
10. Rock CL, Newman V, Flatt SW, Faerber S, Wright FA, Pierce JP: Nutrient intakes from foods and dietary supplements in women at risk for breast cancer recurrence. Nutr Cancer 29:133-139, 1997.
11. Archer SL, Stamler J, Moag-Stahlberg A, et al: Association of dietary supplement use with specific micronutrient intakes among middle-aged American men and women: The INTERMAP Study. J Am Diet Assoc 105:1106-1114, 2005.
12. Reedy J, Haines PS, Campbell MK: Differences in fruit and vegetable intake among categories of dietary supplement users. J Am Diet Assoc 105:1749-1759, 2005.
13. Foote JA, Murphy SP, Wilkens LR, Hankin JH, Henderson BE, Kolonel LN: Factors associated with dietary supplement use among healthy adults of five ethnicities. Am J Epidemiol 157:888-897, 2003.
14. Jasti S, Siega-Rizz AM, Bently ME: Dietary supplement use in the context of health disparities: Cultural, ethnic and demographic determinants of use. J Nutr 133(suppl):2010S-2013S, 2003.
15. Stang J, Story MT, Harnack L, Newmark-Sztainer D: Relationships between vitamin and mineral supplement use, dietary intake, and dietary adequacy among adolescents. J Am Diet Assoc 100:905-910, 2000.
16. Dwyer JT, Garceau AO, Evans M, et al: Do adolescent vitamin-mineral supplement users have better nutrient intakes than nonusers? Observations from the CATCH tracking study. J Am Diet Assoc 101:1340-1346, 2001.
17. Institute of Medicine: Dietary reference intakes for vitamin A, vitamin K, arsenic, boron, chromium, copper, iodine, iron, manganese, molybdenum, nickel, silicon, vanadian and zinc, Washington, D.C., 2001, National Academy Press.
18. Institute of Medicine. Dietary reference intakes for thiamin, riboflavin, niacin, vitamin B_6, folate, vitamin B_{12}, pantothenic acid, biotin, and choline, Washington, D.C., 1998, National Academy Press.
19. Heaney RP: Factors influencing the measurement of bioavailability, taking calcium as a model. J Nutr 131:1244S-1348S, 2001.
20. Srinivasan VS: Bioavailability of nutrients: A practical approach to in vitro demonstration of the availability of nutrients in multivitamin-mineral combination products. J Nutr 1349S-1350S, 2001.
21. Solomons, N, Slavin JL: What impact does stage of physiological development and/or physiological state have on the bioavailability of dietary supplement? Summary of workshop discussion. J Nutr 131:1392S-1395S, 2001.
22. Krebs NF: Bioavailability of dietary supplements and impact of physiologic state: Infants, children and adolescents. J Nutr 1351S-1354S, 2001.
23. Code of Federal Regulations. Bioavailability and bioequivalence requirements. 21 CFR 320.1.
24. Hoag SW, Hussain AS: The impact of formulation on bioavailability: Summary of workshop discussion. J Nutr 131:1389S-1391S, 2001.
25. Yates AA: National nutrition and public health policies: Issues related to bioavailability of nutrients when developing dietary reference intakes. J Nutr 131:1331S-1334S, 2001.
26. King JC: Effect of reproduction on the bioavailability of calcium, zinc and selenium. J Nutr 131:1355S-1358S, 2001.
27. International Nutritional Anemia Consultative Group (INACG): Technical brief on iron compounds for fortification of staple foods, Washington, D.C., 2002, ILSI Press.
28. Finch S, Doyle W, Lowe C, et al: The national diet and nutrition survey: People aged 65 and over, London, 2004, The Stationery Office.
29. Solomon SM, Kirby DF: The refeeding syndrome: A review. J Parenter Enteral Nutr 14:90-97, 1990.
30. Kay RG, Tasman-Jones C, Pybus J, et al: A syndrome of acute zinc deficiency during total parenteral alimentation in man. Ann Surg 183:331-340, 1976.
31. Schnyder G, Rouvinez G: Total plasma homocysteine and restenosis after percutaneous coronary angioplasty: Current evidence. Ann Med 35:156-163, 2003.
32. Wald DS, Law M, Morris JK: Homocysteine and cardiovascular disease evidence on causality from a meta-analysis. BMJ 325:1202, 2002.
33. Lange H, Suryapranata H, De Luca G, et al: Folate therapy and in-stent restenosis after coronary stenting. N Eng J Med 350:2673-2681, 2004.
34. Bonaa K, Njolstad I, Ueland P, et al: Homocysteine lowering and cardiovascular events after acute myocardial infarction. N Engl J Med 354:1578-1588, 2006.
35. The Heart Outcomes Prevention Evaluation (HOPE) 2 Investigators: Homocysteine lowering with folic acid and B vitamins in vascular disease. N Engl J Med 345:1567-1577, 2006.
36. Lascalzo J: Homocysteine trials-clear outcomes for complex reasons. N Engl J Med354:1629-1632, 2006.
37. Heart Outcome Prevention Evaluation Study Investigators: Effects of ramipril on cardiovascular and microvascular outcomes in people with diabetes mellitus: Results of the HOPE study and MICRO-HOPE substudy. Lancet 355:253-259, 2000.
38. Gruppo Italiano per lo Studio della Sopravvivenza nell'infarto miocardico: Dietary supplementation with n-3 polyunsaturated fatty acids and vitamin E after myocardial infarction: Results of the GISSI-Prevension trial. Lancet 354:447-455, 1999.
39. Heart Protection Study Collaborative Group: MRC/BHF heart protection study of antioxidant vitamin supplementation in 20,536 high-risk individuals: A randomized placebo-controlled trial. Lancet 360:23-33, 2002.
40. Kris-Etherton PM, Lichtenstein, AH, Howard BV, et al: Antioxidant vitamin supplements and cardiovascular disease. Circulation 110:637-641, 2004.
41. Prentice RL: Clinical trials and observational studies to assess the chronic disease benefits and risks of multivitamin-mineral supplement. Am J Clin Nutr 85(suppl):308S-313S, 2007.
42. Age-related Eye Disease Study Research Group: A randomized, placebo-controlled clinical trial of high-dose supplementation with vitamins C and E and beta carotene for age-related macular degeneration and vision loss: AREDS report no. 9. Arch Ophthalmol 119:1439-1452, 2001.
43. Age-related Eye Disease Study Research Group: A randomized, placebo-controlled clinical trial of high-dose supplementation with vitamins C and E and beta carotene for age-related

macular degeneration and vision loss: AREDS report no. 8. Arch Ophthalmol 119:1417-1436, 2001.

44. Stephen AI, Avenell A: A systematic review of multivitamin and multimineral supplementation for infection. J Hum Nutr Diet 19:179-190, 2006.
45. Murphy SP, White KK, Sharma S: Multivitamin-multimineral supplements' effect on total nutrient intake. Am J Clin Nutr 85(suppl):280S-284S, 2007.
46. Dror Y, Stern F, Berner YN, et al: Recommended micronutrient supplementation for institutionalized elderly. J Nutr Health Aging 295-300, 2002.
47. Woo JJY: Adverse event monitoring and multivitamin-multimineral dietary supplements. Am J Clin Nutr 85(suppl): 323S-324S, 2007.
48. Maka DA, Murphy LK, Verger JT, Schears G, Lord LM: Drug-nutrient interactions: A review. Advanced Crit Care 11(4):580-589, 2000.
49. Sørensen JM: Herb-drug, food-drug, nutrient-drug, and drug-drug interactions: Mechanisms involved and their medical implications. J Alternat Complement Med 8:293-308, 2002.
50. Chan L-N: Drug-nutrient interaction in clinical nutrition. Curr Opin Clin Nutr Metab Care 5:327-332, 2002.
51. Cheymol G: Effects of obesity on pharmacokinetics. Clin Pharmacokinet 39:215-231, 2000.
52. Boullata JI, Barber JR: A perspective on drug-nutrient interactions. In Boullata JI, Armenti VA, editors: Handbook of drug-nutrient interactions, Totowa, NJ, 2004, Humana Press.
53. Singh BN: Effects of food on clinical pharmacokinetics. Clin Pharmacokinet 37:213-255, 1999.
54. Schmidt LE, Dalhoff K: Food-drug interactions. Drugs 62:1481-1502, 2002.
55. Lennernäs H: Modeling gastrointestinal drug absorption requires more in vivo biopharmaceutical data: Experience from in vivo dissolution and permeability studies in humans. Curr Drug Metab 8:645-657, 2007.
56. Santos CA, Boullata JI: An approach to evaluating drug-nutrient interactions. Pharmacotherapy 25(12):1789-1800, 2005.
57. Lennernäs H, Fager G: Pharmacodynamics and pharmacokinetics of the HMG-CoA reductase inhibitors. Clin Pharmacokinet 32:403-425, 1997.
58. Custodio JM, Wu C-Y, Benet LZ: Predicting drug disposition, absorption/elimination/transporter interplay and the role of food on drug absorption. Adv Drug Delivery Rev 60:717-733, 2008.
59. Welty DF, Siedlik PH, Posvar EL, et al: The temporal effect of food on tacrine bioavailability. J Clin Pharmacol 34:985-988, 1994.
60. Gleiter CH, Schug BS, Herman R, et al: Influence of food intake on the bioavailability of thioctic acid enantiomers. Eur J Clin Pharmacol 50:513-514, 1996.
61. Reppas C, Eleftheriou G, Macheras P, et al: Effect of elevated viscosity in the upper gastrointestinal tract on drug absorption in dogs. Eur J Pharm Sci 6:131-139, 1998.
62. Pao L-H, Zhou SY, Cook C, et al: Reduced systemic availability of an antiarrhythmic drug, bidisomide, with meal co-administration: Relationship with region-dependent intestinal absorption. Pharm Res 15:221-227, 1998.
63. Barnwell SG, Laudanski T, Dwyer M, et al: Reduced bioavailability of atenolol in man: The role of bile acids. Int J Pharm 89:245-250, 1993.
64. Yamaguchi T, Ikeda C, Sekine Y: Intestinal absorption of a β-adrenergic blocking agent nadolol: II. Mechanism of the inhibitory effect on the intestinal absorption of nadolol by sodium cholate in rats. Chem Pharm Bull 34:3836-3843, 1986.
65. Yamaguchi T, Oida T, Ikeda C: Intestinal absorption of a β-adrenergic blocking agent nadolol: III Nuclear magnetic resonance spectroscopic study on nadolol-sodium cholate micellar complex and intestinal absorption of nadolol derivatives in rats. Chem Pharm Bull 34:4259-4264, 1986.
66. Barry M, Gibbons S, Back D, et al: Protease inhibitors in patients with HIV disease. Clinically important pharmacokinetic considerations. Clin Pharmacokenet 32:194-209, 1997.
67. Ingwesen SH, Mant TG, Larsen JJ: Food intake increases the relative oral bioavailability of vanoxerine. Br J Clin Pharmacol 35:308-310, 1993.
68. Welling PG: Effects of food on drug absorption. Pharmacol Ther 43:425-441, 1989.
69. Mao CC, Jacobson ED: Intestinal absorption and blood flow. Am J Clin Nutr 820-823, 1970.
70. McLean AJ, McNamara PJ, DuSouich P, et al: Food, splanchnic blood flow, and bioavailability of drugs subject to first-pass metabolism. Clin Pharmacol Ther 30:31-34, 1978.
71. Abrahamsson B, Alpsten M, Bake B, et al: Drug absorption from nifedipine hydrophilic matrix extended-release (ER) tablet-comparison with an osmotic pump tablet and effect of food. J Control Rel 52:301-310, 1998.
72. Gidal BE, Maly MM, Kowalski JW, et al: Gabapentin absorption: Effect of mixing with foods of varying macronutrient composition. Ann Pharmacother 32:405-409, 1998.
73. Kottke MK, Stetsko G, Rosenbaum SE, et al: Problems encountered by the elderly in the use of conventional dosage forms. J Geriatr Drug Ther 5:77-92, 1990.
74. Williams L, Davis JA, Lowenthal DT: The influence of food on the absorption and metabolism of drugs. Med Clin North Am 77:815-829, 1993.
75. Fleisher D, Li C, Zhou Y, Pao L-H, Karim A: Drug, meal and formulation interactions influencing drug absorption after oral administration. Clin Pharmacokinet 36:233-254, 1999.
76. Brefel C, Thalamas C, Rayet S, et al: Effect of food on the pharmacokinetics of ropinirole in parkinsonian patients. Br J Clin Pharmacol 45:412-415, 1998.
77. Hartshorn EA: Food and drug interactions. J Am Diet Assoc 70:15-19, 1977.
78. Shively CA, Simons RJ, Passananti GT, et al: Dietary patterns and diurnal variations in aminopyrine disposition. Clin Pharmacol Ther 29:65-73, 1981.
79. Uenatsy T, Nagashima S, Niwa M, et al: Effect of dietary fat content on oral bioavailability of menatetrenone in humans. J Pharm Sci 85:1012-1016, 1996.
80. Lau DT, Kalafsky G, Aun RL, et al: The effect of the fat content of food on the pharmacokinetics and pharmacodynamics of SDZ FOX 988, an antidiabetic agent, in the dog. Biopharm Drug Dispo 16:137-150, 1995.
81. Pan HY, DeVault AR, Brescia D, et al: Effect of food on pravastatin pharmacokinetics and pharmacodynamics. Int J Clin Pharmacol Ther Toxicol 31:291-294, 1993.
82. Zhi J, Rakhit A, Patel IH: Effects of dietary fat on drug absorption. Clin Pharmacol Ther58:487-491, 1995.
83. Tam YK: Individualized variation in first-pass metabolism. Clin Pharmacokinet 25:300-328, 1993.
84. Richter WO, Jacob BG, Schwandt P: Interaction between fiber and lovastatin. Lancet 338:706, 1991.
85. Davidson MH, Dugan LD, Burns JH, et al: Cholesterol-lowering effects of soluble-fiber cereals as part of a prudent diet for patients with mild to moderate hypercholesterolemia. Am J Clin Nutr 52:1020-1026, 1990.
86. US Food and Drug Administration. MedWatch (website). http://www.fda.gov/medwatch/report/hcp.htm: Accessed April 17, 2009.
87. Zerwekh JE, Homan R, Tindall R, Pak CY: Decreased serum 24,25-dihydroxyvitamin D concentration during long-term anticonvulsant therapy in adult epileptics. Ann Neurol 12(2):184-186, 1982.
88. Kelly MP, Kight MA, Rodriguez R, Castillo S: A diagnostically reasoned case study with particular emphasis on B6 and zinc imbalance directed by clinical history and nutrition physical examination findings. Nutr Clin Pract 13:32, 1998.

25

Topical Drugs and Treatments Used in Wound Management

Sue Paparella-Pitzel and Leslie-Faith Morritt Taub

This chapter will focus on the topical care of chronic wounds (venous stasis ulcers, arterial ulcers, diabetic foot ulcers, and pressure ulcers), which require the attention, knowledge, and special skills of the health care practitioner. To support evidence-based practice, we present the state of the science in topical chronic wound care. This science is young, and much research still remains to be done. To support clinical practice until a larger body of definitive research is in place, we provide direction from the Cochrane reviews, practice guidelines of major professional organizations, and information from peer-reviewed journals that synthesize the available evidence and expert opinion.

PHYSIOLOGY AND PATHOPHYSIOLOGY OF WOUNDS

Acute wounds are defined as a disruption of tissue, which heals within 21 days and proceeds through the three phases of tissue healing: inflammation, proliferation, and remodeling.[1] The inflammatory phase (phase I) includes vasoconstriction, platelet aggregation, and release of thromboplastin for clotting and achieves homeostasis, vasodilatation, and phagocytosis. Vasodilatation is initiated by the release of cytokines (immunomodulating agents) and growth factors and results in increased blood flow to the wound, which aids in phagocytic activity. The proliferative phase (phase II) includes granulation, in which fibroblasts lay down collagen, new capillaries are produced, and contraction of wound edges and re-epithelialization occur. Re-epithelialization takes place when epithelial cells differentiate into type I collagen and cells migrate across the wound bed. This is a complex and fragile stage, and if this process is disrupted, chronic inflammation may result.[2] The remodeling phase (phase III) is the final phase of tissue healing, in which the new collagen increases its tensile strength, and scar tissue is formed.

Chronic wounds are defined as wounds that have failed to progress through the healing process. More specifically, if a wound has not shown reduction in size by 20% to 40% after 2 to 4 weeks, the wound is considered to be chronic.[3] When the chronic wound's inflammatory phase of healing persists, there is resulting tissue damage from an influx of neutrophils that release cytolytic enzymes and free oxygen radicals. Tissue hypoxia accompanies this persistent inflammatory state and results in the proliferation of bacteria, especially anaerobic organisms.[2]

Venous stasis ulcers (VSUs), arterial leg ulcers (ALUs), diabetic foot ulcers (DFUs), and pressure ulcers (PUs) are all chronic wounds (Figure 25-1, A-D). They are wounds that either have failed to progress through the healing process or have not sustained this process to recover anatomic and functional integrity.[4] Venous ulcers represent 70% of chronic lower extremity ulcers and arterial ulcers about 25%.[5,6] It is important to understand that arterial insufficiency also contributes to ulcers of other etiologies, such as VSU and DFU, and must be considered in wounds that fail to heal.[7] Ischemia impairs wound healing by decreasing available oxygen, leukocytes, other blood-borne factors, and antibiotics.[8] Additionally, in people with diabetes, oxygen to the skin is decreased—which is thought to be caused by a decrease in oxygen exchange due to high levels of glucose—which results in diminished cell membrane deformation and function. Autonomic neuropathy, often a concomitant condition, may cause shunting of blood away from the skin surface.[9] Pressure ulcers result from compression of soft tissue against a bony prominence and are seen most often in older adults, the acutely ill, and those with spinal cord injuries.[10] It has been asserted that PUs, VSUs, and DFUs have some common pathways as a result of prolonged inflammation that leads to internal tissue degradation by proteolytic enzymes and reactive oxygen species, which, in turn, result in wound formation from the breakdown of connective tissue components in the skin.[11] It is this inflammation triggered by alternating ischemia and reperfusion and small vessel hypertension that, in a cascade effect resulting from the release of cytokines, proteolytic enzymes, and inflammatory infiltrate, lead to tissue breakdown. The underlying disease processes, which set the stage for the inflammatory process and skin breakdown remain, and this may explain why even after initial healing, the wound tends to recur.[11]

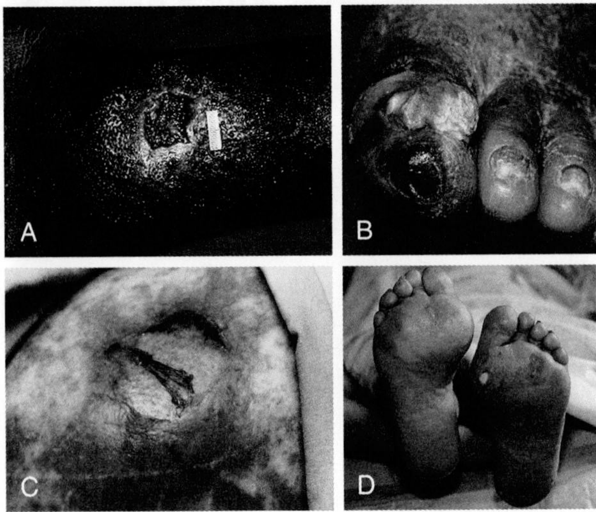

FIGURE 25-1 **A.** Venous ulcer; **B.** arterial ulcer; **C.** diabetic foot ulcer and **D.** Pressure ulcer. (A and C from Bryant R, Nix D: Acute and chronic wounds: current management concepts, 3e, Philadelphia, Saunders, 2007. B from Libby P, Bonow RO, Mann DL: Braunwald's heart disease: a textbook of cardiovasuclar medicine. 8e, Philadelpiha, Saunders, D from Wold GH: Basic geriatric nursing, 4e, St. Louis, Mosby, 2008.)

CREATING THE IDEAL WOUND ENVIRONMENT FOR HEALING

Preparing the Wound Area

The rehabilitation team member must ensure the ideal wound environment that includes the appropriate amount of moisture, cleanliness, and tissue free from stress from pressure and shearing forces. The wound base must be free to heal from the bottom up. Removal of necrotic tissue via débridement ensures a clean wound base and prepares the integument for the three phases of healing to occur. The clinician must work to convert the chronic wound environment into an acute wound bed environment to facilitate the three phases of tissue healing.[12]

In preparing the wound bed, the clinician needs to evaluate the following factors: need for débridement, presence of infection versus inflammation, the status of moisture balance, and wound edge advancement characterized by Sibbald's DIME (D: débridement; I: infection; M: moisture imbalance; and E: edge of wound advancement), the acronym adapted from The International Wound Bed Advisory Board.[12,13] Débridement often occurs as a natural part of the healing process, and assisted débridement enhances that process. Débridement is often necessary to remove devitalized tissue that would support infection. If débridement is indicated, it may take the following forms: autolytic, sharp, enzymatic, mechanical, or biological. Autolytic débridement occurs in the early stages of wound healing through the actions of proteolytic enzymes and macrophages; and this can be a slow process, depending on the state of the body's natural defenses. Autolytic débridement is enhanced by moisture-balanced dressings. Moist wound environments accelerate healing by as much as 50% compared with dry wound environments.[14] However, when autolytic débridement is insufficient to improve wound healing within 72 hours, then other forms of débridement need to be considered.

Considerations about Enzymatic Pharmaceutical Débridement Agents

Use of enzymatic pharmaceutical débridement agents effectively removes necrotic tissue from PUs and leg ulcers and may often enhance autolytic débridement under a dressing.[15] In the case of certain wounds, clinicians choose to combine an enzymatic débridement agent with surgical or sharp débridement. This combination therapy is applied at each dressing change. However, combining two or more enzymatic pharmaceutical débridement agents is not recommended. Other application recommendations with regard to using enzymatic agents include protecting intact wound edges and using a sharp hatching technique on the eschar where necrotic tissue or eschar is very thick in order to facilitate penetration of the enzymatic agent. Examples of enzymatic pharmaceutical agents include collagenase, papain/urea, and trypsin (Box 25-1). The effectiveness and benefits of these agents vary.[16] Collagenase is more effective than placebo for débridement of necrotic tissue from PUs and leg ulcers. Some evidence suggests that papain-urea–based agents remove necrotic tissue more rapidly than does collagenase. The proteolytic enzyme papain cannot be used alone and requires urea as an activator. Both collagenase and papain-urea agents promote wound healing.[12,15,17,18] Trypsin is a milder débriding agent, which dissolves blood clots and does not act against viable tissue.[12,14] More clinical trials to compare the efficacy and safety of

BOX 25-1 Enzymatic Agents

Enzymatic Agents	Selected Products	pH Range Necessary for Activity
Collagenase	Santyl	6–8 (small range)
Papain/urea	Accuzyme, Ethezyme, Gladase, Kovia	3–12 (wider range)
Papain/urea/Chlorophyllin Copper Complex(CCC)	Panafil, Ziox	3–12
Trypsin	Xenaderm, Granulex	3–12

Adapted from Falabella, A: Debridement and wound bed preparation, *Dermatol Ther* 19:317–325, 2006.

these enzymatic agents at the cellular level and at the level of clinical application are needed.

Using the DIME paradigm of wound bed evaluation, after evaluating the wound for necessary débridement (D), clinical observation of the wound will include monitoring for signs and symptoms of an acute inflammatory response, which are pain, erythema, swelling, and increased temperature. With regard to chronic wounds, the clinician must distinguish between chronic inflammation and infection (I). If high levels of bacteria are present causing increased cytokines and proteases and decreased growth factor activity, the recommended clinical action is to apply topical antimicrobials, anti-inflammatories, protease inhibitors, and growth factors in order to restore the healing environment.[12,13] Lack of moisture (M) slows epithelial cell migration, and excessive moisture results in maceration. Applications of moisture-balanced dressings promote wound healing.[12,13] (See the Wound Dressings section later in this chapter.) When poor advancement of the wound edge (E) is evident, the clinician must reassess the cause and consider referral for surgical intervention.

Additional considerations affecting the wound bed environment include intrinsic factors of wound healing, such as adequate nutrition with sufficient protein to support tissue repair, tissue perfusion, and oxygenation.[4,7] Oxygenation of a wound can be impaired due to inadequate tissue perfusion in the presence of dehydration, environmental cold, stress, and pain. Cigarette smoking causes peripheral vasoconstriction and decreases tissue perfusion. Systemic auto immune diseases such as rheumatoid arthritis, uncontrolled vasculitis, and pyoderma gangrenosum delay local wound healing, so these diseases need to be treated first so adequate wound healing is possible.[7] The presence of multiple wounds causes a delay in the rate of healing. Systemic steroids and immunosuppressive drugs interfere with wound healing by altering immune function, metabolism, inflammation, nutrition, and tissue perfusion. Surgical stress also diminishes the capacity for wound healing.[4] Nonsteroidal anti-inflammatory drugs (NSAIDs) such as aspirin and ibuprofen decrease collagen production that is necessary for wound repair.[19] With regard to the wound itself, necrotic tissue, bacterial burden, and cellular debris need to be addressed for adequate wound healing. Colonization of the wound with bacteria is not synonymous with wound infection. These bacteria are usually resident microorganisms, and they may, in fact, serve to protect the wound from virulent pathogens.[8] Lower levels of bacteria can be handled by the immune system. The choice of topical antimicrobials should be based on quantitative tissue biopsy, which will ascertain the identity of the pathogen, sensitivity of the organism, and the concentration of the pathogen per gram of tissue. The goal is to bring the bacterial concentration to $<$100,000 colony-forming units (CFUs) of bacteria per gram of tissue so that remaining bacteria can be eliminated by normal immune defenses.[19]

Agents for Wound Cleansing

Cleansing the wound is the first step in preparing the wound bed for the healing process and is a routine component in the management of any wound. Antiseptic agents inhibit the growth and development of microorganisms and are commonly used to cleanse or irrigate the wound. Semi-solid forms of antiseptics are products that remain in contact with the wound. Although antiseptics inhibit the growth of microorganisms, disruption of the cellular processes of healthy resident microorganisms should be minimized.[20,21] Large, well-designed clinical trials are necessary to demonstrate the safety and efficacy of antiseptics for a number of reasons. The use of iodine-based antiseptics remains controversial.[3] Also, the effects of hydrogen peroxide and povidone–iodine solutions for cleansing of the wound bed result in the disruption of keratinocytes and fibroblasts.[22] In comparison with hydrogen peroxide and povidone-iodine solutions, chlorhexidine and silver-containing compounds are less detrimental to fibroblast activity while still maintaining antibacterial properties and cell proliferation.[22] There is little evidence from controlled studies on humans comparing the solutions for irrigation and cleansing described above. Some researchers contend that depending on the type of wound and it's normal wound flora, antiseptic application should be considered and the assumption that healing is impeded be further investigated.[3,20]

Normal saline is nontoxic to tissue and does not affect the normal skin flora or the flora associated with the acute wound environment. In a review of the evidence comparing saline with normal tap water for cleansing acute wounds, no significant differences were found in the rate of wound healing or infections.[2,23] Saline and tap water are inexpensive cleansing options compared with chlorhexidine and silver-containing compounds. The use of povidone–iodine solutions for cleansing is supported only in the treatment of infected wounds, specifically those infected by *Pseudomonas* and methicillin-resistant *Staphylococcus aureus* (MRSA).[3,14,24]

Cleansing solutions that contain metal (e.g., silver products) should not be used with débriding agents (collagenase and papain-urea), as the former have been shown to decrease the effectiveness of the latter.[25] Other solutions to be avoided, or are no longer in clinical use, include chlorine-releasing hypochlorite, such as bleach and boric acid, which are considered to be disinfectants rather than antiseptics. These solutions are known to be cytotoxic and are excluded from the current practice for wound management.[3]

1. Povidone–iodine (PVP-I): 10% solution, 10% ointment, and 2.5% dry powder spray; antibacterial activity
2. Hydrogen peroxide (H_2O_2): 3% and 6% solutions, and 1% cream; antimicrobial activity
3. Chlorhexidine and silver-containing compounds: available as 0.05% solution and also a constituent

of skin cleansers; high antibacterial activity against gram-negative fungi and viruses
4. Saline solution or tap water

Note: *Solutions* are aqueous formulations and are used for cleansing and/or irrigation. *Creams, gels,* or *ointments* are semisolid formulations and are used as topical applications.

SPECIFIC CONCERNS AND ADJUVANT INTERVENTIONS FOR CHRONIC WOUNDS

Venous Stasis Ulcers

The venous system within the legs comprises deep, superficial, and communicating veins, which depend on the compression of calf muscles during ambulation for venous blood to return to the heart through one-way venous valves. VSUs are thought to occur due to incompetent valves, immobility, poor calf muscle pumping, or a combination of these; the ulcers are caused by the trapping of leukocytes and growth factor within pericapillary fibrin cuffs and the release of cytokines, leading to capillary dysfunction, ischemia, and ultimately to ulceration.[26] The estimate of the prevalence of VSUs in the United States in 2008 was 600,000.[5]

Health care practitioners should be aware of the potential complexity in the presentation of VSUs. While compression treatment for reducing leg edema is well supported in the literature, if arterial disease is also present, venous healing will be impeded, and high-level compression may further compromise circulation.[4]

Clinical Presentation. VSUs typically have irregular but well-defined borders surrounded by erythematous or hyperpigmented skin on the medial leg. Venous hypertension causes large molecules to pass into the dermal layer, which causes the deposition of hemosiderin, an iron complex, and a resultant brawny skin discoloration and induration.[5] Venous ulceration results from distal venous pressure elevation, despite ambulation, causing limb edema and white cell and fibrin elevations, which impede capillary blood flow and entrap growth factors.[4,5] Healing of VSUs is facilitated when adequate compression is applied to the lower extremity.

Topical Treatment. Débridement to remove devitalized tissue is necessary to prevent infection of a venous leg wound. In the presence of any level of beta hemolytic streptococci after débridement or a high wound microbial concentration ($\geq 10^6$ CFU/g of tissue), topical antimicrobials should be used to lower the bacterial burden of the wound. Antimicrobials include antibiotics (chemicals produced by microorganisms to inhibit or kill other microorganisms) and antiseptics (chemicals that inhibit the growth of microorganisms on living tissue). To prevent cell damage and bacterial resistance, this treatment should be discontinued when the bacterial burden has been reduced. Wounds should be cleaned at each dressing change with normal saline or clean tap water to remove loose debris.[4]

The Cochrane review of topical antibiotics and antiseptics enumerates methodologic problems in many primary studies, including the lack of: randomization of study subjects, allocation concealment, blinded outcome assessment, and intention-to-treat analysis. Additionally, pooling of data for a meta-analysis was hindered by differences in treatment regimens, study settings, and baseline criteria such as ulcer size and duration and whether the wound was colonized by bacteria or actually infected. There was also a lack of data to calculate effect sizes in intervention studies, differences among studies as to primary and secondary outcomes, and very small sample sizes that made study results subject to type 1 error (the assumption that differences in study groups exist, when, in actuality, none exist).[21] We present the strongest study results described by the Cochrane review, with the caveat that more research in this area is still required.

One study ($n = 100$) of predominately colonized wounds, in which povidone–iodine (an iodine complex that has microbicidal activity but slow release of free iodine minimizing iodine toxicity in human cells) was compared with dextranomer, a cicatrizant (a hydroscopic dextran polymer, which creates a suction force that moves both microorganisms and high-molecular-weight substances away from the wound). The average healing time was significantly shorter in the group using dextranomer (4.4 weeks versus 5.3 weeks, $p = <0.05$). Additionally, the dextranomer group had a shorter colonization with *Staphylococcus aureus* than did the povidone iodine group (14.7 days versus 18.7 days, $p = 0.01$).[21] In another study ($n = 200$), 10% povidone–iodine was applied to the venous ulcer, and the wound was then covered with paraffin gauze; then this treatment was compared with hydrocolloid dressing. Both groups of patients received a two-layer compression or a compression stocking. Ten percent of the large ulcers healed in less than 4 months, the trial period, in the povidone–iodine group, compared with 34% in the hydrocolloid group ($p = 0.02$). Intergroup difference in terms of dichotomous healing at the study endpoint was not statistically different (51% of VSUs healed in the hydrocolloid group versus 47% in the povidone group, RR 0.92, 95% confidence interval CI 0.69–1.23). The cost, inclusive of the time required to do the respective dressings, was less for povidone–iodine (betadine).[21]

While 10 trials (N= 645) of cadexomer iodine treatment (a water-soluble starch polymer, which absorbs exudate and particulate matter from a granulating wound while releasing bactericidal iodine as the dressing becomes moist) were mentioned in the Cochrane review, failure to report baseline ulcer status, duration, wound infection or colonization, and other methodologic details such as study regimen differences (outpatient care versus inpatient care) and the failure to report complete healing as the endpoint made it difficult to compare data and impossible to pool data from most of the studies. Results from two outpatient trials (Steele, n = 60, Harcup, n = 72) that compared cadexomer plus compression with standard care (Steele compared cadexomer with a heterogeneous group of topical agents, including antibiotics, antiseptics, hydrophilic agents, topical steroids, and bland agents; Harcup compared cadexomer with a dry dressing) were pooled at the 4-week mark with complete healing as the outcome measure. There was a statistically significant result in favor of cadexomer (Iodosorb, Iodoflex) (RR 6.72, 95% CI 1.56–28.95).[21]

Three small trials of peroxides as treatment for VSUs were reported.[21] The first trial (n = 10 patients) compared benzoyl peroxide lotion 10% with normal saline; the second trial (n = 10 patients) compared benzoyl peroxide lotion 20% with normal saline; the third trial compared the vehicle of the lotion (the control) with normal saline. Each patient had two ulcers and served as his or her own control. After 42 days, the 10% benzoyl peroxide lotion was found to be more effective than saline in reducing the ulcer area (the mean wound diameter was reduced by 30.4% more than in the normal saline–treated wound (95% CI 42.12–18.68). The 20% benzoyl peroxide lotion reduced the wound diameter by 34.1% more than did normal saline (95% CI–46.22) to –21.98). The small sample sizes in these trials may reflect a chance occurrence.[21]

In two similar studies comparing hydrogen peroxide 1% cream with placebo in treating VSUs pretreated with systemic antibiotics to eradicate infection, after 10 days, the wound sizes were decreased by a mean of 35% by the hydrogen peroxide cream compared with 11% in the case of placebo-treated ulcers ($p = <0.05$) in the first study (n = 20), and 44.8% versus 32% ($p = <0.005$) in the second study (n = 32). Both these studies included compression in the treatment.[21]

Dressings. Dressings for VSUs should be used in combination with compression systems.[4] Principles of dressing VSUs include maintenance of a moist healing environment in the wound to promote cell migration, matrix formation, and autolytic débridement.[4] Ideal dressings prevent wound border maceration and continuous contact with the wound exudate, both of which cause wound enlargement and impede healing. Dressing should not increase pressure on the wound; use of adhesive, a cause of contact dermatitis, should be avoided, and pressure dressing should be used instead to keep the dressing in place.[4] Recurrence rates of VSUs are as high as 90%, so long-term surveillance of these wounds is required even after they have healed.[5] Exercise to increase calf muscle pumping has been shown to prevent VSUs.[4]

Pressure Dressings. Support hose or elastic bandages with 40 to 60 mm Hg pressure are used when no arterial disease is present.[5] Because venous pressure hypertension is an ongoing process, compression of the extremity should be maintained indefinitely.[4] Compression bandages (single layer: Ace wraps, Comperm, Setopress; triple layer: Dyna-Flex) provide elastic compression that works to create constant compressive forces diminishing filtration of fluid from the venous circulation and increasing the absorption of interstitial fluid into the venous circulation.[27]

Intermittent pneumatic pressure (with or without compression dressings) is used in those who cannot or will not tolerate an adequate compression dressing. Other treatments may include high-pressure systems such as the Unna boot, which comprises dressings impregnated with zinc-oxide, calamine, and glycerine; when dry, they become rigid and function as a support against which the calf muscles contract for effective edema control. This treatment only benefits patients who ambulate.[27] Another system is the Duke boot, which provides 30 mm Hg of compression to the lower extremity. First, a hydrocolloid dressing is applied to the VSU; then a layer of viscopaste, a zinc-impregnated gauze wrap, which keeps the skin supple; and, finally, a layer of Coban. Coban is a stretch-elastic wrap that forms the compression layer. One wrap provides about 30 mm Hg compression, and two wraps provide about 40 mm Hg compression. The Duke boot is left in place for 1 week. Manufacturers have developed prepackaged systems that function similarly to the Duke boot. Two of these are the Profore Four Layer Bandaging System and the Dyna-Flex Multi-Layer Compression System.

Arterial Leg Ulcers

ALUs are the result of poor arterial blood supply to the extremities resulting in inadequate blood supply to the skin. Risk factors for ALUs include smoking, diabetes, hyperlipidemia, hypertension, and elevated homocysteine levels.[7] Surgery is undertaken when possible to improve the blood supply by bypassing areas of blockage or narrowing. Topical treatments such as dressings and topical agents are also utilized to promote wound healing.[6]

Clinical Presentation. The patient typically provides a history of injury prior to the ulceration. The ulceration is pale to black, and the wound borders are clearly delineated. The extremity has weak or absent dorsalis pedis (DP) or posterior tibial (PT) pulses, thin hairless skin, hypertrophic toenails, and delayed capillary refill in the nail bed of >2 seconds. DP pulses are absent in 8.1% and PT pulses absent in 2.9% of the general population related to anatomic differences. Nonetheless, absence of pulses or diminished pulses in an extremity with an ulceration should be referred to the primary care provider for vascular evaluation.[7] The patient may give a history of intermittent claudication or rest pain if the arterial disease is very severe. The practitioner will observe pallor on leg elevation and rubor and edema when the extremity is in the dependent position (Buerger's test).[28] The primary care provider often initiates assessment of the extremity by evaluating the Ankle Brachial Index (ABI), which is a ratio of the systolic blood pressure in the lower extremity to the systolic blood pressure in an arm. A resting ABI of <0.9 should prompt further evaluation for the extent of peripheral vascular disease. An ABI of >1.2 that results from calcification of the vasculature causing incompressible vessels (often seen in those with diabetes) should also lead to further evaluation.[7] In patients with ALUs, revascularization to correct the ischemic condition is the treatment of choice; however, not all patients are candidates for surgery, and these procedures are not always successful or produce sustained results.[7] ALUs should not be débrided until the extremity has been revascularized to prevent enlargement of a nonhealing ulcer.[7]

Topical Treatment. In general, a moist healing environment promotes wound healing by promoting cell migration and matrix formation; however, dry gangrene and eschar should be left dry until the extremity has been revascularized.[7] There is no evidence that favors one dressing over another.[7] Wounds open to the air tend to become heavily colonized with bacteria, and blood flow is impaired; the resulting hypoxia sets the stage for healing impairment. While support from meta-analyses and randomized control trials is lacking, expert opinion supports the use of occlusive topical antimicrobial dressings to aid in the healing of heavily colonized wounds.[7]

Diabetic Foot Ulcers

About 15% of those with diabetes will have a foot ulcer at some time in their life.[29] The risk factors for DFUs include neuropathy, trauma, poor glycemic control, long duration of diabetes, foot deformity, high plantar pressures, smoking, older age, male gender, insulin use, a prior foot ulcer, and peripheral arterial disease.[9,30] The most common precursors to ulceration are neuropathy followed by a traumatic event.[29] The healing of DFUs is influenced by the presence of infection and ischemia, depth of the ulcer, glycemic control, pressure relief, and protective footwear.[31] Healing of DFUs is optimized by good glycemic control.[32] Recurrence rates for DFUs are between 8% and 59%, so use of protective footwear and long-term surveillance are necessary.[32] Up to 3% of those with DFUs go on to have a lower-limb amputation.[31]

Clinical Presentation. Prior to ulcer formation, a callus may be noticed in a high-pressure area such as the plantar area at the second metatarsal head. If the foot is not offloaded properly, ulceration will follow. Ulcers are considered infected if they have a purulent discharge or two local signs, for example, warmth, erythema, lymphangitis, lymphadenopathy, edema, tenderness, and pain.[31,33] Wound depth at the level of bone and signs of local (cellulitis or abscess formation) or systemic infection with radiologic support suggests osteomyelitis.[9] Vascular insufficiency of the extremity is suggested clinically by the absence of pedal pulses in the ulcerated extremity or an ABI of <0.9.[9,30] The presence of neuropathy may be assessed by the lack of vibration perception at the great toe, diminished deep tendon reflexes, impaired pain sensation, or impaired two-point discrimination. Local or extensive areas of gangrene may also be present.[9]

Treatment. Débridement of the wound to remove necrotic and devitalized tissue and to prevent bacterial growth and offloading of the ulcerated foot (with crutches, walkers, wheelchairs, custom shoes, shoe modifications, diabetic boots or casts) serve as the basics of treatment for DFUs.[32] If the ulcer is not epithelializing from the wound border after 2 weeks or if infection is suspected, a tissue biopsy or validated quantitative swabbing should determine the type and level of infection.[32] If the ulcer has $\geq 1 \times 10^6$ colony-forming units (CFUs) of bacteria per gram of tissue or any level of beta-hemolytic streptococci, then application of topical antimicrobial agents should be initiated for a short period to decrease the bacterial load.[32] Systemic antibiotics are only used for acute diabetic wounds; however, they do not decrease the bacterial load in granulating wounds.[32] If the ulcer is surrounded by cellulitis, commonly caused by staphylococcal or streptococcal infection, a systemic antibiotic with gram-positive activity should be initiated.[32] After 4 weeks of treatment, the wound size is expected to be reduced by 40%, or a re-evaluation of the treatment should be initiated.[32] Dressings that maintain a moist wound environment speed healing by promoting cell migration, matrix formation, and autolytic débridement.[32] Only one topical cytokine growth factor, the recombinant human platelet–derived growth factor becaplermin (PDGF, brand name Regranex), has been found to be an effective agent in the healing of diabetic neuropathic ulcer.[32] It works by promoting chemotactic recruitment and proliferation of cells involved in wound repair and by enhancing the formation of granulation tissue. Four randomized, prospective, blinded, placebo-controlled, multicenter trials demonstrated rapid closure and complete healing of chronic diabetic ulcers with once-a-day topical treatment with 100 mcg/g of PDGF.[34] To date, there is insufficient evidence for or against the use of silver-based wound dressings and protease-modulating dressings in the treatment of DFUs.[29,35] There is a lack of scientific evidence to provide guidance as to the superiority of one wound dressing or product over another.[33]

Pressure Ulcers

PUs are seen in those who do not or cannot shift positions on their own when in the sitting position or lying position. Those with spinal cord injuries may be unable to mobilize themselves. Older adults or the acutely ill may suffer from muscular weakness and not experience any discomfort from remaining in one position for long periods. All of these factors predispose to PUs, especially in the presence of impaired nutrition, other disabilities such as contractures, and surfaces that promote shear and friction forces between the skin and the surface of the bed or chair. The basics of prevention and healing of existing PUs is frequent turning and positioning.

Clinical Presentation. See Box 25-2.

Treatment. Management of PUs includes pressure reduction, débridement of necrotic tissue, treatment of infection, adequate nutrition, correction of anemia, and maintenance of adequate fluid volume. To maintain adequate protein for healing, 1 to 2 g/kg/day is recommended. With medical management, stage 1 and 75% of stage 2 ulcers will heal spontaneously. In those who have PUs, a schedule of once-every-hour turning is recommended. Management for stage 3 and stage 4 ulcers include low-air-loss or air-fluidized beds.[10] Stage III and stage IV ulcers often require surgery for closure of the wound.[37]

BOX 25-2 The National Pressure Ulcer Advisory Panels Staging System (2007)

Stage 1	An erythemic area that may also be warm and indurated as a result of hyperemia after the relief of pressure to an area. When the area of erythema is compressed, the tissue will blanch. If pressure continues, the area remains erythemic and will not blanch. Eventually, the skin may appear pale due to the extended ischemia.
Stage 2	The second stage of a pressure ulcer appears as a shallow ulcer with a pink wound bed and involves the loss of epidermal and dermal tissues.
Stage 3	The third stage extends to the loss of subcutaneous tissue, and subcutaneous fat may be visible.
Stage 4	The fourth stage exposes bone, muscle, tendon, or joint capsule. Eschar may be present in the wound. Osteomyelitis and destruction of bone and sinus tracts may also be present.[36,37]
Deep tissue injury	Deep tissue injury, a newer classification, first appears as a bruised or purple area on the skin, which may rapidly go on to become a full-thickness wound. In darker-skinned persons, this injury may not be readily apparent, but as the wound evolves, a thin blister may appear over a dark wound bed, and this wound may further evolve to expose more layers of tissue.[36]
Unstageable ulcer	In an unstageable pressure ulcer, full-thickness tissue loss is seen; however, the base of the ulcer is covered by eschar or slough, so the depth of the wound is not apparent, and therefore the ulcer cannot be staged.

Débriding agents include wet-to-dry normal saline dressing for mechanical débridement and collagenase (Santyl) for enzymatic débridement.[37] With regard to wounds requiring reduction in bacterial load, silver sulfadiazine is bactericidal to many gram-positive and gram-negative organisms as well as yeast.[37] Sulfamylon is a bacteriostatic agent with both gram-positive and gram-negative coverage, and it also includes activity against *Pseudomonas aeruginosa*.[37] Those with infections in other sites (e.g., urinary tract infections) should be treated with appropriate antibiotics because bacteria traveling in the blood or lymphatics can lodge in the compromised tissue of a developing PU.[10]

Wound Dressings

Wound location, size, drainage, condition of the wound border, complaints of pain, and presence of granulation tissue should all be observed and documented in the initial evaluation, subsequent progress notes, and discharge summaries. Wound dressings should be chosen to keep the wound moist, manage the drainage, and protect the surrounding skin from maceration and exudates, which can cause wound enlargement and result in poor healing (Box 25-3).[4,38,39] Wound dressings can assist in managing infection by maintaining the level of antimicrobial agents in the wound bed (cadexomer iodine) and by providing a barrier against harmful microorganisms (semipermeable films). They can also maintain an optimal amount of moisture in the wound bed by absorbing excess exudate from wound beds (hydrocolloid dressings, polyurethane and silicone foams) and promote moisture in dry wound beds (alginate dressings, hydrogel wound fillers, semipermeable films, tulles). Dressings are also used to eliminate dead space (such as deep cavities, tunneling, or undermining) by filling in wound cavities, thus preventing abscess formation and promoting granulation tissue formation (hydrogel wound filler, hydrofiber, foam dressings).

SPECIAL CONSIDERATIONS FOR THE REHABILITATION PROFESSIONAL

Examination and evaluation of the wound area is performed by various members of the rehabilitation team. Acronyms such as DIME (see Preparing the Wound Area section earlier in this chapter) and MEASURE (Measure, Exudate, Appearance, Suffering, Undermining, Re-evaluate, and Edge) guide clinicians in evaluating the wound bed.[2,13] Each member of the rehabilitation team should examine and evaluate the wound using the MEASURE method and also assess the dressing for the adequacy of its role in healing. Additional evaluation of the wound includes management of products directly applied to the wound and observing the role of the exercise and diet plan in the patient's healing.

Rehabilitation includes interventions administered by the various members of the wound care team.

BOX 25-3 Types of Wound Dressings

Hydrocolloid (HCD) Dressings	
Brand names	DuoDERM CGF Extra Thin, Intrasite HCD, Tegasorb, Replicare, CombiDERM, Comfeel, Granuflex
Type of dressing	• Occlusive dressings composed of carboxymethylcellulose, gelatin, pectin, elastomers, and adhesives that turn into a gel and rapidly absorb exudates
Indications	• Pain relief achieved by covering of nerve endings with gel and exudates • Rehydration of dry necrotic eschar and promotion of autolytic débridement • Prevention of friction and shear
Wearing instructions	• May be worn for up to 7 days when wound drainage is moderate • Water-resistant film border adheres to the wound edges
Precautions	• Should not be used on infected wounds or wounds that need frequent inspection, such as diabetic foot ulcers
Alginate Dressings	
Brand names	3MTegagen, Kaltostat, Kaltogel, SorbSan, Tegagel, SeaSorb, Algisite M, Algosteril, Comfeel, Curasorb, SilvaSorb
Type of dressing	• Composed of calcium alginate (a seaweed component) • Contains mannuronic acid (M) and glucuronic acid (G) • Calcium in the dressing is exchanged with sodium from the wound fluid; this interaction turns the dressing into a gel that maintains a moist wound healing environment
Indications	• Highly absorbent and can be used on moderately to severely exudating, sloughing, and granulating wounds • Highly conformable and can be used to treat leg ulcers and pressure ulcers • Débriding agent for necrotic tissue in chronic wounds
Wearing instructions	• High M alginates should be washed from the wound (e.g., Kaltostat), and high G alginates should be removed from the wound intact (e.g., SorbSan) before redressing the wound
Precautions	• Should be changed daily and should not be used for dry or infected wounds
Hydrogel Wound Filler	
Brand names	Tegagel, Intrasite Gel, Aquasorb, Duoderm, Granugel, Normigel, Nu-Gel, Purilon Gel, KY Jelly
Type of dressing	• Composed mainly of water in a complex network of fibers that keeps the starch polymer gel intact
Indications	• Used for dry and minimally draining ulcers • Used for sloughing or necrotic wound beds to rehydrate and remove devitalized tissue • Keeps the wound moist and cool to enhance healing and reduce pain
Wearing instructions	• Cover with a secondary dressing because hydrogels are nonadhesive
Precautions	• May macerate wound borders causing a decrease in keratinocyte re-epithelialization • Should not be used in wounds with gangrenous tissue or where there is a high level of exudates
Semipermeable Film	
Brand names	Opsite, Tegaderm, Bioclusive, Skintact, Release
Type of dressing	• Sheet of polyurethane coated with hypoallergenic acrylic adhesive
Indications	• Transparent cover allows wound observation • Facilitates autolytic débridement
Wearing instructions	• Allows for coverage over joints and other difficult-to-dress anatomic sites
Polyurethane or Silicone Foams[38,39]	
Brand names	Allevyn, Lyofoam
Indications	• Absorbs large amounts of exudates
Precautions	• Not useful for débridement
Hydrofiber	
Brand names	Aquacel, Aquacel-Ag, Versiva
Type of dressing	• Soft pad or ribbon dressing made from sodium carboxymethylcellulose fibers
Indications	• Aquacel-Ag contains 1.2% ionic silver, an antimicrobial, which is effective against methicillin-resistant *Staphylococcus aureus* and vancomycin-resistant enterococci
Wearing instructions	• Used in deep wounds that require packing
Precautions	• Requires a secondary dressing cover
Collagens	
Type of dressing	• Dressings come in particles, gels, or pads
Indications	• Promotes collagen formation in the wound bed • Absorbs exudates and provides a moist environment

BOX 25-3 Types of Wound Dressings—cont'd

Hyaluronic Acid	
Brand names	Hyalograft 3D, Laserskin (HYAFF-11)
Type of dressing	• Composed of a benzyl ester derivative of hyaluronic acid • Semipermeable films
Indications	• Used on diabetic foot ulcers and venous leg ulcers • May be used as a wound cover or as a scaffold to cultivate fibroblasts and keratinocytes
Nonadherent Dressings (Tulles)	
Brand names	Mepore, Skintact, Release
Type of dressing	• Open weave cloth saturated with soft paraffin or chlorhexidine or multilayered perforated plastic films that prevent adherence to the wound bed; allows exudates to pass through into a secondary dressing while maintaining a moist wound bed
Indications	• Pain, maceration, and odor are less on removal of nonadherent dressings
Foam Dressings	
Brand names	LYOfoam, Spyrosorb, Allevyn
Type of dressing	• Polyurethane or silicone foam is used to transmit moisture vapor and oxygen and thermally insulate the wound • Polyurethane foams have two or three layers—one hydrophilic layer that contacts the wound bed and one hydrophobic layer that hold the exudates in the dressing
Indications	• May be used to fill a wound cavity; comes as a membrane of perforated polymeric film with chips of hydrophilic polyurethane foam within • Silicone foam expands to fit the wound by forming a soft foam dressing which absorbs exudates and protects the area around the wound.
Selected Antimicrobial Dressings	
Brand names	Povidine–iodine impregnated tulle Cadexomer iodine (Iodosorb, Iodoflex)
Indications	• 1 g of cadexomer iodine can absorb 7 mL of fluid; iodine is slowly released, lowering the bacterial load and débriding the wound
Precautions	• Systemic uptake of iodine is possible, so caution must be exercised in patients who have thyroid disease
Dextranomer Dressings	
Type of dressing	• A sterile, insoluble powder in the form of circular beads, 0.1 to 0.3 mm in diameter when dry • It is a long-chain polysaccharide constructed in a three-dimensional network of cross-linked dextran molecules • Highly hygroscopic due to its high hydroxyl group content; 1 g of it absorbs 4 mL of water and swells until it is saturated • The suction force generated in vitro is in the range of 200 mm Hg.
Indications	• Dextranomer cleanses by absorbing the wound exudate, protein degradation products, prostaglandins, bacteria, and other contaminants, which results in reduced inflammation and healing

Interventions and treatment approaches administered by the physical therapist for overall wound management includes:

1. Patient/client and/or caregiver education
2. Positioning considerations: for sitting and supine positions, this includes use of positioning devices and positioning for preventive pressure relief and edema control
3. Mobility assessment: prescription of devices for wheelchair seating, ambulation, and/or orthotics:
   - Exercise prescription for edema control, improved circulation, and improved functional mobility[40]
   - Specific physical therapy interventions for DFUs, including patient and caregiver education on foot care, foot inspection, footwear, and exercise
   - Specific physical therapy interventions for pressure ulcers, including patient and caregiver education on pressure relief, bed mobility, and bed positioning and seated positioning
4. Application of mechanical modalities and physical agents:
   - Electrical stimulation
   - Ultrasound
   - Short-wave diathermy
   - Cold laser
   - Vacuum-assisted closure
   - Hyperbaric oxygen tanks

CONCLUSION

Pharmaceutical agents can effectively promote wound healing when the selection of the agent is based on proper examination and evaluation of the patient at each stage of the wound healing process. The pharmaceutical agent is one component of the intervention plan and management of the patient. Creating the ideal wound environment, preparing the wound bed, choosing the proper cleansing agent, and classifying the wound type are essential steps in initiating the wound healing process. Following choice of appropriate pharmaceutical agents and dressings, the effects of all the interventions need to be systematically evaluated and adjusted to optimize the healing and ultimate closure of the wound.

ACTIVITIES 25

Case Study

MB, a 55-year-old female, presents with a venous stasis ulcer (VSU) on her right lower extremity (RLE) and a chronic diabetic foot ulcer (DFU) on the plantar aspect of her left foot. MB has a medical history that includes type 2 diabetes and poorly controlled hypertension. The surgeon has ruled out osteomyelitis. The patient is on antibiotics and is receiving services from a home care company. Nursing care, physical therapy, and occupational therapy have been ordered by the physician.

Social History

Married, with two adolescent children
Teacher (part-time)
Nonsmoker
Coach of her child's soccer league

Medications

Lantus insulin 20 units subcutaneous at bedtime
Metformin 1000 mg twice daily
Enalapril 10 mg twice daily
Toprol XL 50 mg once daily
Acetylsalycylic acid (ASA) 81 mg once daily

Exam Findings

Blood pressure (BP) 160/94, pulse (P) 72, temperature (T) 101, body mass index (BMI) 35
The finger stick before breakfast for the last week >200 mg/dL (last Hgb A_{1C} a month ago 7.8%)
RLE, lateral aspect of leg, 4 inches below the knee: a quarter-size ulcer with irregular borders
Left foot, on the plantar surface, just below the great toe: a 2-cm wide and 1-cm deep ulceration

Questions

1. Based on the exam findings, what are at least two areas of concern that will require further pharmacologic intervention?
2. What specific exam findings will contribute negatively to the healing of the VSU and the DFU?
3. Considering that osteomyelitis has been ruled out, how will you proceed with the wound examination?
4. What specific procedures will need to be performed to investigate the wounds for infection?
5. What intervention/treatment actions will you initiate for each wound?
6. Who should be included in the wound care team in order to manage this patient's care efficiently?
7. What will be the health care provider's order to the team members responsible to clean the wound (povidone–iodine solution, hydrogen peroxide, chlorhexidine/silver compound, or normal saline and/or water)?
8. What are the possible dressings that will be ordered if the VSU and the DFU are presenting with moderate exudate during the first week of consultation? Consider the dressings that are readily available at your particular facility.
9. What primary interventions will be included in the rehabilitation therapist's plans?
10. What are additional modalities that the physical therapist should consider and investigate for the facilitation of healing of each wound?
11. What will be the primary areas for follow-up and re-evaluation? If positive results are not apparent, where is the first place you will begin to readjust the regimen?

REFERENCES

1. Kelly DG: Physical rehabilitation. In O'Sullivan S, Schmitz T, editors: Physical rehabilitation (5th ed.), Philadelphia, 2007, F.A. Davis.
2. Sibbald RG, Orsted H, Schultz GS, Coutts P, Keast D: Preparing the wound bed 2003: Focus on infection and inflammation. Ostomy Wound Manage 49:23-51, 2003.
3. Leaper DJ, Durani P, Leaper DJ, Durani P: Topical antimicrobial therapy of chronic wounds healing by secondary intention using iodine products. Int Wound J 5:361-368, 2008.
4. Robson MC, Cooper DM, Aslam R, et al: Guidelines for the treatment of venous ulcers. Wound Repair Regen 14:649-662. 2006.
5. Stillman RM: Wound care. In eMedicine: WebMD, 2008.
6. Nelson EA, Bradley MD: Dressings and topical agents for arterial leg ulcers. Cochrane Database Syst Rev (1):CD001836, 2007.
7. Hopf HW, Ueno C, Aslam R, et al: Guidelines for the treatment of arterial insufficiency ulcers. Wound Repair Regen 14:693–710, 2006.
8. Lipsky B, Berendt AR, Embil JM, de Lalla F: Diagnosing and treating diabetic foot infections. Diabetes Metab Res Rev 20:S56–S64, 2004.
9. Fard AS, Esmaelzadeh M, Larijani: Assessment and treatment of diabetic foot ulcer. Int J Clin Pract 61:1931–1938, 2007.
10. Whitney J, Phillips L, Aslam R, et al: Guidelines for the treatment of pressure ulcers. Wound Repair Regen 14:663–679, 2006.
11. Chen J, Rogers AA: Recent insights into the causes of chronic leg ulceration in venous diseases and implications on other types of chronic wounds. Wound Repair Regen 15:434–449, 2007.
12. Schultz GS, Sibbald RG, Falanga V, et al: Wound bed preparation: A systematic approach to wound management. Wound Repair Regen 11(suppl 1):S1–S28, 2003.
13. Sibbald RG, Orsted HL, Coutts PM, Keast DH: Best practice recommendations for preparing the wound bed: Update 2006. Adv Skin Wound Care 20:390–405; quiz 6–7, 2007.
14. Falabella AF: Debridement and wound bed preparation. Dermatol Ther 19:317–325, 2006.
15. Ramundo J, Gray M: Enzymatic wound debridement. J Wound Ostomy Continence Nurs 35:273–280, 2008.
16. Smith RG: Enzymatic debriding agents: An evaluation of the medical literature. Ostomy Wound Manage 54:16–34, 2008.
17. Konig M, Vanscheidt W, Augustin M, Kapp H: Enzymatic versus autolytic debridement of chronic leg ulcers: A prospective randomised trial. J Wound Care 14:320–323, 2005.

18. Alvarez OM, Fernandez-Obregon A, Rogers RS, Bergen L, Black M: A prospective randomized comparative study of collagenase and papain-urea for pressure ulcer debridement. Wounds 14:293–301, 2002.
19. Stadelmann WK, Digenis AG, Tobin GR: Impediments to wound healing. Am J Surg 176:39S–47S, 1998.
20. Drosou A, Falabella AF, Kirsner R: Antiseptics on wounds: Area of controversy. Wounds 15:149–166, 2003.
21. O'Meara S, Al-Kurdi D, Ovington LG: Antibiotics and antiseptics for venous leg ulcers. Cochrane Database Syst Rev (1):CD003557, 2008.
22. Thomas GW, Rael LT, Bar-Or R, et al: Mechanisms of delayed wound healing by commonly used antiseptics. J Trauma 66:82–90; discussion-1, 2009.
23. Sasson C, Hennah A, Diner B: Evidence based medicine: Wound Cleaning—water or saline? Israeli J Emerg Med 5:3–7, 2005.
24. Bergstrom N: Pressure ulcer treatment: Clinical practical guidelines. In AHRQ: Quick reference guide for clinicians, Rockville MD, 1994, AHRQ.
25. Kirshen C, Woo K, Ayello EA, Sibbald RG: Debridement: A vital component of wound bed preparation. Adv Skin Wound Care 19:506–517; quiz 17–19, 2006.
26. Phillips TJ, Etufugh CN: Venous stasis ulcers. In Rakel RE, Bope ET, editors: Conn's current therapy, (60th ed.), Philadelphia, 2008, WB Saunders.
27. Ennis JE, Meneses P: Standard, appropriate, and advanced care and medico-legal considerations: Part two—venous ulcerations. Wounds 15:107–122, 2003.
28. Lyden SP, Joseph D: The clinical presentation of peripheral arterial disease and guidance for early recognition. Cleveland Clin J Med 73:S15–S21, 2006.
29. Bergin S, Ross L, Thomas S, Royle P, Waugh N: Protease modulating dressings for treating diabetic foot ulcers. Cochrane Database of Systematic Reviews [CD005361].
30. Frykberg R: Diabetic foot ulcers. Am Fam Physician 66:1655–1662, 2002.
31. Oyibo SO, Jude EB, Tarawneh I, Nguyen HC, Harkless LB, Boulton AJM: A comparison of two diabetic foot ulcer classification systems. Diabetes Care 24:84–88, 2001.
32. Steed DL, Attinger C, Colaizzi T, et al: Guidelines for the treatment of diabetic ulcers. Wound Repair Regen 14:680–692, 2006.
33. Lipsky B, Berendt AR, Deery HG, et al: Diagnosis and treatment of diabetic foot infections. Clinical Infectious Diseases 39:885–910, 2004.
34. Steed DL: Clinical evaluation of recombinant human platelet-derived growth factor for the treatment of lower extremity ulcers. Plast Reconstr Surg 117(7 suppl):143S–149S, 2006.
35. Bergin S, Wraight P: Silver based wound dressings and topical agents for treating diabetic foot ulcers. Cochrane Database Syst Rev (1):CD005082, 2006.
36. Pressure ulcer stages revised by the NPUAP 2007 (website). http://www.npuap.org/pr2.htm. Accessed May 28, 2009.
37. Kirman CN, Molnar: Pressure ulcers, nonsurgical treatment and principles: Treatment and medication, eMedicine: WebMD, 2008.
38. Zibigniew R, Schwartz RA, Joss-Wichman E, Wichman R, Zalewska A: Surgical dressings, eMedicine: WebMD, 2009.
39. Jones V, Grey JE, Harding KG: Wound dressings. BMJ 332:777–780, 2006.
40. Yang D, Vandongen YK, Stacey MC: Effect of exercise on calf muscle pump function in patients with chronic venous disease. Br J Surg 86:338–341, 1999.

26

Complementary and Alternative Medicine in Pharmacology

Lisa Dehner

INTRODUCTION

Pharmacology is important to the practicing therapist because, as the chapters of this book outline, drugs affect the bodies that therapists rehabilitate. Many patients take prescription drugs; those drugs are prescribed for a medical condition by the patient's physician or nurse practitioner. However, some patients also take drugs that used to be prescription-only drugs but are now considered "over-the-counter" drugs, that is, drugs that can be bought by the patients themselves and used safely without medical supervision. Finally, still other patients may take vitamins, supplements, or herbs. A complete knowledge of the effects of all these types of drugs is vital for providing optimal rehabilitation. Any substance that has the ability to affect the patient's physiology is relevant to the therapist who strives to do the same.

The use of herbs and supplements, for the most part, is considered outside the scope of conventional, Western medicine and, as such, is a part of the larger concept of complementary and alternative medicine (CAM). As the name indicates, these practices can be complementary or adjuvant to conventional practices, or they may be used in isolation as an alternative. Beyond the use of herbs and supplements, CAM includes homeopathic medicine, traditional Chinese medicine, mind-body techniques, and energy (biofield) practices, just to name a few examples.

Drug Regulation

In the United States, the U.S. Food and Drug Administration (FDA) is responsible for the approval and monitoring of prescription as well as "over-the-counter" drugs.[1] Ultimately, pharmaceutical companies must go through a rigorous approval process that includes preclinical (animal) trials and clinical (human) trials before a drug is approved for use in this country. Prescription drugs can also be evaluated for their use without medical supervision ("over the counter"). This is the case with gastrointestinal (GI) drugs such as famotidine (Pepcid®) and cimetidine (Tagamet®), which were once available for use only with a prescription. After a drug is released for use in the United States, the FDA has the responsibility for postmarket monitoring of that drug and its effect on consumers. Often, the long-term effects of a drug are unknown and become apparent only after FDA approval and use in the public. Such was the case with the adverse effects of rofecoxib (Vioxx), which was voluntarily withdrawn from the market by the manufacturer after concerns about cardiovascular events emerged.[2] This type of oversight and regulation is crucial to ensuring public health. Unfortunately, the FDA does not have such power or authority over herbs, vitamins, and supplements. The *Dietary Supplement Health and Education Act of 1994* (*DSHEA*) defined a dietary supplement as "a product (other than tobacco) intended to supplement the diet that bears or contains one or more of the following dietary ingredients: vitamin, mineral, amino acid, herb or other botanical."[3] Dietary supplements are considered food, not drugs, and are therefore not subject to the same type of regulation. Manufacturers, not the FDA, are responsible for making sure that a supplement is safe before bringing it to the consumer. Once on the market, like any other food, the FDA is responsible for identifying any potential harm to the public but has the burden of first proving that the supplement is unsafe. Much of the FDA's postmarket monitoring relies on voluntary reporting by manufacturers. Nonetheless, action from the FDA does occur and may include removal of a product from the market for proven safety concerns or warnings about content of a dietary supplement.[4]

An important consideration when investigating the efficacy of supplements is that the FDA has no legal standards for the purity, quality, or contents of dietary supplements sold to consumers. As a result, several studies have demonstrated the variability of the contents of dietary supplement products.[5-7] In 2009, the FDA recalled a dietary supplement because it, in fact, contained a prescription drug.[8] For-profit companies such as ConsumerLab.com have come into existence to provide testing services to the public, some free and some fee based.

Although it currently has no authority to standardize the supplement industry, the US government has formed the National Center for Complementary and Alternative Medicine (NCCAM), a new division of the National Institutes of Health (NIH).[9] The mission of the NCCAM is to facilitate rigorous, high-quality research in the alternative and complementary areas of medicine and disseminate the information to the public. The goal of the NCCAM is to investigate the claims of supplements and provide consumers with scientific evidence delineating which supplements can be a valuable part of medical care and which simply do not work. Unfortunately, the marketing language and advertising of a product can be confusing and misleading. Words such as "natural" and "health" are vague, but they are legally permissible and serve to promote a positive feeling about a product, without necessarily being specific or even true. Legally, anything classified as a dietary supplement cannot claim to diagnose, treat, prevent, or cure a disease (only drugs do these things).[3] Ambiguous claims such as "supports well being" or "helps promote health" can be made, but more specific claims related to physiology or pathology, for example, "lowers cholesterol," are not allowed. Claims are monitored and enforced by both the FDA and the Federal Trade Commission (FTC).

In summary, the supplement industry is largely self-monitored. Ultimately, consumers (including patients and their therapists) are responsible for understanding the actions and effects of the supplements on the body.

Use of CAM

Many adults in the United States are using CAM for general health or for a stated medical condition. The NCCAM and the National Center for Health Statistics gathered data on the use of CAM from over 20,000 American adults through the 2007 National Health Interview Survey (NHIS) and found that 38.3% were using CAM.[10] Barnes and colleagues found approximately 1 in 5 adults (18.9%) had used a herb for a medical condition in the past year.[11] Individuals taking CAM tend to have a health complaint, be female, be Caucasian, have a higher socioeconomic status, be a former smoker, be of normal weight, and have a more physically active lifestyle.[12-14] Four of the top five diagnoses given for the use of CAM were back pain, neck pain, joint pain, and arthritis, all musculoskeletal conditions encountered in the physical therapy clinic.[10] In the United States, complementary medicine is used most often, compared with alternative medicine.[15]

Clearly, the use of CAM occurs in a significant percentage of the American population. Although the implication may be that these "natural" products are harmless, any substance powerful enough to affect human physiology also has the potential to create adverse events. As such, physical therapists should actively question patients about any use of supplements. While physical therapists do not have the burden of prescribing knowledge, they should understand the general effects of these substances on physiology and whether there is potential for any interaction between a prescribed therapeutic activity and a supplement's effect. The chapters of this book that discuss prescription medications and this chapter on supplements are designed to assist the physical therapist in this endeavor.

Reviewing the Literature

The drugs available for use and the way drugs are prescribed change greatly over time. The same can be said for the availability and use of dietary supplements. New formulations and new theories on how to improve health are constantly being developed. Therefore, in order to maintain a base of knowledge in this area, the therapist must be able to efficiently and effectively sift through research articles on any given topic. One of the most efficient ways to learn if a supplement is safe and effective is to read a systematic review or a meta-analysis. These types of articles synthesize relevant individual studies to attempt to answer the clinical bottom-line: What effects, beneficial or adverse, will the product have on the patient? The majority of these articles report their findings using the concept of effect size—which is the strength or magnitude of the difference between those individuals taking the supplement and those individuals not taking the supplement. For example, a group of individuals participates in a study to investigate if black cohosh reduces the number of hot flashes in postmenopausal women. One group is given black cohosh for 4 weeks, and one group is given a placebo for that same period. The participants' frequency of hot flashes before the intervention and after the 4 weeks of the study period is recorded using a patient log. Then each group's total number of hot flashes is calculated. The effect size of these two sets of data can be expressed by the difference in the two means. According to Cohen, the relative value of the effect size can be expressed as follows: 0.2 is a small difference, 0.5 is a moderate difference, and 0.8 is a large difference.[16] Of course, the larger the effect size, the more different the two individual groups are with respect to the dependent variable (number of hot flashes). If the study was well controlled, this would indicate that black cohosh is effective in reducing the number of hot flashes in postmenopausal women.

The concept of an effect size can also be expressed as the standard mean difference (SMD) or weighted mean difference (WMD), both of which express differences between groups. WMD involves assigning some studies more statistical weight (e.g. if there are more subjects or if the study is of better quality) and others less. SMD and WMD can be reported as either a positive or a negative number depending on the pooling favoring the treatment group or the control group. Often, a negative number means the outcome favors the treatment group, but it is important to verify this by looking at the forest plot, which should be included in the article.

Additional statistics that may be used are odds ratios (OR) and relative risk ratios (RR), which are different strategies to determine the probability or incidence of an event (e.g., disease) in a population. Which statistic is used depends on the type and extent of population data. An OR of 1 would mean that both groups have the same probability of the event and, therefore, the treatment did not have a significant effect. An RR of 3 favoring the control group would mean it is three times more likely to experience the event or develop the disease. Finally, the number needed to treat (NNT) and the number needed to harm (NNH) are also frequently used. The NNT reflects the number of individuals that would need to be administered the intervention for one individual to gain benefit. Thus, a NNT of 4 would mean that if four individuals were given the treatment, one of those four individuals would meet a set standard defined by the author (e.g., a 30% reduction in pain from a visual analog scale [VAS]). The NNH is similar but expresses the number of people who would experience an adverse event that would not have occurred if they had been given a placebo. Ultimately, the greater the effect of the intervention, the lower is the NNT and the higher is the NNH.

Unfortunately, systematic reviews and meta-analyses of supplements are not common. More likely, the therapist will find individual clinical trials of a supplement in question. When trying to synthesize several articles, it is important to keep a number of factors in mind: (1) The study's level of control: Did a group receive a placebo? If there is no control group, then there is no way to determine whether the supplement itself caused a beneficial change or some other unknown factor was affecting the outcome. (2) Were the groups randomized into a control group and a supplement group, and were their baseline characteristics compared? For example, was the control group significantly younger than the supplement group? If these factors are not evaluated and controlled, they can dramatically affect the outcome of the study. (3) Most importantly, what are the dependent variables? Dependent variables are the tools used by the researcher to measure change. In the example above for NNT, the dependent variable was pain, and a valid and reliable visual analog scale was used to measure it. The dependent variable is a crucial part of the research process, and, as such, the physical therapist should be critical of the choice. Ask the following questions: Does the tool actually measure the desired change? Is the tool solely reliant on subjective report? Does the tool measure change at an impairment level or a functional level? Many studies claim a significant statistical difference between groups, but the change in the actual dependent variable is so small that the outcome is not clinically meaningful. For example, a study that demonstrates a significant improvement (–3 points) in the score of an arthritis questionnaire, but the study subjects are, however, still having pain and difficulty during activities of daily living (ADLs). The change is statistically significant but not clinically meaningful to therapists or patients. This is the concept of minimal clinically important difference (MCID). Unfortunately, the MCID is difficult to quantify and is not known for all dependent variables.

Another caveat when reviewing the literature on supplements is manufacturer bias. Many of the studies evaluating the effectiveness of a supplement are financially supported by the supplement manufacturer, or the authors of the study are affiliated with the manufacturer and could stand to gain financially based on the outcome of the study. McAlindon and colleagues conducted a meta-analysis of the research for glucosamine sulfate and chondroitin sulfate for the treatment of osteoarthritis (OA) and found that of the 15 eligible studies, 13 had some level of manufacturer bias.[17] Furthermore, a significant portion of supplement research is carried out in Europe, using European-manufactured supplements. These supplements are sometimes available in the United States, but often they are not. Thus, it is unclear whether the outcomes derived from studies of supplements not available in the United States conducted on European subjects can be generalized to the American population. Such findings underscore the importance of the development of the NCCAM and its mission to fund well-controlled trials of dietary supplements in the United States.

In summary, when reviewing the literature to evaluate a supplement's effectiveness, the physical therapist should take into consideration whether the article synthesizes many studies or presents just one experiment, the level of control of extraneous variables (including manufacturer bias and where the study was conducted), and the dependent variable used to report clinical change between groups.

EVIDENCE-BASED REVIEW OF SELECTED SUPPLEMENTS

Supplements for Pain

Complaints of pain are common among patients in physical therapy. The source of pain can be from various causes such as osteoporosis, neuropathic and chronic pain syndromes, and delayed-onset muscle pain. There is a large market of supplements directed at patients with these complaints; these supplements include, but are not limited to, those selected for this chapter: glucosamine, chondroitin sulfate (CS), and S-adenosylmethionine (SAM-e) for the pain and inflammation of OA, and capsaicin and menthol for neuropathic pain and muscle soreness.

For the most part, researchers working with the selected supplements measure success using a visual analog scale (VAS) for pain or standardized functional measures such as the Western Ontario and McMaster Universities Osteoarthritis Index (WOMAC) and the Lequesne Algofunctional Index (LI).[18-21] By using a Likert scale or a VAS form, the WOMAC gathers subjective responses from patients about their pain, stiffness, and their physical, social, and emotional functions. The LI gathers subjective responses from patients about their pain, maximum distance walked, and ADLs. An LI score of ≥14 would indicate the consequences of the pathology to be "extremely severe," and a score of 1 to 4 would be considered "mild."

Glucosamine (Glucosamine Sulfate [GS]; Glucosamine Hydrochloride [GH]) and Chondroitin Sulfate (CS)

Background. According to Wold and colleagues, 17% and 12% of all adults over 65 years of age in the United States are taking glucosamine and CS, respectively.[22] Together, glucosamine and CS generated 300 million dollars of revenue in the year 2000.[22] Both supplements are heavily advertised for their ability to increase flexibility, improve movement, and lubricate joints, clearly targeting patients with OA.

OA is a degenerative joint disease associated with defective articular cartilage, subchondral bony changes, and acute or subacute inflammation.[for review, 23] Patients with OA have an imbalance of cartilage degeneration and adequate repair mechanisms. The osteoarthritic joint is dehydrated, has less cartilage-building chondrocytes, an increased level of degradative enzymes, inflammation of the synovium, and potential collapse of the subchondral bone. Clinically, patients present with joint pain and stiffness, diminished range of motion (ROM), muscle weakness, and crepitus. Unfortunately, joint pain and stiffness limit mobility, which further endangers the joint. Articular cartilage health is directly related to the passage of nutrients and waste via joint movement. GS and CS are both endogenously occurring substances present in the extracellular matrix (ECM) of articular cartilage.[24] The theory behind their supplementation involves their ability to help facilitate cartilage building and repair mechanisms.

Glucosamine is a small, amino-monosaccharide constituent of larger glycosaminoglycans (GAGs) present in the ECM of articular cartilage. Evidence from animal and in vitro studies are controversial as to whether supplementation of glucosamine actually improves GAG levels[25,26] or has no effect.[27,28] However, it does appear to decrease the total levels of degradative enzymes[29-31] and total aggrecan (GAGs + hyaluronic acid) count.[29] CS is a large, negatively charged GAG present in the ECM of articular cartilage. Evidence from animal and in vitro studies demonstrate that CS can stimulate the formation of aggrecan [25,32] and reduce the number of degradative enzymes.[25,33,34] Thus, albeit controversially, there is at least some evidence to support the alteration of cartilage-building mechanisms by glucosamine and CS.

Efficacy. Both glucosamine and CS have been extensively investigated. The outcomes of these studies vary from a strong significant decrease in pain and improvement in function compared with placebo to no difference at all. Several meta-analyses and systematic reviews have attempted to synthesize these conflicting reports.[17,35-41] Most of these articles report favorable results with respect to the ability of glucosamine and CS to reduce the pain of OA and to improve function. Analyzing studies of GS supplementation (1.5 g/day for at least 4 weeks), Poolsup and colleagues reported pooled effect sizes of 0.41 and 0.46 for pain reduction and improvement in function, respectively.[41] Similarly, Towheed et al conducted a systematic review of glucosamine compared with placebo for the Cochrane Library and found improvement to reduce pain (SMD = 0.61) and function (SMD= 0.51), as measured by the LI but not when measured by the WOMAC.[36] Richy reported an NNT of 4.87 for the administration of either glucosamine (0.75 to 1.5 g/day × 4 weeks to 3 years) or CS (800–2000 mg/day × 3 months to 1 year) over placebo.[37] Thus, about five patients would need to be given either glucosamine or CS for one patient to benefit from treatment.

At this point, one may be tempted to stop the discussion and conclude that glucosamine and CS are effective in reducing pain and improving function with a moderate effect size. However, it would not be prudent to take these meta-analyses at face value. While each study had various strategies to attempt to appropriately pool the data, all acknowledge the difficulty of mathematically combining studies that are vastly different, or heterogeneic. The primary sources of heterogeneity include number of subjects, length of study, amount of control and blinding, dependent variables used, and exact formulation of the supplement utilized. Glucosamine supplements come in two main forms, the most common of which is glucosamine sulfate (GS) and, more rarely, glucosamine hydrochloride (GH). Additionally, proprietary formulations of GS from a particular European manufacturer demonstrate more dramatic results than those of other GS formulations.[40]

In their meta-analysis of the effectiveness of glucosamine and CS, McAlindon and colleagues conducted a quality assessment of the pooled studies and found significant manufacturer affiliation (direct or indirect), significant methodologic issues among the studies, and a direct correlation between the quality of the study and the resultant effect size (the lower the quality, the greater was the magnitude of the results).[17] The authors concluded that the effect sizes of the glucosamine and CS studies up to that point were likely exaggerated.

Vlad and colleagues sought to further investigate the issues of heterogeneity in the glucosamine trials by analyzing data based on certain characteristics.[40] When pooling the data from only those studies using GH, the effect size was 0.06, that is, virtually no effect. Industry-funded GS trials ($n = 11$) had a pooled effect size of 0.47 in stark contrast to 0.05 of that of independent trials ($n = 4$). However, heterogeneity was still very high in just the 11 industry-funded trials, further limiting the interpretation of the already moderate effect. The extent of allocation concealment (the process of randomized assignment of subjects to groups, which should be concealed from both the investigators and the subjects) also had dramatic effects on study results. Studies with adequate concealment had a pooled effect size of 0.09, which is dramatically lower than the effect sizes of studies with intermediate or inadequate concealment (0.47, and 0.54, respectively). The authors concluded that there is enough evidence from trials published thus far to state that GH demonstrates no effect above placebo in the treatment of OA. Unfortunately, because of the significant heterogeneity of the trials, the authors concluded that the pooling of GS effect sizes is still problematic and, as such, determinations of efficacy cannot be reached.

Further illustrating the concerns of McAlindon and Vlad, when other authors synthesized the studies more judiciously, the GS and CS effect sizes diminished. When Towheed and colleagues restricted their analysis to those studies with adequate allocation concealment, GS showed no benefit above placebo with regard to pain or function as measured by the WOMAC (a small improvement remained for function as measured by LI).[36] Similarly, Hauselmann (2001) showed that the effect size of GS for pain was 0.56 when all studies were pooled but dropped to 0.26 when only higher-quality studies were used.[35] The effect sizes for CS showed the same trend (effect sizes = 1.37 versus 37).

Several authors have also investigated the effects of CS alone. Leeb et al combined six randomized controlled trials (RCTs) and reported significant pooled effect sizes for CS (1.2 g for at least 4 weeks) to reduce pain and improve function (pain = 0.9, LI = 0.74).[38] However, the authors acknowledged the significantly smaller numbers of subjects in the CS studies compared with those testing any form of glucosamine. Additionally, Leeb et al conducted no formal quality assessment of the studies included in the meta-analysis. Reichenbach and colleagues initially combined 20 CS trials and found a significant effect size of -0.75 for the reduction of pain (representing ~ 1.6 cm on a 10-cm VAS).[39] However, like Vlad et al, Reichenbach and colleagues found a great deal of heterogeneity in the CS trials. Their pooled effect size was reduced to -0.01 when using the largest trials with adequate allocation concealment (representing a 0.2-cm change on a VAS scale). Both Vlad (GS) and Reichenbach (CS) demonstrated a declining effect size based on the year of publication, that is, more recent studies showed that GS and CS have less of an effect than did earlier studies. Both authors supposed that this was due to improved controls and larger sample sizes.

The pooling of data and determining effect sizes are attempts to determine whether patients will experience any clinically meaningful improvement using the drugs under study. Tubach and colleagues determined parameters for improvement in patients with OA (n = 814) as "minimal perceptible improvement," "slight improvement," and "important improvement."[42] Using these categories for the VAS, Bjordal et al determined in their meta-analysis of glucosamine and CS studies that although use of these supplements did show a statistically significant improvement of 4.7 and 3.7 mm on a 20-mm VAS scale, respectively, neither came close to the demarcation of minimal perceptible improvement at 4 weeks (~9 mm).[43]

A potential benefit of CS not addressed in other studies was found following the NIH Glucosamine/Chondroitin Arthritis Intervention (GAIT) Trial.[44,45] Subjects taking 1.2 g/day CS for 6 months had statistically significant reductions in knee joint swelling than those taking placebo. Not all patients with OA have observable swelling, but this study shows that those that do may benefit from taking CS to not only reduce that swelling but also potentially to reduce pain and improve function as well.

Additionally, two recent studies evaluated the effects of combining exercise and these supplements. One hundred and forty-two Japanese women participated in a study that investigated the addition of 1.5 g/day of GH for 18 months to a prescribed home exercise program (HEP) versus HEP alone.[46] Both groups demonstrated significant improvement in WOMAC scores and reductions in VAS pain scores. However, there was no significant difference between the two groups. The authors concluded, on the basis of their results, that if GH were to have an effect on the symptoms of OA, they would not be greater than that of prescribed HEP alone. Similar results were found by Messier et al who administered both 1.5 g/day GH and 1.2 g/day CS for 12 months in addition to exercise to their study subjects.[47] The supplement plus exercise group was not superior to the exercise-alone group in terms of symptoms of OA. However, it is important to note that both studies administered GH, concluded by some meta-analyses to be ineffective at treating symptoms of OA.[36,40] However, no studies in humans have directly compared the effects of GS/GH versus placebo.

Safety. Meta-analyses of studies on glucosamine and CS demonstrate that these supplements are generally safe and that subjects taking them either reported less adverse effects overall than those taking placebo and in a few studies, fewer than those taking nonsteroidal anti-inflammatory drugs (NSAIDs).[36] There were no reports of serious adverse effects in the study populations, who were monitored up to 3 years following the study.[36] The most common complaints of these subjects were related to gastrointestinal (GI) dysfunction (e.g., diarrhea, constipation, nausea, abdominal pain) and joint pain.[36]

Potentially serious adverse effects may occur in patients who are allergic to shellfish, as GS is primarily derived from crustacean shells and CS from bovine and shark cartilage. Indeed, many manufacturers have started including a warning about this on the labels of their products. However, 15 subjects with known shrimp allergies demonstrated no allergic reactions following a single 1.5-g dose of GS, nor did 6 subjects who were given through a prick an extract made from 0.5 g of GS.[48,49] These authors argue that shellfish antigens arise from the meat of the shellfish and not the shells and therefore allergic reactions should not occur when taking glucosamine or CS. Despite this, there is a single case report of an immediate hypersensitive reaction in an individual with no known allergies;[50] and another report that was about the use of a GS/CS combination that exacerbated asthma symptoms in asthmatics.[50,51]

Because CS can be derived from bovine trachea, concerns have also been raised regarding contamination of products by the organism that causes bovine spongiform encephalopathy (BSE, or "mad cow disease"). No reports of any contamination of CS have ever been documented, and one study found no detectable BSE prions in the trachea (which could be used to manufacture CS) of BSE-infected cattle.[52]

Glucosamine can mimic glucose in the metabolic pathway thought to regulate cellular utilization of glucose, leading to the question whether glucosamine would negatively affect insulin mechanisms. While initial animal studies demonstrated conflicting results, several studies in healthy humans and in those with diabetes mellitus have demonstrated no alterations in hemoglobin A_{1c} levels, total glucose uptake, insulin sensitivity, and glycemic control parameters.[53-57] Therefore, glucosamine does not appear to adversely affect the function of glucose or insulin in humans.

Numerous cases report altered coagulation when GS, CS, or the combination is used in patients concomitantly taking warfarin, some requiring hospitalization for bleeding events.[58-61] Therefore, patients on warfarin would be wise to avoid taking GS and/or CS or at least have their international normalized ratio (INR) more closely monitored.

Conclusions. Glucosamine and CS supplements are big business; people all over the United States are spending hundreds of dollars a year in the hope that they will find relief from the painful effects of OA. In fact, placebo effects in the studies reviewed above are typically very high. At best, glucosamine (1.5 g/day) and CS (1.2 g/day) have a modest effect on pain and function. At worst, glucosamine and CS have no effect beyond placebo effect on the symptoms of OA. Deciding whether the magnitude of the placebo effect or something slightly higher is significant enough to justify the cost of supplementation and potential adverse effects is ultimately left to the patient. When held to the bar of meaningful clinical improvement, glucosamine and CS fall short, at least after supplementation of 4 weeks. Admittedly, studies of longer supplementation may come closer to this goal. There is certainly an argument to be made that the safety profiles of glucosamine and CS are better than those of other treatments for OA such as corticosteroids or NSAIDs. However, the purpose of taking these supplements is not their relative safety but their efficacy. The largest, best controlled trials of these supplements show modest, if any, benefits in patients with OA.

The therapist treating patients taking glucosamine and/or CS should be aware of the potential adverse events that can occur. Because of the potential interaction between warfarin and glucosamine and/or CS, the therapist should be more vigilant in monitoring for signs and symptoms of abnormal bleeding, and take care while providing vigorous manual therapies to patients taking these supplements who also have coagulation disorders. Additionally, patients should be monitored for any allergic reaction (skin or respiratory symptoms), and those with asthma should be more carefully monitored, especially when exercising.

S-Adenosylmethionine (SAM-e)

Background. SAM-e, an endogenous sulfur containing compound produced in the liver, has varied physiologic functions, including stimulation of chondrocytes and proteoglycans.[62] Reports of SAM-e's anti-inflammatory and analgesic effects exist, but the exact mechanisms that underlie these effects are unclear.[63]

Efficacy. The Agency for Healthcare Research and Quality (AHRQ) conducted a meta-analysis of SAM-e studies and reported a small but significant effectiveness (effect size = 0.2) over placebo in reducing pain in patients with OA.[64] The primary reason for this positive outcome was a single well-controlled RCT in 1994, which demonstrated a significant improvement in pain after 2 weeks with combined intravenous (for 5 days) and oral dosing (200 mg 3× day, for 18 days) of SAM-e, compared with placebo.[65] Additionally, significant improvement occurred only in those patients with a milder form of OA (Kellegran & Lawrence grade 2).[66]

In the same meta-analysis, there was no significant difference between SAM-e and NSAIDs in the relief of pain. This would indicate that SAM-e is at least as effective as NSAIDs.[64] However, most of the studies contributing to this effect were 20 or more years old and involved small sample sizes (n = 20–45), had short study durations (4 weeks), and did not include a placebo arm.[67-69] More recently, Najm and colleagues completed a double-blind crossover study of 56 patients with OA of the knee.[70] Patients were randomized to receive 1.2 g (600 mg 2× day) of SAM-e or 200 mg (100 mg 2× day) of celecoxib for 8 weeks. Following a 1-week washout period, subjects received the alternate treatment. Celecoxib showed significantly higher reductions in pain in the first 4 weeks over placebo and SAM-e. However, after 4 weeks, subjects taking SAM-e demonstrated significantly better pain relief than those who took placebo and equal pain relief when compared with those taking celecoxib. Clinically, it is important to note that pain was rated on a 1–100 VAS and both treatment groups experienced only about 20% reduction in total pain "today."

Safety. Pooled data from trials comparing SAM-e and NSAIDs showed that subjects were approximately 58% less likely to experience an adverse event when taking SAM-e.[71] In two studies comparing SAM-e with placebo, the experience of adverse events was not statistically different. Because SAM-e is so pervasive in the body, its effects (endogenously or exogenously) are not confined to the musculoskeletal system. SAM-e can affect neurotransmitters, particularly amines such as serotonin, norepinephrine, and dopamine.[72] Because of this, potential neurologic adverse effects could include anxiety, mania, irritability, and, more seriously, interactions with drugs such as antidepressants or drugs for schizophrenia or Parkinson's disease. When combined with drugs that increase serotonin, SAM-e has the potential to cause life-threatening serotonin syndrome. Alteration of neurotransmitters affecting mood could provide a rationale for the analgesia experienced by patients with OA independent of the drug's effects on the musculoskeletal system.[71] However, in their study of 81 patients with OA, Najm et al found no change in scores on the geriatric depression scale or SF-36.[70]

Conclusions. There is evidence from a limited number of older, mostly small studies that SAM-e can reduce the pain of OA, perhaps equal to some NSAIDs. Better quality, larger studies of patients are needed to confirm these effects. Additionally, there are several drawbacks to SAM-e's widespread use. The first is cost, which averages over $100 a month, similar to the cost of NSAIDs, although, admittedly, patients on SAM-e are likely to experience fewer adverse effects than those on NSAIDs. Secondly, SAM-e is inherently an unstable compound. Najm et al reported a 51% loss of potency in SAM-e after about 3 months.[70] Consumers who would like to try SAM-e should take care to buy it from a reputable company and check independent tests of quality (e.g., Consumerlab.com). The Natural Medicines Comprehensive Database suggests the use of butane-disulfonate salt formations of SAM-e because they are more stable.[73]

In the studies reviewed, SAM-e users did not experience any more adverse events than those taking placebo. However, there are potential adverse events that need to be kept in mind by the physical therapist. Primarily, the physical therapist should monitor for any change in neurologic status, including mood changes, sleep disturbances, and serotonin syndrome. Warning signs of serotonin syndrome include, but are not limited to, tachycardia, an irregular heart rhythm, increased blood pressure, increased reflexes, and nausea and vomiting.

Capsaicin

Background. Various topical treatments are currently marketed to consumers for their analgesic properties, including ointments and creams that contain capsaicin. Capsaicin is a component of the fruit of the *Solanaceae* plant family, commonly known as chili *(capsicum)* peppers. Capsaicin can bind to sensory neurons, whether gustatory neurons in the tongue, as in the hot feeling you get when you eat a pepper, or somatosensory neurons in the skin. In the skin, capsaicin interacts specifically with the transient receptor potential vanilloid 1 (TRPV1) present on nociceptors (pain sensing neurons).[74] Activation of C-fibers and the release of substance P is thought to create the prickling and/or burning sensation that occurs shortly after application of capsaicin.[75] Thus, initially, capsaicin actually causes pain. However, after repeated application of capsaicin, neurons become desensitized and ultimately, nerve fibers degenerate creating hypalgesia.[76] Once capsaicin use is discontinued, nerve fibers begin to regenerate over a 6-week period.[76] Capsaicin and its short term ability to desensitize and degenerate some nociceptors may therefore be helpful to patients with OA, rheumatoid arthritis (RA), complex regional pain syndromes, and neuropathy.

Efficacy. A recent systematic review evaluated RCTs of capsaicin to treat patients with chronic pain of musculoskeletal and/or neuropathic origins.[77] The authors defined responders as individuals with a 50% reduction in pain. Capsaicin was significantly better than placebo at reducing subjects' musculoskeletal and neuropathic pain. After 4 weeks (n = 313), 57% of subjects treated with capsaicin (0.075%) versus 42% of those treated with placebo were considered responders. This increased to 60% versus 42% after 8 weeks of treatment (n = 656). For every 6 patients treated with capsaicin for neuropathic pain, 1 individual experienced a 50% (or more) reduction in pain (NNT: 4 weeks = 6.4; 8 weeks = 5.7). Among those with musculoskeletal pain, 38% of subjects treated with capsaicin (0.025%) versus 25% of those treated with placebo were responders. For every 8 patients treated with capsaicin for musculoskeletal pain, 1 individual experienced a 50% (or more) reduction in pain (NNT: 4 weeks = 8.1).

Two case studies on the use of capsaicin in *complex regional pain syndrome* (the older term is *reflex sympathetic dystrophy [RSD]*) demonstrated elimination of symptoms with the use of capsaicin (0.075%) four times per day for 3 to 6 weeks.[78,79]

While pooled results of studies on the use of capsaicin versus placebo are significant, the magnitude of the effect is not. This is surprising given the action of capsaicin in vitro; however, high-dose capsaicin patches or injection protocols are currently being considered.[80] One pilot study using such a protocol demonstrated that capsaicin (5%–10%) injections significantly reduced pain for 1 to 18 weeks in most patients (9 out of 10) with intractable pain.[81] High-dose capsaicin patches were more effective than placebo in reducing the pain of subjects with human immunodeficiency virus (HIV) infection–associated neuropathy, and those with postherpetic neuralgia.[82,83] However, the magnitude of the results was similar to those studies using topical preparations and not greater, as one might expect.

Safety. Because of its stimulation of sensory neurons, capsaicin causes initial discomfort ranging from itching to prickling to burning on contact. In all the studies reviewed, subjects taking capsaicin were far more likely than those taking placebo to experience adverse events and to withdraw from the study.[77] In fact, a systematic review by Mason et al determined that the NNH was only 2.5, that is, of every 2 to 3 patients treated with capsaicin, 1 experienced an adverse event.[77] Capsaicin is also a tussive agent, and thus a common adverse effect can be coughing, especially in those using 0.075% capsaicin.[77]

Conclusions. A criticism of topical treatments, including capsaicin, is that the act of rubbing, which activates mechanoreceptors, is the reason these treatments work, irrespective of the active ingredient. However, Mason and colleagues disputed this claim as placebo agents were also rubbed into the skin and the data still suggested the superiority of capsaicin over placebo.[77]

Capsaicin is significantly better than placebo at reducing the pain from both musculoskeletal and neurologic causes, but because of the unimpressive relative magnitude of its effect, combined with its potential to cause discomfort, it is typically not recommended as a first-line treatment and may be better utilized as an adjuvant treatment or when other treatments have proved unsuccessful.[77]

Salicylates

Background. Like capsaicin, topical salicylates, such as Aspercreme®, and Myoflex®, are also used for the relief of pain. The mechanism of the analgesic action of these products is not fully understood. Possible explanations may include their action as a counter-irritant or as a rubefacient (increasing local blood flow) or their action on prostaglandin synthesis (much like aspirin and NSAIDs).[84] Unfortunately, there is conflicting evidence that these substances are fully absorbed and active in human skin.[85,86] Although it is not known that systemic presence of salicylate is needed for therapeutic benefit, one study found no significant increase in plasma salicylate levels after phonophoretic application of trolamine salicylate.[87] So while topical salicylates have the potential to reduce pain, it is not known whether the topical forms of these substances can also exert this effect.

Efficacy. There are a limited number of clinical trials evaluating the efficacy of topical salicylates. However, a recent systematic review did combine the results of seven studies on their effectiveness in acute and chronic pain in patients with varying diagnoses (e.g., traumatic muscle pain, OA, rheumatic conditions).[84] The authors defined responders as individuals with a 50% reduction in pain. Acute pain response rate (n = 182) in those using topical salicylates was 67%, which was significantly better than the 18% of the placebo group. About 2 subjects needed to be treated with topical salicylates for 1 of them to have a 50% reduction in pain at 7 days (NNT = 2.1). The response rates in individuals with chronic pain (n = 429), although significant, were less dramatic (54% for topical salicylates versus 36% for placebo). About 5 subjects needed to be treated with topical salicylates for 1 of them to have a 50% reduction in pain at 14 days (NNT = 5.3). The authors noted that several studies included in the analysis had low validity (quality) scores and that the lower the score, the less was the analgesic effect. As discussed previously in this chapter, the studies combined in Mason et al were varied with regard to topical salicylates used and study populations. Therefore, these pooled data should be interpreted cautiously.

Two small studies (combined n = 74) on topical salicylates that were not included in the Mason et al systematic review are worth mentioning. Hill and Richardson and Ciccone investigated the effects of 10% trolamine salicylate (Aspercreme) on delayed-onset muscle soreness (DOMS).[88,89] Hill and Richardson reported significant analgesic effects (≥3 on VAS) among college students after using trolamine salicylate (4 times per day for 5 days) versus placebo. In contrast, Ciccone et al did not find any effect of topical trolamine salicylate (once per day for 3 days) on DOMS.[89] However, there was a significant difference in DOMS when ultrasound (US) was applied but not when US was combined with 10% trolamine salicylate.[89] Thus, trolamine salicylate may have ameliorated the soreness caused by the US. However, each treatment group was small, consisting of only 10 individuals.

Safety. According to Mason et al, local adverse events from the use of topical salicylates were rare (4 out of 208, i.e., 2%) and not significantly different from those of placebo (4 out of 210, i.e., 2%).[84] In one study of subjects using copper salicylate, significantly more subjects reported a skin rash and withdrew from the study because of it than those in the placebo group (17% and 1.7%, respectively).[90]

Several cases of topical salicylates potentiating the anticoagulant effects of warfarin have been reported.[91-93] Additionally, all salicylates have the potential to create salicylate poisoning, especially in those using methyl salicylate and in children.[94-96] Finally, one study found that methyl salicylate applied on pregnant hamsters caused failure of the cephalic neural tube to close, resulting in anencephaly in the newborn.[97]

Conclusions. It is yet unknown how topical salicylates may affect the pain induced by exercise, trauma, OA, or rheumatic conditions. This is likely one of the reasons why there is so much variation in the clinical literature. There is some limited evidence that these products may be beneficial in reducing pain, especially acutely.[84] The study by Hill and Richardson would suggest that the use of the salicylate would need to be frequent (four times per day). However, the current evidence is based on a small number of subjects and is quite heterogeneous with respect to the reason for pain and the type of topical salicylate used.

If topical salicylates create analgesia by acting as rubefacients, then their absorption and efficacy are dependent on the local blood flow, itself influenced by heat and activity. Thus, the more active patients are, the more the salicylate is washed out of the local tissue. Activity is imperative in patients with chronic OA and rheumatoid conditions to maintain joint health and ROM, and thus restriction of activity could be counterproductive.

The therapist should be aware of the potential for salicylate poisoning due to high doses, high frequency of use, or long duration of use. Patients with *salicylism* can present with nausea, vomiting, tinnitus, headache, seizure, hyperpnea, and hyperthermia. Additionally, because poisoning can occur more rapidly in the young, care should be taken to keep topical salicylates away from children. Finally, patients who are taking warfarin or are pregnant should only use topical salicylates with the approval of their physician, although this warning is based only on case reports.

Menthol

Background. Menthol is from the *Mentha* family of botanicals and is present in peppermint, citronella, and eucalyptus oils.[98] Menthol-containing products are used as flavoring, digestive, antiseptic, and, most importantly here, analgesic agents. Menthol is an agonist to sensory neurons that are sensitive to temperature, and when applied, it creates a sensation of coolness.[99] This is similar in form but opposite in spectrum to capsaicin, which creates a sensation of heat. Specifically, menthol activates peripheral vasoactive C-fibers.[100] Like capsaicin, menthol initially sensitizes nociceptors, but with continued use, can actually desensitize them, thus acting as a counterirritant.[101] However, it has been suggested that menthol has a shorter-term effect than capsaicin.[102] Menthol has also been shown to have rubefacient activity at concentrations of 5% and above and to activate kappa κ-opioid receptors (oral menthol).[103,104]

Efficacy. Very few studies have investigated the effects of menthol alone on pain. A case report indicated that a 76-year-old woman with postherpetic neuralgia experienced pain relief for 4 to 6 hours after application of 10% menthol.[105] Small clinical trials ($n = <40$) on creams including both menthol and methyl salicylate (Bengay®) have demonstrated decreases in DOMS after 15 minutes.[106,107] However, the benefit in the small number of study subjects cannot be clearly ascribed to menthol, methyl salicylate, or their combination.

Safety. The use of high concentrations of menthol (40% but not 30%) can result in significant skin erythema, burning, and allergic reactions.[98] The combination product containing menthol and methyl salicylate applied to the back and covered with a heating pad created full thickness tissue necrosis and local kidney damage in one patient.[108] Menthol can cause serious toxicity in children, even in small doses.[95]

Conclusions. Although physiologic evidence supports the rubefacient–counterirritant action of menthol, there is little clinical evidence to support the use of menthol-only products in patients. Combinations of menthol and methyl salicylate may attenuate DOMS immediately after application, but the duration of such pain relief is unknown. Menthol used in concentrations of >5% and <40% appear to be well tolerated, but care should be taken to keep these items away from children. The therapist should monitor patients using menthol for signs of toxicity, including, but not limited to, shortness of breath, abdominal pain, nausea and vomiting, tachycardia, and convulsions. Additionally, patients using counterirritant creams containing menthol and methyl salicylate should be advised not to simultaneously use a heating pad over the area.

SUPPLEMENTS FOR CARDIOVASCULAR DISEASE

Many patients receiving rehabilitative services have a medical history that includes one or more cardiovascular pathologies. The inpatient therapist or the home health therapist may be treating a patient following angioplasty or coronary artery bypass surgery. The outpatient therapist often treats common musculoskeletal disorders, for example, bursitis or tendinitis, in patients with cardiovascular comorbidities such as hypertension or atrial fibrillation. In addition to the multitude of drug classes reviewed elsewhere in this text, such patients may also be consuming supplements in the hope of improving their health. Several supplements have been identified for their potential to improve cardiovascular function, including, but not limited to, those selected for this chapter: garlic, coenzyme Q10, and soy products.

Measuring cardiovascular outcomes in research studies is not dissimilar to measuring them in the clinic. Articles in this section will define success as lowered blood pressure or altered serum lipid levels (reduced total cholesterol, low density lipoproteins [LDL], triglycerides [TG], and increased high density lipoproteins [HDL]). Additionally, to address the effect of supplements on the potential for atherosclerosis, many authors evaluate subjects' vascular function by measuring flow-mediated dilatation (FMD). FMD is a measure of the response of a vessel's endothelium to the flow of blood and essentially its ability to alter vasomotor tone.[109] Therefore, altered FMD is reflective of endothelial dysfunction, which itself contributes to the development of arteriosclerosis.[109]

Beyond these measures, it is important to also investigate a drug's or supplement's ability to affect global cardiac outcomes, that is, its ability to prevent major cardiac events. Just as an improvement in balance does not always prevent falls, a reduction of serum lipid levels in someone with hyperlipidemia does not necessarily mean that the person will avoid a future cardiac event. Unfortunately, as is common in the literature on supplements, the reader will see that few articles actually address this important clinical issue.

Garlic

Background. Garlic (*Allium sativum, Allium ursinum*), now most commonly added to enhance the flavor of a dish, has also been used since the time of the ancient Egyptians to improve cardiovascular health. Allicin, the component that gives garlic its odor, has been shown to exert an effect on blood pressure[110] and the production of cholesterol[111] in animal and in vitro studies. High blood pressure and high serum cholesterol levels are themselves risk factors for the development of serious cardiac pathology, including ischemic heart disease, peripheral vascular disease, and cerebrovascular accidents. Because garlic is a frequently used ingredient in the food of many cultures, there is an implied safety in the consumption of garlic; therefore, if it really does have cardioprotective properties, it could be an effective alternative to more traditional pharmaceuticals.

Efficacy. Several meta-analyses have investigated the various cardiovascular effects of garlic. Jepson et al published a Cochrane review of the effectiveness of garlic in patients with peripheral vascular disease.[112] Unfortunately, the authors found only one randomized, placebo-controlled study of 78 patients with peripheral arterial occlusive disease.[113] After 3 months of taking 800 mg garlic powder, the subjects showed no significant difference in their ankle or brachial blood pressures. However, there was a small, but significant, difference in pain-free walking distance in the group taking garlic (46 m) compared with those taking placebo (30 m) in the last weeks of the trial. Jepson et al concluded that more studies, especially of longer duration, would need to occur before the use of garlic could be recommended to patients with peripheral vascular disease.

Both Ried et al and Reinhardt et al conducted meta-analyses of garlic's effects on blood pressure and reported similar results.[110,114] Garlic did not significantly affect blood pressure in normotensive individuals. However, significant decreases in both systolic and diastolic pressures were seen in individuals with existing high blood pressure (>140/90 mm Hg). Reid et al reported a pooled systolic decrease of 8.4 mm Hg and a pooled diastolic decrease of 7.3 mm Hg. Reinhardt et al described more dramatic decreases in systolic (16.3 mm Hg) and diastolic (9.3 mm Hg) pressures. Supplementation of garlic in the analyzed studies, which ran for 3 to 6 months, included garlic powder (600–900 mg), aged garlic extract (2.4 g, 10 mL), and garlic oil (12.3 mg). In the studies with greatest decreases in pressures, the subjects had been administered garlic powder and not aged garlic extract or garlic oil. Both authors reported moderate to low heterogeneity in the studies analyzed but also that very few studies were conducted independent of manufacturer support.

The most recent meta-analysis (n = 13) of garlic's effect on serum cholesterol reported a small, but significant 5.8% decrease in the total cholesterol levels of hyperlipidemic patients.[115] This decrease after supplementation with 600 to 900 mg of garlic powder and 10 mg or 0.25 mg/kg of garlic oil for 2 to 6 months is similar to that achieved from diet alone but much lower than that of HMG (3-hydroxy-3-methyl-glutaryl)-CoA inhibitors (statin) medications.[115] However, as in similar meta-analyses, when the authors pooled data from the highest-quality studies, this small effect was further reduced. None of the studies included in Stevinson's meta-analysis investigated the clinical implications of lowering cholesterol. However, recently, a pilot study of 19 subjects demonstrated that the addition of aged garlic extract to a standard protocol of statins and aspirin in subjects with hyperlipidemia inhibited coronary artery calcification more than the standard protocol alone.[116]

Garlic powder is the most common formulation sold today and the one most studied. However, the amount of allicin differs greatly depending on whether the garlic is eaten raw or taken in powder, oil, or extract forms. As in the meta-analyses by Reid et al and Reinhardt et al, the type of garlic used may influence its effects. Gardner et al attempted to evaluate the effect of formulation on garlic's cholesterol-lowering effects.[111] In a trial of 192 adults with high LDL levels, supplementation of the diet with raw (4 g), powdered (1.4 g) or aged extract (1.8 g) forms of garlic, 6 days per week for 6 months showed no significant reduction in LDL levels or total cholesterol levels compared with placebo. This study highlights the need for future studies for further quantification of the bioavailability of allicin in these various types of supplements. Although this study would suggest that garlic has no effect on those with moderate hyperlipidemia, it does not necessarily rule out the use of garlic in patients at risk for cardiovascular disease.[117,118] To date, no clinical trials have linked the use of garlic and the number of cardiovascular events in the population. However, Hunyh and colleagues have published a Cochrane protocol to investigate the relationship of garlic and morbidity and mortality in hypertensive patients, which may help elucidate the long-term clinical effects of garlic.[119]

Safety. No serious adverse events were reported by any of the above meta-analyses, however, the pooled sample sizes were not large enough to rule out this possibility.[110-112,114,115] Larger studies of longer duration (no study evaluated was longer than 6 months) would further elucidate the long-term effects of garlic supplementation. Most commonly, subjects taking garlic complained of bad breath, body odor, flatulence, and other gastrointestinal distress more than those taking placebo.[110-112,114,115]

Bleeding, a very serious adverse effect, has been reported in patients taking garlic.[113,120-122] In fact, allicin has been shown to inhibit platelet function in vitro.[123,124] However, in a recent study of 18 healthy volunteers, neither a single ingestion of dietary levels of raw garlic nor ingestion over a 1-week period altered platelet function.[125] Also, despite the reported anticoagulant effects of garlic, in two small studies, no alteration was seen in the effects of warfarin when subjects were concomitantly taking aged garlic extract or garlic powder.[126,127]

Conclusions. Garlic supplementation (800 mg for 3 months) may improve pain-free walking in individuals with peripheral vascular disease, but this finding is based on one trial. Garlic in various forms and doses taken for at least 3 months can reduce the blood pressure of hypertensive individuals. However, the long-term cardiovascular outcomes and the adverse effects of garlic have not been evaluated, as they have been for antihypertensive agents. Thus, most authors would not recommend substituting garlic for the more proven methods of blood pressure reduction.[110,114] The evidence for garlic's effects on cholesterol are much more controversial and suggest little to no added benefit to direct reductions in LDLs and total cholesterol levels. Rehabilitative therapists treating patients taking garlic should advise them to speak with their physician about the potential risk of bleeding and/or its interaction with anticoagulant therapies such as aspirin and warfarin.

Coenzyme Q_{10} (CoQ_{10})

Background. CoQ_{10} is an endogenous substance found in all tissues but predominates in the heart, where it plays a key role in mitochondrial energy production and as an antioxidant.[128] Cardiac muscle tissue is replete with mitochondria, producing the necessary levels of energy required for optimal pump performance. The price of such high activity is the creation of destructive reactive oxygen species (ROS) that must be neutralized by antioxidants. In vitro, CoQ_{10} has demonstrated an age-specific cardioprotective effect from ischemic injury.[129] In fact, older individuals and those with cardiovascular disease have lower levels of CoQ_{10}.[128,130] Therefore, in theory, supplementation with CoQ_{10} in older adults or those with cardiovascular disease should help improve cardiovascular function.

Efficacy. Supplementation with CoQ_{10} has been evaluated most commonly in patients with heart failure and hypertension. The most recent meta-analysis in patients with heart failure indicated a significant improvement in resting ejection fraction and stroke volume after taking 60 to 225 mg/day of CoQ_{10} for 1 to 6 months.[131] Patients with less severe heart failure and those not taking angiotensin-converting enzyme (ACE) inhibitors showed the most benefit from supplementation.[131] Administration of CoQ_{10} 2 mg/kg per day reduced the number of hospitalizations in patients with heart failure for 1 year.[132] Berman et al found 60 mg CoQ_{10} for 3 months significantly improved distance in the 6-minute walk test and decreased fatigue levels versus placebo, potentially suggesting its role as a bridge therapy in patients awaiting heart transplantation (n = 27).[133] However, objective clinical measures of heart failure status, such as echocardiography (ECG) and lab values, did not improve significantly.[133] In patients with an ejection fraction of <40% on conventional therapy, the addition of 150 mg CoQ_{10} for 3 months significantly improved performance on the 6-minute walk test and improved the patient's heart failure classification.[134]

CoQ_{10} also appears to reduce systolic and diastolic blood pressures in hypertensive patients. Rosenfeldt and colleagues found a pooled decrease of 16.6 mm Hg systolic and 8.2 mm Hg diastolic in their recent meta-analysis of randomized controlled trials (n = 120).[135] Despite the small number of subjects, the authors concluded that there was enough evidence to recommend the addition of CoQ_{10} to conventional therapy.[135] Hodgson et al reported that CoQ_{10} supplementation (200 mg/day) in individuals with type 2 diabetes mellitus (n = 74) significantly reduced systolic and diastolic blood pressure and glycemic control (HbA_{1C} levels).[136]

The effect of CoQ_{10} on exercise parameters in healthy individuals remains controversial. Although dosage and duration of treatment were similar, 6 out of 11 small trials (n = 18–28) demonstrated positive effects on maximal oxygen consumption and exercise capacity but the remaining 5 trials (n = 10–19) trials showed no significant results.[137] Larger studies of homogeneous healthy subjects are needed to determine the effects of CoQ_{10} on exercise parameters.

Dosage of CoQ_{10} seems an important factor in its efficacy, but to date, dose–response relationships in its use in hypertension and heart failure remain unclear. Because formulation and individual absorption and bioavailability are so varied, Rosenfeldt et al recommended individual monitoring of the patient's therapeutic blood levels (>2.5 mcg/mL) for optimal dosing.[135] Additionally, Langsjoen and Langsjoen reported difficulty in reaching therapeutic plasma CoQ_{10} levels in patients with end-stage congestive heart failure.[138] They switched 7 such patients from supplementation of CoQ_{10} ubiquinone (oxidized form) to ubiquinol (reduced, active form). ECG measurements improved in 4 of 7 patients, and 6 of 7 survived longer than predicted and moved from end-stage classification to a more moderate classification. On the basis of this study and on their experience treating patients with congestive heart failure, the authors recommended the use of the ubiquinol formulation and a plasma level of >3.5 mcg/mL for patients with heart failure.[138]

CoQ_{10} may also be taken by patients on statin medications. Statins such as atorvastatin, pravastatin, rosuvastatin, and lovastatin are prescribed to individuals with hyperlipidemia as they inhibit the HMG-CoA enzyme involved in the synthesis of cholesterol. However, HMG Co-A is also involved in the pathway for the synthesis of CoQ_{10}; this has led to concerns that statin drugs, while significantly lowering cholesterol, may also diminish cardiovascular function, which questions their long-term usefulness.[139,140] Studies in hypercholesterolemic patients taking statins demonstrate a significant decrease in plasma concentrations of CoQ_{10} upon initiation of statin therapy.[141-146] On the one hand, the long-term cardiovascular effects, if any, of this reduction in CoQ_{10} levels by statins is not clear. On the other hand, statin drugs have been shown to significantly reduce cardiovascular events in patients with coronary artery disease and thus are an important part of the treatment regime for these patients. Therefore, CoQ_{10} supplementation may be prescribed in addition to the statin drug.[147]

The therapist should be aware that statin drugs sometimes cause myalgia and, more rarely, rhabdomyolysis (see Chapter 7). Some authors have suggested that these symptoms may be related to the loss of CoQ_{10} that occurs with statin therapy. While the use of various statin drugs clearly demonstrates a reduction in serum CoQ_{10} in humans, the evidence for a drop in intramuscular CoQ_{10} is more controversial. Two recent systematic reviews indicate that there is, at present, insufficient evidence to support a direct link between the loss of CoQ_{10} and the myalgia associated with statin therapy.[146,148] Young et al gave 200 mg/day of CoQ_{10} plus simvastatin or simvastatin alone for 3 months to 44 patients who had been unable to tolerate statin therapy because of myalgia. No significant difference in the incidence of patient-reported myalgia was found between the groups, leading the authors to conclude that there was no influence of CoQ_{10} supplementation on statin-induced myalgia.[149] In contrast, Caso and colleagues supplemented 32 patients with existing statin regimes and myopathic complaints with 100 mg CoQ_{10} per day or 400 international units (IU) per day of vitamin E (control) for 4 weeks.[150] Patients in the CoQ_{10} group reported significantly less pain and less pain interference with daily activities than those in the vitamin E group. Therefore, whether or not CoQ_{10} supplementation can alleviate statin-induced myalgia is still unclear.

Safety. None of the studies reviewed reported serious adverse events nor any difference in overall toxicity between CoQ_{10} and placebo.[128,133-138] In about 2500 patients with heart failure, supplementation with 50 to 150 mg/day of CoQ_{10} for up to 7 years showed no significant increase in adverse effects compared with placebo.[151] Williams et al demonstrated the safety of CoQ_{10} up to 1200 mg/kg/day in rats and developed an acceptable daily intake of 600 mg for individuals weighing 110 lb (50 kg), and Ikematsu et al demonstrated safety in healthy volunteers of up to 900 mg.[152,153]

Despite this evidence, there is still a question as to whether or not supplementation with CoQ_{10} can increase bleeding episodes and/or interact with warfarin. While Shalansky et al noted an increased risk of self-reported bleeding in individuals concurrently taking CoQ_{10} and warfarin, a randomized placebo-controlled crossover study by Engelsen et al demonstrated no interaction between CoQ_{10} and warfarin.[154,155] Nor did Langsjoen and Langsjoen find any adverse event in 4 of the 7 patients in their study who were simultaneously taking warfarin and CoQ_{10}.[138]

Conclusions. In patients with mild heart failure, CoQ_{10} supplementation can improve exercise tolerance and stroke volume and reduce hospitalizations over 1 year. CoQ_{10} can also lower blood pressure in individuals with hypertension and in those with type 2 diabetes mellitus. However, CoQ_{10}'s effect on healthy individuals with regard to cardioprotection or improvement in aerobic exercise capacity is unclear. Although generally considered a safe supplement, patients with a cardiovascular medical history, especially those taking statin drugs, should consult their physicians before beginning a CoQ_{10} regimen in order to develop an optimal dose and to monitor for adverse effects. The therapist working with patients taking CoQ_{10}, whether they have current cardiovascular dysfunction or not, should monitor the vital signs and observe for signs and symptoms of myopathy and hemorrhage.

Soy Products

Background. Soybeans are legumes native to Eastern Asia and are processed to make various foods and supplements. Soy can be consumed as soybeans, soy milk, and soy nuts; as an isolated protein; or in a multitude of other forms. Soybeans contain isoflavones, a subfamily of a larger group of substances called *flavonoids*, which are also found in red wine, chocolate, and green tea.[156] Soy products are purported to affect the cardiovascular system by reducing serum lipids and blood pressure, thereby helping to prevent cardiac pathologies and major cardiac events. This theory grew from data that showed people of Asian origin having a lower incidence of heart disease than those in the Western world.[157] One reason for this difference could be that a typical Asian diet contains a much higher volume of soy protein than does a typical Western diet.[158,159]

Efficacy. The most recent meta-analyses have shown that supplementation of the diet with soy protein (~50 g with isoflavone) consistently but modestly lowers serum LDL levels (about 3%–5%).[160-164] However, authors differ about whether or not soy protein has significant effects on total cholesterol, HDL, and triglyceride levels.[160-164]

Though the beneficial effect of soy protein on LDL levels seems consistent, there is still debate as to whether or not the effect is due to the soy protein, the isoflavone, or both. Some studies of soy protein without isoflavone show similar reductions in LDL levels and others do not.[165] Studies of isolated isoflavone extracts are similarly controversial. Some evidence suggests that isoflavone supplementation of 80 to 100 mg significantly lowers total cholesterol and LDL levels.[161-163] However, other authors contend that the relative isoflavone content does not affect the overall improvement in lipid profiles.[160,164,165]

To put the values of soy protein and isoflavone in perspective, supplementation of 50 g of soy protein makes up about half the daily intake of protein in the United States.[165] Furthermore, daily intake of 100 mg of isoflavone is approximately twice the normal amount consumed by the Japanese population.[161] Alteration of the diet in this way would be a significant change to most individuals in the United States who eat a typical Western diet. The duration of supplementation of soy protein with isoflavone (1–4 months) also affected the overall results, favoring longer supplementation.[163] Certainly, one could argue that these types of dietary changes (increasing soy protein and decreasing animal protein-saturated fat) would be most effective when life long.

Despite evidence that soy can affect lipid profiles, a prospective study of over 30,000 postmenopausal women demonstrated that soy and isoflavone consumption did not significantly reduce cardiovascular morbidity and mortality.[158] Additionally, soy products with or without isoflavones added to the diet do not significantly decrease blood pressure or improve endothelial function.[160,165] However, despite these findings, the American Heart Association (AHA) does suggest that the replacement of animal and dairy products (i.e., saturated fats and cholesterol) in the diet with soy protein–rich foods may indirectly reduce the risk of cardiovascular disease.[166]

Safety. Soybeans are a food staple in many cultures and, as such, pose no serious health risks. However, patients may have unknown allergies to soy or soy products or experience GI symptoms following a change in diet. The isoflavones in soy products have been shown to have an effect on animals and infants with thyroid disorders and may alter the absorption of synthetic thyroid hormone.[167] However, in a recent study of 35 healthy young men, supplementation of soy protein with high (~60 mg) or low isoflavone (~2 mg) levels for 57 days did not significantly alter endogenous thyroid hormone levels.[168]

Isoflavones are considered to be phytoestrogens—plant-derived substances that exert a weak, estrogen-like effect on the body. The benefits and risks of this aspect of soy products will be discussed later in the section on supplements for menopausal symptoms.

Conclusions. Soy protein with isoflavone improves LDL profiles and may affect total cholesterol levels in patients, especially when it replaces animal protein. However, the amount and duration of supplementation is significant and would require a drastic change from a typical Western diet. Despite this promising effect, longitudinal evidence shows soy/isoflavone consumption in women did not affect the incidence of major cardiac events. There is also no current evidence to support soy supplementation to reduce blood pressure.

Although supplementation with soy is generally safe, patients with thyroid dysfunction or those on synthetic thyroid hormone should not drastically increase their soy intake without medical supervision.

Supplements to Improve Cognitive and Affective Function

Many therapists routinely treat patients with cognitive impairments ranging from mild confusion to a loss of orientation to person, place, and time. Patients with dementia, including that of Alzheimer's disease, can be difficult to rehabilitate because of this altered mental status. Supplements that could enhance a patient's daily cognitive function could result in increased independence and quality of life. Similarly, rehabilitation efforts can be derailed in patients with concomitant affective (mood) disorders such as anxiety and depression. Both these diagnoses can affect motivation and willingness to change and may include somatic symptoms such as asthenia and fatigue.

Conventional drugs for cognitive and affective disorders often have several adverse effects, so patients seek other alternatives. In fact, CAM use is higher in patients with psychiatric disorders, especially depression.[169,170] Several supplements have been identified for their potential to improve cognitive and affective disorders, including, but not limited to, those selected for this chapter: valerian and kava for the treatment of anxiety, St. John's wort and SAM-e for the treatment of depression, and ginkgo biloba and dehydroepiandrosterone (DHEA) for the treatment of cognitive impairment.

A variety of tests and tools are employed by researchers to measure the success of pharmacolgic interventions in patients with cognitive and affective disorders. The State-Trait Anxiety Inventory (STAI) and the Hamilton Anxiety Scale (HAM-A) are valid and reliable measures commonly used to assess a patient's level of anxiety. STAI is a subjective report completed by the patient and is designed to take into account temporary "state" anxiety and more chronic "trait" anxieties.[171] The HAM-A is a physician-rated assessment of the patient's anxiety, including the aspects of anxious mood, tension, fears, insomnia, and somatic complaints.[172] HAM-A is typically used as an outcome measure for the success or failure of psychotherapy and pharmacotherapy, which makes it a good choice in experiments evaluating the effectiveness of supplements. Hamilton also developed another physician-rated tool to measure depression (HAM-D); it evaluates a patient's depressed mood, guilty feelings, suicide, sleep disturbances, anxiety levels, and weight loss.[173] The measurement of cognitive status is much more varied in the literature. There are several standardized measures that are utilized, including the Folstein Mini Mental Status Exam (MMSE), the Alzheimer's Disease Assessment Scale-Cognitive (ADAS-cog), and the Syndrome Kurz Test (SKT).[174-176] In general, these are batteries assessing a patient's memory, attention, language, and orientation. The Clinical Global Impression of Change (CGIC) is a physician's impression of the patient's overall improvement, with lower scores indicating more improvement.[177]

Valerian (*Valeriana officinalis, V. edulis, V. wallichii*)

Background. Valerian is a perennial plant native to Europe and Asia and is a top-selling supplement for treating anxiety and anxiety-related insomnia.[178,179] Extracts of valerian root, which contain varying levels of valerenic acids and valepotriates, may have affinity for gamma-aminobutyric acid (GABA) and serotonin receptors depending on the species and extraction methods.[180,181] As in the case of many natural products, the relative concentration of active ingredients and the species of the valerian can differ drastically.

Efficacy. A recent Cochrane Database meta-analysis found only a single double-blind, randomized pilot study (n = 36) testing the effects of valerian (50 mg valepotriate extraction) versus diazepam versus placebo on patients with anxiety disorders.[181,182] This study found no effect of valerian on HAM-A or STAI scores after treatment.

A recent systematic review of the literature on valerian, as treatment for insomnia, attempted to draw conclusions on its efficacy, taking into consideration the species and type of preparation.[179] Ethanolic extracts (300–600 mg for 1–42 nights) of valerian did not significantly improve subjective (e.g., ratings of sleep or reports of improvement) or objective (e.g., onset of sleep [latency], sleep duration, polysomnography) factors. Aqueous extracts (180–900 mg for 1–14 nights) of valerian may significantly improve subjective sleep outcomes but not objective measures of sleep. Valepotriate preparations (60–450 mg for 1–30 nights)—in the manufacture of which high concentrations of ethanol are used to extract the constituent—may reduce sleep disturbances (e.g., waking, restless sleep). Taibi et al do not recommend the global use of valerian in patients with or without diagnosed insomnia but concede that up to now, no rigorously controlled studies with a large number of subjects has been conducted in patients with insomnia.

Safety. No serious adverse effects were reported in a systematic review of 37 studies of valerian.[179] Commonly reported adverse effects were gastrointestinal or neurologic in nature (e.g., headache, irritability) and were not greater in incidence than placebo.[179] However, temporary alteration in liver function was reported in two individuals in 1989.[183] Additionally, high doses of valepotriate caused cell death and DNA damage in vitro.[184]

Conclusions. Though a popular supplement in the United States, valerian has not demonstrated consistent efficacy in improving sleep or anxiety. Some isolated, small studies have shown improvement in subjective and objective measures of sleep after treatment with valerian but differ greatly with respect to the preparation used. Further study into the physiologic effects of valerenic acid and valepotriate, the optimal dose and preparation of valerian root, and the duration of treatment could shed light on the conflicting results of current clinical studies. While generally safe, valerian could be damaging to the liver and should be used only with medical supervision in any patient with liver pathology. Although no serious adverse effects were reported in subjects of studies on valepotriates, in vitro evidence calls into question the safety of this form of valerian.

Kava (*Piper methylsicum*)

Background. Indigenous South Pacific populations have long used the Kava shrub to brew a beverage for relaxation. The active ingredient of this plant is kavalactone extracted from its foliage. Commercially, kava is prepared in pill form by extracting the kavalactones with ethanol (whereas the native beverage is made with water).

Efficacy. Data from two recent meta-analyses indicate that kava supplementation is superior to placebo in patients with nonpsychotic anxiety disorders.[185,186] Pittler and Ernst included 12 studies in their meta-analysis; data from 7 ($n = 305$) were pooled, and the authors reported a modest improvement with kava supplementation (150–450 mg in two doses for 6 months) when compared with placebo (WMD = 3.4) as rated by the HAM-A.[185] Witte et al focused their meta-analysis on a specific extract of kava by a single manufacturer (WS®1490, 150–300 mg for 1–6 months) and reported a pooled improvement ($n = 354$) of 5.94 (0.86–12.8) points on the HAM-A, but it only approached significance ($p = 0.07$).[186] However, when data were pooled on the basis of responders, defined as an increase in HAM-A score by 50% or more, the weighted OR was determined to be 3.3 (2.09–5.22), which indicates that treatment with kava improves the chances of a successful outcome threefold. Witte also analyzed the effect of kava in subpopulations of subjects and found that those taking 300 mg (and not 150 or 200 mg) per day, who were women, and were younger than 53 years demonstrated more dramatic effects when compared with those taking placebo. Additionally, while some trials of shorter duration showed no effect, trials 8 weeks and longer have shown better results.[185,186,187] With evidence that kava has some positive effect on those with anxiety disorders, it could be considered an alternative to conventional treatment with benzodiazepines and other anxiolytic medications. One small study in healthy volunteers showed that, unlike benzodiazepines, a single dose of kava improved performance on several cognitive parameters.[188]

Safety. Adverse effects of kava in clinical trials include GI complaints, restlessness, drowsiness, fatigue, and headache, and skin rash.[185,189] The primary concern with the use of kava is its ability to inhibit cytochrome P450, a liver enzyme that functions to metabolize many conventional drugs.[187,190] Case reports of severe hepatotoxicity were reported; in response, the European Union banned the import of kava in 2002 and the FDA issued an advisory against it.[191] However, subsequent analysis revealed only a single case where a direct relationship between kava and liver damage likely existed, and additional predisposing factors might also have played a role in this case.[192] The European ban on the import of kava was lifted at the end of 2008.[193,194] No liver dysfunction or hepatotoxicity was reported in the clinical trials ($n = 300\text{-}400$) reviewed for meta-analyses, and several studies had, in fact, included monitoring of liver function.[185,186] However, the duration and follow-up of these studies are admittedly short (≤6 months). Even in light of the multitude of case reports, kava's adverse effect profile is still better than that of benzodiazepines.[189]

Conclusions. Current evidence suggests that individuals with nonpsychotic anxiety disorders may benefit from supplementation of kava. Although no serious adverse events were reported in clinical trials, kava physiologically affects the liver and therefore its use should be medically monitored in any individual taking prescription drugs or who has existing liver disease or risk factors for it. The physical therapist treating patients taking kava should be observant for the presence of kava dermopathy (skin rash) and signs and symptoms of liver dysfunction (e.g., jaundice, right upper quarter pain, dark urine, CNS changes).

S-Adenosylmethionine (SAM-e)

Background. SAM-e, as discussed previously, is an endogenous compound involved in various metabolic processes. It is an intermediary product of the pathways ultimately responsible for the production of phospholipids and neurotransmitters. In this way, SAM-e supplementation, may help regulate the activity of neurons and neurotransmitters, specifically those implicated in affective disorders such as depression. In fact, SAM-e levels are decreased in depressed patients.[195]

Efficacy. SAM-e's effect on patients with major depressive disorders has been extensively studied. While most studies were uncontrolled and of small sample size, recent reviews of the literature have reported a general improvement in depressive symptoms after SAM-e supplementation (200 mg to 1.6 g for 2–8 weeks) compared with placebo, as measured by the HAM-D (n = 422), and equal to tricyclic antidepressants (n = 1015) and serotonin selective reuptake inhibitors (SSRI) and venlafaxine (n = 30).[64,196-199] Decreases in HAM-D scores average about 6 points, which is a clinically significant change.[64] Administration of SAM-e was either parenteral (intravenous or intramuscular) or oral, and in most studies the dose was increased, based on homocysteine levels (an indirect measure of SAM-e) and adverse effects, to up to 1.6 g per day. In a recent, large multicenter study (n = 294) comparing SAM-e with imipramine, both parenteral and oral doses of SAM-e were comparable in decreasing scores on the HAM-D.[200] The duration of most clinical trials on SAM-e is 4 weeks, but many showed an effect of SAM-e within 1 week (compared with about 4 weeks with typical antidepressants) and/or the ability of SAM-e to shorten the latency of effect of typical antidepressants.[197,198]

Safety. Complaints of adverse effects in subjects taking SAM-e are similar to those taking placebo and include headache, restlessness, and GI symptoms. Additionally, several authors have reported an increase in manic symptoms with use of SAM-e.[201-203] The results from studies on SAM-e supplementation for depression are similar to those from studies on its supplementation for osteoarthritis; the reader is directed to the discussion on this topic earlier in this chapter.

Conclusions. Evidence from open-label as well as randomized, placebo-controlled studies indicates that SAM-e is effective in reducing the symptoms of those with major depressive disorders. Indeed, SAM-e appears to be as effective as tricyclic antidepressants and potentially SSRIs and venlafaxine in the treatment of depression with far fewer adverse events. Physical therapists treating patients taking SAM-e, especially those with depression, should monitor for any signs of manic behavior.

St. John's Wort (*Hypericum perforatum*)

Background. St. John's wort (SJW) is a flowering plant native to Europe and has been used historically for treating mental disorders and neuropathic pain and as a balm for skin wounds. SJW blooms from June to August, and the flowers are harvested to produce the supplement. SJW contains several ingredients with physiologic function, such as hypericin, hyperforin, and some flavonoids.[204] In vitro effects of these constituents include nonselective reuptake inhibition of amine neurotransmitters and an affinity for their receptors.[205] On the basis of the knowledge that amine and probably other neurotransmitters and receptors are involved in the pathogenesis of several affective disorders (e.g., depression), SJW is used today primarily to improve mood and to treat depression.

Efficacy. Clinical trials of SJW for depression have presented mixed results. One of the primary reasons for the confounding results seems to be the level of depression. Whiskey et al pooled data from 22 RCTs and concluded that there was a statistically significant improvement in depressive symptoms in patients with chronic mild-to-moderate depression at baseline after supplementation with 300 to 900 mg of SJW for at least 4 weeks.[206] Similar results were reported in a meta-analysis by Linde et al.[207]

Similarly, Kasper et al attempted to evaluate the effect of SJW on acute mild depression by pooling data from previous studies and reported that 600 mg (WS®5570) of SJW for 6 weeks significantly lowered HAM-D scores, increased the percentage of responders (≥50% reduction in HAM-D scores), and increased the number of patients in remission (≤7 HAM-D score).[208] The authors argued that in patients with acute mild depression where the adverse effects of typical antidepressants may outweigh the benefits of treatment, SJW could be an excellent alternative.[208]

However, in patients with major depressive disorders, the findings seem less clear. Linde et al reported a relative response ratio of 1.28 (1.10 to 1.49) of SJW (500–1500 mg for at least 4 weeks) compared with placebo in patients with major depression.[209] A relative response rate of 1 would indicate that the number of responders in the treatment group equaled the number of responders in the control group. So, while this reflects a superiority of SJW, the effect is modest. When investigating the subpopulations of the SJW clinical trials, those with major depression, a higher initial HAM-D score, and a longer duration of depression were less likely to respond.[207] Linde et al reiterated their conclusion that the effects of SJW in major depression are negligible.[207] This contention is supported by a recent large US trial of SJW in the treatment of major depressive disorders.[210] Positive outcomes of SJW were more likely to be seen in older, smaller trials of German origin, which may have included patients with more diverse forms of depression.[207]

Comparisons of SJW with conventional antidepressants have added even more controversy. Many, but not all, comparative trials (SJW versus tricyclic antidepressants or SSRIs) involved patients with major depression and demonstrated no statistical difference between the two treatments, indicating that SJW is as effective as conventional medications.[211-216] Because of these results, some authors then concluded that SJW is effective in patients with major depression.[206,217] However, several studies of antidepressant-alone treatments have not shown any significant improvement compared with placebo.[207] A recent study of SJW and fluoxetine demonstrated the significance of SJW compared with fluoxetine but not placebo.[218] Clinically, not all patients respond to certain antidepressants and must go through a period of trial and error with different drug classes before experiencing improvement. Thus, without knowing whether or not the antidepressant studied would have helped the patient, the fact that SJW was not different from the antidepressant is inconclusive. Linde et al also argued that some trials used antidepressant doses in the lower therapeutic range.[207]

An additional trial warrants mention for the physical therapist. Paris et al investigated the effect of a homeopathic treatment that included SJW on the cumulative morphine intake of subjects (n = 158) after anterior cruciate ligament (ACL) reconstruction.[219] They reported no significant difference in subjects' pain (VAS) or total use of morphine from day 0 to day 4 after surgery.

Safety. The commonly reported adverse effects of SJW include GI distress and headache. Data from meta-analyses indicate a trend among subjects taking SJW to report fewer adverse effects and fewer withdrawals compared with placebo and conventional antidepressants.[206,207,217] The primary concern in using SJW is its potential to interact with a multitude of prescription drugs. Like kava, SJW is known to alter cytochrome P450 enzymes and P-glycoprotein, thereby altering the hepatic metabolism of many drugs, including some chemotherapeutic agents, antivirals, antimicrobials, cardiovascular drugs (e.g., digoxin, warfarin, verapamil, and nifedipine), neurologic drugs, oral hypoglycemic drugs, oral contraceptives, proton pump inhibitors, HMG-CoA reductase inhibitors (statins), and anti-inflammatories (e.g., ibuprofen).[205,217,220,221] A study conducted in Germany revealed 12 of 150 patients admitted to the hospital had plasma concentrations of the constituents of SJW that were not familiar to the medical team and, more seriously, that 7 of 12 patients had been treated with medications that are known to have interactions with SJW.[222]

Conclusions. The clinical evidence for SJW's effectiveness on depressive symptoms is controversial. Current best evidence points to a significant effect of supplementation on patients with acute episodes of mild depression and those with chronic mild-to-moderate depression. The effect of SJW on major depression appears to be minimal. When compared with conventional antidepressants (tricyclics, and SSRIs), SJW may be equally effective and is clearly better tolerated. Supplementation with SJW is safe in most people; however, physical therapists should strongly encourage patients to inform their physician if they use SJW, especially if they are also taking any prescription medications.

Ginkgo Biloba (Ginkgo)

Background. The leaves and nuts from the Ginkgo tree, thought to have originated in Asia over 150 million years ago, are routinely used in traditional Chinese medicine.[223] The active components of the ginkgo leaf are flavonoids and terpene lactones (ginkgolides, bilobalide). These active ingredients have varied physiologic effects, including antioxidant activity (see earlier discussion on flavonoids), antiplatelet activity, effects on neurotransmitters, and inhibition of the β-amyloid precursor protein (APP).[223-225] Effects on amyloids signifies a potential therapeutic benefit of ginkgo supplementation, as they are implicated in the pathogenesis of Alzheimer's disease.[226-229] In the last several decades, Western cultures have begun to use extracts from the ginkgo leaves in hopes of improving cognition and memory and preventing dementia and Alzheimer's disease.

Efficacy. In their review of clinical trials, Canter and Ernst concluded that neither single doses nor longer-term use (up to 13 weeks) of ginkgo extracts had significant cognitive or memory effects in healthy individuals under 60 years of age.[230] The authors reviewed clinical trials of ginkgo that had reported positive results; however, those studies tended to be older, less controlled, and underpowered. The authors pointed out that even studies with homogeneous study parameters were contradictory. In healthy individuals, a ceiling effect could occur, that is, ginkgo's physiologic effect may not be observed in individuals with normal cognition and memory. Canter and Ernst noted that their findings in healthy individuals did not rule out ginkgo's effect in individuals with cognitive impairment or dementia.

In their 2009 Cochrane review, Birks and Grimley-Evans evaluated clinical trials using ginkgo to improve the status of patients with acquired cognitive impairment (including dementia).[231] They found inconsistency in the results of the combined trials, even after including more recent, better-quality trials. The benefit of ginkgo supplementation, compared with placebo, was shown (120–300 mg for 6 weeks to 1 year) in CGIC scores (more subjects "improved" or remained "unchanged" and did not get "worse"; OR 1.66), in terms of cognitive function in trials longer than 4 weeks (SMD = 0.65), and on the SKT (SMD = 3.57). No other significant differences were found, and overall measures of heterogeneity were high. The most recent ginkgo trials are also controversial, reporting overall benefit or no significant differences versus placebo. It is interesting to note that in one of these negative studies, a small subgroup of patients with neuropsychiatric symptoms (e.g., agitation, aggression, delusions, hallucinations, wandering) did experience significant improvement compared with those taking placebo, and that one of the positive studies included only patients with neuropsychiatric symptoms.[232-236] Finally, a recent independent study by McCarney and colleagues also found no significant differences in the ADAS-Cog or quality of life after supplementation with ginkgo (120 mg per day for 6 months) in patients older than 55 years who had dementia (n = 176).[237]

Two recent studies have evaluated the preventative effects of ginkgo supplementation. DeKosky et al found that ginkgo supplementation (240 mg per day for an average of 6.1 years) in over 3000 subjects over 75 years of age with normal cognition or mild cognitive impairment did not prevent or reduce the incidence of all-cause dementia or Alzheimer's disease.[238] The overall dementia rate was 3.3/100 in those receiving ginkgo and 2.9/100 in those receiving placebo. Further, the results were not affected by subject gender, age, ethnicity or apolipoprotein E genotype. Similarly, in a smaller study including 118 subjects over 85 years of age Dodge et al found no cognitive protective effects of ginkgo (240 mg per day for 3.5 years) versus placebo.[239] However, when adherence to medication was controlled in a secondary analysis, subjects taking ginkgo had a lower risk of dementia and had a smaller decline in memory scores. The much larger study by DeKosky et al reported no differences between groups with respect to drug adherence, but this may be reflective of the older age of the subjects in the Dodge trial. An additional study of over 2800 subjects, based in Europe, investigating the incidence Alzheimer's disease in older adults taking 240 mg ginkgo per day is currently in progress.[240]

One study investigated the effect of ginkgo supplementation on anxiety. Woelk et al conducted a double-blind RCT on 107 patients with anxiety disorders.[241] Subjects were randomized into two treatment groups (EGb761; 480 mg per day and 240 mg per day for 4 weeks) and a placebo group. The subjects taking high and low doses of ginkgo had significant reductions in anxiety (HAM-A score) compared with those taking placebo (14.3, 12.1, and 7.8 points, respectively, $p = 0.003$).

Safety. Birks and Grimley-Evans reported no significant differences in the incidence of adverse events between subjects taking ginkgo and those taking placebo.[231] Common complaints include GI upset, headache, dizziness, and allergic skin reaction.[73] In the longest studies conducted, by DeKosky et al and by Dodge et al, the adverse event profiles and mortality rates were similar in both ginkgo and placebo groups.[238,239] However, Dodge et al reported higher incidences of cerebrovascular accident (CVA) and transient ischemic attack (TIA)—6 occlusive, 1 hemorrhagic—in those taking ginkgo.[239]

Case reports and in vitro studies have demonstrated the potential of ginkgo to cause excessive bleeding (intracranial, ocular, postsurgical, and other severe and minor cases of bleeding).[73,242] However, Koch et al found platelet inhibition by ginkgo only at levels 100 times the serum levels of ginkgo after oral ingestion.[243] Additionally, ginkgo (EGb761) had no effect on coagulation or platelet function in 32 healthy males or 12 healthy males who were concurrently taking warfarin.[244,245] In her review of controlled trials and case reports, Bone concluded that concerns about bleeding caused by ginkgo, even when combined with aspirin or warfarin, have been greatly exaggerated and that the evidence from the clinical trials using ginkgo would support this notion.[242] In their case report and systematic review of hemorrhage reports of ginkgo, Bent et al came to a different conclusion. Although patients in many of the case reports had other confounding factors related to bleeding, in six individuals, when ginkgo supplementation was withdrawn, the bleeding stopped and did not recur.[246] The authors concluded that a causal relationship might exist between ginkgo and hemorrhage, so patients, especially those with risk factors, should be warned about this. Beyond the serious potential interactions with anticoagulant and/or antiplatelet drugs, ginkgo may also interact with prescription medications (e.g., anticonvulsants, antidepressants, antibiotics, diuretics) due to its effect on liver enzymes.[73]

Conclusions. Current evidence does not support ginkgo supplementation to improve cognitive function in healthy individuals. In patients with normal cognitive function or in those with mild cognitive impairment, ginkgo does not reduce the incidence of dementia or the decline of cognitive function. However, the change in results in the Dodge trial with controlling for medication adherence may leave a small spark of hope that ginkgo may still be helpful in this respect. This hope will be supported or refuted by the results of the ongoing trial by Andrieu and colleagues. Whether ginkgo supplementation improves the cognitive function of those already diagnosed with dementia is more difficult to determine. Recent, large, high-quality studies would suggest that the global mixed population of patients with dementia may show limited to modest improvements in some cognitive measures. A subpopulation of individuals with dementia that may benefit more significantly are those with neuropsychiatric symptoms associated with dementia. A single RCT suggests that ginkgo may also improve symptoms of anxiety.

The physical therapist should strongly urge patients taking ginkgo to take the supplement only after consulting their physicians and to monitor for signs and symptoms of hemorrhage (e.g., pink or red urine, red or black stools, unusual bleeding from gums, chronic headache or abdominal pain that intensifies, nausea or vomiting, petechiae, increased bruising) and for allergic reactions.

Dehydroepiandosterone (DHEA)

Background. DHEA is a steroid hormone produced in the adrenal glands and in the brains of both men and women throughout the lifespan.[247,248] By binding to various receptor types, DHEA appears to exert an overall excitatory effect on neurons.[248-250] DHEA also shows an affinity for brain receptors that bind various antidepressant and antipsychotic drugs and those that function in memory formation and storage.[248] Additionally, animal studies of DHEA have suggested a neuroprotective effect.[251-253] Finally, DHEA levels are known to decline with age leading to the theory that DHEA supplementation could not only prevent age-related declines in cognition but also improve mood and well being and protect older individuals from pathologic dementia such as Alzheimer's disease.[254]

Efficacy. According to some studies, higher DHEA levels in healthy older adults appeared to be related to subjective measures of overall health, function, and well being but not to cognitive performance.[255,256] DHEA levels also did not predict changes in cognitive function or score on the MMSE in healthy older adults.[257-259] Clinical trials for supplementation of DHEA are also largely negative. In their Cochrane review, Grimley-Evans and colleagues found no evidence to support any improvement in cognition after short term (<3 months) DHEA supplementation (50 mg) in healthy individuals.[260] A larger dose of 100 mg also had no effect on cognition in 39 healthy older men.[261] Most recently, Kritz-Silverstein et al found no significant improvement in any cognitive test or in any measures of well being and sexual function in 225 men and women after 50 mg of DHEA supplementation for 1 year.[262] Studying only older postmenopausal women, Parsons et al actually reported a decline in cognitive function after DHEA supplementation of 25 mg for 6 months.[263]

Whether DHEA levels are lower in older adults with Alzheimer's disease is controversial and inconsistent.[248] The largest longitudinal study monitored 883 men for 31 years and found no correlation between DHEA levels and cognitive status or decline.[264] In the only RCT published to date, Wolkowitz and colleagues found no significant difference in any measure of disease progression or cognitive function in 58 individuals with Alzheimer's disease after DHEA supplementation of 100 mg for 6 months.[265]

In line with the relationship between serum DHEA levels and feelings of well being, clinical trials support a more positive effect of DHEA supplementation on mood and affect. The study by Kritz-Silverstein et al mentioned above demonstrated a significant effect in subjects' mood but not overall quality of life (as measured by the SF-36).[262] Wolkowitz et al reported a significant 30% decrease in depression scores after 6 weeks of 30 to 90 mg of DHEA supplementation in 22 depressed adults (mean age 44 years) who were also taking antidepressants.[266] Similarly, Bloch et al found improvement in depressive symptoms after 6 weeks of DHEA supplementation (30–150 mg/day) in 15 adults who were not taking other medications.[267]

Safety. The supplementation of DHEA leads to different physiologic outcomes based on gender. In women, there is an increase in circulating androgens, and in men, an increase in estrogens occurs.[268]

Because of the complicated role of DHEA in the endocrine and nervous systems, adverse effects may be largely individual and appear to be more frequent in women. The most common adverse effects reported include oily skin, acne, facial and body hair, and sweating.[265,268] Several studies have also reported a significant decrease in HDL cholesterol levels, which could have serious cardiovascular consequences.[268] Finally, though no direct evidence exists, DHEA supplementation could potentially increase the risk for the development of hormone-related cancers (e.g., breast cancer, prostate cancer).[268]

Conclusions. While DHEA levels do decrease with age, the complicated relationship of this steroid to other steroids/hormones in the body does not support a simple supplementation solution. In healthy adults, DHEA supplementation does not improve cognitive function; nor does it prevent or treat dementia such as that of Alzheimer's disease. However, there is preliminary clinical evidence that DHEA supplementation may improve mood and help treat patients with depression. However, the magnitude of such improvement may not be superior to current antidepressant treatments, especially in light of the potential risks of supplementation.

Supplements for Menopausal Symptoms

An understanding of menopause and its clinical manifestations is important for any physical therapist treating women between the ages of 40 and 60 years of age. The normal cessation of menstruation and loss of fertility in women of this age is brought about by changing hormone levels, which has major physiologic impacts beyond the reproductive system.[for review 269,270] Women going through menopause experience a multitude of symptoms ranging from those that cause mild discomfort to those that severely limit ADLs. Some of the most common clinical complaints include vasomotor symptoms such as hot flashes (or flushes) and night sweats, vaginal dryness and dyspareunia, arthralgia, myalgia, affective disorders, and fatigue. For relief from these symptoms, it has been estimated that 46% to 79% of women turn to dietary supplements.[271-273] Keenen et al found that hot flashes (~63%) and night sweats (~48%) were the symptoms for which menopausal women most commonly seek treatment.[271] Presumably, the percentage of women seeking "natural" treatment for menopausal symptoms has increased following the Women's Health Initiative report that hormone replacement therapy (estrogen and/or progestin) appears to increase the risk for various cardiovascular events and some cancers.[274-276]

Clinical research investigating the effect of supplements on menopausal symptoms use various strategies to measure success. A daily log of the number, duration, and severity of hot flashes is commonly used in addition to a multitude of standardized scales assessing various physical, social, and emotional effects of menopause. These tools are either scored by the physician, as is the case with the Kupperman Index (KI), or by the subject herself as with the Greene Climacteric Scale (GCS), the Menopause Rating Scale (MRS), and the Women's Health Questionnaire (WHQ).[277-283] In general, these tools attempt to address the severity and impact of a multitude of menopausal symptoms but do not always address the frequency of symptoms.

Various supplements are used frequently for the alleviation of symptoms of menopause, including, but not limited to, the ones selected for this chapter: black cohosh and isoflavones (soy products and red clover).

Black Cohosh (*Actaea racemosa, Cimicifuga racemosa*)

Background. Black cohosh is a plant indigenous to North America historically used by Native Americans for "female complaints" relating to menstruation and childbirth.[284] An extract or powder can be formed from the rhizome of the plant and contains triterpene glycolides (~1 mg per 20–40 mg dose) and flavonoids.[285] The exact mechanism of action in treating the symptoms of menopause is not known, but most authors agree that black cohosh should not be considered a phytoestrogen; it may, instead, affect the symptoms of menopause by binding to estrogen receptors and serotonin receptors in the CNS.[286-289]

Efficacy. Black cohosh has been studied extensively in postmenopausal women and compared not only with placebo but with hormone replacement therapy (HRT), tibolone, and antidepressants such as fluoxetine. These clinical trials reported varied results, which depended on the dose and duration of use of black cohosh, the outcome measure used, and the stage of menopause of the subjects. Black cohosh supplementation of 20 to 160 mg for 4 weeks to 1 year was used in these trials, and the most positive results came from those evaluating success with one of the standardized scales discussed above. After 3 months of 40 mg black cohosh supplementation, compared with placebo, statistically significant improvement in scores on the MRS and KI were reported in four studies, although in one study those results were significant only in women with more severe baseline symptoms.[290-293] A study using the GCS found no significant difference in scores between the black cohosh and placebo groups.[294] However, in studies that also had subjects keep a daily log of hot flashes, two of three trials demonstrated no significant decline in the frequency of hot flashes after black cohosh supplementation.[292,294] It is important to note that the single positive study also reported a negative effect of conjugated equine estrogen (CE) on hot flashes, which raises questions about the validity of the study, since it is estrogen loss that is primarily responsible for the development of hot flashes in the first place.[293] In a longer study (1 year) using 160 mg of black cohosh conducted in the United States, no significant differences were found between black cohosh supplementation and placebo in the number or intensity of hot flashes.[295] However, the authors did report a significant reduction in night sweats at the 3-month testing period.[295]

Several studies have investigated black cohosh in women with breast cancer taking tamoxifen, which is known to increase the number of hot flashes. Similar to the results above, significant differences between placebo and 40 mg black cohosh were found in the scores of the MRS after 12 weeks, but not in the number of hot flashes, after 8 weeks of supplementation.[290,296] In contrast, Hernandez and colleagues did find a significant difference in the number of hot flashes with 20 mg black cohosh per day for 1 year.[297]

Comparing black cohosh with fluoxetine, Oktem and colleagues reported a significant reduction in KI scores and in the number and severity of hot flashes in 120 postmenopausal women in both treatment groups.[298] After 6 months, 40 mg black cohosh was superior to fluoxetine in the reduction of KI scores and hot flashes. It is important to note, however, that this study did not include a placebo group, so it is not known if the reduction in symptoms brought about by black cohosh would have exceeded that by placebo.

Safety. Published case reports have suggested a hepatotoxic effect of black cohosh.[299-302] Both the NIH and the US Pharmacopeia (USP) have investigated the potential of black cohosh.[302,303] Both reports concluded that there was only weak evidence and no known mechanism for the link between black cohosh and liver dysfunction. However, the USP did recommend a warning statement on its monograph on black cohosh.

Because of the determination that black cohosh is not estrogenic, the risk for proliferation or alteration of breast, vaginal, or endometrial tissue is unlikely, and several clinical studies support this notion.[291,304-307] Furthermore, a recent retrospective case-control study (n = ~2500) of women with or without breast cancer demonstrated a protective effect of black cohosh.[308] Although promising, this single study should be interpreted with caution as only ~100 women (25 with breast cancer) in the study reported using black cohosh.

Minciullo et al reported a case of severe asthenia with high levels of creatine phosphokinase, which is of special relevance to the therapist.[309] The 54-year-old postmenopausal woman took 40 mg black cohosh for 1 year, discontinued treatment, and then reinstituted treatment, after which she began to have myopathic symptoms. After discontinuing the black cohosh the second time, the patient's condition returned to normal.

In a recent analysis of the safety of black cohosh, Borelli and Ernst reviewed clinical trials, case reports, and postmarketing surveillance studies and concluded that "adverse events of black cohosh were rare, mild, and reversible."[310] The most common complaints included GI distress and skin rashes. However, the data to this point about the safety of black cohosh are short term in nature (<1 year).

Conclusions. Studies of black cohosh have suggested a general benefit in all menopausal symptoms with supplementation of 40 mg for at least 3 months. While some studies reported a more specific reduction in the frequency of hot flashes, others did not. As is typical, the larger, more rigorous studies demonstrated a more modest benefit compared with placebo. For women who are unable or unwilling to take hormone replacement therapy to alleviate the symptoms of menopause, a personal trial with black cohosh may be beneficial, especially when those symptoms are severe.

With respect to safety, the physical therapist should assist the patient in monitoring for any signs and symptoms of liver dysfunction, such as jaundice, dark urine, abdominal pain, and/or myopathy. Additionally, patients with a history of hormone-related cancer or liver disease should be encouraged to speak with their physician before beginning supplementation with black cohosh.

Isoflavones (soy products and red clover)

Background. As discussed in the previous section on soy products, isoflavones are part of the flavonoid family. In relation to menopausal symptoms, isoflavones are also one of three classes of phytoestrogens, which have documented action on estrogen receptors.[311-313] Thus, a diet high in isoflavones could potentially "replace" the estrogen lost in menopause and thereby reduce the adverse symptoms of menopause. Isoflavones occur naturally in various plant products, notably soy and red clover. Products made from soybeans have varying isoflavone content ranging from high levels (~125–200 mg) in soy flour and dry roasted soy beans to low levels (5–20 mg) in soy milk and soy burgers.[314] Red clover *(Trifolium pretense)* is a perennial plant native to Europe, Asia, and Africa, and its extracts manufactured as tablets typically contain 40 mg of isoflavone.

Efficacy. Lethaby et al conducted a Cochrane review on the efficacy of phytoestrogens, including isoflavones derived from soy food products (dietary soy) and extracted into pill form, on the vasomotor symptoms of menopause.[315] Seven of the nine studies reported no significant difference in the vasomotor symptoms of the subjects after increasing soy content in their diets. The challenge of understanding the effect of dietary soy on menopausal symptoms is that diet is difficult to control and that the isoflavones from soy can come in so many different forms. However, most studies that included supplementation of 42 to 134 mg of isoflavone for 3 months to 2 years indicated no effect on the vasomotor symptoms of menopause. Of the 9 studies reviewed by Lethaby et al that used soy extracts, 4 reported positive results over placebo, and 1 reported no significant difference compared with estrogen supplementation. Half of the studies (3 of 6) that evaluated the frequency of hot flashes reported a significant reduction but with notably high placebo effects (21%–43% reduction). Despite more studies with positive results, the authors stated that there was no conclusive evidence for the effectiveness of soy extracts on vasomotor symptoms.

Nelson et al also conducted a meta-analysis on the effect of isoflavones from soy extracts on vasomotor symptoms.[316] Pooled studies supplementing with 50 to 150 mg of isoflavone for 4 to 6 weeks indicated a small positive effect on the number of hot flushes (WMD = -0.83). This effect was slightly higher for studies supplementing with 50 to 70 mg of isoflavone for 12 to 16 weeks (WMD = 0.97). Both results suggest that supplementation could reduce hot flashes in women by just <1/day. Of note, Nelson et al rated all the studies pooled as "fair to poor," with no studies considered of good quality. Howes et al reported a much smaller effect of soy extract supplementation (d =-0.34) when pooling 12 studies that used 40 to 134 mg of isoflavone for 6 to 26 weeks.[317]

A recent small study (n = 80) of postmenopausal women taking 250 mg of a soy extract (100 mg of isoflavone) for 10 months reported a significant difference in the number of hot flashes at the conclusion of the study but not at the 3- or 6-month period.[318] The women included in this study had severe menopausal symptoms, notably ≥5 hot flushes per day.

Several studies have applied meta-analysis techniques to trials of red clover isoflavone (40 to 80 mg/day) with different results.[315-317,319] Lethaby et al (n = 5), Nelson et al (n = 6), and Howes et al (n = 5) reported similar minimal WMD/effect sizes when pooling studies (WMD = -0.57, -0.44, d=-0.16, respectively). Their reports indicate that, at best, a woman taking red clover extracts would experience half a hot flash less per day. Nelson and colleagues also separated out data based on the dose of isoflavone (40 mg versus 80 mg) and found a slight increase in the effect (WMD =-0.40 versus -0.79) with the higher dose, but it still did not reach the level where a woman would experience one full hot flash less per day.

In contrast to the results of Lethaby et al and Nelson et al, Thompson Coon and colleagues published a meta-analysis with more positive results for red clover supplementation. Using the same five studies as Lethaby et al, Thompson Coon et al reported a WMD of -1.45, that is, a woman taking red clover would experience 1.5 less hot flushes per day. It is not clear why these two studies' results are so different. Of the five studies pooled, the largest (n = 84), best-quality study reported no significant difference in the number of hot flashes per day with 80 mg of isoflavone for 3 months.[320]

Neither Lethaby et al nor Nelson et al found that the actual dose of isoflavone or duration of treatment consistently predicted the magnitude of the effect, leading the authors to conclude that other factors played a role in the outcome. Indeed, several analyses have suggested that a more favorable outcome can be gained in women who have more severe symptoms at baseline (≥5 hot flashes per day).[315,317,318,321]

Studies of isoflavone supplementation in women with breast cancer are uniformly negative. No significant differences, compared with placebo, were reported on the KI or in frequency or severity of hot flashes (with supplementation of up to 114 mg for 3 months).[322-324]

Safety. Analyses of the clinical trials of isoflavones indicate that they are generally safe in peri- and postmenopausal women not allergic to soy products but do have the potential to cause GI discomfort (e.g., bloating, nausea) and weight gain.[315,316,325] This is especially true of dietary soy supplementation. More serious concerns about isoflavone use centers around its effect on estrogen receptors. Unfer et al reported a significantly increased incidence of endometrial hyperplasia after supplementation with 150 mg of soy extract isoflavone per day for 5 years.[326] No change was seen for up to 30 months of supplementation. Subjects in several shorter studies (1 year or less) taking either soy or red clover isoflavone demonstrated no change in endometrial thickness after supplementation with lower doses (<115 mg) of isoflavones.[318,327-330] Isoflavones have been reported to be safe in women with breast cancer but only in the short term (3 months or less).[322-324] Powles et al demonstrated that supplementation with red clover isoflavone (40 mg) was safe for 3 years in women with a first-degree relative with breast cancer.[331] The study demonstrated no difference in breast density, endometrial thickness, or increase in the development of breast cancer among the subjects compared with those taking placebo, which is similar to the results of other shorter trials in breast cancer patients.[322-324]

Conclusions. There is little compelling evidence that isoflavone supplementation through dietary soy or red clover extracts is effective at reducing symptoms of menopause. The evidence for soy extract, although more positive, still indicates a small effect at best. Increasing the diet with soy or taking soy or red clover extracts at 100 mg or less in the short term appears safe. However, the safety of larger doses (150 mg or more) for long periods was considered questionable by Unfers and colleagues.[326] In patients with breast cancer, longer-term supplementation of smaller doses (40 mg) did not cause significant adverse effects.[331] Because the magnitude of the estrogenicity of isoflavones is still unknown, therapists should encourage patients with personal or family histories of hormone-related cancers and patients who are pregnant to consult their physicians before beginning isoflavone supplementation. Other patients should be advised to limit their supplementation to 40 to 80 mg, as there is no evidence that higher doses are more effective.

FINDING SUPPLEMENT INFORMATION AND ADVISING PATIENTS

Patients frequently ask about CAM, and therefore it is important for the therapist to have a base knowledge of what CAM is and where to find valid and reliable information about it. It is a very difficult task to keep up with the volume of supplements that are commercially available claiming to improve health. The first step should be to turn to reference texts, such as this one, that offer general information about a particular supplement. Because this or any other reference will never be comprehensive by itself, the therapist should familiarize himself or herself with other valid and reliable references on such information. The therapist should be adept at searching for clinical literature, such as meta-analyses and randomized controlled trials, in library databases such as the National Library of Medicine's MEDLINE, the Cumulative Index to Nursing and Allied Health Literature (CINAHL), or the Cochrane Library. While a tutorial on how to use these databases is beyond the scope of this text, it is important to always search with a specific question in mind (e.g., whether glucosamine sulfate decreases the pain of osteoarthritis). Focusing the search by using keywords makes the searching more efficient. Sometimes, however, the busy therapist may not have time to find, read, and summarize all of the research on a particular supplement. In this case, there are excellent Internet sites designed to help both health care professionals and patients. However, finding valid and reliable information on the Internet can be tricky. Many Web sites that offer information on health are actually commercial sites with the primary goal of selling a product. The best medical information Web sites have a purely educational purpose, include references, and are updated regularly. Many governmental agencies have made significant educational contributions on the Web, with the most relevant one to this chapter being the NCCAM Web site, which also has helpful guidelines for evaluating the reliability and validity of medical information from other Web sites.

Whatever method the therapist uses to search for information, he/she should keep several things in mind when advising patients who ask questions about supplements. First and foremost, patients must be counseled to speak with their physician *before* beginning any supplementation, especially if they are considering stopping any current drug or other therapies. A few physical therapists in the United States have prescribing power, but most do not. Therefore, they do not have the authority to advise patients to take or not take a particular supplement. However, it is appropriate to inform patients, if you are knowledgeable, about a particular supplement's efficacy or its potential adverse events. Also, many patients may be basing their decisions on suspect information found on the Internet. Here, the physical therapist can help steer patients to valid and reliable Web sites so that the patient is better informed. By doing these two things—(1) educating patients when appropriate and (2) counseling patients to discuss supplementation with their physicians—the therapist is advocating for patients' best health care.

REFERENCES

1. US Food and Drug Administration: What we do (website). http://www.fda.gov/AboutFDA/WhatWeDo/default.htm. Accessed May 7, 2009.
2. Post market drug and safety information for patients and providers—Vioxx® (website). http://www.fda.gov/Drugs/DrugSafety/PostmarketDrugSafetyInformationforPatientsandProviders/ucm106290.htm, Accessed May 7, 2009.

3. National Institutes of Health, Office of Dietary Supplements Public Law 104-417: Dietary Supplement Health and Education Act of 1994. (website). http://ods.od.nih.gov/About/DSHEA_Wording.aspx. Accessed May 7, 2009.
4. US Food and Drug Administration: Laws enforced 9website). http://www.fda.gov/AboutFDA/WhatWeDo/Laws/default.htm. Accessed May 7, 2009.
5. Harkey MR, Henderson GL, Gershwin ME, et al: Variability in commercial ginseng products: An analysis of 25 preparations. Am J Clin Nutr 73:1101–1106, 2001.
6. Ernst E: Toxic heavy metals and undeclared drugs in Asian herbal medicines. Trends Pharmacol Sci 23(3):136–139, 2002.
7. Slifman NR, Obermeyer WR, Aloi BK, et al: Contamination of botanical dietary supplements by Digitalis lanata. N Engl J Med 339:806–811, 1998.
8. US Food and Drug Administration: MedWatch recall steam dietary supplement (website). http://www.fda.gov/Safety/MedWatch/SafetyInformation/SafetyAlertsforHumanMedicalProducts/ucm174339.htm. Accessed May 15, 2009.
9. National Center for Complementary and Alternative Medicine Home Page (website). http://nccam.nih.gov. Accessed May 7, 2009.
10. National Center for Health Statistics: National Health Interview survey 2007. (website). http://www.cdc.gov/nchs/about/major/nhis/quest_data_related_1997_forward.htm. Accessed May 7, 2009.
11. Barnes PM, Bloom B, Nahin R: Complementary and alternative medicine use among adults and children: Natl Health Stat Report. United States, 2007, 12:1–23, 2008.
12. Barnes PM, Powell-Griner E, McFann K, et al: Complementary and alternative medicine use among adults: United States, 2002. Adv Data 343:1–19, 2004.
13. Nahin RL, Dahlhamer JM, Taylor BL, et al: Health behaviors and risk factors in those who use complementary and alternative medicine. BMC Public Health 7:217, 2007.
14. Gardiner P, Graham R, Legedza ATR, et al: Factors associated with herbal therapy use by adults in the United States. Adv Ther 13(2): 22–28, 2007.
15. Wheaton AG, Blanck HM, Gizlice Z, et al: Medicinal herb use in a population-based survey of adults: Prevalence and frequency of use, reasons for use, and use among their children. Ann Epidemiol 15:678–685, 2005.
16. Cohen J: Statistical power analysis for the behavioral sciences, Hillsdale, NJ, 1988, Lawrence Erlbaum Associates.
17. McAlindon TE, Lavalley MP, Gulin JP, Felson DT: Glucosamine and chondroitin for treatment of osteoarthritis. JAMA 283 (11):1469–1475, 2000.
18. Bellamy N, Buchanan WW, Goldsmith H, Campbell J, Stitt LW: Validation study of WOMAC, a health status instrument for measuring clinical important patient relevant outcomes of antirheumatic drug therapy in patients with osteoarthritis of the hip or knee. J Rheumatol 15:1833–1840, 1988.
19. Lequesne M, Mery C, Samson M, Gerard P: Indexes of severity for osteoarthritis of the hip and knee. Validation, value in comparision with other assessment tests. Scand J Rheumatol 65(suppl):85–89, 1987.
20. Lequesne M: Indices of severity and disease activity for osteoarthritis. Semin Arthritis Rheum 20(suppl 2):48–54, 1991.
21. Lequesne M: The Algofunctional indices for hip and knee osteoarthritis. J Rheumatol 24:779–781, 1997.
22. Wold RS, Lopez ST, Yau CL, et al: Increasing trends in elderly persons' use of nonvitamin, nonmineral dietary supplements and concurrent use of medications. J Am Diet Assoc 105(1): 54–63, 2005.
23. Goodman C., Fuller K., and Boissonault W: Pathology: Implications for the Physical Therapist. 2nd ed, St. Louis, MO, 2003, Saunders Elsevier.
24. Culav EM, Clark CH, Merrilees MJ: Connective tissues: Matrix composition and its relevance to physical therapy. Physical Therapy 79:308–319, 1999.
25. Bassleer C, Rovati L, Franchimont P: Stimulation of proteoglycan production by glucosamine sulfate in chondrocytes isolated from human osteoarthritic articular cartilage in vitro. Osteoarthritis Cartilage 6(6):427–434, 1998.
26. Setnikar I, Pacini MA, Revel L: Anti-arthritic effects of glucosamine sulfate studied in animal models. Arzneimittelforshung 41(5):542–545, 1991.
27. Mroz PJ, Silbert JE: Use of 3H-glucosamine and 35S-sulfate with cultured human chondrocytes to determine the effect of glucosamine concentration on formation of chondroitin sulfate. Arthritis Rheum 50(11):3574–3579, 2004.
28. Mroz PJ, Silbert JE: Effects of [3H]glucosamine concentration on [3H]chondroitin sulphate formation by cultured chondrocytes. Biochem J 376(Pt 2):511–515, 2003.
29. Dodge GR, Jimenez SA: Glucosamine sulfate modulates the levels of aggrecan and matrix metalloproteinase-3 synthesized by cultured human osteoarthritis articular chondrocytes. Osteoarthritis Cartilage 11(6):424–432, 2003.
30. Sandy JD, Gamett D, Thompson V, Verscharen C: Chondrocyte mediated catabolism of aggrecan: Aggrecanase dependent cleavage induced by interleukin-1 or retinoic acid can be inhibited by glucosamine. Biochem J 335:59–66, 1998.
31. Gouze JN, Bordji K, Gulberti S, et al: Interleukin-1β downregulates the expression of glucuronosyltransferase I, a key enzyme priming glycosaminoglycan synthesis. Arthritis Rheum 44:351–360, 2001.
32. Verbruggen G, Cornelissen M, Elewaut D, Broddelez C, De Ridder L, Veys EM: Influence of polysulfated polysaccharides on aggrecans synthesized by differentiated human articular chondrocytes. J Rheumatol 26(8):1663–1671, 1999.
33. Bassleer CT, Combal JP, Bougaret S, Malaise M, Effects of chondroitin sulfate and interleukin-1 beta on human articular chondrocytes cultivated in clusters. Osteoarthritis Cartilage 6(3):196–204, 1998.
34. Bucsi L, Poor G: Efficacy and tolerability of oral chondroitin sulfate as a symptomatic slow-acting drug for osteoarthritis (SYSADOA) in the treatment of knee osteoarthritis. Osteoarthritis Cartilage 6 (suppl A):31–36, 1998.
35. Hauselmann HJ: Nutripharmaceuticals for osteoarthritis. Best Pract Res Clin Rheumatol 15(4):595–607, 2001.
36. Towheed TE, Maxwell L, Anastassiades TP, et al: Glucosamine therapy for treating osteoarthritis. Cochrane Database Syst Rev (2):CD002946, 2005.
37. Richy F, Bruyere O, Ethgen O, et al: Structural and symptomatic efficacy of glucosamine and chondroitin in knee osteoarthritis: A comprehensive meta-analysis. Arch Int Med 163(13): 1514–1522, 2003.
38. Leeb BF, Schweitzer H, Montag K, Smolen JS: A meta-analysis of chondroitin sulfate in the treatment of osteoarthritis. J Rheumatol 27(1):205–211, 2000.
39. Reichenbach S, Sterchi R, Scherer M, et al: Meta-analysis: Chondroitin for osteoarthritis of the knee or hip. Ann Inter Med 146:580–590, 2007.
40. Vlad SC, LaValley MP, McAlindon TE, Felson, DT: Glucosamine for pain in osteoarthritis. Why do trial results differ? Arthritis Rheum 56(7):2267–2277, 2007.
41. Poolsup N, Suthisisang C, Channark P, Kittikulsuth W: Glucosamine long term treatment and the progression of knee osteoarthritis: Systematic review of randomized controlled trials. Ann Pharmacother 39(6):1080–1087, 2005.
42. Tubach F, Ravaud P, Baron G, et al: Evaluation of clinically relevant changes in patients reported outcomes in knee and hip osteoarthritis: The minimally clinically important improvement. Ann Rheum Dis 64:29–33, 2005.

43. Bjordal JM, Klovning A, Ljunggren AE, Slordal L: Short-term efficacy of pharmacotherapeutic interventions in osteoarthritic knee pain: A meta-analysis of randomised placebo-controlled trials. Eur J Pain 11:125–138, 2007.
44. Clegg DO, Reda DJ, Harris CL, et al: Glucosamine, chondroitin sulfate, and the two in combination for painful knee osteoarthritis. N Engl J Med 354(8):795–808, 2006.
45. Hochberg MC, Clegg DO: Potential effects of chondroitin sulfate on joint swelling: A GAIT report. Osteoarthritis Cartilage 16:S22–S24, 2008.
46. Kawasaki T, Kurosawa H, Ikeda H, et al: Additive effects of glucosamine or risendronate for the treatment of osteoarthritis of the knee combined with home exercise: A prospective randomized 18 month trial. J Bone Miner Metab 26(3): 279–287, 2008.
47. Messier SP, Mihalko S, Loeser RF, et al: Glucosamine/chondroitin combined with exercise for the treatment of knee osteoarthritis: A preliminary study. Osteoarthritis Cartilage 15:1256–1266, 2007.
48. Villacis J, Rice TR, Bucci LR, et al: Do shrimp-allergic individuals tolerate shrimp-derived glucosamine? Clin Exp Allergy 36:1457–1461, 2006.
49. Gray HC, Hutcheson PS, Slavin RG: Is glucosamine safe in patients with seafood allergy? [letter]. J Allergy Clin Immunol 114(2):459–460, 2004.
50. Matheu V, Gracia Bara MT, Pelta R, et al: Immediate-hypersensitivity reaction to glucosamine sulfate. Allergy 54: 643–650, 1999.
51. Tallia AF, Cardone DA: Asthma exacerbation associated with glucosamine-chondroitin supplement. J Am Board Fam Pract 15: 481–484, 2002.
52. Taylor DM, Ferguson CE, Chree A: Absence of detectable infectivity in trachea of BSE-affected cattle. Vet Rec 38: 160–161, 1996.
53. Scroggie DA, Albright A, Harris MD: The effect of glucosamine-chondroitin supplementation on glycosylated hemoglobin levels in patients with type 2 diabetes mellitus: A placebo controlled, double-blinded, randomized clinical trial. Arch Int Med 163(13): 1587–1590, 2003.
54. Pouwels MH, Jacobs JR, Span PN, Lutterman JA, Smits P, Tacks CJ: Short term glucosamine infusion does not affect insulin sensitivity in humans. J Clin Endocinol Metab 86: 2009–2103, 2001.
55. Yu JG, Boies SM, Olefsky JM: The effect of oral glucosamine sulfate on insulin sensitivity in human subjects. Diabetes Care 26(6):1941–1942, 2003.
56. Muniyappa R, Karne RJ, Hall G, et al: Oral glucosamine for 6 weeks at standard doses does not cause or worsen insulin resistance or endothelial dysfunction in lean or obese subjects. Diabetes 55:3142–3150, 2006.
57. Albert SG, Oiknine RF, Parseghian S: The effect of glucosamine on serum HDL cholesterol and apolipoprotein AI levels in people with diabetes. Diabetes Care 30(11):2800–2803, 2007.
58. Knudsen JF, Sokol GH: Potential glucosamine-warfarin interaction resulting in increased international normalized ratio: Case report and review of the literature and MedWatch database. Pharmacotherapy 28(4):540–548, 2008.
59. Rozenfeld V, Crain JL, Callahan AK: Possible augmentation of warfarin effect by glucosamine-chondroitin. Am J Health Syst Pharm 61:306–307, 2004.
60. Scott GN: Interaction of warfarin with glucosamine-chondroitin. Am J Health Syst Pharm 61(11):1186, 2004.
61. FDA MedWatch (website). http://www.fda.gov/Safety/MedWatch/default.htm. Accessed May 20, 2009.
62. Harmand MF, Vilarhitjana J, Maloche E, et al: Effects of S-adenosylmethionine on human articular chondrocytes differentiation: an in vitro study. Am J Med 83(suppl 5A): 48–54, 1987.
63. Stramentinoli G: Pharmacologic aspects of S-adenosylmethionine, Pharmacokinet pharmacodynam. Am J Med 83: 35–42, 1987.
64. Agency for Healthcare Research and Quality, US Department of Health and Human Services: S-Adenosyl-L-methionine (SAMe) for depression, osteoarthritis, and liver disease. Number 64. Rockville, MD: Agency for Healthcare Research and Quality, 2002. (website). http://www.ahrq.gov/clinic/tp/sametp.htm. Accessed May 15, 2009.
65. Bradley JD, Flusser D, Katz BP, et al: A randomized, double-blind, placebo-controlled trial of intravenous loading with s-adenosylmethionine (SAM) followed by oral SAM therapy in patients with knee osteoarthritis. J Rheumatol 21(N5): 905–911, 1994.
66. Kellegren JH, Lawrence JS: Radiological assessment of osteoarthritis. Ann Rheum Dis 16:494–501, 1957.
67. Domljan Z, Vrhovac B, Dürrigl T, Pucar I: A double-blind trial of ademetionine vs naproxen in activated gonarthrosis. Int J Clin Pharmacol Ther Toxicol 27(7):329–333, 1989.
68. Muller-Fassbender H: Double-blind clinical trial of S-adenosylmethionine versus ibuprofen in the treatment of osteoarthritis. Am J Med 83(5A):81–83, 1987.
69. Vetter G: Double-blind comparative comparative clinical trial with S-adenosylmethionine and indomethacin in the treatment of osteoarthritis. Am J Med 83(5A):78–80, 1987.
70. Najm WI, Reinsch S, Hoehler F, et al: S-Adenosylmethionine (SAMe) versus celecoxib for the treatment of osteoarthritis symptoms: A double blind cross-over trial. BMC Musculoskelet Disord 5:6, 2004.
71. Soeken KL, Lee WL, Bausell RB, et al: Safety and efficacy of S-adenosylmethionine (SAMe) for osteoarthritis. J Fam Pract 51(5):425–430, 2002.
72. Agnoli A, Andreoli V, Casacchia M, et al: Effect of s-adenosyl-l-methionine (SAMe) upon depressive symptoms. J Psychiatr Res13(1):43–54, 1976.
73. Jellin JM, Gregory PJ, Batz F, et al: Pharmacist's letter/prescriber's letter natural medicines comprehensive database (8th ed.), Stockton, CA, 2006, Therapeutic Research Faculty.
74. White PF: Red-hot chili peppers: A spicy new approach to preventing post-operative pain. Anesth Analg 107(1):6–8, 2008.
75. Julius D: From peppers to peppermints: Natural products as probes of the pain pathway. Harvey Lectures 101:89–115, 2006.
76. Nolano M, Simone DA, Wendelschafer-Crabb G, et al: Topical capsaicin in humans: Parallel loss of epidermal nerve fibers and pain sensation. Pain 81:135–145, 1999.
77. Mason L, Moore RA, Derry S, et al: Systematic review of topical capsaicin for the treatment of chronic pain. BMJ (Clinical Research Ed.) 328(7446):991, 2004.
78. Cheshire WP, Synder CR: Treatment of RSD with topical capsaicin. Pain42:307–311, 1990.
79. Ribbers GM, Stam HJ: Complex regional pain syndrome type 1 treated with topical capsaicin: A case report. Arch Phys Med Rehab 82(6):851–852, 2001.
80. Knotkova H, Pappagallo M, Szallasi A: Capsaicin (TRPV1 agonist) therapy for pain relief: Farewell or revival? Clin J Pain 24(2):142–145, 2008.
81. Robbins WR, Staats PS, Levine J, et al: Treatment of intractable pain with topical large-dose capsaicin: Preliminary report. Anesth Analg 86(3):579–583, 1998.
82. Simpson DM, Brown S, Tobias J: NGX-4010 C107 Study Group. Neurology 70(24):2305–2313, 2008.
83. Backonja M, Wallace MS, Blonsky ER, et al: NGX-4010, a high-concentration capsaicin patch, for the treatment of postherpetic neuralgia: A randomised, double-blind study. Lancet Neurol 7(12):1106–1112, 2008.

84. Mason L, Moore RA, Edwards JE, et al: Systematic review of efficacy of topical rubefacients containing salicylates for the treatment of acute and chronic pain. BMJ 328(7446):995, 2004.
85. Cross SE, Anderson C, Thompson MJ, Roberts MS: Is there tissue penetration after application of topical salicylate formulations? Lancet 350(9078):636, 1997.
86. Cross SE, Megwa SA, Benson HAE, Roberts MS: Self promotion of deep tissue penetration and distribution of methyl salicylate after topical application. Pharmaceut Res 16(3): 427–433, 1999.
87. Oziomek RS, Perrin DH, Herold DA, Denegar CR: Effect of phonophoresis on serum salicylate levels. Med Sci Sports Exer 23(4):397–401, 1991.
88. Hill DW, Richardson JD: Effectiveness of 10% trolamine salicylate on muscular soreness induced by a reproducible program of weight training. J Orthop Sports Phys Ther 11(1):19–23, 1989.
89. Ciccone CD, Leggin BG, Callamaro JJ: Effects of ultrasound and trolamine salicylate phonophoresis on delayed-onset muscle soreness. Phys Ther 1991; 71(9): 666–75
90. Shackel NA, Day RO, Kellet B, Brooks PM: Copper-salicylate gel for pain relief in osteoarthritis: a randomized controlled trial. Med J Aust 167:134–136, 1997.
91. Joss JD, LeBlond RF: Potentiation of warfarin anticoagulation associated with topical methyl salicylate. Ann Pharmacother 34 (6):729–733, 2000.
92. Yip AS, Chow WH, Tai YT, Cheung KL: Adverse effect of topical methyl salicylate ointment on warfarin anticoagulation: An unrecognized potential hazard. Postgrad Med J 66(775):367–369, 1990.
93. Chan TY: Potential dangers from topical preparations containing methyl salicylate. Hum Exp Toxicol 15(9):747–750, 1996.
94. Morra P, Bartle WR, Walker SE, et al: Serum concentrations of salicylic acid following topically applied salicylate derivatives. Ann Pharmacother 30(9):935–940, 1996.
95. Liebelt EL, Shannon MW: Small doses, big problems: A selected review of highly toxic common medications. Pediatr Emerg Care 9(5):292–297, 1993.
96. Bell AJ, Duggin G: Acute methyl salicylate toxicity complicating herbal skin treatment for psoriasis. Emerg Med 14:188–190, 2002.
97. Overman DO, White JA: Comparative teratogenic effects of methyl salicylate applied orally or topically to hamsters. Teratology 28(3):421–426, 1983.
98. Patel T, Ishiuji Y, Yosipovitch G: Menthol: A refreshing look at this ancient compound. J Am Acad Dermatol 57:873–878, 2007.
99. Hensel H, Zotterman Y: The effect of menthol on thermoreceptors. Acta Physiol Scand24:27–34, 1951.
100. Wasner G, Schattschneider J, Binder A, Baron R: Topical menthol—a human model for cold pain by activation and sensitization of C nociceptors. Brain 127:1159–1171, 2004.
101. Cliff MA, Green BG: Sensory irritation and coolness produced by menthol: Evidence for selective desensitization of irritation. Physiol Behav 56:1021–1029, 1994.
102. Harris B: Menthol: A review of its thermoreceptor interactions and their therapeutic applications. Int J Aromather 2006; 16: 117–131.
103. Namer B, Seifert F, Handwerker HO, Maihofner C: TRPA1 and TRPM8 activation in humans: Effects of cinnamaldehyde and menthol. Neuroreport 16:955–959, 2005.
104. Galeotti N, Di Cesare Mannelli L, Mazzanti G, et al: Menthol: A natural analgesic compound. Neurosci Lett 322: 145–148, 2002.
105. Davies SJ, Harding LM, Baranowski AP: A novel treatment of postherpetic neuralgia using peppermint oil. Clin J Pain 18(3):200–202, 2002.
106. Haynes DC, Perrin DH: Effect of a counterirritant on pain and restricted range of motion associated with delayed onset muscle soreness. J Sport Rehabil 1(1): 13–18, 1992.
107. Hill JM, Sumida KD: Acute effect of 2 topical counterirritant creams on pain induced by delayed onset muscle soreness. J Sport Rehabil 11:202–208, 2002.
108. Heng MC: Local necrosis and interstitial nephritis die to topical methyl salicylate and menthol. Cutis 39:442–444, 1987.
109. Kelm M: Flow mediated dilation in human circulation: Diagnostic and therapeutic aspects. Am J Physiol Heart Circ Physiol 282:1–5, 2002.
110. Ried K, Frank OR, Stocks NP, et al: Effects of garlic on blood pressure: A systematic review and meta-analysis. BMC Cardiovasc Disord 8:13, 2008.
111. Gardner CD, Lawson LD, Block E, et al: Effect of raw garlic vs. commercial garlic supplements on plasma lipid concentrations in adults with moderate hypercholesterolemia. Arch Int Med 167:346–353, 2007.
112. Jepson RG, Kleijnen J, Leng GC: Garlic for peripheral arterial occlusive disease. Cochrane Database Syst Rev 2: (CD 000095).
113. Kiesewetter H, Jung EM, Mrowietz C, et al: Effect of garlic on platelet aggregation in patients with increased risk of juvenile ischaemic attack. Eur J Clin Pharmacol 45:333–336, 1993.
114. Reinhardt KM, Coleman CI, Teevan C, et al: Effects of garlic on blood pressure in patients with and without systolic hypertension: a meta-analysis. Ann Pharmacother 42:1766–1771, 2008.
115. Stevinson C, Pittler MH, Ernst E: Garlic for treating hypercholesterolemia. Ann Intern Med 133:420–429, 2000.
116. Budoff M: Aged garlic extract retards progression of coronary artery calcification. J Nutr 136:741S–744S, 2006.
117. Charlson M, McFerren M: Garlic: What we know and what we don't know. Arch Int Med 167:325–326, 2007.
118. Maslin D: Effects of garlic on cholesterol: Not down but not out either. Arch Int Med 168:111–113, 2008.
119. Hunyh F, Fowkes C, Tejani A: Garlic for the prevention of cardiovascular morbidity and mortality in hypertensive patients (protocol). Cochrane Database Syst Rev1: (CD 007653).
120. German K, Kumar U, Blackford HN: Garlic and the risk of TURP bleeding. Br J Urol 76:518, 1995.
121. Petry JJ: Garlic and postoperative bleeding. Plast Reconstr Surg 96:483–484, 1995.
122. Burnham BE: Garlic as a possible risk for postoperative bleeding. Plast Reconstr Surg 95:213, 1995.
123. Briggs WH, Xiao H, Parkin KL, et al: Differential inhibition of human platelet aggregation by selected allium thiosulfinates. J Agric Food Chem 48(11):5731–5735, 2000.
124. Lawson LD, Ransom DK, Hughes BG: Inhibition of whole blood platelet aggregation by compounds in garlic clove extracts and commercial garlic products. Thromb Res 65: 141–156, 1992.
125. Scharbert G, Kalb ML, Duris M, et al: Garlic at dietary does not impair platelet function. Anesth Analg 105:1214–1218, 2007.
126. Macan H, Uykimpang R, Alconcel M, et al: Aged garlic extract may be safe for patients on warfarin therapy. J Nutr. – 136:793S–795S, 2006.
127. Abdul MI, Jiang X, Williams KM, et al: Pharmacodynamic interaction of warfarin with cranberry but not with garlic in healthy subjects. Br J Pharmacol 154:1691–1700, 2008.
128. Langsjoen PH, Langsjoen AM: Overview of the use of in cardiovascular disease. Biofactors 9:273–284, 1999.
129. Pepe S, Marasco SF, Haas SJ, et al: Coenzyme Q_{10} in cardiovascular disease. Mitochondrion 7(suppl):S154–S167, 2007.

130. Folkers K, Vadhanavikit S, Mortensen, SA: Biochemical rationale and myocardial tissue data on the effective therapy of cardiomyopathy with coenzyme Q_{10}. Proc Natl Acad Sci USA 82:901–904, 1985.
131. Sander S, Coleman CI, Patel AA, et al: The impact of coenzyme Q_{10} on systolic function in patients with chronic heart failure. J Card Fail 12(6):464–472, 2006.
132. Morisco C, Trimarco B, Condorelli M: Effect of coenzyme Q_{10} therapy in patients with congestive heart failure: A long-term multicenter randomized study. Clin Investig 71(8 suppl): S134–S136, 1993.
133. Berman M, Erman A, Ben-Gal T, et al: Coenzyme Q_{10} in patients with end-stage heart failure awaiting cardiac transplantation: A randomized, placebo controlled study. Clin Cardiol 27(5):295–299, 2004.
134. Keogh A, Fenton S, Leslie C, et al: Randomised double-blind, placebo controlled trial of coenzyme Q_{10} therapy in class II and class III systolic heart failure. Heart Lung Circ 12: 135–141, 2003.
135. Rosenfeldt FL, Haas SJ, Krum H, et al: Coenzyme Q_{10} in the treatment of hypertension: A meta-analysis of the clinical trials. J Hum Hypertens 21:297–306, 2007.
136. Hodgson JM, Watts GF, Playford DA, et al: Coenzyme Q_{10} improves blood pressure and glycaemic control: A controlled trial in subjects with type 2 diabetes. Eur J Clin Nutr 56:1137–1142, 2002.
137. Rosenfeldt FL, Hilton D, Pepe S, Krum H: Systematic review of effect of coenzyme Q_{10} in physical exercise, hypertension and heart failure. BioFactors 18:91–100, 2003.
138. Langsjoen PH, Langsjoen AM: Supplemental ubiquinol in patients with advanced congestive heart failure. BioFactors 32:119–128, 2008.
139. De Pinieux G, Chariot P, Ammi-Said M, et al: Lipid lowering drugs and mitochondrial function: Effects of HMG-CoA reductase inhibitors on serum ubiquinone and blood lactate/pyruvate ratio. Br J Clin Pharmacol 42:333–337, 1996.
140. Laaksonen R, Ojala JP, Tikkanen MJ, Himberg JJ: Serum ubiquinone concentrations after short- and long- term treatment with HMG Co-A reductase inhibitors. Eur J Clin Pharmacol 46:313–317, 1994.
141. Laaksonen R, Jokelainen K, Laakso J, et al: The effect of simvastatin treatment on natural antioxidants in low density lipoproteins and high energy phosphates and ubiquinone in skeletal muscle. Am J Cardiol 77:851–854, 1996.
142. Jula A, Marniemi J, Risto A, et al: Effects of diet and simvastatin on serum lipid, insulin and antioxidants in hypercholesterolemic men: A randomized controlled trial in men. JAMA 287:598–605, 2002.
143. Mabuchi H, Higashikata T, Kawashiri M, et al: Reduction of serum ubiquinol-10 and ubiquinone-10 levels by atorvastatin in hypercholesterolemic patients. J Atheroscler Thromb 12(2):111–119, 2005.
144. Rundek T, Naini A, Sacco R, et al: Atorvastatin decreases the coenzyme Q_{10} level in the blood of patients at risk for cardiovascular disease and stroke. Arch Neurol 61:889–892, 2004.
145. Paiva H, Thelen KM, van Coster R, et al: High-dose statins and skeletal muscle metabolism in humans: A randomized, controlled trial. Clin Pharmacol Ther 78:60–68, 2005.
146. Marcoff L, Thompson PD: The role of coenzyme Q_{10} in statin-associated myopathy: A systematic review. J Am Coll Cardiol 49:22331–22237, 2007.
147. Littarru GP, Langsjoen P: Coenzyme Q_{10} and statins: Biochemical and clinical implications. Mitochondrion 7:S168–S174, 2007.
148. Schaars CF, Stalenhoef AFH: Effects of ubiquinone (coenzyme Q_{10}) on myopathy in statin users. Curr Opin Lipidol 19:553–557, 2008.
149. Young JM, Florkowski CM, Molyneux SL, et al: Effect of coenzyme Q_{10} supplementation on simvastatin-induced myalgia. Am J Cardiol 100:1400–1403, 2007.
150. Caso G, Kelly P, McNurlan MA, Lawson WE: Effect of coenzyme Q_{10} myopathic symptoms in patients treated with statins. Am J Cardiol 99:1409–1412, 2007.
151. Baggio E, Gandini R, Plancher AC, et al: Italian multicenter study on the safety and efficacy of coenzyme Q_{10} as adjunctive therapy in heart failure. CoQ_{10} Drug Surveillance Investigators. Mol Aspects Med 15 (suppl):S287–S294, 1994.
152. Williams KD, Maneke JD, AbdelHameed M, et al: 52 week oral gavage chronic toxicity study with ubiquinone in rats with a 4 week recovery. J Agric Food Chem 47:3756–3763, 1999.
153. Ikematsu H, Nakamura K, Harashima S, et al: Safety assessment of coenzyme Q_{10} (Kaneka Q_{10}) in healthy subjects: A double-blind, randomized, placebo-controlled trial. Regul Toxicol Pharmacol 44:212–218, 2006.
154. Shalansky S, Lynd L, Richardson K, et al: Risk of warfarin-related bleeding events and supratherapeutic international normalized ratios associated with complementary and alternative medicine: A longitudinal analysis. Pharmacotherapy 27(9):1237–1247, 2007.
155. Engelsen J, Nielsen JD, Winther K: Effect of coenzyme Q_{10} and Ginkgo biloba on warfarin dosage in stable, long-term warfarin-treated outpatients. A randomised, double-blind, placebo-crossover trial. Thromb Haemost 87:1075–1076, 2002.
156. USDA-Iowa State University: The isoflavone content of foods, Release 1.3 – 2002. (website). http://www.nal.usda.gov/fnic/foodcomp/Data/isoflav/isoflav.html. Accessed June 1, 2009.
157. World Health Organization: World Data Table (website). http://www.who.int/cardiovascular_diseases/en/cvd_atlas_29_world_data_table.pdf. Accessed June 1, 2009.
158. Mink PJ, Scrafford CG, Barraj LM, et al: Flavonoid intake and cardiovascular disease mortality: A prospective study in post menopausal women. Am J Clin Nutr 85:895–909, 2007.
159. Peeters PHM, Keinan-Boker L, van der Schouw YT, Grobbee DE: Phytoestrogens and breast cancer risk. Breast Cancer Res Treat 77:171–183, 2003.
160. Hooper L, Kroon PA, Rimm EB, et al: Flavonoids, flavonoids-rich foods, and cardiovascular risk: A meta-analysis of randomized controlled trials. Am J Clin Nutr 88:38–50, 2008.
161. Taku K, Umegaki K, Sato Y, et al: Soy isoflavones lower serum total and LDL cholesterol in humans: A meta-analysis of 11 randomized controlled trials. Am J Clin Nutr 85:1148–1156, 2007.
162. Zhuo XG, Melby MK, Watanabe S: Soy isoflavone intake lowers serum LDL cholesterol: A meta-analysis of 8 randomized controlled trials in humans. J Nutr 134:2395–2400, 2004.
163. Reynolds K, Chin A, Lees KA, et al: A meta-analysis of the effect of soy protein supplementation on serum lipids. Am J Cardiol 98:633–640, 2006.
164. Weggemans RM, Trautwein EA: Relation between soy-associated isoflavones and LDL and HDL cholesterol concentrations in humans: A meta-analysis. Eur J Clin Nutr 57:940–946, 2003.
165. Sacks FM, Lichtenstein A, Van Horn L, et al: Soy protein, isoflavones, and cardiovascular health: A summary of a statement for professionals from the American Heart Association Nutrition Committee. Arterioscler Thromb Vasc Biol 26:1689–1692, 2006.
166. Lichtenstein AH, Appel LJ, Brands M, et al: Summary of American Heart Association diet and lifestyle recommendations revision 2006. Arterioscler Thromb Vasc Biol 26:2186–2191, 2006.

167. Xiao CW: Health effects of soy protein and isoflavones in humans. J Nutr 138:1244S–1294S, 2008.
168. Dillingham BL, McVeigh BL, Lampe JW, Duncan AM: Soy protein isolates of varied isoflavone content do not influence serum thyroid hormones in health young men. Thyroid 17(2):131–137, 2007.
169. Ernst E, Rand JI, Stevinson C: Complementary therapies for depression: An overview. Arch Gen Psych 55:1026–1032, 1998.
170. Eisenberg DM, Davis RB, Ettner SL, et al: Trends in the alternative medicine use in the United States, 1990-1997: Results of a follow-up national survey. JAMA 280:1569–1575, 1998.
171. Spielberger C D, Gorsuch RL, Lushene RE: Manual for the State-Trait Anxiety Inventory, Palo Alto, CA, 1970, Consulting Psychologists Press.
172. Hamilton M: The assessment of anxiety states by rating. Br J Med Psychol 32:50–55, 1959.
173. Hamilton M: A rating scale for depression. J Neurol Neurosurg Psychiatry 23:56–62, 1960.
174. Folstein MF, Folstein SE, McHugh PR: "Mini-mental state." A practical method for grading the cognitive state of patients for the clinician. J Psychiatr Res 12(3):189–198, 1975.
175. Rosen WG, Mohs RC, Davis KL: A new rating scale for Alzheimer's disease. Am J Psychiatry 141(11):1356–1364, 1984.
176. Overall JE, Schaltenbrand R: The SKT neuropsychological test battery. J Geriatr Psychiatry Neurol 5(4):220–227, 1992.
177. Guy W, Bonato RR, editors: Manual for the ECDEU Assessment Battery 2, Chevy Chase, MD, 1970, National Institute of Mental Health.
178. Blumenthal M, Ferrier GKL, Cavaliere C: Market report. Total sales of herbal supplements in United States show steady growth: Sales in mass market channel show continued decline. HerbalGram 71:64–66, 2006.
179. Taibi DM, Landis CA, Petry H, Vitiello MV: A systematic review of valerian as a sleep aid: Safe but not effective. Sleep Med Rev 11:209–230, 2007.
180. Kennedy DO, Little W, Haskell CF, Scholey AB: Anxiolytic effects of a combination of Melissa officinalis and Valeriana officinalis during laboratory induced stress. Phytother Res 20:96–102, 2006.
181. Miyasaka LS, Atallah AN, Soares B: Valerian for anxiety disorders. Cochrane Database Syst Rev4:(CD004515), 2006.
182. Andreatnini R, Sartori VA, Seabra MLV, Leite JR: Effect of valepotriates (valerian extract) in generalized anxiety disorder: A randomized, placebo controlled pilot study. Phytother Res 16:650–654, 2002.
183. MacGregor FB, Abernethy VE, Dahabra S, et al: Hepatoxicity of herbal medicines. BMJ 299:1156–1157, 1989.
184. Hui-lan W, Dong-fang Z, Zhao-feng L, et al: In vitro study on the genotoxicity of dichloromethane extracts of valerian (DEV) in human endothelial ECV304 cells and the effect of vitamins E and C in attenuating the DEV-induced DNA damages. Toxicol Appl Pharmacol 188:36–41, 2003.
185. Pittler MH, Ernst E: Kava extract versus placebo for treating anxiety. Cochrane Database Syst Rev1:(CD003383), 2003.
186. Witte S, Loew D, Gaus W: Meta-analysis of the efficacy of the acetonic kava-kava extract WS®1490 in patients with non-psychotic anxiety disorders. Phytother Res 19:183–188, 2005.
187. Saeed SA, Bloch RM, Antonacci DJ: Herbal and dietary supplements for treatment of anxiety disorders. Am Fam Physician 76:549–556, 2007.
188. Thompson R, Ruch W, Hasenöhrl RU: Enhanced cognitive performance and cheerful mood by standardized extracts of Piper methysticum (kava-kava). Hum Psychopharmacol Clin Exp 19:243–250, 2004.
189. Clouatre DL: Kava kava: Examining new reports of toxicity. Toxicol Lett 150:85–96, 2004.
190. Kumar V: Potential medicinal plants for CNS disorders: An overview. Phytother Res 20:1023–1035, 2006.
191. Center for Food Safety and Applied Nutrition, U.S. Food and Drug Administration Consumer Advisory: Kava (website). http://vm.cfsan.fda.gov/~dms/addskava.html. Accessed June 6, 2009.
192. Teschke R, Gaus W, Loew D: Kava extracts: Safety and risk including rare hepatotoxicity. Phytomedicine 10:440–446, 2003.
193. Radio Australia: Kava ban lifted from European countries (website). http://www.radioaustralia.net.au/programguide/stories/200811/s2418909.htm. Accessed June 6, 2009.
194. Fiji Times Online: Europe lifts ban on kava (website). http://www.fijitimes.com/story.aspx?id=106071. Accessed June 6, 2009.
195. Bottiglieri T, Godfrey P, Flynn T, et al: Cerebrospinal fluid S-adenosylmethionine in depression and dementia: Effects of treatment with parenteral and oral S-adenosylmethionine. J Neurol Neurosurg Psychiatry 53(12):1096–1098, 1990.
196. Sarris J, Schoendorfer N, Kavanaugh DJ: Major depressive disorder and nutritional medicine: A review of monotherapies and adjuvant treatments. Nutr Rev 67(3):125–131, 2009.
197. Brown RP, Gerbarg PL, Bottiglieri T: Rx update: S-adenosylmethionine (SAMe) in the clinical practice of psychiatry, neurology, and internal medicine. Int J Integrat Med 3(4): 6–14, 2002.
198. Williams A, Girard C, Jui D, et al: S-adenosylmethionine (SAMe) as treatment for depression: A systematic review. Med Clin Exp 28(3):132–139, 2005.
199. Alpert J, Papakostas G, Mischoulon D, et al: S-adenosylmethionine (SAMe) as an adjunct for resistant major depressive disorder. J Clin Psychopharmacol 24(6):661–664, 2004.
200. Delle Chiaie R, Pancheri P, Scapicchio P: Efficacy and tolerability of oral and intramuscular S-adenosyl-L-methionine 1,4-buanedisulfonate (SAMe) in the treatment of major depression: Comparison with imipramine in 2 multicenter studies. Am J Clin Nutr 76(suppl):1172S–1176S, 2002.
201. Mischoulon D, Fava M: Role of S-adenosyl-L-methionine in the treatment of depression: A review of the evidence. Am J Clin Nutr 76(suppl):1158S–1161S, 2002.
202. Carney MWP, Chari TKN, Bottiglieri T. et al: Switch mechanism in affective illness and oral S-adenosylmethionine (SAM) [letter]. Br J Psychiatry 150:724–725, 1987.
203. Kagan BL, Sultzer DL, Rosenlicht N, Gerner RH: Oral S-adenosylmethionine in depression: A randomized, double-blind, placebo-controlled trial. Am J Psychiatry 147:591–595, 1990.
204. Butterweck V, Nahrstedt A, Evans J, et al: In vitro receptor screening of pure constituents of St. John's wort reveals novel interactions with a number of GPCRs. Psychopharmacol 162(2):193–202, 2002.
205. Zhou SF, Lai X: An update on clinical drug interactions with the herbal antidepressant St. John's wort. Curr Drug Metab 9:394–409, 2008.
206. Whiskey E, Werneke U, Taylor D: A systematic review and meta-analysis of Hypericum perforatum in depression: A comprehensive clinical review. Clin Psychopharmacol 16(5):239–252, 2001.
207. Linde K, Berner M, Egger M, Mulrow C: St. John's wort for depression: Meta-analysis of randomized controlled trials. Br J Psychiatry 186:99–107, 2005.
208. Kaspar S, Gastpar M, Muller WE, et al: Efficacy of St. John's wort extract WS® 5570 in acute treatment of mild depression. Eur Arch Psychiatry Clin Neurosci 258:59–63, 2008.

209. Linde K, Berner MM, Kriston L: St. John's wort for major depression. Cochrane Database Syst Rev4:(CD000448), 2008.
210. Hypericum Depression Trial Study Group: Effect of Hypericum perforatun (St John's wort) in major depressive disorders: A randomized controlled trial. JAMA 287:1807–1814, 2002.
211. Behnke K, Jensen GS, Graubaum HM, Greunwald J, Hypericum perforatum versus fluoxetine in the treatment of mild to moderate depression. Adv Ther19:43–52, 2002.
212. Woelk H: Comparison of St John's wort and imipramine for treating depression: Randomized controlled trial. BMJ321: 536–539, 2000.
213. van Gurp G, Meterissian GB, Haiek LN, et al: St John's wort or sertraline? Randomized controlled trial in primary care. Can Fam Physician 48:905–912, 2002.
214. Phillip M, Kohnen R, Hiller KO: Hypericum extract versus imipramine or placebo in patients with moderate depression: Randomised multicentre study of treatment for eight weeks. BMJ 3319: 1534–1539, 1999.
215. Schrader E: Equivalence of St. John's wort extract (ZE117) and fluoxetine: A randomized controlled study in mild-moderate depression. Clin Psychopharmacol 15:61–68, 2000.
216. Wheatley D: LI 160, an extract of St. John's wort, versus amitriptyline in mildly to moderately depressed outpatients—a controlled 6 week clinical trial. Pharmacopsychiatry 30(suppl 2):77–80, 1997.
217. Rahimi R, Nikfar S, Abdollahi M: Efficacy and tolerability of Hypericum perforatum in major depressive disorder in comparison with selective serotonin reuptake inhibitors: A meta-analysis. Prog Neuropsychopharmacol Biol Psychiatry 33:118–127, 2009.
218. Fava M, Alpert J, Nierenberg AA, et al: A double-blind randomized trial of St. John's wort, fluoxetine, and placebo in major depressive disorder. J Clin Psychopharmacol 25:441–447, 2005.
219. Paris A, Gonnet N, Chaussard C, et al: Effect of homeopathy on analgesic intake following knee ligament reconstruction: A phase III monocentre randomized placebo controlled study. Br J Clin Pharmacol 65(2):180–187, 2007.
220. Knüppel L, Linde K: Adverse effects of St. John's Wort: A systematic review. J Clin Psychiatry 65(11):1470–1479, 2004.
221. Hammerness P, Basch E, Ulbricht C, et al: St John's wort: A systematic review of adverse effects and drug interactions for the consultation psychiatrist. Psychosomatics 44(4):271–282, 2003.
222. Martin-Facklam M, Rieger K, Riedel KD, et al: Undeclared exposure to St. John's wort in hospitalized patients. Br J Clin Pharmacol 58(4):437–441, 2004.
223. Mahadeven S, Park Y: Multifaceted therapeutic benefits of Ginkgo biloba L.: Chemistry, efficacy, safety and uses. J Food Sci 73(1):R14–R19, 2008.
224. Yao ZX, Han Z, Drieu K, Papadopoulos V: Ginkgo biloba extract (EGb 761) inhibits beta-amyloid production by lowering free cholesterol levels. J Nutr Biochem 15:749–756, 2004.
225. Birks J, Grimley-Evans J: Ginkgo biloba for cognitive impairment and dementia. Cochrane Database Syst Rev1: (CD003120), 2009.
226. Glenner, GG, Wong CW: Alzheimer's disease: Initial report of the purification and characterization of a novel cerebrovascular amyloid protein. Biochem Biophys Res Commun120(3):885–890, 1984.
227. Nikolaev A, McLaughlin T, O'Leary D, et al: N-APP binds DR6 to cause axon pruning and neuron death via distinct caspases. Nature 457(7232):981–989, 2009.
228. Selkoe DJ: The molecular pathology of Alzheimer's disease. Neuron 6:487–498, 1991.
229. Hardy J, Allsop D: Amyloid deposition as the central event in the aetiology of Alzheimer's disease. Trends Pharmacol Sci 12(10):383–388, 1991.
230. Canter PH, Ernst E: Ginkgo biloba is not a smart drug: An updated systematic review of randomised clinical trials testing the nootropic effects of G. biloba extracts in healthy people. Hum Psychopharmacol Clin Exp 22:265–278, 2007.
231. Birks J, Grimley-Evans J: Ginkgo biloba for cognitive impairment and dementia. Cochrane Database Syst Rev1: (CD003120), 2009.
232. Napryeyenko O, Borzenko I (GINDEM-NP Study Group): Ginkgo biloba special extract in dementia with neuropsychiatric features. Arzneimittelforschung 57(1):4–11, 2007.
233. Mazza M, Capuano A, Bria P, Mazza S: Ginkgo biloba and donepezil: A comparison in the treatment of Alzheimer's dementia in a randomized placebo-controlled double-blind study. Eur J Neurol 13:981–985, 2006.
234. Schneider LS, DeKosky ST, Farlow MR, et al: A randomized, double-blind, placebo-controlled trial of two doses of gingko biloba extract in dementia of the Alzheimer's type. Curr Alzheimer Res 2:541–551, 2005.
235. van Dongen MCJ, van Rossum E, Kessels AGH, et al: The efficacy of ginkgo for elderly people with dementia and age-associated memory impairment: New results of a randomized clinical trial. J Am Geri Soc 48(10):1183–1194, 2000.
236. van Dongen M, van Rossum E, Kessels A: Ginkgo for elderly people with dementia and age-associated memory impairment: A randomized clinical trial. J Clin Epidemiol56(4):367–376, 2003.
237. McCarney R, Fisher P, Iliffe S, et al: Ginkgo biloba for mild to moderate dementia in a community setting: A pragmatic, randomised, parallel-group, double-blind, placebo-controlled trial. Int J Geriatr Psychiatry 23:1222–1230, 2008.
238. DeKosky ST, Williamson JD, Fitzpatrick A, et al (GEM Study Investigators): Ginkgo biloba for prevention of dementia: A randomized controlled trial. JAMA 300(19):2253–2262, 2008.
239. Dodge HH, Zitzelberger T, Oken BS, et al: A randomized placebo-controlled trial of ginkgo biloba for the prevention of cognitive decline. Neurology 70(19 pt2):1809–1817, 2008.
240. Andrieu A, Ousset PJ, Coley N, et al: GuidAge study: A 5 year double-blind, randomised trial of EGb761 for the prevention of Alzheimer's disease in elderly subjects with memory complaints. Curr Alzheimer Res 5(4):406–415, 2008.
241. Woelk H, Arnoldt KH, Kieser M, Hoerr R: Ginkgo biloba special extract EGb761® in generalized anxiety disorder and adjustment disorder with anxious mood: A randomized, double-blind, placebo-controlled trial. J Psychiatric Res 41:472–480, 2007.
242. Bone KM: Potential interaction of Ginkgo biloba leaf with antiplatelet or anticoagulant drugs: What is the evidence? Mol Nutr Food Res 52:764–771, 2008.
243. Koch E: Inhibition of platelet activating factor (PAF)-induced aggregation of human thrombocytes by ginkgolides: Considerations on possible bleeding complications after oral intake of Ginkgo biloba extracts. Phytomedicine 12:10–16, 2005.
244. Sollier CBD, Caplain H, Drouet L: No alteration in platelet function or coagulation induced by EGb761 in a controlled study. Clin Lab Haem 25:251–253, 2003.
245. Jiang X, Williams KM, Liauw WS, et al: Effect of Ginkgo and ginger on the pharmacokinetics and pharmacodynamics of warfarin in healthy subjects. Br J Clin Pharmacol 59:425–432, 2005.
246. Bent S, Goldberg H, Padula A, Avins AL: Spontaneous bleeding associated with Ginkgo biloba: A case report and systematic review of the literature. J Gen Intern Med 20:657–661, 2005.

247. Fuller SJ, Tan RS, Martins RN: Androgens in the etiology of Alzheimer's disease in aging men and possible therapeutic interventions. J Alzheimers Dis 12:129–142, 2007.
248. Wolf OT, Kirschbaum C: Actions of dehydroepiandrosterone and its sulfate in the central nervous system: Effects on cognition and emotion in animals and humans. Brain Res Rev 30:264–288, 1999.
249. Debonnel G, Bergeron R, de Montigny C: Potentiation by dehydroepiandrosterone of the neuronal response to N-methyl-D-aspartate in the CA3 region of the rat dorsal hippocampus: An effect mediated via sigma receptors. J Endocrinol 150 (suppl):S33–S42, 1996.
250. Majewska MD: Neuronal actions of dehydroepiandrosterone. Ann NY Acad Sci 774:111–120, 1996.
251. Reddy DS, Kulkami SK: Possible role of nitric oxide in the nootropic and antiamnesic effect of neurosteroids on aging and dizocilpine-induced learning impairment. Brain Res 799:215–229, 1998.
252. Shen S, Cooley DM, Glickman LT, et al: Reduction in DNA damage in brain and peripheral blood lymphocytes of elderly dogs after treatment with dehydroepiandrosterone (DHEA). Mutat Res 480:153–162, 2001.
253. Kimonides VG, Spillantini MG, Sofroniew MV, et al: Dehydroepiandrosterone (DHEA) antagonizes the neurotoxic effects of corticosterone and translocation of SAPK3 in hippocampal primary cultures. Neuroscience 89:429–436, 1999.
254. Orentreich N, Brind L, Rizer R, et al: Age changes and sex differences in serum dehydroepiandrosterone sulfate concentrations throughout adulthood. J Clin Endocrinol Metab 59:551–555, 1984.
255. Rudman D, Shetty KR, Mattson DE: Plasma dehydroepiandrosterone sulfate in nursing home men. J Am Geriatr Soc 38:421–427, 1990.
256. Berr C, Lafont S, Debuire B, et al: Relationships of dehydroepiandrosterone sulfate in the elderly with functional, psychological, and mental status, and short-term mortality: A French community-based study. Proc Natl Acad Sci USA 93:13410–13415, 1996.
257. Barrett-Conner E, Edelstein SL: A prospective study of dehydroepiandrosterone sulfate and cognitive function in an older population: The Rancho Bernardo study. J Am Geriatr Soc 42:420–423, 1994.
258. Kalmijn D, Launer LJ, Stolk RP, et al: A prospective study on cortisol, dehydroepiandrosterone sulfate, and cognitive function in the elderly. J Clin Endrocrinol Metab 83:3487–3492, 1998.
259. Yaffe K, Ettinger B, Pressman A, et al: Neuropsychiatric function and dehydroepiandrosterone sulfate in elderly women: A prospective study. Biol Psychiatry 43:694–700, 1998.
260. Grimley-Evans J, Malouf R, Huppert FAH, van Niekerk JK: Dehydroepiandrosterone (DHEA) supplementation for cognitive function in healthy elderly people. Cochrane Database Syst Rev4:(CD006221), 2006.
261. Flynn MA, Weaver-Osterholtz D, Sharpe-Timms KL, et al: Dehydroepiandrosterone replacement in aging humans. J Clin Endocrinol Metab 84:1527–1533, 1999.
262. Kritz-Silverstein D, von Muhlen D, Laughlin GA, Bettencourt R: Effects of dehydroepiandrosterone supplementation on cognitive function and quality of life: The DHEA and Well-Ness (DAWN) trial. J Am Geriatr Soc 56(7):1292–1298, 2008.
263. Parsons TD, Kratz KM, Thompson E, et al: DHEA supplementation and cognition in postmenopausal women. Int J Neurosci 116:141–155, 2006.
264. Moffat SD, Zonderman AB, Harman SM: The relationship between longitudinal declines in dehydroepiandrosterone sulfate concentrations and cognitive performance in older men. Arch Intern Med 160:2193–2198, 2000.
265. Wolkowitz OM, Kramer JH, Reus VI, et al: DHEA treatment of Alzheimer's disease: A randomized, double-blind, placebo-controlled study. Neurology 60:1071–1076, 2003.
266. Wolkowitz OM, Reus VI, Roberts E, et al: Double-blind treatment of major depression with dehydroepiandrosterone. Am J Psychiatry 156:646–649, 1999.
267. Bloch M, Schmidt PJ, Danaceau MA, et al: Dehydroepiandrosterone treatment of midlife dysthymia. Biol Psychiatry 45:1533–1541, 1999.
268. Italian Study Group on Geriatric Endrocrinology (GISEG): Consensus document on substitution therapy with DHEA in the elderly. Aging Clin Exp Res 18(4):277–300, 2006.
269. Sapsford R, Bullock-Saxton J, Markwell S: Women's health: A textbook for physiotherapists, London, 1998, WB Saunders.
270. Stephenson RG, O'Conner LJ: Obstetric and gynecologic care in physical therapy (2nd ed.). Thorofare, NJ, 2000, Slack.
271. Keenan NL, Mark S, Fugh-Berman A, Browne D, Kaczmarczyk J, Hunter C: Severity of menopausal symptoms and use of both conventional and complementary/alternative therapies. Menopause 10(6):507–515, 2003.
272. Mahady GB, Parrot J, Lee C, Yun GS, Dan A: Botanical dietary supplement use in peri- and postmenopausal women. Menopause 10(1):65–72, 2003.
273. Gold EB, Bair Y, Zhang G, et al: Cross-sectional analysis of specific complementary and alternative medicine (CAM) use by racial/ethnic group and menopausal status: The Study of Women's Health Across the Nation (SWAN). Menopause 14 (4):612–623, 2007.
274. Rossouw JE, Anderson GL, Prentice RL, et al; Writing Group for the Women's Health Initiative Investigators: Risks and benefits of estrogen plus progestin in healthy postmenopausal women: Principal results from the Women's Health Initiative randomized controlled trial. JAMA 288(3):321–333, 2002.
275. Chlebowski RT, Hendrix SL, Langer RD, et al; WHI Investigators: Influence of estrogen plus progestin on breast cancer and mammography in healthy postmenopausal women: The Women's Health Initiative randomized trial. JAMA289(22):3243–3253, 2003.
276. Anderson GL, Limacher M, Assaf AR, et al; Women's Health Initiative Steering Committee: Effects of conjugated equine estrogen in postmenopausal women with hysterectomy: The Women's Health Initiative randomized controlled trial. JAMA 291(14):1701–1712, 2004.
277. Blatt MH, Wiesbader H, Kupperman HS: Vitamin E and climacteric syndrome: Failure of effective control as measured by menopausal index. AMA Arch Intern Med 91(6):792–799, 1953.
278. Kupperman HS, Blatt MHG, Wiesbaden H, Filler W: Comparative clinical evaluation of estrogen preparation by the menopausal and amenorrhoeal indices. J Clin Endocrinol13: 688–703, 1953.
279. Greene JG: Constructing a standard climacteric scale. Maturitas 29(1):25–31, 1998.
280. Schneider HPG, Heinemann LAJ, Rosemeier HP, Potthoff P, Behre HM: The menopause rating scale (MRS): Reliability of scores of menopausal complaints. Climacteric 3:59–64, 2000.
281. Schneider HPG, Heinemann LAJ, Rosemeier HP, Potthoff P, Behre HM: The menopause rating scale (MRS): Comparison with Kupperman index and quality of life scale SF–36. Climacteric3:50–58, 2000.
282. Hunter MS: The Women's Health Questionnaire (WHQ): The development, standardization and application of a measure of mid-aged women's emotional and physical health. Quality Life Res 9:733–738, 2000.
283. Hunter MS: The Women's Health Questionnaire: A measure of mid-aged women's perceptions of their emotional and physical health. Psychol Health 7:45–54, 1992.

284. Borrelli F, Ernst E: Black cohosh (Cimicifuga racemosa) for menopausal symptoms: A systematic review of its efficacy. Pharmacol Res 58:8–14, 2008.
285. Jiang B, Kronenberg F, Nuntanakorn P, et al: Evaluation of the botanical authenticity and phytochemical profile of black cohosh products by high-performance liquid chromatography with selected ion monitoring liquid chromatography-mass spectrometry. J Agric Food Chem 54:3242–3253, 2006.
286. Mahady GB: Is black cohosh estrogenic? Nutr Rev 61(5 Pt 1): 183–186, 2003.
287. Burdette JE, Liu J, Chen SN, et al: Black cohosh acts as a mixed competitive ligand and partial agonist of the serotonin receptor. J Agric Food Chem 51(19):5661–5670, 2003.
288. Viereck V, Emons G, Wuttke W: Black cohosh: Just another phytoestrogen? Trends Endocrinol Metab 16(5):214–221, 2005.
289. Seidlova-Wuttke D, Hesse O, Jarry H, et al: Evidence for selective estrogen receptor modulator activity in a black cohosh (Cimicifuga racemosa) extract: Comparison with estradiol-17β. Eur J Endocrinol 149:351–362, 2003.
290. Osmers R, Friede M, Liske E, et al: Efficacy and safety of isopropanolic black cohosh extract for climacteric symptoms. Obstet Gynecol 105:1074–1083, 2005.
291. Wuttke W, Seidlova-Wuttke D, Gorkow C: The cimicifuga preparation BNO 1055 vs. conjugated estrogens in a double-blind placebo controlled study: Effects on menopause symptoms and bone markers. Maturitas 44 (suppl 1):S67–S77, 2003.
292. Frei-Kleiner S, Schaffner W, Rahlfs VW, Bodmer CH, Birkhauser M: Cimicifuga racemosa dried ethanolic extract in menopausal disorders: A double-blind placebo-controlled clinical trial. Maturitas 51(4):397–404, 2005.
293. Stoll W: Phytopharmacon influences atrophic vaginal epithelium: Double-blind study Cimicifuga vs. estrogenic substances. Therapeuticum 1:23–31, 1987.
294. Pockaj BA, Gallagher JG, Loprinzi CL, et al: Phase III double-blind, randomized, placebo-controlled crossover trial of black cohosh in the management of hot flashes: NCCTG Trial N01CC1. J Clin Oncol 24(18):2836–2841, 2006.
295. Newton KM, Reed SD, LaCroix AZ: Treatment of vasomotor symptoms of menopause with black cohosh, multibotanicals, soy, hormone therapy, or placebo. Ann Int Med 145:869–879, 2006.
296. Jacobson JS, Troxel AB, Evans J, et al: Randomized trial of black cohosh for the treatment of hot flashes among women with a history of breast cancer. J Clin Oncol 19(10):2739–2745, 2001.
297. Hernandez-Munoz G, Pluchino S: Cimicifuga racemosa for the treatment of hot flushes in women surviving breast cancer. Maturitas 44 (suppl 1):S59–S65, 2003.
298. Oktem M, Eroglu D, Karahan H, et al: Black cohosh and fluoxetine in the treatment of postmenopausal symptoms: A prospective, randomized trial. Adv Ther 24(2):448–461, 2007.
299. Thomsen M, Vitetta L, Sali A, Schmidt M: Acute liver failure associated with the use of herbal preparations containing black cohosh. Med J Aust180(11):598–599, 2004.
300. Cohen SM, O'Connor AM, Hart J, et al: Autoimmune hepatitis associated with the use of black cohosh: A case study. Menopause 11:575–577, 2004.
301. Lynch CR, Folkers ME, Hutson WR: Fulminant hepatic failure associated with the use of black cohosh: A case report. Liver Transpl 126:989–992, 2006.
302. Mahady GB, Low Dog T, Barrett ML, et al: United States Pharmacopeia review of the black cohosh case reports of hepatotoxicity. Menopause 15(4):628–638, 2008.
303. National Institutes of Health (NIH), National Center for Complementary and Alternative Medicine (NCAAM): Workshop on the Safety of Black Cohosh in Clinical Studies (website). http://nccam.nih.gov/news/events/blackcohosh/blackcohosh_mtngsumm.pdf. Accessed December 1, 2009.
304. Reed SD, Newton KM, LaCroix AZ, et al: Vaginal, endometrial, and reproductive hormone findings: Randomized, placebo-controlled trial of black cohosh, multibotanical herbs, and dietary soy for vasomotor symptoms: The Herbal Alternatives for Menopause (HALT) study. Menopause 15(1): 51–58, 2008.
305. Hirschberg AL, Edlund M, Svane G, et al: An isopropanolic extract of black cohosh does not increase mammographic breast density or breast cell proliferation in postmenopausal women. Menopause 14:89–96, 2007.
306. Wuttke W, Raus K, Gorkow C: Efficacy and tolerability of the black cohosh (Actaea racemosa) ethanolic extract BNO 1055. on climacteric complaints: A double-blind, placebo- and conjugated estrogens controlled study. Maturitas 55S: S83–S91, 2006.
307. Raus K, Brucker C, Gorkow C, Wuttke W: First-time proof of endometrial safety of the special black cohosh extract (Actaea or Cimicifuga racemosa extract) CR BNO 1055. Menopause 13(4):678–691, 2006.
308. Rebbeck TR, Troxel AB, Norman S, et al: A retrospective case-control study of the use of hormone-related supplements and association with breast cancer. Int J Cancer 120:1523–1528, 2007.
309. Minciullo PL, Saija A, Patafi M, et al: Muscle damage induced by black cohosh (Cimicifuga racemosa). Phytomedicine 13(1-2):115–118, 2006.
310. Borrelli F, Ernst E: Black cohosh (Cimicifuga racemosa): A systematic review of adverse effects. Am J Obstet Gynecol 199(5):455–466, 2008.
311. Zava DT, Dollbaum CM, Blen M: Estrogen and progestin bioactivity of foods, herbs, and spices. Exp Biol Med 217:369–378, 1998.
312. Knight D, Eden JA: A review of the clinical effects of phytoestrogens. Obstet Gynecol 87:897–904, 1996.
313. Setchell KDR: Phytoestrogens: The biochemistry, physiology, and implications for human health of soy isoflavones. Am J Clin Nutr68 (suppl):1333–1346, 1998.
314. Consumer Lab.com: Isoflavones (website). http://www.consumerlab.com/tnp.asp?chunkiid=21778. Accessed February 20, 2009.
315. Lethaby A, Marjoribanks J, Kronenberg F, et al: Phytoestrogens for vasomotor menopausal symptoms. Cochrane Database Syst Rev4:(CD001395), 2007.
316. Nelson HD, Vesco KK, Haney E, et al: Nonhormonal therapies for menopausal hot flashes—systematic review and meta-analysis. JAMA 295(17):2057–2071, 2006.
317. Howes LG, Howes JB, Knight DC: Isoflavone therapy for menopausal flushes: A systematic review and meta-analysis. Maturitas 55:203–211, 2006.
318. Nahas EAP, Nahas-Neto J, Orsatti FL, et al: Efficacy and safety of a soy isoflavone extract in postmenopausal women: A randomized, double-blind, and placebo-controlled study. Maturitas 58:249–258, 2007.
319. Thompson-Coon J, Pittler MH, Ernst E: Trifolium pretense isoflavones in the treatment of menopausal hot flushes: A systematic review and meta-analysis. Phytomedicine 14:153–159, 2007.
320. Tice JA, Ettinger B, Ensrud K, et al: Phytoestrogen supplements for the treatment of hot flashes: The Isoflavone Clover Extract (ICE) Study: A randomized controlled trial. JAMA 290(2):207–214, 2003.
321. Huntley AL, Ernst E: Soy for the treatment of perimenopausal symptoms—a systematic review. Maturitas 47:1–9, 2004.
322. Quella SK, Loprinzi CL, Barton DL, et al: Evaluation of soy phytoestrogens for the treatment of hot flashes in breast

cancer survivors: A North Central Cancer Treatment Group trial. J Clin Oncol 18(5):1068–1074, 2000.
323. Nikander E, Kilkkinen A, Metsa-Heikkila M, et al: A randomized placebo-controlled crossover trial with phytoestrogens in treatment of menopause in breast cancer patients. Obstet Gynecol 101(6):1213–1220, 2003.
324. Van Patten CL, Olivotto IA, Chambers GK, et al: Effect of soy phytoestrogens on hot flashes in postmenopausal women with breast cancer: A randomized, controlled clinical trial. J Clin Oncol 15;20(6):1449–1455, 2002.
325. Munro IC, Harwood M, Hlywka JJ, et al: Soy isoflavones: A safety review. Nutr Rev 61(1):1–33, 2003.
326. Unfer V, Casini ML, Costabile L, et al: Endometrial effects of long-term treatment with phytoestrogens: A randomized, double-blind, placebo-controlled study. Fertil Steril 82(1):145–148, 2004.
327. Hale GE, Hughes CL, Robboy SJ, et al: A double-blind randomized study on the effects of red clover isoflavones on the endometrium. Menopause 8:338–346, 2001.
328. Penotti M, Fabio E, Modena AB, et al: Effect of soy-derived isoflavones on hot flushes, endometrial thickness, and the pulsatility index of the uterine and cerebral arteries. Fertil Steril 79(5):1112–1117, 2003.
329. Nikander E, Rutanen EM, Nieminen P, et al: Lack of effect of isoflavonoids on the vagina and endometrium in postmenopausal women. Fertil Steril 83(1):137–142, 2005.
330. Clifton-Bligh PB, Baber RJ, Fulcher GR, et al: The effect of isoflavones extracted from red clover (Rimostil®) on lipid and bone metabolism. Menopause 8(4):259–265, 2001.
331. Powles TJ, Howell A, Gareth Evans D, et al: Red clover isoflavones are safe and well tolerated in women with a family history of breast cancer. Menopause Int 14:6–12, 2008.

27

Drugs of Abuse: Anabolic Steroids and Other Doping Agents

Wolfgang Vogel

DEFINITIONS

Abuse is defined as the excessive use of a drug or substance for purposes for which it was not medically intended. This includes legal as well as illegal drugs or substances. *Addiction*, sometimes referred to as *psychological dependence*, can be defined in various ways. It can be defined as (1) the compulsive use of a drug or substance, despite its negative and sometimes dangerous health and social consequences; (2) as the overwhelming involvement with the drug or substance and the securing of its supply, as well as a high tendency to relapse after cessation of its use; or (3) as an "uncontrollable behavior." The controlled use of a drug or substance is not considered addiction (e.g., social consumption of alcohol or any other drugs). More recently, this definition has also been applied to nondrug abuses such as excessive eating and gambling. Most researchers and health professionals believe that the root cause of addiction lies in the personality of the individual and is not the drug per se, since some individuals can avoid a drug or substance completely or handle a drug or substance "socially" regardless of availability, whereas some cannot and have no control over its use. It is also generally believed that addiction is not an isolated problem but is a comorbidity with other mental problems such as depression and anxiety and that treatment considerations must include these other problems as well. Genetic predispositions as well as environmental factors are implicated as possible causes.

Physical dependence is an altered physiologic state caused by the repeated administration of a drug or substance (legal or illegal), which later on creates a persistent demand for its continued use to prevent "withdrawal or abstinence syndrome." The occurrence of withdrawal syndrome indicates the existence of physical dependence. Physical dependence carries certain health risks, but withdrawal can be dangerous or even life threatening. The degree of physical dependence depends on drug (some drugs will cause it and others will not), dose (usually high doses) and time (usually long periods of continuous use; intermittent excessive use will not cause dependence). The physiologic basis seems to involve the down- or upregulation of receptors caused by chronic stimulation or blockade by the drugs.

Withdrawal occurs only after abrupt cessation of a drug or substance in a physically dependent individual. Signs and symptoms are usually opposite to those of the original drug effects (e.g., morphine causes miosis and constipation, whereas morphine withdrawal causes mydriasis and diarrhea). Withdrawal syndrome can be avoided if the drug is slowly withdrawn by tapering the dose (over a period ranging from a week to months, depending on the drug).

Tolerance is defined as a slow loss of clinical efficacy over time necessitating an increase in dose to maintain clinical efficacy. Again, while some drugs cause tolerance, others do not. Causes can involve pharmacokinetic (e.g., induction of drug-metabolizing enzymes with increased metabolism) or dynamic (e.g., up- or down-regulation of receptors) parameters.

The mesolimbic dopamine system, or the "reward center," in the brain is believed to be ultimately involved in addiction.[1] This system comprises the ventral tegmental area, nucleus accumbens (nucleus and shell), frontal cortex, and prefrontal cortex. All these areas are neuronally interconnected by neurotransmitters such as dopamine, glutamate, acetylcholine (ACh), gamma (γ)-amino butyric acid (GABA), serotonin, and endorphins, and, most likely, other neurotransmitters as well. It is hypothesized that "addictive personalities" possess a dysregulation or underfunctioning of this system, which does not provide the necessary "reward feeling" that is experienced by healthy people. This pathology can be caused by genetic (as shown by studies of identical twins) and environmental factors (improper responses to environmental stresses). Most health care professionals now speak of "addictive" personalities and not of "addictive "drugs. The "addicted person" now is thought to use drugs (or other modalities such as gambling) to directly or indirectly stimulate this system in order to obtain the needed reward feeling.

Addiction, physical dependence, and tolerance are independent phenomena and may or may not occur together. A drug can cause physical dependence but not addiction (e.g., β-blocker) or be used by addicts without producing significant physical dependence (e.g., cocaine).

ALCOHOL

Alcohol or ethanol is one of the oldest "drugs" that dates back to prehistoric times. It is mostly produced by fermenting various fruits with yeast but can also be synthesized. It is metabolized in the body predominantly by two enzymes: alcohol dehydrogenase and aldehyde dehydrogenase. Other routes that have been identified include the cytochrome p450 system, which can be affected by alcohol and subsequently change the metabolism of some drugs. The rate of metabolism is about 150 mg/kg/hr or roughly 5 to 10 mL/hr/person depending on body weight. Females metabolize alcohol more slowly than do males. One glass of wine or beer causes a blood alcohol concentration (BAC) of about 15 to 30 mg of alcohol per 100 mL of blood. BACs of 80 mg/100 mL, or 0.08%, are considered a sign of intoxication in certain states in the United States. It is also partially exhaled by the lungs (the breathalyzer test is based on this fact). Alcohol is evenly distributed throughout the body, and a blood test can predict its levels in the brain and tissues and estimate its pharmacologic effects.

Alcohol causes vasodilatation and heat loss in the body, but its most important site of action is the brain. It is a central nervous system (CNS) depressant and is thought to act by disordering neuronal membranes, enhancing the effects of the inhibitory GABA system as well as other mechanisms in the CNS, such as the cholinergic system. Low CNS concentrations of alcohol seem to inhibit central inhibitory pathways, which results in euphoria, relaxation, loss of inhibitions, and aggressive behavior. As concentrations increase, general CNS depression ensues, along with impaired sensory function and muscular coordination; changes in mood, personality, and behavior; and reduced mental activity. Intoxicated persons often are not aware of these impairments disturbing their sense of reality, that is, they are under the impression that they still can function normally, even though their ability for normal functioning is, in fact, decreased (most often evidenced by automobile accidents). The rewarding action of alcohol is believed to be affected by the stimulation of GABA-A receptors and release of endogenous opioid peptides that cause dopamine release in the nucleus accumbens.

Small amounts of alcohol (one or two drinks or glasses of wine, particularly, red wine) seem to be beneficial in maintaining good health, but large amounts consumed over long periods lead to alcoholism and significant health risks that are often exacerbated by poor diets and vitamin deficiencies (e.g., that of thiamine). Adverse reactions include damage to the liver (hepatitis, cirrhosis), pancreas (pancreatitis), stomach (gastritis, ulcer), heart (cardiomyopathy, dysrhythmias), and brain (Korsakoff/Wernicke syndrome with memory loss and psychotic behavior). Consumption of high doses of alcohol during pregnancy can result in fetal alcohol syndrome (facial/mental abnormalities in the newborn).

Alcohol is the most widely used recreational substance. While most individuals do not use alcohol at all or use it responsibly, a significant number of people abuse this substance and are considered alcoholics (about 5% of the U.S. population age 18 and over are heavy drinkers, and 14.4% are considered moderate drinkers. [http://www.cdc.gov/nchs/data/series/sr_10/sr10_245.pdf accessed 5/20/10]). Alcohol is the leading cause of diseases and deaths (about one third of deaths is caused by or related to alcohol) in the United States. Even among social drinkers, alcohol is responsible for about half the number of serious or fatal car accidents. Recent research into the etiology of alcoholism has implicated environmental and genetic factors; genetic predisposition is becoming a more prominent factor based on studies on fraternal and identical twins, where identical twins showed a twofold higher concordance for alcoholism.

Chronic use of alcohol causes physical dependence as well as withdrawal syndrome (delirium tremens, convulsions) that can be life threatening. Withdrawal can be facilitated with benzodiazepines, which show cross-sensitivity. Subsequently, alcoholism is treated with behavioral modification techniques as well as a number of drugs. Disulfiram (Antabuse) is an aldehyde dehydrogenase inhibitor, which causes increased concentrations of acetaldehyde in the body if alcohol is consumed; these can cause nausea, vomiting, and a throbbing headache; in some cases, however, it can be fatal. Thus, this drug is reserved for strongly motivated individuals, who are not likely to consume alcohol during treatment. Consumption of just 7 mL of alcohol during treatment will cause symptoms that may last from 30 minutes to several hours. There have been some reports of disulfiram reactions occurring even with skin preparations with alcohol as well as with alcohol-containing shampoos. Naltrexone (extended release, Vivitrol) is an opioid receptor antagonist, which seems to reduce the "high" of alcohol and thus reduce the craving; its mechanism of action is, however, not clear. The latest FDA approved drug for the treatment of alcoholism is acamprosate (Campral), which is structurally similar to the endogenous compounds GABA and taurine.[2] It reduces physical and emotional discomforts (sweating, anxiety, and sleep disturbances) experienced by individuals when they stop drinking. Its mechanism is not well understood but might involve effects on central endorphins.

TOBACCO

Tobacco is probably the second most widely used substance in the world, although differences among countries are marked.[3] In the United States, the number of smokers has decreased lately (to about 25% of the population) due to an educational campaign and the restriction of smoking in workplaces and public areas.[4] Smoking is still widespread in Asian and African countries.

The smoker inhales tobacco smoke, which contains a multitude of chemicals, of which nicotine, tar, and carbon monoxide (CO) are the most deleterious.

Nicotine stimulates the nicotinic receptors in the autonomic nervous system and in the brain and releases epinephrine from the adrenals. It is absorbed almost completely in the lungs and passes into the bloodstream. In the body, it can increase blood pressure; increase or decrease heart rate; sweating; increase gastrointestinal (GI) activity; slight tremor; in overdoses, irregular heart rate, a fall in blood pressure, confusion, muscular weakness and paralysis, and respiratory depression; and, at very high doses, death (mostly in cases where pure nicotine used in pesticide has been ingested). Nicotine is implicated in the etiology of hypertension, tachycardia, gastric problems, and cardiovascular pathology. The rewarding action of nicotine is believed to be caused by activation of nicotinic acetylcholine receptors in the ventral tegmental area and in the nucleus accumbens; however, recent research has suggested that other compounds also present in tobacco smoke might contribute to the rewarding effects as well.

Tar is the product of incomplete combustion of organic material and contains irritating and carcinogenic compounds (e.g., benz-alpha-pyrene). The latter can induce P450 enzymes and accelerate the metabolism of some drugs (e.g., opioids, benzodiazepines), which creates the need for higher doses of these drugs. Tar can cause inflammation of the lungs (smoker's cough, bronchitis, emphysema) and throat, lung, and bladder cancers. If a heavy smoker stops smoking, his or her chances of dying from cancer will slowly diminish.

CO is formed by the incomplete combustion of organic materials and will bind to hemoglobin and replace oxygen, which leads to a reduction in the oxygen supply to all tissues (as hemoglobin is converted to carboxyhemoglobin). Although CO is present in the body in small amounts, higher concentrations have been found to affect the cardiovascular system and to slightly diminish mental activities.

In spite of its decline, smoking is still a major factor in premature deaths. Environmental and genetic factors both play a role in the use of tobacco. Nicotine strongly satisfies addictive personality traits of certain individuals, and its withdrawal syndrome (irritation, insomnia, dysphoria) is generally mild. Cessation of smoking is difficult, and only about 7% of smokers who want to quit do succeed. Therapy includes behavioral modification and various drugs. Gums, patches, and lozenges containing nicotine are used as replacement therapy. The antidepressant bupropion (Wellbutrin, Zyban) helps some smokers to resist the urge to smoke. The new drug varenicline (Chantix) is a partial agonist of a subtype of the nicotinic acetylcholine receptor.[5] It blocks the action of nicotine but stimulates the release of dopamine. This drug seems to be most promising at this time, although some individuals have reported experiencing adverse behavioral changes such as aggression, depression, and suicidal tendencies.

MARIJUANA

Marijuana or its more potent form hashish consists of the dried flowers and leaves of cannabis sativa.[6] It is smoked by about 4% of the American population. Populations of other countries such as Ghana, Zambia, and Canada seem to use marijuana more widely, with estimates ranging from 16% to 28% according to the 2007 World Drug Report. When smoked, marijuana has a quick onset of action, with a duration of 1 to 3 hours. When consumed with food, it has poorer penetration into the body and a delayed onset but a slightly longer duration of action. The smoke of marijuana contains a multitude of compounds, including the active and rewarding compound tetrahydrocannabinol (THC), tar, and CO (see previous section on tobacco). THC is highly lipophilic and can be detected in the body weeks after its use.

THC causes increased heart rate, dry mouth, increased appetite, vasodilatation (red eyes), euphoric feeling (high), more intense perception of colors and sounds, a sense of slow passage of time, impairment of short-term memory, and poor reaction time, judgment, and visual activity (leading to more hazardous driving, particularly when used simultaneously with alcohol). Since marijuana smoke contains more carcinogenic compounds than does tobacco smoke, risks of bronchitis, emphysema, and cancer should be increased (although no studies have thus far found a solid correlation between the use of marijuana and cancer). This is further amplified by the fact that marijuana smoke is kept longer in the respiratory tract than tobacco smoke. Marijuana also seems to undermine the immune system, thus increasing the risk for infections. The rewarding effects of marijuana seem to be caused by the stimulation of THC or cannabinoid receptors, referred to as *CB1 receptors* (whose endogenous ligand is a substance called *anandamide*), located in the ventral tegmental area; this causes an increased release of dopamine in the nucleus accumbens but might also activate opioid receptors in other areas of the brain. It also has been found to block voltage-gated calcium channels. The theory that marijuana is a stepping stone to other drugs has been largely abandoned (as the use of inhalants, tobacco, and alcohol usually precedes that of marijuana). Treatment consists mostly of counseling.

In some states, it is legal to use marijuana for medical purposes, for example, to suppress nausea and vomiting and to stimulate appetite in cancer patients. Recently, the federal government stopped prosecuting such individuals, respecting the rights of the individual states to regulate the medical use of marijuana. THC or dronabinol is available as a prescription drug for the same reasons.

HEROIN

Heroin, or diacetylmorphine, is a synthetic opioid. It is usually injected, sniffed, or smoked by users.[7] In the United States, about three million people have used heroin at least once, and about a half million are regular users. Heroin is converted in the body to morphine, which produces both CNS and peripheral effects similar to those of morphine (see the section on opioid analgesics). Users prefer heroin to morphine, since heroin crosses more quickly into the brain and provides a faster and more rewarding feeling ("rush"). Opioids interact with three receptors: mu (μ), delta (δ), and kappa (κ). These receptors are G-protein coupled and cause an inhibition of adenyl cyclase, a decrease in cyclic adenosine monophosphate (cAMP), an increase in potassium conductance, and a decrease in calcium conductance. The endogenous peptides endorphins (often called *endogenous opioids*) bind to the same receptors. The analgesic and euphoric actions are mediated mostly by μ-receptors.

Major effects in the body include pupillary constriction ("pin-point pupils"), constipation, analgesia, respiratory depression, relaxation, and euphoria (sometimes also associated with nausea and vomiting in the beginning of use). In the case of an overdose, fatal respiratory depression occurs. Heroin causes physical dependence, but withdrawal syndrome (irritation, dysphoria, involuntary leg movements, diarrhea) is milder than that seen with alcohol. The reward feeling seems to be mediated by the μ-receptors located on the interneurons in the ventral tegmental area and nucleus accumbens, with dopamine release in the latter.

Therapy for heroin addiction is focused on alleviating withdrawal symptoms and reducing the craving for the drug. Besides psychological and psychiatric interventions, drug therapies are employed with varying success. Methadone (Dolophine), which is a long-acting, orally effective opioid agonist, can alleviate withdrawal symptoms and reduce the craving. This is, in most cases, the preferred therapy. Other drugs include buprenorphine (Buprenex), which is a partial μ-agonist; nalaxone (Narcan) and naltrexone, which are opioid antagonists; and clonidine (Catapress), which is an α_2-agonist. Although not approved in the United States, a new approach has been used in Switzerland recently; this approach is based on the outcome of a public referendum (which, by the way, rejected decriminalization of marijuana) and offers heroin to users as maintenance therapy under medical supervision.

COCAINE

Cocaine occurs naturally in the coca bush (*Erythroxylon coca*), and coca leaves have been chewed and ingested for energy for thousands of years by native Indians in South America living in high altitudes.[8] In Western countries, purified cocaine hydrochloride has been used for more than 100 years. Early on, it was the main active ingredient in many medications and tonics as well as in Coca Cola until it was made illegal. Physicians can, however, still use cocaine hydrochloride as a local anesthetic. The salt is usually snorted or injected, whereas the free base (free basing, crack) is smoked, since cocaine, per se, is volatile. The free base provides a quicker and more intense effect that lasts for about 1 hour. Currently, there are about two million cocaine users, of which approximately 610,000 use crack. Adults aged 18 to 25 years show the highest user rate, with men reporting higher uses; little differences are seen among ethnic groups.

Generally, cocaine produces a euphoric effect and increases energy, talkativeness, and mental alertness (enhanced sensations of sight, sound, and touch) but decreases the need for food and sleep. It constricts blood vessels, dilates pupils, and increases body temperature, heart rate, and blood pressure. Large amounts of cocaine can lead to bizarre, erratic, and violent behaviors as well as to disturbances in heart rhythm and heart attacks, strokes, and seizures, particularly in individuals with pre-existing pathologies. Cocaine-related deaths are often the result of cardiac arrest or seizures followed by respiratory arrest. Research has also shown a dangerous interaction between cocaine and alcohol; this interaction is the cause for most serious drug-related problems and deaths. Pharmacologically, cocaine increases dopamine and norepinephrine levels by blocking their reuptake mechanisms (except analgesic activity). The rewarding effects are caused by increased release of dopamine, apparently mostly in the shell of the nucleus accumbens.[9]

Treatment consists of counseling, but no medications approved by the U.S. Food and Drug Administration (FDA) are currently available. Nevertheless, several medications, including the antidepressant desipramine (Norpramin) or the CNS stimulant modafinil (Provigil), have been used with little to moderate effects. A vaccine that works by binding cocaine in the blood and preventing it from reaching the brain is now under study. Early results indicate that it is effective in about one third of users, in whom it did not avert the craving but effectively prevented relapse.[10]

HALLUCINOGENIC SUBSTANCES

Hallucinogenic substances cause hallucinations, which are profound distortions in a person's perceptions of reality.[11] They include mescaline, or 3,4,5-trimethoxyphenethylamine (naturally occurring in various cacti such as peyote cactus); LSD, or lysergic acid diethylamide (synthetic, extremely potent with effects becoming noticeable with as little as 0.150 mg and lasting up to 12 hours); diethyltryptamine (synthetic); psilocybin (found in certain mushrooms such as psilocybe); PCP, or phencyclidine ("angel dust," synthetic, used at one time as anesthetic); and others. The use of hallucinogens has markedly declined over the last decade, and in a recent survey among students, only about 5% of students have reported ever having tried a hallucinogen, with very few being chronic users. However, mescaline is still being used legally for ritual purposes by some native Indian tribes in the southwest United States.

Users of hallucinogens might see images, hear sounds, and feel sensations that seem real but do not exist. Here, synesthesia occurs often, that is, users claim that they can "hear" colors. Some hallucinogens also produce rapid and intense emotional swings. These experiences can be pleasurable ("good trip") or unpleasant and frightening ("bad trip"). Experiences seem to depend on expectations (e.g., religious expectations may produce religious experiences).

Adverse effects, including unpleasant experiences, mostly occur with phencyclidine ("talking down" is often sufficient as treatment); however, serious, sometimes fatal, misconceptions of the user (who would jump from a high floor thinking he or she could fly) have also been caused by hallucinogens. The mechanisms of hallucinogens are unclear. Based on the similarity between the structures of LSD and other hallucinogens and those of serotonin and catecholamines, it is thought that they might interact with these neurotransmitters. Other evidence implicates the neurotransmitter glutamate and its interaction with a special receptor that is involved in the perception of and responses to the environment. Psychological therapy is the recommended treatment.

INHALANTS

Inhalants can be found in various house products and are mostly volatile solvents (toluene and chlorinated hydrocarbons), aerosol propellants (ethyl chloride, chlorofluorocarbon compounds), and gases (nitrous oxide, butane, propane).[12] In addition, amyl nitrite and nitrous oxide are obtained illegally from medical supplies. These inhalants are mostly used by younger children, with use peaking at eighth grade.

Inhalants are mostly CNS depressants and cause relaxation, sedation, and eventually sleep. Prolonged use can cause CNS damage, blood dyscrasias, and cardiotoxicity (with chlorofluorocarbons). Deaths can occur when users place both the inhalants and their heads into a plastic bag and suffocate when they fall asleep. The mode of action of inhalants is unclear, but since they are highly lipophilic, it is posited that they dissolve in the fatty membranes of nerves and disturb their normal activity.

ANABOLIC STEROIDS

Anabolic steroids are testosterone-related compounds such as oxymetholone, stanozolol, oxandrolone, nandrolone, and tetrahydrogestrinone.[13] They cause or promote the development of male sexual characteristics and increase muscle mass (androgenic effect). The latter is caused by a stimulation of receptor molecules in muscle cells, which activate specific genes to produce proteins that form muscle tissue. Medically, they are used to treat hypogonadism, delayed puberty, some types of sexual dysfunction, and wasting of body mass caused by human immunodeficiency virus (HIV) infection or other diseases. The discovery that anabolic steroids facilitate the growth of skeletal muscle, as was seen in laboratory animals, has led to its abuse by body builders and athletes.

While anabolic steroids are relatively safe at medically used doses, they can produce significant adverse reactions in individuals who use high doses over long periods for their androgenic effects (although their actual effect on muscle building in humans seems to be minimal). Adverse reactions include reduced sperm production, short stature (if taken early in life), tendon rupture, cardiovascular problems with increased incidence of heart attacks, hepatitis, liver cancer, aggressive behavior, and mania.[14] After withdrawal of the drug, the risk of adverse reactions diminishes. The use of these substances is prohibited by the governing bodies of most sports.

"STREET DRUG" TOXICITY

Illegally obtained drugs or substances used by individuals but not in medicine carry risks that can be quite severe or even fatal. The current health status of the user or the presence of undiagnosed or unrecognized health problems can often determine the severity of the adverse reactions experienced. A healthy individual might easily cope with some adverse reactions, but an undiagnosed, underlying medical condition can enhance the adverse reactions of the drugs or substances discussed above. The effects of cocaine on the healthy cardiovascular system might be tolerable, while individuals with untreated hypertension or cardiac rhythm problems can experience serious or even life-threatening episodes. Similarly, the adverse reactions of a drug or substance can be amplified by the simultaneous use of other drugs or substances. Here, alcohol often plays a major role and is often associated with severe or even fatal drug experiences.

The problems with illegally obtained drugs or substances are as follows:

1. The main problem is the uncertainty about what has been obtained and is actually being used.[14] This has been recognized, but is not widely known, as a major contributing factor in the severity of adverse reactions as well as fatal outcomes. The user can never be sure about what he or she is actually buying. Often, phencyclidine is sold as LSD, which is known to cause more "bad trips" than LSD itself.
2. The next problem is the amount sold and bought. Often too little (to increase the profit of the seller) but sometimes too much of the substance is sold (for instance, to introduce a new "brand"). Many deaths have occurred when "high-powered" heroin

(that is much more than the usual amounts) is sold, with the user not being aware of these high amounts or not trusting the claims of the seller. This can cause fatal overdose reactions and is the leading cause of heroin-related deaths.

3. The third problem is the presence of impurities, which are often added on purpose to cut the original substance (to increase profits), to kill the user (strychnine has been added to kill users suspected to be police informers), or due to poorly performed synthesizing procedures (for example, impurities from the synthesis of a designer drug sold in California caused irreversible pseudoparkinson's syndrome in users).
4. The fourth, and probably the most severe, problem is the way such drugs or substances are injected with shared contaminated needles (at one time needles could not be obtained legally by the user), which results in hepatitis and acquired immune deficiency syndrome (AIDS).

All of the above factors also contribute to toxicity and deaths among users.

IMPLICATIONS FOR REHABILITATIVE THERAPISTS

The therapist must be aware that many legal and illegal drugs can cause physical dependence and that it is important for the patients to withdraw these drugs slowly to avoid serious withdrawal reactions.

The therapist must also be aware that addiction is not only associated with illegal drugs but also with excessive and long-term use of alcohol, tobacco, nasal sprays, androgenic steroids, and laxatives.

The therapist can reinforce the warnings that concurrent contraceptive use and smoking increases the risk of strokes and heart attacks, that alcohol enhances the irritating effects of NSAIDs on the stomach, and that the simultaneous use of alcohol and even moderate doses of acetaminophen can increase liver toxicity.

The therapist can inform individuals who are on muscle relaxants that the simultaneous use of even small amounts of alcohol can lead to excessive sedation and incoordination and can make driving an automobile particularly dangerous.

The therapist can advise individuals about the dangers of using or abusing certain substances and encourage them to stop such harmful practices. This is particularly true when cigarette smoke or alcohol is detected on the patient's breath during therapy sessions early in the day.

The therapist can warn the user of an illegal drug—if known—or younger individuals who express thoughts about buying drugs on the street that he/she may experience serious ill effects and even die not only by using the substances they buy but also, more importantly, because of the unsanitary and unprofessional techniques used in their manufacturing and the unscrupulous selling practices.

ACTIVITIES 27

1. Why might it be necessary to monitor alcohol withdrawal in the intensive care unit?
2. An air traffic controller returns to work from a 2-week vacation. He is asked to take a urine drug test, which returns positive for a metabolite of cocaine. The employee claims that he had a novocaine injection for dental work immediately before returning to work. Is it possible for novocaine to produce a positive drug test for cocaine?
3. A 20-year-old man is found unconscious in his college dormitory and transported to the nearest emergency room. The patient exhibits pupil constriction and a depressed respiratory rate. Oxygen and intravenous (IV) fluids are started. In addition, the patient is given IV dextrose, which, however, does not affect the level of consciousness. Naloxone is then given, and the patient begins to wake up. The patient subsequently needs three additional doses of naloxone over the next 48 hours until the drugs are eliminated from the body. A urine drug screen had been performed when the patient arrived at the emergency room and had returned positive for opiates and marijuana. Was the drug screen necessary, and why was the patient given dextrose?

REFERENCES

1. Chapter by Koob GF, Everitt BJ, Robbins TW: Reward, motivation and addiction. In Squire LR, et al (editors): Fundamental Neuroscience Third Edition, 2008.
2. Hammarberg A, Nylander I, Zhou Q, Jayaram-Lindström N, Reid MS, Franck J: The effect of acamprosate on alcohol craving and correlation with hypothalamic pituitary adrenal (HPA) axis hormones and beta-endorphin, Brain Res 305(suppl): S2-S6, 2009.
3. NIDA: Tobacco addiction, NIDA Research Report Series, Mar 31, 2009.
4. Mendez D, Warner KE, Courant PN: Has smoking cessation ceased? Expected trends in the prevalence of smoking in the United States, Am J Epidemiol. 148(3):249-258, 1998.
5. Jorenby DE, Hays JT, Rigotti NA, et l: Efficacy of varenicline, an alpha$_4$-beta$_2$ nicotinic acetylcholine receptor partial agonist, vs placebo or sustained-release bupropion for smoking cessation: A randomized controlled trial, JAMA 296(1):56-63, 2006.
6. NIDA: Marijuana abuse, NIDA Research Report Series, July 1, 2005.
7. NIDA: Heroin abuse and addiction, NIDA Research report Series, September 8, 2009.
8. NIDA: Cocaine: Abuse and addiction, NIDA Research Report Series, May 22, 2009.
9. Ferraro TN, Golden GT, Berrettini WH, et al: Cocaine intake by rats correlates with cocaine-induced dopamine changes in the nucleus accumbens. Pharmacol Biochem Behav 66:397-401, 2000.

10. Martell BA, Orson FM, Poling J, Mitchell E, et al: Cocaine vaccine for the treatment of cocaine dependence in methadone-maintained patients: A randomized, double-blind, placebo-controlled efficacy trial, Arch Gen Psychiatry 66(10):1116-1123, 2009.
11. NIDA: Hallucinogens and dissociative drugs, NIDA Research Report Series, May 5, 2001.
12. NIDA: Inhalant abuse, NIDA Research Report Series, Mar 31, 2009.
13. NIDA: Anabolic steroid abuse, NIDA Research Report Series, April 7, 2008.
14. Di Paolo M, Agozzino M, Toni C, et al: Sudden anabolic steroid abuse-related deaths in athletes, Int J Cardiol 114(1):114-117, 2007.
15. Vogel WH: Toxicity of drugs and "street" drugs: Medical and legal problems, Contemp Drug Prob 125-134, 1972.

28

Exploring Drug–Exercise Interactions

Mary Jane Myslinski

INTERACTIONS BETWEEN SELECTIVE CARDIOPULMONARY AND DIABETIC MEDICATIONS AND EXERCISE

The beneficial effects of exercise in those with cardiac, pulmonary, and metabolic diseases are well documented in the literature.[1-3] The *American Heart Association Scientific Statement on Cardiac Rehab and Secondary Prevention of Coronary Heart Disease* cites the cardioprotective mechanisms of exercise in those with coronary artery disease (CAD).[1] Among these mechanisms are the increased flow-mediated shear stress on artery walls during exercise, the decrease in cross-reactive (C-reactive) proteins, the reduction in rate pressure product, the improvement in coronary artery compliance and endothelium-dependent vasodilatation, and the increase in the luminal area of conduit vessels through arteriogenesis and myocardial capillary density by angiogenesis.

The most recent *Official Statement of the American Thoracic Society on Pulmonary Rehabilitation* states that "the efficacy and scientific foundation of pulmonary rehabilitation have been firmly established."[2] The American Thoracic Society has stated that pulmonary rehabilitation reduces symptoms, increases functional ability, and improves quality of life in individuals with chronic respiratory disease, even in the presence of irreversible abnormalities of lung architecture. According to the report, exercise is the foundation of pulmonary rehabilitation and has a positive effect on dyspnea.

The *Clinical Practice Recommendations 2004: Position Statement of the American Diabetic Association* cites the beneficial influences of physical activity on both type 1 and type 2 diabetes.[3] The benefits include glycemic control, prevention of cardiovascular disease, decrease in triglyceride-rich very-low-density lipoprotein (VLDL), decrease in blood pressure (BP), enhancement of weight loss, and prevention of type 2 diabetes.

The question, therefore, is not whether patients with cardiac, pulmonary, and metabolic diseases should exercise but how these patients can exercise safely and what the effects of medications on exercise responses are.

The basic principles of exercise—overload, specificity, individuality, and reversibility—must be applied when the prescription is formulated to achieve the desired exercise outcomes.[4] *Overload* refers to the application of a load that enhances physiologic function to bring about an exercise response, that is, the exercise prescription. Manipulation of frequency, intensity, and duration will help achieve the appropriate exercise overload. *Specificity* refers to the adaptations in metabolic and physiologic functions that depend on the overload imposed. Exercise outcomes are specific to the muscles and energy systems trained as well as to the type of exercise mode. Specificity focuses on the "how to" of goal achievement. *Individuality* refers to the individual variation in the exercise response. This principle takes into account the person's level of fitness and other specific factors to gear the prescription to the person's needs and capacities. It focuses on the skilled interventions that are required to safely exercise each patient. *Reversibility* focuses on the detraining response, which occurs rapidly when the overload is removed. In a sense, it refers to "use it or lose it." This principle focuses on the need for patient compliance. These basic principles must be followed when the therapist is preparing an effective and safe exercise prescription for a patient.

The normal responses to exercise in a healthy individual are well documented in exercise physiology textbooks as well as in the guidelines for an exercise prescription (Box 28-1).[4] Also, a plethora of research has been done on the responses to exercise in healthy individuals receiving medication. However, the responses to exercise in those receiving medications and who have an actual disease are not well documented. More specifically, data on the responses to long-term exercise, versus a brief bout of exercise, are sparse in the literature. Interpretation of the literature is difficult also because studies vary with respect to drug doses, drugs examined, times

BOX 28-1 Normal Aerobic Exercise Responses in Healthy Sedentary Individuals

Variable	Rest	Exercise
HR	60–90 beats/min	↑10–12 beats/min/MET level
SBP	<120 mm Hg	↑ 7 mm Hg/MET level
DBP	<80 mm Hg	↑↓ 10 mm Hg in entire session
SpO_2	97–98	↔ or ↑
VO_2	3.5 mL/kg/min^{-1}	↑
CO	5 L/min	↑ to 20–22 L/min
SV	71 mL/beat	↑ to 100 mL/beat; but plateaus at 40% to 50%

↑, Increase; ↓, decrease; ↔, no effect; *HR*, heart rate; *MET*, metabolic equivalent; *SBP*, systolic blood pressure; *DBP*, diastolic blood pressure; *SpO_2*, saturation of oxygen with hemoglobin; *VO_2*, oxygen consumption; *CO*, cardiac output; *SV*, stroke volume.

of day when patients exercise, and exercise parameters used as outcome measures. The purpose of this chapter is to discuss responses to exercise in subjects with cardiac, pulmonary, and metabolic diseases who are taking appropriate medications for these conditions.

CARDIAC MEDICATIONS

The *American College of Sports Medicine Guidelines for Exercise Testing and Prescription* delineates the exercise responses that can be expected during treatment with certain cardiac medications.[4] This section focuses on two of the most prescribed medications for those with cardiac disease: β-blockers and calcium channel blockers. These medications are used to treat hypertension and angina pectoris. Their mechanisms of action on cardiac parameters are discussed to explain exercise responses. Different medications produce different responses, depending on the disease. For example, patients with hypertension show a decrease in exercise capacity while taking a β-blocker, but patients with CAD demonstrate an increase in exercise capacity. The population considered here consists of patients with coronary artery disease (CAD).

β-Blockers

β-Blocking drugs, regardless of their selectivity, cause reduction in heart rate (HR), blood pressure (BP), and cardiac output (CO) during rest and exercise; decrease in myocardial contractility; and decrease in coronary and muscle blood flow, all of which increase myocardial efficiency as a result of a reduction in oxygen consumption.[5-7] Studies have shown a reduction in exercising HR by 20% to 30% and CO by 5% to 23%.[8,9] During exercise of moderate intensity (50% to 60% of maximum oxygen consumption [VO_{2max}]), the reduction in HR becomes more pronounced and causes compensatory adjustments in the cardiovascular system, such as an increase in stroke volume to maintain CO and exercise levels.[9,10] HR is a major determinant of myocardial oxygen consumption; this decrease in HR allows for an increase in diastolic filling time of coronary arteries, which, in turn, allows for an increase in myocardial oxygen supply in comparison with the "unblocked" state.[6]

All β-blocking drugs (selective β-blockers more than nonselective β-blockers) produce an increase in exercise capacity in patients who have CAD but may decrease physical work capacity in those who only have hypertension.[11-25] The increase noted in physical work capacity with those who have CAD is documented by an increase in VO_{2max} with a decrease in HR and a lower rate pressure product at maximum levels, suggesting myocardial efficiency (Box 28-2). The oxygen economy of the myocardium may also be influenced by the interference of its cellular metabolism.[17]

Propranolol, a nonselective β-blocker, has been found to decrease the myocardial use of free fatty acids, causing a rise in myocardial carbohydrate utilization.[26] This could indicate an oxygen-saving shift in myocardial energy metabolism.[27] Despite the increase in work capacity with a lower rate pressure product, chest pain has been documented to occur, which suggests myocardial insufficiency.[14,20,21] This mechanism is not fully understood; the explanation may be that an increase in left

BOX 28-2 Central (Cardiac) Responses During Exercise of Patients with Coronary Artery Disease While Taking a β-Blocker

Variable	Response
RHR	↓
MHR	↓ 20%–30%
SBP	↓
RPP	↓
CO	↓ 5%–23%
MVO_2	↑
CBF	↓
TET	↑
DFT	↑
Exercise capacity	↑
VO_2max	↑
SV	↑ Moderate exercise
DF	↑
Myocardial contractility	↓
ST depression	↓
Myocardial efficiency	↑
Ischemic threshold	↓

↑, Increase; ↓, decrease; *RHR*, resting heart rate; *MHR*, maximum heart rate; *SBP*, systolic blood pressure; *RPP*, rate pressure product; *CO*, cardiac output; *MVO_2*, myocardial oxygen consumption; *CBF*, coronary blood flow; *TET*, total exercise time; *DFT*, diastolic filling time; *VO_{2max}*, maximum oxygen consumption; *SV*, stroke volume; *DF*, diastolic function.

ventricular volume and ejection time is caused by the decrease in HR and contractility, which may increase myocardial oxygen demand.[16]

Another finding in the literature is that despite a further decrease in ejection fraction seen with β-blockade during exercise in patients whose ejection fraction is less than 40% at rest, an increase in work capacity is still seen.[13,14,28] This is in keeping with the finding that the left diastolic function, and not the left systolic function, predicts exercise tolerance.[29,30] β-Blockers have the potential to increase exercise tolerance by improving diastolic function.[31] They lengthen the diastolic period and improve subendocardial perfusion, in addition to decreasing left ventricular filling pressure and increasing left ventricular compliance.[13]

β-Blockers, particularly propranolol, may prevent the "coronary steal" phenomenon. Bortone et al found that despite coronary constriction at rest, coronary constriction of the stenosed segments during exercise was prevented with propranolol.[32] Drug administration causes "reverse coronary steal" by the redistribution of the coronary blood flow from normal to ischemic regions, perhaps by way of collaterals.

Selective and nonselective β-blockers have the same effect on cardiac parameters as described previously. However, their differences lie in their pharmacokinetics; in their pulmonary influence; and in their metabolic, thermoregulatory, and vascular resistance effects.[6,7,24,33] Nonselective β-blockers have adverse effects on these parameters, so when medication is prescribed for active patients, β_1 drugs tend to be preferred (Box 28-3). It is important to note that β-blockers with intrinsic sympathomimetic activity confer no advantage during exercise.[6,7,24]

Some of the nonselective drugs are lipophilic and readily cross the blood–brain barrier to enter the central nervous system (CNS).[6,7] This may account for the CNS adverse effects (nightmares, fatigue, depression) seen with use of these agents.[34] It is presumed that these adverse effects can have implications for an individual's perception of the exercise bout and the physical therapist should keep this in mind as he or she is attempting to promote a positive feeling regarding exercise.[6]

BOX 28-3 Nonselective β-Blockade and Metabolic and Thermoregulatory Responses During Exercise

Variable	Responses
Fatigue	↑
Thermoregulation	Accelerated sweating response; dehydration
Fat utilization	Inhibition of intramuscular lipolysis; reduction in adipose tissue lipolysis
Glucose utilization	Inhibitory effect on muscle glycogen breakdown
Decrease in blood glucose levels:	Impaired hepatic glycogenolysis Reduced hepatic gluconeogenesis Possible inhibitory effect on glucose uptake by exercising muscles

Thermoregulation is affected by β-blockers as a result of an accelerated sweating response of approximately 10%.[24] This mechanism is not fully understood because nonselective agents cause peripheral constriction. Nevertheless, dehydration may occur if fluid replacement is not done during exercise. Skin blood flow is also impaired as a result of a reduction in CO during exercise.[25] Even though the stroke volume does increase to compensate for the decrease in HR, which maintains the CO, stroke volume plateaus at 40% of the person's VO_{2max} despite existing disease.[35] Fluid replacement is important during exercise to prevent the decrease in BP that has been seen in patients participating in cardiac rehabilitation programs, especially those taking propranolol (anecdotal findings).

Metabolically, both selective and nonselective β-blockers have effects on fat, glucose, and triglyceride utilization during exercise, but nonselective blockers seem to have a greater effect. Refer to the article by Head for a detailed discussion of this subject.[7] This abnormality of metabolism can contribute to the premature fatigue experienced during exercise and also contributes to the unpleasantness sometimes associated with exercise during treatment with these drugs. The kinetics of drug release can also affect metabolic changes and exercise performance. Exercising at peak plasma concentrations can cause more fatigue and thus decrease exercise performance. Peak concentrations generally occur about 90 minutes after administration of β-blockers.[36] Also, at higher doses, the selectivity appears to decrease, and the benefits of a selective β-blocker are lost.[37]

Exercise Prescription for Patients Taking β-Blockers. It is accepted that patients with CAD are able to attain a physiologic exercise effect, regardless of the type of β-blocker they are taking.[7,24,38] The general principles of exercise and prescription apply to this population as well.[4,35] The only exceptions are due to the pharmacokinetic properties of β-blockers. The exercise prescription needs to be individualized according to the results of an exercise test performed while the person is taking the β-blocker.[6,24] Also, the exercise should take place at the same time each day to avoid differences in the plasma concentrations of the β-blocker and thus different exercise responses. Appropriate action needs to be taken when the patient experiences any of the adverse effects during exercise.[4] An exercise prescription should be based on the factors that are listed in the box below.[39-44]

Type of exercise: aerobic for both upper and lower extremities and anaerobic for both upper and lower extremities if the patient meets the American Association of Cardiovascular and Pulmonary Rehabilitation criteria[39]
Mode: walking, stationary biking, upper extremity endurance training, rowing, dual-action devices
Frequency: 3 to 5 days per week
Duration: 20 to 60 minutes of continuous exercise
Intensity: 40% to 75% of Karvonen's formula ([(max HR − resting HR [RHR]) × %] + RHR) with HR_{max} taken from the peak HR obtained during the stress test
Monitoring:
1. All patients should exercise on the basis of the calculated intensity of their target heart rate (THR).
2. Rate of perceived exertion can only be used as an adjunct to HR monitoring.[6,40-42]

Guidelines:
1. Exercise should occur at the same time each day.
2. Fluid replacement needs to be provided during the exercise session.
3. Pulse rate should be measured by the patient to monitor the THR during exercise.
4. The training HR must always be obtained by the patient's performance during the stress test conducted while he or she is taking medication.
5. If the patient does not take the medication, the exercise intensity is limited to an HR of 20 beats/min above resting value.[4]
6. If the medication is changed to another β-blocker or if the dose is adjusted, then the exercise HR is limited to 20 beats/min above resting value.[4]
7. The patient still requires a THR for skilled physical therapy.
8. The intensity of exercise should be limited to the THR so as not to violate the ischemic threshold during training.[43,44]
9. If nitroglycerin is prescribed, the patient should carry it at all times.

Calcium Channel Blockers

The introduction of calcium channel blockers in the treatment of cardiovascular disease has been considered the most significant advance in therapy since the introduction of β-blockers.[45,46] Calcium ion antagonists are used to decrease myocardial contractility, reduce peripheral vascular resistance, and dilate coronary arteries.[47] The resulting increase in coronary blood flow and reduced pressures is believed to decrease myocardial oxygen demand during exercise and thus prevent exertional angina pectoris.[48] Calcium channel blockers are not equal in their reactions and differ in their primary antianginal mechanisms because of their different chemical structures.[49-51] This results in different exercise effects based on the type of calcium channel blocker administered.

Dihydropyridines (amlodipine, nicardipine, nifedipine) increase HR at rest and at maximal exercise levels but are more vascular selective with less effect on nodal tissue than other calcium channel blockers.[47] This increase in HR can, in turn, increase myocardial oxygen consumption and possibly induce angina pectoris.[52] However, in general, this class of drugs will increase exercise time, increase the time before ST-segment depression, increase time to angina, and decrease the incidence of angina.[47,53,54]

Dihydropyridines are also known for decreasing BP—both the systolic and diastolic readings—in normotensive as well as hypertensive individuals. In some individuals, when BP is lowered to a great extent, the heart compensates by producing a reflex tachycardia.[53,55,56] The ensuing increase in myocardial oxygen consumption, caused by the increase in HR, creates additional angina. Amlodipine and nifedipine are the two drugs in this class that produce this adverse effect. Amlodipine is also known for producing lower extremity edema as a result of local effects on microcirculation.[47,52,57] Another serious adverse effect with this group is the coronary steal phenomenon.[58,59] This occurs because blood is shunted away from the ischemic region to the nonischemic region, which worsens myocardial ischemia and thus increases episodes of angina.[60] This phenomenon will occur only in patients with good collateral blood flow.

Other commonly used calcium channel blockers such as diltiazem and verapamil influence cardiac muscle and nodal activity to a greater degree than do dihydropyridines. This property makes diltiazem and verapamil more effective than dihydropyridines in the treatment of exertional angina.[54] They reduce HR at rest and during exercise because of their nonspecific inhibition of sympathetic drive. They are effective in the treatment of supraventricular tachycardia and atrial fibrillation because they slow conduction through the atrioventricular node, thereby increasing the PR interval.[47,48,53,57] The reduction in HR reduces myocardial oxygen consumption in these patients and the incidence of exertional angina, thus having a greater impact on effort-induced indices of myocardial ischemia. Diltiazem and verapamil therefore reduce myocardial oxygen demand better than the dihydropyridines.[53] They also dilate the coronary arteries and have negative chronotropic and mild inotropic effects, while also reducing peripheral vascular resistance to a lesser extent, compared with dihydropyridines.[47,53] Diltiazem and verapamil will decrease submaximal and maximal BP but not resting BP, thus preventing the reflex tachycardia seen with dihydropyridines.[48] Calcium channel blockers also increase exercise time, increase the time before ST-segment depression, increase time to angina, and decrease the incidence of angina.[47,48,53]

Therefore, given the varying effects of calcium channel blockers, it seems logical that an active patient with mild-to-moderate hypertension would probably perform better with a dihydropyridine, whereas a lower-functioning patient with exertional angina would do better with either verapamil or diltiazem. Because emerging evidence indicates that many patients with exertional angina have both CAD and increased vasomotor tone, these patients may perform better with diltiazem.[61,62] This "dynamic obstruction" is superimposed on a fixed obstruction, which results in variability of the anginal threshold during exercise, and may be a contributing factor to the pathogenesis of myocardial ischemia.[63] Diltiazem has also been shown to increase resting coronary blood flow, increase resting and exercise levels of the left ventricular ejection fraction, and produce less depression of ventricular muscle.[57,64] Box 28-4 presents a summary of the hemodynamic responses produced by calcium channel blockers.

Exercise Prescription for Patients Taking Calcium Channel Blockers. The guidelines for patients taking calcium channel blockers are similar to those for patients taking β-blockers. The general principles of exercise apply as well to patients taking calcium ion antagonists. The most important consideration would be the class of calcium blockers the patient is taking. This would provide a general idea of what to expect during rest as well as during the exercise session. If the patient experiences any adverse effects of exercise, appropriate action must be taken immediately (see box below).[1]

Type of exercise: aerobic for both upper and lower extremities and anaerobic for both upper and lower extremities if the patient meets the American Association of Cardiovascular and Pulmonary Rehabilitation criteria[39]

Mode: walking, stationary biking, upper extremity endurance training, rowing, dual-action devices

Frequency: 3 to 5 days per week

Duration: 20 to 60 minutes of continuous exercise

Intensity: 40% to 75% of Karvonen's formula ([(max HR – RHR) × %] + RHR) with HR max taken from the peak HR obtained during the stress test

Monitoring:

1. All patients should exercise on the basis of the calculated intensity of their THR.
2. Rate of perceived exertion can only be used as an adjunct to HR monitoring.[6,40-42]

Guidelines:

1. Exercise should occur at the same time each day.
2. Pulse rate should be measured by the patient to monitor HR during exercise.
3. Adverse effects are more common with dihydropyridines: reflex tachycardia, edema of the ankles, increase in RHR, and possible increase in angina during exercise.
4. If the patient does not take his or her medication, the exercise intensity should be limited to an HR of 20 beats/min above RHR.[4]
5. If the medication is changed to another calcium channel blocker or if the dose is adjusted, then the exercise HR is limited to 20 beats/min above resting HR.[4]
6. The patient still requires a THR for skilled physical therapy.
7. The intensity of exercise should be limited to the THR so as not to violate the ischemic threshold during training.[43,44]
8. If nitroglycerin is prescribed, the patient should carry it at all times.

BOX 28-4 Hemodynamic Responses of Calcium Channel Blockers

Variable	Dihydropyridines	Benzothiazepines
RHR	↑	↓
MHR	↑	↓
MVO_2	↑	↓
TET	↑	↑
Time to ST depression	↑	↑
Time to angina	↑	↑
Anginal incidence	↓	↔
RSBP	↓	↔
RDBP	↓	↔
Reflex tachycardia	θ	↔
Edema (LEs)	θ	↔
Coronary steal	θ	↔
Dilatation of coronary arteries	↔	θ

↑, Increase; ↓↓ decrease; ↔, no effect; θ, has an effect; *RHR*, resting heart rate; *MHR*, maximum heart rate; *MVO_2*, myocardial oxygen consumption; *TET*, total exercise time; *RSBP*, resting systolic blood pressure; *RDBP*, resting diastolic blood pressure; *LEs*, lower extremity.

β-Blockers or Calcium Channel Blockers for the Exercising Patient with Cardiac Disease. In a meta-analysis, Heidenreich et al compared the relative efficacy and tolerability of treatment with β-blockers and calcium channel blockers in patients with stable angina pectoris.[56] A total of 143 articles were identified by MEDLINE and EMBASE searches, of which 90 fulfilled the inclusion criteria of the authors. Their results showed the following: (1) There was no significant difference in the cardiac death and myocardial infarction rates between patients taking β-blockers and those taking calcium channel blockers; (2) significantly fewer episodes of angina were observed per week in patients taking β-blockers than in those taking calcium channel blockers; (3) calcium channel blockers were discontinued significantly more often than were β-blockers because of adverse events; and (4) no significant differences were found between the drugs in time to ischemia or in exercise time to ischemia. Heidenreich et al concluded: "β-Blockers should be considered first-line agents because they are as effective as and better tolerated than calcium antagonists and have been shown to improve prognosis in other populations with coronary disease."[56]

PULMONARY MEDICATIONS

Chronic obstructive pulmonary disease (COPD) is a major cause of morbidity and mortality in the United States. Currently, it is ranked as the fourth major cause of death, affecting an estimated 11.2 million people. It is estimated that 24 million more adults have some evidence of impaired lung function, indicating an underdiagnosis of the disease.[65] The projected economic cost of lung disease is expected to be $177 billion in 2009—$144 billion in direct health expenditures and $64 billion in the indirect cost of morbidity and mortality—according to estimates made by the National Heart, Lung, and Blood Institute. Currently, there is no cure for COPD, although two treatments—smoking cessation and long-term oxygen therapy—will increase survival.[66,67] Bronchodilators will increase exercise capacity, but there is no evidence that this will increase the survival rate. However, an increase in exercise capacity will improve quality of life and the patient's ability to perform activities of daily living (ADLs). The focus of this section is bronchodilators and their effect on exercise capacity.

Bronchodilator Therapy

A main goal of bronchodilator therapy is to reduce the airflow limitation in the airways, thereby decreasing dyspnea and improving exercise tolerance.[68] Dyspnea can be caused by many factors, including airway obstruction, impaired gas exchange, thoracic hyperinflation, impaired ventilatory mechanics and diaphragmatic function, loss of elastic lung recoil, respiratory and peripheral muscle weakness, and deconditioning.[67] Despite these differences in physiology, according to the literature, it is fairly clear that dyspnea is relieved by bronchodilators, regardless of the cause of impairment or class of bronchodilators administered. However, the reductions in dyspnea during exercise noted in response to these drugs appear to be closely related to the reduction in dynamic hyperinflation.[69]

Although bronchodilators seemingly improve exercise capacity, it is difficult to determine from the literature which type is best for which patient. Comparisons between studies are often difficult to make. Liesker et al present the following five reasons for this confusion: (1) failure to clarify whether the patients were limited in exercise because of their ventilatory capacity or limited by nonventilatory reasons such as cardiovascular limitations, decrease in muscle performance or motivation, or diminished diffusion capacity; (2) exclusion, in some studies, of patients with reversible airway disease such as asthma; (3) variability in dosing of the bronchodilator; (4) administration of tests that were sensitive to a learning effect; and (5) the small number of patients in the studies.[68] Oga et al added to this list by reporting on the variability of exercise tests used to measure the outcome of improved exercise capacity.[70] They discovered that a cycle endurance test was much more sensitive in detecting the effects of an anticholinergic drug on exercise capacity than was the 6-minute walk test or a progressive cycle ergometry test. Other researchers have criticized the use of forced expiratory volume in 1 second (FEV_1) as a measure of exercise capacity, stating that it is not a sensitive marker of bronchodilator responsiveness.[71] Instead, they use inspiratory capacity as a marker of responsiveness because dynamic hyperinflation is considered to be responsible for the dyspnea noted during exercise. Moreover, inspiratory capacity is predictive of an improvement in exercise tolerance and a reduction in dyspnea, and FEV_1 is not.[72]

In a systematic review of the effects of bronchodilators on exercise capacity by Liesker et al, 33 double-blind, randomized, placebo-controlled studies were selected and reviewed.[68] Exercise capacity was measured by either a steady-state or an incremental exercise test, both of which measure cardiorespiratory endurance. Dyspnea was measured by using the Borg scale slope (ΔBorg score/ΔVO_{2max}). This parameter indicates the rise in dyspnea when patients increase their oxygen consumption during exercise. Only half the studies reviewed demonstrated a significant positive effect of bronchodilation on exercise capacity. Anticholinergics showed the most significant effects, with high-dose therapies tending to show better results than low-dose therapies. Short-acting β_2 sympathomimetics also produced significant positive effects on exercise capacity, but this was not the case with the longer-acting ones. Methylxanthines showed negative effects on exercise capacity. The review also indicated that the addition of a second bronchodilator showed no proven advantage in improving exercise capacity. Finally, the majority of the studies demonstrated a reduction in dyspnea, even in the absence of improvement in exercise capacity.

In a newer study by Oga et al, the effects of salbutamol (a short-acting β_2 sympathomimetic) on exercise endurance were compared with those of ipratropium (an anticholinergic bronchodilator).[73] Improvement in exercise capacity, as measured by time on a cycle endurance test, was equal with both types of bronchodilators. Oga et al concluded that both types could be used as first-line drugs in the treatment of patients with COPD who want to exercise.[73] They also found that the effects on exercise capacity varied within individuals, possibly because of a complex mechanism responsible for the different effects of bronchodilators on exercise capacity versus airflow limitation.

Weiner et al investigated the cumulative effects of the long-acting bronchodilator (LABD) salmeterol, exercise, and inspiratory muscle exercise on the perception of dyspnea in patients with advanced COPD.[74] The LABD had no effect on exercise capacity, FEV_1, or the perception of dyspnea. The nonsignificant results of FEV_1 are in keeping with the conclusion of Newton et al who found that this was not a sensitive measure for airway responsiveness.[71] The significant results, however, indicated that inspiratory muscle exercise decreased the perception of dyspnea and that the endurance exercise increased the 6-minute-walk test time.

Brusasco et al examined health outcomes after treatments with tiotropium (anticholinergic) and salmeterol (LABD) in patients with COPD.[75] The outcome measures consisted of exacerbations, health resource use, dyspnea, health-related quality of life, and spirometry. Results showed that anticholinergics had more significant effects on all these measures. Exacerbations and health resource use were significantly less, and there were significant improvements in responses to the health-related quality-of-life survey, demonstration of an improved FEV_1 by spirometric test results, and the improved perception of dyspnea.

It appears that anticholinergics and short-acting β_2 sympathomimetics improve exercise capacity and reduce dyspnea in patients with COPD. Anticholinergics also improve quality-of-life measures as compared with an LABD. Methylxanthines appear to have negative effects on exercise capacity in patients with COPD. Their adverse effects appear to be significantly deleterious as well. They include tachycardia, hypertension, palpitations, chest pain, agitation, dizziness, and headache.[76] The adverse effects of β_2 sympathomimetics include tremor, palpitation, headache, nervousness, dizziness, nausea, and hypertension; and anticholinergics appear to have fewer adverse effects, which include delirium, hallucinations, and decreased gastrointestinal (GI) activity.[76]

Anticholinergics are used more frequently than are β-agonists in patients with COPD because of their more effective bronchodilator properties and fewer adverse effects.[77,78] β-agonists are also known to cause adverse effects at rest after administration (i.e., a significant drop in PaO_2) by inhalation through the mechanism of a worsening ventilation/perfusion ratio.[79] Saito et al looked at the effects of an anticholinergic (oxitropium) and a β_2 sympathomimetic (fenoterol) on pulmonary hemodynamics at rest and during exercise in patients with COPD.[80] The purpose of this study was to determine whether the resting effects of the β_2 sympathomimetic improved or worsened during exercise. Fenoterol caused a significant increase in HR, CO, mixed venous oxygen tension, and oxygen delivery and a significant decrease in pulmonary vascular resistance, PaO_2, and $PaCO_2$. During rest, oxitropium caused a significant decrease in HR and oxygen delivery. These differences between these drugs were not seen during exercise. Both classes of drugs significantly attenuated exercise-induced increases in pulmonary artery pressure, pulmonary capillary wedge pressure, and right arterial pressure. Thus both classes of drugs were equally effective in attenuating right heart afterloads during exercise in patients with COPD, with the main differences in pulmonary hemodynamics occurring at rest. This is an important consideration because these values have a tendency to stay at resting levels in most patients.

In summary, compared with other classes of bronchodilators, anticholinergics are more effective in increasing exercise capacity and decreasing dyspnea, have fewer central effects at rest, better improve quality of life and attenuate right heart afterloads during exercise, and have fewer adverse effects when they are used for the treatment of COPD. These drugs are taken by a metered-dose inhaler (MDI) or a dry powder inhaler (DPI). The DPI is easier for the patient to use because there is no need for coordination with breathing as with the MDI. See Box 28-5 for the summary of rest and exercise responses of the bronchodilators.

COPD is now considered a systemic disease, with cardiovascular and musculoskeletal impairments starting early in the disease process.[81] Exercise performance

BOX 28-5 Responses of Bronchodilators at Rest and During Exercise

Variable	β-Mimetics	Xanthines	Anticholinergics
Dyspnea	↓	↓	↓
Exercise capacity	↓ (LABD)	Ø	↑↑↑ (SABD)
Exacerbations	↔	NS	↓
Health resource usage	↔	NS	↓
Quality of life	↔	NS	↑
Adverse effects	↑	↑↑	↓
RHR	↑	↑	↓
$RPaO_2$	↓	NS	↔
$EpaO_2$	↑	↑	↑
BP	↑	↑↓	↔

↑, Increase; ↓, decrease; ↔, no effect; ↑↓, increase or decrease; Ø, negative effects; *LABD*, long-acting bronchodilator; *SABD*, short-acting bronchodilator; *RHR*, resting heart rate; *$RPaO_2$*, resting partial pressure of oxygen; *$EPaO_2$*, exercising partial pressure of oxygen; *BP*, blood pressure.

is limited because of physical deconditioning, even in patients with only mild degrees of airway obstruction.[82] It is vital that all patients with COPD start an exercise program that is safe, with due consideration of their impairments and the effects of their medications on their exercise response.

Exercise Prescription for the Patient Taking Bronchodilators. It is a well-accepted fact that patients with COPD benefit from exercise, even though it has not resulted in measurable effects on the respiratory system.[4,83] Its positive effects on dyspnea and the importance of physical deconditioning as a comorbid factor in advanced lung disease make exercise a very important factor in the treatment of patients with COPD. Some of the benefits of exercise include increased exercise capacity, increased functional ability, decreased severity of dyspnea, and improved quality of life. The prescription follows the basics of exercise and is based on the individual patient's severity of disease, exercise test results, and impairments.[4,83] If a patient experiences any adverse effects during exercise, appropriate action must be taken immediately.[4]

Type of exercise: aerobic for both upper and lower extremities and anaerobic for both upper and lower extremities
Mode: walking, stationary biking, upper extremity endurance training, rowing, dual-action devices
Specific respiratory techniques: pursed lip breathing, respiratory muscle training, supplemental oxygen therapy, breathing exercises, ventilatory strategies, energy conservation techniques, posture re-education, airway clearance techniques if necessary
Frequency: 3 to 5 days per week
Duration: 20 to 30 minutes of continuous exercise; initially, intermittent training may be necessary with rest periods of 3 to 5 minutes between bouts
Intensity: 60% of Karvonen's formula ([(max HR – RHR) × %] + RHR) with HR_{max} taken from the peak HR obtained during the stress test
Monitoring:
1. All patients should exercise on the basis of the calculated intensity of their THR.
2. Symptoms must be monitored (e.g., shortness of breath, paradoxical breathing pattern, leg fatigue).
3. SpO_2 saturation of oxygen with hemoglobin should be monitored.

Guidelines:
1. Paradoxical breathing is the first clinical sign of respiratory muscle fatigue.
2. RHR will be elevated in patients taking β-agonists and methylxanthines.
3. More serious adverse effects will occur with the methylxanthines.
4. Monitor for signs of right ventricular failure.
5. Patients should exercise at the same drug plasma levels by exercising at the same time each day.
6. If a rescue inhaler is prescribed, the patient should carry it, especially during physical therapy.

DIABETES MEDICATIONS

Diabetes mellitus (DM) is a metabolic disorder characterized by hyperglycemia resulting from defects in insulin secretion, insulin action, and glucose sensing by the pancreas.[84] Complications of DM include heart disease, stroke, hypertension, blindness, kidney disease, nervous system disease, amputations, dental disease, complications of pregnancy, and susceptibility to illness, and biochemical imbalances.[85] Disturbances in fat, protein, and carbohydrate metabolism also occur, causing additional complications during exercise. The most lethal potential complication is hypoglycemia, which occurs more frequently in type 1 (T1) DM than in type 2 (T2) DM. Microvascular and macrovascular complications are directly related to the level of glycemic control, and patients with tightly controlled T1DM exhibit more frequent episodes of hypoglycemia. Patients with DM, regardless of the type, also demonstrate endothelial dysfunction, decrease in baroreflex sensitivity, autonomic dysfunction of the parasympathetic nervous system or of both parasympathetic and sympathetic nervous systems, impaired cardiac function, and altered energetic properties of both skeletal and cardiac muscles—all of which potentially alter exercise capacity. These will be explored later in relation to their effects on exercise response. The focus of this section is the interaction between exercise and drug therapy.

Antidiabetic Medications, Exercise, and Glucose Utilization Pathways

The use of exercise as a treatment for diabetes is critical to the well-being of patients who have this metabolic disorder. Although there are not many rules to follow, some very specific guidelines must be followed with patients taking antidiabetic medications.

The main class of oral antidiabetic medications that produce hypoglycemia is the sulfonylureas. These drugs increase insulin production and subsequently lower plasma glucose concentrations.[86-88] Exercise is also known to cause a decrease in plasma glucose and insulin concentrations in the postabsorptive as well as postprandial states.[89] The important question is whether the combined effect of exercise and a sulfonylurea will cause an increase in the hypoglycemic response. Three recent studies have attempted to examine this response, but design flaws weaken their conclusions.[90-92] Riddle et al examined the effect of exercise in 25 moderately obese subjects with T2DM. Subjects underwent an exercise test consisting of treadmill walking at 2.5 mph for 90 minutes before and after 9 weeks of either glipizide or placebo treatment. Outcome measures included plasma glucose, insulin, and C-peptide concentrations.[90] No real conclusions could be drawn with regard to the effect of the drug on exercise performance or plasma glucose concentration from this study because testing had been conducted at too low an intensity, and "exercise only" and "medication only" treatment groups were not included. Massi et al demonstrated that greater decrease in plasma glucose levels occurred when exercise was combined with either glibenclamide or glimepiride than when exercise was done alone; however, a "drug-only" treatment group was not included in this study.[91] A third study by Larsen et al did succeed in demonstrating an enhanced hypoglycemic response with the combination of exercise and glibenclamide.[92] In this study, the design flaws were minimized, the exercise intensity was individualized for each patient, and the appropriate guidelines were followed. Glibenclamide increased plasma insulin concentrations, thus lowering hepatic glucose production, while glucose clearance remained unchanged. Exercise, on the other hand, decreased plasma glucose concentrations by increasing glucose clearance. This is in keeping with the fact that patients with T2DM have defective insulin-stimulated glucose uptake and insulin-stimulated GLUT 4 translocation but have normal contraction-stimulated glucose uptake and GLUT 4 translocation.[93-95] Patients with T2DM retain the capacity to translocate GLUT 4 to the sarcolemma in response to exercise. The actual risk of developing serious hypoglycemia will depend on the pharmacokinetics and pharmacodynamics of the particular sulfonylurea and the increase in the plasma insulin levels before the start of exercise.

Concerns have been expressed about the safety of sulfonylureas, especially in combination with exercise, with regard to cardiac mortality.[96-99] In the University Groups Diabetes Program and the Bypass Angioplasty Revascularization Investigation, patients taking sulfonylureas experienced a higher mortality rate as a result of cardiac dysfunction than those taking alternatives.[100,101] One explanation may be that sulfonylureas cause loss of ischemic preconditioning. Ischemic preconditioning refers to a protective mechanism in the heart that reduces ischemia and subsequent myocardial damage after temporary blockage of coronary blood flow or after short-term increase in myocardial oxygen demand, as in exercise. Essentially, this is the heart's "warm-up." In terms of exercise, this phenomenon reduces ischemia during a closely followed second bout of exercise.[102] The adenosine triphosphate (ATP)–sensitive potassium channel located in cardiomyocytes and in vascular smooth muscle is believed to mediate this ischemic preconditioning. The open channel has a role in the regulation of coronary blood flow and also in protecting cardiac muscle from ischemia.[103] Therefore, when this channel is blocked by the sulfonylureas, there is "no flow" after ischemia.[104-106] Övünç studied this phenomenon in 18 patients with T2DM.[107] Subjects underwent two consecutive treadmill tests with a 15-minute rest period between each test, with and without the sulfonylurea. It was found that glibenclamide eliminated the warm-up phenomenon and diminished the improvement in the ischemic threshold and exercise tolerance during the second bout of exercise. The author concluded that this drug should be used carefully in patients with CAD.

Glimepiride, a third-generation sulfonylurea, differs from the other sulfonylureas in that it is associated with a lower risk of hypoglycemia and less weight gain.[108] There is also evidence that myocardial preconditioning is preserved with this drug because glimepiride was shown to have less influence on the cardiovascular mitochondrial ATP-sensitive potassium (KATP) channels.[109] Other oral antidiabetic agents do not produce such serious adverse effects, especially when they are combined with exercise. Generally, if hypoglycemia results from other agents besides sulfonylureas, it is due to the patient taking an increased dose to offset his or her "sugar" intake.

As discussed previously, patients with T2DM still have normal contraction-stimulated glucose uptake and GLUT 4 translocation.[12] A study by Musi et al demonstrated that an acute bout of exercise in patients with T2DM increases glucose uptake via the insulin-independent pathway mediated by the activation of adenosine monophosphate–activated protein kinase (AMPK).[110] AMPK is a protein consisting of one catalytic subunit and two regulatory subunits.[111,112] Two isoforms of the catalytic subunit have been identified—α_1 and α_2. AMPK-α_1 is widely distributed; AMPK-α_2 is predominantly localized in the skeletal muscle, heart, and liver.[113] Musi et al found that exercise significantly increased AMPK-α_2 activity 2.7-fold over basal activity; this protein expression was also found in those without diabetes.[110] In another study, Musi et al also demonstrated a significant increase in AMPK-α_2 activity in the skeletal muscle after 10 weeks of treatment with metformin.[114] The increase in AMPK activity results in the stimulation of glucose uptake in muscle, fatty acid oxidation in muscle and liver, and inhibition of hepatic glucose production. In a 26-week double-blind trial in which patients received rosiglitazone or metformin, metformin was shown to improve contraction-stimulated glucose uptake via the AMPK pathway but had no effect on the insulin-stimulated glucose uptake.[115] Activation of AMPK-α_2 enhances GLUT 4 translocation and hence increases glucose utilization during exercise. Rosiglitazone (a thiazolidinedione), however, improved insulin responsiveness via the insulin receptor in resting skeletal muscle and doubled the insulin-stimulated glucose uptake during physical exercise by improving insulin-stimulated glucose uptake.

Patients with T1DM, who are also insulin resistant, appear to have a defect in both pathways for glucose uptake, insulin-stimulated and contraction-stimulated.[116] In a study by Peltoniemi et al., it was shown that patients with T1DM had a blunted effect with the two pathways; thus, even exercise did not increase glucose uptake in these patients.[116] The authors hypothesized that the increase in free fatty acids seen in this population could account for the diminished ability of exercise to stimulate glucose uptake. The higher free fatty acid concentrations might have caused a lower rate of glucose uptake, either through impaired insulin signaling or substrate competition.[117,118] Insulin resistance can be reversed in patients with T1DM if glycemic control is normalized.[119,120]

Much of the research surrounding insulins examines their effect with regard to hypoglycemia and glycemic control with either aerobic exercise (see Chapter 14) or no exercise component at all. However, metabolic responses to intermittent high intensity exercise are different from those to moderately intense aerobic exercise. Several studies conducted recently have attempted to determine glucoregulatory responses to exercise that closely resembles a variety of sports and also mimics child's play. One study utilized a work-recovery interval of 4 seconds of high intensity bouts (sprints) with 2 minutes of rest, for 20 minutes.[121] Patients were administered their usual morning insulin dose followed by a typical breakfast with exercise commencing 2 hours later. As expected, there was a decrease in glucose levels compared with the control (inactive) group, but during the post-workout hour, glucose levels in the exercise group remained the same, whereas the control group's continued to decline. Overall, the total declines in blood sugar levels in the exercise group and in the control group were similar. A similar study was conducted subsequently, but in this study the rest periods were replaced by lower-intensity continuous exercise (active recovery performed at 40% VO_{2max}), and the control group received continuous moderate-intensity exercise.[122] Even though the treatment group performed more total work, there was less of a decline in glucose compared with the group performing continuous aerobic exercise; and this decline extended into the post-exercise period. The conclusion drawn from both these studies was that intermittent high-intensity exercise designed to mimic sports such as soccer lessened the decline in glucose level compared with continuous aerobic exercise. This indicates that young adults who are physically active may not need to lower their pre-exercise insulin dose as much as previously recommended.[123] However, these studies did not explore any late-onset hypoglycemia and also did not look at subjects of varying ages or subjects with varying physical conditions.

Since some types of exercise have been shown to increase the rate and amount of absorption of insulin when it is injected near active exercise sites, it has long been recommended that it be injected in the abdomen or in the deltoid area before lower extremity activity. However, a recent study using glargine, the new long-acting, peakless insulin, demonstrated no increase in the rate of absorption when it was injected into the thigh prior to continuous aerobic exercise for 30 minutes at a 65% VO_{2max}.[124] These results are in contrast to what has previously been reported with the short-acting insulins, and further study is needed.

Exercise Implications for the Patient with T1DM. It is important to note that exercise will increase glucose utilization several-fold; thus hypoglycemia is a frequent problem in patients with insulin-treated diabetes and one of the most common reasons for patients not exercising. Insulin dosage may need to be adjusted, or carbohydrate ingestion before exercise may be needed. The physician needs to be consulted when hypoglycemia limits a patient's ability to exercise.

Children and adolescents are prone to a greater variability in blood glucose levels, which has prompted the American Diabetes Association (ADA) to issue a statement recommending that physical activity is a vital part of managing youth T1DM but that careful supervision is necessary for the prevention or management of hypoglycemia.[125] The following guidelines were established after a review of the literature by Rachmiel et al.[126]

1. School-aged children should be encouraged to engage in 30 to 60 minutes of moderate or vigorous physical activity daily.
2. Blood glucose (BG) should be monitored before, during, and after exercise. *After* is defined as 2 hours after the stoppage of activity as well as in the middle of the night if the activity occurred in late afternoon. BG level prior to exercise is the most important factor predicting exercise-induced hypoglycemia—with a level lower than 6.6 mmol/L, the risk is very high.
3. Insulin injection and insulin pump insertion sites should be located in a non-exercising limb to prevent the increase in insulin flow due to the increase in blood flow.
4. A reduction of insulin by 30% to 50% is recommended for planned activity that is mild to moderate.
5. An increase in carbohydrate (CHO) consumption is recommended for nonplanned activity during and after exercise. An extra 15 to 30 g of CHO per every 60 minutes of moderate activity should occur and an added 15 to 30 g after the activity ends.
6. To treat hypoglycemia during exercise, add an extra 30 to 45 g of oral simple glucose.
7. To prevent nocturnal hypoglycemia, pre-bedtime glucose should be higher than 7.2 mmol/L on days of activity. The young person should eat a complex CHO meal and a large bedtime snack that comprises foods with a low glycemic index.

The athlete with T1DM also requires guidelines, since firm contraindications to certain sports no longer exist. These guidelines will focus on managing hypoglycemia and hyperglycemia. Other guidelines will be discussed later, since they apply to both types of DM. Simply stated, athletes with T1DM may engage in vigorous activity if they are in good metabolic control. That generally means the A_{1C} is below 7%. If the A_{1C} is above 9%, the athlete is at risk for hyperglycemia and diabetic ketoacidosis (DK), which could result in coma; thus, in this case, exercise will worsen metabolic control or increase the complications of diabetes. The athlete must also know the signs of hypoglycemia. These general guidelines are based on a review by Lisle et al and from the research of Grimm et al and focus more on endurance-type exercises, that is, aerobic exercises.[126,127]

1. Generally, the athlete should eat a meal 1 to 3 hours before exercise, exercise only after peak action of insulin, and delay exercise until glucose and ketones are under control.
2. BG monitoring should occur every 30 minutes if the exercise lasts beyond an hour.
3. Late-onset hypoglycemia should be anticipated, and monitoring of BG should occur even into the late evening.
4. After exercise, ingestion of 30 to 40 g of CHO for every 30 minutes of intensive exercise is required.
5. Insulin is reduced by 20% to 50% based on duration and intensity.
6. CHO ingestion is 15 to 100 g based on duration and intensity.
7. The most important factor is that each athlete will exhibit different metabolic responses to exercise, and insulin and CHO intake need to be adjusted on the basis of their individual responses.

Athletes who perform more of the high-intensity type of exercise—>80% VO_{2max}—have the opposite problem from that of the endurance athlete. These athletes can become hyperglycemic with exercise. This intensity of exercise will utilize the first two energy systems for fuel as the dominant systems—adenosine triphosphate–phosphocreatine (ATP-CP) and anaerobic metabolism. This will cause an increase in the catecholamine response, producing an outpouring of glucose from the liver in excess of glucose uptake. Since in recovery, there is an absence of the normal insulin rise to combat the increase in glucose, prolonged hyperglycemia results. In a review by Guelfi et al, it was concluded that the risk of hypoglycemia is not increased during or immediately following high-intensity exercise; rather, hyperglycemia results. They recommended a small, additional dose of insulin to prevent hyperglycemia.[128]

In summary, the glycemic response will depend on the action of insulin, injection site used, intensity of exercise, metabolic response of the athlete, and other factors that may not be identified at this point in time. Illness will also cause a change in the glycemic response. The best advice for the athlete is to keep himself or herself in good metabolic control; to monitor the BG before, during, and after exercise; and to adjust the insulin dose and CHO ingestion in relation to the BG response.

Diabetic Autonomic Neuropathy and Its Implications for Exercise. Some other factors related to exercise must be considered before the exercise prescription is discussed. Microvascular and macrovascular complications of DM are well known and can have implications for exercise. What is least known is the complication known as diabetic autonomic neuropathy (DAN). This is a neuropathy of the autonomic nervous system (ANS) and can involve every system in the body, especially those systems that receive dual innervation from the parasympathetic and sympathetic fibers. The following discussion is based on reviews by Maser and Lehhard, Boulton et al, and Vinik et al.[129-131]

DAN is among the least recognized and understood complications despite its significant negative impact on survival and quality of life. Hypotheses concerning the etiology of DAN include a metabolic insult to the nerve fibers, neurovascular insufficiency, autoimmune damage, and neurohormonal growth factor deficiency. The result of this multifactorial process may be activation of poly-ADP-ribosylation depletion of ATP, resulting in cell necrosis and activation of genes involved in neuronal damage. The symptoms of DAN are listed in Box 28-6. As can be seen, its effects are widespread and diffuse. DAN is assessed by focusing on the symptoms or dysfunction. The most studied form of DAN is cardiac autonomic neuropathy (CAN) and, by far, the most serious complication. CAN causes abnormalities of HR control, as well as defects in central and peripheral vascular dynamics. The prevalence of CAN varies widely, depending on the cohort studied and the methods of assessment used. Vinik et al found the prevalence to be 80% in people with DM.[131] It is recommended that screening for DAN be done at the time of diagnosis in those with T2DM and within 5 years after diagnosis in those with T1DM.

The clinical manifestations of CAN are listed in Box 28-7. The major ones for our consideration here are exercise intolerance, orthostatic hypotension, hypoglycemia unawareness, and silent myocardial ischemia. Often, it is therapists who recognize this neuropathy from the inappropriate exercise responses of patients. Exercise intolerance will present with blunted HR and BP responses due to a decreased cardiac output and ejection fraction

BOX 28-6 Symptoms of Diabetic Autonomic Neuropathy (DAN)

Cardiovascular	Gastrointestinal	Genitourinary	Metabolic	Pseudomotor
Resting tachycardia	Esophageal dysmotility	Neurogenic bladder	Hypoglycemia unawareness	Anhidrosis
Exercise intolerance	Gastroparesis	Erectile dysfunction	Abnormal and delayed response to hypoglycemia	Heat intolerance
Orthostatic hypotension	Constipation	Female sexual dysfunction	—	Gustatory sweating
Silent myocardial infarction	Diarrhea	—	—	Dry skin

BOX 28-7 Clinical Manifestations of Cardiac Autonomic Neuropathy (CAN)

Exercise intolerance
Intraoperative cardiovascular liability
Orthostatic hypotension
Increased risk of mortality
Autonomic dysfunction
Hypoglycemia unawareness
Silent myocardial ischemia

BOX 28-8 Symptoms of Silent Myocardial Ischemia

Unexplained fatigue	Dysrhythmias
Confusion	Cough
Tiredness	Dyspnea
Edema	Nausea
Hemoptysis	Vomiting
Diaphoresis	

caused by systolic dysfunction and diastolic filling dysfunction. Orthostatic hypotension occurs due to damage to the efferent sympathetic vasomotor fibers, particularly in the splanchnic vasculature. It is defined as a fall in BP >20 mm Hg for systolic or >10 mm Hg for diastolic in response to postural change from the supine position to the standing position. Some may exhibit symptoms, but many will remain asymptomatic with postural changes. Silent myocardial ischemia is defined as impaired timely recognition of myocardial ischemia or infarction. The person will continue to exercise due to the delay in recognizing angina. This is one of the many reasons why rating of perceived exertion (RPE) cannot be used alone as a measure of exercise exertion. Signs and symptoms of silent myocardial ischemia are listed in Box 28-8. It is important to recognize these and stop the person from continuing the exercise. People with DAN do have an increased risk of mortality. According to Vinik et al, the mortality rate among patients with CAN after 5 years is 53%.[131] Sudden death may be caused by severe but asymptomatic ischemia leading to lethal arrhythmias, and mortality rates after an MI are higher. Hypoglycemia unawareness is defined as a hypoglycemic episode that occurs without warning, in which the person does not feel any symptoms. This is believed to be associated with lack of epinephrine release. Frequent BG monitoring is a must to avoid the serious consequences of low blood sugar, and is associated with lack of epinephrine release.

It is important to remember that poor glycemic control plays a central role in the development and progression of CAN. CAN is detected using the tests for autonomic dysfunction, HR variability (HRV), valsalva maneuver, and postural BP testing. HRV is the test that can measure parasympthetic as well as sympathetic nervous system outflow noninvasively. To determine if the autonomic function is returning to normal, HRV is used as a marker for such a change. An increase in PNS tone is positive and shows normalization of autonomic tone.

Medications are used to decrease the effects of CAN, but the results are equivocal. In the review by Maser et al, angiotensin-converting enzyme (ACE) inhibitors, angiotensin type 1 blockers, aldosterone blockers, and calcium channel blockers all had conflicting results—some of the medications, regardless of their class, would decrease the autonomic dysfunction (Δ in HRV) in some patients but not in others and actually worsen it in still others.[129] They concluded that the effect of medications might not be homogeneous, even within the same class. The medications should be tried and the patients monitored to measure the outcomes. Of interest is the effect of β-blockers on mortality and parasympathetic tone.[132,133] In the Cooperative Cardiovascular Project, after an MI, patients with DM had a 36% reduction in mortality, while in the Heart Attack Trial, propranolol improved the recovery of parasympathetic tone and decreased morning sympathetic predominance, leading to an improvement in autonomic function.[132,133] This is counterintuitive to the use of β-blockers, since it is well known that β-blockers mask the signs and symptoms of hypoglycemia. Again, the best treatment for CAN is keeping tight glycemic control—A_{1C} below 7%.

The symptoms of CAN are a late complication, but other complications of exercise can occur and are listed in Box 28-9. All of these must be taken into consideration when prescribing the exercise for patients with CAN. Objective outcomes must be used to evaluate their response to exercise. HR and BP as well as BG levels must be taken before, during, and after exercise.

Screening Prior to an Exercise Program for Those with DM. Before starting an exercise program, the patient is required to obtain clearance from his or her physician with regard to his or her macrovascular or microvascular disease. An ECG stress test is recommended if the individual meets any of the following criteria:[4]

1. Age >35 years, with or without cardiovascular disease risk factors other than diabetes
2. Age >30 years and
   - Type 1 or type 2 diabetes of >10 years' duration
   - Hypertension
   - Cigarette smoking
   - Dyslipidemia
   - Proliferative or preproliferative retinopathy
   - Nephropathy, including microalbuminuria
3. Any of the following, regardless of age:
   - Known or suspected CAD, cerebrovascular disease, and/or peripheral vascular disease
   - Autonomic neuropathy
   - Advanced nephropathy with renal failure
4. Initiating an exercise program >60% of max HR.

Exercise Prescription for those with DM. See the box below for a description of prescription for patients with diabetes mellitus.

Type of exercise: aerobic for both upper and lower extremities and anaerobic for both upper and lower extremities; stretching is very important due to limited joint mobility (LJM)
Mode: walking, stationary biking, upper extremity endurance training, rowing, dual-action devices
Frequency: 4 to 7 days per week of aerobic because the duration of increased insulin sensitivity is 72 hours, thus the time between the sessions should not be more than 72 hours; resistance training is generally 2 to 3 days per week
Duration: 20 to 60 minutes of continuous exercise; add the warm-up and cool-down periods 150 min/wk of moderate intensity aerobic exercise (40% to 60% of Karvonen); 90 min/wk of vigorous intensity aerobic exercise (60% to 75% of Karvonen)
Intensity: 40% to 75% of Karvonen's formula ([(max HR – RHR) × %] + RHR) with HR_{max} taken from the peak HR obtained during the stress test
Monitoring:

1. All patients should exercise on the basis of the calculated intensity of their THR.
2. Rate of perceived exertion can only be used as an adjunct to HR monitoring.

Guidelines:

1. Proper footwear must be worn, and foot inspection needs to occur.
2. Proper identification must be carried by the patient at all times.
3. Fast-acting carbohydrate must be carried by the patient at all times.
4. No exercise should be done if fasting glucose levels are >280 mg/dL.
5. Patient should ingest a carbohydrate if glucose levels are <70 mg/dL before exercise.
6. Glucose level needs to be monitored before, during, and after exercise in those with T1DM and before and after exercise in those with T2 DM.
7. Glucose needs to be monitored 4 to 8 hours after an exercise bout in those with T1DM.
8. Fluid ingestion should occur before, during, and after exercise.
9. For patients with retinopathy:
   a. head jarring activities should be avoided
   b. valsalva should be avoided
   c. position with the head below the waist should be avoided
   d. SBP should not rise above 20–30 mm Hg above RBP
10. For those with nephropathy:
    a. SBP should not rise above 180 mm Hg
    b. weight lifting, breath holding, or high-intensity aerobic exercise should be avoided
11. For those with autonomic neuropathy:
    a. BG signs should be monitored more closely
    b. signs and symptoms of silent ischemia should be monitored for
    c. BP and HR response to exercise may be blunted
12. The patient should not exercise at peak insulin levels (see Table 14-11).
13. Insulin injection sites should be rotated away from active muscles.
14. Exercise should be avoided during illness; illness can increase glucose levels.
15. Alcohol should be avoided 3 hours before exercise and after exercise.
16. Vigorous exercise above 80% of Karvonen can cause hyperglycemia after exercise.
17. Exercise should be avoided prior to bedtime.
18. Patients should be aware of their A_{1C}—a value of 7% is good control.

BOX 28-9 Complications of Exercise

Systemic	Cardiovascular	Metabolic	Musculoskeletal
Retinal hemorrhage	Cardiac dysrhythmias	Increased hyperglycemia	Foot ulcers
Increased proteinuria	Ischemic heart disease	Increased ketosis	Orthopedic injury
Acceleration of microvascular lesions	Hypertensive blood pressure response during exercise	Dehydration	Accelerated joint disease
—	Postexercise orthostatic hypertension	—	—

Adapted from McArdle WD, Katch FI, Katch VL: *Exercise physiology: Energy, nutrition, and human performance* (6th ed.), New York, 2007, Lippincott Williams & Wilkins.

ACTIVITIES 28

Case Study

In this section, you will be given a case study and asked to prescribe an exercise program. This section will also teach you how to actually prescribe on the basis of data from a stress test. A stress test gives objective information regarding exercise responses. Since all patients have a pathology, the normal formula for target HR cannot be used due to medication effect, disease effect, and general deconditioning that is more than their aged-matched controls. Basic answers will be given to assist the reader in this case.

Mrs. S is a 44-year-old woman with a diagnosis of T2DM and CAD. She had a stent placed 1 year ago to treat CAD in one vessel. Since that time she has been diagnosed with T2DM and hypertension. She is a single mother of 3 children ranging in age from 16 to 19 years. She works 50 to 60 hours per week as a paralegal. She reports that she is starting to feel tired and complains of joint pain. Her physician has told her that it was important that she lose weight for health reasons and become more fit. She is eager and motivated to get started. She has no time for a gym but does own a bike and some free weights. She lives in an apartment complex with walkways throughout that are well lit. She has been put on oral medications for diabetes (metformin) and for hypertension and CAD (amlodipine). She has just had another stress test to assess her status. She presents with the following:

Anthropometric Measurements:

Height – 5'4"
Weight – 192 lb
Body fat – 39% (calipers)
BMI – 33

Blood Chemistry:

Triglycerides – 230 mg/dL
HDL – 30 mg/dL
Cholesterol – 260 mg/dL
LDL – 150 mg/dL
Hemoglobin (Hb) – 13 mg/dL
A_{1C} – 15%
BG – 220 mg/dL

Stress Test Results:

Resting HR – 90 beats/min
Resting BP – 140/90 mm Hg
PHR – 140 beats/min
PBP – 180/90 mm Hg
Dysrhythmias – occasional PVCs
Metabolic equivalent (MET) level – 6.8 METs
Reason for stopping – fatigue, shortness of breath (SOB)

Questions

1. Evaluate the information given above.
2. List the risk factors for CAD and T2DM in this patient.
3. Write the exercise prescription.
4. What referrals would you make?
5. Examine the patient.
6. What drug and exercise interactions would you look for?

(The answers given are basic and are meant to help the student stay on the right track. More elaboration is necessary to fully complete the case study.)

REFERENCES

1. Leon AS (Chair), Franklin BA, Costa F, et al: Cardiac rehabilitation and secondary prevention of coronary heart disease. AHA Scientific Statement. Circulation 111:369–376, 2005.
2. American Thoracic Society: Pulmonary rehabilitation: 1999. 1666–1682, 1999.
3. American Diabetes Association: Clinical Practice Recommendations 2004. Position Statement. Physical activity/exercise and diabetes. Diabetes Care 27(1): S58-S62, 2004.
4. Myers J, Nieman D, editors: ACSM's guidelines for exercise testing and prescription (8th ed.), New York, 2009, Lippincott Williams & Wilkins.
5. Lands AM, Arnold A, McAuliff JP, et al: Differentiation of receptor systems activated by sympathomimetic amines. Nature 214:597-598, 1967.
6. Eston R, Connolly D: The use of ratings of perceived exertion for exercise prescription in patients receiving β-blocker therapy. Sports Med 21(3):176-190, 1996.
7. Head A: Exercise metabolism and β-blocker therapy. Sports Med 27(2):81-96, 1999.
8. Joyner MF, Freund BJ, Jilka SM, et al: Effects of beta adrenergic blockade on exercise capacity of trained and untrained men: Haemodynamic comparison. J Appl Physiol 60:1429-1434, 1986.
9. Reybrouck T, Amery A, Fagard R, et al: Haemodynamic responses to graded exercise after chronic beta adrenergic blockade. J Appl Physiol 42:133-138, 1977.
10. Lund-Johansen P: Haemodynamic changes at rest and during exercise in long-term beta-blockade therapy of essential hypertension. Acta Med Scand 195:117-121, 1974.
11. Todd IC, Ballantyne D: Antianginal efficacy of exercise training: A comparison with β-blockade. Br Heart J 64(1):14-19, 1990.
12. Kaski JC, Rodriguez-Plaza L, Brown J, et al: Efficacy of carvedilol in exercise-induced myocardial ischemia. J Cardiovasc Pharmacol 10(suppl.11):S137-S140, 1987.
13. Poulsen SH, Jensen SE, Egstrup K: Improvement of exercise capacity and left ventricular diastolic function with metoprolol XL after acute myocardial infarction. Am Heart J 140(1): 6e-11e, 2000.
14. Steele P, Gold F: Favorable effects of acebutolol on exercise performance and angina in men with coronary artery disease. Chest 82(1):40-43, 1982.
15. Magder S, Sami M, Ripley R, et al: Comparison of the effects of pindolol and propranolol on exercise performance in patients with angina pectoris. Am J Cardiol 59:1289-1294, 1987.
16. Lee G, DeMaria A, Favrot L, et al: Efficacy of acebutolol in chronic stable angina using single-blinded and randomized double-blinded protocol. J Clin Pharmacol 22:371-378, 1982.
17. Uusitalo A, Keyriläinen O, Johnsson G: A dose-response study on metoprolol in angina pectoris. Ann Clin Res 13(suppl.30): 54-57, 1981.
18. Thadani U, Davidson C, Chir B, et al: Comparison of the immediate effects of five β-adrenoreceptor-blocking drugs with different ancillary properties in angina pectoris. N Engl J Med 300(14):750-755, 1979.
19. Shapiro W, Park J, DiBianco R, et al: Comparison of nadolol, a new long-acting beta-receptor blocking agent, and placebo in the treatment of stable angina pectoris. Chest 80(4):425-430, 1981.
20. Thadani U, Parker JO: Propranolol in angina pectoris: Duration of improved exercise tolerance and circulatory effects after acute oral administration. Am J Cardiol 44:118-125, 1979.
21. Biron P, Tremblay G: Acebutolol: Basis for the prediction of effect on exercise tolerance. Clin Pharmacol Ther 19(3):333-338, 1975.
22. Tzivoni D, Medina A, David D, et al: Effect of metoprolol in reducing myocardial ischemic threshold during exercise and during daily activity. Am J Cardiol 81(6):775-777, 1998.

23. Miller L, Crawford M, O'Rourke R: Nadolol compared to propranolol for treating chronic stable angina pectoris. Chest 86(2):189-193, 1984.
24. Gordon NF, Duncan JJ: Effect of beta-blockers on exercise physiology: Implications for exercise training. Med Sci Sports Exerc 23(6):668-676, 1991.
25. Gordon NF, Van Rensburg JP, Van Den Heever DP, et al: Effect of dual β-blockade and calcium antagonism on endurance performance. Med Sci Sports Exerc 19(1):1-6, 1987.
26. Marchetti G, Merlo L, Noseda V: Myocardial uptake of free fatty acids and carbohydrates after β-adrenergic blockade. Am J Cardiol 22:370-374, 1968.
27. McKenna DH, Curliss RJ, Sialer S, Zarnstorff WC, Crumpton CW, Rowe GG: Effect of propranolol on systemic and coronary haemodynamics at rest and during stimulated exercise. Circ Res 19:520-527, 1966.
28. Steele PP, Maddoux G, Kirch DL, et al: Effects of propranolol and nitroglycerin on left ventricular performance in patients with coronary arterial disease. Chest 73:19-23, 1978.
29. Finkelhor RS, Sun J-P, Bahler RC: Left ventricular filling shortly after an uncomplicated myocardial infarction as a predictor of subsequent exercise capacity. Am Heart J 119:85-91, 1990.
30. Yuasa F, Sumimoto T, Hattori T, et al: Effects of left ventricular peak filling rate on exercise capacity 3 to 6 weeks after acute myocardial infarction. Chest 111:590-594, 1997.
31. Mueller HS: Propranolol in acute myocardial infarction in man: Effects of hemodynamics and myocardial oxygenation. Acta Med Scand 587(suppl):177-183, 1976.
32. Bortone AS, Hess OM, Gaglione A, et al: Effect of intravenous propranolol on coronary vasomotion at rest and during dynamic exercise in patients with coronary artery disease. Circulation 81:1225-1235, 1990.
33. Chick TW, Halperin AK, Gacek EM: The effect of antihypertensive medications on exercise performance: A review. Med Sci Sports Exerc 20(5):447-454, 1988.
34. Van Camp S: Pharmacologic factors in exercise and exercise testing. In ACSM: Resource manual for guidelines for exercise testing and prescription, Philadelphia, 1988, Lea and Febiger.
35. McArdle WD, Katch FI, Katch VL: Exercise physiology: Energy, nutrition, and human performance (6th ed.), New York, 2007, Lippincott Williams & Wilkins.
36. Brown HC, Carruthers SG, Johnstone GB, et al: Clinical pharmacologic observations on atenolol, a beta-adrenoceptor blocker. Clin Pharmacol Ther 20:524-534, 1976.
37. Silas JH, Freestone S, Leard MS, et al: Comparison of two slow release preparations of metoprolol with conventional metoprolol and atenolol. Br J Clin Pharmacol 20:387-391, 1985.
38. Blood SM, Ades PA: Effects of beta-adrenergic blockade on exercise conditioning in coronary patients: A review. J Cardiopulm Rehab 8:141-144, 1988.
39. Robertson L, Reel K, Crist R, et al, editors: Guidelines for cardiac rehabilitation and secondary prevention programs (3rd ed.), Champaign, IL, 2000, Human Kinetics.
40. Dunbar C, Glickman-Weiss E, Bursztyn D, et al: A submaximal treadmill test for developing target ratings of perceived exertion for outpatient cardiac rehabilitation. Percept Mot Skills 87:755-759, 1998.
41. Eston RG, Thompson M: Use of ratings of perceived exertion for predicting maximal work rate and prescribing exercise intensity in patients taking atenolol. Br J Sports Med 31:114-119.
42. Joo KC, Brubaker PH, MacDougall A, et al: Exercise prescription using heart rate plus 20 or perceived exertion in cardiac rehabilitation. J Cardiopulm Rehabil 24(3):178-184, 2004.
43. Mittleman MA, Maclure M, Tofler GH, et al: Triggering of acute myocardial infarction by heavy physical exertion: Protection against triggering by regular exertion. N Engl J Med 329:1677-1683, 1993.
44. Hassock K, Hartwig R: Cardiac arrest associated with supervised cardiac rehabilitation. J Cardiopulm Rehabil 2:402-408, 1982.
45. Schamroth L: The philosophy of calcium ion antagonists. In Zanchetti A, Krikler DM, editors: Calcium antagonism in cardiovascular therapy. Exercise with verapamil, Amsterdam, 1981, Excerpta Medica.
46. Zelis R, Flaim SF: Calcium blocking drugs for angina pectoris. Annu Rev Med 33:465-478, 1982.
47. Khurmi NS, Raftery EB: A comparison of nine calcium ion antagonists and propranolol: Exercise tolerance, heart rate, and ST-segment changes in patients with chronic stable angina pectoris. Eur J Clin Pharmacol 32:539-548, 1987.
48. Hossack KF, Bruce RA: Improved exercise performance in persons with stable angina pectoris receiving diltiazem. Am J Cardiol 47:95-101, 1981.
49. Henry PD: Comparative pharmacology of calcium antagonists: Nifedipine, verapamil and diltiazem. Am J Cardiol 46:1047-1058, 1980.
50. Millard RW, Lathrop DA, Grupp G, et al: Differential cardiovascular effects on calcium channel blocking agents: Potential mechanisms. Am J Cardiol 49:499-506, 1982.
51. Fleckenstein A: Specific pharmacology of calcium in myocardium, cardiac pacemakers and vascular smooth muscle. Annu Rev Pharmacol Toxicol 17:149-166, 1977.
52. Davies RF, Habibi H, Klinke WP, et al: Effect of amlodipine, atenolol and their combination on myocardial ischemia during treadmill exercise and ambulatory monitoring. J Am Coll Cardiol 25:619-625, 1995.
53. Chugh SK, Digpal K, Hutchinson T, et al: A randomized, double-blind comparison of the efficacy and tolerability of once-daily modified-release diltiazem capsules with once-daily amlodipine tablets in patients with stable angina. J Cardiovasc Pharmacol 38(3):356-364, 2001.
54. Van der Vring JA, Daniëls MC, Holwerda NJ, et al: Combination of calcium channel blockers and beta-adrenoceptor blockers for patients with exercise-induced angina pectoris: A double-blind parallel-group comparison of different classes of calcium channel blockers. Br J Clin Pharmacol 47(5):493-498, 1999.
55. Hung J, Lamb IH, Connoly ST, et al: The effect of diltiazem and propranolol, alone and in combination, on exercise performance and left ventricular performance in patients with stable effort angina: A double-blind, randomized, and placebo-controlled study. Ther Prev- Coron Artery Dis 68(3):560-566, 1983.
56. Heidenreich PA, McDonald KM, Hastie T, et al: Meta-analysis of trials comparing beta-blockers, calcium antagonists, and nitrates for stable angina. JAMA 281(20):1927-1936, 1999.
57. Opie LH: Pharmacological differences between calcium antagonists. Eur Heart J 18(suppl A):A71-A79, 1997.
58. Egstrup K, Andersen PJ: Transient myocardial ischemia during nifedipine therapy in stable angina pectoris, and its relation to coronary collateral flow and comparison with metoprolol. Am J Cardiol 71:177-183, 1993.
59. Schultz W, Jost S, Kober G, et al: Relation of antianginal efficacy of nifedipine to degree of coronary arterial narrowing and to presence of coronary collateral vessels. Am J Cardiol 55:26-32, 1985.
60. Kaufmann PA, Mandinov L, Seiler C, et al: Impact of exercise-induced coronary vasomotion on anti-ischemic therapy. Coron Artery Dis 11(4):363-369, 2000.
61. Maseri A, Chierchia S: A new rationale for the clinical approach to the patient with angina pectoris. Am J Med 71:639-644, 1981.
62. Maseri A, L'Abbate A, De Nes M, et al: "Variant" angina: One aspect of a continuous spectrum of vasospastic myocardial ischemia. Am J Cardiol 42:1019-1035, 1978.

63. Boden WE, Bough EW, Reichman MJ, et al: Beneficial effects of high-dose diltiazem in patients with persistent effort angina on β-blockers and nitrates: A randomized, double-blind, placebo-controlled cross-over study. Circulation 71(6):1197–1205, 1985.
64. Millard RW, Lathrop DA, Grupp G, et al: Differential cardiovascular effects of calcium channel blocking agents: Potential mechanisms. Am J Cardiol 49:499-506, 1982.
65. National Center for Health Statistics: National Health Interview Survey, 1997–2002. Information cited in: American Lung Association, Epidemiology and Statistics Unit: Trends in chronic bronchitis and emphysema: Morbidity and Mortality, April 2004. (website). http://www.lungusa.org/site/pp.asp?c=dvLUK9O0E&b=35019. Accessed May 3, 2005.
66. The COPD Guidelines Group of the Standards of Care Committee of the BTS: BTS guidelines for the management of chronic obstructive pulmonary disease. Thorax 52(suppl 5): S1-S28, 1997.
67. Roche N: Recent advances: Pulmonary medicine. BMJ 318; 171–176, 1999.
68. Liesker JJW, Wijkstra PJ, Ten Hacken NHT, et al: A systematic review of the effects of bronchodilators on exercise capacity in patients with COPD. Chest 121(2):597-608, 2002.
69. Belman MJ, Botnick WC, Shin JW, et al: Inhaled bronchodilators reduce dynamic hyperinflation during exercise in patients with chronic obstructive pulmonary disease. Am J Respir Crit Care Med 153:967-975, 1996.
70. Oga T, Nishimura K, Tsukino M, et al: The effects of oxitropium bromide on exercise performance in patients with stable chronic obstructive pulmonary disease: A comparison of three different exercise tests. Am J Respir Crit Care Med 161: 1897-1901, 2000.
71. Newton MF, O'Donnell DE, Forkert L: Response of lung volumes to inhaled salbutamol in large population of patients with severe hyperinflation. Chest 121(4):1042-1050, 2002.
72. O'Donnell DE, Lam M, Webb KA: Measurement of symptoms, lung hyperinflation and endurance during exercise in chronic obstructive pulmonary disease. Am J Respir Crit Care Med 158:1557-1565, 1998.
73. Oga T, Nishimura K, Tsukino M, et al: A comparison of the effects of salbutamol and ipratropium bromide on exercise endurance in patients with COPD. Chest 123(6):1810-1816, 2003.
74. Weiner P, Magadle R, Berar-Yanay N, et al: The cumulative effects of long-acting bronchodilators, exercise, and inspiratory muscle training on the perception of dyspnea in patients with advanced COPD. Chest 118(3):672-678, 2000.
75. Brusasco V, Hodder R, Miravittles M, et al: Health outcomes following treatment for six months with once daily tiotropium compared with twice daily salmeterol in patients with COPD. Thorax 58(5):399-404, 2003.
76. Cahalin LP, Sadowsky HS: Pulmonary medications. Phys Ther 75(5):397-414, 1995.
77. Chapman KR: The role of anticholinergic bronchodilators in adult asthma and chronic obstructive pulmonary disease. Lung 168(suppl):295-303, 1990.
78. Chapman KR: Anticholinergic bronchodilators for adult obstructive airway disease. Am J Med 91(suppl):13S-16S, 1991.
79. Wagner PD, Dantzker DR, Iacovoni VE, et al: Ventilation-perfusion inequality in asymptomatic asthma. Am Rev Respir Dis 118:511-524, 1978.
80. Saito S, Miyamoto K, Nishimura M, et al: Effects of inhaled bronchodilators on pulmonary hemodynamics at rest and during exercise in patients with COPD. Chest 115(2):376-382, 1999.
81. Petty TL: COPD in perspective. Chest 121(5 suppl):116S-120S, 2002.
82. Carter R, Nicrota B, Blevins W, et al: Altered exercise gas exchange and cardiac function in patients with mild chronic obstructive pulmonary disease. Chest 103:745-750, 1993.
83. Lareau SC, ZuWallack R, Carlin B, et al: Pulmonary rehabilitation: 1999. Official Statement of The American Thoracic Society. Am J Respir Crit Care Med 159: 1666-1682, 1999.
84. The Expert Committee on the Diagnosis and Classification of Diabetes Mellitus: Report of the Expert Committee on the Diagnosis and Classification of Diabetes Mellitus. Diabetes Care 20:1183-1197, 1997.
85. Centers for Disease Control and Prevention: National Diabetes Fact Sheet 2002, Atlanta, GA, 2003, U.S. Department of Health and Human Services, Centers for Disease Control and Prevention.
86. Jennings AM, Wilson RM, Ward JD: Symptomatic hypoglycemia in NIDDM patients treated with oral hypoglycemic agents. Diabetes Care 12:203-208, 1989.
87. Seltzer HS: Drug-induced hypoglycemia: A review of 1,418 cases. Endocrinol Metab Clin North Am 18:163-183, 1989.
88. Ferner RE, Neil HA: Sulphonylureas and hypoglycemia. BMJ Clin Res Ed 296:949-950, 1998.
89. Martin IK, Katz A, Wahren J: Splanchnic and muscle metabolism during exercise in NIDDM patients. Am J Physiol 269:E583-E590, 1995.
90. Riddle MC, McDaniel PA, Tive LA: Glipizide-GITS does not increase the hypoglycemic effect of mild exercise during fasting in NIDDM. Diabetes Care 20(6):992-994, 1997.
91. Massi B, Herz M, Pfeiffer C: The effects of acute exercise on metabolic control in type II diabetic patients treated with glimepiride or glibenclamide. Horm Metab Res 28:451-455, 1996.
92. Larsen JJ, Dela F, Madsbad S, et al: Interaction of sulfonylureas and exercise on glucose homeostasis in type 2 diabetic patients. Diabetes Care 22(10):1647-1654, 1999.
93. Zierath JR, He L, Guma A, et al: Insulin action on glucose transport and plasma membrane GLUT4 content in skeletal muscle from patients with NIDDM. Diabetologia 39: 1180-1189, 1996.
94. Garvey WT, Maianu L, Zhu JH, et al: Evidence for the defects in the trafficking and translocation of GLUT4 glucose transporters in skeletal muscle as a cause of human insulin resistance. J Clin Invest 101:2377-2386, 1998.
95. Kennedy JW, Hirshman MF, Gervino EV, et al: Acute exercise induces GLUT4 translocation in skeletal muscle of normal human subjects with type 2 diabetes. Diabetes 48:1192-1197, 1999.
96. Willett LL, Albright ES: Achieving glycemic control in type 2 diabetes: A practical guide for clinicians on oral hypoglycemics. South Med J 97(11):1088-1092, 2004.
97. Panunti B, Kunhiraman B, Fonseca V: The impact of antidiabetic therapies on cardiovascular disease. Curr Atheroscler Rep 7:50-57, 2005.
98. Jadhav S, Petrie J, Ferrell W, et al: Insulin resistance as a contributor to myocardial ischemia independent of obstructive coronary atheroma: A role for insulin sensitization? Heart 90:1379-1383, 2004.
99. Jia EZ, Yang ZJ, Chen SW, et al: Significant association of insulin and proinsulin with clustering of cardiovascular risk factors. World J Gastroenterol 7:149-153, 2005.
100. Klimt CR, Knatterud GL, Meinert CL, et al: A study of the effects of hypoglycemic agents on vascular complications in patients with adult onset diabetes. Diabetes 19:744-830, 1970.
101. The BARI (Bypass Angioplasty Revascularization Investigation) Investigators: Influence of diabetes on 5 year mortality and morbidity in a randomized trial comparing CABG and PTCA in patients with multivessel disease. The Bypass

Angioplasty Revascularization Investigation (BARI). Circulation 96:1761-1769, 1997.

102. Noma A: ATP-regulated K channels in cardiac muscle. Nature 305:147-148, 1983.
103. Farouque HM, Worthley SG, Meredith IT: Effect of ATP-sensitive potassium channel inhibition on coronary metabolic vasodilation in humans. Arterioscler Thromb Vasc Biol 5: 905-910, 2004.
104. Miura T, Miki T: ATP-sensitive K+ channel openers: Old drugs with new clinical benefits for the heart. Curr Vasc Pharmacol 1(3):251-258, 2003.
105. Huizar JF, Gonzalez LA, Alderman J, Smith HS: Sulfonylureas attenuate electrocardiographic ST-segment elevation during an acute myocardial infarction in diabetics. J Am Coll Cardiol 42(6):1017-1021, 2003.
106. Leibowitz G, Cerasi E: Sulphonylurea treatment of NIDDM patients with cardiovascular disease: A mixed blessing? Diabetologia 5:503-514, 1996.
107. Övünç K: Effects of glibenclamde, a KATP channel blocker on warm up phenomenon in type II diabetic patients with chronic stable angina pectoris. Clin Cardiol 23:535-539, 2000.
108. Massi-Benedetti M: Glimepiride in type 2 diabetes mellitus: A review of the worldwide therapeutic experience. Clin Ther 25(3):799-816, 2002.
109. Smits P, Bijlstra PJ, Russel FG, et al: Cardiovascular effects of sulphonylurea derivatives. Diabetes Res Clin Pract 31(suppl):S55-S59, 1996.
110. Musi N, Fujii N, Hirshman MF, et al: AMP-activated protein kinase (AMPK) is activated in muscle of subjects with type 2 diabetes during exercise. Diabetes 50(5):921-927, 2001.
111. Hardie DG, Carling D, Carlson M: The AMP-activated/SNF1 protein kinase subfamily: Metabolic sensors of the eukaryotic cell? Annu Rev Biochem 67:821-855, 1998.
112. Kemp BE, Mitchelhill KI, Stapleton D, et al: Dealing with energy demand: The AMP-activated protein kinase. Trends Biochem Sci 24:22-25, 1999.
113. Stapleton D, Mitchelhill KI, Gao G, et al: Mammalian AMP-activated protein kinase subfamily. J Biol Chem 271:611-614, 1996.
114. Musi N, Hirshman MF, Nygren J, et al: Metformin increases AMP-activated protein kinase activity in skeletal muscle of subjects with type 2 diabetes. Diabetes 51(7):2074-2081, 2002.
115. Hällsten K, Virtanen KA, Lönnqvist F, et al: Rosiglitazone but not metformin enhances insulin- and exercise-stimulated skeletal muscle glucose uptake in patients with newly diagnosed type 2 diabetes. Diabetes 51(12):3479-3485, 2002.
116. Peltoniemi P, Yki-Järvinen H, Oikonen V, et al: Resistance to exercise-induced increase in glucose uptake during hyperinsulinemia in insulin-resistant skeletal muscle of patients with type 1 diabetes. Diabetes 50:1371-1377, 2001.
117. Nuutila P, Koivisto VA, Knuuti J, et al: Glucose-free fatty acid cycle operates in human heart and skeletal muscle in vivo. J Clin Invest 89:1767-1774, 1992.
118. Yki-Järvinen H, Koivisto VA: Continuous subcutaneous insulin infusion therapy decreases insulin resistance in type 1 diabetes. J Clin Endocrinol Metab 58:659-666, 1984.
119. Revers RR, Kolterman OG, Scarlett JA, et al: Lack of in vivo insulin resistance in controlled insulin-dependent, type 1 diabetic patients. J Clin Endocrinol Metab 58:353-358, 1984.
120. Guelfi KJ, Jones TW, Fournier PA: Intermittent high-intensity exercise does not increase the risk of early post-exercise hypoglycaemia in individuals with type 1 diabetes. Diabetes Care 28(6):416-418, 2005.
121. Guelfi KJ, Jones TW, Fournier PA: The decline in blood glucose levels is less with intermittent high-intensity compared with moderate exercise in individuals with type 1 diabetes. Diabetes Care 28:1289-1294, 2005.
122. Guelfi KJ, Jones TW, Fournier PA: New insights into managing the risk of hypoglycaemia associated with intermittent high-intensity exercise in individuals with type 1 diabetes mellitus. Sports Med 37:937-946, 2007.
123. Peter R, Luzio SD, Dunseath G, et al: Effects of exercise on the absorption of insulin glargine in patients with type 1 diabetes. Diabetes Care 28:560-565, 2005.
124. Silverstein J, Klingensmith G, Copelan K, et al: Care of children and adolescents with type 1 diabetes: A statement of the American Diabetes Association. Diabetes Care 28:186-212, 2005.
125. Rachmiel M, Buccino J, Daneman D: Exercise and type 1 diabetes mellitus in youth: Review and recommendations. Pediatr Endocrinol Rev 5:656-665, 2007.
126. lisle DK, Trojian TH: Managing the athlete with type 1 diabetes. Curr Sports Med Rep 5:93-98, 2006.
127. Grimm JJ, Ybarra J, Berne C, et al: A new table for prevention of hypoglycemia during physical activity in type 1 diabetic patients. Diabetes Metab 30:465-470, 2004.
128. Guelfi KJ, Jones TW, Fournier PA: New Insights into managing the risk of hypoglycemia associated with intermittent high-intensity exercise in individuals with type 1 diabetes mellitus. Sports Med 37:937-946, 2007.
129. Maser RE, Lenhard MJ: Review: Cardiovascular autonomic neuropathy due to diabetes mellitus: Clinical manifestations, consequences, and treatment. J Clin Endocrinol Metab 90:5896-5903, 2005.
130. Boulton AJ, Vinik AI, Arezzo JC, et al: Diabetic neuropathies: A statement by the American Diabetes Assòciation. Diabetes Care 28;770–776, 2005.
131. Vinik AI, Maser RE, Mitchell BD, Freeman R: Diabetic autonomic neuropathy. Diabetes Care 26:1553-1579, 2003.
132. Chen J, Marciniak TA, Radford MJ, et al: Beta blocker therapy for secondary prevention of myocardial infarction in elderly diabetic patients. Results from the National Cooperative Cardiovascular Project. J Am Coll Cardiol 34:1388-1394, 1999.
133. Lampert R, Ickovics JR, Viscoli CJ, Horwitz RI, Lee FA: Effects of propranolol on recovery of heart rate variability following acute myocardial infarction and relation to outcome in the beta-blocker heart attack trial. Am J Cardiol 2003. 137-142, 2003.

A

Page numbers followed by *f* refer to illustrations; page numbers followed by *t* refer to tables; page numbers followed by *b* refer to boxes.

C

M

N

O

P